W9-CZR-184

Glickman's
Clinical
Periodontology

PREVENTION, DIAGNOSIS AND TREATMENT OF PERIODONTAL DISEASE IN THE PRACTICE OF GENERAL DENTISTRY

FERMIN A. CARRANZA, JR., Dr. Odont.

Professor and Chairman, Section of Periodontology
School of Dentistry, Center for the Health Sciences
Member, Dental Research Institute
University of California, Los Angeles

WITH CONTRIBUTIONS BY 14 AUTHORITIES

W. B. SAUNDERS COMPANY
Philadelphia   London   Toronto

W. B. Saunders Company: West Washington Square
Philadelphia, PA   19105

1 St. Anne's Road
Eastbourne, East Sussex BN21 3UN, England

1 Goldthorne Avenue
Toronto, Ontario M8Z 5T9, Canada

Listed here is the latest translated edition of this book, together
with the language of the translation and the publisher.

Italian (2nd Edition) – Editrice Scientifica, Milan, Italy

French (4th Edition) – Julien Prelat, Paris, France

Spanish (4th Edition) – NEISA, Mexico City, Mexico

Library of Congress Cataloging in Publication Data

Glickman, Irving.

Glickman's Clinical periodontology.

Includes bibliographies.

1. Periodontics.   I. Carranza, Fermin A.   II. Title.
   III. Title: Clinical periodontology. [DNLM:
   1. Periodontal diseases. WU240 G559c]

RK361.G58 1978   617.6'32   77–16991

ISBN 0–7216–2440–5

Glickman's Clinical Periodontology   ISBN   0-7216-2440-5

Print No.   9   8   7   6   5   4   3

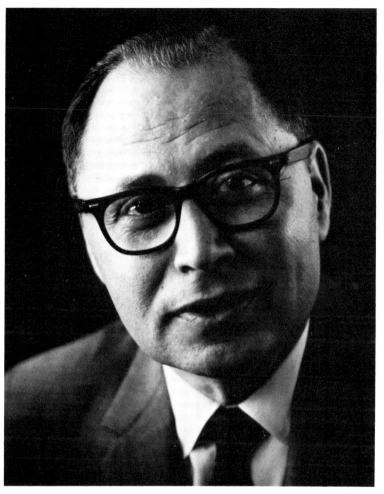

DEDICATED TO THE MEMORY OF IRVING GLICKMAN
BRILLIANT RESEARCHER, INSPIRED TEACHER, DEAR FRIEND

CONTRIBUTORS

JUAN J. CARRARO, Dr. Odont.
Chief of Dental Service
Hospital Fiorito
Avellaneda, Argentina
Chapter 29

JOHN E. FLOCKEN, B.S., D.M.D.
Clinical Professor of Restorative Dentistry
School of Dentistry
University of California at Los Angeles
Chapter 36

E. BARRIE KENNEY, B.D.Sc., D.D.S., M.S.
Professor of Periodontics
School of Dentistry
University of California at Los Angeles
Chapter 56

ROBERT L. MERIN, D.D.S., M.S.
Lecturer in Periodontics
School of Dentistry
University of California at Los Angeles
Chapters 58 and 59

MICHAEL G. NEWMAN, B.A., D.D.S.
Associate Professor of Periodontics
School of Dentistry
University of California at Los Angeles
Chapters 13, 23, 24, 25, and 45

ANNA MATSUISHI PATTISON, M.S., R.D.H.
Assistant Professor of Dental Hygiene and Periodontics
School of Dentistry
University of Southern California, Los Angeles
Chapters 37, 38, and 39

GORDON PATTISON, D.D.S.
Assistant Professor of Periodontics
School of Dentistry
University of Southern California, Los Angeles
Chapters 37, 38, and 39

MAX O. SCHMID, B.A., D.M.D.
Assistant Professor of Periodontics
School of Dentistry
University of California at Los Angeles
Chapters 42 and 43

GERALD SHKLAR, B.Sc., D.D.S., M.S., M.A. (Hon.)
Charles A. Brackett Professor of Oral Pathology and
Head of the Department of Oral Medicine and Oral Pathology
Harvard University, School of Dental Medicine, Boston
Chapter 12

THOMAS N. SIMS, D.D.S.
Lecturer in Periodontics
School of Dentistry
University of California at Los Angeles
Director of Graduate Periodontics
Wadsworth Veterans Administration Hospital
Los Angeles
Chapter 51

WILLIAM K. SOLBERG, B.A., D.D.S., M.S.D.
Associate Professor of Restorative Dentistry and
Chairman, Section of Gnathology and Occlusion
School of Dentistry
University of California at Los Angeles
Chapters 27 and 55

VLADIMIR W. SPOLSKY, B.S., D.M.D., M.P.H.
Associate Professor of Public Health and Preventive Dentistry
School of Dentistry
University of California at Los Angeles
Chapter 22

HENRY H. TAKEI, D.D.S., M.S.
Associate Clinical Professor of Periodontics
School of Dentistry
University of California at Los Angeles
Chapters 36 and 50

ALFRED WEINSTOCK, D.D.S., Ph.D.
Clinical Professor of Periodontics and Clinical Professor of Anatomy
School of Dentistry, School of Medicine
University of California at Los Angeles
Chapters 1, 2, 3, 4, 5, and 6

NOTE: The extent of each individual's contribution to the chapter(s) listed
under his name is briefly described in the Preface to this edition.

PREFACE
to the Fifth Edition

Dr. Irving Glickman was a distinguished researcher and teacher whose dynamic personality, clear judgment, and profound knowledge of all areas of periodontics and related fields marked him as a leader in the progress of our discipline for three decades. This revision of his major work *Clinical Periodontology* has attempted to respect his basic concepts and approaches to the problems while incorporating new information and including recent findings that have shed light on previously obscure subjects.

This new edition of *Clinical Periodontology* incorporates all the major advances that have taken place in periodontics since the last edition while remaining a text aimed at the student and the practitioner.

After careful consideration, a major rearrangement of chapters was done in an attempt to coordinate the existing material and the new being added. In many cases, the new material made extensive revisions and rewriting of chapters necessary.

Fortunately, I was able to obtain the valuable help of a group of periodontists with remarkable expertise and knowledge in different clinical and research areas, to whom I am extremely grateful. Their excellent work, reflected in their contributions to the fifth edition of *Clinical Periodontology*, has been brought to fruition on the rich soil offered by the monumental task accomplished by Irving Glickman.

The group of distinguished collaborators to this fifth edition of *Clinical Periodontology* have contributed to different degrees in the various chapters.

Dr. Alfred Weinstock revised and updated the section on "The Tissues of the Periodontium" and also assisted in rewriting Chapter 6 on "Gingivitis." *Dr. Gerald Shklar* revised the chapter on "The Oral Manifestations of Dermatologic Disease," which now includes chronic desquamative gingivitis. *Dr. Vladimir Spolsky* revised and largely rewrote the chapter on epidemiology.

Dr. Michael G. Newman contributed to Chapter 13 on "Classification of Periodontal Disease" and rewrote the chapters on host response, the role of microorganisms, saliva, calculus, etc. He also wrote the section on antimicrobial therapy, included in Chapter 45. *Dr. William K. Solberg* revised and rewrote the chapters dealing with principles of occlusion and occlusal adjustment. *Dr. J. J. Carraro* revised the section on diabetes in Chapter 29.

Dr. Henry H. Takei, in collaboration with *Anna* and *Gordon Pattison*, prepared the chapters in Section III, Part II, dealing with instrumentation. *Dr. John Flocken* rewrote the section on electrosurgery. *Dr. Max O. Schmid* revised the chapter on plaque control and contributed Chapter 42 on tooth surface preparation. *Dr. Thomas N. Sims* updated the bibliography on bone grafts and reattachment. *Dr. E. Barrie Kenney* revised and rewrote extensive parts of the chapter on "Restorative-Periodontal Interrelationships." *Dr. Robert Merin* wrote Chapter 59 on "Results of Periodontal Treatment" and revised with extensive additions the chapter on "Maintenance Care."

I am indebted particularly to Drs. E. Barrie Kenney, Michael G. Newman, Max O. Schmid, and Henry H. Takei for their constructive criticism and constant support.

I also gratefully acknowledge the collaboration of Dr. Russell J. Nisengard, who read the chapter on host response and offered valuable suggestions; Dr. Sigmund S. Socransky, whose advice and guidance in the microbiology chapter were most helpful; and Dr. Sidney Finegold, who offered constructive criticism on the section on antimicrobial therapy.

Thanks are also due to the following colleagues who have contributed unpublished information or illustrations: Drs. R. Barbanell, R. G. Caffesse, R. Genco, R. Gibbons, A. G. Hannum, T. Hansson, L. Hirschfeld, T. Inage, J. Klingsberg, M. Listgarten, T. Oberg, R. Page, M. Ruben, Z. Skobe, J. Smulow, J. Sottosanti, J. VanHoute, and J. Yee.

I am also indebted to Mr. Alfred Strohlein; to Ms. Irene Petravicius for her excellent art work and untiring efforts to follow our ideas; to Ms. Catherine Boris, Mr. Richard L. Friske, and Mrs. Liliane Kennedy for the photographic material; to Ms. Ana Silberman and to Ms. Rhoda Freeman and the UCLA Word Processing Center (Ms. Michelle Kirsch, Ms. Mickey Kluchnik, and Ms. Barbara Mersini) for their excellent typing assistance; to the Hu-Friedy Company for supplying us with the instruments used for the illustrations in the section on instrumentation.

Special appreciation goes to Dr. Violeta Glickman for her confidence and her support, and to Mr. Carroll Cann, Ms. Laura Tarves, and Mr. Raymond Kersey and the W. B. Saunders Company for their trust and expertise.

Last but not least, my thanks go to my wife, Rita, and my three children, Fersy, Patricia, and Laura, for bearing with me through the period during which this work was done.

FERMIN A. CARRANZA, JR.
Los Angeles, California

PREFACE
to the First Edition

This is a textbook for practitioners of general dentistry and students preparing to be general practitioners. It was the author's desire to create an analytical text, fostered by a critical objectivity. An effort has been made to differentiate between fact and unsubstantiated hypothesis. This constitutes a challenge, especially when it means parting with tradition. However, difficult though it may be, it is sometimes necessary to guard against the hampering influence of habit which tends to nudge us along the well-traveled pathways of thought.

This book is predicated on the premise that the periodontal care of the American public is primarily the concern of the practitioner of general dentistry. The establishment of periodontia as a specialty should be a stimulus for improved periodontal care by the general practitioner. The existence of a group of dentists who desire to limit their practices or specialize in periodontia cannot be hailed as a sign that the obligation of the general practitioner in regard to periodontal problems is diminished. If anything, the opposite is true. The existence of individuals with a primary interest in cardiology who limit their practices accordingly has not meant that medical schools have diminished their teaching of the anatomy and physiology of the heart and the diagnosis and management of cardiac dysfunction—or that practitioners of general medicine have discarded their stethoscopes.

The need for training the general practitioner so that he can fulfill his responsibility to provide periodontal care for all his patients has stimulated a reorientation in the philosophy of dental education and intensification in the teaching of periodontology at both the undergraduate and postgraduate levels. The general practitioner should know enough to handle most periodontal problems which confront him. The availability of a well-trained group of specialists for unusual problems should serve to supplement the dental care available to our population. The establishment of periodontia as a specialty and continued improvement in the ability of the general practitioner to cope with periodontal problems are interdependent movements—mutually dependent upon each other for continued stimulation and progress.

Much information is available regarding the nature of periodontal disease and its treatment. Many problems are as yet unsolved. The existing status of knowledge does not warrant an attitude of complacency. On the other hand, a sizable accumulation of knowledge has resulted from the industry of clinicians and research workers. A considerable portion of this information is applicable in the practice of dentistry. It is the purpose of this textbook to present existing knowledge regarding periodontal problems in such a manner that it can be incorporated in the practice of general dentistry. It was planned with the following objectives in mind:

> The application of basic principles of periodontology in the prevention, diagnosis and treatment of periodontal disease.
>
> An appreciation of the extent to which the initiation of periodontal disease and tooth loss from pathological destruction of the periodontal tissues can be prevented.
>
> An evaluation of the interrelation of local and systemic factors in the causation of periodontal disease.
>
> An appreciation of the effect of treatment procedures upon the tissue changes underlying clinical disease.
>
> The presentation of treatment techniques that can be performed with the degree of skill possessed by every qualified practitioner of general dentistry.
>
> An explanation of the application of various treatment techniques to specific clinical periodontal problems.
>
> The clarification of the interrelation of clinical periodontal procedures with the other aspects of general dentistry.

It has been the experience of the author that the type of preparation which dental students and dentists engaged in graduate and postgraduate training find most useful in the clinical management of periodontal problems is an understanding of clinical phenomena in terms of underlying tissue changes. All clinical periodontal problems are basically gross expressions of microscopic tissue changes. The microscopic changes underlying clinical periodontal disease are essentially manifestations of the composite effects of disease-causing factors. The effectiveness of treatment procedures is reflected in terms of microscopic tissue changes. It is understandable why the interpretation of clinical phenomena in terms of tissue changes is of such practical value in the periodontal field. Crystallization of the clinical management of periodontal problems in terms of microscopic tissue changes is therefore the keynote of this book.

Terminology in the periodontal field is still in a somewhat unsettled state. Conscientious efforts are in progress to clarify this situation. Disagreement over terminology tends to divert attention from more basic considerations. Emphasis is therefore placed upon the explanation of the nature of various conditions, rather than upon the terms by which they are designated.

IRVING GLICKMAN
Boston, Massachusetts
1953

CONTENTS

Section 3

THE TREATMENT OF PERIODONTAL DISEASE

Part I Diagnosis; Determination of the Prognosis;
         The Treatment Plan

Introduction

THE HISTORICAL BACKGROUND OF PERIODONTOLOGY

THE PAST

Periodontal disease is a major problem in modern dental practice. Paleopathological studies indicate that man has been subject to periodontal disease since prehistoric times, and our earliest historical records reveal an awareness of periodontal disease and the need for treating it.

Periodontal disease was the commonest of all diseases of which there was evidence in the embalmed bodies of the **Egyptians** of 4000 years ago.[6] Much of the present-day knowledge of Egyptian medicine comes from the Ebers and Edwin Smith Surgical Papyri.[1] The Ebers papyrus contains many references to gingival disease and prescriptions for strengthening the teeth, and also makes mention of specialists in the care of the teeth.

Oral hygiene was practiced by the **Sumerians** of 3000 B.C., and elaborately decorated **golden toothpicks** found in the excavations at Ur in Mesopotamia suggest an interest in cleanliness of the mouth.[7] The **Babylonians** and **Assyrians** following the earlier Sumerian civilization apparently suffered from periodontal conditions, and a clay tablet of the period tells of treatment by gingival massage combined with various

herbal medications. Medicinal mouthwashes were also used, and Jastrow[4] refers to a tablet where six different drugs are suggested for the treatment of "sickness of the mouth," presumably periodontal disease.

In the oldest known **Chinese** medical work, written about 2500 B.C. by **Hwang-Fi,** oral disease is divided into three types, as follows: (1) Fong Ya, or inflammatory conditions. (2) Ya Kon, or diseases of the soft investing tissues of the teeth. (3) Chong Ya, or dental caries.[7] Gingival inflammations, periodontal abscesses, and gingival ulcerations are described in accurate detail. One gingival condition is described as follows: "The gingivae are pale or violet red, hard and lumpy, sometimes bleeding; the toothache is continuous." Herbal remedies, "Zn-hine-tong," are mentioned for the treatment of these conditions. The Chinese were among the earliest people to use the "**chew stick**" as a **toothpick and toothbrush** to clean the teeth and massage the gingival tissues.

The importance of oral hygiene was recognized by the early **Hebrews.** Many pathologic conditions of the teeth and their surrounding structures are described in the Talmudic writings. Vestiges of the **Phoeni-**

cian civilization include a specimen of wire splinting apparently constructed to stabilize teeth loosened by chronic destructive periodontal disease.

Among the ancient **Greeks, Hippocrates of Cos (460–335 B.C.)** was the father of modern medicine, the first to institute a systematic examination of the patient's pulse, temperature, respiration, excreta, sputum, and pains. He discussed the function and eruption of the teeth and also the etiology of periodontal disease. He believed that inflammation of the gums could be produced by accumulations of pituita or calculus with gingival hemorrhage occurring in cases of persistent disease. He described different varieties of splenic maladies, to one of which he assigned the following symptoms: "The belly becomes swollen, the spleen enlarged and hard, the patient suffers from acute pain. The gums are detached from the teeth and smell bad."[7]

The **Etruscans,** much before 735 B.C., were adept in the art of constructing artificial dentures, but there is no evidence of their awareness of the existence of periodontal disease or its treatment.

Among the **Romans, Aulus Cornelius Celsus (first century A.D.)** referred to diseases which affect the soft parts of the mouth and their treatment as follows: "If the gums separate from the teeth, it is beneficial to chew unripe pears and apples and keep their juices in the mouth." He described looseness of the teeth caused by the weakness of their roots or by flaccidity of the gums and noted that in these cases it is necessary to touch the gums lightly with a red hot iron and then smear them with honey. The Romans were very interested in oral hygiene. Celsus believed that stains on the teeth should first be removed and the teeth then rubbed with a **dentifrice.** The use of the **toothbrush** is mentioned in the writings of many of the Roman poets. Gingival massage was an integral part of oral hygiene. **Paul of Aegina** during the seventh century differentiated between epulis, a fleshy excrescence of gums in the neighborhood of a tooth, and parulis, which he described as an abscess of the gums. He wrote that tartar incrustations must be removed either with scrapers or a small file, and that the teeth should be carefully cleansed after the last meal of the day.

Rhazes (850–923), an Arabian of the Middle Ages, recommended opium, oil of roses, and honey in the treatment of periodontal disease. To strengthen loosened teeth he recommended **astringent mouth washes** and **dentifrice powders.** He described a procedure of scarification of the gingiva, and strong counterirritants in the treatment of disease of the gums. A voluminous writer, he has seven chapters in his "Al-Fakkir" on the teeth. They are entitled *"The Teeth, Teeth on Edge, Decay of the Teeth, Looseness of the Gums, Suppuration of the Gums, Pyorrhea and Bleeding Gums,* and *Halitosis."* **Avicenna (980–1037)** discussed the filing of elongated teeth and reported that "in order to have loosened teeth become firm again, one must avoid using same in mastication." He wrote extensively on diseases of the gingiva such as ulcers, suppuration, recession, and fissures.

Albucasis (936–1013) stressed the care and treatment of the supporting structures. He recognized an interrelation between tartar and disease of the gums. Albucasis referred to the treatment of periodontal disease as follows:[3] **"Sometimes on the surface of the teeth, both inside and outside, as well as under the gums, are deposited rough scales, of ugly appearance, and black, green or yellow in colour; thus corruption is communicated to the gums, and so the teeth are in the process of time denuded. It is necessary for thee to lay the patient's head upon thy lap and to scrape the teeth and molars, on which are observed either true incrustations, or something similar to sand, and this until nothing more remains of such substance, and until also the dirty colour of the teeth disappears, be it black or green, or yellowish, or of any other colour. If a first scraping is sufficient, so much the better; if not, thou shalt repeat it on the following day, or even on the third or fourth day, until the desired purpose is obtained. Thou must know however, that the teeth need scrapers of various shapes and figures, on account of the very nature of this operation. In fact the scalpel with which the teeth must be scraped on the inside, is unlike that with which thou shalt scrape the outside; and that with which thou shalt scrape the interstices between the teeth shall likewise have another shape. Therefore thou must have all this series of scalpels ready if so it pleases God."**

A set of instruments was designed by

Albucasis for scaling the teeth. These instruments were crude but their role in the heritage of the modern periodontal instrumentarium is quite apparent.

In the fifteenth century, **Valescus of Montpellier (1382–1417)** stated that in order to treat disease of the gums tartar must be removed little by little either with iron instruments or with dentifrices. In the fourteenth and fifteenth centuries reference is also made to white wine, roasted salt, and aromatic substances as adjuncts in periodontal therapy.

Bartholomeus Eustachius, in a book published in **Venice (1563),** explained the firmness of teeth in the jaws as follows: "There exists besides a very strong ligament, principally attached to the roots by which these latter are tightly connected with the alveoli." The gums also contribute to their firmness, and here he compares it to the joining of the skin to the finger nails.

With the beginning of the eighteenth century dentistry developed the early signs of scientific curiosity which were the precursors of present-day research disciplines. **Pierre Fauchard (1678–1761),** the father of modern dentistry, in the first and second editions of his epochal treatise *"Le Chirurgien Dentiste"* discussed many aspects of the subject of periodontology. He described chronic periodontal disease as a "kind of scurvy" which attacked the gums, the alveoli, and the teeth. The clinical acuity of the observation of Fauchard is shown by his statement, **"Not only are the gums affected by it (periodontal disease) which are livid, swollen, and inflamed, but those which do not show these symptoms as yet are not immune from this affliction. It is recognized by a yellowish almost white pus and by a little glutinous material which is emitted from the gums when a rather heavy pressure is applied by the finger."** * Fauchard believed that internal remedies were not effective in treating periodontal disease. He recommended careful scaling of the teeth to remove the calculus deposits, and he developed many instruments for this purpose; dentifrices, mouthwashes, and splinting of loose teeth were included in his therapeutic procedures.

John Hunter, the eighteenth century English physiologist and surgeon, published two books on dentistry in which he discussed diseases of the alveolar process which he believed to be the site of suppurative periodontal disease. The nineteenth century brought new names and developments to the periodontal field, such as **Kunstmann** and his surgical measures for the treatment of periodontal disease, and **Robiscek** and the "flap operation." **John M. Riggs,** the first of many North American contributors, was credited by his contemporaries with "originating and first publicly describing a new treatment for the cure of . . . absorption of the alveolar process . . . thereby saving and restoring to firmness the loosened teeth." His treatment consisted of **subgingival curettage.** He described periodontal disease in detail, and chronic destructive disease of the supporting tissues was for many years called "Riggs' disease."[5]

With the beginning of the twentieth century there developed a prolific group of clinicians and scientists throughout the world with a major interest in the periodontal field. Their names and contributions are documented throughout the pages of this book.

PRESENT-DAY PERIODONTICS IN THE PRACTICE OF DENTISTRY

Before undertaking a detailed study of periodontal disease, it is important to have a proper perspective regarding the role of periodontics in the practice of dentistry.

Periodontal disease is the major cause of tooth loss in adults, and for many years periodontics was thought of as a conglomeration of treatment techniques for the purpose of trying to save teeth suffering from advanced disease.

It gradually became apparent that the periodontal disease which caused tooth loss in adults was the terminal stage of processes which started, but were untreated, in youth. Attention shifted to early treatment because it is simpler, produces more predictable results, and spares the patient unnecessary loss of tooth-supporting tissues.

Today the emphasis is upon preventing periodontal disease, because most periodontal disease is preventable. No longer confined within the limitations of an

---

*Darby, quoted in Weinberger.[7]

autonomous branch of dentistry, periodontics has become a philosophy underlying all dental practice.

Every dental procedure is performed with concern for its effect upon the periodontium, and effective chairside measures for preventing periodontal disease are part of the total dental care of all patients. In addition, educational programs are being developed to alert the public to the importance of periodontal disease and to motivate them to take advantage of available methods of preventing it. **The priority of periodontics in the practice of dentistry has shifted from repairing damage done by preventable disease to keeping healthy mouths healthy.**[2]

REFERENCES

1. Castiglione, A.: History of Medicine, 2nd ed. New York, Alfred A. Knopf, 1941.
2. Glickman, I.: Preventive periodontics—A blueprint for the periodontal health of the American public. J. Periodontol., 38:361, 1967.
3. Guerini, V.: History of Dentistry. Philadelphia, Lea & Febiger, 1909.
4. Jastrow, N.: The medicine of the Babylonians and Assyrians. Proc. Soc. Med., London, 7:109, 1914.
5. Merritt, A. H.: The historical background of periodontology. J. Periodontol., 10:7, 1939.
6. Ruffer, M. A.: Studies in the Palaeopathology of Egypt. Chicago, University of Chicago Press, 1921.
7. Weinberger, B. W.: An Introduction to the History of Dentistry. St. Louis, The C. V. Mosby Co., 1948.

THE TISSUES OF THE PERIODONTIUM

The periodontium is the investing and supporting tissues of the tooth, and consists of the *periodontal ligament,* the *gingiva, cementum,* and *alveolar bone.* The cementum is considered a part of the periodontium because, with the bone, it serves as the support for the fibers of the periodontal ligament. The periodontium is subject to morphologic and functional variations as well as changes with age. This section deals with the normal features of the tissues of the periodontium, knowledge of which is necessary for an understanding of periodontal disease.

The Gingiva

The *oral mucosa* consists of the following three zones: the gingiva and the covering of the hard palate, termed the masticatory mucosa; the dorsum of the tongue, covered by specialized mucosa; and the oral mucous membrane lining the remainder of the oral cavity. The *gingiva* is that part of the oral mucosa that covers the alveolar processes of the jaws and surrounds the necks of the teeth.

NORMAL CLINICAL FEATURES

The gingiva is divided anatomically into the marginal, attached, and interdental areas.

The Marginal Gingiva (Unattached Gingiva)

The marginal ("unattached") gingiva is the terminal edge or border of the gingiva surrounding the teeth in collar-like fashion (Fig. 1–1) and demarcated from the adjacent attached gingiva by a shallow linear depression, the *free gingival groove*.[1] Usually slightly more than a millimeter wide, it forms the soft tissue wall of the gingival sulcus. It may be separated from the tooth surface with a periodontal probe.

THE GINGIVAL SULCUS. The gingival sulcus is the shallow crevice or space around the tooth bounded by the surface of the tooth on one side and the epithelium lining the free margin of the gingiva on the other. It is V-shaped and barely permits the entrance of a periodontal probe. The average depth of the normal sulcus has been reported as 1.8 mm., with a variation of from 0 to 6 mm.[93] Other studies show 2 mm.,[12] 1.5 mm.,[149] and 0.69 mm.[38] Gottlieb considered the "ideal" sulcus depth to be zero.[46]

The Attached Gingiva

The attached gingiva is continuous with the marginal gingiva. It is firm, resilient,

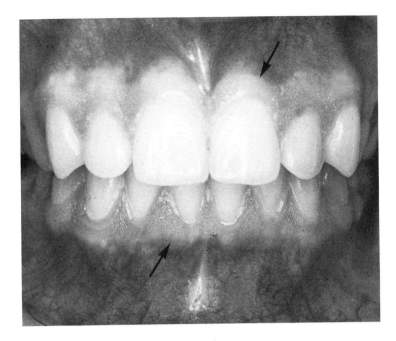

Figure 1–1 Normal Gingiva in Young Adult. Note the demarcation (mucogingival line) between the attached gingiva and darker alveolar mucosa.

and tightly bound to the underlying periosteum of alveolar bone. The facial aspect of the attached gingiva extends to the relatively loose and movable *alveolar mucosa* from which it is demarcated by the *mucogingival junction* (Fig. 1–2). The width of the attached gingiva on the facial aspect in different areas of the mouth varies from less than 1 mm. to 9 mm.[11] On the lingual aspect of the mandible, the attached gingiva terminates at the junction with the lingual alveolar mucosa, which is continuous with the mucous membrane lining the floor of the mouth. The palatal surface of the attached gingiva in the max-illa blends imperceptibly with the equally firm, resilient palatal mucosa.

The Interdental Gingiva

The interdental gingiva occupies the *gingival embrasure*, which is the interproximal space beneath the area of tooth contact. It usually consists of two papillae, one facial and one lingual, and the *col*.[20] The latter is a valley-like depression which connects the papillae and conforms to the shape of the interproximal contact area (Figs. 1–3 and 1–4). When teeth are

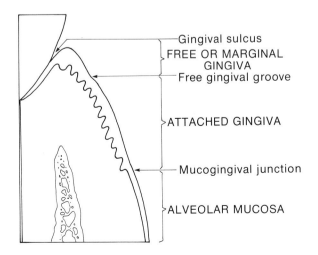

Gingival sulcus
FREE OR MARGINAL GINGIVA
Free gingival groove

ATTACHED GINGIVA

Mucogingival junction

ALVEOLAR MUCOSA

Figure 1–2 Diagram showing anatomical landmarks of the gingiva.

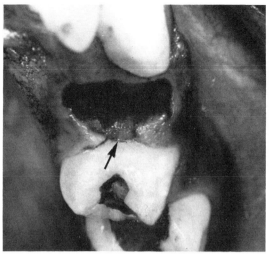

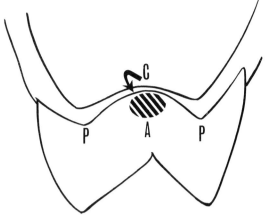

Figure 1–4 Interdental papillae (P), col (C), and relationship to contact area (A) on mesial surface.

Figure 1–3 Site of extraction showing the facial and palatal interdental papillae and the intervening col (*arrow*).

not in contact, the col is often absent. Even when teeth contact, the col may be absent in some individuals (Fig. 1–5).

Each interdental papilla is pyramidal; the facial and lingual surfaces are tapered toward the interproximal contact area, and the mesial and distal surfaces are slightly concave. The lateral borders and tip of the interdental papillae are formed by a continuation of the marginal gingiva from the adjacent teeth. The intervening portion consists of attached gingiva (Fig. 1–6).

Figure 1–5 Diagram comparing anatomical variations of the interdental col in the normal gingiva (left side) and after gingival recession (right side). *A* and *B*, Mandibular anterior segment, facial and buccolingual views, respectively. *C* and *D*, Mandibular posterior region, facial and buccolingual views, respectively. Tooth contact points are shown in *B* and *D*.

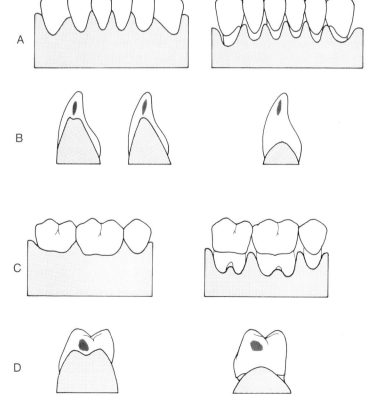

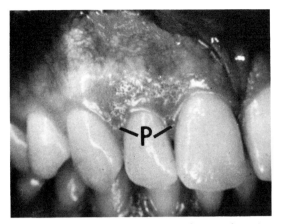

Figure 1–6   Interdental Papillae with Central Portion Formed by Attached Gingiva. The shape of the papillae (P) varies according to the dimension of the gingival embrasure.

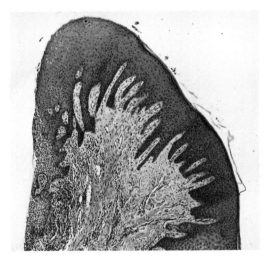

Figure 1–8   Section of Clinically Normal Gingiva, showing inflammation which is almost always present near the base of the sulcus. Keratin strands are visible on the outer surface, where they have been displaced due to artifact.

In the absence of proximal tooth contact, the gingiva is firmly bound over the interdental bone and forms a smooth rounded surface without interdental papillae (Fig. 1–7).

NORMAL MICROSCOPIC FEATURES

The Marginal Gingiva (Unattached Gingiva)

The marginal gingiva consists of a central core of connective tissue covered by stratified squamous epithelium (Fig. 1–8). The epithelium on the crest and outer surface of the marginal gingiva is keratinized, parakeratinized or both, contains prominent rete pegs or ridges and is continuous with the epithelium of the attached gingiva. The epithelium along the inner surface (facing the tooth) is devoid of rete pegs, is neither keratinized nor parakeratinized, and forms the lining of the gingival sulcus.

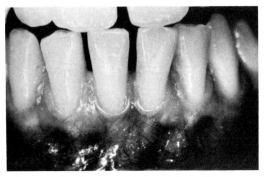

Figure 1–7   Absence of interdental papillae and col where proximal tooth contact is missing.

The gingival fibers

The connective tissue of the marginal gingiva is densely collagenous, containing a prominent system of **collagen fiber bundles** called the gingival fibers. The gingival fibers have the following functions: to brace the marginal gingiva firmly against the tooth; to provide the rigidity necessary to withstand the forces of mastication without being deflected away from the tooth surface; and to unite the free marginal gingiva with the cementum of the root and the adjacent attached gingiva. The gingival fibers are arranged in three groups: gingivodental, circular, and transseptal.[3, 35]

GINGIVODENTAL GROUP.   These are the fibers of the facial, lingual, and interproximal surfaces. They are embedded in the cementum just beneath the epithelium at the base of the gingival sulcus. On the facial and lingual surfaces they project from the cementum in fanlike conformation toward the crest and outer surface of the marginal gingiva and terminate short of the epithelium (Figs. 1–9 and 1–10). They also extend external to the periosteum of the facial and lingual alveolar bone and terminate in the attached gingiva or blend with the periosteum of the bone. Interproximally, the gingivodental fibers extend toward the crest of the interdental gingiva (Fig. 1–8).

ment in the gingival connective tissue is the fibroblast. Numerous fibroblasts are found between the fiber bundles. As in connective tissue elsewhere in the body, fibroblasts synthesize and secrete the collagen fibers, as well as elastin, the non-collagenous proteins, glycoproteins, and glycosaminoglycans. The renewal of collagen fibers and other chemical constituents, and possibly their degradation, is regulated by fibroblasts. Wound healing following gingival surgery or as a result of injury or pathological processes is also regulated by gingival fibroblasts.

Mast cells, which are distributed throughout the body, are numerous in the connective tissue of the oral mucosa and

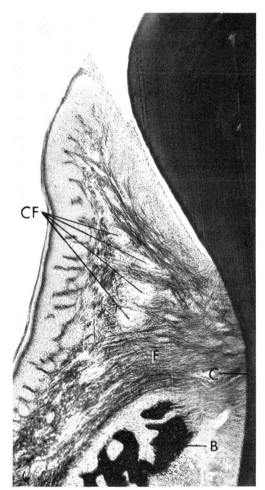

Figure 1–9 Faciolingual Section of Marginal Gingiva, showing gingival fibers (F) extending from the cementum (C) to the crest of the gingiva, to the outer gingival surface, and external to the periosteum of the bone (B). Circular fibers (CF) are shown in cross section between the other groups. (Courtesy of Dr. Sol Bernick.)

CIRCULAR GROUP. These fibers course through the connective tissue of the marginal and interdental gingiva and encircle the tooth in ringlike fashion.

TRANSSEPTAL GROUP. Located interproximally, the transseptal fibers form horizontal bundles that extend between the cementum of approximating teeth into which they are embedded. They lie in the area between the epithelium at the base of the gingival sulcus and the crest of the interdental bone and are sometimes classified with the principal fibers of the periodontal ligament.

CONNECTIVE TISSUE CELLULAR ELEMENTS. The preponderant cellular ele-

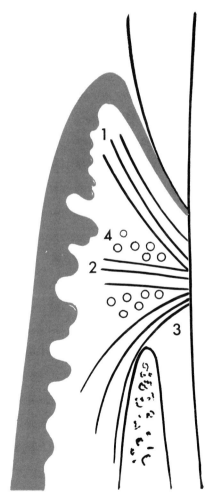

Figure 1–10 Diagrammatic Illustration of the Gingivodental Fibers extending from the cementum (1) to the crest of the gingiva, (2) to the outer surface, and (3) external to the periosteum of the labial plate. Circular fibers (4) are shown in cross section.

the gingiva.[18, 145] They contain a variety of **biologically active substances** such as histamine, proteolytic-esterolytic enzymes, "slow-reacting substances," and lipolecithins all of which may be involved in the development and progress of gingival inflammation, and heparin which is a factor in bone resorption in vitro. Other products such as serotonin, unsaturated fatty acids, β-glucuronidase, ascorbic acid, and phosphatase are also found.[155]

The active chemicals are liberated by degranulation of the mast cells. Although some disagree,[109] it is believed that mast cells are increased in chronic gingival inflammation, except in areas of dense leukocytic infiltration and ulceration.[111, 154]

In clinically normal gingiva, small foci of plasma cells and lymphocytes are almost always found in the connective tissue near the base of the sulcus. They represent a chronic inflammatory response to irritation from constantly present bacteria and their products in the sulcus area.

Gingival plasma cells[141] are numerous in the lamina propria in the vicinity of blood vessels. These cells produce antibodies (i.e., IgG, IgA, or IgM) directed against local antigens. They are present in large quantities in chronically inflamed gingiva.

Lymphocytes are also found in the lamina propria of the gingiva. Both thymus-derived (T) lymphocytes and bone-marrow–derived (B) lymphocytes are involved in the immunological defense mechanism. Although lymphocytes and plasma cells are most abundant in inflamed gingiva, they have also been detected in small quantities in clinically healthy gingiva, and even in the lamina propria of gingiva from gnotobiotic (germ-free) animals. Their presence is believed to be related to the penetration of antigenic substances from the oral cavity via the sulcular and junctional epithelium.

Neutrophils can be seen in relatively high numbers in both the gingival connective tissue and the sulcus. It is common to see them migrating through the sulcular and junctional epithelium. These cells perform a protective role by phagocytizing bacteria and other foreign substances. They contain lysosomes which in turn contain a variety of hydrolytic enzymes that kill bacteria after phagocytosis. When neutrophils die these enzymes are released and may contribute to tissue destruction.

Macrophages are large phagocytic cells that are also numerous in the gingival lamina propria. These cells may also have a role in the immune system.

These inflammatory cells are usually present in small amounts in clinically normal gingiva. They are not present, however, if gingival normalcy is judged by very strict clinical criteria.[92a] Therefore, in spite of the frequency of their occurrence, the inflammatory infiltrate cells are not a normal component of the gingival tissue.

The Gingival Sulcus, Sulcus Epithelium and Junctional Epithelium

The marginal gingiva forms the soft tissue wall of the gingival sulcus, and is joined to the tooth at the base of the sulcus by the junctional epithelium (Fig. 1–11). The sulcus is lined with thin, non-keratinized stratified squamous epithelium without rete pegs. It extends from the coronal limit of the junctional epithelium at the base of the sulcus to the crest of the gingival margin. The sulcus epithelium is extremely important, because it may act as a **semipermeable membrane** through which injurious bacterial products pass into the gingiva and tissue fluid from the gingiva seeps into the sulcus.[125]

The **junctional epithelium** consists of a collar-like band of stratified squamous epithelium. It is three to four layers thick in early life, but the number of layers increases to 10 or even 20 with age; its length ranges from 0.25 to 1.35 mm.

The epithelial attachment of the junctional epithelium consists of a **basal lamina (basement membrane)**[72] that is comparable to that which attaches epithelium to connective tissue elsewhere in the body. The basal lamina consists of a **lamina densa** (adjacent to the enamel) and a **lamina lucida** to which **hemidesmosomes** are attached (Figs. 1–12 to 1–14). Organic strands from the enamel appear to extend into the lamina densa.[120] The junctional epithelium attaches to **afibrillar cementum** when it is present (usually restricted to an area within 1 mm. of the cemento-enamel junction)[105] on the crown (Figs. 1–12 to 1–14) and to **root cementum** in a similar

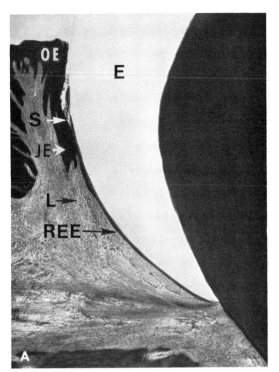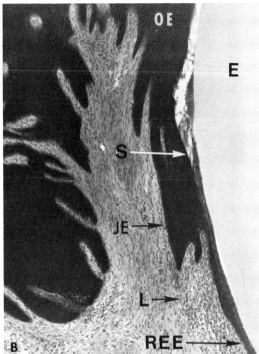

Figure 1–11 Gingival Sulcus in an Erupting Monkey Tooth. *A,* Gingival sulcus (S), the enamel (E), and the junctional epithelium (JE). Note the oral epithelium (OE), the reduced enamel epithelium (REE), and the leukocytic infiltration (L). *B,* High power section showing the base of the sulcus (S), the enamel (E), and the junctional epithelium (JE). Leukocytic infiltration (L) usually present in clinically normal gingiva is shown beneath the base of the sulcus. Tissue within the sulcus is artifact and debris.

manner. Histochemical evidence for the presence of neutral polysaccharides in the zone of the epithelial attachment has been reported.[130]

The attachment of the junctional epithelium to the tooth is reinforced by the gingival fibers, which brace the marginal gingiva against the tooth surface. For this reason the junctional epithelium and the gingival fibers are considered a functional unit, referred to as the *dentogingival unit.*

Development of the Junctional Epithelium and Gingival Sulcus

Gottlieb's initial description of the origin of the epithelial attachment apparatus was based upon observations made with the light microscope. Additional information has evolved from subsequently developed research techniques such as histochemistry, radioautography,[32] and electron microscopy.[59, 105, 116] To understand the development of the junctional epithelium

and its relationship to the teeth, it is best to start with the unerupted tooth.

After enamel formation is complete, the enamel is covered with reduced enamel epithelium and is attached to the tooth by a basal lamina. Hemidesmosomes can be seen on the apical plasma membrane of the reduced ameloblasts.[73, 121] When the tooth penetrates the oral mucosa, the reduced enamel epithelium unites with the oral epithelium to form what Gottlieb termed the *epithelial attachment*[44, 47] and described as organically attached to the enamel. According to current terminology,[105] the united epithelium is called the "junctional epithelium," whereas the epithelial attachment refers to the union of the epithelial cells with the tooth surfaces. As the tooth erupts, this united epithelium condenses along the crown. The reduced (shortened) ameloblasts, which form the inner layer of the reduced enamel epithelium (Fig. 1–15), disappear and are gradually replaced by squamous epithelial cells. The junctional epithelium forms a collar around

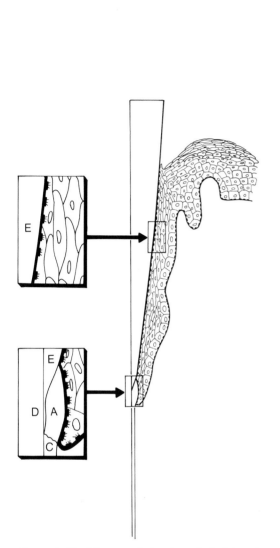

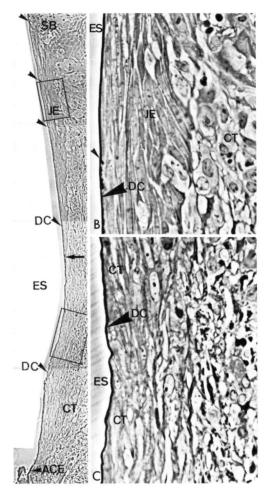

Figure 1–13 Phase contrast micrographs of the dento-epithelial junction from a demineralized tooth showing the junctional epithelium and dental cuticle.

On the left is a low power micrograph in which most of the enamel space (ES) has been cut away except for a thin border along the enamel surface. The gingival sulcus bottom (SB) is located at the top, and root cementum at the cemento-enamel junction can be seen as a dark structure at lower left. The dental cuticle (DC) appears as a single, thin, dark line extending from the small zone of afibrillar cementum (ACE) at the cemento-enamel junction to the base of the gingival sulcus. The cuticle is a relatively continuous layer overlying the enamel surface, although irregularities or interruptions can be detected (arrowheads). The arrow at right center indicates the apical termination of the junctional epithelium (JE). Below this arrow the connective tissue (CT) of the gingiva is in direct contact with the cuticle. Magnification × 125.

At upper right is an enlargement of the rectangular area in the upper portion of the figure on the left. Note that the dental cuticle (DC) is of relatively even thickness, and is interposed between the junctional epithelium (JE) and enamel space (ES). CT, connective tissue. Magnification × 950. (From Schroeder, H. E., and Listgarten, M. A.: Fine structure of the developing epithelial attachment of human teeth. *In* Wolsky, A. (ed.): Monographs in Developmental Biology, vol. 2. Basel, S. Karger, 1971.)

Figure 1–12 Diagram of the dentogingival junction showing the junctional epithelium adhering to the tooth surface. At upper left, an enlarged view of epithelial cells showing hemidesmosomes in those cells along the enamel (E) surface. Intervening between the epithelial cells and the enamel are the basal lamina and dental cuticle, respectively; both of these structures are represented by the single, thick line along the enamel. At lower left, an enlarged view of the cemento-enamel junction showing a small area of afibrillar cementum (A). C, cementum; D, dentin.

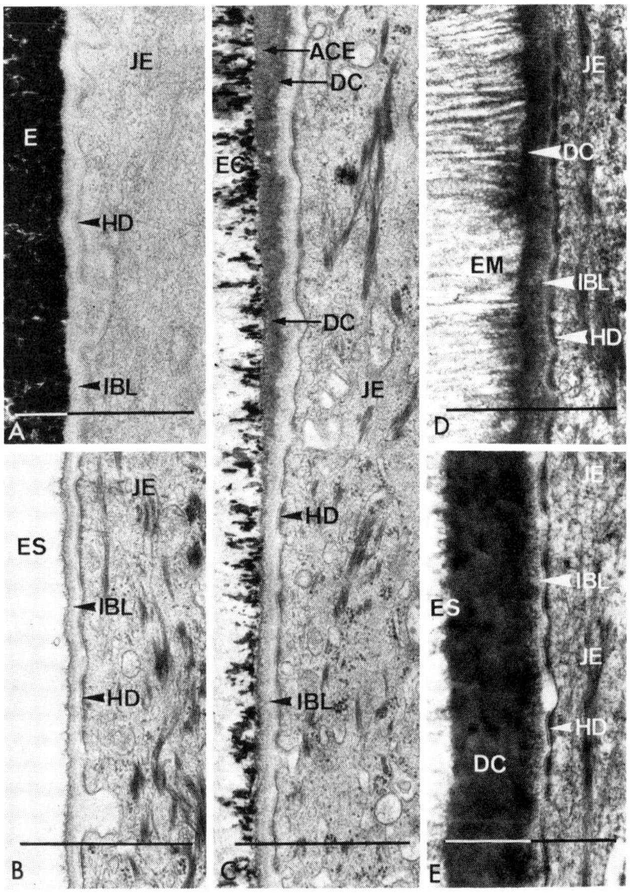

Figure 1–14 High power electron micrographs of portions of the junctional epithelium showing the epithelial attachment to the enamel surface and dental cuticle, when present.

At upper left, an undemineralized preparation showing a junctional epithelial cell (JE) attached to the enamel (E) surface via hemidesmosomes (HD) and the basal lamina (IBL). The dark portion of enamel represents apatite crystals packed closely together.

At lower left, a preparation similar to that at upper left, but after demineralization. Since the apatite crystals have been removed, the enamel space (ES) appears empty. A portion of a junctional epithelial cell (JE), the basal lamina (IBL), and hemidesmosomes (HD) can be seen in proper relationship. This is the epithelial attachment.

The center micrograph represents a partially demineralized tooth in which some of the enamel apatite crystals (EC) are still present. The upper half shows a region in which an electron-dense dental cuticle (DC) is situated between the basal lamina (IBL) and the enamel surface. At the top some afibrillar cementum (ACE) intervenes between the cuticle and enamel surface. The lower half of the micrograph shows the epithelial attachment against the enamel surface with no intervening dental cuticle. JE, junctional epithelial cell; HD, hemidesmosome.

At upper right, a demineralized specimen in which an electron-dense dental cuticle (DC) can be seen overlying the enamel surface. In this preparation there is some organic enamel matrix (EM) present which is represented by the horizontal lines. Note that these matrix components become continuous with the dental cuticle. IBL, basal lamina; JE, junctional epithelial cell; HD, hemidesmosome.

At lower right, a demineralized preparation showing a portion of a thick dental cuticle (DC). The specimen is otherwise similar to the one above it. ES, enamel space; IBL, basal lamina; JE, junctional epithelial cell; HD, hemidesmosome.

Magnification × 41,000 (approx.) (From Schroeder, H. E., and Listgarten, M. A.: Fine structure of the developing epithelial attachment of human teeth. *In* Wolsky, A. (ed.): Monographs in Developmental Biology, vol. 2. Basel, S. Karger, 1971.)

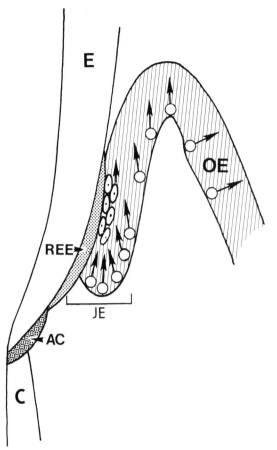

Figure 1–15 Junctional epithelium on an erupting tooth. The junctional epithelium (JE) is formed by the joining of the oral epithelium (OE) and the reduced enamel epithelium (REE). Afibrillar cementum, sometimes formed on enamel after degeneration of the reduced enamel epithelium, is shown at AC. The arrows indicate the coronal movement of the regenerating epithelial cells, which multiply more rapidly in the junctional epithelium than in the oral epithelium (OE). Enamel, E; root cementum, C. (From Dr. Max A. Listgarten.[71])

A similar cell turnover pattern exists in the fully erupted tooth.

the fully erupted tooth, which is attached to the enamel in the same manner as the ameloblasts it displaced.

The junctional epithelium is a continually **self-renewing structure** with mitotic activity occurring in all cell layers[82] (Fig. 1–16). The regenerating epithelial cells move toward the tooth surface and along it in a coronal direction to the gingival sulcus, where they are shed[9] (Fig. 1–15). The migrating daughter cells provide a continuous attachment to the tooth surface. Although the epithelial attachment, comprised of hemidesmosomes and the basal lamina, represents the biological bond of the junctional

epithelium to the tooth surface, the strength of the attachment has not been measured.

The gingival sulcus is formed when the tooth erupts into the oral cavity. At that time the junctional epithelium and reduced enamel epithelium together form a broad band that is attached to the tooth surface from near the tip of the crown to the cemento-enamel junction. The gingival sulcus is the shallow V-shaped space or groove between the tooth and gingiva that encircles the newly erupted tip of the crown. In the fully erupted tooth, only the junctional epithelium persists. The sulcus consists of the shallow space that is coronal to the attachment of the junctional epithelium and is bounded by the tooth on one side and the sulcular epithelium on the other. The coronal extent of the gingival sulcus is the gingival margin.

A historical note is perhaps interesting to consider at this point. Gottlieb's concept of the formation of the gingival sulcus and the epithelial attachment was challenged: Weski,[149] Gross,[51] and Wodehouse[153] contended that the gingival sulcus was formed by a split in the epithelial attachment (intraepithelial split) rather than by separation from the tooth. Becks (1929) and Skillen (1930) maintained that the reduced enamel epithelium degenerated and disappeared when the gingival sulcus was formed and that it did not persist as an epithelial attachment. Waerhaug[137, 138] claimed that the epithelial attachment was not attached to the enamel but was in close apposition to it, and therefore should be called the epithelial cuff. According to this belief, the bottom of the sulcus is at the deepest (apical) point of the epithelial cuff rather than at its most superficial (coronal) level (Fig. 1–17). However, other investigators[8, 72, 77, 128, 136] have reaffirmed the concept that the epithelium is attached to the tooth, and one of them[94] proposed the term attached epithelial cuff. (See ref. 105 for a summary on this topic.)

Dental Cuticle

A dental cuticle is often seen on various tooth surfaces, including enamel, afibrillar

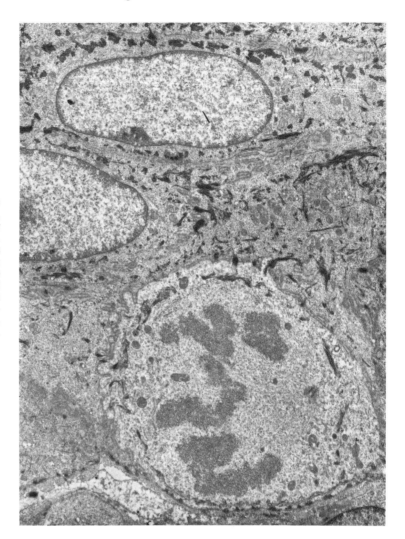

Figure 1–16 Electron micrograph of gingival epithelium from a rat, showing a cell in the basal cell layer undergoing mitosis (lower center). Note that the nuclear envelope has disappeared and that the chromatin has condensed into clusters. These clusters represent sectional coiled chromosomes. Connective tissue is located at the bottom of the micrograph. Magnification × 12,000. Courtesy of Drs. A. Weinstock and T. Inage.

cementum, and radicular (fibrillar) cementum near the cemento-enamel junction. It is an organic, non-mineralized thin layer that may or may not be present between the junctional epithelium and the tooth surface.[64, 105] It is believed to be a product of reduced (shortened) ameloblasts. The cuticle that is visible with the light microscope can be resolved further with the electron microscope into either a single structural component as described above, or in certain instances (i.e., near the cemento-enamel junction) two layers, the innermost one being afibrillar cementum which is mineralized.

Gingival Fluid (Crevicular Fluid)

The gingival sulcus contains a fluid which seeps into it from the gingival connective tissue through the thin sulcular wall.[13, 19, 78] The gingival fluid is believed to (1) cleanse material from the sulcus; (2) contain plasma proteins which may improve adhesion of the epithelial attachment to the tooth; (3) possess antimicrobial properties; and (4) exert antibody activity in defense of the gingiva.

The gingival fluid and its significance in health and disease will be discussed in detail in a subsequent chapter.

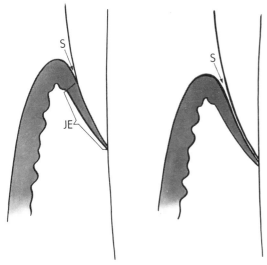

Figure 1–17 *Left,* **Gottlieb's Concept** of "broad epithelial attachment" and shallow gingival sulcus (S). The base of the sulcus is at the most superficial (coronal) level of the attached epithelium which, according to current terminology, is called the junctional epithelium (JE). *Right,* **Waerhaug's Concept** of a broad nonattached epithelial cuff with a deep gingival sulcus (S) with its base at the most apical level of the epithelium.

The Attached Gingiva

The attached gingiva is continuous with the marginal gingiva and consists of stratified squamous epithelium (Fig. 1–18) and an underlying connective tissue stroma. The epithelium is differentiated into (1) a cuboidal or columnar basal layer, (2) a spinous layer comprised of polygonal cells, (3) a multilayered granular component consisting of flattened cells with prominent basophilic keratohyaline granules in the cytoplasm and somewhat shrunken hyperchromic nucleus, and (4) a cornified layer that may be keratinized, parakeratinized, or both (Figs. 1–19 and 1–20).

The gingival epithelium is similar in structure to epidermis. In the female, a large Feulgen-positive particle has been found adjacent to the nuclear membrane in 75 per cent of the examined cases; in the male, a similar but smaller particle is present in 1 to 2 per cent of the cells.[80]

Electron microscopy reveals that the

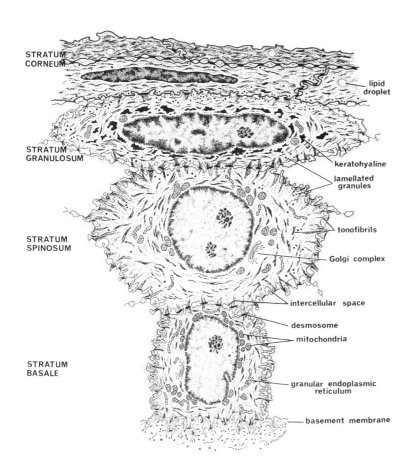

STRATUM CORNEUM

lipid droplet

STRATUM GRANULOSUM

keratohyaline

lamellated granules

STRATUM SPINOSUM

tonofibrils

Golgi complex

intercellular space

desmosome

mitochondria

STRATUM BASALE

granular endoplasmic reticulum

basement membrane

Figure 1–18 Diagram showing representative cells from the various layers of stratified squamous epithelium as seen by electron microscopy. (From Dr. A. Weinstock. *In* Ham, A. W.: Histology, 7th ed. Philadelphia, J. B. Lippincott Co., 1974.)

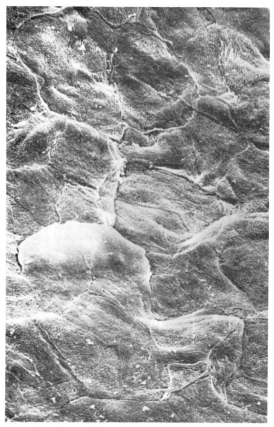

Figure 1–19 Scanning electron micrograph of keratinized gingiva showing the flattened keratinocytes and their boundaries on the surface of the gingiva. Magnification × 1000. (From Kaplan, G. B., Pameijer, C. H., and Ruben, M. P.: J. Periodontol., 48:446, 1977.)

cells of the gingival epithelium are connected to each other by structures along the cell periphery called *desmosomes*.[74] These desmosomes have a typical structure consisting of two dense *attachment plaques* into which tonofilaments insert, and an intermediate electron-dense line in the extracellular space. *Tonofibrils* radiate in brushlike fashion from the attachment plaques into the cytoplasm of the cells (Figs. 1–18 and 1–21). The space between the cells shows cytoplasmic projections resembling *microvilli* that extend into the intercellular space and often interdigitate.

Less frequently observed forms of epithelial cell connections[126, 144, 150] have been reported to represent *tight junctions* (zonula occludens), areas where the membranes of adjoining cells are believed to be fused; nevertheless, experimental evidence that verifies this hypothesis in gingival epithelium is lacking. It is possible that these structures represent patches of membrane fusion (rather than a zonula) or else gap junctions. There is evidence that suggests that these structures allow ions and small molecules to pass from one cell to another.

The epithelium is joined to the underlying connective tissue by a basal lamina 300 to 400 Å thick, which lies approximately 400 Å beneath the basal epithelial

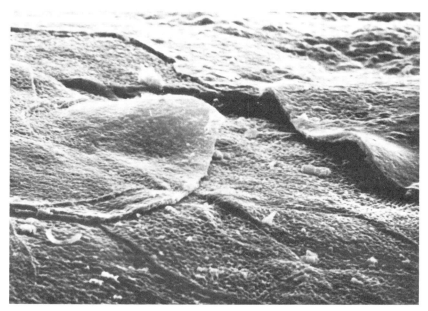

Figure 1–20 Scanning electron micrograph of gingival margin at edge of gingival sulcus showing at close-up view several keratinocytes about to be exfoliated. Magnification × 3000. (From Kaplan, G. B., Pameijer, C. H., and Ruben, M. P.: J. Periodontol., 48:446, 1977.)

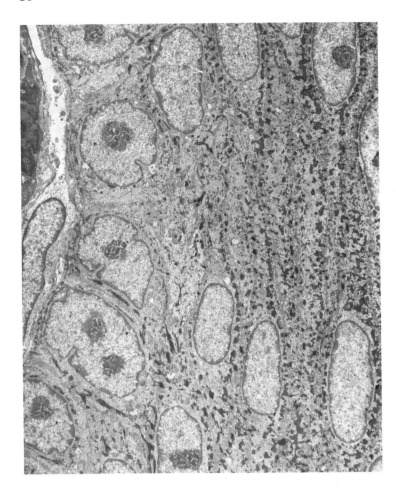

Figure 1–21 Electron micrograph of a portion of the sulcular epithelium from a rat incisor. At the extreme left is connective tissue. Next is a vertical row of cells in the basal cell layer, each with one or more prominent nucleoli. (The basal lamina is not visible at this magnification.) To the right of the basal cells are several layers of cells in the stratum spinosum. Out of view on the far right is the tooth. Magnification × 5000 (approximate). (Courtesy of Drs. A. Weinstock and T. Inage.)

layer.[66, 106, 119] The basal lamina consists of lamina lucida and lamina densa. The lamina densa is composed in part of glycoprotein.[64a] Hemidesmosomes of the basal epithelial cells abut on the lamina lucida.

The basal lamina is synthesized by the basal epithelial cells and consists of a **polysaccharide-protein complex and collagen (reticulin) fibers.**[91] *Anchoring fibrils* (also a component of what is believed to be reticulin) extend from the underlying connective tissue into the basal lamina, some of which penetrate through the lamina densa and lamina lucida to the membrane of the basal epithelial cells.[122] The basal lamina is permeable to fluids but acts as a barrier to particulate matter.

The Lamina Propria

The connective tissue of the gingiva is known as the lamina propria. It is densely collagenous with few elastic fibers. Argyrophilic reticulin fibers ramify between the collagen fibers and are continuous with reticulin in the blood vessel walls.[83] The lamina propria consists of two layers: (1) a **papillary layer** subjacent to the epithelium which consists of papillary projections between the epithelial rete pegs, and (2) a **reticular layer** contiguous with the periosteum of the alveolar bone.

Blood Supply, Lymphatics, and Nerves

There are *three sources of blood supply to the gingiva* (Fig. 1–22): (1) *Supraperiosteal arterioles* along the facial and lingual surfaces of the alveolar bone, from which capillaries extend along the sulcus epithelium and between the rete pegs of the external gingival surface.[28, 63] Occasional branches of the arterioles **pass through the alveolar bone to the periodontal ligament,**

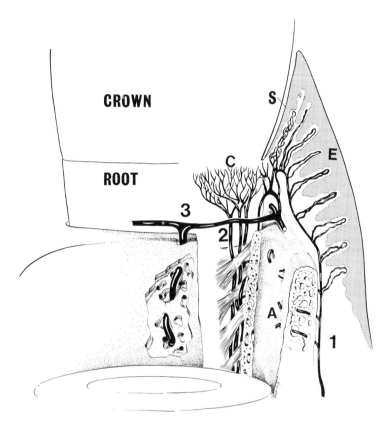

Figure 1–22 Periodontal Blood Supply. Diagrammatic, three dimensional representation of the three sources of blood supply to the gingiva as follows: (1) Supraperiosteal arterioles along the facial and lingual bone surfaces supply capillaries along the gingival sulcus (S) and external surface (E). Supraperiosteal branches also enter and pass through the bone to reach the periodontal ligament as alveolar penetrating vessels (A). (2) Longitudinal vessels of the periodontal ligament supply the col (C) and anastomose with capillaries in the sulcus area (S). (3) Arterioles penetrate the crest of the interdental septa and run along the crest of the bone to anastomose with vessels of the periodontal ligament and capillaries of the sulcus area (S) and with other vessels along the crest of the bone.

or run over the crest of the alveolar bone (Fig. 1–23). (2) *Vessels of the periodontal ligament*, which extend into the gingiva and anastomose with capillaries in the sulcus area. (3) *Arterioles, which emerge from the crest of the interdental septa*[36] and extend parallel to the crest of the

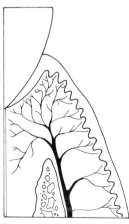

Figure 1–23 Diagrammatic representation of arteriole penetrating the interdental alveolar bone to supply the interdental tissues (left), and a supraperiosteal arteriole overlying the facial alveolar bone, sending branches to the surrounding tissue (right).

bone to anastomose with vessels of the periodontal ligament, with capillaries in the gingival crevicular areas, and with vessels which run over the alveolar crest.

Beneath the epithelium on the outer gingival surface, capillaries extend into the papillary connective tissue between the epithelial rete pegs in the form of terminal hairpin loops with efferent and afferent branches,[53, 63] spirals and varices (Fig. 1–24). The loops are sometimes linked by cross communications,[34] and there are also flattened capillaries which serve as reserve vessels when the circulation is increased in response to irritation.[41] Along the sulcus epithelium, capillaries are arranged in a flat anastomosing plexus which extends parallel to the enamel from the base of the sulcus to the gingival margin.[17] In the col area there is a mixed pattern of anastomosing capillaries and loops.

The *lymphatic drainage* of the gingiva begins in the lymphatics of the connective tissue papillae. It progresses into the collecting network external to the periosteum of the alveolar process and then to the regional lymph nodes (particularly the submaxillary group).[110] In addition, lym-

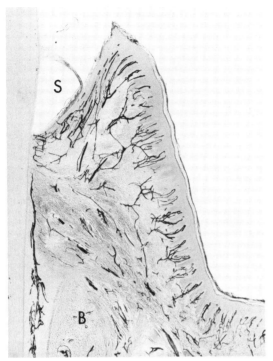

Figure 1-24   Blood Supply and Peripheral Circulation of the Gingiva. Tissues perfused with India ink. Note the capillary plexus parallel to the sulcus (S) and the capillary loops in the outer papillary layer. Note also the supraperiosteal vessels external to the bone (B) which supply the gingiva and a periodontal ligament vessel anastomosing with the sulcus plexus. (See also Fig. 2–6.) (Courtesy of Dr. Sol Bernick.)

phatics just beneath the epithelial attachment extend into the periodontal ligament and accompany the blood vessels.

Gingival innervation is derived from fibers arising from nerves in the periodontal ligament and from the labial, buccal, and palatal nerves.[10] The following nerve structures are present in the connective tissue: a meshwork of *terminal argyrophilic* fibers, some of which extend into the epithelium; *Meissner-type tactile corpuscles; Krause-type end bulbs*, which are temperature receptors; and *encapsulated spindles.*[66]

The Interdental Gingiva and the Col

As the proximal tooth surfaces contact in the course of eruption, the oral mucosa between the teeth is separated into the facial and lingual interdental papillae joined by the col.[20] Each interdental papilla consists of a central core of densely collagenous connective tissue covered by thinly keratinized stratified squamous epithelium. The so-called *oxytalan* fibers in the connective tissue of the col[65] as well as in other areas of the gingiva[36] are believed by some authorities to represent elastin.

At the time of eruption and for a period

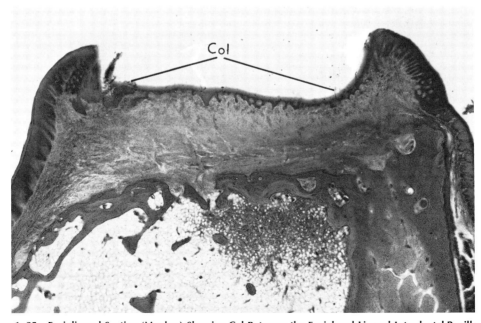

Figure 1-25   Faciolingual Section (Monkey) Showing Col Between the Facial and Lingual Interdental Papillae. The col is covered with non-keratinized stratified squamous epithelium.

thereafter, the col is covered by *reduced enamel epithelium* derived from the approximating teeth. This is gradually replaced by non-keratinized *stratified squamous epithelium* from the adjacent interdental papillae (Fig. 1–25). It has been suggested that during the period that the col is covered by reduced enamel epithelium it is highly susceptible to injury and disease because the protection provided by this type of epithelium is inadequate.[84] However, the significance of this hypothesis has yet to be determined. The fact that keratin is lacking in the adult col epithelium probably renders it more susceptible to bacterial injury and disease. As described in detail in another chapter, this is the site of the initial lesion in gingivitis.

CORRELATION OF THE NORMAL CLINICAL AND MICROSCOPIC FEATURES

To understand the normal clinical features of the gingiva, one must be able to interpret them in terms of the microscopic structures they represent.

Color

The color of the attached and marginal gingiva is generally described as coral pink, and is produced by the vascular supply, the thickness and degree of keratinization of the epithelium, and the presence of pigment-containing cells. The color varies in different persons and appears to be correlated with the cutaneous pigmentation. It is lighter in blond individuals with a fair complexion than in swarthy brunettes.

The attached gingiva is demarcated from the adjacent alveolar mucosa on the buccal aspect by a clearly defined mucogingival line. The alveolar mucosa is red, smooth, and shiny rather than pink and stippled. Comparison of the microscopic structure of the attached gingiva and alveolar mucosa affords an explanation for the difference in appearance. The epithelium of the alveolar mucosa is thinner, non-keratinized, and contains no rete pegs (Fig. 1–26). The connective tissue of the alveolar mucosa is loosely arranged and the blood vessels are more numerous.

PHYSIOLOGIC PIGMENTATION (MELANIN). Melanin, a non-hemoglobin–derived brown pigment, is responsible for the normal pigmentation of the skin, gingiva, and remainder of the oral mucous membrane. It is present in all individuals, often not in sufficient quantities to be detected clinically, but is absent or severely diminished in albinism. Melanin pigmentation in the oral cavity is prominent in blacks (Plate I).

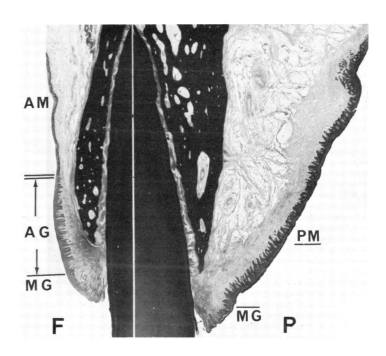

Figure 1–26 Oral Mucosa, Facial and Palatal Surfaces. *F,* Facial surface showing the marginal gingiva (MG), attached gingiva (AG), and alveolar mucosa (AM). The double line (⇒) marks the mucogingival junction. Note the differences in the epithelium and connective tissue in the attached gingiva and alveolar mucosa. *P,* Palatal surface showing the marginal gingiva (MG) and thick keratinized palatal mucosa (PM).

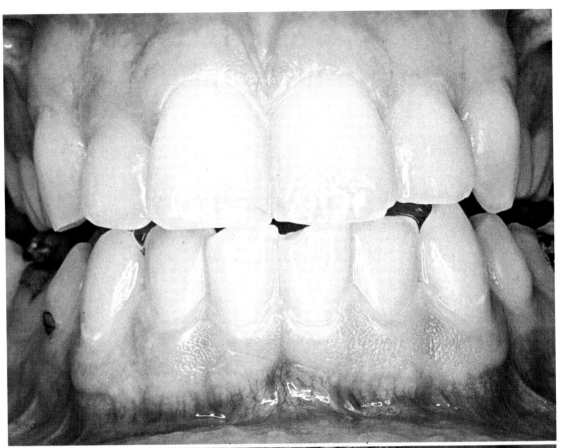

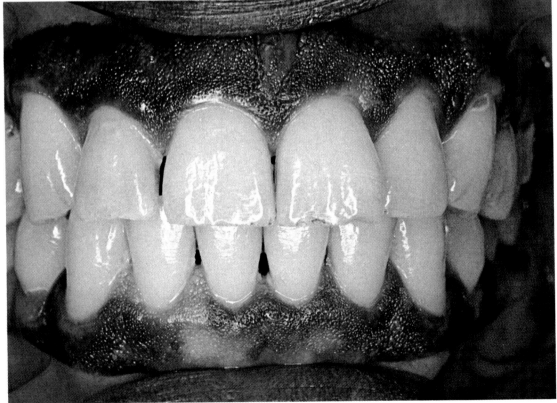

Plate I *See legend on opposite page*

20

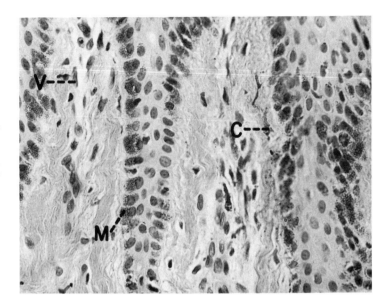

Figure 1–27 Pigmented Gingiva, showing melanocytes (M) in the basal epithelial layer and melanophores (C) in the connective tissue. Also shown is a capillary (V) in the papillary connective tissue.

Melanin is formed by dendritic *melanocytes* in the basal and spinous layers of the gingival epithelium (Fig. 1–27). It is synthesized in *organelles* within the cells called *premelanosomes* or *melanosomes*.[22, 104, 117] These contain tyrosinase, which hydroxylates tyrosine to dihydroxyphenylalanine (dopa), which in turn is progressively converted to melanin. Melanin granules are phagocytosed by and contained within other cells of the epithelium and connective tissue called *melanophages* or *melanophores*.

According to Dummett,[27] the distribution of oral pigmentation in blacks is as follows: gingiva, 60 per cent; hard palate, 61 per cent; mucous membrane, 22 per cent; and tongue, 15 per cent. Gingival pigmentation occurs as a diffuse, deep purplish discoloration or as irregularly shaped brown and light brown patches. It may appear in the gingiva as early as three hours after birth, and often is the only evidence of pigmentation.

Size

The size of the gingiva corresponds to the sum total of the bulk of cellular and intercellular elements and their vascular supply. Alteration in size is a common feature of gingival disease.

Contour

The contour or shape of the gingiva varies considerably, and depends upon the shape of the teeth and their alignment in the arch, the location and size of the area of proximal contact, and the dimensions of the facial and lingual gingival embrasures. The marginal gingiva envelops the teeth in collar-like fashion, and follows a scalloped outline on the facial and lingual surfaces. It forms a straight line along teeth with relatively flat surfaces. On teeth with pronounced mesiodistal convexity (e.g., maxillary canines), or in labial version, the

Plate I *A,* Clinically normal gingiva in young adult. *B,* Heavily pigmented (melanotic) gingiva in middle-aged adult. (From Glickman, I., and Smulow, J. B.: Periodontal Disease: Clinical, Radiographic, and Histopathologic Features. Philadelphia, W. B. Saunders Company, 1974.)

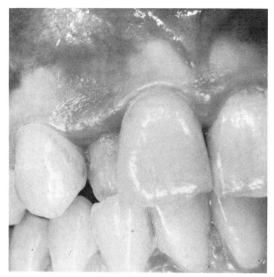

Figure 1–28 Thickened shelflike contour of gingiva on tooth in lingual version aggravated by local irritation caused by plaque accumulation.

normal arcuate contour is accentuated and the gingiva is located further apically. On teeth in lingual version the gingiva is horizontal and thickened (Fig. 1–28).

The *shape* of the *interdental gingiva* is governed by the contour of the proximal tooth surfaces, the location and shape of the contact area, and the dimensions of the gingival embrasures. When the proximal surfaces of the crowns are relatively flat faciolingually, the roots are close together, the interdental bone is thin mesiodistally, and the gingival embrasures and interdental gingiva are narrow mesiodistally. Conversely, with proximal surfaces that flare away from the area of contact, the mesiodistal diameter of the interdental gingiva is broad (Fig. 1–29). The height of the interdental gingiva varies with the location of the proximal contact.

Consistency

The gingiva is firm and resilient and, with the exception of the movable free margin, tightly bound to the underlying bone. The collagenous nature of the lamina propria and its contiguity with the mucoperiosteum of the alveolar bone determines the firm consistency of the attached gingiva. The gingival fibers contribute to the firmness of the gingival margin.

Surface Texture

The gingiva presents a textured surface like an orange peel, and is referred to as being *stippled*. Stippling is best viewed

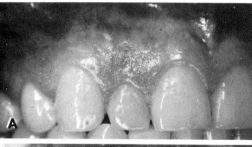

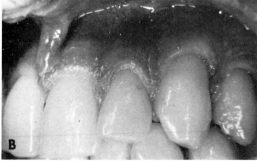

Figure 1–29 Shape of interdental gingival papillae correlated with shape of teeth and embrasures. *A,* Broad interdental papillae; *B,* narrow interdental papillae.

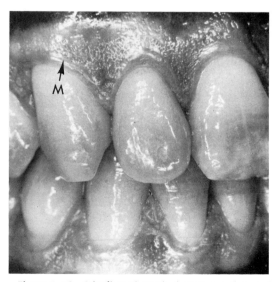

Figure 1–30 **Stippling** of attached gingiva and central portions of interdental papillae. The gingival margin (M) is smooth.

by drying the gingiva (Fig. 1–30). The attached gingiva is stippled; the gingival margin is not. The central portion of the interdental papillae is usually stippled, but the margin borders are smooth. The pattern and extent of stippling vary from person to person, and in different areas of the same mouth.[49, 101] It is less prominent on lingual than on facial surfaces, and may be absent in some patients.

Stippling varies with age. It is absent in infancy, appears in some children at about five years of age, increases until adulthood, and frequently begins to disappear in old age.

Microscopically, stippling is produced by alternate rounded protuberances and depressions in the gingival surface. The papillary layer of the connective tissue projects into the elevations, and both the elevated and depressed areas are covered by stratified squamous epithelium (Fig. 1–31). The degree of keratinization and the prominence of stippling appear to be related.

Stippling is a form of adaptive specialization or reinforcement for function. It is a feature of healthy gingiva, and **reduction or loss of stippling is a common sign of gingival disease.** When the gingiva is restored to health following treatment, the stippled appearance returns.

Keratinization

The epithelium covering the outer surface of the marginal gingiva and the attached gingiva is keratinized or parakeratinized or presents varied combinations of both conditions.[103] The surface layer is shed in thin strands and replaced by cells from the underlying granular layer. Keratinization is considered to be a protective adaptation to function which increases when the gingiva is stimulated by toothbrushing.

Keratinization of the oral mucosa varies in different areas in the following order: palate (most keratinized), gingiva, tongue, and cheek (least keratinized).[87] The degree of gingival keratinization is not necessarily correlated with the different phases of the menstrual cycle,[61, 88] and diminishes with age and the onset of menopause.[96]

Gingival keratin has been examined by means of scanning electron microscopy.[62] Its morphology varies slightly depending on its anatomical location.

Renewal of Gingival Epithelium

The oral epithelium undergoes continuous renewal. Its thickness is maintained by a balance between new cell formation in the basal and spinous layers and the

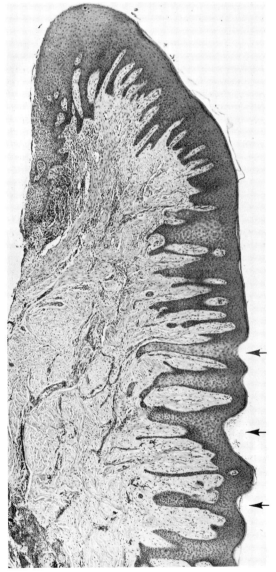

Figure 1–31 Gingival biopsy of patient shown in Figure 1–30, demonstrating alternate elevations and depressions (arrows) in the attached gingiva responsible for stippled appearance.

shedding of old cells at the surface. The *mitotic activity* exhibits a 24-hour periodicity, with highest and lowest rates occurring in the morning and evening respectively.[132] The mitotic rate is higher in non-keratinized gingival epithelium than in keratinized areas, and is increased in gingivitis, without significant sex differences. Opinions differ as to whether the mitotic rate is increased[76, 85] or decreased[6] with age.

The mitotic rate in experimental animals varies in different areas of the oral epithelium in the following descending order: buccal mucosa, hard palate, sulcus epithelium, junctional epithelium, outer surface of the marginal gingiva, and attached gingiva.[2, 52, 76, 132] The following have been reported as the turnover times for different areas of the oral epithelium in experimental animals: palate, tongue, and cheek, 5 to 6 days; gingiva, 10 to 12 days, with the same or more time required with age; and junctional epithelium, 1 to 6 days.[9, 114]

Position

The position of the gingiva refers to the level at which the **gingival margin is attached to the tooth.** When the tooth erupts into the oral cavity, the margin and sulcus are at the tip of the crown; as eruption progresses, they are seen closer to the root. During this eruption process, as described earlier, the junctional epithelium, oral epithelium, and reduced enamel epithelium undergo extensive alterations and remodeling, while at the same time maintaing the shallow physiologic depth of the sulcus.[121] Without this remodeling of the epithelia, an abnormal anatomical relationship between the gingiva and tooth would result.

Continuous Tooth Eruption

According to the *concept of continuous eruption* (Gottlieb[48]), eruption does not cease when teeth meet their functional antagonists, but continues throughout life. It consists of an *active* and *passive* phase. *Active eruption* is the movement of the teeth in the direction of the occlusal plane, whereas *passive eruption* is the exposure of the teeth by separation of the junctional epithelium from the enamel and migration onto the cementum.

Inherent in the concept is the distinction between the *anatomic crown* (the portion of the tooth covered by enamel) and the *anatomic root* (the portion of the tooth covered by cementum), and the *clinical crown* and *clinical root*. The clinical crown is the part of the tooth that has been denuded of epithelium and projects into the oral cavity; the clinical root is that portion of the tooth covered by periodontal tissues.

When the teeth reach their functional antagonists, the gingival sulcus and junctional epithelium are still on the enamel,[93] and the clinical crown is approximately two thirds of the anatomic crown.

Active and passive eruption were believed by Gottlieb to proceed together.

ACTIVE ERUPTION. Active eruption is coordinated with attrition. The teeth erupt to compensate for tooth substance worn away by attrition. Attrition reduces the clinical crown and prevents it from becoming disproportionately long in relation to the clinical root, thus avoiding excessive leverage on the periodontal tissues. Ideally, the rate of active eruption keeps pace with tooth wear, preserving the *vertical dimension* of the dentition.

As the teeth erupt, cementum is deposited at the apices and furcations of the roots, and bone is formed along the fundus of the alveolus and at the crest of the alveolar bone. In this way part of the *tooth substance lost by attrition is replaced by lengthening of the root, and socket depth is maintained to support the root.*

PASSIVE ERUPTION. Passive eruption is divided into four stages (Fig. 1–32). While this was originally thought to be a normal physiological process, it is now recognized to be a *pathological* process.

Stage One. The teeth reach the line of occlusion. The junctional epithelium and base of the gingival sulcus are on the enamel.

Stage Two. The junctional epithelium proliferates so that part is on the cementum and part on the enamel. The base of the sulcus is still on the enamel.

Stage Three. The entire junctional epi-

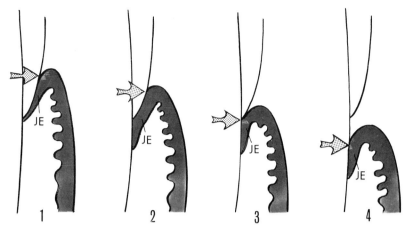

Figure 1–32 Diagrammatic representation of the four steps in passive eruption according to Gottlieb.[48] 1, Base of the gingival sulcus (arrow) and the junctional epithelium (JE) are on the enamel. 2, Base of the gingival sulcus (arrow) is on the enamel, and part of the junctional epithelium is on the root. 3, Base of the gingival sulcus (arrow) is at the cemento-enamel line, and the entire junctional epithelium is on the root. 4, Base of the gingival sulcus (arrow) and the junctional epithelium are on the root.

thelium is on the cementum, and the base of the sulcus is at the cemento-enamel junction. As the junctional epithelium proliferates from the crown onto the root, it remains no longer at the cemento-enamel junction than at any other area of the tooth.

Stage Four. The junctional epithelium has proliferated further on the cementum. The base of the sulcus is on the cementum, a portion of which is exposed.

Proliferation of the junctional epithelium onto the root is accompanied by degeneration of gingival and periodontal ligament fibers and their detachment from the tooth. The cause of this degeneration was not understood, but at the present time authorities believe that it is the result of chronic inflammation.

As noted above, apposition of bone accompanies active eruption. The distance between the apical end of the epithelial attachment and the crest of the alveolus remains constant throughout continuous tooth eruption (1.07 mm.).[38]

Gingival Recession (Gingival Atrophy)

According to the concept of continuous eruption, the gingival sulcus may be located on the crown, cemento-enamel junction, or root, depending upon the age of the patient and the stage of eruption. **Exposure of the root by the apical migration of the gingiva is called gingival recession,** or atrophy. Some root exposure is considered normal with age and is referred to as *physiologic recession;* excessive exposure is termed *pathologic recession* (see Chap. 8). The distinction is one of degree. Investigators who do not accept the concept of continuous eruption maintain that the cemento-enamel junction is the normal location of the gingiva and that any exposure of the root is pathological.[151, 152]

Cuticular Structures on the Tooth

The term cuticle is used to describe a thin acellular structure with a homogeneous matrix, sometimes enclosed within clearly demarcated linear borders. The following cuticular structures have been described on the teeth: (For a complete summary and review on this subject, see ref. 118.)

1. *Acquired pellicle (acquired cuticle, salivary pellicle).* This is an acquired rather than anatomical structure deposited on the tooth surface by the saliva as a *thin, acellular, translucent film.* It is believed to represent the adsorption of salivary glycoproteins onto hydroxyapatite crystals.

2. *Primary cuticle (enamel cuticle, Nasmyth's membrane).* Originally described by Nasmyth[92] ("persistent dental capsule") and subsequently by Gottlieb, this cuticle is present *on the enamel* of the unerupted tooth. Nasmyth unknowingly described

the reduced enamel epithelium, and since that time the "persistent dental capsule," also termed "Nasmyth's membrane," has produced much confusion. Gottlieb later described the "primary enamel cuticle" which he considered to be the final product of degenerating ameloblasts after completion of enamel formation.

Electron microscopy reveals that the structure designated as "primary cuticle" consists of **ameloblasts of the reduced enamel epithelium attached to the enamel by a basal lamina (basement lamina).**[71, 74, 121] This consists of a lamina densa (adjacent to the enamel) and a lamina lucida to which hemidesmosomes of the ameloblasts are attached. Thus, as a result of the high resolution afforded by electron microscopy, the confusing results of numerous light microscopists have now been clarified. It can be concluded that the so-called "primary cuticle" is not a cuticle.

3. *Secondary cuticle or dental cuticle (cuticula dentis, transposed crevicular cuticle).*[44] This cuticle was believed to be deposited upon the enamel (external to the primary enamel cuticle, with which it combines) and on the nearby cementum. It was thought to be deposited by the "epithelial attachment" as it migrated along the tooth and separated from crown and root during eruption stages (Fig. 1–33). It was not present on cementum to which the periodontal ligament is attached. It was originally described as keratinized,[45] but this observation has not been supported by subsequent histochemical studies.[147, 148]

As described earlier, electron microscopy has shown that the dental cuticle consists of a layer of homogeneous organic material of variable thickness (ca. 0.25 micron) overlying the enamel surface. It is non-mineralized and is not always present. In some instances near the cemento-enamel junction, it is deposited over a layer of afibrillar cementum which, in turn, overlays enamel. The cuticle may or may not be present between the junctional epithelium and the tooth. It is believed to be deposited, at least in part, by reduced ameloblasts (Figs. 1–12 to 1–14), but its origin is still uncertain.[105] It has been shown that reduced ameloblasts have a secretory function.[142, 143] Some investiga-

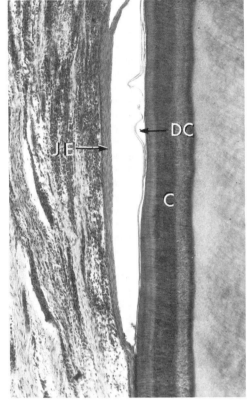

Figure 1–33 "Secondary" cuticle or dental cuticle. In this paraffin section the dental cuticle (DC) consists of both the amorphous, homogeneous layer seen in the electron microscope and surface epithelial cells torn away from the sulcus epithelium. This structure is similar to that which Gottlieb described. C, cementum.

tors believe that the dental cuticle is a pathologic product of inflamed gingiva,[86] or a pathologic conglutinate of erythrocytes.[55]

HISTOCHEMICAL ASPECTS OF NORMAL GINGIVA

Cellular and Intercellular Substances

Histochemical techniques provide useful information regarding the chemical components and enzyme systems of normal gingiva. In addition to adding to our understanding of physiologic processes in the gingiva, this information may provide **guidelines for interpreting the changes which occur in gingival disease.**

The connective tissue of normal gingiva

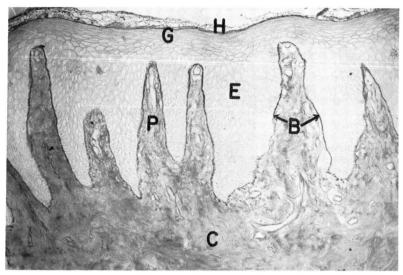

Figure 1–34   Normal Human Gingiva Stained with the Periodic Acid-Schiff (P.A.S.) Histochemical Method. The basement membrane (B) is seen between the epithelium (E) and underlying connective tissue (C). In the epithelium there is glycoprotein material between the cells and in the cell membrane of the superficial hornified (H) and underlying granular layers (G). The connective tissue presents a diffuse amorphous ground substance and collagen fibers. The blood vessel walls stand out clearly in the papillary projections of the connective tissue (P).

contains a *PAS-positive (periodic acid-Schiff stain) heteropolysaccharide intercellular ground substance*[31] that is also present in the walls of the blood vessels and between the cells of the epithelium.[109] A thin PAS-positive basement membrane demarcates the connective tissue from the epithelium (Fig. 1–34). Electron microscopy reveals this to be a band of thin collagen fibers (reticulin) on the connective tissue side of the lamina densa of the basal lamina, rather than the basal lamina itself which is not involved in the PAS reaction.[123]

PAS-negative acid mucopolysaccharides, hyaluronic acid, and *chondroitin sulfate A, C, and B*[108, 129] demonstrated between the epithelial cells are considered by some[127] to be intercellular cementing substances and by others[42] to be stained portions of the intercellular attachment apparatus. *Neutral mucopolysaccharides* also occur intercellularly in the epithelium.

Glycogen, which is PAS-positive, is an intracellular component seen throughout the connective tissue and in the smooth muscle of the arterioles.[135] In the epithelium, glycogen occurs intracellularly, in concentrations inversely related to the degree of keratinization. Some consider it a normal component of epithelium;[107, 140]

others find it only in acanthosis, usually associated with inflammation.[26] *Phosphorylase activity* generally occurs in the epithelium where glycogen is located.[100]

RNA is found in large quantities in the basal cells of normal gingival epithelium, decreasing toward the superficial layers, and in lowest concentration in the crevicular epithelium.[69] *DNA,* normally present in the nucleus of all gingival cells, is increased in gingival hyperplasia. The DNA and RNA activity of the epithelium at the gingival margin and junctional epithelium is greater than in the remaining oral mucosa.[39, 50]

Sulfhydryls and *disulfides* are normal components of the gingival epithelium and connective tissue.[133] In the keratinization process sulfhydryls are oxidized to disulfides and both are significant in a wide range of biologic activities such as enzymatic and antibody reactions, cell growth and division, and cell permeability and detoxification. Sulfhydryls and disulfides are present throughout the gingival epithelium; the former is increased in keratinized and parakeratinized layers,[133] and the latter in the surface keratinized cells.[81] In the connective tissue, sulfhydryls and disulfides occur intercellulary and in the fibroblasts and endothelial cells. The *phospholipid* and *cholesterol* content of the gingiva is comparable to that of skin,[54] and lipids have been demonstrated in keratohyaline granules in the epithelium.[25]

Enzymes

Alkaline phosphatase is present in the endothelial cells, in the capillary walls, and possibly in the fibers of the connective tissue. It has been described in keratinized and parakeratinized surface layers,[21] but there is some doubt that it occurs in epithelium.[16]

Acid phosphatase, found in the epithelium in greatest concentration in the surface and prickle cell layers,[139] is related to keratinization.[15] It is not present in the junctional epithelium or sulcus lining. Different patterns of distribution have been described in different animal species for acid and alkaline phosphatases.[57] *Diphospho and triphosphopyridine nucleotide reductases,* present in all epithelial cells except keratin and parakeratin, in desmosomes, tonofibrils and nucleoli, suggest an oxidative metabolic pathway for the formation of the keratin precursor substance and keratin.[30] In tissue culture mucopolysaccharides and acid phosphatase are present in epithelial and fibroblast-like gingival cells, but the amount of alkaline phosphatase is negligible.[115]

Acetylcholinesterase and nonspecific *cholinesterase* are present in gingival connective tissue.[5] *Endogenous reducing enzymes, succinic dehydrogenase, glucose-6-phosphate dehydrogenase, lactic dehydrogenase,*[29] *beta-D-glucuronidase, beta-glucosidase, beta-galactosidase,*[70] and *aminopeptidase*[90, 99] have been observed in gingiva. *Esterase*[58, 70] occurs in the basal and granular layers of the epithelium and in the connective tissue near periodontal pockets.[16]

In a quantitative histochemical study of human gingival epithelium,[59] glucose-6-phosphate dehydrogenase was found to have its maximum content in epithelium of marginal gingiva and lower content in oral mucosal epithelium, sulcular epithelium, and junctional epithelium. Succinic dehydrogenase content was found to be greater in attached gingiva. Glucose-6-

phosphate dehydrogenase increased its concentration from the basal to the superficial layers in attached and marginal gingiva, remained stable in all strata of oral mucosal epithelium and sulcular epithelium, and reduced its activity toward the surface in junctional epithelium. Succinic dehydrogenase decreased its concentration from the basal to the superficial layers in all zones.[59]

These findings have suggested that the basal layer has an oxidative activity of the Krebs cycle type that tends to switch to the pentose shunt as it approaches the surface.[59]

Collagenase is produced in epithelium and connective tissue of normal gingiva as well as in the periodontal ligament and alveolar bone.[37] *Cytochrome oxidase* activity occurs in the sulcular and junctional epithelium, in the basal layers of marginal and attached gingiva, and in the connective tissue.[98] *5-Nucleotidase* occurs in the blood vessels and surface epithelial cells of keratinized gingiva and only in the blood vessels of non-keratinized and parakeratinized gingiva.[24] *Lysosomes* have been demonstrated in exfoliated cells of the junctional epithelium.[68]

The *oxygen consumption of normal gingiva* (QO_2 1.6 ± 0.37) is comparable to that of skin (QO_2 1.48 ± 0.48).[43] The respiratory activity of the epithelium is approximately three times greater than that of the connective tissue,[89] and the sulcular epithelium is approximately twice that of whole gingiva.[67]

REFERENCES

1. Ainamo, J., and Löe, H.: Anatomical characteristics of gingiva. A clinical and microscopic study of the free and attached gingiva. J. Periodontol., 37:5, 1966.
2. Anderson, G. S., and Stern, I.: The proliferation and migration of the attachment epithelium on the cemental surface of the rat incisor. Periodontics, 4:115, 1966.
3. Arnim, S. S., and Hagerman, D. A.: The connective tissue fibers of the marginal gingiva. J. Am. Dent. Assoc., 47:271, 1953.
4. Avery, J. K., and Rapp, R.: Pain conduction in human dental tissues. Dent. Clin. North Am., July 1959, p. 489.
5. Avery, J. K., and Rapp, R.: Presence of acetylcholinesterase in human gingiva. J. Periodontol., 30:152, 1959.

6. Barakat, N. J., Toto, P. D., and Choukas, N. C.: Aging and cell renewal of oral epithelium. J. Periodontol., 40:599, 1969.

7. Bass, C. C.: A demonstrable line in extracted teeth indicating the location of the outer border of the epithelial attachment. J. Dent. Res., 25:401, 1946.

8. Baume, J. L.: The structure of the epithelial attachment revealed by phase contrast microscopy. J. Periodontol, 24:99, 1953.

9. Beagrie, G. S., and Skougard, M. R.: Observations in the life cycle of the gingival epithelial cells of mice as revealed by autoradiography. Acta Odontol. Scand., 20:15, 1962.

10. Bernick, S.: Innervation of the teeth and periodontium. Dent. Clin. North Am., July 1959, p. 503.

11. Bowers, G. M.: A study of the width of the attached gingiva. J. Periodontol., 34:201, 1963.

12. Box, H. K.: Treatment of the Periodontal Pocket. Toronto, The University of Toronto Press, 1928.

13. Brill, N., and Björn, H.: Passage of tissue fluid into human gingival pockets. Acta Odontol. Scand., 17:11, 1959.

14. Burnett, G. M., Gouge, S., and Toye, A. E.: Lysozyme content of human gingiva and various rat tissues. J. Periodontol., 30:148, 1959.

15. Cabrini, R. L., and Carranza, F. A., Jr.: Histochemical distribution of acid phosphatase in human gingiva. J. Periodontol., 29:34, 1958.

16. Cabrini, R. L., and Carranza, F. A., Jr.: Histochemistry of periodontal tissues. A review of the literature. Int. Dent. J., 16:466, 1966.

17. Carranza, F. A., Jr., Itoiz, M. E., Cabrini, R. L., and Dotto, C. A.: A study of periodontal vascularization in different laboratory animals. J. Periodont. Res., 1:120, 1966.

18. Carranza, F. A., Jr., and Cabrini, R. L.: Mast cells in human gingiva. Oral Surg., 8:1093, 1955.

19. Cimasoni, G.: The Crevicular Fluid. Monographs in Oral Science, Vol. 3. H. M. Meyer, ed., Basel, S. Karger, 1974.

20. Cohen, B.: Morphological factors in the pathogenesis of periodontal disease. Br. Dent. J., 107:31, 1959.

21. Cohen, L.: Alkaline phosphatase activity in human gingival epithelium. Periodontics, 6:23, 1968.

22. Cohen, L.: ATPase and dopa oxidase activity in human gingival epithelium. Arch. Oral Biol., 12:1241, 1967.

23. Cohen, L.: Keratinization of the gingivae. Dent. Pract., 18:134, 1967.

24. Cohen, L.: Presence of 5-nucleotidase in human gingiva. J. Dent. Res., 46:757, 1967.

25. Cohen, L.: Presence of lipids in keratohyaline granules of human gingiva. J. Dent. Res., 46:630, 1967.

26. Dewar, M. R.: Observations on the composition and metabolism of normal and inflamed gingivae. J. Periodontol, 26:29, 1955.

27. Dummett, C. O.: Physiologic pigmentation of the oral and cutaneous tissues in the Negro. J. Dent. Res., 25:422, 1946.

28. Egelberg, J.: The topography and permeability of blood vessels at the dentinogingival junction in dogs. J. Periodont. Res., 2(Suppl. 1), 1967.

29. Eichel, B.: Oxidation enzymes of gingiva. Ann. N.Y. Acad. Sci., 85:479, 1960.

30. Eichel, B., Shahrik, H. A., and Lisanti, V. F.: Cytochemical demonstration and metabolic significance of reduced diphospho-pyridine-nucleotide and triphospho-pyridinenucleotide reductases in human gingiva. J. Dent. Res., 43:92, 1964.

31. Engel, M. B.: Water-soluble mucoproteins of the gingiva. J. Dent. Res., 32:779, 1953.

32. Engler, W. O., Ramfjord, S. P., and Hiniker, J. J.: Development of epithelial attachment and gingival sulcus in Rhesus monkeys. J. Periodontol., 36:44, 1965.

33. Folke, L. E. A., and Stallard, R. E.: Periodontal microcirculation as revealed by plastic microspheres. J. Periodont. Res., 2:53, 1967.

34. Forsslund, G.: Structure and function of capillary system in the gingiva in man. Development of stereophotogrammetric metnod and its application for study of the subepithelial blood vessels in vivo. Acta Odontol. Scand., 17:9 (Suppl. 26), 1959.

35. Frohlich, E.: Veränderungen im Gefüge des Zahnfleischbindegewebes bei den entzündlichen marginalen Zahnbetterkrankungen. Dtsch. Zahnärz, Z., 7:477, 1952.

36. Fullmer, H. M.: Critique of normal connective tissue of the periodontium and some alterations with periodontal disease. J. Dent. Res., 41 (Suppl. 1):223, 1962.

37. Fullmer, H. M., et al.: The origin of collagenase in periodontal tissues of man. J. Dent. Res., 48:636, 1969.

38. Gargiulo, A. W., Wentz, F. M., and Orban, B.: Dimensions and relations of the dentogingival junction in humans. J. Periodontol., 32:261, 1961.

39. Gimenez, I. B., and Carranza, F. A., Jr.: Microspectrophotometric study of DNA in gingival epithelium. J. Dent. Res., 52:1345, 1973.

40. Glickman, I., and Bibby, B. G.: The existence of cuticular structures on human teeth. J. Dent. Res., 22:91, 1943.

41. Glickman, I., and Johannessen, L.: Biomicroscopic (slit-lamp) evaluation of the normal gingiva of the albino rat. J. Am. Dent. Assoc., 41:521, 1950.

42. Glickman, I., and Smulow, J. B.: Histopathology and histochemistry of chronic desquamative gingivitis. Oral Surg., 21:325, 1966.

43. Glickman, I., Turesky, S., and Hill, R.: Determination of oxygen consumption in normal and inflamed human gingiva using the Warburg manometric technic. J. Dent. Res., 28:83, 1949.

44. Gottlieb, B.: Der Epithelansatz am Zahne. Dtsch. Monatschr. Zahnhk., 39:142, 1921.

45. Gottlieb, B.: Tissue changes in pyorrhea. Trans. 7th Int. Dent. Congress, 1:421, 1926.

46. Gottlieb, B.: What is a normal pocket? J. Am. Dent. Assoc., 13:1747, 1926.

47. Gottlieb, B.: Zur Biologie des Epithelansatzes und des Alveolarrandes. Dtsch. Zahnärztl. Wochenschr., 25:434, 1922.

48. Gottlieb, B., and Orban, B.: Active and passive eruption of the teeth. J. Dent. Res., 13:214, 1933.

49. Greene, A. H.: A study of the characteristics of stippling and its relation to gingival health. J. Periodontol., 33:176, 1962.

50. Greulich, R. C.: Epithelial DNA and RNA synthetic activities of the gingival margin. J. Dent. Res., 40:682, 1961.

51. Gross, H.: Zur Genese der vertieften Zahnfleischtasche Paradentium, 3:69, 1930.

52. Hansen, E. R.: Mitotic activity of the gingival epithelium in colchicinized rats. Odont. T., 74:229, 1966.

53. Hansson, B. O., Lindhe, J., and Branemark, P. I.: Microvascular topography and function in clinically healthy and chronically inflamed dentogingival tissues—A vital microscopic study in dogs. Periodontics, 6:265, 1968.

54. Hodge, H. C.: Gingival tissue lipids. J. Biol. Chem., 101:55, 1933.

55. Hodson, J.: The distribution, structure, origin, and nature of the dental cuticle of Gottlieb. Periodontics, 5:295, 1967.

56. Ito, H., Enomoto, S., and Kobayashi, K.: Electron microscopic study of the human epithelial attachment. Bull. Tokyo Med. Dent. Univ., 14:267, 1967.

57. Itoiz, M. E., Carranza, F. A., Jr., and Cabrini, R. L.: Histotopographic distribution of alkaline and acid phosphatase in periodontal tissues of laboratory animals. J. Periodontol., 38:470, 1964.

58. Itoiz, M. E., Carranza, F. A., Jr., and Cabrini, R. L.: Histotopographic study of esterase and 5-nucleotidase in periodontal tissues of laboratory animals. J. Periodontol., 38:130, 1967.

59. Itoiz, M. E., Carranza, F. A., Jr., Gimenez, I., and Cabrini, R. L.: Microspectrophotometric analysis of succinic dehydrogenase and glucose-6-phosphate dehydrogenase in human oral epithelium. J. Periodont. Res., 7:14, 1972.

60. Itoiz, M. E., Carranza, F. A., Jr., Neira, V., and Cabrini, R. L.: Fine structural localization of thiamine pyrophosphatase in normal human gingiva. J. Periodontol., 45:579, 1974.

61. Iusem, R.: A cytological study of the cornification of the oral mucosa in women. Oral Surg., 3:1516, 1950.

62. Kaplan, G. B., Pameijer, C. H., and Ruben, M. P.: Scanning electron microscopy of sulcular and junctional epithelia correlated with histology (Part 1). J. Periodontol., 48:446, 1977.

63. Karring, T., and Löe, H.: Blood supply of the periodontium. J. Periodont. Res., 2:74, 1967.

64. Kindlova, M.: The blood supply of the marginal periodontium in Macaccus Rhesus. Arch. Oral Biol., 10:869, 1965.

64a. Kobayashi, K., Rose, G., and Mahan, C. J.: Ultrastructural histochemistry of the dento-epithelial junction. J. Periodont. Res., 12: 351, 1977.

65. Kohl, J., and Zander, H. A.: Fibres conjunctive oxytalan dans le tissue gingival interdentaire. Paradontol., 16:23, 1962.

66. Kurahashi, Y., and Takuma, S.: Electron microscopy of human gingival epithelium. Bull. Tokyo Dent. Col., 3:29, 1962.

67. Lainson, P. A., and Fisher, A. K.: Endogenous oxygen consumption rates of bovine attached gingiva. J. Periodont. Res., 3:132, 1968.

68. Lange, D., and Camelleri, G. E.: Cytochemical demonstration of lysosomes in the exfoliated epithelial cells of the gingival cuff. J. Dent. Res., 46:625, 1967.

69. Leng, A., et al.: Determination of the nucleic acids in normal and pathologic gingiva. Rev. Dent. Chile, 45:809, 1955.

70. Lisanti, V. F.: Hydrolytic enzymes in periodontal disease. Ann. N.Y. Acad. Sci., 85:461, 1960.

71. Listgarten, M. A.: Changing concepts about the dento-epithelial junction. J. Can. Dent. Assoc., 36:70, 1970.

72. Listgarten, M. A.: Electron microscopic study of the gingivo-dental junction of man. Am. J. Anat., 119:147, 1966.

73. Listgarten, M. A.: Phase contrast and electron microscopic study of the junction between reduced enamel epithelium and enamel in unerupted human teeth. Arch. Oral Biol., 11:999, 1966.

74. Listgarten, M. A.: The ultrastructure of human gingival epithelium. Am. J. Anat., 114:49, 1964.

75. Löe, H., and Karring, T.: A quantitative analysis of the epithelium-connective tissue interface in relation to assessments of the mitotic index. J. Dent. Res., 48:634, 1969.

76. Löe, H., and Karring, T.: Mitotic activity and renewal time of the gingival epithelium of young and old rats. J. Periodont. Res., Suppl., 4:18, 1969.

77. Macapanpan, L. C.: Union of the enamel and gingival epithelium. J. Periodontol., 25:243, 1954.

78. Mandel, J. I., and Weinstein, E.: The fluid of the gingival sulcus. Periodontics, 2:147, 1964.

79. Manhold, J. H., and Volpe, A. P.: Effect of inflammation in the absence of proliferation on the oxygen consumption of gingival tissue. J. Dent. Res., 42:103, 1963.

80. Marwah, A. S., and Weinmann, J. P.: A sex difference in epithelial cells of human gingiva. J. Periodontol., 26:11, 1955.

81. McHugh, W. D.: Keratinization of gingival epithelium in laboratory animals. J. Periodontol., 35:338, 1964.

82. McHugh, W. D., and Zander, H. A.: Cell division in the periodontium of developing and erupted teeth. D. Pract., 15:451, 1965.

83. Melcher, A. H.: Gingival reticulin: Identification and role in histogenesis of collagen fibers. J. Dent. Res., 45:426, 1966.

84. Melcher, A. H.: Pathogenesis of chronic gingivitis. II. The effect of inflammatory changes in the corium on the overlying epithelium. Dent. Pract., 13:50, 1962.

85. Meyer, J., Marwah, A. S., and Weinmann, J. P.:

Mitotic rate of gingival epithelium in two age groups. J. Invest. Dermatol., *27*:237, 1956.

86. Meyer, W.: Controversial questions regarding the histology of the enamel cuticle. Vierteljhschr. Zahnheilk., *46*:42, 1930.

87. Miller, S. C., Soberman, A., and Stahl, S.: A study of the cornification of the oral mucosa of young male adults. J. Dent. Res., *30*:4, 1951.

88. Montgomery, P. W.: A study of exfoliative cytology of normal human oral mucosa. J. Dent. Res., *30*:12, 1951.

89. Morgan, R. E., and Wingo, W. J.: The oxygen consumption of gingival crevicular epithelium. Oral Surg., *22*:257, 1966.

90. Mori, M., and Kishiro, A.: Histochemical observation of aminopeptidase activity in the normal and inflamed oral epithelium. J. Osaka Univ. Dent. Sch., *1*:39, 1961.

91. Moss, M. L.: Phylogeny and comparative anatomy of oral ectodermal-ectomesenchymal inductive interactions. J. Dent. Res., *48*:732, 1969.

92. Nasmyth, A.: On the structure, physiology, and pathology of the persistent capsular investments and pulp of the tooth. Medico-Chirurgical Transactions of the Royal Medical & Chirurgical Society of London, *22*:310, 1839.

92a. Oliver, R. C., Holm-Pedersen, P., and Löe, H.: The correlation between clinical scoring, exudate measurements and microscopic evaluation of inflammation in the gingiva. J. Periodontol., *40*:201, 1969.

93. Orban, B., and Kohler, J.: The physiologic gingival sulcus. Z. Stomatol., *22*:353, 1924.

94. Orban, B., et al.: The epithelial attachment (The attached epithelial cuff). J. Periodontol., *27*:167, 1956.

95. Ostrom, C. A., Skillen, W. G., and Fosdick, L. S.: Chemical studies in periodontal disease VIII. Gingival glycogen concentration in experimental occlusal trauma. J. Dent. Res., *29*:55, 1950.

96. Papic, M., and Glickman, I.: Keratinization of the human gingiva in the menstrual cycle and menopause. Oral Surg., *3*:504, 1950.

97. Pelzer, R. H.: A method for plasma phosphatase determination for the differentiation of alveolar crest bone types in periodontal disease. J. Dent. Res., *19*:73, 1940.

98. Person, P., Felton, J., and Fine, A.: Biochemical and histochemical studies of aerobic oxidative metabolism of oral tissues. III. Specific metabolic activities of enzymatically separated gingival epithelium and connective tissue components. J. Dent. Res., *44*:91, 1965.

99. Quintarelli, G.: Histochemistry of the gingiva III. The distribution of aminopeptidase in normal and inflammatory conditions. Arch. Oral Biol., *2*:271, 1960.

100. Quintarelli, G., and Cheraskin, E.: Histochemistry of the gingiva VI. Distribution and localization of phosphorylase. J. Periodontol., *32*:339, 1961.

101. Rosenberg, H., and Massler, M. J.: Gingival stippling in young adult males. J. Periodontol., *38*:473, 1967.

102. San Martín Sánchez, A.: Spectrographic Analysis of the Normal and Pyorrhetic Mucosa. Santiago, University of Chile Press, 1946.

103. Schilli, W.: The most superficial zone of the stratum corneum of the gingiva. Oral Surg., *25*:896, 1968.

104. Schroeder, H. E.: Melanin containing organelles in cells of the human gingiva. J. Periodont. Res., *4*:1, 1969.

105. Schroeder, H. E., and Listgarten, M. A.: Fine Structure of the Developing Epithelial Attachment of Human Teeth. Monographs in Developmental Biology, Vol. 2. A. Wolsky, (ed.). Basel, S. Karger, 1971.

106. Schroeder, H. E., and Theilade, J.: Electron microscopy of normal human gingival epithelium. J. Periodont. Res., *1*:95, 1966.

107. Schultz-Haudt, S. D., and From, S.: Dynamics of periodontal tissues. I. The epithelium. Odont. Tskr., *69*:431, 1961.

108. Schultz-Haudt, S. D., From, S. H. J., and Nordbo, H.: Histochemical staining properties of isolated polysaccharide components of human gingiva. Arch. Oral Biol., *9*:17, 1964.

109. Schultz-Haudt, S. D., Paus, S., and Assev, S.: Periodic acid-Schiff reactive components of human gingiva. J. Dent. Res., *40*:141, 1961.

110. Schweitzer, G.: Lymph vessels of the gingiva and teeth. Arch. Mik. Anat. Ent., *69*:807, 1907.

111. Shapiro, S., Ulmansky, M., and Scheuer, M.: Mast cell population in gingiva affected by chronic destructive periodontal disease. J. Periodontol., *40*:276, 1969.

112. Shelton, L., and Hall, W.: Human gingival mast cells. J. Periodont. Res., *3*:214, 1968.

113. Skillen, W. G.: The morphology of the gingivae of the rat molar. J. Am. Dent. Assoc., *17*:645, 1930.

114. Skougaard, M. R., and Beagrie, G. S.: The renewal of gingival epithelium in marmosets (Callithrix jacchus) as determined through autoradiography with thymidine-H_3. Acta Odontol. Scand., *20*:467, 1962.

115. Smulow, J. B., and Glickman, I.: In vitro cultural and histochemical characteristics of human oral mucosa. Arch. Oral Biol., *11*:1143, 1966.

116. Soni, N. N., Silberkweit, M., and Hayes, R. L.: Pattern of mitotic activity and cell densities in human gingival epithelium. J. Periodontol., *36*:15, 1965.

117. Squier, C. A., and Waterhouse, L. P.: The ultrastructure of the melanocyte in human gingival epithelium. J. Dent. Res., *46*:112, 1967.

118. Stallard, R. E., Diab, M. A., and Zander, H. A.: The attaching substance between enamel and epithelium—a product of the epithelial cells. J. Periodontol., *36*:40, 1965.

119. Stern, I. B.: Electron microscopic observations of oral epithelium. I. Basal cells and the basement membrane. Periodontics, *3*:224, 1965.

120. Stern, I. B.: Further electron microscopic observations of the epithelial attachment. Int. Assoc. Dent. Res. Abstr., 45th General Meeting, 1967, p. 118.

121. Stern, I. B.: The fine structure of the amelo-

blast—enamel junction in rat incisors, epithelial attachment and cuticular membrane. 5th Internat. Congress for Electron Micros., 2:6, 1966.

122. Susi, F.: Histochemical autoradiographic and electron microscopic studies of keratinization in oral mucosa. Ph.D. Thesis. Tufts University, 1967.

123. Swift, J. A., and Saxton, C. A.: The ultrastructural location of the periodate-Schiff reactive basement membrane of the dermoepidermal junctions of human scalp and monkey gingiva. J. Ultrastruct. Res., 17:23, 1967.

124. Talbot, E.: Histopathology of the jaws and apical dental tissues: The so-called Nasmyth's membrane. Dent. Cosmos, 1920.

125. Thilander, H.: Permeability of the gingival pocket epithelium. Int. Dent. J., 14:416, 1964.

126. Thilander, H., and Bloom, G. D.: Cell contacts in oral epithelia. J. Periodont. Res., 3:96, 1968.

127. Thonard, J. C., and Scherp, H. W.: Histochemical demonstration of acid mucopolysaccharides in human gingival epithelial intercellular spaces. Arch. Oral Biol., 7:125, 1962.

128. Toller, J. R.: The organic continuity of the dentine, the enamel and the epithelial attachment in dogs. Br. Dent. J., 67:443, 1939.

129. Toto, P. D., and Grundel, E. R.: Acid mucopolysaccharides in the oral epithelium. J. Dent. Res., 45:211, 1966.

130. Toto, P. D., and Sicher, H. J.: Mucopolysaccharides in the epithelial attachment. J. Dent. Res., 44:451, 1965.

131. Trott, J. R.: An investigation into the glycogen content of the gingivae. Dent. Pract., 7:234, 1957.

132. Trott, J. R., and Gorenstein, S. L.: Mitotic rates in the oral and gingival epithelium of the rat. Arch. Oral Biol., 8:425, 1963.

133. Turesky, S., Crowley, J., and Glickman, I.: A histochemical study of protein-bound sulfhydryl and disulfide groups in normal and inflamed human gingiva. J. Dent. Res., 36:225, 1957.

134. Turesky, S., Glickman, I., and Fisher, B.: The effect of physiologic and pathologic processes upon certain histochemically detectable substances in the gingiva. J. Periodontol., 30:116, 1959.

135. Turesky, S., Glickman, I., and Litwin, T.: A histochemical evaluation of normal and inflamed human gingivae. J. Dent. Res., 30:792, 1951.

136. Ussing, M. J.: The development of the epithelial attachment. Acta Odontol. Scand., 13:123, 1956.

137. Waerhaug, J.: Current views on the epithelial cuff. Periodontics, 4:278, 1966.

138. Waerhaug, J.: The gingival pocket. Odont. Tskr. 60. Suppl. 1, 1952, Oslo.

139. Waterhouse, J. P.: The gingival part of the human periodontium. Its ultrastructure and the distribution in it of acid phosphatase in relation to cell attachment and the lysosome concept. Dent. Pract., 15:409, 1965.

140. Weinmann, J. P., et al.: Occurrence and role of glycogen in the epithelium of the alveolar mucosa and of the attached gingiva. Am. J. Anat., 104:381, 1959.

141. Weinstock, A.: Plasma cells in human gingiva. An electron microscope study. Anat. Rec., 162:289, 1968.

142. Weinstock, A.: Uptake of ³H-galactose label by "resorptive" ameloblasts and its secretion into a periodic acid (PA)-Schiff-positive surface layer during the phase of enamel maturation. Anat. Rec. (Proc.), 166:395, 1970.

143. Weinstock, A.: Secretory function of "postsecretory" ameloblasts as shown by electron microscope radioautography. J. Dent. Res., 50:82, 1972.

144. Weinstock, A., and Albright, J. T.: Electron microscopic observations on specialized structures in the epithelium of the normal human palate. J. Dent. Res. (Suppl.), 45:79, 1966.

145. Weinstock, M., and Wilgram, G. F.: Fine-structural observations on the formation and enzymatic activity of keratinosomes in mouse tongue filiform papillae. J. Ultrastruct. Res., 30:262, 1970.

146. Weinstock, A., and Albright, J. T.: The fine structure of mast cell in normal human gingiva. J. Ultrastruct. Res., 17:245, 1967.

147. Wertheimer, F. W.: A histologic comparison of apical cuticles, secondary dental cuticles and hyaline bodies. J. Periodontol., 37:5, 1966.

148. Wertheimer, F. W., and Fullmer, H. M.: Morphologic and histochemical observations on the human dental cuticle. J. Periodontol., 33:29, 1962.

149. Weski, O.: Die chronischen marginalen Entzündungen des Alveolar-fortsatzes mit besonderer Berücksichtigung der Alveolarpyorrhoe. Vierteljahrschr. Zahnheilk., 38:1, 1922.

150. Wilgram, G. F., and Weinstock, A.: Advances in genetic dermatology: Acantholysis, hyperkeratosis, and dyskeratosis. Arch. Dermatol., 94:456, 1966.

151. Wilkinson, F. C.: A patho-histological study of the tissue of tooth attachment. D. Rec., 55:105, 1935.

152. Williams, C. H. M.: Present status of knowledge regarding the etiology of periodontal disease. Oral Surg., 2:729, 1949.

153. Wodehouse, W. B.: The gingival trough—Its early development. Australian J. Dent., 33:139, 1929.

154. Zachrisson, B. U.: Mast cells of the human gingiva. IV. Experimental Gingivitis. J. Periodont. Res., 4:46, 1969.

155. Zachrisson, B. U., and Schulz-Haudt, S. D.: Biologically active substances of the mast cell. J. Periodont. Res., 2:21, 1967.

156. Zander, H. A.: The distribution of phosphatase in gingival tissue. J. Dent. Res., 20:347, 1941.

The Periodontal Ligament

The periodontal ligament is the connective tissue structure that surrounds the root and connects it with the bone. It is continuous with the connective tissue of the gingiva and communicates with the marrow spaces through vascular channels in the bone.

NORMAL MICROSCOPIC FEATURES

Principal Fibers

The most important elements of the periodontal ligament are the principal

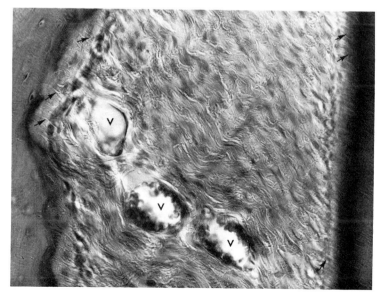

Figure 2–1 Principal Fibers on the Periodontal Ligament Follow a Wavy Course When Sectioned Longitudinally. The formative function of the periodontal ligament is illustrated by the newly formed osteoid and osteoblasts along a previously resorbed bone surface (left) and the cementoid and cementoblasts (right). Note the fibers embedded in the forming calcified tissues (arrows). V, vascular channels.

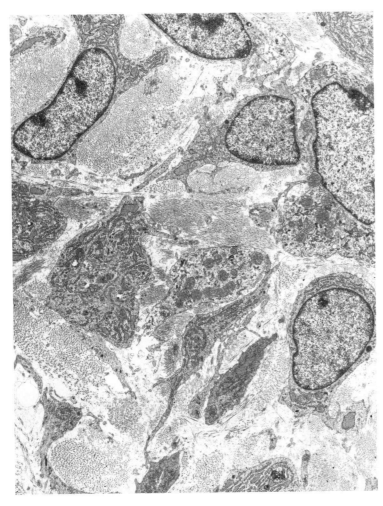

Figure 2–2 Cross section through the periodontal ligament of a rat molar as seen by electron microscopy at low power. Portions of fibroblasts are seen between bundles of collagen fibers on end. Note the intimate association of the bundles of collagen fibers and the fibroblast processes; each cell appears to have a domain occupied by collagen. Magnification × 4350. (Courtesy of Dr. Jack Yee.)

Figure 2–3 Electron micrograph of attachment of periodontal ligament collagen fibers to cementum as seen in longitudinal section at high power. The collagen fibers generally run parallel and insert at varying angles into the electron-opaque cementum matrix (far right). The fibers have a periodic crossbanding pattern typical of collagen. Rat molar. Magnification × 66,250. (Courtesy of Dr. Jack Yee.)

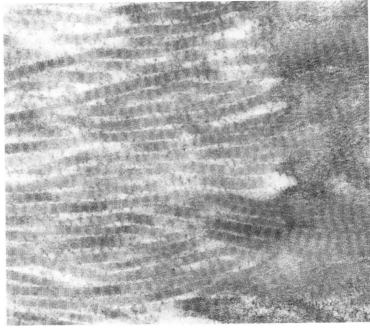

fibers, which are collagenous, arranged in bundles, and follow a wavy course when viewed in longitudinal section (Fig. 2–1). Electron microscopy has shown an intimate relationship between the collagen fibers and fibroblasts (Fig. 2–2). Terminal portions of the principal fibers that insert into cementum (Fig. 2–3) and bone are termed Sharpey's fibers.

PRINCIPAL FIBER GROUPS OF THE PERIODONTAL LIGAMENT. The principal fibers are arranged in the following groups: transseptal, alveolar crest, horizontal, oblique, and apical (Figs. 2–4 and 2–5).

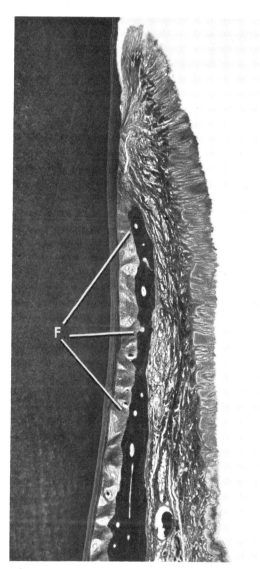

Figure 2–4 Principal Fiber Bundles (F) of the Periodontal Ligament on the facial surface of a mandibular premolar (silver stain).

Transseptal Group. These fibers extend interproximally over the alveolar crest and are embedded in the cementum of adjacent teeth (Fig. 2–6). The transseptal fibers are a remarkably constant finding. They are reconstructed even after destruction of the alveolar bone has occurred in periodontal disease.

Alveolar Crest Group. These fibers extend obliquely from the cementum just beneath the junctional epithelium to the alveolar crest. Their function is to counterbalance the coronal thrust of the more apical fibers, thus helping to retain the tooth within its socket and resist lateral tooth movements.

Horizontal Group. These fibers extend at right angles to the long axis of the tooth from the cementum to the alveolar bone. Their function is similar to those of the alveolar crest.

Oblique Group. These fibers, the largest group in the periodontal ligament, extend from the cementum in a coronal direction obliquely to the bone. They bear the brunt of vertical masticatory stresses and transform them into tension on the alveolar bone.

Apical Group. The apical group of fibers radiate from the cementum to the bone at the fundus of the socket. They do not occur on incompletely formed roots.

Other Fibers

Other well-formed fiber bundles interdigitate at right angles or splay around and between regularly arranged fiber bundles.

Less regularly arranged *collagen fibers* are found in the interstitial connective tissue between the principal fiber groups which contains the blood vessels, lymphatics, and nerves. Other fibers of the periodontal ligament are the *elastic fibers,*[50] which are relatively few, and the so-called oxytalan[20, 24] (acid-resistant) fibers, which are distributed mainly around the blood vessels and embedded in cementum in the cervical third of the root. Their function is not understood, but many investigators believe that they represent an immature form of elastin. In the electron microscope, mature elastin has a homogeneous, amorphous appearance, whereas immature elastin appears as bundles of microfilaments.

Small collagen fibers have been detected in association with the larger principal collagen fibers. These fibers appear to

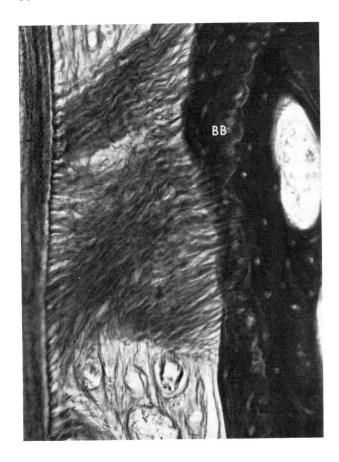

Figure 2–5 Detailed view of Figure 2–4 showing continuous collagen fibers embedded in the cementum *(left)* and bone *(right)* (silver stain). Note the Sharpey's fibers within the bundle bone (BB) overlying lamellar bone.

form a plexus and have been termed "indifferent" fibers.[42]

THE INTERMEDIATE PLEXUS. The principal fiber bundles consist of individual fibers which form a continuous anastomos-ing network between tooth and bone.[11, 47] It has been suggested that instead of being continuous the individual fibers consist of two separate parts spliced together midway between cementum and bone in a

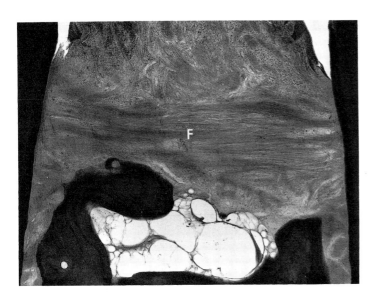

Figure 2–6 Transseptal Fibers (F) at the crest of the interdental bone.

zone called the *intermediate plexus.* The plexus has been reported in the periodontal ligament of continuously growing incisors of animals,[29, 34, 43] but not in the posterior teeth;[57] and in actively erupting human and monkey[26] teeth, but not after they reach occlusal contact. Rearrangement of the fiber ends in the plexus is supposed to accommodate tooth eruption, without necessitating the embedding of new fibers into tooth and bone.[34] There are doubts regarding the existence of such a plexus;[6, 51] some consider it a microscopic artefact,[21] and no evidence of its existence has been found when collagen fiber formation is traced with radioactive proline.[15]

Cellular Elements

The cellular elements of the periodontal ligament are fibroblasts, endothelial cells, cementoblasts, osteoblasts, osteoclasts, tissue macrophages, and strands of epithelial cells termed the "epithelial rests of Malassez" or "resting epithelial cells."[54]

Recent investigations have shown that fibroblasts synthesize collagen by first producing a precursor molecule called procollagen. Procollagen is believed to be carried within the cell in small, elongated secretory granules.[56] Upon discharge from the cell, the procollagen molecules become chemically modified, and collagen fibers then arise. Periodontal ligament fibroblasts have been shown to possess the capacity to phagocytose "old" collagen fibers and degrade them[17, 49] by enzyme hydrolysis (Fig. 2–7). Thus, collagen turnover appears to be regulated by the same cell type.

The *epithelial rests* form a latticework in the periodontal ligament and appear as either isolated clusters of cells or interlacing strands, depending on the plane in which the microscopic section is cut. Continuity with the junctional epithelium in experimental animals has been suggested.[25] They are considered to be remnants of the Hertwig root sheath, which disintegrates during root development after cementum is formed on the dentin surface, but this concept has been questioned.[18]

Epithelial rests are distributed close to the cementum throughout the periodontal ligament of most teeth, and are most numerous in the apical[41] and cervical areas.[55] They diminish in number with age[44] by degenerating and disappearing or undergoing calcification to become cementicles.

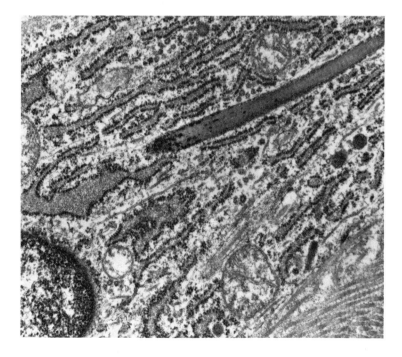

Figure 2–7 Electron micrograph of a portion of a periodontal ligament fibroblast showing part of the nucleus (lower left) and abundant rough endoplasmic reticulum. The endoplasmic reticulum surrounds a large elongated phagosome (upper right) containing collagen fibers (note the crossbanding pattern within the phagosome). This preparation was processed to demonstrate the hydrolytic enzyme acid phosphatase; thus, a dense precipitate of lead can be seen within the left portion of the phagosome, indicating the presence of this enzyme. This evidence suggests that the collagen within the phagosome is being digested and is associated with the normal collagen turnover process within the periodontal ligament. At lower right, collagen fibers in the extracellular space may be seen. Magnification × 33,125. (Courtesy of Dr. Jack Yee.)

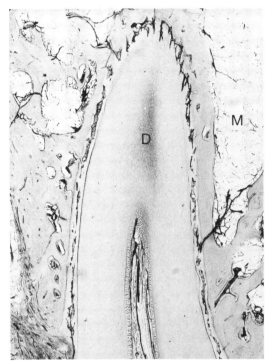

Figure 2–8 Vascular Supply of the Periodontium (monkey perfused with India ink). Note the longitudinal vessels in the periodontal ligament, and alveolar arteries passing through channels between the bone marrow (M) and periodontal ligament. D, dentin. (Courtesy of Dr. Sol Bernick.)

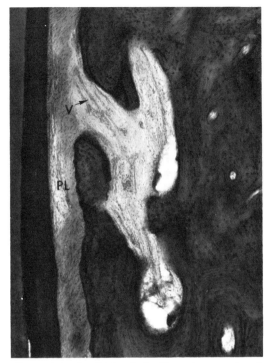

Figure 2–9 Small Vessels in Channel connecting the periodontal ligament (PL) and alveolar bone.

They are surrounded by a PAS-positive, argyrophilic, fibrillar, sometimes hyaline capsule from which they are separated by a distinct basement lamina or membrane. Epithelial rests proliferate when stimulated[48, 52] and participate in the formation of periapical cysts and lateral root cysts.

The periodontal ligament may also contain calcified masses called cementicles which are adherent to, or detached from, the root surfaces.

Vascular Supply

The blood supply is derived from the *inferior* and *superior alveolar arteries* and reaches the periodontal ligament from three sources: *apical vessels, penetrating vessels from the alveolar bone,* and *anastomosing vessels from the gingiva.*[12] The apical vessels enter the periodontal ligament at the apical region and extend to the gingiva, giving off lateral branches in

the direction of the cementum and bone. The vessels within the periodontal ligament are connected in a net-like plexus which receives its principal supply from alveolar perforating arteries and small vessels which penetrate through channels in the alveolar bone[19] (Figs. 2–8 and 2–9). The blood supply from this source increases from the incisors to molars; is greatest in the gingival third of single-rooted teeth, less in the apical third, and least in the middle; is equal in the apical and middle thirds of multirooted teeth; is slightly greater on the mesial and distal surfaces than on the facial and lingual; and is greater on the mesial surfaces of mandibular molars than on the distal.[8] The vascular supply from the gingiva is derived from branches of deep vessels in the lamina propria. The venous drainage of the periodontal ligament accompanies the arterial supply.

Lymphatics

Lymphatics supplement the venous drainage system. Those draining the region just beneath the junctional epithelium pass into the periodontal ligament and accompany the blood vessels into the periapical region.[9] From there they pass through the alveolar bone to the inferior dental canal in the mandible, or the infraorbital canal in the maxilla, and to the submaxillary group of lymph nodes.

Innervation

The periodontal ligament is abundantly supplied with sensory nerve fibers capable of transmitting *tactile, pressure,* and *pain* sensations by the trigeminal pathways.[2, 5] Nerve bundles pass into the periodontal ligament from the periapical area and through channels from the alveolar bone. The nerve bundles follow the course of the blood vessels and divide into single myelinized fibers, which ultimately lose their myelin sheath and terminate either as free nerve endings or elongate spindle-like structures. The latter are *proprioceptive receptors* that account for the sense of localization when the tooth is touched.

Development of the Periodontal Ligament

The periodontal ligament develops from the *dental sac,* a circular layer of fibrous connective tissue surrounding the tooth bud. As the developing tooth erupts, the loose connective tissue of the sac differentiates into three layers: an outer layer adjacent to the bone, an inner layer along the cementum, and an intermediate layer of unorganized fibers.[37] The principal fiber bundles are derived from the intermediate layer and arranged according to functional requirements when the tooth reaches occlusal contact. Studies on the squirrel monkey[26] have shown that during eruption cemental fibers are first observed, followed by Sharpey's fibers emerging from bone. When the tooth reaches occlusal function, fiber bundles become thicker and soon become organized into classical principal fiber arrangements. Nevertheless, the transseptal and alveolar crest fibers develop upon emergence of the tooth into the oral cavity.

FUNCTIONS OF THE PERIODONTAL LIGAMENT

The functions of the periodontal ligament are *physical, formative, nutritional,* and *sensory.*

Physical Function

The physical functions of the periodontal ligament entail the following:[35] transmission of occlusal forces to the bone; attachment of the teeth to the bone; maintenance of the gingival tissues in their proper relationship to the teeth; resistance to the impact of occlusal forces (shock absorption); and provision of a "soft tissue casing" to protect the vessels and nerves from injury by mechanical forces.

RESISTANCE TO THE IMPACT OF OCCLUSAL FORCES (SHOCK ABSORPTION). According to Parfitt[38] the initial responsibility

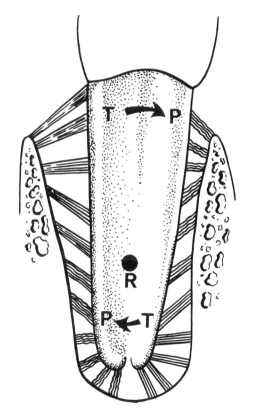

Figure 2–10 Distribution of Faciolingual Forces (arrows) around the axis of rotation (R) in a mandibular premolar. The periodontal ligament fibers are compressed in areas of pressure (P) and taut in areas of tension (T).

for resisting occlusal forces rests in four systems of the periodontal ligament rather than in the principal fibers. The fibers serve a secondary role of restraining the tooth against lateral movement and preventing deformity of the periodontal ligament under compressive force. The four systems that initially resist occlusal forces are (1) the *vascular system*, which acts as a shock absorber and takes up strains of sudden occlusal forces; (2) the *hydrodynamic system*, consisting of tissue fluid and fluid which passes through small vessel walls[7] and is squeezed into the surrounding areas through foramina in the alveoli to resist axial forces; (3) the *pitch system*, which is probably closely related to the hydrodynamic system and controls the pitch or level

of the tooth in the socket, and (4) the *resilient system*, which causes the tooth to spring back into position when the occlusal forces are removed. These systems are phenomena of the blood vessels and the ground substance–collagen complex of the periodontal ligament.

TRANSMISSION OF OCCLUSAL FORCES TO THE BONE. The arrangement of the principal fibers is similar to a suspension bridge or a hammock. When an axial force is applied to a tooth, there is a tendency toward displacement of the root into the alveolus. The oblique fibers alter their wavy untensed pattern, assume their full length, and sustain the major part of the axial force.

When a horizontal or tipping force is

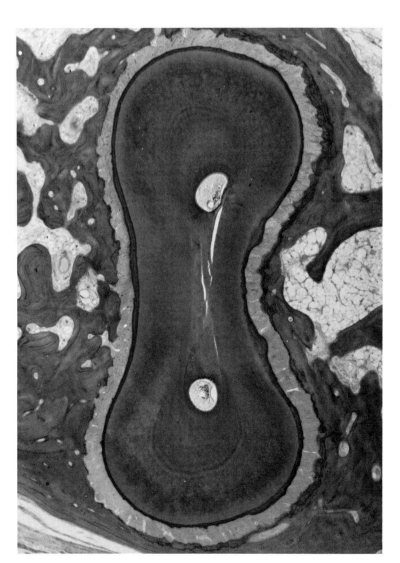

Figure 2–11 Physiologic Mesial Migration. Horizontal section through molar root. The periodontal ligament is thinner on the side toward which the tooth is migrating (mesial surface, *left*) than on the distal surface *(right)*. The distal fibers are taut.

TABLE 2–1   THICKNESS OF PERIODONTAL LIGAMENT OF 172 TEETH FROM FIFTEEN HUMAN JAWS (COOLIDGE[14])

	Average of Alveolar Crest	Average of Midroot	Average of Apex	Average of Tooth
Ages 11–16				
83 teeth from 4 jaws	0.23	*0.17*	0.24	0.21
Ages 32–50				
36 teeth from 5 jaws	0.20	*0.14*	0.19	0.18
Ages 51–67				
35 teeth from 5 jaws	0.17	*0.12*	0.16	0.15
Age 25 (1 case)				
18 teeth from 1 jaw	0.16	*0.09*	0.15	0.13

applied, there are **two characteristic phases** of tooth movement: the first is **within the confines of the periodontal ligament,** and the second produces a **displacement of the facial and lingual bony plates.**[16] The tooth rotates about an axis which may change as the force is increased. The apical portion of the root moves in a direction opposite to the coronal portion. In areas of tension the principal fiber bundles are taut rather than wavy. In areas of pressure the fibers are compressed, the tooth is displaced, and there is a corresponding distortion of bone in the direction of root movement.[39]

In single-rooted teeth the axis of rotation is located slightly apical to the middle third of the root (Fig. 2–10). The root apex[35] and the coronal half of the clinical root have been suggested as other locations of the axis of rotation. The periodontal ligament, shaped like a hourglass, is narrowest in the region of the axis of rotation[14, 32] (Table 2–1). In multirooted teeth the axis of rotation is located in the bone between the roots.

In compliance with the physiologic mesial migration of the teeth, the periodontal ligament is thinner on the mesial root surface than on the distal surface (Figs. 2–11 and 2–12).

OCCLUSAL FUNCTION AND THE STRUCTURE OF THE PERIODONTAL LIGAMENT. Just as the tooth depends upon the **periodontal ligament to support it during function, so does the periodontal ligament depend upon stimulation provided by occlusal function to preserve its structure.** Within physiologic limits the periodontal ligament can accommodate increased function by an increase in width (Table 2–2), a thickening of the fiber bundles, and an increase in diameter and number of Sharpey's fibers. Occlusal forces which exceed what the periodontal ligament can withstand produce injury called *trauma from occlusion* (see Chapter 19).

When fuction is diminished or absent, the periodontal ligament atrophies. It is thinned, and the fibers are reduced in number and density, become disoriented,[1] and ultimately are arranged parallel to the root surface (Fig. 2–13). In addition, the cementum is either unaffected[13] or thickened, and the distance from the cementoenamel junction to the alveolar crest is increased.[40]

TABLE 2–2   COMPARISON OF PERIODONTAL WIDTH OF FUNCTIONING AND FUNCTIONLESS TEETH IN A MALE AGED 38 (KRONFELD[32])

	Heavy Function Left Upper 2nd Bicuspid	Light Function Left Lower 1st Bicuspid	Functionless Left Upper 3rd Molar
Average width of periodontal space at entrance of alveolus	0.35 mm.	0.14 mm.	0.10 mm.
Average width of periodontal space at middle of alveolus	0.28 mm.	0.10 mm.	0.06 mm.
Average width of periodontal space at fundus of alveolus	0.30 mm.	0.12 mm.	0.06 mm.

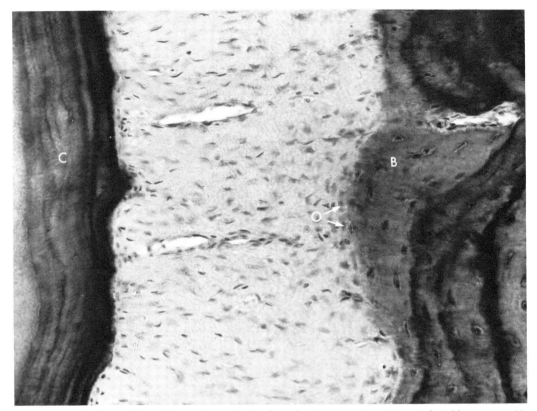

Figure 2–12   High Power View of Figure 2–11; distal surface, showing cementum (C), periodontal ligament, and bone. The tooth is migrating mesially (toward the left). Note the osteoblasts (O) and new bone formation (B) (*right*).

Destruction of the periodontal ligament and alveolar bone by periodontal disease disrupts the balance between the periodontium and occlusal forces. When supporting tissues are reduced by disease, the burden upon the tissue which remains is increased. Occlusal forces which were beneficial to the intact periodontal ligament may now become injurious.

Formative Function

The periodontal ligament serves as the periosteum for cementum and bone. Cells of the periodontal ligament participate in the formation and resorption of these tissues which occur in physiologic tooth movement, in the accommodation of the periodontium to occlusal forces, and in the repair of injuries. Variations in cellular enzyme activity (certain dehydrogenases[21] and nonspecific esterase[23]) are correlated with the remodeling process. In areas of

bone formation, osteoblasts, fibroblasts, and cementoblasts stain intensely, suggesting the presence of nonspecific alkaline phosphatase, glucose-6-phosphatase, and thiamine pyrophosphatase.[22] In areas of bone resorption osteoclasts, fibroblasts, osteocytes, and cementocytes show a staining reaction for nonspecific acid phosphatase. Cartilage formation in the periodontal ligament, although unusual may represent a metaplastic phenomenon in the repair of the periodontal ligament following injury.[3]

Like all structures of the periodontium, the periodontal ligament is constantly undergoing remodeling. Old cells and fibers are broken down and replaced by new ones, and mitotic activity can be observed in the fibroblasts and endothelial cells.[36] Fibroblasts form the collagen fibers and may also develop into osteoblasts and cementoblasts. The rate of formation and differentiation of fibroblasts affects the rate of formation of collagen cementum and bone. Collagen formation increases with the rate of eruption.[45]

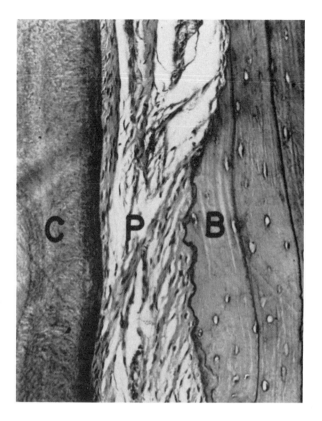

Figure 2–13 Atrophic Periodontal Ligament (P) of Tooth Devoid of Function. Note the scalloped edge of the alveolar bone (B), suggesting that resorption had occurred. Cementum (C).

Radioautographic studies with radioactive thymidine, proline, and glycine indicate a high rate of collagen metabolism in the periodontal ligament. Formation of new fibroblasts and collagen is most active adjacent to the bone and in the middle of the ligament and least active on the cementum side.[15, 46] Collagen turnover is greatest at the crest and apex.[10] There is also rapid turnover of sulfated mucopolysaccharides in the cells and amorphous ground substance of the periodontal ligament.[4]

Nutritional and Sensory Functions

The periodontal ligament supplies nutrients to the cementum, bone, and gingiva by way of the blood vessels and provides lymphatic drainage. The innervation of the periodontal ligament provides *proprioceptive* and *tactile sensitivity*,[31, 53] which detects and localizes external forces acting upon the individual teeth and serves an important role in the neuromuscular mechanism controlling the masticatory musculature.

REFERENCES

1. Anneroth, G., and Ericsson, S. G.: An Experimental histological study of monkey teeth without antagonist. Odont. Revy, 18:345, 1967.
2. Avery, J. K., and Rapp, R.: Pain conduction in human dental tissues. Dent. Clin. North Am., July 1959, p. 489.
3. Bauer, W. H.: Effect of a faulty constructed partial denture on a tooth and its supporting tissue, with special reference to formation of fibrocartilage in the periodontal membrane as a result of disturbed healing caused by abnormal stresses. Am. J. Orthod. Oral Surg., 27:640, 1941.
4. Baumhammers, A., and Stallard, R.: S35-sulfate utilization and turnover by connective tissues of the periodontium. J. Periodont. Res., 3:187, 1968.
5. Bernick, S.: Innervation of the teeth and periodontium. Dent. Clin. North Am., July 1959, p. 503.
6. Bevelander, G., and Nakara, H.: The fine structure of the human periodontal ligament. Anat. Rec., 162:313, 1968.
7. Bien, S. M.: Hydrodynamic damping of tooth movement. J. Dent. Res., 45:907, 1966.
8. Birn, H.: The vascular supply of the periodontal membrane. J. Periodont. Res., 1:51, 1966.
9. Box, K. F.: Evidence of lymphatics in the periodontium. J. Can. Dent. Assoc., 15:8, 1949.
10. Carneiro, J., and Fava de Moraes, F.: Radioauto-

graphic visualization of collagen metabolism in the periodontal tissues of the mouse. Arch. Oral Biol., 10:833, 1955.

11. Ciancio, S. C., Neiders, M. E., and Hazen, S. P.: The principal fibers of the periodontal ligament. Periodontics, 5:76, 1967.

12. Cohen, L.: Further studies into the vascular architecture of the mandible. J. Dent. Res., 39:936, 1960.

13. Cohn, S. A.: Disuse atrophy of the periodontium in mice. Arch. Oral Biol., 10:909, 1965.

14. Coolidge, E. D.: The thickness of the human periodontal membrane. J. Am. Dent. Assoc., 24:1260, 1937.

15. Crumley, P. J.: Collagen formation in the normal and stressed periodontium. Periodontics, 2:53, 1964.

16. Davies, R., and Picton, D. C. A.: Dimensional changes in the periodontal membrane of monkey's teeth with horizontal thrusts. J. Dent. Res., 46:114, 1967.

17. Deporter, D. A., and Ten Cate, A. R.: Fine structural localization of acid and alkaline phosphatase in collagen-containing vesicles of fibroblasts. J. Anat. (Lond.), 114:457, 1973.

18. Diab, M. A., and Stallard, R. E.: A study of the relationship between epithelial root sheath and root development. Periodontics, 3:10, 1965.

19. Folke, L. E. A., and Stallard, R. E.: Periodontal microcirculation as revealed by plastic microspheres. J. Periodont. Res., 2:53, 1967.

20. Fullmer, H. M.: A critique of normal connective tissues of the periodontium and some alterations with periodontal disease. J. Dent. Res., 41 (Suppl. to No. 1):223, 1962.

21. Gibson, W., and Fullmer, H.: Histochemistry of the periodontal ligament. I. The dehydrogenases. Periodontics, 4:63, 1966.

22. Gibson, W., and Fullmer, H.: Histochemistry of the periodontal ligament: II. The phosphatases. Periodontics, 5:226, 1967.

23. Gibson, W., and Fullmer, H.: Histochemistry of the periodontal ligament. III. The esterases. Periodontics, 6:71, 1968.

24. Goggins, J. F.: The distribution of oxytalan connective tissue fibers in periodontal ligaments of deciduous teeth. Periodontics, 4:182, 1966.

25. Grant, D., and Bernick, S.: A possible continuity between epithelial rests and epithelial attachment in miniature swine. J. Periodontics, 40:87, 1969.

26. Grant, D., and Bernick, S.: The formation of the periodontal ligament. J. Periodontol., 43;17, 1972.

27. Griffin, J. C.: Fine structure of the synthetizing periodontal fibroblasts and the maturation of periodontal collagen. J. Dent. Res., 46:1311, 1967.

28. Grupe, H. E., Ten Cate, A. R., and Zander, H. A.: A histochemical and radiobiological study of in vitro and in vivo human epithelial cell rest proliferation. Arch. Oral Biol., 12:1321, 1967.

29. Hindle, M. C.: Quantitative differences in periodontal membrane fibers. J. Dent. Res., 43:953, 1964.

30. Inoue, M., and Akiyoshi, M.: Histologic investigation on Sharpey's fibers in cementum of teeth in abnormal function. J. Dent. Res., 41:503, 1962.

31. Kizior, J. E., Cuozzo, J. W., and Bowman, D. C.: Functional and histologic assessment of the sensory innervation of the periodontal ligament of the cat. J. Dent. Res., 47:59, 1968.

32. Kronfeld, R.: Histologic study of the influence of function on the human periodontal membrane. J. Am. Dent. Assoc., 18:1242, 1931.

33. Levy, B. M., and Bernick, S.: Studies on the biology of the periodontium of marmosets: II. Development and organization of the periodontal ligament of deciduous teeth in marmosets (Callithrix jacchus). J. Dent. Res., 47:27, 1968.

34. Melcher, A. H.: Remodelling of the periodontal ligament during eruption of the rat incisor. Arch. Oral Biol., 12:1649, 1967.

35. Muhlemann, H. R.: The determination of tooth rotation centers. Oral Surg., 7:392, 1954.

36. Muhlemann, H. R., Zander, H. A., and Halberg, F.: Mitotic activity in the periodontal tissues of the rat molar. J. Dent. Res., 33:459, 1954.

37. Orban, B.: Embryology and histogenesis. Fortschr. Zahnheilk., 3:749, 1927.

38. Parfitt, G. H.: The physical analysis of tooth supporting structures. In The Mechanism of Tooth Support. Bristol, J. Wright and Sons, Ltd., 1967, p. 154.

39. Picton, D. C. S., and Davies, W. I. R.: Dimensional changes in the periodontal membrane of monkeys (Macaca irus) due to horizontal thrusts applied to the tooth. Arch. Oral Biol., 12:1635, 1967.

40. Pihlstrom, B. L., and Ramfjord, S. P.: Periodontal effects of nonfunction in monkeys. J. Periodontol., 42:748, 1971.

41. Reeve, C. M., and Wentz, F. J.: The prevalence, morphology and distribution of epithelial rests in the human periodontal ligament. Oral Surg., 15:785, 1962.

42. Shackleford, J. M.: The indifferent fiber plexus and its relationship to principal fibers of the periodontium. Am. J. Anat., 131:427, 1971.

43. Sicher, H.: The axial movement of continuously growing teeth. J. Dent. Res., 21:201, 1942.

44. Simpson, H. E.: The degeneration of the rests of Malassez with age as observed by the apoxestic technique. J. Periodontol., 36:288, 1965.

45. Stallard, R. E.: The effect of occlusal alterations on collagen formation within the periodontal ligament. Periodontics, 2:49, 1964.

46. Stallard, R. E.: The utilization of H_3-proline by the connective tissues of the periodontium. J. Am. Soc. Periodontol., 1:185, 1963.

47. Stern, I. B.: An electron microscopic study of the cementum, Sharpey's fibers and periodontal ligament in the rat incisor. Am. J. Anat., 115: 377, 1964.

48. Ten Cate, A. R.: The histochemical demonstration of specific oxidative enzymes and glycogen in the epithelial cell of Malassez. Arch. Oral Biol., 10:207, 1965.

49. Ten Cate, A. R., and Deporter, D. A.: The degradative role of the fibroblast in the remodelling and turnover of collagen in soft connective tissue. Anat. Rec., 182:1, 1975.

50. Thomas, N. G.: Elastic fibers in periodontal

membrane and pulp. J. Dent. Res., *7*:325, 1927.

51. Troth, J. R.: The development of the periodontal attachment in the rat. Acta Anat., *51*:313, 1962.

52. Trowbridge, H. O., and Shibata, F.: Mitotic activity in epithelial rests of Malassez. Periodontics, *5*:109, 1967.

53. Tryde, G., Frydenberg, O., and Brill, N.: An assessment of the tactile sensibility in human teeth. An evaluation of a quantitative method. Acta Odontol. Scand., *20*:233, 1962.

54. Valderhaug, J. P., and Nylen, M. U.: Function of epithelial rests as suggested by their ultrastructure. J. Periodont. Res., *1*:69, 1966.

55. Valderhaug, J. P., and Zander, H.: Relationship of "epithelial rests of Malassez" to other periodontal structures. Periodontics, *5*:254, 1967.

56. Weinstock, M.: Collagen formation-observations on its intracellular packaging and transport. Z. Zellforsch., *129*:455, 1972.

57. Zwarych, P. D., and Quigley, M. B.: The intermediate plexus of the periodontal ligament: History and further observations. J. Dent. Res., *44*:383, 1965.

The Cementum

NORMAL MICROSCOPIC FEATURES

Cementum is the calcified mesenchymal tissue that forms the outer covering of the anatomic root. It may exert a far more critical role in the development of periodontal disease than has thus far been demonstrated.

There are two main forms of root cementum: *acellular* (primary) and *cellular* (secondary). Both consist of a calcified interfibrillar matrix and collagen fibrils. Afibrillar cementum was discussed in Chapter 1, and will be mentioned briefly below. The cellular type contains cementocytes in individual spaces (lacunae) which communicate with each other through a system of anastomosing canaliculi. There are two sources of collagen fibers in cementum: Sharpey's fibers, the embedded portion of principal fibers of the periodontal ligament[40, 51] which are formed by the fibroblasts, and a second group of fibers belonging to cementum matrix per se produced by the cementoblasts.[48] Cementoblasts also form the glycoprotein interfibrillar ground substance.

Acellular and cellular cementum are arranged in *lamellae* separated by incremental lines parallel to the long axis of the root (Figs. 3–1 and 3–2). They represent rest periods in cementum formation and are more mineralized than the adjacent cementum.[57] Sharpey's fibers make up most of the structure of *acellular cementum*, which has a principal role in supporting the tooth. Most of the fibers are inserted at approximately right angles into the root surface and penetrate deep into the cementum (Figs. 3–3 and 2–3), but others enter from several different directions.[9] Their size, number, and distribution increase with function.[21] Sharpey's fibers are completely calcified with the mineral crystals oriented parallel to the fibrils, as they are in dentin and bone, except in a 10 to 50 micron wide zone near the cemento-dentinal junction where they are partly calcified. The peripheral portions of Sharpey's fibers in actively mineralizing cementum tend to be more calcified than the interior regions according to evidence obtained by scanning electron microscopy.[25] Acellular cementum also contains other collagen fibrils which are calcified and irregularly arranged or parallel to the surface.[44]

Cellular cementum is less calcified than the acellular type.[22] Sharpey's fibers occupy a smaller portion of cellular cemen-

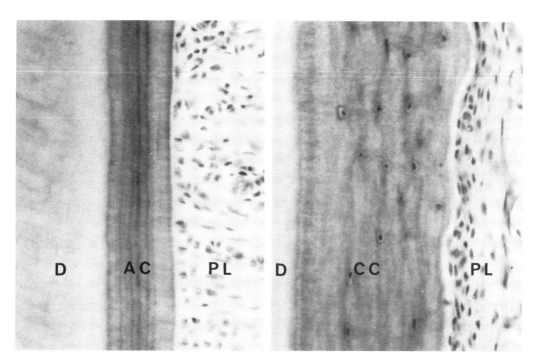

Figure 3–1 A light micrograph of acellular cementum (AC) showing incremental lines running parallel to the long axis of the tooth. These lines represent the appositional growth of cementum. Note the thin light lines running into the cementum perpendicular to the surface; these represent Sharpey's fibers of the periodontal ligament (PL). D, dentin. Magnification ×300.

Figure 3–2 Cellular cementum (CC) showing cementocytes lying within lacunae. The cellular cementum is thicker than acellular cementum (cf. Fig. 3–1). There is also evidence of incremental lines, but they are less distinct than in acellular cementum. The cells adjacent to the surface of the cementum in the periodontal ligament (PL) space are cementoblasts. D, dentin. Magnification × 300.

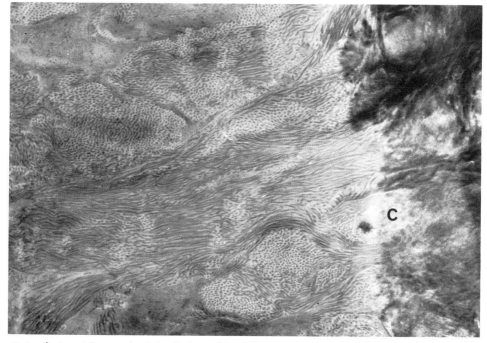

Figure 3–3   Electron Micrograph of the Surface of Acellular Cementum. Bundles of densely packed collagen fibrils of the periodontal ligament (left) are inserted into the cementum (C) surface. ×10,000. (From Dr. Knut A. Selvig.[47])

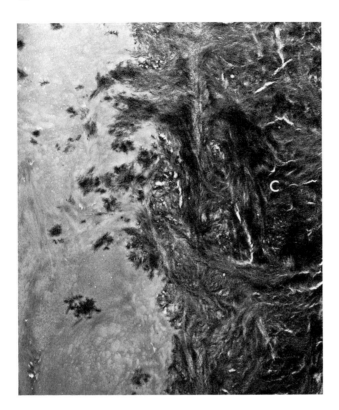

Figure 3–4   Electron Micrograph of the Surface of Mineralized Cellular Cementum. The cementum (C) contains irregularly arranged bundles of collagen fibrils covered with apatite crystals. Calcification foci are present in the precementum (left, unmineralized) within a 5-micron wide zone at the surface of the cementum. ×10,000. (From Dr. Knut A. Selvig.[47])

tum and are separated by other fibers which are arranged either parallel to the root surface or at random (Fig. 3–4). Some of Sharpey's fibers are completely calcified, others are partially calcified, and in some there is a central uncalcified core surrounded by a calcified border.[25, 48]

The distribution of acellular and cellular cementum varies. The coronal half of the root is usually covered by the acellular type, and cellular cementum is more common in the apical half. With age the greatest increase in cementum is of the cellular type in the apical half of the root and in the furcation areas.

Intermediate cementum is an ill-defined zone near the cemento-dentinal junction of certain teeth which appears to contain cellular remnants of Hertwig's sheath embedded in calcified ground substance.[12, 30]

The *inorganic content* of cementum (hydroxyapatite, $Ca_{10} (PO_4)_6 (OH)_2$) is 45 to 50 per cent, which is less than that of bone (65 per cent), enamel (97 per cent) or dentin (70 per cent).[60] The calcium and magnesium-phosphorus ratio is higher in api-

cal than in cervical areas.[49] Opinions differ as to whether the microhardness increases[34] or decreases with age,[55] and no relationship has been established between aging and the mineral content of cementum.

Histochemical studies indicate that the *matrix of cementum* contains a *carbohydrate-protein complex. Neutral and acid mucopolysaccharides* are present in the matrix and cytoplasm of some cementoblasts. The lining of the lacunae, the incremental lines, and the precementum are rich in *acid mucopolysaccharides, possibly chondroitin sulfate B*.[43] Precementum stains metachromatically,[18] and the ground substance of acellular and cellular cementum is orthochromatic.

The Cemento-enamel Junction

The cementum at and immediately subjacent to the cemento-enamel junction is of particular clinical importance in root scaling procedures.[39] Three types of rela-

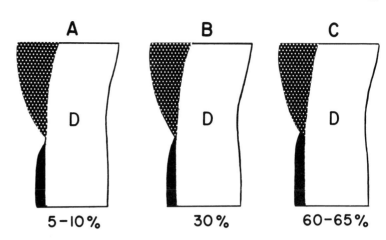

Figure 3–5 Statistical Representation of Normal Variations in Tooth Morphology at the Cemento-Enamel Junction. *A,* Space between enamel and cementum with dentin exposed (D). *B,* End-to-end relationship of enamel and cementum. *C,* Cementum overlapping the enamel. (After Hopewell-Smith.)

tionships involving the cementum may exist at the cemento-enamel junction.[35] Cementum *overlaps the enamel* in about 60 to 65 per cent of the cases (Fig. 3–5). In about 30 per cent there is an *edge-to-edge butt joint,* and in 5 to 10 per cent, the *cementum and enamel fail to meet.* In the latter instance gingival recession may be accompanied by an accentuated sensitivity because the dentin is exposed.

A layer of *afibrillar cementum* sometimes extends a short distance onto the enamel at the cemento-enamel junction (see Chap. 1). It contains acid mucopolysaccharides and possibly a nonfibrillar form of collagen, in contrast with root cementum which is rich in collagen fibers. It has been hypothesized that this material is deposited on the enamel by connective tissue following degeneration and shrinkage of the reduced enamel epithelium.[32] The afibrillar cementum may be partially covered by root cementum.

Cementum occurs on the crown of the tooth overlying the enamel in swine, covering more of the surface than in humans,[31] and over the entire enamel of bovine teeth.[14, 45]

Thickness of Cementum

The thickness of cementum on the coronal half of the root varies from 16 to 60 microns, or about the thickness of a hair. It attains its greatest thickness of up to 150 to 200 microns in the apical third, and also in the bifurcation and trifurcation

areas.[37] Between the ages of 11 and 70 the average thickness of the cementum increases threefold, with the greatest increase in the apical region. Average thickness of 95 microns at age 20 and 215 microns at age 60 have been reported.[58]

Permeability of Cementum

In very young animals, both cellular and acellular cementum are very permeable and permit the diffusion of dyes from the pulp canal and from the external root surface. In cellular cementum the canaliculi in some areas are contiguous with the dentinal tubuli. Devitalized teeth take up about one tenth as much radioactive phosphorus (^{32}P) through the cementum as vital teeth.[56]

With age, the permeability of cementum diminishes.[10] There is also a relative diminution in the contribution of the pulp to the nutrition of the tooth, which increases the importance of the periodontal ligament as a pathway for metabolic exchange.[54] In the very aged, the phosphate exchange in the tooth by way of the periodontal ligament and cementum increases to 50 per cent of the total.[53]

CEMENTOGENESIS

Cementum formation starts, as does bone and dentin, with the deposition of a meshwork of irregularly arranged collagen fibrils sparsely distributed in an interfibrillar ground substance or matrix called precementum or cementoid.[45, 46] It increases in thickness by the apposition of matrix by cementoblasts. The progressive mineralization of matrix begins at the cemento-dentin junction, and advances in the direction of the cementoblasts. Hydroxyapatite crystals are deposited first within and on the surface of the fibers and then in the ground substance. Periodontal ligament fibers being incorporated into the cementum at approximately right angles to the surface (Sharpey's fibers) become mineralized and appear under the scanning electron microscope as a series of mineralized spurs from which a fiber projects into the periodontal ligament.[25] Cementoblasts, initially separated from the cementum by uncalcified cementoid, sometimes become enclosed within the matrix and become trapped. Once enclosed they are referred to as cementocytes, and they remain viable in a similar fashion to osteocytes. Cementum formation is a continuous process which proceeds at a varying rate, but it is usually much slower than bone or dentin formation.

Continuous Deposition of Cementum

Cementum deposition continues after the teeth have erupted into contact with their functional antagonists and throughout life. This is part of the over-all process of continuous tooth eruption. The teeth erupt in an effort to keep pace with tooth substance lost by occlusal and incisal wear. As they erupt, less of the root remains in the socket, weakening the support of the teeth. This is compensated for by continuous deposition of cementum on the root surface, in greatest amounts in the apices and furcation areas,[28] plus the formation of bone at the crest of the alveolus. The combined effect is to lengthen the root and deepen the socket. The physiologic width of the periodontal ligament is preserved by continuous deposition of cementum, and bone formation along the inner socket wall as the tooth continues to erupt.

An uncalcified surface layer of precementum, part of the process of continuous cementum deposition, was considered by Gottlieb[15] to be the natural barrier to excessive apical migration of the epithelial attachment. Impaired cementum formation ("cementopathia") was thought to be a cause of pathologic periodontal pocket formation because it reduced the restraint on epithelial migration.

Function and Cementum Formation

No clear-cut correlation has been established between occlusal function and cementum deposition.[27] From the findings of well-developed cementum on the roots of teeth in dermoid cysts, and from the presence of thicker cementum on embedded teeth than on teeth in function,[17] it has been inferred that function is not necessary for cementum formation. Cementum is thinner in areas of injury caused by excessive occlusal forces,[4] but thickening of cementum may also occur in these areas.

The biological role of afibrillar cementum and its clinical implications are not understood at the present time.

Hypercementosis

The term *hypercementosis* (cementum hyperplasia) refers to a prominent thickening of the cementum. It may be localized to one tooth or may affect the entire dentition. Because of considerable physiologic variation in the thickness of cementum among different teeth of the same person and among teeth of different persons, it is sometimes difficult to distinguish between hypercementosis and physiologic thickening of cementum.

Hypercementosis occurs as a generalized thickening of the cementum, with nodular enlargement of the apical third of the root. It also appears in the form of spikelike excrescences (cemental spikes) created by either the coalescence of cementicles that adhere to the root[17] or the calcification of periodontal fibers at the sites of insertion into the cementum.[29]

The etiology of hypercementosis varies and is not completely understood. The spikelike type of hypercementosis generally

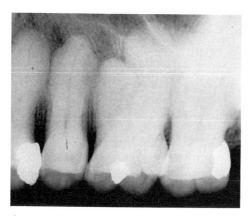

Figure 3–6 Hypercementosis in Paget's Disease.

results from excessive tension from orthodontic appliances or occlusal forces. The generalized type occurs in a variety of circumstances. In teeth without antagonists, it is interpreted as an effort to keep pace with excessive tooth eruption. In teeth subject to low-grade periapical irritation arising from pulp disease, it is considered as compensation for the destroyed fibrous attachment to the tooth. The cementum is deposited adjacent to the inflamed periapical tissue. Hypercementosis of the entire dentition may be hereditary,[59] and also occurs in Paget's disease[42] (Fig. 3–6). Localized hypercementosis occurs at the insertion of the transseptal fibers in experimental lathyrism.[13] Cementum formation is diminished in hypophosphatasia.[3]

Cementicles

Cementicles are globular masses of cementum arranged in concentric lamellae that lie free in the periodontal ligament or adhere to the root surface (Fig. 3–7). Cementicles may develop from calcified epithelial rests, around small spicules of cementum or alveolar bone traumatically displaced into the periodontal ligament, from calcified Sharpey's fibers, and from calcified thrombosed vessels within the periodontal ligament.[33]

Cementoma

Cementomas are masses of cementum generally situated apical to the teeth to which they may or may not be attached. They are considered as either odontogenic neoplasms or developmental malformations. Cementomas occur more frequently in females than in males, more often in the mandible than in the maxilla,[7] and may occur singly or multiply.[44] Usually harmless, they are generally discovered upon radiographic examination. In some cases they produce deformity of jaw contour.

The microscopic structure of the cementoma varies with regard to the proportions of connective tissue and cementum. The cementum may be arranged either as numerous coalescent cementicles or as an irregular mesh-work

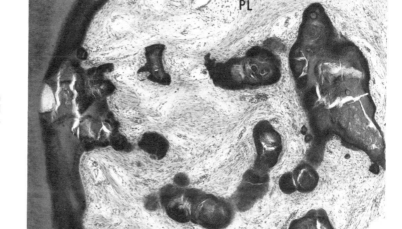

Figure 3–7 Cementicles free in the periodontal ligament (PL) and adherent to the root surface. C, cementum; D, dentin.

of trabeculae separated by fibrous connective tissue.[15]

The surface of the cementoma is generally formed by a layer of newly formed incompletely calcified cementoid lined by cementoblasts and surrounded by a connective tissue capsule. With continued deposition of cementum, the proportion of connective tissue within the lesion is reduced.

The radiographic appearance of the cementoma varies, depending upon the proportion of calcified cementum and fibrous connective tissue in the lesion. When composed principally of cementum, the lesion appears as a discrete, circumscribed, dense, radiopaque mass within which isolated radiolucent markings may be seen.

CEMENTUM RESORPTION AND REPAIR

The cementum of erupted as well as unerupted teeth is subject to resorption. The resorptive changes may be of microscopic proportions or sufficiently extensive to present a radiographically detectable alteration in the root contour. Cementum resorption is extremely common. In a microscopic study of 261 teeth it occurred in 236 (90.5 per cent).[20] The average number

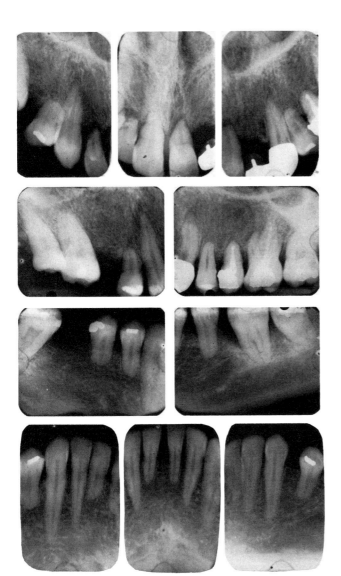

Figure 3–8 Idiopathic Root Resorption without unusual medical findings or history of orthodontic treatment.

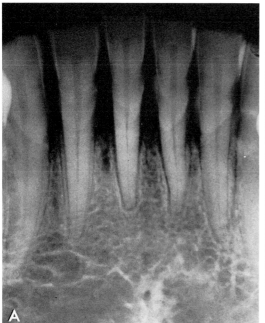

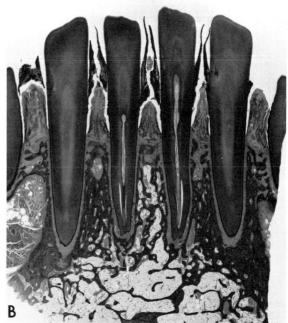

Figure 3–9 Cemental Resorption Associated With Excessive Occlusal Forces. *A,* Radiograph of mandibular anterior teeth. Note the thickening of the periodontal ligament space and lamina dura with blunting of the apices of the central incisors. *B,* Low power histological section of the mandibular anterior teeth. *C,* Higher power micrograph of left central incisor shortened by resorption of cementum and dentin. Note partial repair of the eroded areas (arrows), and cementicle at upper right.

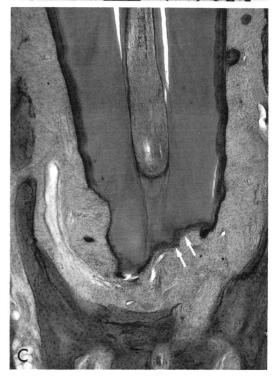

of resorption areas per tooth was 3.5. Of the 922 areas of resorption, 708 (76.8 per cent) were located in the apical third of the root, 177 (19.2 per cent) in the middle third, and 37 (4.0 per cent) in the gingival third of the root. Seventy per cent of all resorption areas were confined to the cementum without involving the dentin.

Cementum resorption may be due to local or systemic causes or may occur without the etiology being apparent (idiopathic) (Fig. 3–8). Among the local conditions under which it occurs are trauma from occlusion[38] (Fig. 3–9), orthodontic movement,[19, 26, 36, 41] pressure from maligned erupting teeth, cysts and tumors,[27]

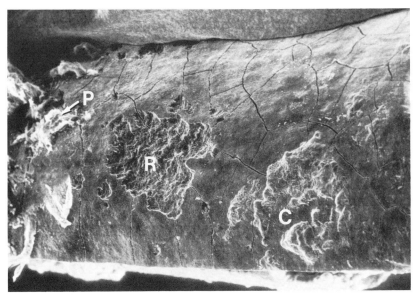

Figure 3–10   Scanning electron micrograph of root exposed by periodontal disease showing large resorption bay (R). Remnants of the periodontal ligament are seen at P and calculus at C. Cracking of the tooth surface occurs as a result of the preparation technique. × 160. (Courtesy Dr. John Sottosanti, San Diego, Cal.)

teeth without functional antagonists, embedded teeth, replanted and transplanted teeth,[1] periapical disease, and periodontal disease. Peculiar susceptibility of the cervical area to resorption has been attributed to the absence of either uncalcified precementum or reduced enamel epithelium.[50] Among the systemic conditions suspected as predisposing to or inducing cemental resorption are debilitating infections such as tuberculosis and pneumonia;[16] deficiencies of calcium,[24] vitamin D[6] and vitamin A;[11] hypothyroidism,[5] hereditary fibrous osteodystrophy,[52] and Paget's disease.[42]

Cementum resorption appears microscopically as baylike concavities in the root surface (Fig. 3–10). Multinucleated giant cells and large mononuclear macrophages are generally found adjacent to cementum undergoing active resorption (Fig. 3–11). Several sites of resorption may coalesce to form a large area of destruction. The resorptive process may extend into the underlying dentin and even into the pulp, but it is usually painless.

Cementum resorption is not necessarily continuous and may alternate with periods of repair and the deposition of new cementum. The newly formed cementum is demarcated

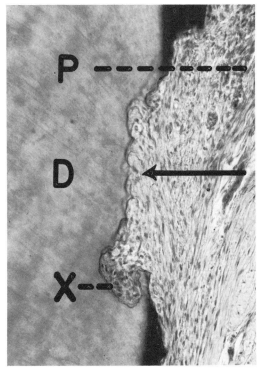

Figure 3–11   Resorption of Cementum and Dentin.   A multinuclear osteoclast is seen at (X). The direction of resorption is indicated by the arrow. Note the scalloped resorption front in the dentin (D). The cementum is the darkly stained band at upper and lower right. P, Periodontal ligament.

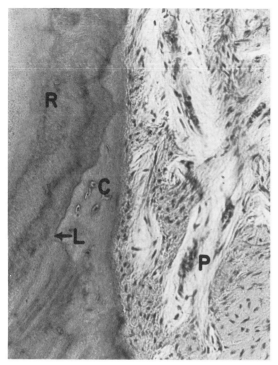

Figure 3–12 Section Showing Repair of Previously Resorbed Root. The defect is filled in with cellular cementum (C), which is separated from the older cementum (R) by an irregular line (L), which indicates the preexistent outline of the resorbed root. Periodontal ligament (P).

from the root by a deeply staining irregular line, termed a reversal line, which designates the border of the previous resorption (Fig. 3–12). Embedded fibers of the periodontal ligament re-establish a functional relation-

ship in the new cementum. Cementum repair requires the presence of viable connective tissue. If epithelium proliferates into an area of resorption, repair will not take place. Cementum repair can occur in devitalized as well as vital teeth.

Fusion of the cementum and alveolar bone with obliteration of the periodontal ligament is termed *ankylosis*. Ankylosis invariably occurs in teeth with cemental resorption, suggesting that it may represent a form of abnormal repair. Ankylosis may also develop following chronic periapical inflammation, tooth replantation, occlusal trauma, and around embedded teeth.

INJURIES TO CEMENTUM

Fracture

When a tooth is subjected to a severe external force, such as a blow or biting on a hard object, fracture of the root (Fig. 3–13) or "tearing" of the cementum may occur. Complete horizontal or oblique fractures may be followed by repair, which includes the deposition of calcified tissues and the embedding of new periodontal fibers. Several factors influence the likelihood of such repair. Exposure of the site of fracture to the oral cavity with subsequent infection will interfere with repair. Even in unexposed fractures, the deposition of calcified tissue is reduced

Figure 3–13 Root Repair After Traumatic Fracture. Detached fragments of cementum are shown at F′ at upper left. The apical section of cementum (F) is separated from the remainder of the root (R) by dense connective tissue (P′) and attached to the bone (B) by the periodontal ligament (P). A filled-in root defect is indicated by L.

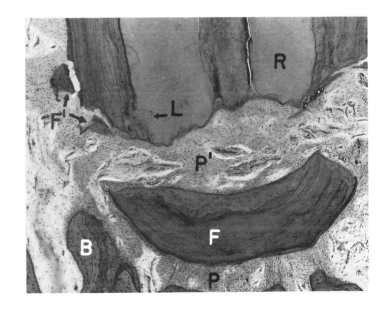

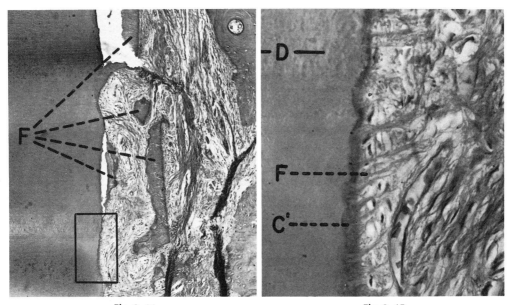

Fig. 3–14   **Fig. 3–15**

Figure 3–14 Traumatic "Cemental Tear" with fragments of cementum (F) free in the periodontal ligament.
Figure 3–15 High-power section of area within rectangle in Figure 3–14. New cementum (C′) is shown along dentin (D). Collagen fibers (F) are embedded in the new cementum.

upon *proximity of the fracture to the oral cavity.*[8] The distance between the fractured root ends and the inherent reparative capacity of the individual also influence repair of complete horizontal or oblique root fractures.

Cemental tear

Detachment of a fragment of cementum from the root surface is known as a *cemental tear.* The separation of cementum may be complete, with displacement of a fragment into the periodontal ligament, or it may be incomplete, with the cementum fragment remaining partially attached to the roots (Figs. 3–14 and 3–15).

Cementum fragments displaced into the periodontal ligament may undergo a variety of changes. New cementum may be deposited at the periphery, and periodontal fibers may become embedded in it, so as to establish a functional relationship between the tooth on one aspect and alveolar bone on the other. The detached cementum may be reunited to the root surface by new cementum. Detached cementum fragments may be completely re- **sorbed or may undergo partial resorption followed by addition of new cementum and embedding of collagen fibers.**

REFERENCES

1. Agnew, R. G., and Fong, C. C.: Histologic studies on experimental transplantation of teeth. Oral Surg., 9:18, 1956.
2. Albright, J. T., and Flanagan, J. B.: Electronmicroscopy of cementum. I.A.D.R. Abstracts of the 40th Meeting, 1962, p. 77.
3. Baer, P., Brown, N., and Hamner, J. E.: Hypophosphatasia. J. Am. Soc. Periodontol., 2:209, 1964.
4. Balbe, R., Carranza, F. A., Sr., and Erausquin, R.: Los paradencios del caso 8. Rev. Odontol., Buenos Aires, July, 1938.
5. Becks, H.: Root resorptions and their relation to pathologic bone formation. Int. J. Orthod. Oral Surg., 22:445, 1936.
6. Becks, H., and Weber, M.: The influence of diet on the bone system with special reference to the alveolar process and the labyrinthine capsule. J. Am. Dent. Assoc., 18:197, 1931.
7. Bernier, J. L., and Thompson, H. C.: The histogenesis of the cementoma. Am. J. Orthod., 32:543, 1946.
8. Bevelander, G.: Tissue reactions in experimental tooth fracture. J. Dent. Res., 21:481, 1942.
9. Bevelander, G., and Nakahara, H.: The fine structure of the human periodontal ligament. Anat. Rec., 162:313, 1968.

10. Blayney, J. R., Wasserman, F., Groetzinger, G., and DeWitt, T. G.: Further studies in mineral metabolism of human teeth by the use of radioactive isotopes. J. Dent. Res., 29:559, 1941.

11. Burn, C. G., Orten, A. I., and Smith, A. H.: Changes in the structure of the developing tooth in rats maintained on a diet deficient in vitamin A. Yale J. Biol. Med., 13:817, 1940–1.

12. El Mostehy, M. R., and Stallard, R. E.: Intermediate cementum. J. Periodont. Res., 3:24, 1968.

13. Gardner, A. F.: Alterations in mesenchymal and ectodermal tissues during experimental lathyrism. Apposition and calcification of cementum. Parodontol., 20:111, 1966.

14. Glimcher, M., Friberg, U., and Levine, P.: The identification and characterization of a calcified layer of coronal cementum in erupted bovine teeth. J. Ultrastruct. Res., 10:76, 1964.

15. Gottlieb, B.: Biology of the cementum. J. Periodontol., 17:7, 1942.

16. Gottlieb, B.: Tissue changes in pyorrhea. J. Am. Dent. Assoc., 14:2178, 1927.

17. Gottlieb, B., and Orban, B.: Biology and Pathology of the Tooth and Its Supporting Mechanism. Trans. by M. Diamond, New York, The Macmillan Co., 1938, p. 70.

18. Haim, G.: Histochemische Untersuchungen des Zementgewebes. Dtsch. Zahnärtzl. Z., 16:71, 1962.

19. Hemley, S.: The incidence of root resorption of vital permanent teeth. J. Dent. Res., 20:133, 1941.

20. Henry, J. L., and Weinmann, J. P.: The pattern of resorption and repair of human cementum. J. Am. Dent. Assoc., 42:271, 1951.

21. Inoue, M., and Akiyoshi, M.: Histological investigation on Sharpey's fibers in cementum of teeth in abnormal function. J. Dent. Res., 41:503, 1962.

22. Ishikawa, J., Yamamoto, H., Ito, K., and Masuda, M.: Microradiographic study of cementum and alveolar bone. J. Dent. Res., 43:936, 1964.

23. Jande, S. S., and Belanger, L. F.: Fine structural studies of rat molar cementum. Anat. Rec., 167:349, 1970.

24. Jones, M. R., and Simonton, F. V.: Mineral metabolism in relation to alveolar atrophy in dogs. J. Am. Dent. Assoc., 15:881, 1928.

25. Jones, S. J., and Boyde, A.: A study of human root cementum surfaces as prepared for and examined in the scanning electron microscope. Z. Zellforsch., 130:318, 1972.

26. Ketcham, A. H.: A progress report of an investigation of apical root resorption of permanent teeth. Int. J. Orthod., 15:310, 1929.

27. Kronfeld, R.: Biology of the cementum. J. Am. Dent. Assoc., 25:1451, 1938.

28. Kronfeld, R.: Die Zementhyperplasien und Nicht-Functionierenden Zähne. Z. Stomatol., 25:1218, 1927.

29. Kronfeld, R.: Cementum and Sharpey's fibers. Z. Stomatol., 26:714, 1928.

30. Lester, K.: The incorporation of epithelial cells by cementum. J. Ultrastruct. Res., 27:63, 1969.

31. Listgarten, M. A.: A light and electron microscopic study of coronal cementogenesis. Arch. Oral Biol., 13:93, 1968.

32. Listgarten, M. A.: Changing concepts about the dento-epithelial junction. J. Can. Dent. Assoc., 36:70, 1970.

33. Mikola, O. J., and Bauer, W. H.: Cementicles and fragments of cementum in the periodontal membrane. Oral Surg., 2:1063, 1949.

34. Nihei, I.: A study of the hardness of human teeth. J. Osaka Univ. Dent. Soc., 4:1, 1959.

35. Noyes, F. B., Schour, I., and Noyes, H. J.: A Textbook of Dental Histology and Embryology, 5th ed. Philadelphia, Lea & Febiger, 1938, p. 113.

36. Oppenheim, A.: Human tissue response to orthodontic intervention of short and long duration. Am. J. Orthod. Oral Surg., 28:263, 1942.

37. Orban, B.: Oral Histology and Embryology, 2nd ed. St. Louis, C. V. Mosby Co., 1944, p. 161.

38. Orban, B.: Tissue changes in traumatic occlusion. J. Am. Dent. Assoc., 15:2090, 1928.

39. Riffle, A. B.: Cemento-enamel junction. J. Periodontol., 23:41, 1952.

40. Romaniuk, K.: Some observations of the fine structure of human cementum. J. Dent. Res., 46:152, 1967.

41. Rudolph, C. E.: An evaluation of root resorption occurring during orthodontic therapy. J. Dent. Res., 19:367, 1940.

42. Rushton, M. A.: Dental tissues in osteitis deformans. Guys Hosp. Rep., 88:163, 1938.

43. Sasso, W.: Histochemical study of human dental cementum. Rev. Fac. Odont., 4:189, 1966.

44. Scannell, J. M.: Cementoma. Oral Surg., 2:1169, 1949.

45. Selvig, K. A.: An ultrastructural study of cementum formation. Acta Odontol. Scand., 22:105, 1964.

46. Selvig, K. A.: Electron Microscopy of Hertwig's epithelial sheath and early dentin and cementum formation in the mouse incisor. Acta Odontol. Scand., 21:175, 1963.

47. Selvig, K. A.: Studies on the Genesis, Composition and Fine Structure of Cementum. Bergen-Oslo-Tromsö, Universitetsforlaget, 1967.

48. Selvig, K.: The fine structure of human cementum. Acta Odontol. Scand., 23:423, 1965.

49. Selvig, K. A., and Selvig, S. K.: Mineral content of human and seal cementum. J. Dent. Res., 41:624, 1962.

50. Southam, J.: Clinical and histological aspects of peripheral cervical resorption. J. Periodontol., 38:534, 1967.

51. Stern, I. B.: An electron-microscopic study of the cementum, Sharpey's fibrils and periodontal ligament in the rat incisor. Am. J. Anat., 115:377, 1964.

52. Thoma, K. H., Sosman, M. C., and Bennett, G. A.: An unusual case of hereditary fibrous osteodystrophy (fragilitas ossium) with replacement of dentine by osteocementum. Am. J. Orthod. Oral Surg., 29:1, 1943.

53. Volker, J. F.: The phosphate metabolism of the erupted tooth as indicated by studies utilizing the radioactive isotope. Tufts Outlook, 16:3, 1942.

54. Volker, J. F., Gilda, J. E., and Ginn, J. T.: Radio-

phosphorus metabolism of pulpless teeth. J. Dent. Res., 21:322, 1942.

55. Warren, E. B., et al.: Effects of periodontal disease and of calculus solvents on microhardness of cementum. J. Periodontol., 35:505, 1964.

56. Wasserman, F., Blayney, J. R., Groetzinger, G., and DeWitt, T. G.: Studies on the different pathways of exchange of minerals in teeth with the aid of radioactive phosphorus. J. Dent. Res., 20:389, 1941.

57. Yamamoto, H., et al.: Microradiographic and his-

topathological study of the cementum. Bull. Tokyo Dent. Univ., 9:141, 1962.

58. Zander, H. A., and Hurzeler, B.: Continuous cementum apposition. J. Dent. Res., 37:1035, 1958.

59. Zemsky, J. L.: Hypercementosis and heredity: An introduction and plan of investigation. Dent. Items Int., 53:355, 1931.

60. Zipkin, I.: The inorganic composition of bones and teeth. In Schraer, H. (ed.): Biological Calcification. New York, Appleton-Century-Crofts, 1970.

Chapter 4

The Alveolar Bone

NORMAL MICROSCOPIC FEATURES

The *alveolar process* is the bone which forms and supports the tooth sockets (alveoli). It consists of the inner socket wall of thin compact bone called the *alveolar bone proper (cribriform plate)*, the *supporting alveolar bone* which consists of cancellous trabeculae and the facial and lingual plates of compact bone. The interdental septum consists of cancellous supporting bone enclosed within a compact border (Fig. 4–1).

The alveolar process is divisible into separate areas on an anatomic basis, *but it functions as a unit. All parts are interrelated in the support of the teeth.* Occlusal forces which are transmitted from the periodontal ligament to the inner wall of the alveolus are supported by the cancellous trabeculae, which in turn are buttressed by the labial and lingual cortical plates. Designation of the entire alveolar process as alveolar bone is more consistent with its functional unity.

Cells and Intercellular Matrix

Alveolar bone is formed during fetal growth by intramembranous ossification, and consists of a calcified matrix with osteocytes enclosed within spaces called lacunae. The osteocytes extend processes into canaliculi which radiate from the lacunae. The canaliculi form an anastomosing system through the intercellular matrix

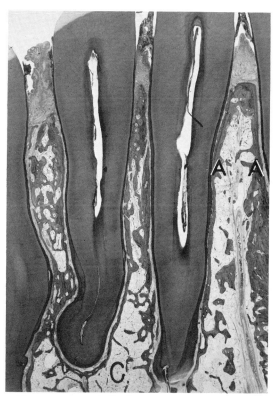

Figure 4–1 Mesiodistal Section Through Mandibular Canine and Premolars Showing Interdental Bony Septa. The dense bony plates (A) represent the alveolar bone proper (cribriform plates) and are supported by cancellous bony trabeculae (C). Note the vertical blood vessels within a nutrient canal in the interdental septum at the right.

of the bone, which brings oxygen and nutrients via the blood to the osteocytes and removes metabolic waste products. Blood vessels branch extensively and travel through the periosteum. The endosteum lies adjacent to the marrow vasculature. Bone growth occurs by apposition of an organic matrix that is deposited by osteoblasts. For a detailed account of bone histology the reader is referred to any current standard textbook of histology.

Bone is composed principally of the minerals calcium and phosphate, along with hydroxyl, carbonates, citrate, and trace amounts of other ions such as sodium, magnesium, and fluorine. The mineral salts are in the form of hydroxyapatite crystals of ultramicroscopic size and constitute approximately 65 to 70 per cent of the bone structure. The organic matrix[6] consists mainly (90 per cent) of collagen (type I),[19] with small amounts of noncollagenous proteins, glycoproteins, phosphoproteins, lipids, and proteoglycans. The apatite crystals are generally aligned with their long axes parallel to the long axes of collagen fibers, and appear to be deposited upon and within the collagen fibers. In this fashion bone matrix is able to withstand heavy mechanical stresses applied to it during function.

Although the alveolar bone tissue is constantly changing in its internal organization, it retains approximately the same form from childhood through adult life. Bone deposition by osteoblasts is balanced by resorption by osteoclasts during the processes of tissue remodelling and renewal.

The bone matrix that is laid down by osteoblasts is not mineralized and is referred to as prebone or osteoid. While new prebone is being deposited, the older prebone located below the surface becomes mineralized as the mineralization front advances. Recent investigations have revealed the morphologic and biochemical steps that are involved during the elaboration of bone matrix collagen.[20, 32] Briefly, procollagen molecules are synthesized and assembled by the rough endoplasmic reticulum and Golgi apparatus respectively within osteoblasts[31, 32] (Fig. 4–2). Secretory granules then carry the procollagen aggregates to the cell surface for secretion to take place (Fig. 4–3). At some time prior or subsequent to discharge from the cell, the procollagen molecules interact with a peptidase and become converted to tropocollagen molecules which then have the capacity to assemble into typical collagen fibrils.

Prior to becoming mineralized, bone matrix collagen becomes coated or associated with a glycoprotein (or proteoglycan) material which, in the electron microscope, appears as an opaque granular substance. It is conceivable that this glycoprotein has

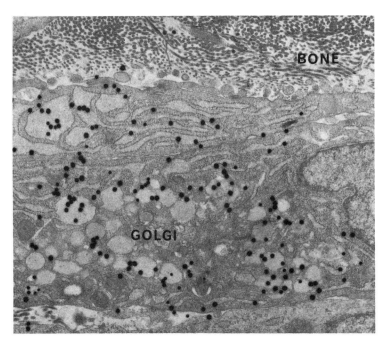

Figure 4–2 Electron microscope radioautograph of osteoblasts obtained 20 minutes after incubation in medium containing ³H-proline. Silver grains (black dots) may be seen over the rough endoplasmic reticulum (RER) throughout the cytoplasm and over the content of the distended portions of the RER (upper left). Also visible at this time after incubation are grains overlying the round, distended, condensing vacuoles located at the periphery of the Golgi apparatus and encircling the Golgi. The collagen fibers in the prebone matrix (top) are unlabeled at this time. A portion of a nucleus can be seen on the right.

These results indicate that radioactively labeled material is located in both organelles after 20 minutes of exposure to ³H-proline. Biochemical analysis showed that 75 to 80 per cent of the radioactivity was in bone procollagen. Magnification ×15,000. (From Weinstock, A. et al.[32])

Figure 4–3 High power electron microscope radioautograph taken 35 minutes after incubation in a medium containing ³H-proline. A peripheral portion of an osteoblast may be seen showing secretory granules (SG) with overlying silver grains (black dots). The secretory granules have approached the plasma membrane, and the elongated one on the left may be in the midst of discharging its content of procollagen filaments by exocytosis. Some of the collagen fibers within the prebone matrix (upper half of micrograph) show overlying grains, indicating that they contain radioactive filaments discharged from the cell a few minutes prior to fixing the tissue. Magnification × 60,000. (From Weinstock, A. et al.³²)

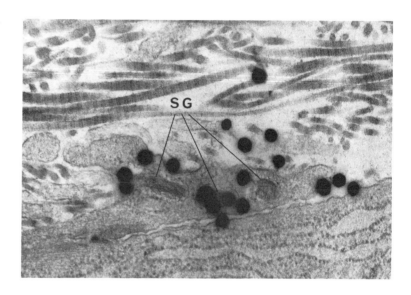

an important role in the mineralization process. Osteoblasts produce this material together with other matrix constituents. A similar series of events is believed to occur during dentin matrix production and mineralization.³²

Osteoclasts are large, multinucleated cells that are often seen on the surface of bone within eroded bony depressions referred to as Howship's lacunae. The main function of these cells is considered to be resorption of bone. When they are active, as opposed to resting, they possess an elaborately developed ruffled border from which hydrolytic enzymes are believed to be secreted. These enzymes digest the organic portion of bone. The activity of osteoclasts and the morphology of the ruffled border can be modified and regulated by hormones such as parathormone and calcitonin.¹⁴ The origin of osteoclasts is still a matter of speculation and controversy.

The Socket Wall

The principal fibers of the periodontal ligament which anchor the tooth in the socket are embedded for a considerable distance into the alveolar bone where they are referred to as *Sharpey's fibers*. Some Sharpey's fibers are completely calcified,

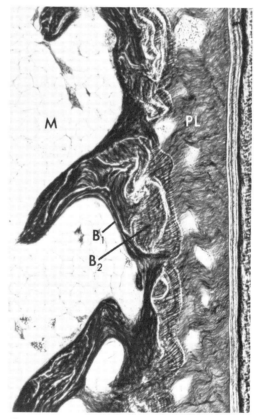

Figure 4–4 Deep penetration of Sharpey's fibers into bundle bone. The darkly stained bone (B₁) is lamellar bone. Bundle bone (B₂) takes up less stain and shows numerous white lines running more or less parallel to each other; these lines correspond to Sharpey's fibers. M, fatty marrow; PL, periodontal ligament.

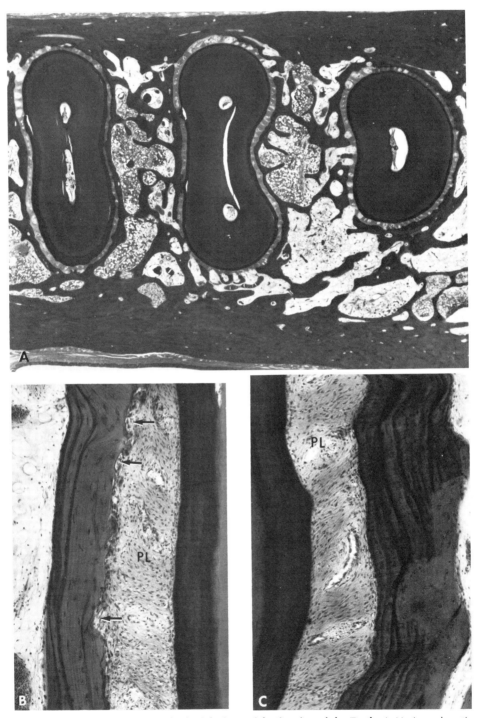

Figure 4–5   Bundle Bone Associated With Physiologic Mesial Migration of the Teeth. *A,* Horizontal section through molar roots in the process of mesial migration (mesial, *left;* distal, *right*). *B,* Mesial root surface showing osteoclasis of bone (arrows). *C,* Distal root surface showing bundle bone which has been partially replaced with dense bone on the marrow side. PL, Periodontal ligament.

but most contain an uncalcified central core within a calcified outer layer.[8, 26] The socket wall consists of dense lamellated bone, some of which is arranged in Haversian systems and *"bundle bone."* Bundle bone is the term given to bone adjacent to the periodontal ligament because of its content of Sharpey's fibers[30] (Fig. 4–4). It is arranged in layers with intervening appositional lines, parallel to the root (Fig. 4–5). Bundle bone is not unique to the jaws; it occurs throughout the skeletal system where ligaments and muscles are attached. Bundle bone is gradually resorbed on the side of the marrow spaces and replaced by lamellated bone.

The *cancellous portion of the alveolar bone* consists of trabeculae which enclose irregularly shaped marrow spaces lined with a layer of thin, flattened endosteal cells. There is wide variation in the trabecular pattern of the cancellous bone,[22] which is affected by occlusal forces. The matrix of the cancellous trabeculae consists of irregularly arranged lamellae separated by deeply staining incremental and resorption lines indicative of previous bone activity, with an occasional Haversian system.

Vascular Supply, Lymphatics, and Nerves

The cribriform plate of the tooth socket appears radiographically as a thin, radio-paque line, termed the *lamina dura.* However, it is perforated by numerous channels containing blood, lymph vessels, and nerves, which link the periodontal ligament with the cancellous portion of the alveolar bone (Fig. 4–6). The vascular supply of the bone is derived from blood vessels branching off of the superior or inferior alveolar arteries. These arterioles enter the interdental septa within nutrient canals together with veins, nerves, and lymphatics. Dental arterioles, also branching off of the alveolar arteries, send tributaries through the periodontal ligament, and some small branches enter the narrow spaces of the bone via the perforations in the cribriform plate. Small vessels emanating from the facial and lingual compact bone also enter the marrow and spongy bone.

The Interdental Septum

The interdental septum consists of cancellous bone bordered by the socket walls of approximating teeth and the facial and lingual cortical plates (Fig. 4–7).

The mesiodistal angulation of the crest of the interdental septum usually parallels a line drawn between the cemento-enamel junctions of the approximating teeth.[24] The average distance between the crest of the alveolar bone and the cemento-enamel junction in the mandibular anterior region

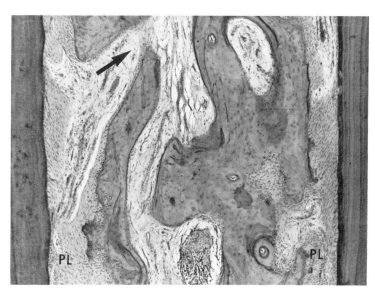

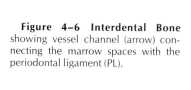

Figure 4–6 Interdental Bone showing vessel channel (arrow) connecting the marrow spaces with the periodontal ligament (PL).

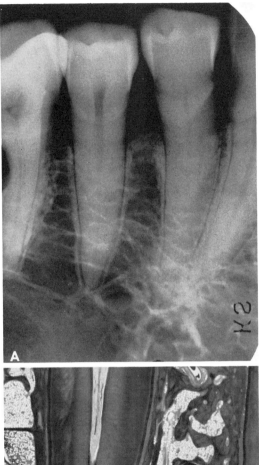

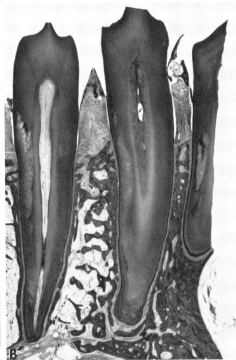

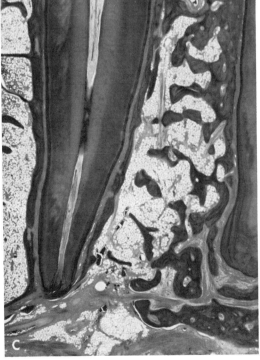

Figure 4–7 Interdental Septa. *A,* Mandibular premolar area. Note the prominent lamina dura. *B,* Interdental septa between the canine *(right)* and premolars. The central cancellous portion is bordered by the dense bony cribriform plates of the socket. (This forms the lamina dura around the teeth in the radiograph.) *C,* Interdental septum between the premolars, showing central cancellous bone and dense cribriform plate around the roots.

of young adults varies between 0.96 mm. and 1.22 mm.[12] With age, the distance between the bone and the cemento-enamel junction increases throughout the mouth (1.88 mm. to 2.81 mm.).[9] However, this phenomenon may not be as much a function of age as of periodontal disease.

The Marrow

In the embryo and newborn, the cavities of all the bones are occupied by red hematopoietic marrow. The red marrow gradually undergoes a physiologic change to the fatty or yellow inactive type of marrow. In the adult, the marrow of the jaw is normally of the latter type, and red marrow is found only in the ribs, sternum, vertebrae, skull, and humerus. However, foci of red bone marrow are occasionally seen in the jaws, often accompanied by resorption of bone trabeculae.[3] Common locations are the maxillary tuberosity (Fig. 4–8) and the maxillary and mandibular molar and premolar areas, which may be visible radiographically as zones of radiolucence. It has been suggested that they may be (1) remnants of the original marrow that has not undergone physiologic change to the fatty state, (2) localized manifestations of a generalized increase in red blood cell formation or of systemic disease such as tuberculosis,[4] or (3) the response to local injury or dental infection.

Bone is the calcium reservoir of the body, and the alveolar bone participates in the maintenance of the body calcium balance. *Calcium is constantly being deposited and withdrawn from the alveolar bone to provide for the needs of other tissues and to maintain the calcium level of the blood.* The calcium in the cancellous trabeculae is more readily available than that in compact bone. Conversely, easily mobilizable calcium is deposited in the trabeculae rather than the cortex of adult bone. The hormonal control of calcium metabolism is complex, and information may be obtained from textbooks specifically on this subject.

So persistent is the effort to maintain a normal calcium level in the blood, that even in cases of skeletal osteoporosis the blood calcium may be normal. In experimental animals the rate of metabolism of alveolar bone is more rapid than that of the diaphysis of the femur, but it is slower than the metaphysis or "growth zone."[25]

THE EXTERNAL CONTOUR OF ALVEOLAR BONE

The bone contour normally conforms to the prominence of the roots, with intervening vertical depressions which taper toward the margin (Fig. 4–9). For a detailed anatomical account of the structure and relations of the alveolar processes, the

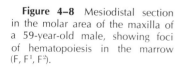
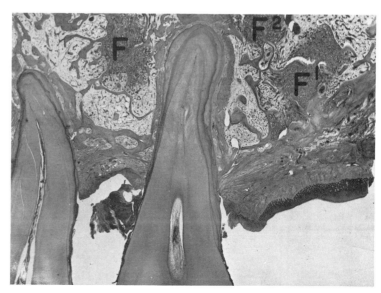

Figure 4–8 Mesiodistal section in the molar area of the maxilla of a 59-year-old male, showing foci of hematopoiesis in the marrow (F, F[1], F[2]).

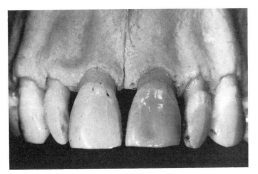

Figure 4–9 Normal Bone Contour conforms to the prominence of the roots.

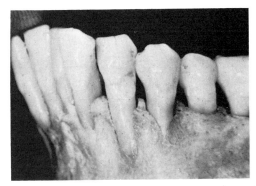

Figure 4–10 Apical location of bone on the labially placed mandibular canine and first premolars. Compare with higher level and thicker margin of the bone on the second premolar.

reader is referred elsewhere.[24, 28] Alveolar bone anatomy varies from patient to patient and has important clinical implications.

The height and thickness of the facial and lingual bony plates are affected by the alignment of the teeth and angulation of the root to the bone and by occlusal forces. On teeth in labial version, the margin of the labial bone is located farther apically than on teeth in proper alignment. The bone margin is thinned to a knife edge and presents an accentuated arc in the direction of the apex (Fig. 4–10). On teeth in lingual version, the facial bony plate is thicker than normal. The margin is blunt and rounded, and horizontal rather than arcuate. The effect of the *root to bone angulation* upon the height of alveolar bone is most noticeable on the palatal roots of maxillary molars. *The bone margin is located farther apically on the roots, which form relatively acute angles with the palatal bone.*[13] The cervical portion of the alveolar plate is sometimes consider-

ably thickened on the facial surface, apparently as reinforcement against occlusal forces (Fig. 4–11).

Fenestrations and Dehiscences

Isolated areas in which the root is denuded of bone and the root surface is covered only by periosteum and overlying gingiva are termed *fenestrations.* In this instance the marginal bone is intact. When the denuded areas extend through the marginal bone, the defect is called a dehiscence (Fig. 4–12). Such defects occur on approximately 20 per cent of the teeth; they occur more often on the facial bone than on the lingual, are more commonly on anterior teeth than on posterior teeth, and are frequently bilateral. There is microscopic evidence of lacunar resorption at the margins. The cause is not clear, but trauma from occlusion may be suspected.[29]

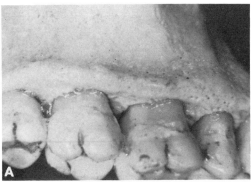
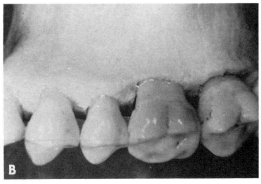

Figure 4–11 Variation in the cervical portion of the buccal alveolar plate. *Left,* Shelf-like conformation. *Right,* Comparatively thin buccal plate.

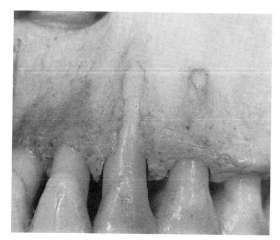

Figure 4–12 **Dehiscence** on the canine and **Fenestration** of the first premolar.

dontal tissues; its structure is in a constant state of flux.[17] The physiologic lability of alveolar bone is maintained by a sensitive balance between bone formation and bone resorption, regulated by local and systemic influences (Fig. 4–13). Bone is resorbed in areas of pressure and formed in areas of tension. The cellular activity which affects the height, contour, and density of alveolar bone is manifested in three areas: (1) *adjacent to the periodontal ligament,* (2) *in relation to the periosteum of the facial and lingual plates,* and (3) *along the endosteal surface of the marrow spaces.*

Prominent root contours, malposition, and labial protrusion of the root combined with a thin bony plate are predisposing factors.[7] Fenestration and dehiscences are important because they may complicate the outcome of periodontal surgery.

THE LABILITY OF ALVEOLAR BONE

In contrast to its apparent rigidity, alveolar bone is the least stable of the perio-

Mesial Migration of the Teeth and Reconstruction of Alveolar Bone

With time and wear the proximal contact areas of the teeth are flattened and the teeth tend to move mesially. This is referred to as *physiologic mesial migration,* a gradual process with intermittent periods of activity, rest, and repair. By age 40, it effects a reduction of 0.5 cm. in the length of the dental arch from the midline to the third molars.[2] Alveolar bone is reconstructed in compliance with the physiologic mesial migration of the teeth. Bone resorption is increased in areas of pressure

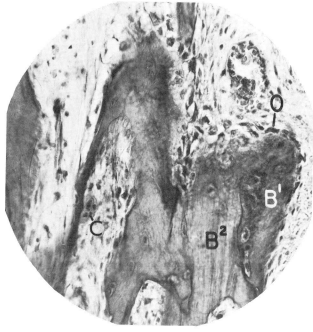

Figure 4–13 **Bone Formation and Bone Resorption in Close Proximity in Alveolar Bone.** Osteoblast (O) at the periphery of new bone (B¹) formed on older lamellated bone (B²) at site of previous resorption, indicated by irregular reversal line. Note osteoclast (C) along adjacent partially resorbed trabecula.

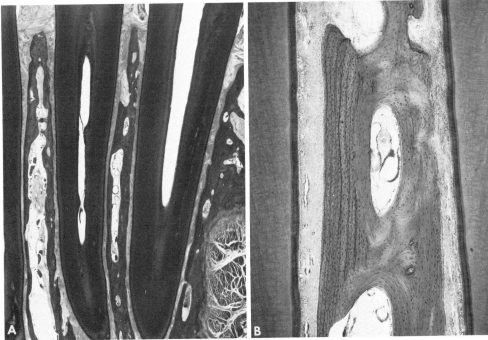

Figure 4–14   Bone Response to Physiologic Mesial Migration. *A*, Interdental septa between the canine *(left)* and first and second premolars. *B*, Interdental septum between the first and second premolars, showing lamellae of newly apposed bone opposite the distal of the first premolar *(left)* and resorption opposite the mesial of the second *(right)*.

along the mesial surfaces of the teeth, and new layers of bundle bones are formed in areas of tension on the distal surfaces (Figs. 4–5 and 4–14).

Occlusal Forces and Alveolar Bone

There are two aspects to the relationship between occlusal forces and alveolar bone. **The bone exists for the purpose of supporting teeth during function,** and, in common with the remainder of the skeletal system, **depends upon the stimulation it receives from function for the preservation of its structure.** There is therefore a constant and sensitive balance between occlusal forces and the structure of alveolar bone.[16]

Alveolar bone undergoes constant physiological remodeling in response to occlusal forces. Osteoclasts and osteoblasts redistribute bone substance to meet new functional demands most efficiently. Bone is removed from where it is no longer needed and added where new needs arise.

When an occlusal force is applied to a tooth either through a food bolus or by contact with opposing teeth, several things happen, depending upon the direction, intensity, and duration of the force. The tooth is displaced against the resilient periodontal ligament, in which it creates areas of tension and compression. The facial and lingual walls of the socket stretch somewhat in the direction of the force.[24] When the force is released, the tooth, liga-

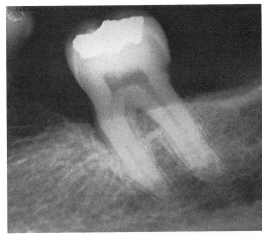

Figure 4–15   Bone Trabeculae realigned perpendicular to the mesial root of tilted molar.

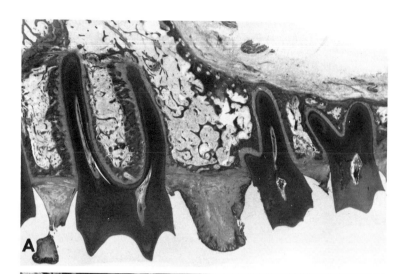

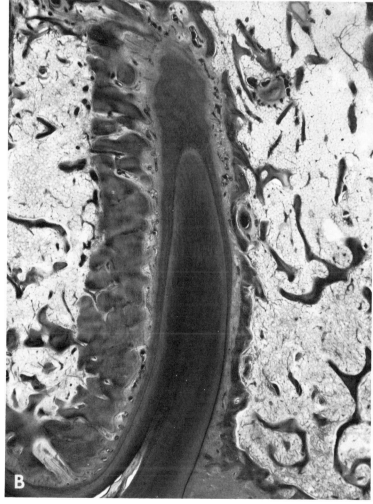

Figure 4–16 Bone Response to Increased Occlusal Forces. *A,* Mesiodistal section through maxillary molar and premolars subjected to increased occlusal forces. *B,* Mesiobuccal root of the second molar, showing thickening of bone along the distal surface in response to increased tension and thinning of the bone on the mesial aspect caused by increased pressure.

ment, and bone spring back to their original positions.

The socket wall reflects the responsiveness of alveolar bone to traumatic occlusal forces. Osteoblasts and newly formed osteoid line the socket in areas of tension; osteoclasts and bone resorption occur in areas of pressure.[2, 21]

The number, density, and alignment of cancellous trabeculae are also influenced by occlusal forces (Fig. 4–15). Experimental systems utilizing photoelastic analysis indicate alterations in stress patterns in the periodontium created by changes in the direction and intensity of occlusal forces.[10] The bone trabeculae are aligned in the path of the tensile and compressive stresses so as to provide maximum resistance to the occlusal force with a minimum of bone substance (Fig. 4–16).[27] Forces which exceed the adaptive capacity of the bone produce injury called trauma from occlusion (see Chap. 19).

When occlusal forces are increased, the cancellous trabeculae are increased in number and thickness, and bone may be added to the external surface of the labial and lingual plates (Fig. 4–11). When occlusal forces are reduced, bone is resorbed, bone height is diminished, and the number and thickness of the trabeculae are reduced.[15] This is termed *disuse or afunctional atrophy*. Although occlusal forces are extremely important in determining the internal architecture and external contour of alveolar bone, other factors such as local physiochemical conditions, vascular anatomy, and the individual systemic condition are also involved.[1]

REFERENCES

1. Anderson, B. G., Smith, A. H., Arnim, S. S., and Orten, A. V.: Changes in molar teeth and their supporting structures in rats following extraction of the upper right first and second molars. Yale J. Biol. Med., 9:189, 1936.
2. Black, C. V.: Pathology of the Hard Tissues of the Teeth. Oral Diagnosis, 8th ed. Woodstock, Ill., Medico-Dental Publishing Co., 1948, p. 389.
3. Box, H. K.: Bone resorption in red marrow hyperplasia in human jaws. Bull. 21, Can. Dent. Res. Found, 1936.
4. Cahn, L. R.: Red marrow in the jaws. J. Am. Dent. Assoc., 27:1056, 1940.
5. Cohn, S. A.: Disuse atrophy of the periodontium in mice. Arch. Oral Biol., 10:909, 1965.
6. Eastoe, J. E.: The organic matrix of bone. In Bourne, G. H. (ed.): The Biochemistry and Physiology of Bone, New York, Academic Press, 1956, p. 81.
7. Elliot, J. R., and Bowers, G. M.: Alveolar dehiscence and fenestration. Periodontics, 1:245, 1963.
8. Frank, R., Lindemann, G., and Vedrine, J.: Structure sub-microscopique de l'os alveolaire des maxillaires à l'etat normal. Rev. Franc. Odont., 5:1507, 1958.
9. Gargiulo, A. W., Wentz, F. M., and Orban, B.: Dimensions and relations of the dentogingival junction in humans. J. Periodontol., 32:216, 1961.
10. Glickman, I., Roeber, F. W., Brion, M., and Pameijer, J. H. N.: Photoelastic analysis of internal stresses in the periodontium created by occlusal forces. J. Periodontol. 41:30, 1970.
11. Glickman, I., and Wood, H.: Bone histology in periodontal disease. J. Dent. Res., 21:35, 1942.
12. Herulf, G.: On det marginala alveolarbenet hos ungdom i studiealder-nenrontgenstudie. Svensk Tandklakare-Tidsskrift., 43:42, 1950.
13. Hirschfeld, I.: A study of skulls in the American Museum of Natural History in relation to periodontal disease. J. Dent. Res., 5:241, 1923.
14. Holtrop, M. E., Raisz, L. G., and Simmons, H. A.: The effects of parathyroid hormone, colchicine and calcitonin on the ultrastructure and the activity of osteoclasts in organ culture. J. Cell Biol., 60:346, 1974.
15. Kellner, E.: Histologic findings on teeth without antagonists. Z. Stomatol., 26:271, 1928.
16. MacMillan, H. W.: A consideration of the structure of the alveolar process, with special reference to the principle underlying its surgery and regeneration. J. Dent. Res., 6:251, 1924–26.
17. Manson, J. D.: Age Changes in Bone Activity in the Mandible. Proceedings of the First European Bone and Tooth Symposium. Oxford, Pergamon Press, 1964, pp. 343–349.
18. McLean, F. C., and Urist, M. R.: Bone, 2nd ed. Chicago, University of Chicago Press, 1961, p. 38.
19. Miller, E. J.: A review of biochemical studies on the genetically distinct collagens of the skeletal system. Clin. Orthop. Relat. Res., 92:260, 1973.
20. Morris, N. P., Fessler, L. I., Weinstock, A., and Fessler, J. H.: Procollagen assembly and secretion in embryonic chick bone. J. Biol. Chem., 250:5719, 1975.
21. Orban, B.: Tissue changes in traumatic occlusion. J. Am. Dent. Assoc., 15:2090, 1928.
22. Parfitt, G. J.: An investigation of the normal variations in alveolar bone trabeculation. Oral Surg., 15:1453, 1962.
23. Picton, D. A.: On the part played by the socket in tooth support. Arch. Oral Biol., 10:945, 1965.
24. Ritchey, B., and Orban, B.: The crests of the interdental alveolar septa. J. Periodontol., 24:75, 1953.
25. Rogers, H. J., and Weidman, S. M.: Metabolism of alveolar bone. Br. Dent. J., 90:7, 1951.

26. Selvig, K. A.: The fine structure of human cementum. Acta Odontol. Scand., 23:423, 1965.

27. Sepel, C. M.: Trajectories of jaws. Acta Odontol. Scand., 8:81, 191, 1948.

28. Sicher, H.: Oral Anatomy. St. Louis, The C. V. Mosby Co., 1949, p. 385.

29. Stahl, S. S., Cantor, M., and Zwig, E.: Fenestrations of the labial alveolar plate in human skulls. Periodontology, 1:99, 1963.

30. Stein, G., and Weinmann, J. P.: The physiologic movement of the teeth. Z. Stomatol., 23:733, 1925.

31. Weinstock, A., and Burgeson, R. E.: Identification of procollagen in isolated chick embryo calvarial osteoblasts after incubation in vitro with proline-^{3}H. Anat. Rec. (Proc.), 178:485, 1974.

32. Weinstock, A., Bibb, C., Burgeson, R. E., Fessler, L. I., and Fessler, J. H.: Intracellular transport and secretion of procollagen in chick bone as shown by E. M. radioautography and biochemical analysis. In Slavkin, H. C., and Greulich, R. C. (eds.): Extracellular Matrix Influence on Gene Expression. New York, Academic Press, 1975, p. 101.

Aging and the Periodontium

Disease of the periodontium occurs in childhood, adolescence and early adulthood, but the prevalence of periodontal disease and the tissue destruction and tooth loss it causes increase with age. Many tissue changes occur with aging, some of which may affect the disease experience of the periodontium. *It is sometimes difficult to draw a sharp line between physiologic aging and the cumulative effects of disease.*

Aging is a slowing down of natural function, a disintegration of the balanced control and organization that characterize the young.[33] It is a process of physiologic and morphologic disintegration, as distinguished from infancy and adolescence, which are processes of integration and coordination. Aging is described in detail in texts devoted to the subject.[6, 9, 19] Some general age changes and alterations in the periodontium will be considered here.

GENERAL EFFECTS OF AGING

Aging is manifested to a different degree and in a different manner in various tissues and organs, but it includes general changes,[42, 45, 46] such as tissue desiccation, reduced elasticity, diminished reparative capacity, altered cell permeability, and increased calcium content in the cells of many organs.[29]

In the skin, the dermis and epidermis are thinned, keratinization is diminished,[22] the blood supply is decreased, and there is degeneration of the nerve endings. Capillaries appear to become more fragile with age, which may result in large hematomas from small traumas. Patchy peripheral anesthesia, indicative of central nervous system deterioration, is common in senility. Tissue elasticity is reduced with aging,[24] and there is degeneration of the elastic tissue fibers of the corium. The atrophic skin changes are less marked in females, and may be reversed in local areas by application of estrogen.

Bone undergoes osteoporosis with aging.[11] The bone is rarefied, trabeculae are reduced in number, the cortical plates are thinned, vascularity is reduced, lacunar resorption is more prominent, and susceptibility to fracture is increased. Resorption on the endosteal surface of long bones is relatively greater than the slight apposition that occurs on the periosteal surface; thus, total bone mass becomes reduced with age. Generalized osteoporosis occurs in aged females more commonly than in males, and has been associated with sex hormone dysfunction.[23] With age, water content of bone is reduced, the mineral crystals are increased in size, and collagen fibrils are thickened.[18, 19]

AGE CHANGES IN THE PERIODONTIUM

Gingiva and other areas of the oral mucosa

In the gingiva the following changes have been identified with aging: recession, diminished keratinization both in males[45] and females,[36] stippling reduced[17] or unchanged,[38] increased width of attached gingiva,[1a] decreased connective tissue cellularity, increased intercellular substances,[50] and reduced oxygen consumption, a measure of metabolic activity.[49] In menopausal patients the gingiva is less keratinized than in patients of comparable age with active menstrual cycles.

Changes in other areas of the oral mucosa include atrophy of the epithelium and connective tissue with loss of elasticity;[40] decrease in protein-bound hexoses and mucoproteins,[7] which may reduce resilience and increase susceptibility to trauma;[12] increase in mast cells;[8] atrophy of the papillae of the tongue, with the filiform papillae more severely affected; decrease in the number of taste buds in the circumvallate papillae,[6] nodular varicose enlargement of veins on the ventral surface of the tongue; and increase in the sebaceous glands in the lip and cheek.

Periodontal ligament

In the periodontal ligament, aging results in an increase in elastic fibers;[18] decrease in vascularity, mitotic activity,[47] fibroplasia,[21, 30] collagen fibers and mucopolysaccharides,[37, 43, 48] increase in arteriosclerotic changes;[16] and both an increase[25] and a decrease[10] in width have been described in aging. In instances where there is a decrease in width, it may be accounted for by a lower functional demand due to the decrease in strength of the masticatory musculature. The decreased width may also result from encroachment upon the ligament by continuous deposition of cementum and bone.[28]

Alveolar bone

In addition to reduction in height[14] (senile atrophy), changes occur in alveolar bone with aging that are similar to changes in the remainder of the skeletal system. These include osteoporosis,[2, 23] decreased vascularity, and a reduction in metabolism and healing capacity.[46] Resorption activity is increased,[32] bone formation is decreased[15, 44] and bone porosity may result. Bone density may increase or decrease depending on location and animal species.[26, 31]

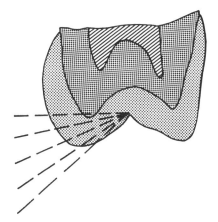

Figure 5–1 **Diminution in Cuspal Inclination** with increasing age.

Tooth-periodontium relationships

The most obvious change in the teeth with aging is a loss of tooth substance caused by attrition. Occlusal wear reduces cusp height and inclination (Fig. 5–1), with a resultant increase in the food table area and loss of sluiceways. The degree of attrition is influenced by the musculature, consistency of the food, tooth hardness, occupational factors and habits such as bruxism and clenching.[27, 39]

The rate of attrition may be coordinated with other age changes such as continuous tooth eruption and gingival recession (Fig. 5–2). As the tooth erupts, cementum is usually deposited in the apical region of the root. Reduction in bone height which occurs with aging is not necessarily related to occlusal wear.[3] In those cases in which bone support is reduced, the clinical crown tends to become disproportionately long and creates excessive leverage upon the bone. **By reducing the clinical crowns, attrition appears to preserve the balance between the teeth and their bony support.**

Wear of teeth also occurs on the proximal surfaces, accompanied by mesial migration of the teeth.[35] Proximal wear reduces the anteroposterior length of the dental arch by approximately 0.5 cm. by age 40.[51] Anteroposterior narrowing from proximal wear is greater in teeth that taper toward the cervical such as the incisors.[51] Progressive attrition and proximal wear result in a reduced maxillary-mandibular overjet in the molar area and an edge-to-edge bite anteriorly.

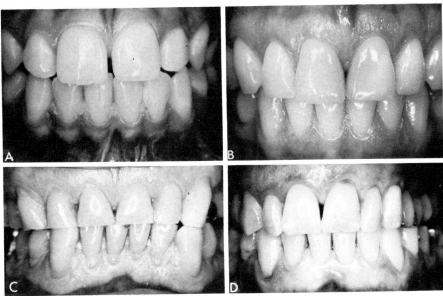

Figure 5–2   Tooth-Periodontium Relationships at Different Ages. *A,* Age 12. The gingiva is located on the enamel and the clinical crown is shorter than the anatomic crown. *B,* Age 25. The gingiva is attached close to the cemento-enamel junction. *C,* Age 50. Slight occlusal wear and slight recession. *D,* Age 72. Moderate attrition and slight to moderate recession. These variations may not be due to an aging process but to the cumulative effect of injurious factors.

Other effects of aging

Regressive changes in the salivary glands with retention cyst formation and associated xerostomia have been identified with aging.[40] Decrease in salivary flow and in the amount of ptyalin have been described as the causes of inadequate lubrication of food during mastication and poor starch digestion. Fatty degeneration of the parotid gland occurs in aged experimental animals.[1] There appears to be a reduction in the number of secretory units with age, as well as an increase in the amount of fibrous tissue.

Masticatory efficiency

Slight atrophy of the buccal musculature has been described as a physiologic feature of aging.[13] However, reduction in masticatory efficiency in aged individuals is more likely to be the result of unreplaced missing teeth, loose teeth, poorly fitting dentures, or an unwillingness to wear dentures. Reduced masticatory efficiency leads to poor chewing habits and the possibility of associated digestive disturbances. Aged persons select carbohydrates and foods requiring less chewing effort when masticatory efficiency is impaired.

Avitaminosis is common in aged persons, but the extent to which it results from impaired masticatory efficiency has not been established. The vitamin requirement of older persons may be increased because of their dietary habits. Long-standing calcium deficiency has been considered by some to be a causative factor in senile osteoporosis.[13] The advisability of increased calcium intake in aged individuals is doubtful, but a diet high in protein and vitamins and comparatively low in carbohydrates and fat may be beneficial.

AGING AND THE CUMULATIVE EFFECTS OF ORAL DISEASE

With time, chronic disease can produce many oral changes, and it is difficult to determine how much physiologic aging contributes to the total picture. Some contend that gingival recession, attrition, and reduction in bone height in the aged result more from disease and factors in the oral

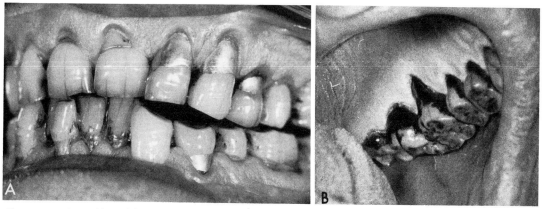

Figure 5–3 *A,* **Attrition of the Teeth** and gingival recession in a 65-year-old male. Note the elliptical contour of the tooth wear associated with biting the stem of a pipe while smoking. *B,* Lingual view showing accentuated recession on the first molar.

environment than from physiologic aging.[4] Although gingival recession, attrition, and bone loss commonly occur with age, they are not present in all patients, and vary considerably in the same age group. An aged individual with marked attrition may present relatively little alveolar bone loss (Figs. 5–3 and 5–4). Marked attrition may also be produced in young and middle-aged adults by bruxing and clenching habits (Figs. 5–5 and 5–6).

Increased alveolar bone loss in the aged has been related to less efficient oral hygiene.[41] Bone loss, pathologic migration of the teeth, and loss of vertical dimension in the aged may be the results of periodontal disease and failure to replace missing teeth.

Leukoplakia of the oral mucosa and staining of the teeth are common in aged individuals who are inveterate smokers. Wearing artificial dentures for years without

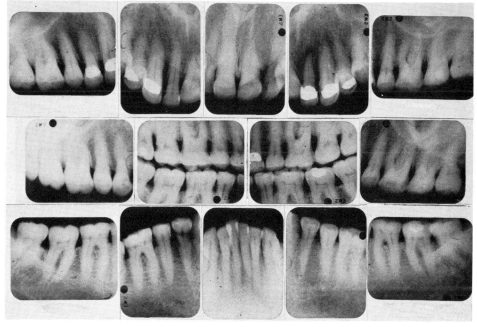

Figure 5–4 Radiographs of the patient shown in Figure 5–3. Aside from a few localized areas of bone loss there is little evidence of reduced bone height considered by some to be a physiologic feature of aging.

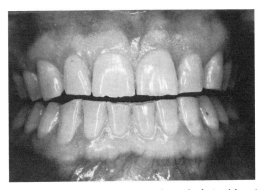

Figure 5–5   **Bruxing Habit and Marked Attrition** in 25-year-old woman.

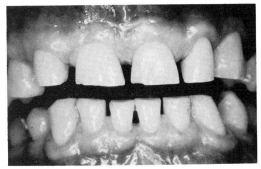

Figure 5–6   **Bruxing Habit and Marked Attrition** in 43-year-old man.

rebasing, with a resultant reduction in vertical dimension, is a common cause of angular cheilosis in the aged.

REFERENCES

1. Andrew, W.: Age changes in salivary glands of Wistar Institute rats with particular reference to the submandibular glands. J. Gerontol., 4: 95, 1949.
1a. Ainamo, J., and Talan, A.: The increase with age of the width of attached gingiva. J. Periodont. Res., 11:182, 1976.
2. Atkinson, P. J., and Woodhead, C.: Changes in human mandibular structure with age. Arch. Oral Biol., 13:1453, 1968.
3. Baer, P. N., et al.: Alveolar bone loss and occlusal wear. Periodontics, 1:45, 1963.
4. Baer, P. N., and Bernick, S.: Age changes in the periodontium of the mouse. Oral Surg., 10:430, 1957.
5. Birren, J. E.: Handbook of Aging and the Individual. Psychological and Biological Aspects. Chicago, University of Chicago Press, 1959.
6. Bourne, S. H.: Structural Aspects of Aging, New York, Hafner Publishing Company, Inc., 1961.
7. Burzynski, N. J.: Relationship between age and palatal tissue and gingival tissue in the guinea pig. J. Dent. Res., 46:539, 1967.
8. Carranza, F. A., Jr., and Cabrini, R. L.: Age variations in the number of mast cells in oral mucosa and skin of albino rats. J. Dent. Res., 38: 631, 1959.
9. Comfort, A.: Aging: The Biology of Senescence. New York, Holt, Rinehart and Winston, Inc., 1964.
10. Coolidge, E.: The thickness of the periodontal membrane. J. Am. Dent. Assoc., 24:1260, 1937.
11. Cowdry, E. V.: Problems of Aging, 2nd ed. Baltimore, Williams and Wilkins Co., 1942; Chapter 12, T. Wingate Todd, p. 322 (Skeleton and Locomotor System).
12. Flieder, D. E.: Cytochemistry of human oral mucosa: Determination of phospholipids, protein-bound hexoses, mucoproteins, colla-genous and non-collagenous proteins. J. Dent. Res., 41:112, 1962.
13. Freeman, J. T.: The basic factors of nutrition in old age. Geriatrics, 2:41, 1947.
14. Froehlich, E.: Periodontal changes in aging, Dtsch. Zahnärtzl. Z., 9:1005, 1965.
15. Gilmore, N., and Glickman, I.: Some age changes in the periodontium of the albino mouse. J. Dent. Res., 38:1195, 1959.
16. Grant, D., and Bernick, S.: Arteriosclerosis in periodontal vessels of aging humans. J. Periodontol., 41:170, 1970.
17. Greene, A. J.: Study of the characteristics of stippling and its relation to gingival health. J. Periodontol., 33:176, 1962.
18. Haim, G., and Baumgartel, R.: Alterations in the periodontal ligament due to age. Dtsch. Zahnärtzl. Z., 23:340, 1968.
19. Hall, D. A.: The Aging of Connective Tissue. London, Academic Press, 1976.
20. Ham, A. W., and Leeson, T. S.: Histology. 4th ed. Philadelphia, J. B. Lippincott Co., 1961, p. 279.
21. Jensen, J. L., and Toto, P. D.: Radioactive labeling index of the periodontal ligament in aging rats. J. Dent. Res., 47:149, 1968.
22. Joseph, N. R., Molimard, R., and Bourliere, F.: Aging of skin I. Titration curves of human epidermis in relation to age. Gerontologia, 1:18, 1957.
23. Kesson, C. M., Morris, N., and McCutcheon, A.: Generalized osteoporosis in old age. Ann. Rheumat. Dis., 6:146, 1947.
24. Kirk, E., and Kvorning, S. A.: Quantitative measurements of the elastic properties of the skin and subcutaneous tissue in young and old individuals. J. Gerontol., 4:273, 1949.
25. Klein, A.: Systemic investigations concerning the thickness of the periodontal membrane. Z. Stomatol., 26:417, 1928.
26. Klingsberg, J., and Butcher, E. O.: Comparative histology of age changes in oral tissues of rat, hamster and monkey. J. Dent. Res., 39:158, 1960.
27. Kronfeld, R.: Structure, Function, and Pathology of the Human Periodontal Membrane. N. Y. J. Dent., 6:112, 1936.

28. Kronfeld, R.: Biology of cementum. J. Am. Dent. Assoc., 25:1451, 1938.

29. Lansing, A. I.: Calcium growth in aging and cancer. Science, 106:187, 1947.

30. Lavelle, C. L. B.: The effect of age on the proliferative activity of the periodontal membrane of the rat incisor. J. Periodont. Res., 3:48, 1968.

31. Lopez Otero, R., Carranza, F. A., Jr., and Cabrini, R. L.: Histometric study of age changes in interradicular bone of Wistar rats. J. Periodont. Res., 2:40, 1967.

32. Manson, J. D., and Lucas, R. B.: A microradiographic study of age changes in the human mandible. Arch. Oral Biol., 7:761, 1962.

33. Muller, H. S., Little, C. C., and Snyder, L. H.: Genetics, Medicine and Man. Ithaca, N.Y., Cornell University Press, 1947. Chapter IV, Growth and Individuality by C. C. Little, p. 104.

34. Murphy, T. R.: A biometric study of the helicoidal occlusal plane of the worn Australian dentition. Arch. Oral Biol., 9:255, 1964.

35. Murphy, T. R.: Reduction of the dental arch by approximal attrition. Br. Dent. J., 116:483, 1964.

36. Papic, M., and Glickman, I.: Keratinization of the human gingiva in the menstrual cycle and menopause. Oral Surg., 3:504, 1950.

37. Paunio, K.: The age change of acid mucopolysaccharides in the periodontal membrane of man. J. Periodont. Res., Suppl. 4, Inter. Conf. Periodont. Res., 32, 1969.

38. Riethe, P.: Surface changes in the attached gingiva in young and old people. Dtsch. Zahnärztl. Z., 9:1028, 1965.

39. Robinson, H. B. G.: Some clinical aspects of intraoral age change. Geriatrics, 2:9, 1947.

40. Robinson, H. B. G., Boling, L. R., and Lischer, B.: Chapter XIII in Cowdry, E. V.: Problems of Aging. Baltimore, Williams and Wilkins Co., 1942, p. 384.

41. Schei, O., Waerhaug, J., Lovdal, A., and Arno, A.: Alveolar bone loss as related to oral hygiene and age. J. Periodontol., 30:7, 1959.

42. Simms, H. S., and Stolman, A.: Changes in human tissue electrolytes in senescence. Science, 86:269, 1937.

43. Skougaard, M. R., Levy, B. M., and Simpson, J.: Collagen metabolism in skin and periodontal membrane of the marmoset. J. Periodont. Res., Suppl. 4, Inter. Conf. Periodont. Res., 28, 1969.

44. Soni, N. N.: Quantitative study of bone activity in alveolar and femoral bone of the guinea pig. J. Dent. Res., 47:584, 1968.

45. Stone, A.: Keratinization of human oral mucosa in the aged male. J. Dent. Med., 8:69, 1953.

46. Thomas, B. O. A.: Gerodontology. The study of changes in oral tissue associated with aging. J. Am. Dent. Assoc., 33:207, 1946.

47. Toto, P. D., and Borg, M.: Effect of age changes on the premitotic index in the periodontium of mice. J. Dent. Res., 47:70, 1968.

48. Toto, P., Jensen, J., and Sawinski, J.: Sulfate uptake and cell kinetics in teeth and bone of aging mice. Periodontics, 5:292, 1967.

49. Volpe, A. R., Manhold, J. H., and Manhold, B. S.: Effect of age and other factors upon normal gingival tissue respiration. J. Dent. Res., 41:1060, 1962.

50. Wentz, F. W., Maier, A. W., and Orban, B.: Age changes and sex differences in the clinically normal gingiva. J. Periodontol., 23:13, 1952.

51. Wood, H. E.: Causal factors in shortening tooth series with age. J. Dent. Res., 17:1, 1938.

PERIODONTAL PATHOLOGY

The term *periodontal disease* has received different meanings and is used rather ambiguously. It is used in a general sense to encompass all diseases of the periodontium in much the same way as are terms such as *liver disease* and *kidney disease*. It may be considered synonymous with *periodontopathia*, although this term is not in current use.

Periodontal diseases may be of different types. The most common by far is also called *periodontal disease;* in old textbooks and papers it was called *pyorrhea, periodontoclasia, periclasia,* etc. This disease is initiated by plaque accumulation in the gingivo-dental area and is basically inflammatory in character. Initially it is confined to the gingiva and is termed gingival disease; later the supporting structures become involved and the disease receives the name of *periodontal disease;* in early editions of this book the term *chronic destructive periodontal disease*, which very accurately describes the condition, was used.

Periodontal disease (synonym not currently used: periodontopathia)
— Periodontal disease
—— Chronic destructive periodontal disease
——— Periodontitis
——— Trauma from occlusion
——— Periodontal atrophy
—— Gingival disease
— Other diseases of the periodontium

The above classification illustrates the different meanings currently assigned to the term *periodontal disease*.

This Section will deal with the clinical and microscopic pathology of all types of periodontal disease, divided into the following parts:

Part I. Gingival disease

Part II. Periodontal disease (chronic destructive periodontal disease)

Part III. The etiology of periodontal disease

Part I

Gingival Disease

Gingivitis

THE ROLE OF INFLAMMATION IN GINGIVAL DISEASE

Gingivitis, inflammation of the gingiva, is the most common form of gingival disease. Inflammation is almost always present in all forms of gingival disease because bacterial plaque, which causes inflammation, and irritational factors that favor its accumulation are very often present in the gingival environment. The inflammation caused by dental plaque gives rise to associated degenerative, necrotic, and proliferative changes in the gingival tissues. There is a tendency to designate all forms of gingival disease as gingivitis, as if inflammation were the only disease process involved. However, pathologic processes not caused by local irritation, such as atrophy, hyperplasia, and neoplasia, also occur in the gingiva. All cases of gingivitis are not necessarily the same because they present inflammatory changes, and it is often necessary to differentiate between inflammation and other pathologic processes that may be present in gingival disease.

The *role of inflammation* in individual cases of gingivitis varies as follows:

1. Inflammation may be the *primary* and *only* pathologic change. This is by far the most prevalent type of gingival disease.

2. Inflammation may be a *secondary* feature, superimposed upon systemically caused gingival disease. For example, inflammation commonly complicates gingival hyperplasia caused by the systemic administration of phenytoin.

3. Inflammation may be the precipitating factor responsible for clinical changes in patients with systemic conditions that of themselves do not produce clinically detectable gingival disease. Gingivitis in pregnancy is an example.

TYPES OF GINGIVAL DISEASES

The most common type of gingival disease is the simple inflammatory involvement caused by bacterial plaque attached to the tooth surface. This type of gingivitis, sometimes called chronic marginal gingivitis or simple gingivitis, may remain stationary for indefinite periods of time or may proceed to destruction of the supporting structures (periodontitis). The reasons for these different behaviors are not clearly understood.

In addition, the gingiva can be involved in other diseases, sometimes but not always related to the usual periodontal problems. An attempt to classify these diseases is difficult and its usefulness doubtful. We prefer to list some of the other types of gingival diseases.

1. Acute necrotizing ulcerative gingivitis (see Chap. 11).

2. Acute herpetic gingivostomatitis (see Chap. 11) and other viral diseases (see Chap. 21).

3. Allergic gingivitis, caused by different allergies (see Chap. 12).

4. Many dermatoses will attack the gingival tissues, inducing characteristic types of gingival disease, such as that seen in

lichen planus, pemphigus, erythema multiforme, etc. They are described in detail in Chapter 12.

5. Some gingivitis may be initiated by bacterial plaque, but the tissue response may be conditioned by some systemic factors. Such is the case in pregnancy, puberty gingivitis (see Chap. 29), and vitamin C deficiency (see Chap. 30).

6. The gingival response to a variety of pathogenic agents may include an increase in volume, termed gingival enlargement. This is described in Chapter 9.

7. Different benign and malignant tumors may appear in the gingiva, either as primary tumors or as metastatic ones. They are discussed in Chapter 9.

PATHOLOGY OF GINGIVITIS

It is generally agreed that the pathologic changes that accompany gingivitis are associated with the presence of oral microorganisms in the gingival sulcus (see Chap. 24). These organisms are capable of synthesizing potentially harmful products that produce cellular damage to epithelial and connective tissue cells, as well as to intercellular constituents, i.e., collagen, ground substance, glycocalyx (cell coat), etc. The widening of the intercellular spaces between the junctional epithelial cells during early gingivitis may permit injurious agents derived from bacteria to gain access to the connective tissue and possibly to penetrate it. Nevertheless, it remains to be demonstrated experimentally that this sequence of events does, in fact, occur.

Vascular changes have been described as the first response to initial gingival inflammation (stage I gingivitis). Clinically, the initial response of the gingiva to bacterial plaque is not apparent. This vascular response is essentially the dilatation of capillaries and increased blood flow.

As time goes on, clinical signs of erythema may appear, mainly owing to the proliferation of capillaries and increased formation of capillary loops between rete pegs or ridges (stage II gingivitis). Bleed-

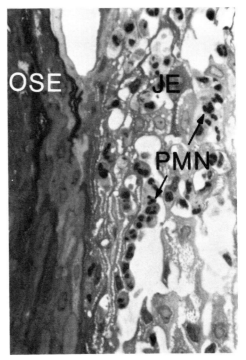

Figure 6–1 Biopsy from a human subject in an experimental gingivitis study. After four days of plaque accumulation the blood vessels immediately adjacent to the junctional epithelium (JE) are distended and contain polymorphonuclear neutrophils (PMN). Neutrophils have also migrated between the cells of the junctional epithelium. OSE, oral sulcular epithelium. Magnification ×500. (From Payne, W. A., et al.: J. Periodont. Res., *10*:51, 1975.)

ing upon probing may also be an early clinical sign.

In chronic gingivitis (stage III) the blood vessels become engorged and congested, venous return is impaired, and the blood flow becomes sluggish. The result is localized gingival anoxemia, which superimposes a somewhat bluish hue upon the reddened gingiva. Extravasation of red blood cells into the connective tissue and breakdown of hemoglobin into its component pigments can also deepen the color of the chronically inflamed gingiva.

Histologically, stage I gingivitis shows some classic features of acute inflammation in the connective tissue beneath the junctional epithelium. Changes in blood vessel morphology, such as widening of small capillaries or venules and adherence

Figure 6–2 Biopsies from human subjects in an experimental gingivitis study. *A,* Control biopsy from a patient with good oral hygiene and no detectable plaque accumulation. The junctional epithelium (JE) is at the left. The connective tissue (CT) shows few cells other than fibroblasts, blood vessels, and a dense background of collagen fibers. Magnification

Legend continued on opposite page

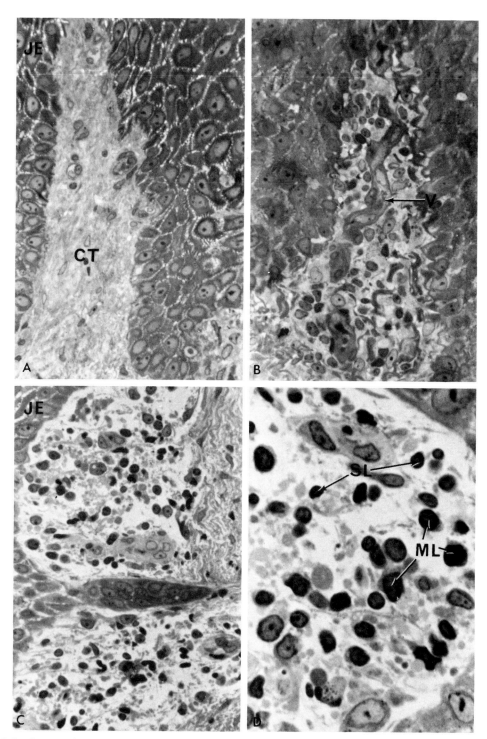

Figure 6–2 *Continued*
×500. *B,* Biopsy taken after eight days of plaque accumulation. The connective tissue is infiltrated with inflammatory cells, which displace the collagen fibers. A distended blood vessel (V) is seen in the center. Magnification ×500. *C,* After 8 days of plaque accumulation the connective tissue next to the junctional epithelium (JE) at the base of the sulcus shows a mononuclear cell infiltrate, and evidence of collagen degeneration (clear spaces around cellular infiltrate). Magnification ×500. *D,* The inflammatory cell infiltrate at higher magnification. After eight days of plaque accumulation numerous small (SL) and medium size (ML) lymphocytes are seen within the connective tissue. Most of the collagen fibers around these cells have disappeared, presumably due to enzymatic digestion. Magnification ×1250. (From Payne, W. A., et al.: J. Periodont. Res., *10:*51, 1975.)

of neutrophils to their walls, occurs within a week and sometimes as early as two days after plaque has been allowed to accumulate.[28] (Fig. 6–1). Leukocytes, mainly polymorphonuclear neutrophils, leave the capillaries by migrating through their walls. They can be seen in increased quantities in the connective tissue, junctional epithelium, and gingival sulcus.[1, 21, 26, 28, 32] Subtle changes can also be detected in the junctional epithelium and perivascular connective tissue at this early stage of development. Lymphocytes soon begin to accumulate (Fig. 6–2). The increase in the migration of leukocytes and their accumulation within the gingival sulcus can be correlated with an increase in the flow of gingival fluid into the sulcus.[2]

Mildly inflamed gingiva can generally be classified as stage II gingivitis. At this stage the lesion is still early in its development. Histologic examination of gingiva reveals a leukocyte infiltration in the connective tissue beneath the junctional epithelium, consisting mainly of lymphocytes (75 per cent)[33] but also some migrating neutrophils, as well as macrophages, plasma cells, and mast cells. There is an intensified overall inflammatory cell response as compared with the stage I initial lesion.[15, 17, 22, 24, 28, 33] The junctional epithelium becomes densely infiltrated with neutrophils, as does the gingival sulcus, and the junctional epithelium may begin to show development of rete pegs or ridges. There is an increase in the amount of collagen destruction as determined both histologically[33] and biochemically;[8] 70 per cent of the collagen is destroyed around the cellular infiltrate. The main fiber groups that are affected appear to be the circular and dentogingival fiber assemblies. Alterations in blood vessel morphology and vascular bed patterns have also been described.[13, 16, 35]

The stage III lesion can be described as moderately to severely inflamed gingiva. In histologic sections of this tissue an intense, chronic inflammatory reaction is observed. Detailed cytologic studies have been carried out on chronically inflamed gingiva.[7, 9, 11, 12, 15, 27, 30, 34, 36] A key feature that differentiates this lesion from the stage II lesion is the increase in number of plasma cells, which become the predominant inflammatory cell type. Plasma cells invade the connective tissue not only immediately below the junctional epithelium, but also deep into the connective tissue, around blood vessels, and between bundles of collagen fibers. The junctional epithelium reveals widened intercellular spaces filled with granular cellular debris, lysosomes derived from disrupted neutrophils, lymphocytes, and monocytes (Fig. 6–3). The lysosomes contain acid hydrolases that can destroy tissue components. The junctional epithelium develops rete pegs or ridges that protrude into the connective tissue, and the basal lamina is destroyed in some areas. In the connective tissue, collagen fibers are destroyed around the infiltrate of intact and disrupted plasma cells, neutrophils, lymphocytes, monocytes, and mast cells. There appears to be an inverse relationship between the number of intact collagen bundles and the number of inflammatory cells.[31] Collagenolytic activity is increased in inflamed gingival tissue.[3, 10] The enzyme collagenase, normally present in gingival tissues,[4] is produced by some oral bacteria, but also by polymorphonuclear neutrophils.

Enzyme histochemistry has shown that chronically inflamed gingiva has elevated levels of acid and alkaline phosphatase,[38] beta-glucuronidase, beta-glucosidase, beta-galactosidase, esterases,[23] aminopeptidase,[25, 29] and cytochrome oxidase.[5] Neutral mucopolysaccharides are decreased,[37] presumably as a result of degradation of the ground substance.

COURSE, DURATION, AND DISTRIBUTION OF GINGIVITIS

Course and duration

Acute Gingivitis. A painful condition which comes on suddenly and is of short duration.

Subacute Gingivitis. A less severe phase of the acute condition.

Recurrent Gingivitis. Disease that reappears after having been eliminated by treatment, or that disappears spontaneously and reappears.

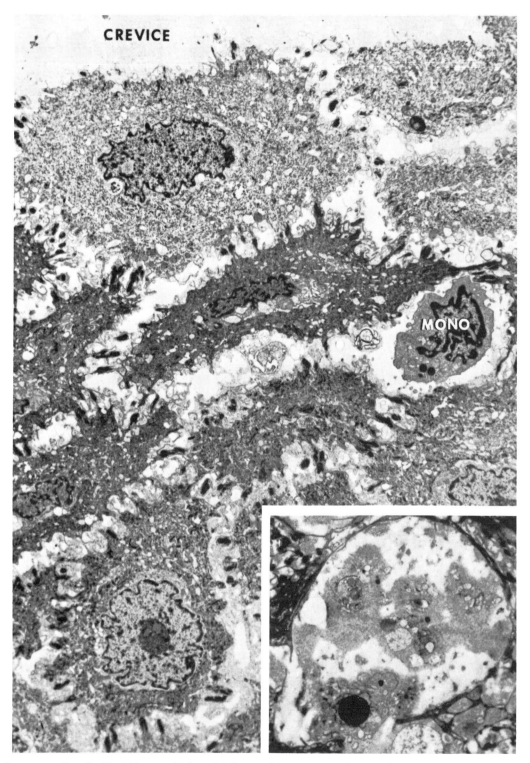

Figure 6–3 Chronic Gingivitis—Crevicular Epithelium. The crevice is at the top. The intercellular spaces are dilated and contain a granular precipitate and cellular fragments. An emigrating monocyte (MONO) is shown between the epithelial cells. ×4400. *Insert,* Cellular fragments and precipitated material in a dilated intercellular space of the crevicular epithelium. Bacteria are not present. ×4036. (From Freedman, H. L., Listgarten, M. A., and Taichman, N. S. J. Periodont. Res., 3:313, 1968.)

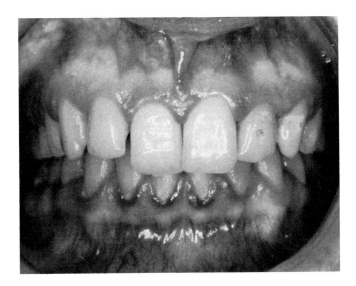

Figure 6–4 Chronic Gingivitis. The marginal and interdental gingivae are smooth, edematous, and discolored.

Chronic Gingivitis. Disease which comes on slowly, is of long duration, and is painless unless complicated by acute or subacute exacerbations. Chronic gingivitis is the type most commonly encountered (Fig. 6–4). Patients seldom recollect having had any acute symptoms. Chronic gingivitis is a fluctuating disease in which inflamed areas persist or become normal and normal areas become inflamed.[14, 18]

Distribution

Localized. Confined to the gingiva in relation to a single tooth or group of teeth.

Generalized. Involving the entire mouth.

Marginal. Involving the gingival margin, but may include a portion of the contiguous attached gingiva.

Papillary. Involving the interdental papillae, and often extending into the adjacent portion of the gingival margin. Papillae are more frequently involved than is the gingival margin, and the earliest signs of gingivitis most often occur in the papillae.[19]

Diffuse. Involving the gingival margin, attached gingiva, and interdental papillae.

The distribution of gingival disease in

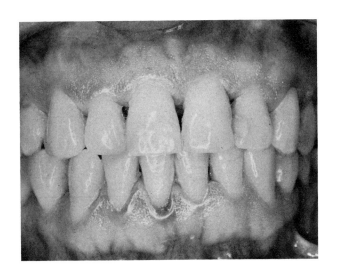

Figure 6–5 Localized Marginal Gingivitis in the mandibular anterior region.

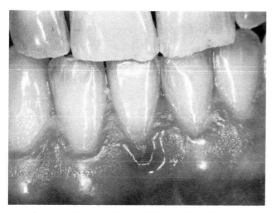

Figure 6–6 Localized Diffuse Gingivitis involving both the marginal and attached gingiva.

individual cases is described by combining the above terms as follows:

Localized Marginal Gingivitis. Confined to one or more areas of the marginal gingiva (Fig. 6–5).

Localized Diffuse Gingivitis. Extending from the margin to the mucobuccal fold, but limited in area (Fig. 6–6).

Papillary Gingivitis. Confined to one or more interdental spaces in a limited area (Fig. 6–7).

Generalized Marginal Gingivitis. Involvement of the gingival margin in relation to all the teeth. The interdental papillae are usually also involved in generalized marginal gingivitis (Fig. 6–8).

Generalized Diffuse Gingivitis. Involving the entire gingiva. The alveolar mucosa is usually also affected so that the demarcation between it and the attached gingiva is obliterated (Fig. 6–9). Systemic conditions are involved in the etiology of generalized diffuse gingivitis except in cases caused by acute infection or generalized chemical irritation.

CLINICAL FEATURES OF GINGIVITIS

As a result of the inflammatory state in chronic gingivitis, the altered epithelial–connective tissue relationship contributes to the color changes seen clinically. The epithelium proliferates and the rete ridges lengthen into the connective tissue. At the same time, the increasing mass of the inflamed connective tissue presses against the overlying epithelium, causing it to stretch and become thin. The engorged blood vessels of the connective tissue extend to within one or two epithelial cells from the surface.[20] The extensions of inflamed connective tissue close to the surface, separated by deepened epithelial rete ridges, create focal areas of accentuated redness.

In chronic gingivitis tissue destruction and repair occur simultaneously. Persistent local irritants injure the tissue, prolong inflammation, and provoke vascular permeability and exudation.[6] At the same time, however, new connective tissue

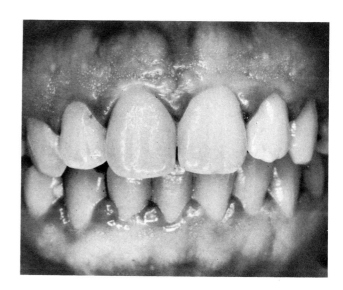

Figure 6–7   Papillary Gingivitis.

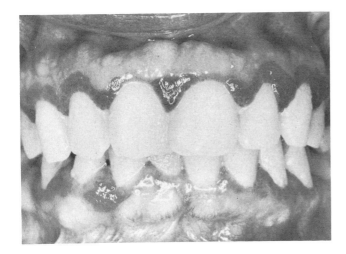

Figure 6–8 Generalized Marginal Gingivitis. The interdental papillae are also involved.

cells, collagen fibers, ground substance, and blood vessels are formed in a continuous effort to repair the tissue damage. This interaction between destruction and repair affects color, size, consistency, and surface texture of the gingiva. If increased vascularity, exudation, and tissue degeneration predominate, then color changes become strikingly apparent. On the other hand, if the dominant feature is fibrosis due to chronic inflammation, the gingiva appears more normal in color despite the existence of a long-standing gingivitis.

In evaluating the clinical features of gingivitis, it is necessary to be systematic. Attention should be focused on very subtle tissue alterations from the norm, since these may be of great diagnostic significance. A systematic clinical approach requires an orderly examination of the gingiva for the following features: color, size and shape, consistency, surface texture and position, ease of bleeding, and pain. These clinical characteristics and the microscopic changes responsible for each are discussed in the chapters that follow.

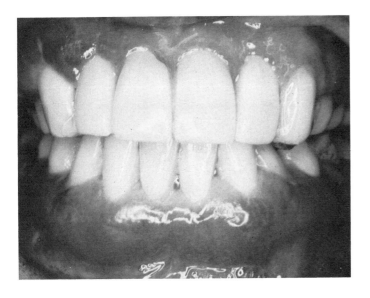

Figure 6–9 Generalized Diffuse Gingivitis. The marginal, interdental, and attached gingivae are involved in chronic desquamative gingivitis.

REFERENCES

1. Attstrom, R.: Studies on neutrophil polymorphonuclear leukocytes at the dento-gingival junction in gingival health and disease. J. Periodont. Res., 6:(Suppl. 8), 1971.
2. Attstrom, R., and Egelberg, J.: Emigration of blood neutrophils and monocytes into the gingival crevices. J. Periodont. Res., 5:48, 1970.
3. Bennick, A., and Hunt, A. M.: Collagenolytic activity in oral tissues. Arch. Oral Biol., 12:1, 1967.
4. Beutner, E. H., Triftshauser, C., and Hazen, S. P.: Collagenase activity of gingival tissue from patients with periodontal disease. Proc. Soc. Exp. Biol. Med., 121:1082, 1966.
5. Burstone, M. S.: Histochemical study of cytochrome oxidase in normal and inflamed gingiva. Oral Surg., 13:1501, 1960.
6. Egelberg, J.: The topography and permeability of vessels at the dento-gingival junction in dogs. J. Periodont. Res., Suppl. 1, 1967.
7. Fish, E. W.: Parodontal disease: The pathology and treatment of chronic gingivitis. Br. Dent. J., 58:531, 1935.
8. Flieder, D. E., and Sun, C. N.: Chemistry of normal and inflamed human gingival tissues. Periodontics, 4:302, 1966.
9. Freedman, H. L., Listgarten, M. A., and Taichman, N. S.: Electron microscopic features of chronically inflamed human gingiva. J. Periodont. Res., 3:313, 1968.
10. Fullmer, H., and Gibson, W.: Collagenolytic activity in gingivae of man. Nature, 209:728, 1966.
11. Garant, P. R., and Mulvihill, J. E.: The fine structure of gingivitis in the beagle. III. Plasma cell infiltration of the subepithelial connective tissue. J. Periodont. Res., 7:161, 1971.
12. Gavin, J. R.: Ultrastructural features of chronic marginal gingivitis. J. Periodont. Res., 5:19, 1970.
13. Hock, J., and Nuki, K.: A vital microscopy study of the morphology of normal and inflamed gingiva. J. Periodont. Res., 6:81, 1971.
14. Hoover, D. R., and Lefkowitz, W.: Fluctuation in marginal gingivitis. J. Periodontol., 36:310, 1965.
15. James, W. W., and Counsell, A.: A histologic investigation into "so-called pyorrhea alveolaris." Br. Dent. J., 48:1237, 1927.
16. Kindlova, M.: Changes in the vascular bed of the marginal periodontium in periodontitis. J. Dent. Res., 44:456, 1965.
17. Lange, D., and Schroeder, H. E.: Cytochemistry and ultrastructure of gingival sulcus cells. Helv. Odontol. Acta, 15(Suppl. 6):65, 1971.
18. Larato, D. C., Stahl, S. S., Brown, R., Jr., and Witkin, G. J.: The effect of a prescribed method of toothbrushing on the fluctuation of marginal gingivitis. J. Periodontol., 40:142, 1969.
19. Levin, M. A.: The interdental papillae in gingivitis: A review survey. J. Periodontol., 37:230, 1966.
20. Levy, B. M., Taylor, A. C., and Bernick, S.: Relationship between epithelium and connective tissue in gingival inflammation. J. Dent. Res., 48:625, 1969.
21. Lindhe, J., Hamp, S. E., and Löe, H.: Experimental periodontitis in the beagle dog. J. Periodont. Res., 8:1, 1973.
22. Lindhe, J., Schroeder, H. E., Page, R. C., Munzel-Pedrazzoli, S., and Hugoson, A.: Clinical and stereologic analysis of the course of early gingivitis in dogs. J. Periodont. Res., 9:314, 1974.
23. Lisanti, V. F.: Hydrolytic enzymes in periodontal tissues. Ann. N. Y. Acad. Sci., 85:461, 1960.
24. Listgarten, M. A., and Ellegaard, B.: Experimental gingivitis in Rhesus monkeys. J. Periodont. Res., 8:199, 1973.
25. Mori, M., and Kishiro, A.: Histochemical observation of aminopeptidase activity in the normal and inflamed oral epithelium. J. Osaka Univ. Dent. Sch., 1:39, 1961.
26. Oliver, R. C., Holm-Pedersen, P., and Löe, H.: The correlation between clinical scoring, exudate measurements, and microscopic evaluation of inflammation of the gingiva. J. Periodontol., 40:201, 1969.
27. Page, R. C., Ammons, W. F., and Simpson, D. M.: Host tissue response in chronic inflammatory periodontal disease. IV. The periodontal and dental status of a group of aged great apes. J. Periodontol., 46:144, 1975.
28. Payne, W. A., Page, R. C., Ogilvie, A. L., and Hall, W. B.: Histopathologic features of the initial and early stages of experimental gingivitis in man. J. Periodont. Res., 10:51, 1975.
29. Quintarelli, G.: Histochemistry of gingiva. III. The distribution of amino-peptidase in normal and inflammatory conditions. Arch. Oral Biol., 2:271, 1960.
30. Schectman, L. R., Ammons, W. F., Simpson, D. M., and Page, R. C.: Host tissue response in chronic periodontal disease. II. Histologic features of the normal periodontium, and histopathologic and ultrastructural manifestations of disease in the marmoset. J. Periodont. Res., 7:195, 1972.
31. Schroeder, H. E.: Extraneous cell surface coat in human inflamed crevicular epithelium. Helv. Odont. Acta, 12:14, 1968.
32. Schroeder, H. E., Graf-de Beer, M., and Attstrom, R.: Initial gingivitis in dogs. J. Periodont. Res., 10:128, 1975.
33. Schroeder, H. E., Munzell-Pedrazzoli, S., and Page, R. C.: Correlated morphological and biochemical analysis of gingival tissue in early chronic gingivitis in man. Arch. Oral Biol., 18:899, 1973.
34. Simpson, D. M., and Avery, B. E.: Histopathologic and ultrastructural features of inflamed gingiva in the baboon. J. Periodontol., 45:500, 1974.
35. Soderholm, G., and Egelberg, J.: Morphological

changes in gingival blood vessels during developing gingivitis in dogs. J. Periodont. Res., 8:16, 1973.

36. Thilander, H.: Epithelial changes in gingivitis. An electron microscopic study. J. Periodont. Res., 3:303, 1968.

37. Turesky, S., Glickman I., and Fisher, B.: The effect of physiologic and pathologic processes upon certain histochemically detectable substances in the gingiva. J. Periodontol., 30: 116, 1959.

38. Winer, R. A., et al.: Enzyme activity in periodontal disease. J. Periodontol., 41:449, 1970.

Gingival Fluid and Bleeding

The two earliest symptoms of gingival inflammation preceding established gingivitis are (1) increased gingival fluid rate and (2) bleeding from the gingival sulcus upon gentle probing.[25]

GINGIVAL FLUID*

The gingival sulcus contains a fluid which seeps into it from the gingival connective tissue through the thin sulcular wall.[4, 21] The gingival fluid (1) cleanses material from the sulcus; (2) contains sticky plasma proteins which may improve adhesion of the junctional epithelium to the tooth; (3) possesses antimicrobial properties; and (4) may exert antibody activity in defense of the gingiva. It may also serve as a medium for bacterial growth and contribute to the formation of dental plaque and calculus.

METHODS OF COLLECTION. Gingival fluid can be collected by means of: (a) Absorbing paper strips placed into the sulcus ("intrasulcular method"); or at its entrance ("extrasulcular method"). The amount of fluid in the strip is measured by microscopic examination of the stained sample. (b) Microcapillary pipets placed in the sulcus whereby fluid is recovered by capillarity. (c) Gingival washings using a special plastic appliance that covers the hard palate and the vestibulum. Fluid is obtained by rinsing the sulci from one side to the other through palatal and facial channels with syringes or a pump. (d) An electronic fluid-meter that measures the volume of fluid on a paper strip. This latter method has been suggested as a procedure to diagnose early gingival inflammation, before overt clinical signs are present.

AMOUNT. Gingival fluid was found in minute amounts in the sulci of normal gingiva,[1, 33] suggesting that it is a physiologic filtration product from the blood vessels, modified as it seeps through the sulcus epithelium. However, it is the prevalent opinion that gingival fluid is an inflammatory exudate.[20] Its presence in normal sulci is considered an artifact caused by increased permeability of capillaries damaged when the fluid is collected by inserting filter paper strips to the base of the sulcus instead of confining them to the crest of the gingival margin.[9] The question of whether gingival fluid is a product of normal gingiva is complicated by the fact that, with few exceptions,[26] gingiva which appears normal clinically invariably exhibits inflammation when examined microscopically.

The *amount of gingival fluid* increases with inflammation,[12, 26] sometimes proportional to its severity.[8, 12, 27] Gingival fluid is also increased by chewing coarse foods, by toothbrushing and massage, by ovulation,[15] and by hormonal contraceptives.[18] Progesterone and estrogen increase the permeability of gingival vessels and the flow of

---

*For a detailed description and literature review on gingival fluid, see the excellent monograph by Cimasoni.[5]

gingival fluid in animals with and without gingivitis.[16, 17, 19] Gingival fluid is not increased by trauma from occlusion.[22]

COMPOSITION. The composition of gingival fluid is similar to that of blood serum except in the proportions of some of its components. Thus far reported as included in gingival fluid are electrolytes (K+, Na+, Ca++), amino acids, plasma proteins, fibrolytic factors, gamma G globulin, gamma A globulin, gamma M globulin (immunoglobulins), albumin and lysozyme, fibrinogen, and a variety of enzymes of bacterial and lysosomal origin.[2, 3, 5, 6, 30] In gingival fluid from nearly normal gingiva the level of sodium is below that of serum, calcium approximately equals the serum level, and potassium is more than three times higher. In inflamed gingiva the sodium content of gingival fluid equals the serum level, and calcium and phosphorus are more than three times higher;[13] the potassium:sodium ratio is elevated and the acid phosphatase content is increased. Also contained in gingival fluid are microorganisms, desquamated epithelial cells, and leukocytes (polymorphonuclears, lymphocytes, and monocytes) which migrate through the sulcal epithelium.[7, 10, 29] Bacteria and leukocytes increase in inflammation.

GINGIVAL BLEEDING CAUSED BY LOCAL FACTORS

Bleeding upon probing is clinically easily detectable and therefore of great value for the early diagnosis and prevention of further involvement. It precedes clinical signs of inflammation.[14] Gingival bleeding varies in severity, duration, and the ease with which it is provoked.

Chronic and Recurrent Bleeding

The most common cause of abnormal gingival bleeding is chronic inflammation.[24] The bleeding is chronic or recurrent and is provoked by mechanical trauma such as that from toothbrushing, toothpicks, or food impaction, or by biting into solid foods such as apples, or by grinding the teeth (bruxism).

Histopathology

The blood vessels of the gingiva are contained in the papillary connective tissue. On the outer surface they are protected from injury by a considerable thickness of keratinized or parakeratinized stratified squamous epithelium. Adjacent to the tooth a plexus of capillaries lies close to the sulcus space, separated from it by a thin layer of semipermeable epithelium.

In gingival inflammation the following alterations result in abnormal gingival bleeding:

Dilation and engorgement of the capillaries increase the susceptibility to injury and bleeding. Injurious agents which initiate the inflammation increase the permeability of the sulcus epithelium by degrading intercellular cement substance and widening the intercellular spaces. As the inflammation becomes chronic, the sulcal epithelium undergoes ulceration. The cellular and fluid exudate and the proliferation of new blood vessels and connective tissue cells create pressure upon the epithelium on the crest and external surface of the marginal and interdental gingiva. The epithelium is thinned and presents varying degrees of degeneration (Figs. 7–1 and 7–2). Because the capillaries are engorged and closer to the surface and the thinned, degenerated epithelium is less protective, stimuli that are ordinarily innocuous cause rupture of the capillaries and gingival bleeding.

The severity of the bleeding and the ease with which it is provoked depend upon the intensity of the inflammation. After the vessels rupture, a complex of mechanisms induces hemostasis.[31] The vessel walls contract and blood flow is diminished; blood platelets adhere to the edges of the tissue; a fibrous clot is formed, which contracts and results in approximation of the edges of the injured area. Bleeding recurs, however, when the area is irritated.

Acute Bleeding

Acute episodes of gingival bleeding are caused by injury or occur spontaneously in acute gingival disease. Laceration of the

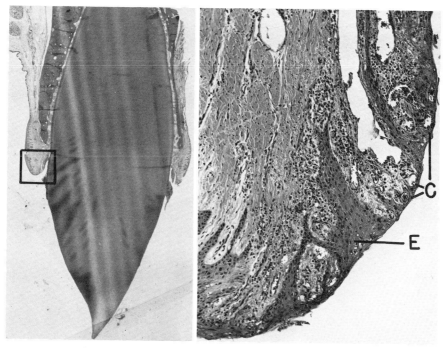

Fig. 7–1　　　　　　　　　　　　　　　　　　**Fig. 7–2**

Figure 7–1　Survey section of maxillary canine in situ.

Figure 7–2　High power study from area marked in Figure 7–1 showing the **Inflamed Marginal Gingiva** in relation to the tooth surface. Note the proximity of the capillaries (C) to the surface. There is some thickening of the epithelium (E) but for the most part it is thinned.

gingiva by aggressive toothbrushing or sharp pieces of hard food causes gingival bleeding even in the absence of gingival disease. Gingival burns from hot foods or chemicals increase the ease of gingival bleeding.

Spontaneous bleeding or bleeding upon slight provocation occurs in *acute necrotizing ulcerative gingivitis.* **In this condition, engorged blood vessels in the inflamed connective tissue are exposed by desquamation of necrotic surface epithelium.**

GINGIVAL BLEEDING ASSOCIATED WITH SYSTEMIC DISTURBANCES

There are systemic disorders in which gingival hemorrhage, unprovoked by mechanical irritation, occurs spontaneously, or in which gingival bleeding following irritation is excessive and difficult to control. These are called *hemorrhagic diseases,* and represent a wide variety of con-

ditions that vary in etiology and clinical manifestations.[34] Such conditions have one feature in common; namely, abnormal bleeding in the skin, internal organs, and other tissues as well as the oral mucous membrane.

In individual patients the hemorrhagic tendency may be due to failure of one or more of the hemostatic mechanisms.[32] **Hemorrhagic disorders in which abnormal gingival bleeding is encountered include the following:** vascular abnormalities (vitamin C deficiency or allergy such as Henoch-Schönlein purpura), platelet disorders (idiopathic thrombocytopenic purpura or thrombocytopenic purpura secondary to diffuse injury to the bone marrow), hypoprothrombinemia (vitamin K deficiency resulting from liver disease or sprue), other coagulation defects (hemophilia, leukemia, Christmas disease), deficient platelet thromboplastic factor (PF$_3$) secondary to uremia,[23] and post-rubella purpura.[11] Bleeding may follow the administration of excessive amounts of drugs such as salicylates and the administration of anticoagulants such as Dicumarol and heparin. (Periodontal involvement in hematologic disorders is considered in Chapter 30).

Cyclical episodes of abnormal gingival bleeding occasionally occur associated with the menstrual period (Chap. 29), and comparatively poor general health and nutritional status have been associated with gingival bleeding following toothbrushing.[28]

REFERENCES

1. Bjorn, H. L., Koch, G., and Lindhe, H.: Evaluation of gingival fluid measurements. Odontol. Revy, 16:300, 1965.
2. Brandtzaeg, P.: Immunochemical comparison of proteins in human gingival pocket fluid, serum and saliva. Arch. Oral. Biol., 10:795, 1965.
3. Brandtzaeg, P., and Mann, W.: A comparative study of the lysozyme activity of human gingival pocket fluid. Acta Odontol. Scand., 22:441, 1964.
4. Brill, N., and Bjorn, H.: Passage of tissue fluid into human gingival pockets. Acta Odontol. Scand., 17:11, 1959.
5. Cimasoni, G.: The crevicular fluid. Monographs in Dental Science, vol. 3. Basel, S. Karger, 1974.
6. Cowley, G. C.: Fluorescence studies of crevicular fluid. J. Dent. Res., 45:655, 1966.
7. Egelberg, J.: Cellular elements in gingival pocket fluid. Acta Odontol. Scand., 21:283, 1963.
8. Egelberg, J.: Gingival exudate measurements for evaluation of inflammatory changes of the gingivae. Odontol. Revy, 15:381, 1964.
9. Egelberg, J.: Permeability of the dento-gingival vessels. II. Clinically healthy gingivae. J. Periodont. Res., 1:276, 1966.
10. Egelberg, J., and Attstrom, R.: Presence of leukocytes within crevices of healthy and inflamed gingiva and their immigration from the blood. J. Periodont. Res. [Suppl.], 4:23, 1969.
11. Haeb, H. P.: Post-rubella thrombocytopenic purpura. A report of cases with discussion of hemorrhagic manifestations of rubella. Clin. Pediatr., 7:350, 1968.
12. Jacoby, R., and Ketterl, W.: Quantitative measurements of gingival pocket exudate in normal and inflamed gingiva. Dtsch. Zahnaerztl. Z., 27:485, 1972.
13. Kaslick, R. S., et al.: Quantitative analysis of sodium, potassium and calcium in gingival fluid from gingiva in varying degrees of inflammation. J. Periodontol., 41:93, 1970.
14. Lenox, J. A., and Kopczyk, R. A.: A clinical system for scoring a patient's oral hygiene performance. J. Am. Dent. Assoc., 86:849, 1973.

15. Lindhe, J., and Attström, R.: Gingival exudation during the menstrual cycle. J. Periodont. Res., 2:194, 1967.
16. Lindhe, J., Attström, R., and Björn, A. L.: Influence of sex hormones on gingival exudation in dogs with chronic gingivitis. J. Periodont. Res., 3:279, 1968.
17. Lindhe, J., Attström, R., and Björn, A. L.: Influence of sex hormones on gingival exudation in gingivitis-free female dogs. J. Periodont. Res., 3:273, 1968.
18. Lindhe, J., and Björn, A. L.: Influences of hormonal contraceptives on the gingiva of women. J. Periodont. Res., 2:1, 1967.
19. Lindhe, J., and Branemark, P. I.: Changes in vascular proliferation after local application of sex hormones. J. Periodont. Res., 2:266, 1967.
20. Loe, H., and Holm-Pedersen, P.: Absence and presence of fluid from normal and inflamed gingivae. Periodontics, 3:171, 1965.
21. Mandel, J. I., and Weinstein, E.: The fluid of the gingival sulcus. Periodontics, 2:147, 1964.
22. Martin, L. P., and Noble, W. H.: Gingival fluid in relation to tooth mobility and occlusal interferences. J. Periodontol., 45:444, 1974.
23. Merril, A., et al.: Gingival hemorrhage secondary to uremia. Review and report of a case. Oral Surg., 29:530, 1970.
24. Milne, A. M.: Gingival bleeding in 848 army recruits. An assessment. Br. Dent. J., 122:111, 1967.
25. Muhlemann, H. R., and Son, S.: Gingival sulcus bleeding, a leading symptom in initial gingivitis. Helv. Odontol. Acta, 15:107, 1971.
26. Oliver, R. C., Holm-Pedersen, P., and Loe, H.: The correlation between clinical scoring, exudate measurements and microscopic evaluation of inflammation in the gingiva. J. Periodontol., 40:201, 1969.
27. Orban, J. E., and Stallard, R. E.: Gingival crevicular fluid: A reliable predictor of gingival health? J. Periodontol., 40:231, 1969.
28. Ringsdorf, W., Cheraskin, E., and Clark, J.: Gingival bleeding and general health. Dent. Survey, 44:49, 1968.
29. Skougaard, M. R., Bay, I., and Klinkhamer, J. M.: Correlation between gingivitis and orogranulocytic migratory rate. J. Res., 48:716, 1969.
30. Sueda, T., and Cimasoni, G.: The origins of acid phosphatase in human gingival fluid. Arch. Oral Biol., 13:553, 1968.
31. Sodeman, W. A., Jr., and Sodeman, W. A.: Pathologic Physiology. Mechanisms of Disease. 5th ed. Philadelphia, W. B. Saunders Company, 1974.
32. Stefanini, M., and Dameshek, W.: The Hemorrhagic Disorders. 2nd ed. New York, Grune and Stratton, Inc., 1962, p. 78.
33. Weinstein, E., Mandel, I. D., Salkind, A., Oshrain, H. I., and Pappas, G. D.: Studies of gingival fluid. Periodontics, 5:161, 1967.
34. Wintrobe, M. M.: Clinical Hematology. 5th ed. Philadelphia, Lea & Febiger, 1961, p. 816.

Chapter 8

Changes in the Color of the Gingiva

COLOR CHANGES IN CHRONIC GINGIVITIS

Change in color is a very important clinical sign of gingival disease, and chronic gingivitis is its most common cause. The normal gingival color is "coral pink." This is due to the tissue's vascularity, modified by the overlying epithelial layers. For this reason, the color of the gingiva will become redder when (a) there is an increase in vascularization, or (b) when the degree of epithelial keratinization becomes reduced or disappears. The color will in turn become paler when (a) vascularization is reduced (associated with fibrosis of the corium), or (b) epithelial keratinization increases. Therefore, chronic inflammation will intensify the red or bluish red color owing to vascular proliferation and to reduction of keratinization due to epithelial compression by the inflamed tissue. Venous stasis will add a bluish hue. Originating as a light redness, the color changes through varying shades of red, reddish blue, and deep blue with increasing chronicity of the inflammatory process. The changes start in the interdental papillae and gingival margin and spread to the attached gingiva (Fig. 8–1). Proper diagnosis and treatment require an understanding of the tissue changes which alter the color of the gingiva at the clinical level. They have been discussed in Chapter 6.

"TRAUMATIC CRESCENTS." These are small, crescent-shaped, bluish red areas in

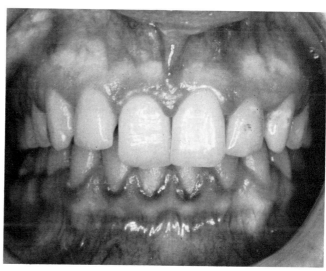

Figure 8–1 Chronic Gingivitis. The marginal and interdental gingivae are smooth, edematous, and discolored.

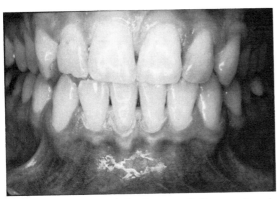

Figure 8-2 "Traumatic Crescents." Crescent-shaped marginal areas of gingival erythema in the mandibular anterior region. Vascular changes produced by trauma from occlusion are the suspected but not proved cause.

the marginal gingiva attributed to trauma from occlusion (Fig. 8-2). *They are chronic inflammatory lesions caused by local irritants.* The suspected contributory role of excessive occlusal forces has not been demonstrated.

COLOR CHANGES IN ACUTE GINGIVITIS

Color changes in acute gingival inflammation differ somewhat from those in chronic gingivitis in nature and distribution. The color changes may be marginal, diffuse, or patch-like, depending upon the acute condition. In *acute necrotizing ulcerative gingivitis* the involvement is marginal; in *herpetic gingivostomatitis* it is diffuse, and in *acute reactions to chemical irritation* it is patch-like or diffuse.

Color changes vary with the intensity of the inflammation. In all instances there is an initial bright red erythema. If the condition does not worsen, this represents the only color change until the gingiva reverts to normal. In severe acute inflammation, the red color changes to a shiny slate-gray, which gradually becomes a dull whitish gray. The gray discoloration produced by tissue necrosis is demarcated from the adjacent gingiva by a thin, sharply defined erythematous zone. Detailed descriptions of the clinical features and pathology of the various forms of acute gingivitis are found in Chapter 11.

METALLIC PIGMENTATION

Heavy metals absorbed systemically from therapeutic use or occupational environments may discolor the gingiva and other areas of the oral mucosa.[2] This is different from tattooing produced by the accidental embedding of amalgam or other metal fragments (Fig. 8-3). Bismuth, arsenic, and mercury produce a black line in the gingiva which follows the contour of the margin (Fig. 8-4). The pigmentation may also appear as isolated black blotches involving marginal, interdental, and attached gingiva. Lead results in a bluish red or deep blue linear pigmentation of the gingival margin (Burtonian line),[1] and silver (argyria) in a violet marginal line, often accompanied by a diffuse bluish gray discoloration throughout the oral mucosa.[3]

Gingival pigmentation from systemically absorbed metals results from **perivascular**

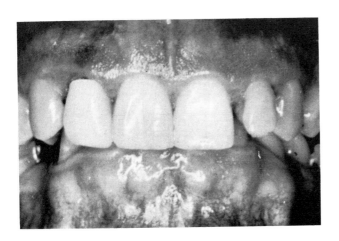

Figure 8-3 Discoloration of Gingiva over lateral incisor caused by embedded metal particles.

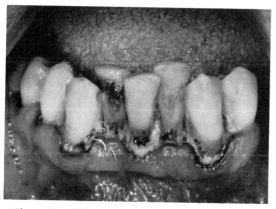

Figure 8–4   Bismuth Line. Linear discoloration of the gingiva in relation to local irritation in a patient receiving bismuth therapy.

taining drugs required for therapeutic purposes. **Temporary correction** is obtained by topical application of concentrated peroxide or by insufflating the gingiva with oxygen to oxidize the dark metallic sulfides. The discoloration reappears unless the procedures are repeated.

CHANGES ASSOCIATED WITH OTHER LOCAL AND SYSTEMIC FACTORS

In Addison's disease the gingiva often presents isolated patches of discoloration, varying from brown to black (Figs. 8–5 and 8–6). Comparable changes are seen in other areas of the oral mucous membrane subject to irritation. The gingiva of patients with blood dyscrasias presents color changes. In *anemia*, the gingiva assumes a diffuse dusky pallor. Diffuse redness of the gingiva is associated with polycythemia. In leukemia the gingiva is often a deep cyanotic purplish blue. When one realizes that gingival tissues in leukemic individuals are crowded with leukocytes, often with varying degrees of reduction of the red blood cells necessary to supply oxygen to the tissues, the cyanotic appearance of the gingiva is understandable. In hemochromatosis, distinct bronze discoloration of the gingiva is associated with comparable pigmentation of the skin. Yellowish gray discoloration of the gingiva may be a feature of xanthomatous disease.

precipitation of metallic sulfides in the sub-epithelial connective tissue. Gingival pigmentation is not an effect of systemic toxicity. It occurs only in areas of inflammation, where the increased permeability of irritated blood vessels permits seepage of the metal into the surrounding tissue. In addition to inflamed gingiva, mucosal areas irritated by biting or abnormal chewing habits such as the inner surface of the lips, the cheek at the level of the occlusal line and the lateral border of the tongue are common pigmentation sites.

Gingival or mucosal pigmentation is eliminated by **removing the local irritating factors and restoring tissue health,** without necessarily discontinuing the metal-con-

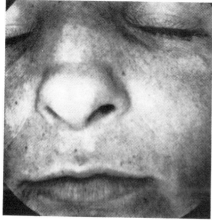

Fig. 8–5   **Fig. 8–6**

Figure 8–5   Addison's Disease. Diffuse pigmentation of the skin.
Figure 8–6   Addison's Disease. Palate of patient shown in Figure 8–5 with spotty distribution of pigment.

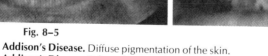

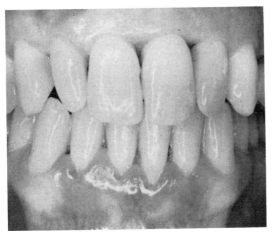

Figure 8-7 **Vertical Discoloration** of marginal and attached gingiva associated with periodontal pockets.

spotty red discoloration occurs in desquamative gingivitis, menopausal gingivostomatitis, and benign mucous membrane pemphigus (pemphigoid).

Exogenous factors capable of producing color changes in the gingiva include atmospheric irritants, such as coal and metal dust, and coloring agents in food. Green staining of the gingiva and diffuse metallic discoloration are seen in workers dealing with brass and silver respectively. Tobacco causes a gray hyperkeratosis of the gingiva. Isolated zones of discoloration of the gingiva are commonly associated with periodontal pocket formation (Fig. 8-7).

Deficiencies in components of the vitamin B complex may give rise to diffuse bluish red or fiery red discoloration of the gingiva as well as the remainder of the oral mucosa. Violaceous discoloration of the gingiva has been described in *diabetes*,[4] and raspberry red or diffuse bluish red discoloration is seen in *pregnancy*. Diffuse or

REFERENCES

1. Dummett, C. O.: Abnormal color changes in gingivae. Oral Surg., 2:649, 1949.
2. McCarthy, F. P., and Dexter, S. O., Jr.: Oral manifestations of bismuth. N. Engl. J. Med., *213*: 345, 1935.
3. Prinz, H.: Pigmentations of oral mucous membrane. Dent. Cosmos, 74:554, 1932.
4. Ziskin, D. E., Loughlin, W. C., and Siegel, E. H.: Diabetes in relation to certain oral and systemic problems. Part II. Am. J. Orthod., *30*: 758, 1944.

Chapter 9

Changes in the Consistency, Surface Texture, and Position of the Gingiva

necrotizing ulcerative gingivitis is primarily a destructive process and acute herpetic gingivostomatitis is characterized by vesicle formation. *The clinical alterations in consistency of the gingiva and the microscopic changes which produce them are summarized in Table 9–1.*

CALCIFIED MASSES IN THE GINGIVA

Calcified microscopic masses are frequently seen in the gingiva.[2] They occur singly or in groups, and vary in size, location, shape, and structure. Such masses may be calcified material removed from the tooth and traumatically displaced into the gingiva during scaling,[8] root remnants, cementum fragments, or cementicles (Fig. 9–3). Chronic inflammation and fibrosis and occasionally foreign body giant cell activity occur in relation to these masses.

CHANGES IN CONSISTENCY

Both chronic and acute inflammation produce changes in the normal firm resilient consistency of the gingiva. As noted earlier, chronic gingivitis is a conflict between destructive and reparative changes, with the consistency of the gingiva determined by the relative balance between the two (Figs. 9–1 and 9–2). Of the most common types of acute inflammation, acute

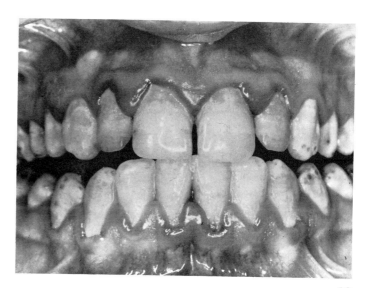

Figure 9–1 Chronic Gingivitis, showing swelling and discoloration produced when inflammatory exudate and tissue degeneration are the predominant microscopic changes. The gingiva is soft, friable, and bleeds easily. Note the mottled teeth.

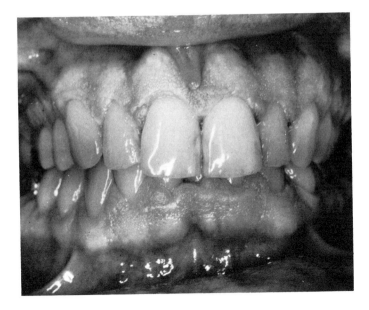

Figure 9–2 **Chronic Gingivitis,** showing firm gingiva with minutely nodular surface produced when fibrosis predominates in the inflammatory process.

They are sometimes enclosed in an osteoid-like matrix. Crystalline foreign bodies have also been described in the gingiva, but their origin has not been determined.[11]

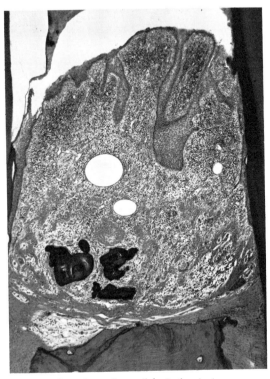

Figure 9–3   **Cementicles** in the gingiva.

CHANGES IN SURFACE TEXTURE

Loss of surface stippling is an early sign of gingivitis. In chronic inflammation the surface is either smooth and shiny, or firm and nodular, **depending upon whether the dominant changes are exudative or fibrotic.** Smooth surface texture is also produced by epithelial atrophy in *senile atrophic gingivitis,* and peeling of the surface occurs in *chronic desquamative gingivitis. Hyperkeratosis* results in a leathery texture, and noninflammatory gingival hyperplasia produces a minutely nodular surface.

CHANGE IN POSITION (RECESSION, GINGIVAL ATROPHY)

The "Actual" and "Apparent" Positions of the Gingiva

Recession is the *exposure of the root surface by an apical shift in the position of the gingiva.* To understand what is meant by recession one must distinguish between the "actual" and "apparent" positions of the gingiva. The *actual position* is the level of the epithelial attachment on the tooth (Fig. 9–4); whereas the *apparent position* is the level of the crest of the gingival margin. It is the actual position of the gingiva, not the apparent position, which determines the severity of reces-

TABLE 9–1   CLINICAL AND HISTOPATHOLOGIC CHANGES IN GINGIVAL CONSISTENCY

Chronic Gingivitis
Clinical Changes

Underlying Microscopic Features

1. Soggy puffiness that pits on pressure	1. Infiltration by fluid and cells of the inflammatory exudate
2. Marked softness and friability, with ready fragmentation upon exploration with a probe and pinpoint surface areas of redness and desquamation	2. Degeneration of connective tissue and epithelium associated with injurious substances which provoke the inflammation and the inflammatory exudate. Change in the connective tissue–epithelium relationship, with the inflamed, engorged connective tissue expanding to within a few epithelial cells of the surface. Thinning of the epithelium and degeneration associated with edema and leukocytic invasion, separated by areas in which the rete pegs are elongated into the connective tissue
3. Firm, leathery consistency	3. Fibrosis and epithelial proliferation associated with long-standing chronic inflammation

Acute Gingivitis
Clinical Changes

Underlying Microscopic Features

1. Diffuse puffiness and softening	1. Diffuse edema of acute inflammatory origin; fatty infiltration in xanthomatosis
2. Sloughing with grayish flake-like particles of debris adhering to the eroded surface	2. Necrosis with the formation of a pseudomembrane composed of bacteria, polymorphonuclear leukocytes and degenerated epithelial cells in a fibrinous meshwork
3. Vesicle formation	3. Inter- and intracellular edema with degeneration of the nucleus and cytoplasm and rupture of the cell wall

sion. There are two types of recession: visible, which is clinically observable; and hidden, which is covered by gingiva and can only be measured by inserting a probe to the level of epithelial attachment (Fig. 9–4). For example, in periodontal disease part of the denuded root is covered by the inflamed pocket wall; some of the recession is hidden, and some is visible (Fig. 9–4). The total amount of recession is the sum of the two.

Recession refers to the location of the gingiva, not its condition. Receded gingiva is often inflamed (Figs. 9–5 and 9–6) but

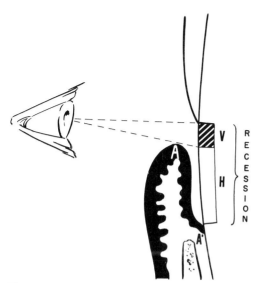

Figure 9–4   Diagram illustrating **Apparent Position of the Gingiva (A), Actual position of the Gingiva (A′), Visible Recession (V),** and **Hidden Recession (H).**

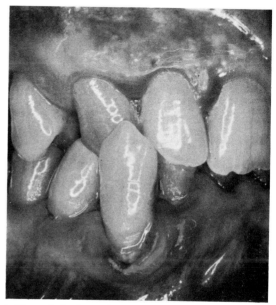

Figure 9–5   Recession on Prominent Canine. Note the severe inflammatory reaction to local irritation.

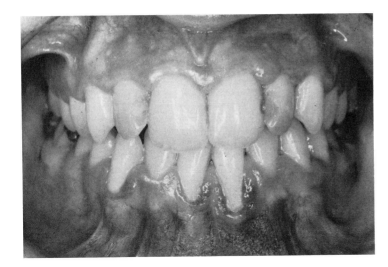

Figure 9–6 Recession around malposed anterior teeth. The gingiva is markedly inflamed.

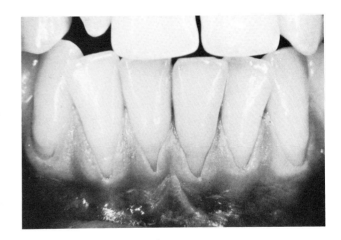

Figure 9–7 Recession on malposed teeth. Note excellent condition of the gingiva.

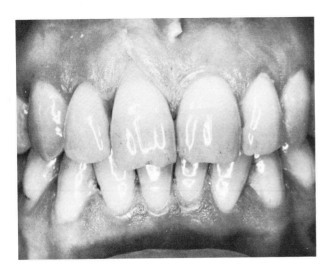

Figure 9–8 Localized Recession on maxillary central incisor associated with aggressive toothbrushing.

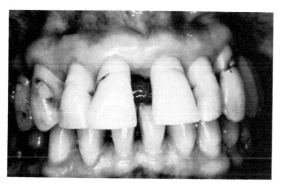

Figure 9–9 **Generalized Recession** resulting from chronic periodontal disease.

may be normal except for its position (Fig. 9–7). Recession may be localized to a tooth (Fig. 9–8) or group of teeth, or generalized throughout the mouth (Fig. 9–9).

Etiology

Gingival recession increases with age; the incidence varies from 8 per cent in children to 100 per cent after the age of 50.[14] This had led some authors to the assumption that recession may be a physiologic process related to aging. Convincing evidence for a physiologic shift of the gingival attachment has never been presented.[5] The gradual apical shift is most probably the result of the cumulative effect of minor pathologic involvement and/or repeated minor direct trauma to the gingiva.

The following factors have been implicated in the etiology of gingival recession: **faulty tooth brushing (gingival abrasion), tooth malposition, friction from soft tissues (gingival ablation),**[12] **gingival inflammation, high frenum attachment.** Trauma from occlusion has also been suggested, but its mechanism of action has never been demonstrated.

While toothbrushing is important for gingival health, **faulty toothbrushing may cause gingival recession.** Recession tends to be more frequent and severe in patients with comparatively healthy gingiva, little bacterial plaque, and good oral hygiene.[3, 9, 10]

Susceptibility to recession is influenced by the position of teeth in the arch,[13] the angle of the root in the bone, and the

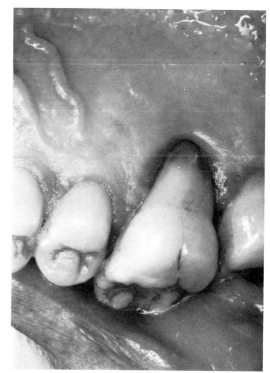

Figure 9–10 **Accentuated Recession** on a maxillary first molar aggravated by the angulation of the prominent palatal root in the bone.

mesiodistal curvature of the tooth surface.[7] On rotated, tilted, or facially displaced teeth, the bony plate is thinned or reduced in height. Pressure from mastication or moderate toothbrushing wears away the unsupported gingiva and produces recession. The effect of the angle of the roots in the bone upon recession is often observed in the maxillary molar area (Fig. 9–10). If the lingual inclination of the palatal root is prominent or the buccal roots flare outward, the bone in the cervical area is thinned or shortened and recession results from wear of the unsupported marginal gingiva (Fig. 9–11). On maxillary molars with flared roots, recession is aggravated by occlusal wear. Occlusal wear is accompanied by eruption of the tooth and accentuation of its normal buccal inclination. This increases the angulation of the lingual root in the palate, reduces the bone level, and furthers recession by lessening the gingival support (Fig. 9–11).

The effect of cheek and lip muscle action on the gingival tissue may also lead to gingival recession; Sognnaes has de-

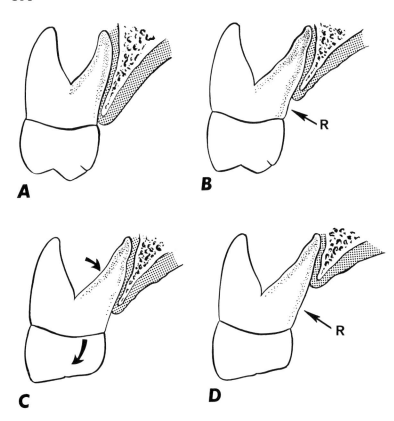

Figure 9–11   Prominent Palatal Root and Occlusal Wear Aggravating Gingival Recession. *A,* Maxillary first molar with gingiva close to the cervical line. *B,* Maxillary molar with prominent palatal root. The altered root-bone angle results in shortened bone support and gingival recession (R). *C,* Occlusal wear is accompanied by tooth eruption with increase in the normal occlusofacial inclination of the tooth (arrow) and worsening of the palatal root-bone angle (arrow). *D,* Altered palatal root-bone angle following occlusal wear lessens bone support and aggravates gingival recession (R).

scribed this effect on artificial dentures and on natural dentitions and has coined the term "dento-alveolar ablation" to describe it.[12]

The role of inflammation in the production of gingival recession has been investigated by Baker and Seymour in rats.[1] They suggest that gingival recession involves a localized inflammatory process which causes breakdown of connective tissue and proliferation of the epithelium into the site of connective tissue destruction. Proliferation of epithelial cells into the connective tissue brings about a subsidence of the epithelial surface which is manifest clinically as recession.[1]

Clinical Significance

Several aspects of gingival recession make it clinically significant. Exposed root surfaces are susceptible to caries. Wearing away of the cementum exposed by recession leaves an underlying dentinal surface that is extremely sensitive, particularly to touch. Hyperemia of the pulp and asso-

ciated symptoms may also result from exposure of the root surface.[6] Interproximal recession creates spaces in which plaque, food, and bacteria accumulate.

REFERENCES

1. Baker, D. L., and Seymour, G. J.: The possible pathogenesis of gingival recession. J. Clin. Periodontol., 3:208, 1976.
2. Barnfield, W. F.: Pathological calcification in the gingivae. Am. J. Pathol., 22:1307, 1946.
3. Gorman, N. J.: Prevalence and etiology of gingival recession. J. Periodontol., 38:316, 1967.
4. Hirschfeld, I.: A study of skulls in the American Museum of Natural History in relation to periodontal disease. J. Dent. Res., 5:241, 1923.
5. Loe, H.: The structure and physiology of the dentogingival junction. *In* Miles, A. E. (ed.): Structural and Chemical Organization of Teeth, vol. 2. New York, Academic Press, 1967.
6. Merritt, A. A.: Hyperemia of the dental pulp caused by gingival recession. J. Periodontol., 4:30, 1933.
7. Morris, M. L.: The position of the margin of the gingiva. Oral Surg., 11:969, 1958.
8. Moskow, B. S.: Calcified material in human gingival tissues. J. Dent. Res., 40:644, 1961.
9. O'Leary, T. J., Drake, R. V., Jividen, G. J., and

Allen, N. F.: The incidence of recession in young males: Relationship to gingival and plaque scores. U.S.A.F. School Aerosp. Med., SAM-TR-67–97:1, November 1967.

10. O'Leary, T. J., Drake, R. V., Crump, P., and Allen, N. F.: The incidence of recession in young males — a further study. J. Periodontol., 42:264, 1971.

11. Orban, B.: Gingival inclusions. J. Periodontol., 16:16, 1945.

12. Sognnaes, R. F.: Periodontal significance of intra-oral frictional ablation. J. Western Soc. Periodontol., 25:112, 1977.

13. Trott, J. R., and Love, B.: An analysis of localized gingival recession in 766 Winnipeg High School Students. D. Practit., 16:209, 1966.

14. Woofter, C.: The prevalence and etiology of gingival recession. Periodontal Abstr., 17:45, 1969.

Gingival Enlargement

Gingival enlargement, increase in size, is a common feature of gingival disease. There are many types of gingival enlargement which vary according to the etiologic factors and pathologic processes that produced them.[29]

The term *hypertrophic gingivitis* is not appropriate for pathologic increases in the size of the gingiva. Hypertrophy means "increase in the size of an organ as a result of increase in size of its individual component cells in order to meet increased functional requirements for useful work."[77] Enlargement of the gingiva in gingival disease is not primarily the result of an increase in size of component cells; nor does it generally occur in response to an increased functional requirement for useful work.

CLASSIFICATION OF GINGIVAL ENLARGEMENT

Gingival enlargement is classified according to etiology and pathology as follows:

  I. **Inflammatory enlargement**
    A. Chronic
      1. Localized or generalized
      2. Discrete (tumor-like)
    B. Acute
      1. Gingival abscess
      2. Periodontal abscess
  II. **Noninflammatory hyperplastic enlargement (gingival hyperplasia)**
    A. Gingival hyperplasia associated with phenytoin (Dilantin) therapy
    B. Familial, hereditary, or idiopathic hyperplastic gingival enlargement
 III. **Combined enlargement**
 IV. **Conditioned enlargement**
    A. Hormonal
      1. Enlargement of pregnancy
      2. Enlargement of puberty
    B. Leukemic
    C. Associated with vitamin C deficiency
    D. Nonspecific enlargement
  V. **Neoplastic enlargement**
 VI. **Developmental enlargement**

Location and Distribution

Using the criteria of location and distribution, gingival enlargement is designated as follows:

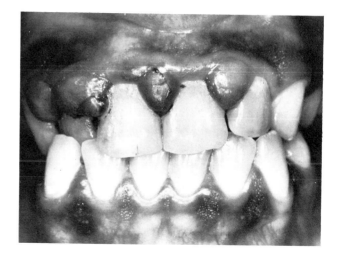

Figure 10–1 Chronic Inflammatory Gingival Enlargement localized to the anterior region, associated with irregularity of teeth.

Localized: Limited to the gingiva adjacent to a single tooth or group of teeth.

Generalized: Involving the gingiva throughout the mouth.

Marginal: Confined to the marginal gingiva.

Papillary: Confined to the interdental papilla.

Diffuse: Involving the marginal and attached gingiva and papillae.

Discrete: An isolated sessile or pedunculated "tumor-like" enlargement.

Gingival enlargement is *classified* on the basis of underlying histopathologic changes and etiology as follows:

I. INFLAMMATORY ENLARGEMENT

Gingival enlargement may result from chronic or acute inflammatory changes. The former is by far the more common cause.

Chronic Inflammatory Enlargement

LOCALIZED OR GENERALIZED

Chronic inflammatory gingival enlargement originates as a slight ballooning of the interdental papilla, marginal gingiva, or both. In the early stages it produces a

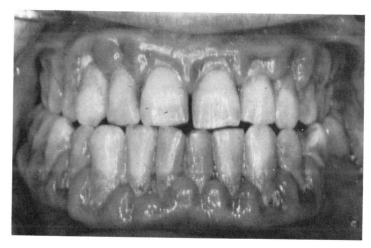

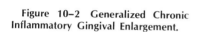

Figure 10–2 Generalized Chronic Inflammatory Gingival Enlargement.

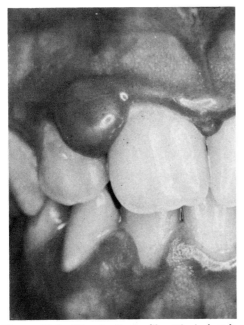

Figure 10-3 Discrete Tumor-like Gingival Enlargement.

lifesaver-like bulge around the involved teeth. This bulge increases in size until it covers part of the crowns. The enlargement is generally papillary or marginal, and may be localized (Fig. 10-1) or generalized (Fig. 10-2). It progresses slowly and painlessly unless it is complicated by acute infection or trauma.

DISCRETE (TUMOR-LIKE)

Occasionally, chronic inflammatory gingival enlargement occurs as a discrete sessile or pedunculated mass resembling a tumor. It may be interproximal or on the marginal or attached gingiva (Fig. 10-3). The lesions are slow-growing and usually painless. They may undergo spontaneous reduction in size, followed by reappearance and continued enlargement. Painful ulceration in the fold between the mass and the adjacent gingiva sometimes occurs.

Histopathology

The following features produce chronic inflammatory gingival enlargement (Figs. 10-4 and 10-5): inflammatory fluid and cellular exudate, degeneration of epithelium and connective tissue, new capillary formation, vascular engorgement, hemorrhage, proliferation of epithelium and connective tissue, new collagen fibers.

The microscopic components determine the clinical features of the enlargement such as color, consistency, and texture. Lesions that consist of a preponderance of inflammatory cells and fluid with associated degenerative changes are deep red or bluish red, soft and friable with a smooth shiny surface; they

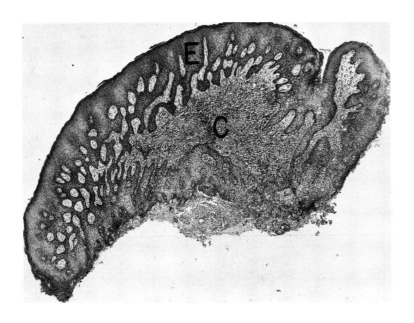

Figure 10-4 Survey Section of Chronic Inflammatory Gingival Enlargement showing the central connective tissue core (C) and thickened epithelium at the periphery (E). Note the ulceration of the epithelial surface at the lower border of the mass that was adjacent to the tooth surface.

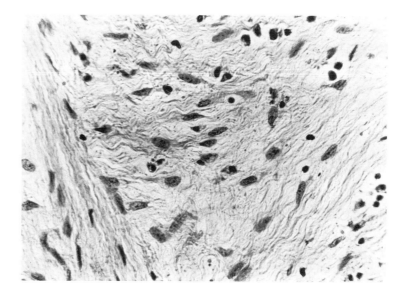

Figure 10–5 High Power Study Showing Young Fibroblasts and collagen fibrils that contribute to the increase in size in chronic inflammatory gingival enlargement.

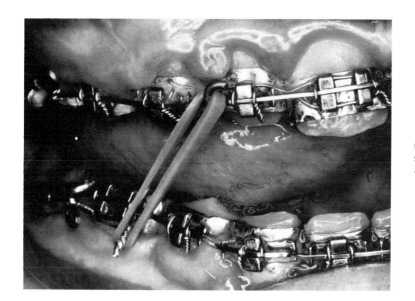

Figure 10–6 Chronic Inflammatory Gingival Enlargement associated with plaque accumulation around orthodontic appliance.

Figure 10–7 Chronic Inflammatory Gingival Enlargement Associated with Irregularity in Tooth Alignment. The difference in the color intensity of the enlarged gingiva and the adjacent comparatively uninvolved attached gingiva is shown in the mandible.

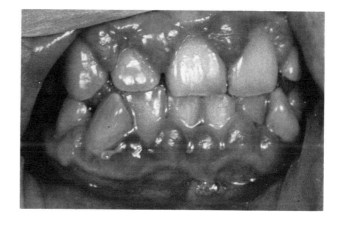

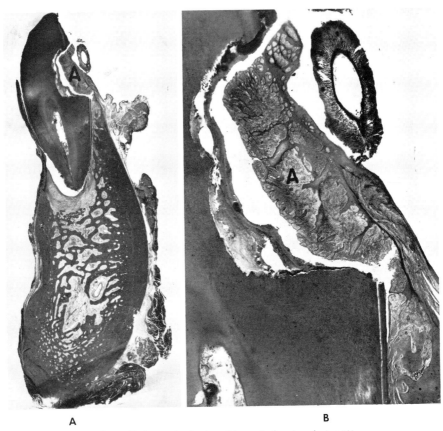

Figure 10–8*A*   Survey section of mandibular canine in situ with cervical carious lesion (A).
Figure 10–8*B*   Detail of Figure 10–8 showing a **Chronic Inflammatory Enlargement** of the gingiva (A) in the carious lesion. Note the continuity between the enlarged mass and the facial gingiva at the lower right.

bleed easily. Lesions predominantly fibrotic with an abundance of fibroblasts and collagen bundles are relatively firm, resilient, and pink.

Etiology

Chronic inflammatory gingival enlargement is caused by prolonged local irritation. The following are typical etiologic factors: [36] poor oral hygiene (Fig. 10–6), abnormal relationships of adjacent teeth (Fig. 10–7) and opposing teeth, lack of function, cervical cavities (Fig. 10–8), overhanging margins of dental restorations, improperly contoured dental restorations or pontics, food impaction (Fig. 10–9), irritation from clasps or saddle areas of removable prostheses, mouth breathing, nasal obstruction, repositioning of teeth by orthodontic therapy, and habitual pressing of the tongue against the gingiva.[2]

GINGIVAL CHANGES ASSOCIATED WITH MOUTH BREATHING. Gingivitis and gingival enlargement are often seen in mouth breathers.[52] The gingiva appears red and edematous with a diffuse surface shininess of the exposed area. The maxillary anterior region is the common site of such involvement. In many cases the altered gingiva is clearly demarcated from the adjacent unexposed normal gingiva (Fig. 10–10). The exact manner in which mouth breathing affects gingival changes has not been demonstrated. Its harmful effect is generally attributed to irritation from surface dehydration. However, comparable changes could not be produced by "air drying" the gingiva of experimental animals.[49]

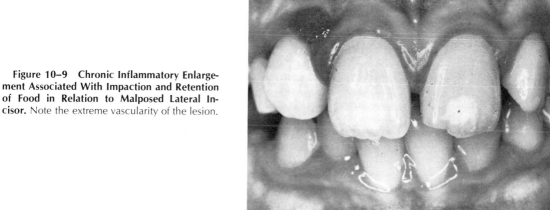

Figure 10–9   Chronic Inflammatory Enlargement Associated With Impaction and Retention of Food in Relation to Malposed Lateral Incisor. Note the extreme vascularity of the lesion.

Acute Inflammatory Enlargement

GINGIVAL ABSCESS

A gingival abscess is a localized, painful, rapidly expanding lesion usually of sudden onset. It is generally limited to the marginal gingiva or interdental papilla (Fig. 10–11). In its early stages it appears as a red swelling with a smooth shiny surface. Within 24 to 48 hours, the lesion is usually fluctuant and pointed, with a surface orifice from which a purulent exudate may be expressed. The adjacent teeth are often sensitive to percussion. If permitted to progress, the lesions generally rupture spontaneously.

Histopathology

The gingival abscess consists of a purulent focus in the connective tissue surrounded by diffuse infiltration of polymorphonuclear leukocytes, edematous tissue, and vascular engorgement. The surface epithelium presents varying degrees of intra- and extracellular edema, invasion by leukocytes, and ulceration.

Etiology

Acute inflammatory gingival enlargement is a response to irritation from foreign substances such as a toothbrush bristle, apple core, or lobster shell forcefully embedded into the gingiva. This lesion is confined to the gingiva, and should not be confused with periodontal or lateral abscesses.

PERIODONTAL (LATERAL) ABSCESS

Periodontal abscesses generally produce enlargement of the gingiva but also in-

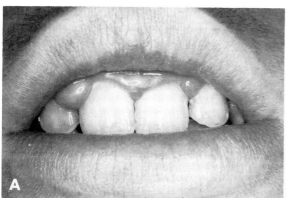
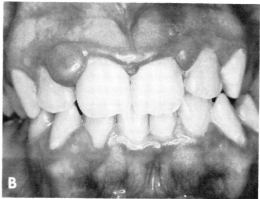

Figure 10–10   Gingivitis in Mouth Breather. A, High lip line in mouth breather. B, Gingivitis and inflammatory gingival enlargement in exposed area of gingiva.

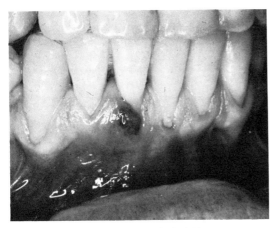

Figure 10–11   Acute Gingival Abscess.

Gingival Hyperplasia Associated with Phenytoin Therapy

Enlargement of the gingiva caused by phenytoin,* an anticonvulsant used in the treatment of epilepsy, occurs in some of the patients receiving the drug. Its reported incidence varies from 3 to 84.5 per cent,[3, 30, 62] with the greater frequencies in younger patients.[4] Its occurrence and severity are not necessarily related to the dosage, concentration of phenytoin in serum or saliva,[18] or duration of drug therapy, although some reports indicate a definite relation between dosage of the drug and degree of gingival hyperplasia.[43, 48]

volve the supporting periodontal tissues. For a detailed description of periodontal abscesses, see Chapter 18.

II. NONINFLAMMATORY HYPERPLASTIC ENLARGEMENT (GINGIVAL HYPERPLASIA)

The term *hyperplasia refers to an increase in the size of tissue or an organ produced by an increase in the number of its component cells. Noninflammatory gingival hyperplasia is produced by factors other than local irritation. It is not common, and occurs most often associated with phenytoin (Dilantin) therapy.*

Clinical Features

The primary or basic lesion starts as a painless, beadlike enlargement of the facial and lingual gingival margin and interdental papillae (Figs. 10–12 to 10–14). As the condition progresses, the marginal and papillary enlargements unite, and they may develop into a massive tissue fold covering a considerable portion of the crowns and may interfere with occlusion (Fig. 10–15). When uncomplicated by inflammation, the lesion is mulberry-shaped,

---

*Commonly known in the United States by its trade name, Dilantin; in other countries, Epanutin.

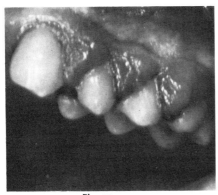

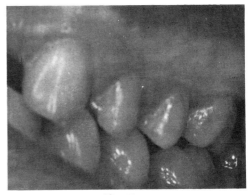

Fig. 10–12   Fig. 10–13

Figure 10–12   **Gingival Enlargement Associated With Dilantin Therapy.** Note the minutely lobulated surface of the enlarged gingiva.
Figure 10–13   Same patient as in Figure 10–12 showing disappearance of the gingival enlargement one month after the cessation of the Dilantin therapy.

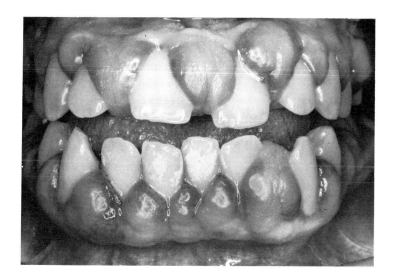

Figure 10–14 Gingival Enlargement Associated With Dilantin Therapy. Note the prominent papillary lesions. The gingiva is firm and nodular. There is marginal inflammation along the crevices deepened by the gingival overgrowth.

firm, pale pink, and resilient, with a minutely lobulated surface and no tendency to bleed. The enlargement characteristically appears to project from beneath the gingival margin, from which it is separated by a linear groove.

Phenytoin-induced hyperplasia may occur in mouths devoid of local irritants, and may be absent in mouths in which local irritants are profuse.

The hyperplasia is usually generalized throughout the mouth, but is more severe in the maxillary and mandibular anterior regions. It occurs in areas in which teeth are present — not in edentulous spaces — and the enlargement disappears in areas from which teeth are extracted. Hyperplasia of

the mucosa in edentulous mouths has been reported, but it is rare.[22]

The enlargement is chronic, and slowly increases in size until it interferes with occlusion or becomes unsightly. When surgically removed, it recurs. Spontaneous disappearance occurs within a few months after the drug is discontinued.

Local irritants (materia alba, calculus, overhanging margins of restorations, food impaction) favor plaque accumulation, thereby causing inflammation which often complicates gingival hyperplasia caused by the drug. *It is important to distinguish between the increase in size caused by the phenytoin-induced hyperplasia and the complicating inflammation caused by local*

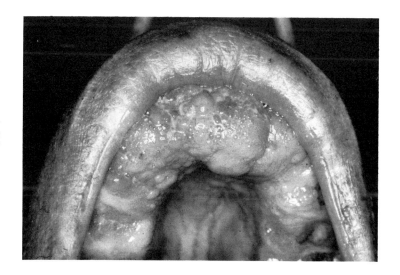

Figure 10–15 Massive Hyperplasia Associated With Dilantin Therapy. The teeth are completely covered. The gingiva is firm and dense with a nodular surface.

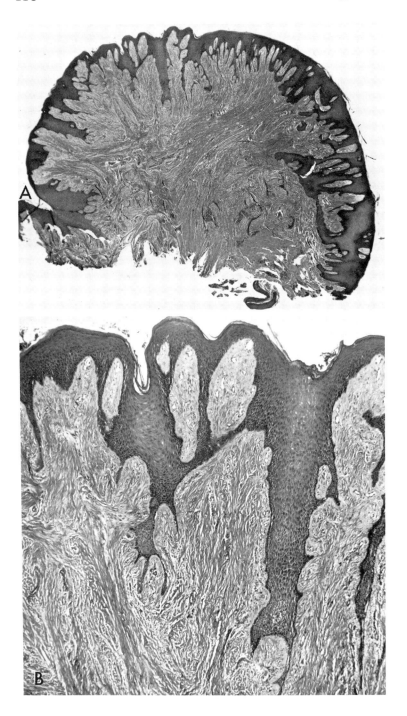

Figure 10–16 Gingival Enlargement Associated With Dilantin Therapy. *A,* Survey section, showing bulbous gingival enlargement. *B,* Detailed view, showing hyperplasia and acanthosis of the epithelium with extension of deep rete pegs into the connective tissue. The connective tissue is densely collagenous. There is little evidence of inflammation.

irritation. Secondary inflammatory changes add to the size of the lesion caused by phenytoin, produce red or bluish red discoloration, obliterate the lobulated surface demarcations, and create an increased tendency toward bleeding.

Histopathology

The enlargement presents pronounced hyperplasia of connective tissue and epithelium (Fig. 10–16). There is acanthosis of the epithelium, and elongated rete pegs extend deep

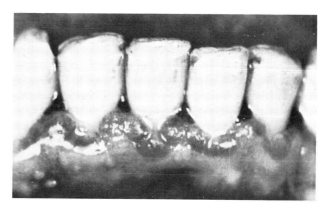

Figure 10–17 Early Recurrence following surgical removal of enlarged gingiva in patient receiving Dilantin therapy.

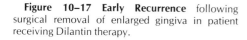

into the connective tissue, which presents densely arranged collagen bundles with an increase in fibroblasts and new blood vessels. Oxytalan fibers are numerous beneath the epithelium and in areas of inflammation.[7] Inflammation is common along the sulcal surfaces of the gingiva. Ultrastructural changes in the epithelium include widening of the intercellular spaces in the basal layer, cytoplasmic edema, and rarefaction of desmosomes.[88] The mitotic index is reduced.

Recurrent enlargements appear as granulation tissue composed of numerous young capillaries and fibroblasts and irregularly arranged collagen fibrils with occasional lymphocytes (Figs. 10–17 and 10–18).

Nature of the lesion

The enlargement is basically a hyperplastic reaction initiated by the drug, with inflammation a secondary complicating factor. Some feel that inflammation is a prerequisite for development of the hyperplasia and that it can be prevented by removal of local irritants and fastidious oral hygiene.[33, 50, 61] Others find that toothbrushing reduces the inflammation but does not lessen the hyperplasia or prevent it.[23]

Except in one study,[38] tissue culture experiments indicate that phenytoin stimulates proliferation of fibroblast-like cells[71] and epithelium.[59] Two analogues of Dilantin (1-allyl, 5-phenylhydantoinate and 5-methyl, 5-phenylhydantoinate) have a similar effect on

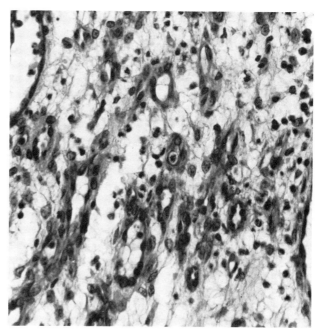

Figure 10–18 Biopsy of Recurrent Gingival Enlargement shown in Figure 10–17. Note the abundance of new blood vessels.

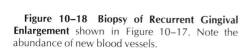

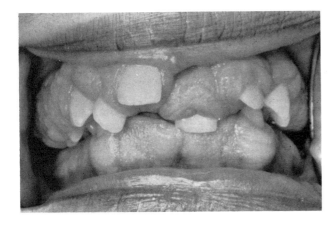

Figure 10–19 Idiopathic Hyperplastic Gingival Enlargement. The gingiva is firm with a nodular pebbled surface. The hyperplastic gingiva deflects the erupting teeth from proper alignment. (From Ball, E. I.[6])

fibroblast-like cells.[70] Stimulation by phenytoin is inhibited in irradiated cells.[72]

In experimental animals phenytoin causes gingival enlargement independent of local inflammation. It starts as hyperplasia of the connective tissue core of the marginal gingiva, which is followed by proliferation of the epithelium.[41] The enlargement increases by proliferation and expansion of the central core beyond the crest of the gingival margin.

Phenytoin occurs in the saliva in amounts correlated with the severity of gingival hyperplasia and the patient's age.[5] But in animals extirpation of the parotid glands does not affect the occurrence of hyperplasia.[7] There is no consensus on whether the severity of the hyperplasia is related to the levels of phenytoin in plasma or saliva.[3]

Systemic administration of phenytoin accelerates the healing of gingival wounds in nonepileptic humans[74] and increases the tensile strength of healing abdominal wounds in rats.[73] The administration of phenytoin may precipitate a megaloblastic anemia[54] and a folic acid deficiency.[79]

Familial, Hereditary, or Idiopathic Hyperplastic Enlargement

This is a rare condition of undetermined etiology which has been designated by such terms as gingivomatosis elephantiasis,[6, 45] diffuse fibroma,[17] familial elephantiasis, idiopathic fibromatosis,[94] hereditary or idiopathic hyperplasia,[68, 86] hereditary gingival fibromatosis[92] and congenital familial fibromatosis.

Clinical features

The enlargement affects the attached gingiva as well as the gingival margin and interdental papillae, in contrast with phenytoin-induced hyperplasia, which is often limited to the gingival margin and interdental papillae. The facial and lingual surfaces of the mandible and maxilla are generally affected, but the involvement may be limited to either jaw. The enlarged gingiva is pink, firm, almost leathery in consistency, and presents a characteristic minutely "pebbled" surface (Fig. 10–19). In severe cases the teeth are almost completely covered, and the enlargement projects into the oral vestibule. The jaws appear distorted because of the bulbous enlargement of the gingiva. Secondary inflammatory changes are common at the gingival margin.

Histopathology

There is a bulbous increase in the amount of connective tissue (Fig. 10–20) that is relatively avascular and consists of densely arranged collagen bundles and numerous fibroblasts. The surface epithelium is thickened and acanthotic with elongated rete pegs.

Etiology

Some cases have been explained on a hereditary basis,[24, 92-94] but the etiology is unknown, and the hyperplasia is appropriately designated as *idiopathic*. The genetic mechanisms involved are not well understood. A study of several families has

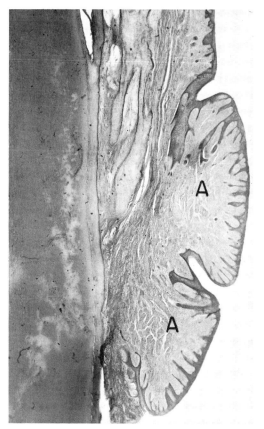

Figure 10–20 **Nodular Noninflammatory Hyperplastic Gingival Enlargement** (A) involving the attached gingiva.

found the mode of inheritance to be autosomal recessive in some cases and autosomal dominant in others.[44] The enlargement usually begins with the eruption of the primary or secondary dentition and may regress after extraction, suggesting the possibility that the teeth (or the plaque attached to them) may be initiating factors. Nutritional and hormonal etiologies have been explored but have not been substantiated.[60] Local irritation is a complicating factor.

Diffuse gingival hyperplasia should be differentiated from the bulbous distortion in the contour of the jaws associated with marked malocclusion. In the latter condition, the gingiva may be essentially unaltered or may present chronic inflammation of the gingival margin in relation to the malposed teeth (Figs. 10–21 and 10–22). The combination of inflamed marginal gingiva and unaltered attached gingiva on the deformed bone creates the erroneous impression of diffuse gingival enlargement. The dense fibrous consistency and accentuated stippling seen in diffuse hyperplastic enlargement are absent.

III. COMBINED ENLARGEMENT

This condition results when gingival hyperplasia is complicated by secondary in-

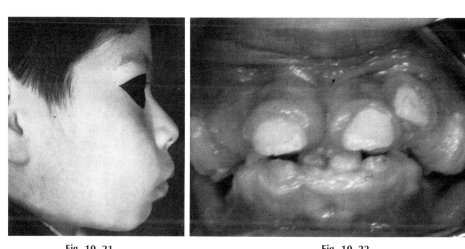

Fig. 10–21   Fig. 10–22

Figure 10–21 Prominent contour of the mouth in a patient with malocclusion.
Figure 10–22 Bulbous distortion of the maxilla and mandible in patient shown in Figure 10–21, aggravated by chronic inflammatory gingival enlargement.

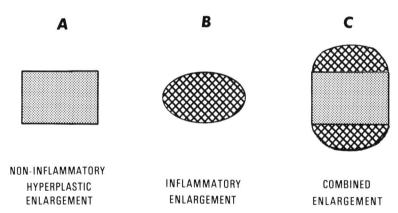

A

B

C

NON-INFLAMMATORY
HYPERPLASTIC
ENLARGEMENT

INFLAMMATORY
ENLARGEMENT

COMBINED
ENLARGEMENT

Figure 10–23 Combined Gingival Enlargement. Diagrammatic representation showing non-inflammatory hyperplastic enlargement (A) complicated by inflammatory enlargement (B) to produce combined gingival enlargement (C).

flammatory changes. The development of the combined type of gingival enlargement is depicted in Figure 10–23. Gingival hyperplasia creates conditions favorable for the accumulation of plaque and materia alba by accentuating the depth of the gingival sulcus, by interfering with effective hygienic measures, and by deflecting the normal excursive pathways of food. The secondary inflammatory changes (Fig. 10–23B) accentuate the size of the pre-existing gingival hyperplasia (Fig. 10–23A) and produce the combined gingival enlargement (Fig. 10–23C). *In many instances, secondary inflammation obscures the features of the preexistent noninflammatory hyperplasia to the extent that the entire lesion appears to be inflammatory* (Fig. 10–24).

It is essential that the nature of combined gingival enlargement be understood. It consists of two components: **a primary or basic hyperplasia of connective tissue and epithelium — the origin of which is unrelated to inflammation — and a secondary complicating inflammatory component.** The removal of local irritation eliminates the secondary inflammatory component and the size of the lesion proportionately, but the noninflammatory hyperplasia remains (Fig. 10–23A). Elimination of the noninflammatory hyperplasia requires correction of the causative factors when possible.

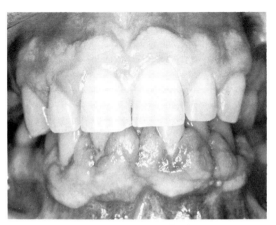

Figure 10–24 Combined Gingival Enlargement in a patient receiving phenytoin therapy. The basic hyperplasia is complicated by secondary inflammatory involvement. Note the edema and discoloration produced by the inflammation.

IV. CONDITIONED ENLARGEMENT

This type of enlargement occurs when the systemic condition of the patient is such as to exaggerate or distort the usual gingival response to local irritation, and produces a corresponding modification of the usual clinical features of chronic gingivitis. The specific manner in which the clinical picture of conditioned gingival enlargement differs from chronic gingivitis depends upon the nature of the modifying systemic influence. *Local irritation is necessary for the initiation of this type of enlargement.* The irritation does not, however, solely determine the nature of its clinical features.

There are three types of conditioned gingival enlargement: hormonal, leukemic, and that associated with vitamin C deficiency.

Hormonal Enlargement

ENLARGEMENT IN PREGNANCY

In pregnancy, gingival enlargement may be marginal and generalized or occur as single or multiple tumor-like masses.

Marginal enlargement

The prevalence of marginal gingival enlargement in pregnancy has been reported as 10 per cent[18] and 70 per cent.[93] It results from the aggravation of previously inflamed areas. However, the gingival enlargement does not occur without clinical evidence of local irritation. **Pregnancy does not cause the condition;** the altered tissue metabolism in pregnancy accentuates the response to local irritants.[39]

CLINICAL FEATURES. The clinical picture varies considerably. The enlargement is usually generalized, and tends to be more prominent interproximally than on the facial and lingual surfaces. The enlarged gingiva is bright red or magenta, soft and friable, and has a smooth shiny surface. Bleeding occurs spontaneously or upon slight provocation.[69]

Tumor-like gingival enlargement

The so-called pregnancy tumor is not a neoplasm; it is an inflammatory response to local irritation, and is modified by the patient's condition. It usually appears after the third month of pregnancy, but may occur earlier,[51] and has a reported incidence of 1.8 to 5 per cent.[55]

CLINICAL FEATURES. It appears as a discrete mushroom-like, flattened spherical mass protruding from the gingival margin, or more frequently, from the interproximal space, attached by a sessile or pedunculated base (Figs. 10–25 and 10–26). It tends to expand laterally, and pressure from the tongue and cheek perpetuate its flattened appearance. Generally dusky red or magenta, it has a smooth glistening surface that frequently presents numerous deep red pinpoint markings. It is a superficial lesion and ordinarily does not invade the underlying bone. The consistency varies, is usually semifirm, but may present varying degrees of softness and friability. It is usually painless unless its size and shape are such as to foster accumulation of debris under its margin or interfere with the occlusion, in which case painful ulceration may occur.

Histopathology

Both the marginal and tumor-like enlargement consist of a central mass of connective tissue, the periphery of which is outlined by stratified squamous epithelium. The connective tissue consists of numerous diffusely arranged, newly formed and engorged capillaries lined by cuboidal endothelial cells (Fig. 10–27). Between the capillaries there is a moderately fibrous stroma that presents vary-

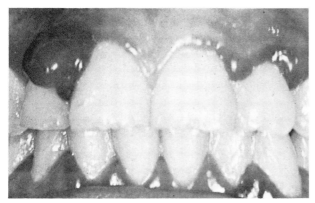

Fig. 10–25

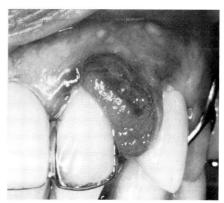

Fig. 10–26

Figure 10–25 Conditioned Gingival Enlargement in pregnancy.
Figure 10–26 Conditioned Gingival Enlargement in pregnancy associated with local irritation and food impaction.

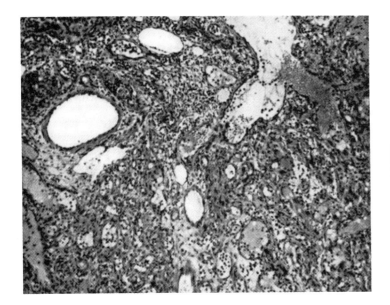

Figure 10–27 Conditioned Gingival Enlargement in pregnancy showing abundance of blood vessels and interspersed inflammatory cells.

ing degrees of edema and leukocytic infiltration. The stratified squamous epithelium is thickened with prominent rete pegs. The basal epithelium presents some degree of intra- and extracellular edema; there are prominent intercellular bridges and leukocytic infiltration. The surface of the epithelium is generally keratinized. There is generalized chronic inflammatory involvement, usually with a surface zone of acute inflammation.

Gingival enlargement in pregnancy is termed angiogranuloma, which avoids the implication of neoplasm implicit in such terms as fibrohemangioma or pregnancy tumor. Prominent endothelial proliferation with capillary formation and associated inflammation are its characteristic features. The capillary formation exceeds the usual gingival response to chronic irritation and accounts for the enlargement. Although the microscopic findings are characteristic of gingival enlargement in pregnancy, they are not pathognomonic in the sense that they can be used to differentiate between pregnant and nonpregnant patients.[55]

Most gingival disease during pregnancy can be prevented by removal of local irritants and institution of fastidious oral hygiene at the outset. In pregnancy treatment of the gingiva that is limited to the removal of tissue without complete elimination of local irritants is followed by recurrence. Although spontaneous reduction in the size of gingival enlargement com-

monly follows the termination of pregnancy, the complete elimination of the residual inflammatory lesion requires the removal of all forms of local irritation.

ENLARGEMENT IN PUBERTY

Enlargement of the gingiva is frequently seen during puberty. It occurs in both males and females, and appears in areas of local irritation.

Clinical features

The size of the gingival enlargement is far in excess of that usually seen associated with comparable local factors. It is marginal and interdental, and characterized by prominent bulbous interproximal papillae (Fig. 10–28). Frequently, only the facial gingivae are enlarged; the lingual surfaces are relatively unaltered. This occurs when the mechanical action of the tongue and the excursion of food prevent a heavy accumulation of local irritants on the lingual surface.

In addition to an increase in size, gingival enlargement during puberty presents all of the clinical features generally associated with chronic inflammatory gingival disease. *It is the degree of enlargement and tendency toward massive recurrence in the presence of relatively little local irritation that distinguishes the gingival*

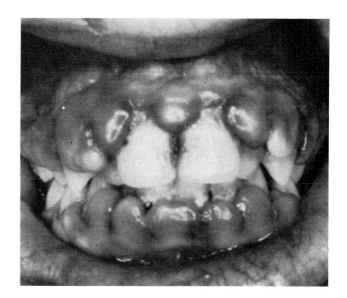

Figure 10–28 Conditioned Gingival Enlargement in puberty in a 13-year-old male.

enlargement of puberty from uncomplicated chronic inflammatory gingival enlargement. After puberty, the enlargement undergoes spontaneous reduction, but does not disappear until local irritants are removed.

A longitudinal study of 127 children, 11 to 17 years of age, showed a high initial prevalence that tended to decline with age.[81] When the mean number of inflamed gingival sites per child are arranged according to the time of maximum number of inflamed sites observed and superimposed on the oral hygiene index at the time, it can be clearly seen that a pubertal peak in gingival inflammation occurs and that it is unrelated to oral hygiene.[81]

Histopathology

Because the condition is predominantly inflammatory in nature, it is difficult to discern the conditioning systemic influence in terms of specific histologic changes. The microscopic picture is that of chronic inflammation with prominent edema and associated degenerative changes.

Leukemic Enlargement

Clinical features

Leukemic gingival enlargement may represent an exaggerated response to local irritation manifested by a dense infiltration of immature and proliferating leukocytes or a neoplastic lesion. The clinical picture is more severe than that of simple chronic inflammation. In some leukemic patients gingival enlargement results from chronic inflammation without involvement of leukemic cells and presents the same clinical and microscopic features as in nonleukemic patients.

True leukemic enlargement occurs in acute or subacute leukemia in the presence of local irritation—seldom in chronic leukemia. Clinically, true leukemic enlargement may be diffuse or marginal, localized or generalized. It may appear as a diffuse enlargement of the gingival mucosa (Fig. 10–29), an oversized extension of the marginal gingiva, or a discrete tumor-like interproximal mass. In true leukemic enlargement the gingiva is generally bluish red and has a shiny surface. The consistency is moderately firm, but there is a tendency toward friability and hemorrhage either spontaneously or upon slight irritation. Acute painful necrotizing ulcerative inflammatory involvement frequently occurs in the crevice formed at the junction of the enlarged gingiva and the contiguous tooth surfaces.

Histopathology

The connective tissue is infiltrated with a dense mass of immature and proliferating

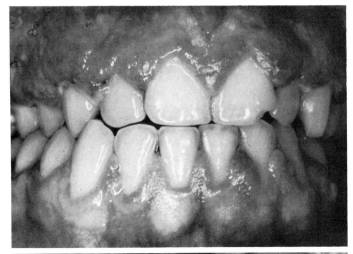

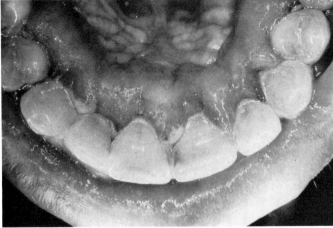

Figure 10-29   Leukemic Gingival Enlargement. *Top,* Leukemic gingival enlargement in a patient with acute myelocytic leukemia. Note that the enlargement is more prominent in the maxilla associated with greater local irritation. *Bottom,* Lingual view of gingival enlargement in a patient with subacute monocytic leukemia, showing bulbous increase in size with discoloration and smooth shiny surface. Note the difference between the enlarged gingiva and the adjacent palatal mucosa.

leukocytes, the specific nature of which varies with the type of leukemia. Mature leukocytes associated with chronic inflammation are also seen. The capillaries are engorged; the connective tissue is for the most part edematous and degenerated. The epithelium presents varying degrees of leukocytic infiltration with edema. Isolated surface areas of acute necrotizing inflammation with a pseudomembranous meshwork of fibrin, necrotic epithelial cells, polymorphonuclear leukocytes and bacteria are frequently seen.

Enlargement Associated with Vitamin C Deficiency

Enlargement of the gingiva is generally included in classic descriptions of scurvy. It is important to recognize that such enlargement is essentially a conditioned response to local irritation. Acute vitamin C deficiency does not of itself cause gingival inflammation,[27] but it does cause hemorrhage, collagen degeneration, and edema of the gingival connective tissue. These changes modify the response of the gingiva to local irritation to the extent that the normal defensive delimiting reaction is inhibited and the extension of the inflammation exaggerated.[28] The combined effect of acute vitamin C deficiency and inflammation produces the massive gingival enlargement in scurvy (Fig. 10-30A).

Clinical features

Gingival enlargement in vitamin C deficiency is marginal; the gingiva is bluish red, soft and friable, and has a smooth

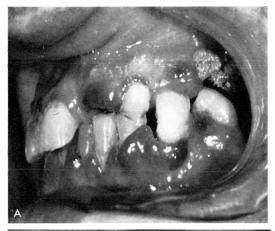

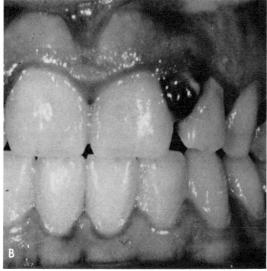

Figure 10–30   *A,* **Conditioned Gingival Enlargement** in vitamin C deficiency. Note the prominent hemorrhagic areas. *B,* **Pyogenic granuloma** in a young adult female.

Nonspecific Conditioned Enlargement (Granuloma Pyogenicum)

Granuloma pyogenicum is a tumor-like gingival enlargement considered to be an exaggerated conditioned response to minor trauma (Fig. 10–30*B*). The exact nature of the systemic conditioning factor has not been identified.[47]

Clinical features

The lesion varies from a discrete spherical tumor-like mass with a pedunculated attachment to a flattened keloid-like enlargement with a broad base. It is bright red or purple, and either friable or firm, depending upon its duration; in the majority of cases it presents surface ulceration and purulent exudation. The lesion tends to involute spontaneously to become a fibroepithelial papilloma, or persists relatively unchanged for years. Treatment consists of removal of the lesions plus the elimination of irritating local factors. The recurrence rate is about 15 per cent.[14] Granuloma pyogenicum is similar in clinical and microscopic appearance to the conditioned gingival enlargement seen in pregnancy.[51] Differential diagnosis depends upon the patient's history.

Histopathology

Granuloma pyogenicum appears as a mass of granulation tissue with chronic inflammatory cellular infiltration. Endothelial proliferation and the formation of numerous vascular spaces are the prominent features. The surface epithelium is atrophic in some areas and hyperplastic in others. Surface ulceration and exudation are common features.

shiny surface. Hemorrhage, either spontaneous or upon slight provocation, and surface necrosis with pseudomembrane formation are common features.

Histopathology

The gingiva presents a chronic inflammatory cellular infiltration with a superficial acute response. There are scattered areas of hemorrhage with engorged capillaries. Marked diffuse edema, collagen degeneration, and scarcity of collagen fibrils or fibroblasts are striking findings.

V. NEOPLASTIC ENLARGEMENT (GINGIVAL TUMORS)

Benign Tumors of the Gingiva

Epulis is a generic term used clinically to designate all tumors of the gingiva. It serves to locate the tumor, but not to describe it. (Most lesions referred to as epulis are inflammatory rather than neoplastic.) Neoplasms account for a comparatively small proportion of the gingival enlargements, and comprise a small percentage of the total number of oral neoplasms. In a survey of 257 oral tumors,[57] approximately 8 per cent occurred on the gingiva. In another study of 868 growths of the gingiva[10] and palate of which 57 per cent were neoplastic and the remainder inflammatory, the following incidence of tumors was noted: carcinoma, 11.0 per cent; fibroma, 9.3 per cent; giant cell tumor, 8.4 per cent; papilloma, 7.3 per cent; leukoplakia, 4.9 per cent; mixed tumor (salivary gland type), 2.5 per cent; angioma, 1.5 per cent; osteofibroma, 1.3 per cent; sarcoma, 0.5 per cent; melanoma, 0.5 per cent; myxoma, 0.45 per cent; lipoma, 0.3 per cent; fibropapilloma, 0.4 per cent; and adenoma, 0.4 per cent.

FIBROMA

Fibromas of the gingiva arise from the gingival connective tissue or from the periodontal ligament. They are slowly growing, spherical tumors that tend to be firm and nodular but may be soft and vascular. Fibromas are usually pedunculated.

Histopathology

The hard fibroma is composed of densely arranged bundles of well-formed collagen fibers with a scattering of flattened elliptical fibrocytes. It is a relatively avascular tumor. In the soft fibroma, fibroblasts are comparatively more numerous and stellate in shape. Collagen is present but is less densely arranged. Varying degrees of vascularity are also seen. Bone formation within the fibromas is a frequent finding. The bone appears as irregularly arranged trabeculae with osteoblasts and osteoid along the margins. Lipofibroma[56] and myxofibroma[11] of the gingiva and alveolar mucosa have also been described.

NEVUS

The nevus may be pigmented or nonpigmented. It occurs commonly on the skin, but a few cases of gingival nevus have been reported. The lesion is benign and slow growing, varying in color from pale gray to dark brown. It may be flat or raised slightly above the gingival surface, sessile or nodular.[12]

Histopathology

The tumor presents discrete clumps of nevus cells in the submucosa directly beneath the basal cell layer of epithelium and separated from it by connective tissue. The cells may contain melanin or may be pigment-free. In either instance, the nevus cells are demonstrable when stained with dihydroxyphenylalanine (DOPA).

MYOBLASTOMA

Myoblastoma is a benign lesion that is nodular and slightly raised beyond the gingival surface.[32, 46]

Histopathology

It appears as a mass of polyhedral or spindle-shaped cells with prominent acidophilic granular cytoplasm. There is a marked pseudo-epitheliomatous hyperplasia of the covering epithelium. Congenital myoblastoma is sometimes referred to as congenital epulis.

HEMANGIOMA

These are benign blood vessel tumors occasionally seen on the gingiva. They occur as a *capillary* or *cavernous* type, more commonly the former. These tumors are soft, sessile or pedunculated, and painless. They may be smooth or irregularly bulbous in outline. The color varies from deep red to purple, and blanches on the

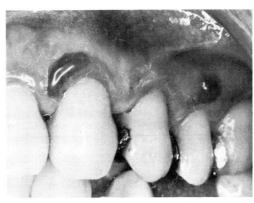

Figure 10–31 **Hematomas** produced by trauma.

application of pressure. These lesions often appear to arise from the interdental gingival papilla and spread laterally to involve the adjacent teeth.[9] They may give rise to hemorrhagic episodes producing secondary ferropenic anemia.[83] A flat, irregularly outlined, diffuse *congenital form of hemangioma* is also seen, either with or without comparable involvement of the face. Hematomas sometimes occur on the gingiva as the result of trauma (Fig. 10–31).

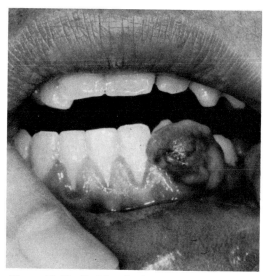

Figure 10–33 **Peripheral Giant Cell Reparative Granuloma.** Comparison of this lesion with the one shown in Figure 10–36 indicates the importance of biopsy for definitive diagnosis.

PAPILLOMA

Papilloma of the gingiva appears as a hard, wart-like protuberance from the gingival surface (Fig. 10–32). The lesion may be small and discrete, or may appear as broad, hard elevations of the gingiva with minutely irregular surfaces.

Histopathology

The lesion presents a central core of connective tissue with a marked proliferation and hyperkeratosis of the epithelium.

PERIPHERAL GIANT CELL REPARATIVE GRANULOMA

Giant cell lesions of the gingiva arise interdentally or from the gingival margin, occur more frequently on the labial surface, and may be sessile or pedunculated.

They vary in appearance from a smooth, regularly outlined mass to an irregularly shaped, multilobulated protuberance with surface indentations (Fig. 10–33). Ulceration of the margin is occasionally seen. The lesions are painless, vary in size, and may cover several teeth. They may be firm or spongy, and the color varies from pink to deep red or purplish blue. There are no pathognomonic clinical features whereby these lesions can be differentiated from other forms of gingival enlargement. Microscopic examination is required for definitive diagnosis (Figs. 10–34 to 10–37).

In the past, giant cell lesions of the gingiva have been referred to as *giant cell epulis* or *peripheral giant cell tumor.* Most often, however, these gingival lesions are essentially responses to local injury and not neoplasms. When they occur on the gingiva they should be referred to as *peripheral giant cell reparative granulomas*[65, 68] to differentiate them from comparable lesions that originate within the jaw bone (central reparative giant cell granuloma).[42]

In some instances, the giant cell reparative granuloma of the gingiva is locally invasive and causes destruction of the underlying bone (Fig. 10–38). Complete removal leads to uneventful recovery.

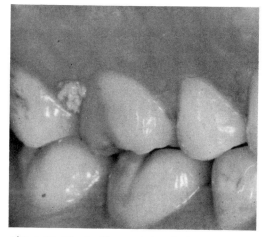

Figure 10–32 **Papilloma** of the gingiva appears as a hard wart-like mass. (Courtesy of Dr. Neal Chilton.)

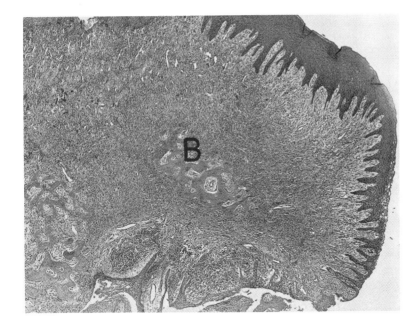

Figure 10–34 Microscopic survey of lesion shown in Figure 10–33. Trabeculae of newly formed bone (B) are contained within the mass.

Figure 10–35 High power study of the above lesion demonstrating the giant cells and intervening stroma which comprise the major portion of the mass.

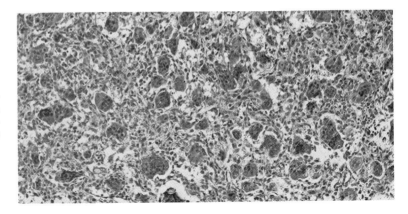

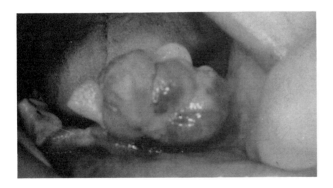

Figure 10–36 Localized gingival enlargement. Microscopic examination reveals it to be a chronic inflammatory lesion. (Compare with Figure 10–33.)

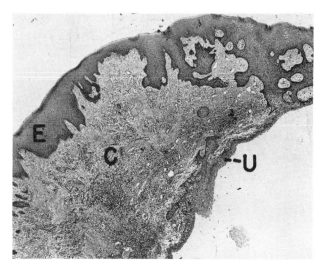

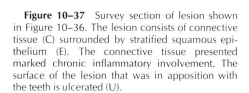

Figure 10–37 Survey section of lesion shown in Figure 10–36. The lesion consists of connective tissue (C) surrounded by stratified squamous epithelium (E). The connective tissue presented marked chronic inflammatory involvement. The surface of the lesion that was in apposition with the teeth is ulcerated (U).

Histopathology

The giant cell reparative granuloma presents numerous foci of multinuclear giant cells and hemosiderin particles in a connective tissue stroma. Areas of chronic inflammation are scattered throughout the lesion with acute involvement at the surface. The overlying epithelium is usually hyperplastic with ulceration at the base. Bone formation occasionally occurs within the lesion.

CENTRAL GIANT CELL REPARATIVE GRANULOMA

These lesions arise within the jaws and produce central cavitation. They occasionally create deformity of the jaw such that the gingiva appears enlarged (Fig. 10–39).

Mixed tumors, salivary gland type tumors, eosinophilic granulomas,[84] and *plasmacytomas* of the gingiva have also been described but are not often seen.

PLASMA CELL GRANULOMA

This is a benign lesion of the marginal interdental or attached gingiva,[15] it usually occurs as a localized mass but may be generalized. It is red, friable, sometimes granular, bleeds easily, and is accompanied by focal distribution of adjacent bone. **Microscopically it appears as a dense almost exclusively plasma cell accumulation in solid sheets or a lobular pattern.** Elimination of local irritants by scaling usually suffices as treatment, but surgical removal may be necessary.

LEUKOPLAKIA

Leukoplakia of the gingiva varies in appearance from that of a grayish white flattened scaly lesion to a thick, irregularly shaped, keratinous plaque (Fig. 10–40).

Histopathology

It presents thickening of the epithelium with hyperkeratosis, acanthosis, and some de-

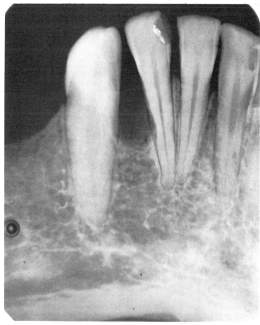

Figure 10–38 Bone Destruction in the interproximal space between the canine and lateral incisor caused by the extension of a peripheral giant cell reparative granuloma of the gingiva. (Courtesy of Dr. Sam Toll.)

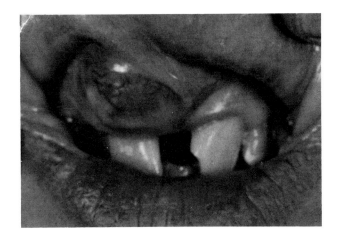

Figure 10–39 Localized Bone Deformity in relation to the maxillary central incisor (*left*) produced by a central giant cell reparative granuloma.

gree of dyskeratosis. **Inflammatory involvement of the underlying connective tissue is a commonly associated finding. Leukoplakia is caused by chronic irritation. Its capacity for malignant transformation must be borne in mind.**

GINGIVAL CYST

Gingival cysts of microscopic proportions are common in the gingiva but they seldom reach a clinically significant size.[58] When they do, they appear as localized enlargements that may involve the marginal and attached gingiva.[66] They occur in the mandibular canine and premolar areas, most often on the lingual surface. They are painless but with expansion may cause erosion of the surface of the alveolar bone. The cysts develop from odontogenic epithelium or from surface or sulcal epithelium

traumatically implanted in the area. Removal is followed by uneventful recovery.

Microscopically they present a cyst cavity lined by stratified squamous epithelium. Small daughter cysts lined with columnar or squamous epithelium may be located in the cyst wall.

Mucus-secreting cysts (mucocele)[37] and *mucous cell metaplasia*[89] have been described as rare findings in the gingiva.

Malignant Tumors of the Gingiva

CARCINOMA

The gingiva is not a common site of oral malignancy. *Squamous cell carcinoma is the most common malignant tumor of the gingiva*. Only 1.9[26] to 5.4 per cent[1a] of oral carcinomas occur on the gingiva, with the mandible, usually the molar area, being the most common site. There is often an associated leukoplakia. In patients with multiple primary oral carcinomas, 25 per cent of the tumors were present on the gingiva.[75]

Carcinomas may be *exophytic* or *verrucous*, both of which are outgrowths from the gingival surface, or *ulcerative*, which appear as flat erosive lesions. They are locally invasive, involving the underlying bone and adjacent mucosa. Often symptom-free, they are frequently unnoticed until complicated by painful inflammation. The inflammatory changes may mask the neoplasm. Metastasis is usually confined to the region above the clavicle; however,

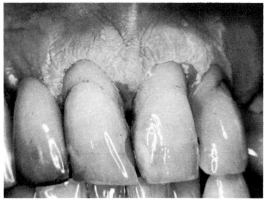

Figure 10–40   Leukoplakia of the Gingiva.

more extensive involvement may include the lung, liver, or bone. A five-year survival rate of 24 per cent has been reported for gingival carcinomas.[76]

MALIGNANT MELANOMA

Malignant melanoma is a rare oral tumor that tends to occur in the gingiva of the anterior maxilla.[8] The malignant melanoma is usually darkly pigmented and is often preceded by the occurrence of localized pigmentation.[20] It may be flat or nodular and is characterized by rapid growth and early metastasis. It arises from melanoblasts in the gingiva, cheek, or palate. An unpigmented malignant melanoma of the gingiva has been reported.[53] Infiltration into the underlying bone and metastasis to cervical and axillary lymph nodes are common.

Histopathology

The malignant melanoma shows some resemblance to the benign nevus; however, the malignant cells vary in morphology. The distribution is irregular and invasive, lacking the clear-cut grouping of the benign lesions, and in some areas they are continuous with the surface epithelium. The connective tissue stroma is more often delicate and relatively scarce.

SARCOMA

Fibrosarcoma, lymphosarcoma, and *reticulum cell sarcoma* of the gingiva are rare; only isolated cases have been described in the literature.[21, 31, 63] Thoma et al.[85] have described a case of *malignant lymphoma* of the gingiva in a 19-year-old female. The lesion was first noticed in an alveolar socket that failed to heal after extraction. The lesion appeared as a persistent raspberry-like protuberance from the surface of the socket associated with suppuration, superficial ulceration, and progressive necrosis of the gingiva and underlying bone. Subsequent lesions occurred in other areas of the gingiva followed by denudation of the root surfaces and tooth loss (Figs. 10–41 and 10–42).

METASTASIS

Tumor metastasis to the gingiva is not common. Hardman[34] describes two gingival tumors that metastasized from a *primary chondrosarcoma in the femur.* The gingival tumors resembled fibromas in appearance, and presented secondary inflammatory involvement associated with local irritation. Microscopically, the tumors of the gingiva consisted of a vascular loose network of spindle cells consistent with a diagnosis of *spindle cell sarcoma.* Among other reported cases of metastasis to the gingiva are *adenocarcinoma from the colon,*[40,] *carcinoma from the lung,*[91] *chondromyxosarcoma from the axilla,*[67] and *hypernephroma.*[64, 80]

One must not be misled by the low incidence of malignancy of the gingiva. Ulcerations that do not respond to therapy in the usual manner and all gingival

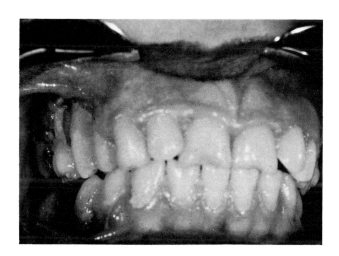

Figure 10–41 Malignant Lymphoma of the Gingiva in a Young Female. The tumor appears as bead-like masses of granulation tissue in the maxillary molar area (*left*).

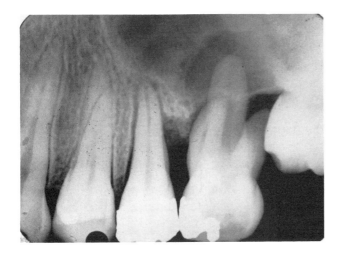

Figure 10–42 Radiograph of patient with malignant lymphoma shown in Figure 10–41. There is extensive loss of bone in relation to the molar and premolar as a result of progressive invasion of the tumor. Note the thickening of the periodontal space around the premolar.

tumors and tumor-like lesions must be biopsied (Chap. 32) and submitted for microscopic diagnosis.

VI. DEVELOPMENTAL GINGIVAL ENLARGEMENT

Clinical Features

This type of enlargement appears as a bulbous distortion of the labial and marginal contours of the gingiva of teeth in various stages of eruption. It is caused by superimposition of the bulk of the gingiva upon the normal prominence of the enamel in the gingival half of the crown. The enlargement often persists until the junctional epithelium has migrated from the enamel to the cemento-enamel junction.

In a strict sense, developmental gingival enlargement is physiological and ordinarily presents no problem. However, when it is complicated by marginal inflammation, the composite picture gives the impression of extensive gingival enlargement (Fig. 10–43). Treatment to alleviate the marginal inflammation rather than resection of the "enlargement" is sufficient in these cases.

Histopathology

When uncomplicated by inflammation, developmental enlargement presents no notable pathologic changes. A zone of chronic inflammation at the gingival margin is, however, a common finding.

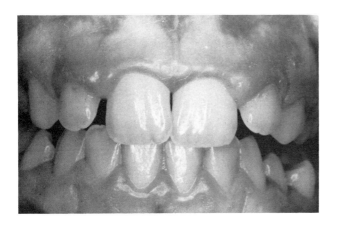

Figure 10–43 Developmental Gingival Enlargement. The normal bulbous contour of the gingiva around the incompletely erupted anterior teeth is accentuated by chronic inflammation.

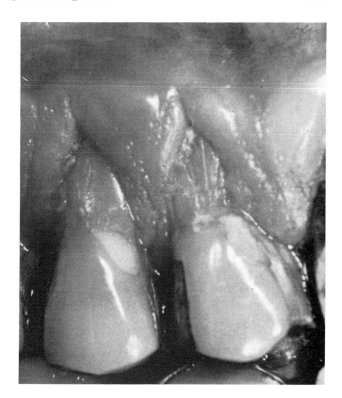

Figure 10–44 "Stillman's Clefts" in the gingiva.

CHANGES IN GINGIVAL CONTOUR

Changes in gingival contour are for the most part associated with gingival enlargement, but changes in gingival contour may occur in other conditions.

Stillman's clefts

Stillman's clefts are apostrophe-shaped indentations extending from and into the gingival margin for varying distances. The clefts generally occur on the facial surface (Fig. 10–44). One or two may be present in relation to a single tooth. The margins of the clefts are rolled underneath the linear gap in the gingiva and the remainder of the gingival margin is blunt instead of knife-edge. Originally described by Stillman[82] and considered to be the result of occlusal trauma, these clefts were subsequently described by Box[16] as pathologic

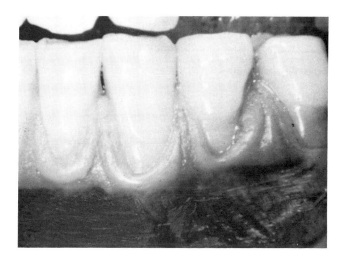

Figure 10–45 "McCall's Festoons" showing characteristic rimlike enlargement of the gingival margin.

pockets in which the ulcerative process had extended through to the facial surface of the gingiva. The clefts may repair spontaneously or persist as surface lesions of deep periodontal pockets that penetrate into the supporting tissues. Their association with trauma from occlusion has not been substantiated.

The clefts are divided into: *simple,* cleavage in a single direction (most common); and *compound,* cleavage in more than one direction (Tishler[87]). The length of the clefts varies from a slight break in the gingival margin to a depth of 5 to 6 mm. or more.

McCall's festoons

McCall's festoons are lifesaver-shaped enlargements of the marginal gingiva that occur most frequently in the canine and premolar areas on the facial surface. In the early stages, the color and consistency of the gingiva are normal. Accumulation of food debris leads to secondary inflammatory changes (Fig. 10–45). Trauma from occlusion and mechanical stimulation are suggested etiologic factors.[25] However, festoons occur on teeth without occlusal antagonists.

REFERENCES

1. Aas, E.: Hyperplasia gingivae diphenylhydantoinea. Universitetsforlaget, 1963.
1a. Ackerman, L. V., and del Regato, J. A.: Cancer, diagnosis, treatment and prognosis. St. Louis, The C. V. Mosby Co., 1947.
2. Aiguer, J.: Localized hypertrophic gingivitis due to tongue habit. J. Periodontol., 9:59, 1938.
3. Angelopoulos, A. P., and Goaz, P. W.: Incidence of diphenyl hydantoin gingival hyperplasia. Oral Surg. Med. Pathol., 34:898, 1972.
4. Babcock, J. R.: Incidence of gingival hyperplasia associated with dilantin therapy in a hospital population. J. Am. Dent. Assoc., 71:1447, 1965.
5. Babcock, J. R., and Nelson, G. H.: Gingival hyperplasia and dilantin content of saliva. J. Am. Dent. Assoc., 68:195, 1964.
6. Ball, E. I.: Case of gingivomatosis or elephantiasis of the gingiva. J. Periodontol., 12:96, 1941.
7. Baratieri, A.: The oxytalan connective tissue fibers in gingival hyperplasia in patients treated with sodium diphenylhydantoin. J. Periodont. Res., 2:106, 1967.
8. Baxter, H. A., Brown, J. B., and Byars, L. T.: Malignant melanomas. Am. J. Orthod., 27:90, 1941.
9. Bellinger, D. H.: Blood and lymph vessel tumors involving the mouth. J. Oral Surg., 2:141, 1944.
10. Bernick, S.: Growth of the gingiva and palate. II. Connective tissue tumors. Oral Surg., 1:1098, 1948.
11. Bernier, J. L., and Ash, J. E.: Atlas of dental and oral pathology. Washington, D. C., Registry Press, 1948.
12. Bernier, J. L., and Tiecke, R. W.: Nevus of the gingiva. J. Oral Surg., 8:165, 1950.
13. Bhaskar, S. N., Bernier, J. L., and Godby, F.: Aneurysmal bone cyst and other giant cell lesions of the jaws. Report of 104 cases. J. Oral Surg., 17:30, 1959.
14. Bhaskar, S. N., and Jacoway, J. R.: Pyogenic granuloma—clinical features, incidence, histology and result of treatment. J. Oral. Surg., 24:391, 1966.
15. Bhaskar, S. N., Levin, M. P., and Frisch, J.: Plasma cell granuloma of periodontal tissues. Report of 45 cases. Periodontics, 6:272, 1968.
16. Box, H. K.: Gingival clefts and associated tracts. N. Y. State Dent. J., 16:3, 1950.
17. Buckner, H. J.: Diffuse fibroma of the gums. J. Am. Dent. Assoc., 24:2003, 1937.
18. Burket, L. W.: Oral Medicine. Philadelphia, J. B. Lippincott Co., 1946, p. 295.
19. Ciancio, S. G., Yaffe, S. J., and Catz, C. C.: Gingival hyperplasia and diphenylhydantoin. J. Periodontol., 7:411, 1972.
20. Chaudry, A. P., Hampel, A., and Gorlin, R. J.: Primary malignant melanoma of the oral cavity: A review of 105 cases. Cancer, 11:923, 1958.
21. Cook, H. P.: Oral lymphomas. Oral Surg. 14:690, 1961.
22. Dallas, B. M.: Hyperplasia of the oral mucosa in an edentulous epileptic. New Zealand Dent. J., 59:54, 1963.
23. Elzay, R. P., and Swenson, H. M.: Effect of an electric toothbrush on dilantin sodium induced gingival hyperplasia. N. Y. J. Dent., 34:13, 1964.
24. Emerson, T. G.: Hereditary gingival hyperplasia. A family pedigree of four generations. Oral Surg., 19:1, 1965.
25. Fuchs, M., and Kurnatowski, A.: Klinische und mikroskopische Untersuchungen der McCall-Girlander. Dtsch. Zahnaerztl., 17:1125, 1962.
26. Gardner, A. F., Schwartz., F. L., and Pallen, H. S.: Carcinoma of the oral regions. Ann. Dent., 21:80, 1962.
27. Glickman, I.: The periodontal tissues of the guinea pig in vitamin C deficiency. J. Dent. Res., 27:9, 1948.
28. Glickman, I.: The effect of acute vitamin C deficiency upon the response of the periodontal tissues of the guinea pig to artificially induced inflammation. J. Dent. Res., 27:201, 1948.
29. Glickman, I.: A basic classification of gingival enlargement. J. Periodontol., 21:131, 1950.
30. Glickman, I., and Lewitus, M.: Hyperplasia of the gingiva associated with dilantin (sodium diphenyl hydantoinate) therapy. J. Am. Dent. Assoc., 28:199, 1941.
31. Goldman, H. M.: Sarcoma. Am. J. Orthod., 30:311, 1944.
32. Hagen, J. D., Soule, E. H., and Gores, R. J.:

Granular-cell myoblastoma of the oral cavity. Oral Surg., *14*:454, 1961.

33. Hall, W. B.: Dilantin hyperplasia: A preventable lesion. J. Periodont. Res. [Suppl.], *4*:36, 1969.
34. Hardman, F. G.: Secondary sarcoma presenting clinical appearance of fibrous epulis. Br. Dent. J., *86*:109, 1949.
35. Henefer, E. P., and Kay, L. A: Congenital idiopathic gingival fibromatosis in the deciduous dentition. Oral Surg., *24*:65, 1967.
36. Hirschfeld, I.: Hypertrophic gingivitis—its clinical aspects. J. Am. Dent. Assoc., *19*:799, 1932.
37. Hodson, J. J.: Mucous cell metaplasia in human gingival epithelium and its relation to certain mucous secreting tumors. Arch. Oral Biol., *5*:174, 1961.
38. Hoess, T.: The effect of 5,5 diphenylhydantoin (Dilantin) on fibroblast-like cells in culture. J. Periodont. Res., *4*:163, 1969.
39. Hugoson, A.: Gingival inflammation and female sex hormones. J. Periodont. Res. [Suppl. 5], 1970.
40. Humphrey, A. A., and Amos, N. H.: Metastatic gingival adenocarcinoma from primary lesion of colon. Am. J. Cancer, *28*:128, 1936.
41. Ishikawa, J., and Glickman, I.: Gingival response to the systemic administration of sodium diphenyl hydantoinate (Dilantin) in cats. J. Periodontol., *32*:149, 1961.
42. Jaffe, H. L.: Giant cell reparative granuloma, traumatic bone cyst, and fibrous (fibro-osseous) dysplasia of the jaw bones. Oral Surg., *6*:159, 1953.
43. Kapur, R. N., Grigis, S., Little, T. M., and Masotti, R. E.: Diphenylhydantoin-induced gingival hyperplasia: Its relation to dose and serum level. Dev. Med. Child Neurol., *15*:483, 1973.
44. Jorgenson, R. J., and Cocker, M. E.: Variation in the inheritance and expression of gingival fibromatosis. J. Periodontol., *45*:472, 1974.
45. Kerageorgis, B. P.: Elephantiasis of the gingivae (Elephantiasis des Gengives). Rev. Chir. Par., *68*:308, 1949. Abst. Surg. Gynecol. Obstet., *90*:461, 1950.
46. Kerr, D. A.: Myoblastic myoma. Oral Surg., *2*:41, 1949.
47. Kerr, D. A.: Granuloma pyogenicum. Oral Surg., *4*:158, 1951.
48. Klar, L. A.: Gingival hyperplasia during dilantin therapy; a survey of 312 patients. J. Public Health Dent., *33*:180, 1973.
49. Klingsberg, J., Cancellaro, L. A., and Butcher, E. O.: Effects of air drying in rodent oral mucous membrane. A histologic study of simulated mouth breathing. J. Periodontol., *32*:38, 1961.
50. Larmas, L. A., Mackinen, K. K., and Paunio, K. U.: A histochemical study of amylaminopeptidase in hydantoin induced hyperplastic, healthy and inflamed human gingiva. J. Periodont. Res., *8*:21, 1973.
51. Lee, K. W.: The fibrous epulis and related lesions. Granuloma pyogenicum, "pregnancy tumor"; fibro-epithelial polyp and calcifying fibroblastic granuloma. A clinico-pathological study. Periodontics, *6*:277, 1968.
52. Lite, T., et al.: Gingival patterns in mouth breathers. A clinical and histopathologic study and a method of treatment. Oral Surg., *8*:382, 1955.
53. Loscalzo, L. J.: Unpigmented melanocarcinoma of the gingivae. Report of a case. Oral Surg., *11*:646, 1958.
54. Lustberg, A., Goldman, D., and Dreskin, O. H.: Megaloblastic anemia due to dilantin therapy. Ann. Int. Med., *54*:153, 1961.
55. Maier, A. W., and Orban, B.: Gingivitis in pregnancy. Oral Surg., *2*:334, 1949.
56. Marfino, N. R.: Developing fibrolipoma of the free gingiva. Oral Surg., *12*:489, 1959.
57. McCarthy, F. P.: A clinical and pathological study of oral disease. J.A.M.A., *116*:16, 1941.
58. Moskow, B. S.: The pathogenesis of the gingival cyst. Periodontics, *4*:23, 1966.
59. Nease, W. J.: Effect of sodium diphenylhydantoinate on tissue cultures of human gingiva. J. Periodontol., *36*:22, 1965.
60. Newby, C. D.: A report on a case of hypertrophied gum tissue. J. Can. Dent. Assoc., *6*:183, 1940.
61. Nuki, K., and Cooper, S. H.: The role of inflammation in the pathogenesis of gingival enlargement during the administration of diphenylhydantoin sodium in cats. J. Periodont. Res., *7*:91, 1972.
62. Panuska, H. J., Gorlin, R. J., Bearman, J. E., and Mitchell, D. F.: The effect of anticonvulsant drugs upon the gingiva. A series of 1048 patients. II. J. Periodontol., *32*:15, 1961.
63. Partsch, C.: Atlas der Zahnheilkunde in Stenokopischen Bilde. Berlin, Julius Springer, 1912.
64. Persson, P. A., and Wallenino, K.: Metastatic renal carcinoma (hypernephroma) in the gingiva of the lower jaw. Acta Odont. Scand., *19*:289, 1961.
65. Phillips, R. L., and Shafer, W. G.: An evaluation of the peripheral giant cell tumor. J. Periodontol., *26*:216, 1955.
66. Rickles, N. H., and Everett, F. G.: Gingival and lateral periodontal cysts. Parodontology, *14*:41, 1960.
67. Robinson, H. B. G.: A clinic on the differential diagnosis of oral lesions. Am. J. Orthod., *32*:720, 1946.
68. Rushton, M. A.: Hereditary or idiopathic hyperplasia of the gums. Dent. Practit., *7*:136, 1957.
69. Setia, A. P.: Severe bleeding from a pregnancy tumor. Oral Surg., *36*:192, 1973.
70. Shafer, W. G.: Effect of dilantin sodium analogues on cell proliferation in tissue culture. Proc. Soc. Exp. Biol. Med., *106*:205, 1960.
71. Shafer, W. G.: Effect of dilantin sodium on various cell lines in tissue culture. Proc. Soc. Exp. Biol. Med., *108*:694, 1961.
72. Shafer, W. G.: Response of radiated human gingival fibroblast-like cells to dilantin sodium in tissue culture. J. Dent Res., *44*:671, 1965.
73. Shafer, W. G., Beatty, R. E., and Davis, W. B.: Effect of dilantin sodium on tensile strength of healing wounds. Proc. Soc. Exp. Biol. Med., *98*:348, 1958.
74. Shapiro, M.: Acceleration of gingival wound healing in non-epileptic patients receiving diphenylhydantoin sodium. Exp. Med. Surg., *16*:41, 1958.
75. Sharp, G. S., Bullock, W. K., and Helsper, J. T.:

Multiple oral carcinomas. Cancer, *14*:512, 1961.

76. Sharp, G. S.: Carcinoma of the gingivae. J. Tenn. S. Dent. Assoc., 29:236, 1959.

77. Smith, L. W., and Gault, E. S.: Essentials of pathology. 3rd ed. New York, Appleton-Century Co., 1948, p. 1925.

78. Soni, N. N., et al.: Mitotic activity in human gingival epithelium associated with dilantin sodium therapy. Periodontics, 5:70, 1967.

79. Stein G. M., and Lewis, H.: Oral changes in a folic acid deficient patient precipitated by anticonvulsant drug therapy. J. Periodontol., *44*:645, 1973.

80. Stein, G.: Hypernephrommetastase als Epulis. Dtsch Ztschr. Chir., *219*:318, 1929.

81. Sutcliffe, P.: A longitudinal study of gingivitis and puberty. J. Periodont. Res., 7:52, 1972.

82. Stillman, P. R.: Early clinical evidences of disease in the gingiva and pericementum. J. Dent. Res., 3:25, 1921.

83. Sznajder, N., Dominguez, F. V., Carraro, J. J., and Lis, G.: Hemorrhagic hemangioma of the gingiva: Report of a case. J. Periodontol., *44*:579, 1973.

84. Taddei, G.: Gingival eosinophilic granuloma. Arch. Ital. Mal. App. Diger., *19*:280, 1953.

85. Thoma, K. H., Holland, D. J., Woodbury, H. W., Burrow, J. G., and Sleeper, E. I.: Malignant lymphoma of the gingiva. Oral Surg., *1*:57, 1948.

86. Thukral, P. P.: Idiopathic gingival hyperplasia. J. Indian Dent. Assoc., *44*:109, 1972.

87. Tishler, B.: Gingival clefts and their significance. Dent. Cosmos, *49*:1003, 1927.

88. Tollaro, I.: Clinical statistical contribution on gingival hyperplasia caused by anticonvulsants. Riv. Ital. Stomat., *23*:1519, 1968.

89. Traeger, K. A.: Cyst of the gingiva (mucocele): Report of a case. Oral Surg., *14*:243, 1961.

90. Westphal, P.: Salivary secretion and gingival hyperplasia in diphenylhydantoin-treated guinea pigs. Svensk. Tandläkane-Tidsskrift, *62*:505, 1969.

91. Willis, R. A.: Pathology of tumors. St. Louis, The C. V. Mosby Co., 1948, p. 376.

92. Zackin, S. J., and Weisberger, D.: Hereditary gingival fibromatosis. Oral Surg., *14*:828, 1961.

93. Ziskin, D. E., Blackberg, S. M., and Stout, A. P.: The gingivae during pregnancy. Surg. Gynecol. Obstet., 57:719, 1933.

94. Ziskin, D. E., and Zegarelli, E.: Idiopathic fibromatosis of the gingivae. Ann. Dent., *2*:50, 1943.

Chapter 11

Acute Gingival Infections

ACUTE NECROTIZING ULCERATIVE GINGIVITIS (ANUG)

The term *acute necrotizing ulcerative gingivitis* (ANUG) connotes an inflammatory destructive disease of the gingiva which presents characteristic signs and symptoms. Other terms by which this condition is known are Vincent's infection, acute ulceromembranous gingivitis, trench mouth, trench gums, phagedenic gingivitis, acute ulcerous gingivitis, acute ulcerative gingivitis, ulcerative gingivitis, ulcerative stomatitis, Vincent's stomatitis, Plaut-Vincent's stomatitis, stomatitis ulcerosa, stomatitis ulcero-membranacea, fusospirillary gingivitis, fusospirillary marginal gingivitis, fusospirillary periodontal gingivitis, fusospirillary peridental gingivitis, fusospirillary periodontitis, fetid stomatitis, putrid stomatitis, putrid sore mouth, stomatocace, stomacace, acute septic gingivitis, pseudomembranous angina, and spirochetal stomatitis.

The disease was recognized as far back as the fourth century B.C. by Xenophon, who mentioned that Greek soldiers were affected with "sore mouth" and foul-smelling breath. John Hunter in 1778 described the clinical findings and differentiated it from scurvy and chronic destructive periodontal disease. It occurred in epidemic form in the French army in the nineteenth century, and in 1886 Hersch discussed some of the features associated with the disease, such as enlarged lymph nodes, fever, malaise, and increased salivation. In the 1890's Plaut[36] and Vincent[56] described the disease and attributed its origin to fusiform and spirochete bacteria. It was commonly known as *Vincent's infection* during the first half of the twentieth century, but the current designation is acute necrotizing ulcerative gingivitis.

Clinical features

CLASSIFICATION. Necrotizing ulcerative gingivitis most often occurs as an *acute* disease. Its relatively mild and more persistent form is referred to as *subacute*. *Recurrent* disease is marked by periods of remission and exacerbation. Reference is sometimes made to *chronic* necrotizing ulcerative gingivitis. However, it is difficult to justify this designation as a separate entity because most periodontal pockets with ulceration and destruction of gingival tissue present comparable microscopic and clinical features.

HISTORY. Acute necrotizing ulcerative gingivitis is characterized by *sudden onset,* frequently following an episode of debilitating disease or acute respiratory in-

135

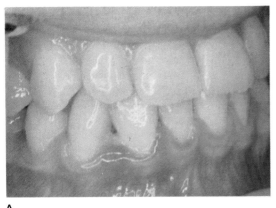

A

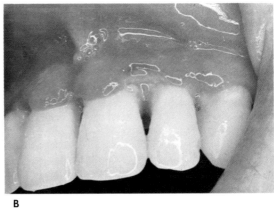

B

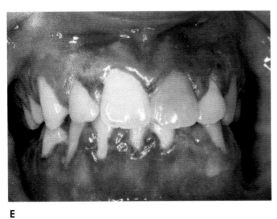

C

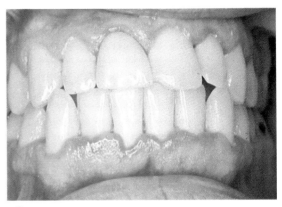

D

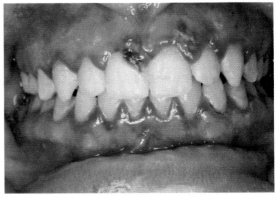

E

F

Plate II

A, **Acute necrotizing ulcerative gingivitis:** typical punched out interdental papilla between mandibular canine and lateral incisor.

B, **Acute necrotizing ulcerative gingivitis:** typical lesions with progressive tissue destruction.

C, **Acute necrotizing ulcerative gingivitis:** typical lesions with spontaneous hemorrhage.

D, **Acute necrotizing ulcerative gingivitis:** typical lesions have produced irregular gingival contour.

E, **Acute herpetic gingivostomatitis:** typical diffuse erythema.

F, **Acute herpetic gingivostomatitis:** vesicles on the gingiva.

fection. Occasionally, patients report that it appeared shortly after they had their teeth cleaned. Change in living habits, protracted work without adequate rest, and psychological stress are frequent features of the patient's history.

ORAL SIGNS. *Characteristic lesions are punched-out, crater-like depressions at the crest of the gingiva that involve the interdental papillae, the marginal gingiva, or both.* The surface of the gingival craters is covered by a gray, pseudomembranous slough demarcated from the remainder of the gingival mucosa by a pronounced linear erythema (Color Plate 2A). In some instances, the lesions are denuded of the surface pseudomembrane, exposing the gingival margin, which is red, shiny, and hemorrhagic. The characteristic lesions progressively destroy the gingiva and underlying periodontal tissues (Color Plate 2B).

A fetid odor, increased salivation, and spontaneous gingival hemorrhage or pronounced bleeding upon the slightest stimulation are additional characteristic clinical signs (Color Plate 2C).

Acute necrotizing ulcerative gingivitis occurs in otherwise disease-free mouths or superimposed upon chronic gingivitis (Color Plate 2D) or periodontal pockets. Involvement may be limited to a single tooth or group of teeth (Fig. 11–1), or be widespread throughout the mouth. It is rare in edentulous mouths, but isolated spherical lesions occasionally occur on the soft palate.

ORAL SYMPTOMS. The lesions are extremely sensitive to touch, and the patient complains of a constant radiating, gnawing pain that is intensified by spicy or hot foods and mastication. There is a metallic foul taste and the patient is conscious of an excessive amount of "pasty" saliva. **The teeth are characteristically described as feeling like "wooden pegs."**

EXTRA-ORAL AND SYSTEMIC SIGNS AND SYMPTOMS. Patients are usually ambulatory, with a minimum of systemic complications. **Local lymphadenopathy and slight elevation in temperature** are common features of the mild and moderate stages of the disease. In severe cases there are marked systemic complications such as

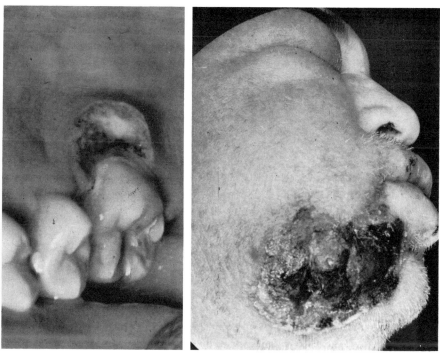

Fig. 11–1   Fig. 11–2

Figure 11–1   Localized Zone of Acute Necrotizing Ulcerative Gingivitis.
Figure 11–2   Noma Following Acute Necrotizing Ulcerative Gingivitis in a 50-year-old male with severe anemia.

high fever, increased pulse rate, leukocytosis, loss of appetite, and general lassitude. Systemic reactions are more severe in children. Insomnia, constipation, gastrointestinal disorders, headache, and mental depression sometimes accompany the condition.

In very rare cases severe sequelae such as the following may occur: noma or gangrenous stomatitis[25] (Fig. 11–2), fusospirochetal meningitis and peritonitis, pulmonary infections,[33] toxemia, and fatal brain abscess.[51]

CLINICAL COURSE. The clinical course is indefinite. If untreated, it may result in progressive destruction of the periodontium and denudation of the roots, accompanied by an increase in the severity of toxic systemic complications. It often undergoes a diminution in severity leading to a subacute stage with varying degrees of clinical symptomatology. *The disease may subside spontaneously without treatment.* Such patients generally present a history of repeated remissions and exacerbations. Recurrence of the condition in previously treated patients is also frequent.

Acute necrotizing ulcerative gingivitis and chronic destructive periodontal disease

It is important to understand the relationship between acute necrotizing ulcerative gingivitis and chronic destructive periodontal disease. As pointed out earlier, acute necrotizing ulcerative gingivitis may occur in a mouth devoid of pre-existing gingival disease, or it may be superimposed upon underlying chronic gingivitis and periodontal pockets. However, it does not usually lead to periodontal pocket formation. It causes rapid destruction of tissue, in contrast to the chronic inflammatory and proliferative changes which give rise to pocket formation.

Histopathology of the characteristic lesion

Microscopically, the lesion appears as a nonspecific acute, necrotizing inflammation at the gingival margin involving both the stratified squamous epithelium and the underlying connective tissue. The surface epithelium is destroyed and replaced by a pseudomembranous meshwork of fibrin, necrotic epithelial cells, polymorphonuclear leukocytes, and various types of microorganisms (Fig. 11–3). This is the zone that appears clinically as the surface pseudomembrane. The underlying connective tissue is markedly hyperemic with numerous engorged capillaries and a dense infiltration of polymorphonuclear leukocytes. This acutely inflamed hyperemic zone appears clinically as the linear erythema beneath the surface pseudomembrane.

The epithelium and connective tissue present alterations in appearance as the distance from the necrotic gingival margin increases. There is a gradual blending of the epithelium from the uninvolved gingiva to the necrotic lesion. At the immediate border of the necrotic pseudomembrane the epithelium is edematous and the individual cells present varying degrees of hydropic degeneration. In addition, there is an infiltration of polymorphonuclear leukocytes in the intercellular spaces. The inflammatory involvement in the connective tissue diminishes as the distance from the necrotic lesion increases until it blends in appearance with the uninvolved connective tissue stroma of the normal gingival mucosa.

It is noteworthy that the microscopic appearance of acute necrotizing ulcerative gingivitis is nonspecific. Comparable changes result from trauma, chemical irritation, or the application of escharotic drugs.

The relation of bacteria to the characteristic lesion has been studied with the light microscope and electron microscope. With the former it appears that the exudate on the surface of the necrotic lesion contains microorganisms which morphologically resemble cocci, fusiform bacilli, and spirochetes.[53] The layer between necrotic and living tissue contains enormous numbers of fusiform bacilli and spirochetes in addition to leukocytes and fibrin. Spirochetes invade the underlying living tissue;[7, 12, 53] other organisms seen on the surface are not found there. Some investigators feel that the spirochetes are pushed into the tissue when gingival specimens are removed for microscopic study.[15]

Electron microscopic examination reveals that in acute necrotizing ulcerative gingivitis, the gingiva is divisible into the following four zones, which blend with

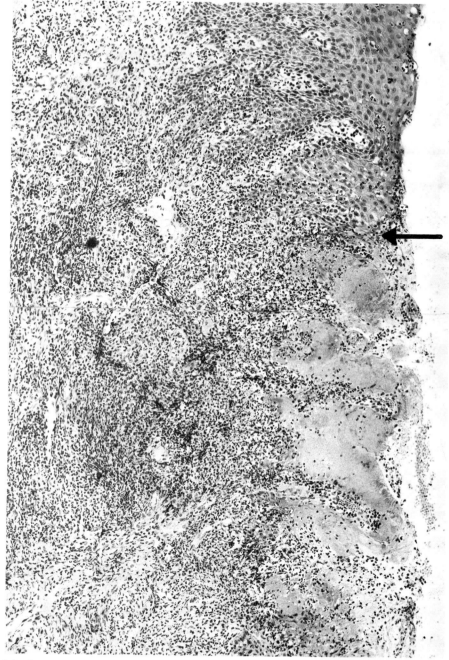

Figure 11–3 Survey Section of the Gingiva in Acute Necrotizing Ulcerative Gingivitis. The portion of the section below the arrow is the accumulation of leukocytes, fibrin, and necrotic tissue which form the gray marginal pseudomembrane.

each other and may not all be present in every case:[29]

Zone 1: *Bacterial zone*, most superficial, consists of varied bacteria, including a few spirochetes of small, medium, and large types.

Zone 2: *Neutrophil-rich zone*, contains numerous leukocytes, predominantly neutrophils, with bacteria, including many spirochetes of various types between the leukocytes.

Zone 3: *Necrotic zone*, consists of disintegrated tissue cells, fibrillar material, remnants of collagen fibers, numerous spirochetes of the intermediate and large type, with few other organisms.

Zone 4: *Zone of spirochetal infiltration,* consists of well-preserved tissue infiltrated with intermediate and large spirochetes, without other organisms.

In no instance are spirochetes deeper than 300 microns from the surface. The majority of spirochetes in the deeper zones are morphologically different from cultivated strains of *Treponema microdentium.* They occur in non-necrotic tissue ahead of other types of bacteria and may be present in high concentrations intercellularly in the epithelium adjacent to the ulcerated lesion and in the connective tissue.

The bacterial flora

Smears taken of the lesions (Fig. 11–4) present scattered bacteria, predominantly spirochetes and fusiform bacilli, desquamated epithelial cells, and occasional polymorphonuclear leukocytes. A smear consisting of only spirochetes and fusiform bacilli is rarely seen. Usually these two organisms are seen together with other oral spirochetes, vibrios, streptococci, and filamentous organisms. The spirochetal organisms form a light-staining, conspicuous, interlacing network throughout the microscopic field.

Electron microscopic studies indicate that **the spirochetes may be classified into three morphologic groups:** "small," 7 to 39 per cent of the total spirochetes present; "intermediate," 43.9 to 90 per cent, and "large," 0 to 20 per cent.[30] It was also suggested that "intermediate" spirochetes are present in greater numbers in pooled scrapings from acute necrotizing ulcerative gingivitis, and are found in greater percentages in the deeper portion of the lesions.

The mean fusiform count in the saliva of patients with acute necrotizing ulcerative

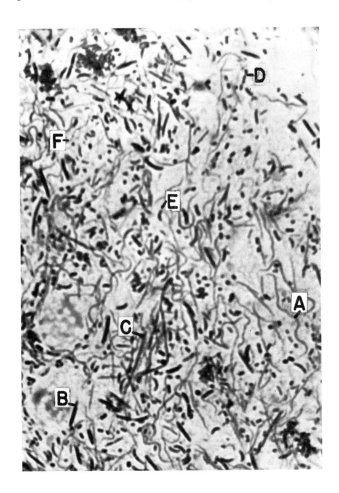

Figure 11–4 Bacterial Smear from Lesion in Acute Necrotizing Ulcerative Gingivitis. *A,* Spirochete. *B,* Bacillus fusiformis. *C,* Filamentous organism (Actinomycetes or Leptotrichia). *D,* Streptococcus. *E,* Vibrio. *F,* Treponema microdentium.

gingivitis is higher than in "normal" patients. Fusobacterium species account for the majority of the total fusiforms in both groups.

Diagnosis

Diagnosis is based upon clinical findings. A bacterial smear may be used to corroborate the clinical diagnosis, but it is not necessary or definitive because the bacterial picture is not appreciably different from that in marginal gingivitis, periodontal pockets, pericoronitis, or herpetic gingivostomatitis.[41] Bacterial studies are useful, however, in the differential diagnosis between acute necrotizing ulcerative gingivitis and specific infections of the oral cavity such as diphtheria, thrush, actinomycosis, and streptococcal stomatitis.

Microscopic examination of the biopsied tissue is not sufficiently specific to be diagnostic. It can be used to differentiate acute necrotizing ulcerative gingivitis from specific infections such as tuberculosis or from neoplastic disease, but it does not differentiate between acute necrotizing ulcerative gingivitis and other acute necrotizing conditions of nonspecific origin such as those produced by trauma or escharotic drugs.

Differential diagnosis

Necrotizing ulcerative gingivitis should be differentiated from other conditions that resemble it in some respects, such as acute herpetic gingivostomatitis (Table 11–1), chronic periodontal pockets, desquamative gingivitis (Table 11–2), streptococcal gingivostomatitis, aphthous stomatitis, gonococcal gingivostomatitis, diphtheritic and syphilitic lesions (Table 11–3), tuberculous gingival lesions, moniliasis, agranulocytosis, dermatoses (pemphigus, erythema multiforme, lichen planus), and stomatitis venenata.

STREPTOCOCCAL GINGIVOSTOMATITIS, GONOCOCCAL STOMATITIS, AGRANULOCYTOSIS, VINCENT'S ANGINA. *Streptococcal gingivostomatitis* is a rare condition characterized by a diffuse erythema of the gingiva and other areas of the oral mucosa. In some instances it is confined as a marginal erythema with marginal hemorrhage. Necrosis of the gingival margin is not a feature of this disease, nor is there a notably fetid odor. Bacterial smears show a predominance of streptococcal forms, which upon culture appear as *Streptococcus viridans*.

Gonococcal stomatitis is rare and is caused by *Neisseria gonorrheae*. The oral mucosa is covered with a grayish membrane that sloughs off in areas exposing an underlying raw bleeding surface.[17] It is most common in the newborn, caused by infection from the maternal passages; but cases in adults caused by direct contact have been described.

Agranulocytosis is characterized by ulceration and necrosis of the gingiva, which resemble that of acute necrotizing ulcerative gingivitis. The oral condition in agranulocytosis is primarily necrotizing. Because of the diminished defense

TABLE 11–1 DIFFERENTIATION BETWEEN ACUTE NECROTIZING ULCERATIVE GINGIVITIS AND ACUTE HERPETIC GINGIVOSTOMATITIS

Acute Necrotizing Ulcerative Gingivitis	Acute Herpetic Gingivostomatitis
Etiology: interaction between host and bacteria, most probably fusospirochetes	Specific viral etiology
Necrotizing condition	Diffuse erythema and vesicular eruption
Punched-out gingival margin. Pseudomembrane that peels off leaving raw areas. Marginal gingiva affected, other oral tissues rarely	Vesicles rupture and leave slightly depressed oval or spherical ulcer
	Diffuse involvement of gingiva, may include buccal mucosa and lips
Relatively uncommon in children	Occurs more frequently in children
No definite duration	Duration of 7 to 10 days
No demonstrated immunity	An acute episode results in some degree of immunity
Contagion not demonstrated	Contagious

TABLE 11–2 DIFFERENTIATION BETWEEN ACUTE NECROTIZING ULCERATIVE GINGIVITIS, CHRONIC DESQUAMATIVE GINGIVITIS AND CHRONIC PERIODONTAL DISEASE

Acute Necrotizing Ulcerative Gingivitis	Desquamative Gingivitis	Chronic Destructive Periodontal Disease
Bacterial smears show fusospirochetal complex	Bacterial smears reveal numerous epithelial cells, few bacterial forms	Bacterial smears are variable
Marginal gingiva affected	Diffuse involvement of the marginal and attached gingiva and other areas of the oral mucosa	Marginal gingiva affected
Acute history	Chronic history	Chronic history
Painful	May or may not be painful	Painless if uncomplicated
Pseudomembrane	Patchy desquamation of the gingival epithelium	No desquamation generally but purulent material may appear from pockets
Papillary and marginal necrotic lesions	Papillae do not undergo necrosis	Papillae do not undergo notable necrosis
Affects adults of both sexes, occasionally children	Affects adults, most often females	Generally in adults, occasionally in children
Characteristic fetid odor	None	Some odor present but not strikingly fetid

mechanism in agranulocytosis, the clinical picture is not marked by the severe inflammatory reaction seen in acute necrotizing ulcerative gingivitis. Blood studies serve to differentiate between necrotizing ulcerative gingivitis and the gingival necrosis in agranulocytosis.

Vincent's angina is a fusospirochetal infection of the oropharynx and throat, as distinguished from acute necrotizing ulcerative gingivitis, which affects the marginal gingiva. In Vincent's angina there is a painful membranous ulceration of the throat with edema and hyperemic patches breaking down to form ulcers covered with pseudomembranous material. The process may extend to the larynx and middle ear.

ACUTE NECROTIZING ULCERATIVE GINGIVITIS IN LEUKEMIA. Leukemia, per se, does not produce acute necrotizing ulcerative gingival inflammation. However, acute necrotizing ulcerative gingivitis may occur superimposed upon gingival tissues altered by leukemia.

The differential diagnosis consists not in

TABLE 11–3 DIFFERENTIATION BETWEEN ACUTE NECROTIZING ULCERATIVE GINGIVITIS, DIPHTHERIA AND SECONDARY STAGE OF SYPHILIS

Acute Necrotizing Ulcerative Gingivitis	Diphtheria	Secondary Stage of Syphilis (Mucous Patch)
Etiology: interaction between host and bacteria, possibly fusospirochetes	Specific bacterial etiology: *Corynebacterium diphtheriae*	Specific bacterial etiology: *Treponema pallidum*
Affects marginal gingiva	Very rarely affects marginal gingiva	Rarely affects marginal gingiva
Membrane removal very easy	Membrane removal difficult	Membrane not detachable
Painful condition	Less painful	Not very painful
Marginal gingiva affected	Throat, fauces, tonsils affected	Any part of mouth affected
Serology negative	Serology negative	Serology positive (Wassermann, Kahn, VDRL)
Immunity not conferred	Immunity conferred by an attack	Immunity not conferred
Doubtful contagiousness	Very contagious	Only direct contact will communicate the disease
Antibiotic therapy relieves symptoms	Antibiotic treatment has little effect	Antibiotic therapy has excellent results

distinguishing between acute necrotizing ulcerative gingivitis and leukemic gingival changes, but rather in determining whether leukemia is a *predisposing factor* in a mouth in which acute necrotizing ulcerative gingivitis is present. For example, if a patient with acute necrotizing involvement of the gingival margin also presents generalized diffuse discoloration and edema of the attached gingiva, the possibility of an *underlying, systemically induced gingival change* should be considered. Leukemia is one of the conditions which would have to be ruled out.

ERYTHEMA MULTIFORME, EROSIVE LICHEN PLANUS, LUPUS ERYTHEMATOSUS, PEMPHIGUS, TUBERCULOUS ULCER, MONILIASIS, STOMATITIS VENENATA, AND CHEMICAL BURNS. For descriptions of the above conditions that may be useful in differentiating between them and acute necrotizing ulcerative gingivitis, see Chapter 12.

Etiology

THE ROLE OF BACTERIA. Plaut[36] and Vincent,[56] in 1894 and 1896 respectively, introduced the concept that acute necrotizing ulcerative gingivitis was caused by specific bacteria, namely, a fusiform bacillus and a spirochetal organism.

Opinions still differ regarding whether bacteria are the primary causative factors in acute necrotizing ulcerative gingivitis. Several observations encourage the concept of primary etiology: **Spirochetal organisms and fusiform bacilli are always found in the disease;** other organisms are also involved. Rosebury, MacDonald and Clark[41] described a fusospirochetal complex consisting of *Treponema microdentium*, intermediate spirochetes, vibrios, fusiform bacilli, and filamentous organisms in addition to several species termed *Borrelia*. The fact that necrotizing ulcerative gingivitis occurs in groups, suggesting contagion, encourages the concept of bacterial origin. The pathogenic mechanism of bacteria, however, remains unclear. An immune pathogenesis has been postulated on the basis of differences in patients and controls in cell-mediated immunity as measured by the lymphocyte transformation test.[59]

Acute necrotizing ulcerative gingivitis has not been produced experimentally in humans or animals by inoculation of bacterial exudates from the lesions. Exudates from acute necrotizing ulcerative gingivitis produce fusospirochetal abscesses when inoculated subcutaneously in experimental animals, and the infection is freely transmissible in series.[40] Local intracutaneous injection of a hyaluronidase and chondroitinase-containing cell-free filtrate of an oral microaerophilic diphtheroid bacillus aggravated spirochetal lesions produced by oral treponemes.[23] Only in one animal experiment has the transmission of lesions comparable to those seen in man been reported.[2]

The specific etiology of acute necrotizing ulcerative gingivitis has not been established. The prevalent opinion is that it is caused by a complex of bacterial organisms, but requiring underlying tissue changes to facilitate the pathogenic activity of the bacteria. In addition to fusiform bacilli, spirochetes, vibrios, and streptococci are invariably included in the complex of bacteria isolated from the lesions in this group of diseases. The other diseases in the group are Vincent's angina, cancrum oris, genital fusospirochetosis, pulmonary fusospirochetosis, tropical ulcer, gangrenous stomatitis, and noma.

LOCAL PREDISPOSING FACTORS. **Preexisting gingivitis, injury to the gingiva and smoking are important predisposing factors.** Although necrotizing ulcerative gingivitis may appear in an otherwise disease-free mouth, it most often occurs *superimposed upon pre-existing chronic gingival disease and periodontal pockets.* Chronic inflammation entails circulatory and degenerative alterations that increase the susceptibility to infection. Any local factors capable of inducing chronic gingival inflammation may predispose to acute necrotizing ulcerative gingivitis. Deep periodontal pockets and pericoronal flaps are particularly vulnerable areas for the occurrence of the disease because they offer a favorable environment for the proliferation of the anaerobic fusiform bacilli and spirochetes. Box[5] refers to such locations as *"incubation zones."*

Areas of the gingiva traumatized by opposing teeth in malocclusion, such as the palatal surface behind maxillary incisors and the labial gingival surface of mandibular incisors, are frequent sites of acute necrotizing ulcerative gingivitis.

SYSTEMIC PREDISPOSING FACTORS. Acute necrotizing ulcerative gingivitis is often superimposed upon gingiva altered by severe systemic disease.

Nutritional Deficiency. Necrotizing gingivitis has been produced by placing animals on nutritionally deficient diets. Goldberger and Wheeler[20] described a deficiency state in dogs simulating human pellagra with oral symptoms consisting of erythema progressing to superficial necrosis of the mucosa of cheeks, tongue, soft palate, and gingiva. Underhill and Mendel[55] produced a similar ulcerative condition in dogs on diets deficient in vitamin A and carotene. The fusospirochetal bacterial complex was found in the oral lesions induced by nutritional deficiency by Smith,[47] Miller and Rhoads,[33] and others.[26] The theory offered to explain their finding was invasion by oral fusospirochetal organisms secondary to lowered tissue resistance caused by deficiency of niacin or vitamin A.

Topping and Fraser[52] found that necrotizing gingivitis occurred in monkeys deficient in vitamin C or B complex with or without nicotinic acid and riboflavin supplements. However, only the animals in the B complex–deficient group developed ulceration at the gingival margin. Fusospirochetal organisms were found in all the experimental animals, but no correlation was made between the bacteria and the clinical lesions. Chapman and Harris[8] confirmed the findings of Topping and Fraser that monkeys maintained on vitamin-deficient diets develop a tendency to oral lesions including necrotizing gingivitis. Animals on diets deficient in vitamin B complex in particular developed severe oral ulcerating lesions. They also found an accompanying increase in the fusospirochetal flora in the mouths of the experimental animals, but the bacteria were regarded as opportunists, proliferating only when the tissues were altered by the vitamin deficiency. Clinical observations have been presented that suggest that low vitamin intake[28] or vitamin C deficiency[38] predisposes to acute necrotizing ulcerative gingivitis.

The Conditioning Effect of Nutritional Deficiency Upon Bacterial Pathogenicity.

Nutritional deficiencies (vitamin C) accentuate the severity of the pathologic changes induced when the fusospirochetal bacterial complex is injected into animals.[47] Necrotizing lesions have been produced by injecting fusospirochetal organisms into vitamin B_2-deficient rats.[27] A correlation between vitamin C deficiency and intestinal fusospirochetosis has been reported in humans and animals.[60] Fusospirochetes may gain a foothold in the intestines in small breaks in the mucosa caused by vitamin C–deficiency–induced mucosal hemorrhages.

Debilitating Disease. Debilitating systemic disease may predispose the gingiva to acute necrotizing ulcerative gingivitis. Included among such systemic disturbances are metallic intoxication, cachexia caused by such chronic diseases as syphilis or cancer, severe gastrointestinal disorders such as ulcerative colitis, blood dyscrasias such as the leukemias and anemia, influenza, and the common cold.[9] Nutritional deficiency secondary to debilitating disease may be an additional predisposing factor. Fusospirochetal abscesses and gingival bleeding[57] have been produced in experimental animals by injecting scillaren B, a mixture of glucosides derived from squill which lowers tissue resistance by reducing the leukocytes.[50, 54] An ulcerative gangrenous stomatitis occurred in animals with experimentally induced leukopenia.[33, 49] Necrotizing gingivitis and stomatitis occurred in 74 per cent of animals with experimentally produced renal insufficiency.[21] Mayo et al.[31] have produced ulceronecrotic lesions in the gingival margin of hamsters exposed to total body irradiation; these lesions could be prevented by systemic antibiotics.

PSYCHOSOMATIC FACTORS. Psychological factors appear to be important in the etiology of acute necrotizing ulcerative gingivitis. The disease often occurs under stress situations such as induction into the army and school examinations.[13, 19] Psychological disturbances are common in patients with the disease,[21] along with increased adrenocortical secretion.[44] Significant correlation between two personality traits, dominance and abasement, suggests the presence of an acute necrotizing ulcerative gingivitis–prone personality.[16] The mechanisms whereby psychologic factors create or predispose to gingival damage have not been established, but alterations in digital and gingival capillary responses suggestive of increased autonomic nervous activity have been demonstrated in patients with acute necrotizing ulcerative gingivitis.[18]

Epidemiology and prevalence

Acute necrotizing ulcerative gingivitis often occurs in groups in an epidemic pattern. At one time it was considered contagious, but this has not been substantiated.[42]

The prevalence of acute necrotizing ulcerative gingivitis appears to have been rather low in the United States and Europe prior to 1914. In World Wars I and II there were numerous "epidemics" among the Allied troops, but Germans did not seem to be similarly affected. There have also been epidemic-like outbreaks among civilian populations. In individuals attending a dental clinic, the following prevalence was reported: 0.08 per cent between 15 and 19 years of age, 0.05 per cent between 20 and 24, and 0.02 per cent between 25 and 29 years.[46]

Acute necrotizing ulcerative gingivitis occurs at all ages,[10] with the highest prevalence reported between ages 20 and 30[11, 48] and between ages 15 and 20.[27] It is not common in children in the United States, Canada, and Europe, but it has been reported in children from low socio-economic groups in underdeveloped countries.[25] In India 54[32] and 58 per cent[35] of the patients in two studies were under 10 years old. In a random school population in Nigeria it occurred in 11.3 per cent of children between the ages of 2 and 6,[45] and in a Nigerian hospital population it was present in 23 per cent of children under 10 years old.[13] In low socio-economic groups it has been reported in several members of the same family. It is more common in mongoloid than in non-mongoloid retarded children.[4]

Opinions differ as to whether it is more common during the winter,[34, 37] summer, or fall,[27, 46] or whether there are no peak seasons.[11, 58]

COMMUNICABILITY. Distinction must be made between communicability and transmissibility when referring to the characteristics of disease. The term *transmissible* denotes a capacity for the maintenance of an infectious agent in successive passage through a susceptible animal host.[39] The term *communicable* signifies a capacity for the maintenance of infection by natural modes of spread such as direct contact through drinking water, food, and eating utensils, via the airborne route, or by means of arthropod vectors. A disease that is communicable is described as contagious. It has been demonstrated that disease associated with the fusospirochetal bacterial complex is transmissible; *however, it has not been shown to be communicable or contagious.*

Attempts have been made to spread acute necrotizing ulcerative gingivitis from human to human without success.[43] King[26] traumatized an area in his gingiva and introduced debris from a severe case of acute necrotizing ulcerative gingivitis. There was no response until he happened to fall ill shortly thereafter, and subsequent to his illness observed the characteristic lesion in the experimental area. It may be inferred with reservation from this experiment that systemic debility is a prerequisite for the contagion of acute necrotizing ulcerative gingivitis.

It is a common impression that, because acute necrotizing ulcerative gingivitis often occurs in groups using the same kitchen facilities, the disease is spread by bacteria on eating utensils. Growth of fusospirochetal organisms requires extremely carefully controlled conditions and an anaerobic environment; they do not ordinarily survive on eating utensils.[23]

The occurrence of the disease in epidemic-like outbreaks does not necessarily mean that it is contagious. The affected groups may be afflicted by the disease because of common predisposing factors rather than because of its spread from person to person. In all likelihood both a predisposed host and proper bacteria are necessary for the production of this disease.

REFERENCES TO ACUTE NECROTIZING ULCERATIVE GINGIVITIS

1. Barnes, G. P., Bowles, W. F., III, and Carter, H. G.: Acute necrotizing ulcerative gingivitis: A

survey of 218 cases. J. Periodontol., *44*:35, 1973.

2. Berke, J. D.: Experimental study of acute ulcerative stomatitis. J. Am. Dent. Assoc., 63:86, 1961.

3. Berman, K. S., and Gibbons, R. J.: Bacteriologic census of debris obtained from Vincent's infection. I.A.D.R. Abstract 267, Forty-Third General Meeting, 1965.

4. Brown, R. H.: Necrotizing ulcerative gingivitis in mongoloid and non-mongoloid retarded individuals. J. Periodont. Res., 8:290, 1973.

5. Box, H. K.: Necrotic Gingivitis. Toronto, University of Toronto Press, 1930.

6. Cadham, F. T.: Vincent's disease; Infection due to fuso-spirillary invasion. J. Can. Med. Assoc., 17:556, 1927.

7. Cahn, L. R.: The penetration of the tissue by Vincent's organisms. A report of a case. J. Dent. Res., 9:695, 1929.

8. Chapman, O. D., and Harris, A. E.: Oral lesions associated with dietary deficiencies in monkeys. J. Infect. Dis., 69:7, 1941.

9. Coutley, R. L.: Vincent's infection. Br. Dent. J., 74:34, 1943.

10. Daley, F. H.: Studies of Vincent's infection at the clinic of Tufts College Dental School from October, 1926 to February, 1928. J. Dent. Res., 8:408, 1928.

11. Dean, H. T., and Singleton, J. E., Jr.: Vincent's infection—A wartime disease. Am. J. Public Health, 35:433, 1945.

12. Ellerman: Vincent's organisms in tissue. Z. Hyg. Infekt. Pr., 56:453, 1907.

13. Emslie, R. D.: Cancrum oris. Dent. Practit., *13*: 481, 1963.

14. Enwonwu, C. O.: Epidemiological and biochemical studies of necrotizing ulcerative gingivitis and noma (cancrum oris) in Nigerian children. Arch. Oral Biol., 17:1357, 1972.

15. Fish, E. W.: Parodontal Disease. London, Eyre and Spottiswoode, Ltd., 1946.

16. Formicola, A. J., Witte, E. T., and Curran, P. M.: A study of personality traits and acute necrotizing ulcerative gingivitis. J. Periodontol., *41*:36, 1970.

17. Frazer, A. D., and Menton, J.: Gonococcal stomatitis. Br. Med. J., 1:1020, 1931.

18. Giddon, D. B.: Psychophysiology of the oral cavity. J. Dent. Res. (suppl. to #6), 45:1627, 1966.

19. Giddon, D. B., Zackin, S. J., and Goldhaber, P.: Acute necrotizing gingivitis in college students. J. Am. Dent. Assoc., 68:381, 1964.

20. Goldberger, J., and Wheeler, G. A.: Experimental black tongue of dogs and its relation to pellagra. U.S. Public Health Report, *43*:172, 1928.

21. Goldhaber, P., and Giddon, D. B.: Present concepts concerning the etiology and treatment of acute necrotizing ulcerative gingivitis. Int. Dent. J., *14*:468, 1964.

22. Hadi, A. W., and Russell, C.: Quantitative estimations of fusiforms in saliva from normal individuals and cases of acute ulcerative gingivitis. Arch. Oral Biol., *13*:1371, 1968.

23. Hampp, E. G., and Mergenhagen, S. E.: Experimental infection with oral spirochetes. J. Infect. Dis., *109*:43, 1961.

24. Holman, R. L.: Necrotizing arteritis in dogs related to diet and renal insufficiency. Am. J. Pathol., *19*:993, 1943.

25. Jimenez, M., and Baer, P. N.: Necrotizing ulcerative gingivitis in children: A 9 year clinical study. J. Periodontol., 46:715, 1975.

26. King, J. D.: Nutritional and other factors in trench mouth with special reference to the nicotinic acid component of vitamin B complex. Br. Dent. J., 74:113, 1943.

27. Kirkpatrick, R. M., and Clements, F. W.: Diet in relation to Vincent's infection. Dent. J. Australia, 6:371, 1934.

28. Lapira, E.: Ulcerative stomatitis associated with avitaminosis in Malta. Br. Dent. J., *74*:257, 1943.

29. Listgarten, M. A.: Electron microscopic observations on the bacterial flora of acute necrotizing ulcerative gingivitis. J. Periodontol., *36*: 328, 1965.

30. Listgarten, M. A., and Lewis, D. W.: The distribution of spirochetes in the lesion of acute necrotizing ulcerative gingivitis: An electron microscopic and statistical survey. J. Periodontol., *38*:379, 1967.

31. Mayo, J., Carranza, F. A., Jr., Epper, C. E., and Cabrini, R. L.: The effect of total-body irradiation on the oral tissues of the Syrian hamster. Oral Surg., *15*:739, 1962.

32. Miglani, D. C., and Sharma, O. P.: Incidence of acute necrotizing gingivitis and periodontosis among cases seen at the government hospital, Madras. J. All Ind. Dent. Assoc., *37*:183, 1965.

33. Miller, D. K., and Rhoads, C. P.: The experimental production in dogs of acute stomatitis associated with leukopenia and a maturation defect of the myeloid elements of the bone marrow. J. Exp. Med., *61*:173, 1935.

34. Pedler, J. A., and Radden, B. G.: Seasonal influence of acute ulcerative gingivitis. Dent. Pract. Dent. Rec., 8:23, 1957.

35. Pindborg, J. J., et al.: Occurrence of acute necrotizing gingivitis in South Indian children. J. Periodontol., 37:14, 1966.

36. Plaut, H. C.: Studien zur bakteriellen Diagnostik der Diphtherie und der Anginen. Dtsch. Med. Wochnschr., 20:920, 1894.

37. Proske, H. O., and Sayers, R. R.: Pulmonary fusospirochetal infection. U.S. Public Health Reports, 49:839, 1934.

38. Radusch, D. F.: Nutrition and dental health. J. Periodontol., *17*:27, 1946.

39. Rosebury, T.: Is Vincent's infection a communicable disease? J. Am. Dent. Assoc., 29:823, 1942.

40. Rosebury, T., and Foley, G.: Experimental Vincent's infection. J. Am. Dent. Assoc., 26:1798, 1939.

41. Rosebury, T., MacDonald, J. B., and Clark, A.: A bacteriologic survey of gingival scrapings from periodontal infections by direct examination, Guinea pig inoculation and anaerobic cultivation. J. Dent. Res., 29:718, 1950.

42. Schluger, S.: Necrotizing ulcerative gingivitis in the army. Incidence, communicability, and treatment. J. Am. Dent. Assoc., 38:174, 1949.

43. Schwartzman, J., and Grossman, L.: Vincent's ul-

ceromembranous gingivostomatitis. Arch. Pediatr., 58:515, 1941.

44. Shannon, I. L., Kilgore, W. G., and Leary, T. J.: Stress as a predisposing factor in necrotizing ulcerative gingivitis. J. Periodontol., 40:240, 1969.

45. Sheiham, A.: An epidemiological study of oral disease in Nigerians. J. Dent. Res., 44:1184, 1965.

46. Skach, M., Zabrodsky, S., and Mrklas, L.: A study of the effect of age and season on the incidence of ulcerative gingivitis. J. Periodont. Res., 5:187, 1970.

47. Smith, D. T.: Spirochetes and related organisms in fusospirochetal disease. Baltimore, The Williams & Wilkins Company, 1932.

48. Stammers, A. F.: Vincent's infection. Br. Dent. J., 76:171, 1944.

49. Swenson, H. M.: Induced Vincent's infection in dogs. J. Dent. Res., 23:190, 1944.

50. Swenson, H. M., and Muhler, J. C.: Induced fusospirochetal infection in dogs. J. Dent. Res., 26:161, 1947.

51. Thompson, L. E.: A fatal case of brain abscess from Vincent's angina. Dent. Digest, 35:821, 1929.

52. Topping, N. H., and Fraser, H. F.: Mouth lesions associated with dietary deficiencies in monkeys. U.S. Public Health Reports, 54:431, 1939.

53. Tunnicliff, R., Fink, E. B., and Hammond, C.: Significance of fusiform bacilli and spirilla in gingival tissue. J. Am. Dent. Assoc., 23:1959, 1936.

54. Tunnicliff, R., and Hammond, C.: Abscess production by fusiform bacilli in rabbits and mice by the use of Scillaren-B or Mucin. J. Dent. Res., 16:479, 1937.

55. Underhill, F. P., and Mendel, L. B.: Further experiments on the pellagra-like syndrome in dogs. Am. J. Physiol., 83:589, 1928.

56. Vincent, H.: Sur l'étiologie et sur les lésions anatomopathologiques de la pourriture d'hôpital. Ann. de l'Inst. Pasteur, 10:448, 1896.

57. Wallace, H., Wallace, E. W., and Robertson, O. H.: The production of experimental Plaut-Vincent's angina in the dog. J. Clin. Invest., 12:909, 1933.

58. Wilkie, R.: An etiology of Vincent's gingivitis. Br. Dent. J., 78:65, 1945,

59. Wilton, J. M. A., Ivanyi, A., and Lehner, T.: Cell-mediated immunity and humoral antibodies in acute ulcerative gingivitis. J. Periodont. Res., 6:9, 1971.

60. Woolsey, F. M., and Black, S. R.: Vitamin C deficiency and intestinal fusospirochetoses. Arch. Pathol., 28:503, 1939.

ACUTE HERPETIC GINGIVOSTOMATITIS

Etiology

Acute herpetic gingivostomatitis is an infection of the oral cavity caused by the herpes simplex virus.[7, 13, 17] Secondary bacterial infection frequently complicates the clinical picture. Acute herpetic gingivostomatitis occurs most frequently in infants and children below the age of 6,[17] but it is also seen in adolescents and adults. It occurs with equal frequency in males and females.

Clinical features

ORAL SIGNS. The condition appears as a diffuse, erythematous, shiny involvement of the gingiva and the adjacent oral mucosa with varying degrees of edema and gingival bleeding (Color Plate 2E). In its initial stage, it is characterized by the presence of discrete spherical gray vesicles (Color Plate 2F), which may occur on the gingiva, the labial and buccal mucosa, the soft palate, the pharynx, the sublingual mucosa, and the tongue (Fig. 11–5). After

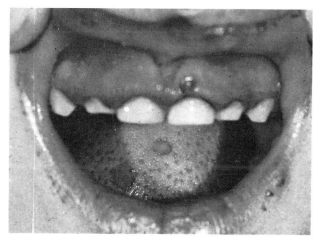

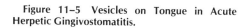
Figure 11–5 Vesicles on Tongue in Acute Herpetic Gingivostomatitis.

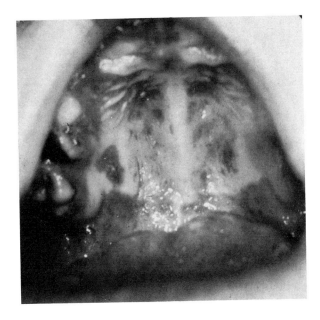

Figure 11–6 Involvement of the Palate in Acute Herpetic Gingivostomatitis.

approximately 24 hours the vesicles rupture and form painful small ulcers with a red, elevated halo-like margin and a depressed yellowish or grayish white central portion. These occur either in widely separated areas or in clusters where confluence occurs (Fig. 11–6).

Occasionally, acute herpetic gingivitis may occur without overt vesiculation. Diffuse erythematous shiny discoloration and edematous enlargement of the gingivae with a tendency toward bleeding comprise the clinical picture.

The course of the disease is limited to 7 to 10 days. The diffuse gingival erythema and edema that appear early in the disease persist for several days after the ulcerative lesions have healed. Scarring does not occur in the areas of healed ulcerations.

Acute herpetic gingivostomatitis may appear in a *localized* form following operative procedures in the oral cavity. Surfaces of the oral mucosa traumatized by cotton rolls or vigorous application of digital pressure in the course of operative procedures are the sites of predilection. The condition appears one or two days after the trauma, and the involvement presents

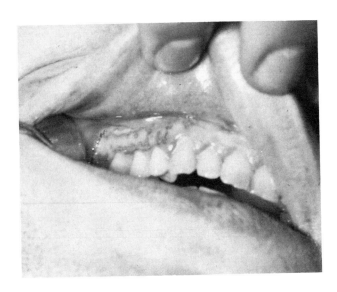

Figure 11–7 Acute Herpetic Involvement Following Surface Trauma With a Cotton Roll.

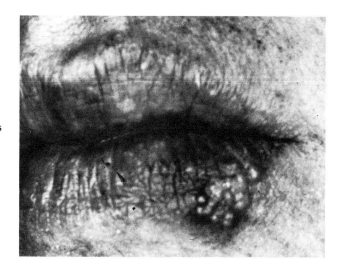

Figure 11–8 Cluster of Herpetic Vesicles ("Cold Sore").

a diffuse shiny erythema with numerous pinpoint vesicles confined to an area that can be clearly demarcated from adjacent uninvolved mucosa (Fig. 11–7). The vesicles rupture and form painful ulcerations. The duration of the involvement is 7 to 10 days, followed by uneventful healing.

ORAL SYMPTOMS. The disease is accompanied by generalized "soreness" of the oral cavity, which interferes with eating or drinking. The ruptured vesicles are the focal sites of pain, and are particularly sensitive to touch, thermal changes and condiments, fruit juices, and the excursive action of coarse foods. In infants the disease is marked by irritability and refusal to take food.

EXTRA-ORAL AND SYSTEMIC SIGNS AND SYMPTOMS. Herpetic involvement of the lips or face (herpes labialis, "cold sore") with vesicles and surface scab formation may accompany the intraoral disease (Fig. 11–8). Cervical adenitis, fever as high as 101 to 105° F. (38.3 to 40.6° C), and generalized malaise are common.

HISTORY. Recent acute infection is a common feature of the history of patients with acute herpetic gingivostomatitis.[7] The condition frequently occurs during and immediately after an episode of such febrile disease as pneumonia, meningitis, influenza, and typhoid. It also tends to occur in periods of anxiety, strain, or exhaustion and during menstruation. A history of exposure to patients with herpetic infection of the oral cavity or lips may also be elicited. Acute herpetic gingivostomatitis often occurs in the early stage of infectious mononucleosis.[14]

Histopathology

The discrete ulcerations of herpetic gingivostomatitis that result from rupture of the vesicles present a central portion of acute inflammation with ulceration and varying degrees of purulent exudate surrounded by a zone rich in engorged blood vessels. The microscopic picture of the vesicles is characterized by extra- and intracellular edema and degeneration of the epithelial cells. The cell cytoplasm appears liquefied and clear; the cell membrane and nucleus stand out in relief. The nucleus later degenerates, loses its affinity for stain, and finally disintegrates. The vesicle formation results from fragmentation of the degenerated epithelial cells.

The fully developed vesicle is a cavity in the epithelial cells with occasional polymorphonuclear leukocytes. The base of the vesicle is formed by edematous epithelial cells of the basal and prickle cell layers. The superficial surface of the vesicle is formed by compressed upper layers of prickle cells of the stratum granulosum and the stratum corneum. Occasionally, rounded eosinophilic inclusion bodies[12] are found in the nuclei of epithelial cells bordering vesicles. According to present theories, inclusion bodies may be either a colony of virus particles, degenerated protoplasm remnants of the affected cell, or a combination of both.[15]

Diagnosis

The diagnosis is usually established from the patient's history and the clinical findings.[11] Material may be obtained from the lesions and submitted to the laboratory for confirmatory tests.

DIRECT SMEARS. If the vesicle is intact, the top is removed and the fluid allowed to escape. The base of the lesion is scraped with a sharp instrument and the material obtained is smeared on a glass, allowed to dry, and stained. The finding of multinuclear cells with swelling, ballooning, and degeneration is adequate for diagnosis; negative findings owing to too early or too late sampling constitute a serious limitation.[4] Electron microscopy of fresh or formalin-fixed material can also be used for diagnosis of herpetic infections.[16] Immunofluorescent antibody techniques have also been used successfully.[8]

ISOLATION OF THE VIRUS. This can be done in tissue culture or in the chorio-allantoic membrane of a chick embryo. For the analysis in *tissue culture*, material obtained from the lesion on a sterile cotton-tipped applicator is sent to the laboratory in skimmed milk. This is then inoculated into cultures of susceptible cells and incubated for 24 hours. Degenerative cellular changes preventable by antibody to herpes simplex constitute a positive finding.

For the analysis in *chick embryo*, the material removed from the suspected lesion is placed in salivary solution or thioglycollate media. Small amounts of the material are injected into 10-day-old embryo-nated eggs; after 48 hours the egg is opened and the chorioallantoic membrane inspected for pocks or viral colonies.

ANTIBODY TITRATIONS. If a specimen of blood is collected when the patient is first seen and examined for neutralizing antibodies, none will be found. Successive specimens taken during the convalescent period will show a rising titer of neutralizing antibodies that will remain high permanently.

BIOPSY. Stained sections of the vesicles of acute herpetic gingivostomatitis, herpes zoster, and varicella (chicken pox) reveal eosinophilic intranuclear inclusion bodies in the peripheral cells (Fig. 11–9).

HEMATOLOGIC STUDIES. It has not been possible to demonstrate alterations in the hematologic picture of patients with acute herpetic gingivostomatitis.

Differential diagnosis

Acute herpetic gingivostomatitis should be differentiated from the following conditions:

1. ACUTE NECROTIZING ULCERATIVE GINGIVITIS. (See page 141.)

2. ERYTHEMA MULTIFORME. The vesicles in erythema multiforme are generally more extensive than those in acute herpetic gingivostomatitis and upon rupture

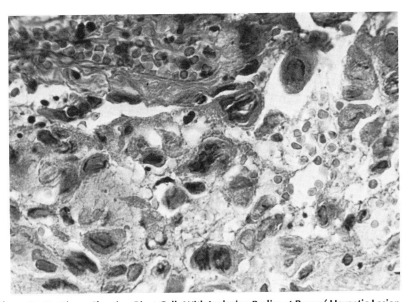

Figure 11–9   Biopsy Showing Giant Cells With Inclusion Bodies at Base of Herpetic Lesion.

present a tendency toward pseudomembrane formation. In addition, the tongue in the former condition usually is markedly involved, with infection of the ruptured vesicles resulting in varying degrees of ulceration. Oral involvement in erythema multiforme may be accompanied by skin lesions. The duration of erythema multiforme may be comparable to that of acute herpetic gingivostomatitis, but prolonged involvement for a period of weeks is not uncommon.

The Stevens-Johnson Syndrome. This is a comparatively rare form of erythema multiforme, characterized by vesicular hemorrhagic lesions in the oral cavity, hemorrhagic ocular lesions, and bullous skin lesions.

3. BULLOUS LICHEN PLANUS. This painful condition, characterized by large blisters on the tongue and cheek that rupture and undergo ulceration, runs a prolonged, indefinite course. Patches of linear gray lace-like lesions of lichen planus are often interspersed among the bullous eruptions. Coexistent involvement of the skin affords a basis of differentiation between bullous lichen planus and acute herpetic gingivostomatitis.

4. DESQUAMATIVE GINGIVITIS. This condition is characterized by diffuse involvement of the gingiva with varying degrees of "peeling" of the epithelial surface and exposure of the underlying tissue. It is a chronic condition.

5. APHTHOUS STOMATITIS (CANKER SORE). This is a condition characterized by the appearance of discrete spherical vesicles that rupture after one or two days and form depressed spherical ulcers. The ulcers consist of a saucer-like red or grayish red central portion and an elevated rim-like periphery (Fig. 11–10). The lesions may occur anywhere in the oral cavity, the mucobuccal fold and the floor of the mouth being common sites. Aphthous stomatitis is painful. It may occur as single lesions or scattered throughout the mouth. The duration of each lesion is 7 to 10 days. As a rule, the lesions are larger than those seen in acute herpetic gingivostomatitis.

Aphthous stomatitis occurs in the following forms:

Occasional Aphthae. In this condition a single lesion occurs occasionally, at inter-

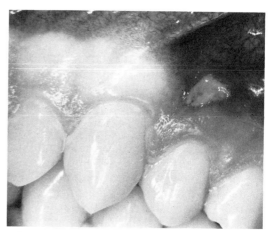

Figure 11–10 Aphthous Lesion in the Mucobuccal Fold. The depressed gray center is surrounded by an elevated red border.

vals that vary from months to years. Healing of the lesion is followed by uneventful recovery.

Acute Aphthae. This condition is characterized by an acute episode of aphthae, which may persist for weeks. During this period, lesions appear in different areas of the mouth, replacing others that are healing or healed. Such acute episodes are often seen in children with acute gastrointestinal disorders and may also occur in adults under comparable conditions. Remission of the gastrointestinal disturbance is generally accompanied by cessation of the acute episode of aphthae.

Chronic Recurrent Aphthae. This is a perplexing condition in which one or more oral lesions are always present. The involvement may extend over a period of years. In rare instances, lesions on the genital, anal, and conjunctival mucosa accompany the oral aphthae. One or more oral lesions are always present. The duration of involvement with chronic aphthae may be a period of years.

The etiology of aphthous stomatitis is unknown. Herpes simplex virus was suspected to be the cause, but antibody[20] and tissue culture[18] studies discourage this opinion. Other factors suggested as causing or predisposing to aphthous stomatitis include hormonal disturbances, allergic phenomena,[2] gastrointestinal disorders, and psychosomatic factors.[1]

Aphthous stomatitis is a different clinical entity from acute herpetic gingivostomatitis.[6, 21] The ulcerations may appear the same in both conditions, but diffuse erythematous involvement of the gingiva and acute toxic systemic symptoms do not occur in aphthous stomatitis.

Communicability

Acute herpetic gingivostomatitis is contagious.[5, 12] Most adults have developed immunity to herpes simplex virus as the result of infection during childhood,[3] which in most instances is subclinical. For this reason acute herpetic gingivostomatitis occurs most often in infants and children. Although recurrent herpetic gingivostomatitis has been reported,[10] it does not ordinarily recur unless immunity is destroyed by debilitating systemic disease. Herpetic infection of the skin such as herpes labialis does recur.[19]

REFERENCES TO ACUTE HERPETIC GINGIVOSTOMATITIS

1. Alexander, F., and French, W.: Studies in Psychosomatic Medicine. Chicago. University of Chicago Press, 1948.
2. Brinck, O.: Clinical observations on the etiology of stomatitis aphthosa. Paradentium, 11:192, 1939.
3. Burnet, F. M., and Williams, S. W.: Herpes simplex: New point of view. Med. J. Australia, 1:637, 1939.
4. Cawson, R. A.: Infections of the oral mucous membrane. In Cohen, B., and Kramer, I.R.H.: Scientific Foundations of Dentistry. Chicago, Year Book Medical Publishers, 1976.
5. Chilton, N. W.: Herpetic stomatitis. Am. J. Orthod. Oral Surg., 30:335, 1944.
6. Dodd, R., and Ruchman, J.: Herpes simplex virus not the etiologic agent of recurrent stomatitis. Pediatrics, 5:833, 1950.
7. Dodd, K., Johnston, L. M., and Buddingh, G. J.: Herpetic stomatitis. J. Pediatr., 12:95, 1938.
8. Gardner, P. S., McQuillin, J., Black, M. M., and Richardson, J.: Rapid diagnosis of herpesvirus hominis infections in superficial lesions by immunofluorescent antibody techniques. Br. Med. J., 4:89, 1968.
9. Greenberg, M. S., Brightman, V. J., and Ship, I. I.: Clinical and laboratory differentiation of recurrent intraoral herpes simplex virus infections following fever. J. Dent. Res., 48:385, 1969.
10. Griffin, J. W.: Recurrent intraoral herpes simplex virus infection. Oral Surg., 19:209, 1965.
11. Grinspan, D.: Enfermedades de la Boca. Vol. 2: Patologia Clinica y Terapeutica de la Mucosa Bucal. Buenos Aires, Ed. Mundi, 1972.
12. Levine, H. D., et al.: Vesicular pharyngitis and stomatitis. J.A.M.A., 112:2020, 1939.
13. McNair, S. T.: Herpetic stomatitis. J. Dent. Res., 29:647, 1950.
14. Nathanson, I., and Morin, G. E.: Herpetic stomatitis. An aid in the early diagnosis of infectious mononucleosis. Oral Surg., 6:1284, 1953.
15. Nicolau, S., and Kopciowska, L.: Inclusion bodies in experimental herpes. Ann. Inst. Pasteur, 60:401, 1938.
16. Roy, S., and Wolman, L.: Electron microscopic observations on the virus particles in herpes simplex encephalitis. J. Clin. Pathol., 22:51, 1969.
17. Scott, T. F. M., Steigman, A. S., and Convey, J. H.: Acute infectious gingivostomatitis: Etiology, epidemiology, and clinical picture of common disorders caused by virus of herpes simplex. J.A.M.A., 117:999, 1941.
18. Ship, I. I., Ashe, W. K., and Scherp, H. W.: Recurrent "fever blister" and "canker sore": Test for herpes simplex and other viruses with mammalian cell cultures. Arch. Oral Biol., 3:117, 1961.
19. Ship, I. I., Brightman, V. J., and Laster, L. L.: The patient with recurrent aphthous ulcers and the patient with recurrent herpes labialis: A study of two population samples. J. Am. Dent. Assoc., 75:645, 1967.
20. Stark, M. M., Kibbrick, S., and Weisberger, D.: Studies on recurrent aphthae. Evidence that herpes simplex is not the etiologic agent with further observations on the immune responses in herpetic infection. J. Lab. Clin. Med., 44:261, 1954.
21. Weathers, D. R., and Griffin, J. W.: Intraoral ulcerations of recurrent herpes simplex and recurrent aphthae: Two distinct clinical entities. J. Am. Dent. Assoc., 81:81, 1970.

PERICORONITIS

The term *pericoronitis* refers to inflammation of the gingiva in relation to the crown of an incompletely erupted tooth (Fig. 11–11). It occurs most frequently in the mandibular third molar area.[1, 4, 5] Pericoronitis may be acute, subacute, or chronic.

Clinical features

The partially erupted or impacted mandibular third molar is the most common site of pericoronitis. The space between the crown of the tooth and the overlying gingival flap is an ideal area for the accumulation of food debris and bacterial growth (Fig. 11–12). Even in patients with no clinical signs or symptoms, the gingival flap is often chronically inflamed and infected and presents varying degrees of ul-

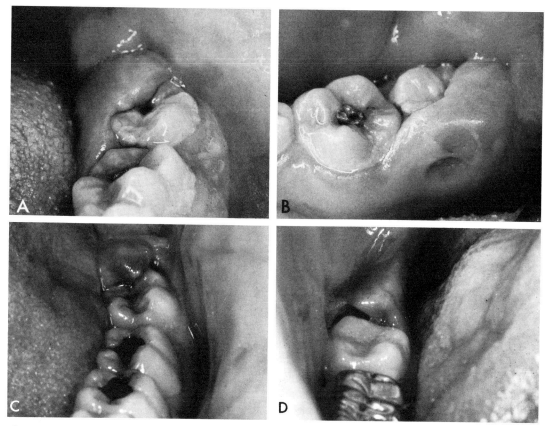

Figure 11–11   Pericoronitis. A, Third molar partially covered by infected flap. B, Lingual view showing sinus draining from infected flap. C, Swollen flap with suppuration at the tip. D, Opening into pericoronal abscess.

ceration along its inner surface. Acute inflammatory involvement is a constantly imminent possibility.

Acute pericoronitis is identified by varying degrees of involvement of the pericoronal flap and adjacent structures as well as systemic complications. Influx of inflammatory fluid and cellular exudate results in an increase in the bulk of the flap, which interferes with complete closure of the jaws. The flap is traumatized by contact with the opposing jaw and the inflammatory involvement is aggravated. **The resultant clinical picture is that of a markedly red, swollen, suppurating lesion that is exquisitely tender, with radiating pains to the ear, throat, and floor of the mouth.** In addition to the pain, the patient is extremely uncomfortable because of a foul taste and an inability to close the jaws. Swelling of the cheek in the region

of the angle of the jaw and lymphadenitis are common findings. The patient may also present toxic systemic complications such as fever, leukocytosis, and malaise.

Complications

The involvement may become localized in the form of a pericoronal abscess. It may spread posteriorly into the oropharyngeal area and medially to the base of the tongue, making it difficult for the patient to swallow. Depending upon the severity and extent of the infection, there is lymph node involvement of the submaxillary, posterior cervical, deep cervical, and retropharyngeal lymph nodes.[2, 3] Peritonsillar abscess formation, cellulitis, and Ludwig's angina are infrequent but nevertheless potential sequelae of acute pericoronitis.

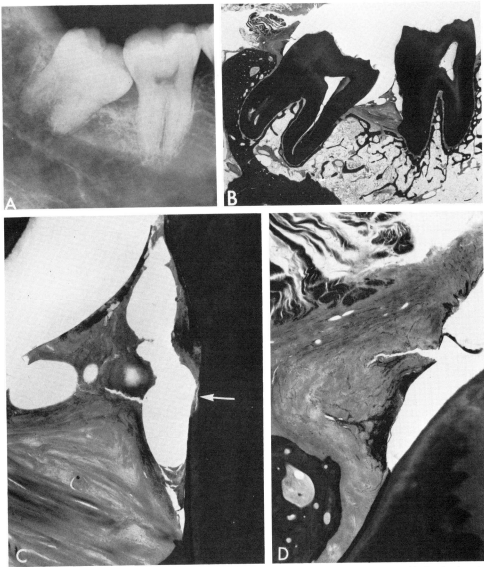

Figure 11–12 Pericoronitis Around Impacted Third Molar. *A,* Radiograph of impacted *mandibular* third molar. *B,* Survey section of molar area. *C,* Plaque, bacteria, and calculus between the second and third molars. Note the resorption of cementum and dentin on the distal surface of the second molar *(arrow)*. *D,* Inflamed gingiva on the distal surface of the third molar.

REFERENCES TO PERICORONITIS

1. Blair, V. P.: The gingival operculum and the erupting lower third molar. Arch. Clin. Oral Pathol., *4*:283, 1940.
2. Jacobs, M. H.: Pericoronal and Vincent's infections: Bacteriology and treatment. J. Am. Dent. Assoc., *30*:392, 1943.
3. Perkins, A. E.: Acute infections around erupting mandibular third molar. Br. Dent. J., *76*:199, 1944.
4. Robinson, R. A.: Clinical aspects of diseases associated with impacted mandibular third molars. Arch. Clin. Oral Pathol., *4*:348, 1940.
5. Salman, I.: Pericoronal infection. Dent. Outlook, *26*:460, 1939.

Chapter 12

The Oral Manifestations of Dermatologic Disease

Oral and skin lesions often occur together in dermatologic disease.[33] Furthermore, changes in the oral cavity may mark the onset of the disease and precede the skin lesions by months or years. In many conditions such as lichen planus, erythema multiforme, and pyostomatitis vegetans, oral lesions may constitute the only manifestation. Oral manifestations in the absence of skin involvement often result from drugs capable of causing dermatoses. Gingival involvement in dermatologic disorders presents a challenging diagnostic and therapeutic problem.

LICHEN PLANUS (LICHEN RUBER PLANUS)

Lichen planus is an inflammatory disease of skin and mucous membrane characterized by the eruption of papules. The papules are violaceous and pointed on skin, but tend to be white and flattened on mucosa. When the disease is confined to the skin, it may be acute, subacute, or chronic; oral involvement is usually chronic. The etiology is generally considered to be psychosomatic.

Oral lesions

Lichen planus may be confined to skin or oral mucosa, or may develop in both locations.[49] However, it has become apparent that a large percentage of cases remain confined to the oral cavity, and the lesions often present a diagnostic problem because of their variability in clinical appearance.

Frictional factors play a role in determining the location of lesions of lichen planus, and the most common oral sites are the buccal mucosa in relation to the occlusal plane of the teeth, the lateral borders of the tongue, the labial and buccal surfaces of the attached gingiva, the hard palate, and the lower lip. The lesions are often symmetrical and tend to be dendritic and papular. The dendritic or reticulated lesions consist of grayish white, linear, lacelike elevations composed of large numbers of small individual papules. Isolated papules of pin-head size may also be observed (Figs. 12–1 to 12–3). In addition to the raised dendritic lesions there may also be raised plaque-like lesions and reddened areas of erosion and ulceration. Vesicles and bullae may also appear in lichen planus and will confuse the clinical picture by suggesting the possibility of a vesiculobullous dermatosis such as pemphigus or pemphigoid. The bullae eventually rupture, leaving areas of ulceration and erosion or desquamation. The great variability in the clinical appearance of the oral lesions of lichen planus depends upon the unique microscopic alterations and the severity of the degenerative changes in the basal layer of the epithelium.

The skin involvement of lichen planus usually results in a pruritus, but the oral lesions tend to be asymptomatic, except if erosion or ulceration is present. These areas may be sensitive to hot, acid, or spicy foods, and extensive areas of ulcerations may be painful. The disease tends to run a chronic or subacute course with the duration varying from several months to many years. Periods of exacerbation of lesions tend to relate to episodes of emotional stress.

Gingival lesions

The gingival tissue is often involved in oral lichen planus and the pattern is extremely variable.[1, 23] Lesions may represent one or more types of four distinctive patterns.

1. *Keratotic lesions.* These raised white

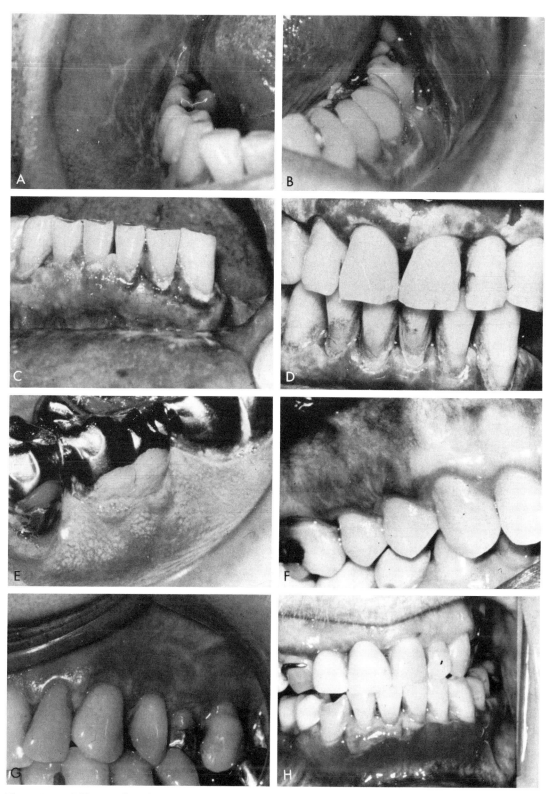

Figure 12-1 Different Clinical Patterns of Oral Lichen Planus: *A,* Reticulate lesions on buccal mucosa. *B,* Reticulate lesions on gingiva. *C,* Reticulate and plaque-like lesions on gingiva and labial mucosa. *D,* Plaque-like and erosive lesions on gingiva. *E,* Papular lesions on gingiva. *F,* Erosive and striated lesions on gingiva. *G,* Erosive and desquamative lesions on gingiva. *H,* Bullous involvement of mandibular gingiva. A large bulla has ruptured, leaving extensive ulceration.

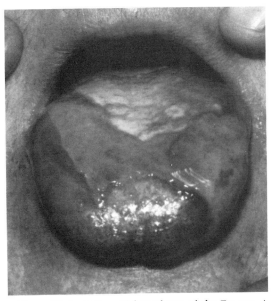

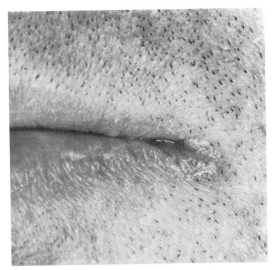

Figure 12-3 Lichen Planus at the labial commissure showing typical papules.

Figure 12-2 Bullous Lichen Planus of the Tongue. A ruptured bulla appears anteriorly and plaque-like lesions posteriorly.

lesions may present as groups of individual papules, as linear or reticulated lesions, or as plaque-like configurations (Fig. 12–1B to E).

2. *Erosive or ulcerative lesions.* These red areas may present as a patchy distribution among keratotic lesions or as extensive involvement. There may be hemorrhage upon slight trauma such as toothbrushing (Fig. 12–1F and G).

3. *Vesicular or bullous involvement.* Raised fluid-filled lesions will rupture, leaving ulceration (Fig. 12–1H).

4. *Atrophic involvement.* Atrophic forms of lichen planus usually occur on tongue or gingiva. Atrophic involvement of the dorsum of the tongue is characterized by loss of filiform and fungiform papillae, resulting in a smooth, reddened dorsal surface. Atrophic involvement of the gingiva results in a thinning of epithelium and a resulting erosive or "desquamative" gingivitis. Since lichen planus is a common disease of the oral mucosa, most cases of so-called "desquamative" gingivitis are in reality cases of erosive gingival lichen planus. If the mouth is carefully examined, lesions in sites other than the gingiva are usually found. In a small number of cases of oral lichen planus (less than 10 per cent), the involvement is confined to the gingiva and the clinical pattern is one of erosion and desquamation.

Histopathology

Microscopically, lichen planus is characterized by three main features—hyperkeratosis or parakeratosis, hydropic degeneration of the basal layer of stratum germinativum, and a dense infiltration of lymphocytes as a broad band in the upper corium adjacent to the epithelium (Figs. 12–4 and 12–5). Occasionally, there may be extension of rete pegs in a saw-tooth pattern, but this feature is more typical of lesions on skin. The hydropic degeneration of the basal layer of the epithelium may be sufficiently extensive that the epithelium becomes thin and atrophic or lifts off the underlying corium and produces either a subepithelial vesicle or an ulcer. The nature of the clinical lesion depends upon the microscopic pattern. The white papular or reticulate lesions demonstrate hyperkeratosis or parakeratosis and lymphocytic infiltration. Erosive or ulcerative lesions demonstrate extensive degeneration of basal layer and patchy loss of epithelium. Vesicular lesions show degenerative and epithelial separation from underlying connective tissue. Atrophic lesions show a thin degenerating epithelium. A microscopic diagnosis can usually be made of oral lesions of lichen planus, but the characteristic pattern is found in the keratotic lesions, and biopsy

Fig. 12–4

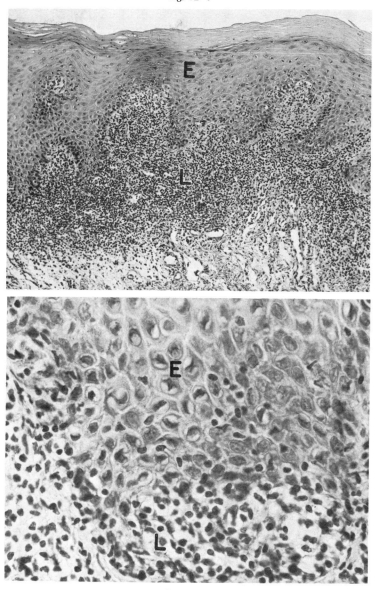

Fig. 12–5

Figure 12–4   Microscopic Appearance of Lichen Planus. Biopsy from lesion on the gingiva showing hyperkeratosis and acanthosis of the epithelium *(E),* as well as extension of rete pegs. There is dense lymphocytic infiltration of the lamina propria *(L)* confined to a broad zone immediately beneath the epithelium.

Figure 12–5   High power view of Fig. 12–4 showing hydropic degeneration in the basal layer of the epithelium *(E)* with lymphocytic infiltration in the lamina propria *(L).*

specimens should be taken in these areas if possible. Oral lesions of lichen planus change in pattern and occasionally a second or even third biopsy may be necessary before a definitive diagnosis can be made in certain unusual cases.

Electron microscopic studies indicate that li-

chen planus can be divided into three stages. The earliest stage is degeneration of the cytoplasm of the epithelial cells with aggregation of particulate material. The intercellular spaces are enlarged, accompanied by lymphocytic infiltration. In the second stage there is loss of collagen fibers in the superficial lamina

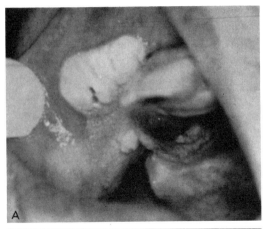

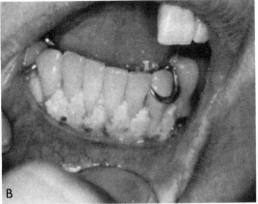

Figure 12–6   Leukoplakia of Buccal Mucosa *(A)* **and of Gingiva** *(B)* in a 53-year-old female. Microscopic examination revealed evidence of dysplasia.

propria. The final stage shows degeneration and necrosis of the basal and lower spinous layers of the epithelium with the exception of the desmosomes, which are for the most part structurally unaltered. The superficial lamina

propria is also degenerated and necrotic and the basement lamina is no longer visible. Secondary bacterial involvement of the necrotic tissue is often observed.[55]

Differential diagnosis

Among the conditions to be considered in the differential diagnosis of oral lichen planus are leukoplakia, chronic discoid lupus erythematosus, white sponge nevus, pemphigus, and mucous membrane pemphigoid.

LEUKOPLAKIA. Leukoplakia usually appears on the oral mucosa as raised plaques of variable size (Fig. 12–6). Linear lesions of oral leukoplakia can resemble the reticulate lesions of lichen planus, and the more common discrete lesions of leukoplakia can resemble plaque-like configurations of lichen planus. However, in lichen planus lesions, the papular structure can usually be discerned grossly. Microscopic study will differentiate the two diseases. Leukoplakia usually occurs in heavy smokers.

WHITE SPONGE NEVUS (WHITE FOLDED GINGIVOSTOMATITIS). This is a benign genetic disease, manifested at birth or during childhood by the development of white plaque-like areas on oral mucosa (Fig. 12–7). Microscopic examination shows a thickened epithelium characterized by extensive spongiosis.

DISCOID LUPUS ERYTHEMATOSUS. Coexistent skin lesions on the face are present in almost all cases, so that the oral lesions, when present, do not present a significant diagnostic problem. They ap-

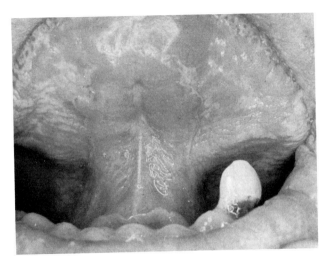

Figure 12–7 White Sponge Nevus (white folded gingivostomatitis), showing thickened epithelium with minute surface folds on the tongue and lips.

pear as slightly raised white plaques or white linear configurations and present a characteristic histopathologic pattern. Biopsy reveals parakeratosis or hyperkeratosis, hydropic degeneration of the basal layer, collagen degeneration, and a perivascular lymphocytic infiltrate.

PEMPHIGUS. Pemphigus may resemble bullous or ulcerative lesions of oral lichen planus. However, the characteristic clinical white striations of lichen planus are usually evident even in cases of bullous lichen planus. Diagnosis of pemphigus can be made by the microscopic finding of acantholysis and usually confirmed by immunofluorescent antibody studies.

MUCOUS MEMBRANE PEMPHIGOID. Mucous membrane pemphigoid may resemble oral lichen planus of the bullous type. In addition, pemphigoid invariably presents an erosive or desquamative gingivitis, and this type of gingival reaction may also appear in lichen planus. Microscopic evaluation of the oral lesions of pemphigoid reveal a subepithelial vesiculation without hydropic degeneration of the basal layer. In oral lichen planus of bullous or ulcerative varieties, the keratotic white striations can usually be found at the periphery of the ulcerated areas.

Therapy

The most important aspect of the management of oral lichen planus is definitive diagnosis so that the patient can be given a specific diagnosis for the disease and reassured that the condition is neither infectious, contagious, nor precancerous. If the oral lesions are of the keratotic variety, no therapy is required. Skin lesions of lichen planus are often characterized by a pruritis, but oral keratotic lesions usually present no discomfort. If the oral lesions are erosive, bullous, or ulcerative, they may be painful and uncomfortable. Peroxide mouthwashes are recommended two or three times per day. If the ulcerative areas are well defined and reasonably localized, they may be dried with a sterile sponge and covered with a corticosteroid ointment or cream several times daily. The ointment can be rubbed gently into the lesions. Intralesional injections of corticosteroids are occasionally beneficial. In severe discomfort, topical anesthetics or a Kaopectate-

Benadryl rinse can be used. In severe, widespread lesions, systemic corticosteroids may be helpful, such as 20 to 30 mg. prednisone daily, reduced to a 5 to 10 mg. maintenance dose after one week. This low maintenance dose, daily or even every second day, can be used for many months without evidence of steroid side effects.

PEMPHIGUS

Pemphigus is a chronic vesiculobullous lesion involving skin and mucous membrane. The oral mucosa is invariably affected and oral lesions usually precede the extensive skin involvement. Early diagnosis of pemphigus is of considerable value, since therapy tends to be simplified if the disease is still confined to the mouth. Systemic corticosteroid therapy at this point in the natural history of the disease may prevent the development of skin lesions, and a lower maintenance dose of steroids may be successfully utilized. Pemphigus has a distinctive microscopic appearance, and a definitive diagnosis can usually be made from an oral biopsy specimen.

The etiology of pemphigus is now considered to be autoimmune, and antibodies can be demonstrated by the use of immunofluorescent techniques.

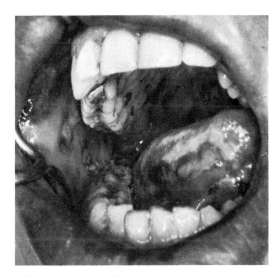

Figure 12–8 Pemphigus of the oral cavity. (Courtesy of Dr. Kurt H. Thoma.)

Oral lesions

Oral lesions of pemphigus range from small vesicles to large bullae (Fig. 12–8). The bullae then rupture, leaving extensive areas of ulceration. Any region of the mouth can be involved, but lesions often develop at sites of irritation or trauma such as the occlusal line of the buccal mucosa or edentulous alveolar ridges. An erosive or desquamative type of gingivitis is occasionally seen as a manifestation of oral pemphigus.

Histopathology

Lesions of pemphigus demonstrate acantholysis, a separation of epithelial cells of the lower stratum spinosum.[13, 30] The upper layers of the epithelium separate from the basal layer, which remains attached to the underlying corium. The intraepithelial vesiculation begins as a microscopic alter- ation (Fig. 12–9) and gradually results in a **grossly visible lesion as a fluid-filled bulla is formed. The separating cells of the stratum spinosum present degenerative changes — the cell outlines are round rather than polyhedral, the intercellular bridges are lost, and the nuclei are large and hyperchromatic. Many of these acantholytic cells are found within the clear fluid of the vesicle. The underlying connective tissue is densely infiltrated with chronic inflammatory cells and these may also enter the vesicular fluid. As the vesicle or bulla ruptures, the ulcerated lesion becomes infiltrated with polymorphonuclear leukocytes and the surface may show suppuration.**

Cytology

Cytologic smears of oral pemphigus lesions may be used as corroborating evidence for a definitive diagnosis. A positive

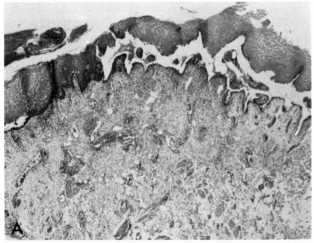

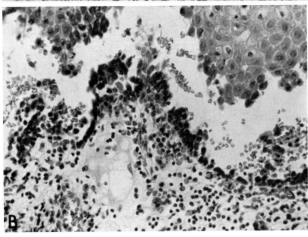

Figure 12–9 Pemphigus Vulgaris. *A,* Oral mucosa showing acantholysis and intra-epithelial vesicle. *B,* Detailed view of intra-epithelial vesicle in pemphigus.

smear will show large numbers of rounded acantholytic cells with serrated borders and large hyperchromatic nuclei.

Electron microscopy

Electron microscopic studies indicate breakdown of the epithelial intercellular cement substance as the first stage in the development of acantholysis.[22] Others feel that the destruction starts in the tonofilaments[56] or the desmosomes[9] (Fig. 12–10).

Immunofluorescence

The presence of antibodies can be demonstrated in the oral mucosa of patients with oral pemphigus by the use of immunofluorescent techniques.[7] In the direct fluorescent techniques, an oral biopsy specimen is incubated with fluorescein-labeled IgG from the patient's serum. An indirect technique can be used but is less sensitive than the direct technique. In the indirect technique a piece of oral or esophageal mucosa from a laboratory animal such as a Rhesus monkey is first incubated with the patient's serum to attach the serum antibodies to the mucosal tissue. The tissue is then incubated with fluorescein-labeled antihuman IgG serum. If the test is positive, the immunofluorescence is observed in the intercellular spaces of the stratified squamous epithelium of the mucosa.

Varieties of pemphigus

The common form of pemphigus is referred to as pemphigus vulgaris. A variant, pemphigus vegetans, may be considered a subacute form of pemphigus vulgaris with comparable but somewhat less severe clinical features. This form of the disease may be confined to the oral cavity for several weeks or months before the skin is involved. In the vegetative type of pemphigus, oral lesions dominate the picture, with crusted lesions of the skin being seen in intertriginous areas. However, the vegetating or hyperplastic lesions do not occur in the mouth. The oral lesions are of the common vesiculobullous and ulcerative form.

Differential diagnosis

The oral lesions of erythema multiforme are frequently similar to those seen in pemphigus. In the former condition, however, there are recurrent active episodes of comparatively short duration followed by long intervals without skin or oral lesions. Erythema multiforme affects the lips with considerable severity. Biopsy studies can differentiate between oral lesions of pemphigus and erythema multiforme, since both have a characteristic histopathology. (Benign) mucous membrane pemphigoid may resemble pemphigus when the latter condition is confined to the mouth. Biopsy studies will demonstrate subepithelial vesiculation with "lifting off" of epithelium from underlying corium instead of the acantholysis characteristic of pemphigus.

Bullous lichen planus must also be considered in the differential diagnosis. The primary lesion of pemphigus may be of a bullous character, followed by erosion with associated pain and discomfort. In lichen planus, however, the characteristic dendritic lesions are invariably found associated with the bullae. Biopsy studies are usually sufficient to differentiate this condition from pemphigus, with its acantholytic changes.

Therapy

Therapy of pemphigus involves the use of systemic corticosteroids, usually with a moderate to high dosage. If the patient responds well to the corticosteroid agent, the dosage can be gradually reduced, but a low maintenance level of the drug is usually necessary in order to prevent recurrence of lesions. In some patients the steroid can be withdrawn completely. In patients who do not respond to corticosteroids or who gradually adapt to them, antimetabolite agents such as methotrexate are used. In general, oral lesions of pemphigus are more resistant to therapy than are skin lesions. The minimization of any irritation in the mouth is essential in patients with oral pemphigus. Optimal oral hygiene is essential, since there is usually widespread involvement of the marginal and attached gingiva as well as other areas of the mouth, and the gingival disease

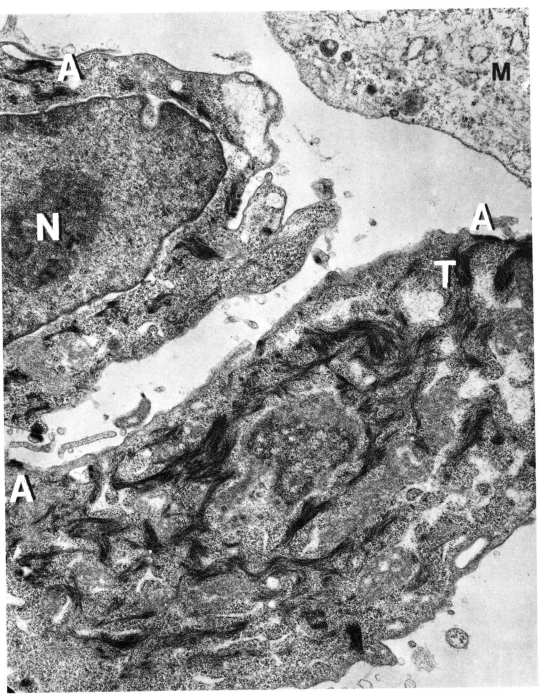

Figure 12–10 Oral Pempighus Vulgaris. Acantholyzed keratinocytes. In spite of disruption of cell to cell junction and detachment of desmosomes, cell membranes are intact and tonofibrils (T) are still attached to the attachment plaques (A) of acantholyzed desmosomes. M = Migrating macrophage; N = nucleus. ×20,000. (Courtesy of Dr. K. Hashimoto.)

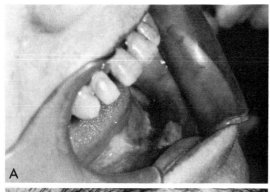

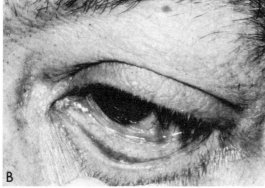

Figure 12–11   *A,* **Bullae on Floor of Mouth** and edentulous mucosa in mucous membrane pemphigoid. *B,* **Conjunctivitis** with symblepharon in mucous membrane pemphigoid.

represents an exaggerated response to local irritation. Periodontal care is an important part of the overall management of patients with pemphigus. Attention should be given to the fit and design of remov-

able prosthetic appliances, since even slight irritation from these prostheses can result in severe inflammation with vesiculation and ulceration.

Local medication for cases of oral pemphigus may include corticosteroid ointments or creams in order to reduce the painful symptomatology. Topical anesthetics such as dyclonine hydrochloride (Dyclone) diluted 50 per cent with water may be used as a mouth rinse several times daily. The anesthetic effect may last for 40 minutes or longer.[54]

BULLOUS PEMPHIGOID

Bullous pemphigoid is a chronic vesiculobullous dermatosis with oral involvement in a small percentage of cases.[47] The skin lesions resemble those of pemphigus clinically, but the microscopic picture is quite distinct from that of pemphigus. There is no evidence of acantholysis, and the developing vesicles are subepithelial rather than intraepithelial. The epithelium separates from the underlying connective tissue at the basement membrane zone. Electron microscopic studies show an actual horizontal splitting or replication of the basal lamina. The separating epithelium remains relatively intact and the basal layer is present and appears regular.

Bullous pemphigoid is also considered to be an autoimmune disease. Antibodies can be demonstrated by immunofluores-

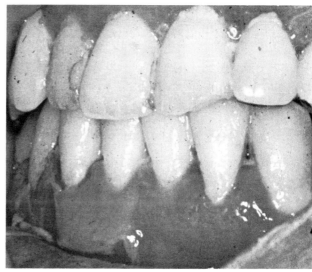

Figure 12–12 **Benign Mucous Membrane Pemphigoid.** Note remnant of ruptured bullous lesion in lower left area.

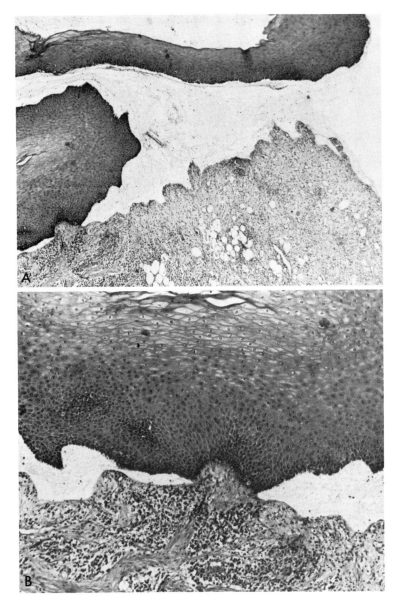

Figure 12–13 Biopsy from oral lesion of **Mucous Membrane Pemphigoid.** Low-power view *(A)* shows clean separation of epithelium from underlying connective tissue. High-power view *(B)* shows intact basal layer as the epithelium separates from connective tissue at the basement membrane zone. Inflammatory infiltration is noted.

cent techniques and they are seen in the basement membrane area.

Oral lesions

Oral lesions are seen in about 10 per cent of cases. There is an erosive or desquamative gingivitis and occasional vesicular or bullous lesions.

Therapy

Therapy involves the systemic use of corticosteroids in moderate dosage.

MUCOUS MEMBRANE PEMPHIGOID (BENIGN MUCOUS MEMBRANE PEMPHIGOID)

This is an unusual chronic vesiculobullous disease with involvement of oral mucosa and other mucosal tissues. Skin is usually not affected. The oral mucous membrane is usually involved, and other sites of predilection are conjunctiva, nasal mucosa, vaginal mucosa, rectal mucosa, and urethra. The ocular lesions can be severe and may result in scarring and eventual blindness.

Oral lesions

The mouth is affected in almost all cases of mucous membrane pemphigoid. The most characteristic feature of the oral involvement is an erosive or "desquamative" gingivitis, with notable erythema of the attached gingiva and areas of desquamation, ulceration, and often vesiculation.[48] Lesions may occur elsewhere in the mouth, and these are vesiculobullous in nature. The bullae tend to have a relatively thick roof, and they rupture in two to three days, leaving irregularly shaped areas of ulceration. Healing of the lesions may take up to three weeks.

Histopathology

The microscopic appearance of the oral lesions, while not completely diagnostic for mucous membrane pemphigoid, is sufficiently distinctive so that a tentative diagnosis can be considered. There is a striking subepithelial vesiculation, with the epithelium lifting off from the underlying corium with an intact basal layer. The separation of epithelium and connective tissue is at the basement membrane zone, and electron microscopic studies have shown a split in the basal lamina.

Varying amounts of chronic inflammatory infiltration are found in the connective tissue. The epithelium remains intact until the bulla ruptures, and then degenerates. The "desquamative" or erosive gingivitis presents a thin epithelium with some evidence of degeneration and occasional ulceration. Inflammatory infiltration may be notable.

Immunofluorescence

Positive immunofluorescence localized to the basement membrane area has been reported in occasional cases of mucous membrane pemphigoid.[44]

Ocular lesions

The eyes are affected in many cases of mucous membrane pemphigoid. There is a conjunctivitis with the development of fibrous adhesions between palpebral and bulbar conjunctivas. There may be adhesions of eyelid to eyeball (symblepharon).

Adhesions at the edges of the eyelids (ankyloblepharon) may result in narrowing of the palpebral fissure. Small vesicular lesions may develop on the conjunctiva. Eventually the conjunctival involvement may lead to scarring, corneal damage, and blindness.

Differential diagnosis

In the differential diagnosis one must consider the vesiculobullous diseases, such as pemphigus, erythema multiforme, and bullous lichen planus. Pemphigus may be confined to the oral cavity in its early stage and the vesicular and ulcerative lesions may resemble those of mucous membrane pemphigoid. An erosive or desquamative gingivitis may also be seen in pemphigus as a rare manifestation. Biopsy studies can quickly rule out pemphigus by the absence of acantholytic changes. In erythema multiforme there are obvious vesiculobullous lesions, but the onset is usually acute rather than chronic, the labial involvement is severe, and the gingiva are usually not affected. A desquamative gingivitis is not seen in erythema multiforme, although occasional vesicular lesions may develop. A biopsy of an oral lesion will reveal an unusual degeneration of the upper stratum spinosum, characteristically seen in oral erythema multiforme lesions.

Therapy

Mucous membrane pemphigoid can be treated with systemic corticosteroids, using moderate daily or every-other-day doses and gradually lowering the dose to a very small maintenance dose (5 to 10 mg. prednisone or comparable doses of other corticosteroids). Topical corticosteroids have limited value, but occasionally applications of corticosteroid ointment may ameliorate the severe desquamative gingivitis and help to promote healing. Optimal oral hygiene is essential, since local irritants on the tooth surface will result in an exaggerated gingival inflammatory response. A soft toothbrush and oxidizing mouthwashes are helpful in maintaining good oral hygiene. If the disease is not severe and the symptomatology is mild, systemic corticosteroids may be omitted. If ocular involvement exists, then systemic corticosteroids are indicated.

ERYTHEMA MULTIFORME

Erythema multiforme is an acute inflammatory eruptive disease involving the skin and oral cavity. More than 80 per cent of the patients with skin involvement present oral lesions,[8] and in rare instances it may be confined to the mouth.[35] **The pathognomonic skin lesions are of a target or iris variety with a** *central vesicle* **or** *bulla* **surrounded by an** *urticarial zone.*

Erythema multiforme is usually a *recurrent disease*. It may be ushered in with fever preceded by a chill, and the duration of the average episode is from 10 days to several weeks. The frequency of involvement varies from three or more attacks per year to a single attack every few years.

Erythema multiforme is probably not an entity etiologically, but a symptom complex or reaction pattern representing many possible causative factors, such as drugs, emotional stress, systemic disease, etc.

Oral lesions

The oral lesions consist of *purplish red macules* or *papules* with interspersed *bullous lesions*. The *tongue* often presents *severe involvement*, with erosion of the bullae followed by ulceration. The lesions are painful so that chewing and swallowing are impaired.

The lips are invariably involved and usually with considerable severity so that extensive bullous and ulcerative lesions are present on the mucosal surface and secondary crusting on the dry skin surface. The extensive labial lesions are often helpful in arriving at a clinical diagnosis.

Histopathology

Microscopically, there is liquefaction degeneration of the upper epithelium with the development of intra-epithelial vesicles, without acantholysis which occurs in pemphigus. Degenerative changes also occur in the basement membrane.[46]

Treatment

There is no specific treatment. Systemic steroid therapy suppresses the symptoms while the disease runs its course.

The Stevens-Johnson Syndrome

The Stevens-Johnson syndrome is a rare form of erythema multiforme, characterized by *erythematous, hemorrhagic,* and *bullous lesions*. The oral cavity, conjunctivae, and genitals are involved as well as other areas of the skin (Fig. 12–14). This hemorrhagic type of erythema multiforme is associated with high fever and prostration, and may be fatal in a small percentage of cases. The oral lesions appear as

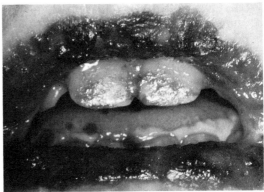

Fig. 12–14

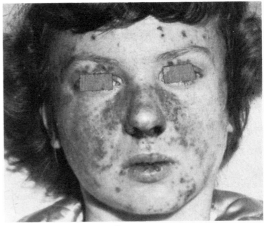

Fig. 12–15

Figure 12–14 Stevens-Johnson Syndrome. Note the crusting of the lips and vesicular eruption on the tongue.

Figure 12–15 Lupus Erythematosus showing butterfly distribution of lesions on the face and crusting of the lips.

purpuric vesicles or bullae. Suppurating superficial and deep erosions of the gingiva are also seen.

Treatment

Steroid therapy is the treatment of choice.

LUPUS ERYTHEMATOSUS

Lupus erythematosus used to be considered one of the so-called collagen diseases,[25] but is now interpreted as an autoimmune disease.[50] It is classified into two forms, a chronic discoid type and a systemic type. The incidence of oral involvement in lupus erythematosus varies, depending upon the acuteness of the disease. Although not more than 10 per cent of the chronic discoid type present oral lesions, as many as 75 per cent of the acute systemic type have some oral manifestation before death. The *characteristic "butterfly" distribution* of the lesions *on the face* is a diagnostic aid in this disease (Fig. 12–15). Lupus erythematosus may occur on the oral mucous membrane without skin lesions in extremely rare instances.

Chronic discoid type

In the oral cavity the disease appears as *well-defined, slightly elevated,* and *infiltrated white lesions* with an erythematous periphery. The lesions are usually localized and are seen more often on the buccal mucosa. At the border of the lesion there may be numerous dilated blood vessels having a radial arrangement extending into the surrounding tissue, coupled with whitish pin-head papules. In the early stages, the center of the lesion is slightly depressed and eroded, and covered with a bluish red epithelial surface showing scarring. In older lesions, the erythematous border becomes less elevated and is transformed into a whitish or bluish white peripheral zone of thickened epithelium. The dilated vessels are replaced by white lines having the same diverging radial arrangement. On the tongue the disease occurs as circumscribed, smooth, reddened areas in which the papillae are lost, or as patches with whitish sheen resembling leukoplakia.

On the lip, the lesions are somewhat similar to those in the mouth and, in most cases, the lip is involved by direct extension from perioral skin lesions. Localized patches may be present, or the entire lip may be involved. Early in the disease, the lip is swollen, bluish red, and often everted. The lip lesions may be covered with adherent scales and crusts remaining localized and rarely diffuse (Fig. 12–15). At the margins of the patches, dilated capillaries or fine branching radial lines may be seen. The lip is tender and sensitive and on removal of the adherent scales, bleeding from the raw surface is noted. Depressed scars may follow the healed deeper lesions.

Microscopically, the epithelial changes in the chronic discoid type consist of keratinization, keratotic plugging, acanthosis, atrophy, pseudocarcinomatous hyperplasia, and liquefaction degeneration of the basal cell layer.[2]

The histopathology of oral lesions is characteristic and consists of hyperkeratosis or parakeratosis, hydropic degeneration of the basal layer of the epithelium, collagen degeneration in the corium, and a perivascular infiltration of lymphocytes. The collagen degeneration shows up clearly with a periodic acid–Schiff stain for mucopolysaccharides.

Periods of activity and quiescence occur. The lesions enlarge by peripheral extension, accompanied by the occurrence of fresh erosions and superficial ulcerations, followed by atrophic changes. Some burning sensation occurs in the erosions and deeper ulcerations.

Acute systemic type

In the systemic variety, the oral lesions are more *acute,* and *greater destruction* occurs. The lesions are characterized by soft, irregular, superficial, or moderately deep erosions, usually covered with a necrotic, grayish pseudomembrane.

Differential diagnosis

Diagnosis usually depends upon the identification of the accompanying skin lesions. The diagnosis of discoid lupus erythematosus confined to the oral cavity is very difficult to make, but microscopic studies usually reveal the characteristic histopathology.[2] The acute systemic variety may present a variety of oral lesions that are essentially nonspecific and erosive in nature. *Erythema multiforme* and *pemphigus* may sometimes appear quite similar. Biopsy will aid in differentiating between *lupus erythematosus* and other erosive diseases.

Treatment

The treatment of lupus erythematosus is nonspecific. Systemic bismuth and gold have been used in the past. Corticotropin (ACTH) and corticosteroids are used currently for the systemic varieties of the disease, and the antimalarial drugs are very successful in controlling the chronic discoid variety, but in systemic lupus erythematosus these drugs have no effect.

SCLERODERMA

Scleroderma is characterized by a primary induration and edema of the skin in localized patches or diffuse areas, and later with atrophy and pigmentation (Fig. 12–16). There are three distinct forms: diffuse scleroderma, acrosclerosis, and circumscribed scleroderma (morphea).[41, 53] The etiology is obscure, although it is considered by many investigators to be of autoimmune origin. In all types of the disease the first sign is usually a moderate induration of the skin gradually followed by the atrophic stage, which results in permanent disfiguration. Ulceration can occur, but it is rare and is seen only in advanced cases. Hemiatrophy is fairly common in cases of facial involvement, sometimes being accompanied by false ankylosis of the temporomandibular joint.

Oral lesions

The diffuse and acrosclerotic types frequently involve the oral cavity.[4, 10] Although the entire mucous membrane may be involved, it is the tongue that is most commonly observed to show pathologic changes, followed in frequency by the

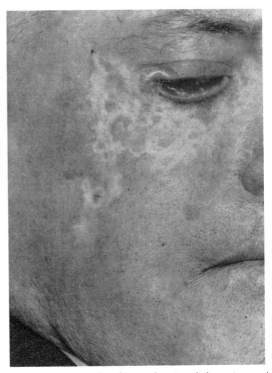

Figure 12–16　Scleroderma showing disfiguration and induration of the skin.

buccal mucosa and gingiva. There may be painful induration of the tongue and gingiva.[45] The usual symptom is a minor speech defect due to impaired mobility of the tongue. The progress of scleroderma of the mucous membrane is chronic, but reportedly more rapid than that of the skin lesions.

In the acrosclerotic variety, the lips become thin and rigid, and their movements are greatly restricted. The opening of the oral cavity is usually materially reduced. Difficulty in eating and talking may follow. Obliterative endarteritis may result in avascularity with increased susceptibility to infection.[17]

In acrosclerosis and diffuse scleroderma, Stafne and Austin[51] have described a characteristic roentgenographic picture consisting of an increase in the width of the periodontal space. This widening was found in 8 of 127 cases of acrosclerosis and in one case of diffuse scleroderma, with the findings much less marked in the latter condition. In acrosclerosis the authors noted that the amount of widening varies. All of the teeth may not be affected, and the posterior teeth are involved more often than the anterior teeth. Radiographically the periodontal space in relation to the entire root is widened to an almost uniform thickness.[38] The increase in width of the periodontal spaces occurs at the expense of the alveolar bone. The lamina dura is obliterated. Clinically the teeth are firm. **Microscopically, the continuity of the periodontal fibers from the cementum to the alveolar bone is broken near the cementum.**

Treatment

There is no effective treatment; however, use of an immunosuppressive agent (Azathioprine) has been described.[24]

PYOSTOMATITIS VEGETANS

This rare disease may be confined to the oral cavity or associated with skin lesions.

Oral lesions

In the oral cavity the primary lesions appear as *multiple small pustules* with a *yellowish tip* and a *reddened base*[34] (Fig. 12–17). The process spreads within a very few weeks to involve the entire oral cavity and creates a diffuse granular surface. As the oral lesions become chronic, the buccal mucosa proliferates to form folds, and the miliary abscesses are found on the summits of the rugae and in the deep invaginations. Oral involvement is accompanied by a mild degree of pain.

Histopathology

Microscopically, there is pronounced hyperkeratosis and acanthosis with broadening and elongation of the rete pegs (Fig. 12–18). The connective tissue presents a granulomatous inflammatory process with unruptured miliary abscesses. Degeneration of the epithelium and focal areas of surface necrosis are also seen.

Treatment

The disease tends to be chronic and resistant to therapy. Because it is frequently associated with an ulcerative colitis, both of these conditions must be treated simultaneously. Iron, liver, and vitamin therapy are of value, but no specific therapy has been discovered to date.

EPIDERMOLYSIS BULLOSA DYSTROPHICA

This is a rare genetic disease characterized by a generalized bullous eruption in-

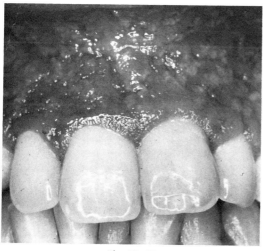

Fig. 12–17

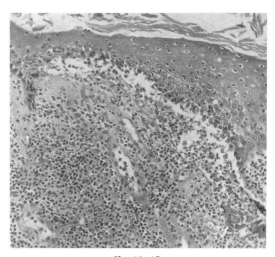

Fig. 12–18

Figure 12–17   Pyostomatitis Vegetans. Multiple small abscesses create granular appearance of the gingiva and adjacent mucosa.

Figure 12–18   Pyostomatitis Vegetans, section showing hyperkeratosis of the epithelium and granulomatous inflammation in the connective tissue.

volving the skin and oral mucosa. Dystrophic changes occur in the nails, and enamel formation is defective.

The slightest friction or trauma is followed by the development of large bullae, which rupture, ulcerate, and form a scar. The oral lesions are apt to be constant, serious, and complicated by inflammatory periodontal changes. Toothbrushing, hard foods, and dental care precipitate the eruption of bullae. Mobility of the tongue may be impaired by scar tissue, and cicatricial bands in the oropharynx may interfere with deglutition. Several variants of the disease have been described.[31]

Microscopically, bullae occur deep in the epidermis or at the junction with the underlying connective tissue. Elastic tissue is reduced or absent, and the connective tissue is moderately inflamed. Leukoplakia and carcinoma are described as possible sequelae of mucous membrane bullae.[41]

Treatment

There is no specific treatment.

DERMATOMYOSITIS

Dermatomyositis is a rare acute or chronic disease of probable autoimmune etiology characterized by muscle pains and weakness, edema, dermatitis, and inflammation and degeneration of muscles. Any skeletal muscle may become involved, including the tongue, and extreme tenderness, pain, and weakness may be noted. Edema may be a prominent feature during the early stages of the disease; atrophy is a late manifestation. **Various forms of stomatitis have been described, ranging from diffuse erosive processes to lesions indistinguishable from lupus erythematosus.** The course of the disease is extremely variable, ranging from a rapidly fatal variety to chronic forms that may undergo spontaneous remission.

Treatment

Corticosteroid therapy is used for the disease.

SYPHILIS

Syphilis is a chronic, specific infection of the body by the spirochete, *Treponema pallidum*, which results in many cutaneous and mucous membrane manifestations. The disease is divided into the following stages.

Primary Stage

This stage is marked by the appearance of the chancre and ends with its disappearance. The chancre or primary lesion of syphilis develops at the point of inoculation, usually in a period of two to six weeks after entrance of the spirochete.

From 5 to 10 per cent of chancres are found in places other than on the genitalia, and about 70 per cent of these extragenital lesions are found on the lips or within the oral cavity. The lips are more frequently involved and multiple primary lesions may occur.

Oral lesions

Lip and intra-oral chancres *vary from small, slightly indurated lesions to deep indolent ulcerations*. Chancres of the oral cavity may be divided into two general types: erosive and ulcerative. Lymph node enlargement is noted in the cervical region, and if the lesion is in or near the median line, the cervical adenopathy may be bilateral. The ulcerative type of mucous membrane chancre may vary from a relatively small ulcer the size of a fingernail, to a large ulcerating nodule. The base and border of the lesion are markedly indurated, and there may be evidence of secondary pyogenic infection.

These lesions tend to have an adherent crust when present on the lip, but within the oral cavity they show a broad, ulcerating, granulating surface. **As a rule, the primary lesion is relatively painless, but those with associated secondary infection may be very tender and painful.**

On the *tongue* the chancre is more often located near the tip and is usually markedly indurated and shows early ulceration.

Chancre of the gingiva is comparatively rare. It appears as an indurated ulcer, which may be covered with a pseudomembrane (Fig. 12–19). Recession of the gingival tissue exposing the tooth root occurs if the lesions begin at the gingival margin. Chancres of the gingiva may also be of the nodular type, with superficial erosion varying in size from that of a split pea to larger lesions, involving the gingiva in relation to several teeth.

Differential diagnosis

In *differential diagnosis* one should consider the possibility of an *aphthous lesion* that has been secondarily infected or aggravated by overtreatment with chemical irritants. *Epidermoid carcinoma* also may resemble a chancre, but these lesions do not show cervical lymph node enlargement in the early stage.

Darkfield examination of the deep serum from the chancre reveals *Treponema pallidum* if no specific medication has previously been given. One should not rely on darkfield examination of intra-oral lesions, as normally occurring spirochetes may be very difficult to differentiate from *T. pallidum*. Chancre of the gingiva tends to grow rapidly and is apt to be more painful than the slower growing tubercular lesions.

Secondary Stage

The secondary stage is characterized by *cutaneous eruption* and *mucous patches* in the *oral cavity*. The mucous patch is the most *contagious lesion of syphilis*, as its surface is covered with an abundance of spirochetes. Mucous patches are slightly elevated, well-demarcated, gray-white lesions with a smooth glistening surface surrounded by an erythematous margin.

There is a *macular type of syphilid* involving the oral cavity early in the secondary stage, which represents a manifestation of the generalized skin eruption.[36] The tongue and palate are most commonly involved, but the *tongue shows the more classic picture of this type of lesion* (Fig. 12–20). These lesions are seen on the tongue as *reddish, round, multiple, symmetrical nonindurated plaques*. Slow denudation of the normal coating of the tongue occurs with shedding of the filiform papillae. The lesions are usually smooth and nonerosive early in their development, and may assume a grayish color and either disappear or develop into a true mucous patch.

A papular type of syphilid is a rare form seen on the dorsum of the tongue or the external commissures of the labial orifice. These lesions are about the size of a split pea, and at the angles of the mouth show a split arrangement with one half of the papule on the upper lip and the other half on the lower lip. Such lesions must be differentiated from the common intertrigo labialis or maceration due to other causes.

Fig. 12–19

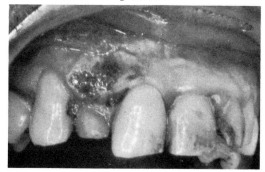

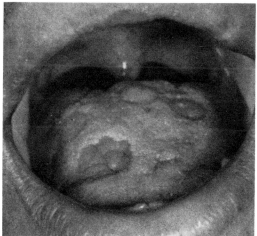

Fig. 12–20

Figure 12–19 Primary Stage of Syphilis. Chancre of the gingiva.

Figure 12–20 Secondary Stage of Syphilis. Patchy denudation of the tongue.

Differential diagnosis

Among the lesions to be considered in the differential diagnosis of mucous patches are the denuded areas found on the tongue in *glossitis areata migrans (geographic tongue)*. In this condition, the individual lesions are characterized by a slight, yellowish, peripheral margin, and tend to clear and reappear at new areas from day to day. *Acute necrotizing ulcerative inflammation* produces localized necrotic and ulcerative lesions. In rare cases, acute necrotizing ulcerative inflammation may be superimposed upon a secondary syphilitic mucous patch and confuse the diagnosis. Severe *aphthous stomatitis* with deep lesions is found in the *periadenitis necrotica* type, which may simulate erosive secondary syphilis.

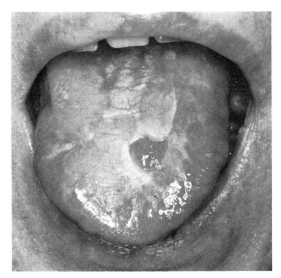

Figure 12–21   Atrophic Glossitis and Leukoplakia of the Tongue.

Tertiary Stage

The tertiary stage of syphilis includes visceral, cutaneous, and oral lesions. The two types of tertiary luetic infection in the oral cavity are gummatous and interstitial. Both conditions tend to leave secondary changes, namely, perforations of the hard and soft palate and atrophic interstitial glossitis respectively.

THE GUMMATOUS REACTION. The *tongue* is a common site of a single or multiple gummatous process. **The gumma is characterized by a growth of epithelioid (granulomatous) tissue in which the spirochete is absent. It usually develops slowly as a relatively painless nodule that may grow to a rather large mass. It tends to ulcerate,** with the production of a thick sanguineous secretion. Healing of the gumma results in the formation of cicatricial tissue, producing a lobulated appearance of the tongue, known as *lingua lobulata*. Other locations of gummata are the *hard and soft palate*.

THE INTERSTITIAL REACTION. More commonly, the tongue is involved in a *sclerosing process*, with the development of the atrophic glossitis of tertiary syphilis referred to as "bald tongue." **The tongue is smooth, red, and glistening in its entirety or may present isolated patches of normal papillae.** The tongue may be shriveled, owing to replacement of the musculature by connective tissue (Fig. 12–21).

The production of this lesion may be explained by a sequence of related pathologic changes. The tongue, a mobile organ subject to mild trauma, receives a large dose of spirochetes in the secondary stage, and if the disease is untreated or inadequately treated, **endarteritis of the smaller vessels results. Later, owing to the interstitial sclerosing process, together with the resulting decrease in the blood supply, the papillae undergo atrophy with the production of patchy smooth bald areas on the surface.** *Leukoplakia* is a common secondary feature, usually as the result of irritation from the products of combustion and heat from smoking. Because the leukoplakic lesions may undergo malignant change, the incidence of carcinoma of the tongue in patients with syphilitic glossitis is high (Fig. 12–22).

Histopathology

Lesions of primary and secondary stages present ulceration and necrosis of surface epithelium with a dense inflammatory infiltration of the underlying connective tissue. The deeper corium presents a characteristic pattern of endarteritis with a perivascular localization of lymphocytes.[36]

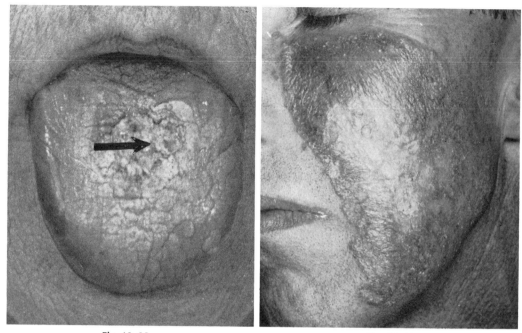

Fig. 12–22   Fig. 12–23

Figure 12–22   **Tertiary Stage of Syphilis.** Interstitial glossitis with verrucous epidermoid carcinoma (*arrow*).
Figure 12–23   **Lupus Vulgaris.** Tuberculosis of skin.

The gumma appears microscopically as a granulomatous process with epithelioid tissue (histiocytes), multinucleate giant cells, and areas of coagulation necrosis. The *T. pallidum* is not demonstrable in the lesion. The diagnosis is confirmed by serologic tests.

Biopsy of syphilitic interstitial glossitis reveals a wide subepithelial zone in which there is disorganization of the musculature caused by an interstitial proliferation of connective tissue. Marked narrowing of the lumina of the efferent arteries is also noted. Atrophy of the epithelial surface and filiform papillae is pronounced in the smooth areas noted clinically on the surface of the tongue. A perivascular lymphocytic infiltration is found in the deeper corium.

Prenatal Syphilis

In prenatal syphilis, acute moist papules with fissuring may occur at the external labial commissures with subsequent healing and scarring and the formation of *radiating "rhagades."* The Hutchinson incisor with the characteristic notching is another oral feature of prenatal syphilis. The *deformed central incisor, interstitial keratitis,* and *deafness* comprise *Hutchinson's triad of congenital syphilis.* These do not always occur together but one or more features are usually demonstrable with other manifestations of congenital syphilis such as "saddle nose" or "saber shins."

TUBERCULOSIS

Tuberculous involvement of the oral cavity is relatively rare and seen more often in males. Although the lesions may involve any area of the oral mucous membrane, the site of involvement is usually the tongue.

Tuberculous lesions of the oral cavity include (1) lupus vulgaris, (2) tuberculous ulcer, (3) disseminated miliary tuberculosis, and (4) tuberculosis cutis orificialis.

Lupus Vulgaris

Lupus vulgaris usually begins before adolescence and tends to be chronic. The face is the most common site of involvement. The small, soft, yellowish or brownish nodules coalesce to form a single lesion. On pressure with the diascope, a characteristic "apple jelly" color is seen which is pathognomonic of the disease. There is a tendency for the lesion to ulcerate, forming an indolent granulomatous ulcer with cicatrizing areas and crusting (Fig. 12–23).

Oral lesions

The oral cavity is rarely involved and, if so, usually by *continuity from the lips.* When the upper lip is involved, it first becomes swollen, fissured, and crusted, with the formation of granulation tissue extending into the cavity. After healing, marked deformity from the resulting scars may occur. In the oral cavity, lupus vulgaris begins as a *soft nodule with subsequent ulceration.* The nodules are soft, slightly elevated, red or yellowish white. The confluent nodules tend to form livid plaques, which are apt to bleed readily.

Histopathology

Microscopically, lupus vulgaris presents typical tubercle formation consisting of nests of epithelioid cells (histiocytes) and multinucleated giant cells of the Langhans type and a peripheral zone of lymphocytes.

Differential diagnosis

As primary involvement of the oral cavity with lupus vulgaris is extremely rare, the diagnosis is usually made by the characteristic lesions on the skin or lip which, by continuity, involve the oral mucosa. Definitive diagnosis is made by biopsy.

Treatment

Treatment with calciferol (vitamin D), and more recently with streptomycin, isonicotinic acid hydrazide (isoniazid) and para-aminosalicylic acid, has revolutionized the treatment of all tuberculous skin, mucous membrane, and lymph node lesions. The use of these preparations, either singly or combined, has been particularly effective in lupus vulgaris.

Tuberculous Ulcer

Two types of tuberculous ulcers are seen in the oral cavity, primary and secondary. The primary type of lesion occurs in nontuberculous individuals, principally children, and involves the lip or tongue. The lesion resembles the primary lesion of syphilis, beginning as an *indurated, sharply defined lesion,* followed by ulceration with lymph node involvement. The diagnosis is made by a biopsy showing typical granulomatous process, with the demonstration of tubercle bacilli in the tissues.

Fig. 12–24

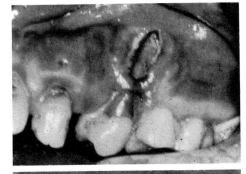

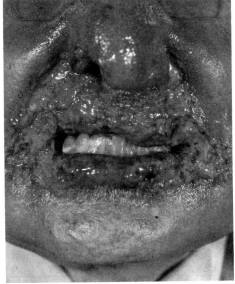

Fig. 12–25

Figure 12–24 Ulcerative Tuberculous Lesion on the Gingiva. (Courtesy Dr. Irving Meyer.)
Figure 12–25 Tuberculosis Cutis Orificialis.

The secondary type of tuberculous ulcer is seen more frequently. It occurs in individuals with tuberculosis and may be subdivided into *nodular, ulcerative, and verrucous types* (Fig. 12–24). The nodular type is more often found at the tip of the tongue, although it may occur elsewhere in the oral cavity. It is characterized by a slowly developing, relatively painless nodule, which may enlarge to a considerable size without showing any appreciable evidence of ulceration. This lesion resembles a syphilitic gumma, especially if located on the tongue. Considering the number of cases of pulmonary tuberculosis, this type of lesion is rare.

The verrucous type of tuberculous lesion in the oral cavity is the rarest of this group. Its usual location is on the dorsum of the tongue in the region of the circumvallate papillae, or on the lips. The lesion may simulate the verrucous type of epidermoid carcinoma.

Histopathology

The tuberculous ulcer is characterized microscopically by tubercle formation. Caseation necrosis is usually seen in addition to the granulomatous reaction of histiocytes and Langhans giant cells. Tubercle bacilli can occasionally be demonstrated within the Langhans giant cells, using special stains.

Disseminated Miliary Tuberculosis

Oral involvement in disseminated miliary tuberculosis occurs in the terminal stage of the disease. The oral lesions tend to break down and produce multiple painful shallow ulcerations, which occur anywhere in the oral cavity. Systemic streptomycin has been particularly effective in the relief of this type of involvement.

Tuberculosis Cutis Orificialis

This type of tubercular process is usually secondary to pulmonary tuberculosis of many years' standing. It tends to involve the nasal, oral, and genital regions,

beginning as a *localized granulation tissue with ulceration*. It is generally complicated by secondary infection with pyogenic organisms. The process is slow but progressive and involves the lips, tongue, gingiva, and buccal mucosa (Fig. 12–25). The involvement may be superficial or deep. It is generally painful and appears as an irregularly outlined mass of granulation tissue bathed in a mucopurulent exudate.

Histopathology

Microscopically, tuberculosis cutis orificialis presents numerous miliary tubercles deep in the cutis. Necrosis and ulceration occur early, and numerous tubercle bacilli are present in the lesions.

Treatment

The chemotherapeutic agents referred to under lupus vulgaris are also used in the treatment of this condition.

ORAL MANIFESTATIONS OF VIRUS DISEASES

Recurrent Herpes Labialis

This is a recurrent herpetic infection that takes the form of the so-called "coldsore" or "fever blister." The lips are the most common site but any part of the integument may be involved. The individual lesions last from 7 to 10 days. The over-all duration of the disease varies from a few months to two years or more. Diagnosis is established by the presence of virally modified epithelial cells in cytologic smear or biopsy of lesion.

Recurrent Intraoral Herpes

Recurrent herpetic infection can occur in the mouth but is rare. It appears as an eruption of small vesicles which rupture rapidly, leaving small punctate ulcers with marginal erythema. The development of these lesions may be stimulated by trauma.

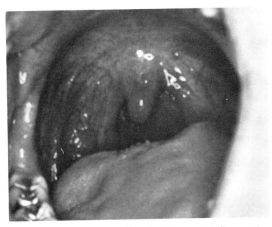

Figure 12–26 **Herpangina** showing acute inflammation of the oropharynx with vesicle formation.

Acute Herpetic Gingivostomatitis

This is an acute infection of the oral cavity produced by the herpes simplex virus. (This disease is described in Chapter 11.)

Herpangina

Herpangina is a relatively common form of oropharyngitis caused by an infection with Coxsackie virus, group A, strain 4. First described in 1920 by Zahorsky,[57] the disease runs a brief course of 7 to 10 days with few complications and mild symptoms. Young adults are affected as well as children, but the symptomatology and the degree of systemic involvement is more severe in children and may result in fever up to 102 to 103° F. (38.9 to 39.4° C), headache, nausea, and abdominal pains.

Oral lesions

The clinical picture is characteristic. Following the initial fever and malaise, there is an acute inflammation of the oropharynx and posterior areas of the mouth such as soft palate, uvula, and the posterior part of the hard palate. Numerous small vesicles develop in these areas and quickly rupture, leaving small ulcers. The anterior part of the mouth is rarely involved. The oropharyngeal involvement may be relatively painful, and there may be dysphagia if the inflammatory involvement results in a significant amount of edema.

Diagnosis

Diagnosis is made on the basis of the characteristic clinical picture. The viral etiology can be confirmed by the finding of virally modified epithelial cells on cytologic smears of ulcerated lesions. Herpangina has often been misdiagnosed clinically as "strep throat."

Treatment

There is no specific treatment. Supportive measures include soft foods and mild oxidizing mouthwashes such as diluted hydrogen peroxide. In patients with high fever, systemic antibiotics may relieve

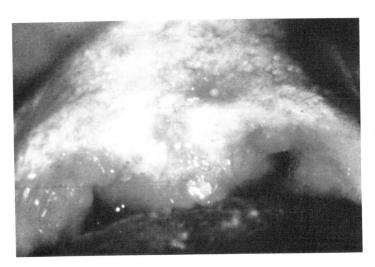

Figure 12–27 Palatal erythema and vesiculation in **Hand-foot-and-mouth Disease.**

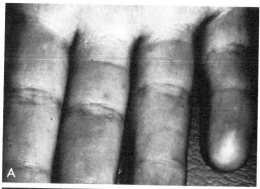

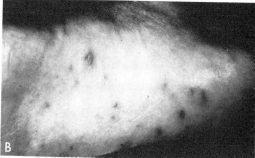

Figure 12–28 Vesicular lesions on palm of hand (A) and sole of foot (B) in **Hand-Foot-and-Mouth Disease.**

some of the severe manifestations by acting on secondary bacterial invaders.

Hand-Foot-and-Mouth Disease

This new viral disease is caused by an infection with several variant strains of the Coxsackie group A virus (strains 5, 10, and 16 have been isolated).[32] The disease first appeared in the 1960's, and occasional outbreaks have occurred since that time. There are oral and oropharyngeal lesions similar to those of herpangina as well as vesiculopapular lesions on the palms of the hands and fingers as well as on the heels and soles of the feet (Figs. 12–27 and 12–28). Systemic involvement tends to be mild, and temperature is usually not elevated. The course of the disease is five to seven days.

Oral lesions

The oropharynx and posterior regions of the mouth are inflamed, and there is an eruption of small vesicles on oropharynx, tonsillar region, and soft palate. Occasional lesions occur on hard palate and tongue.

Diagnosis

Diagnosis is made on the basis of the highly characteristic clinical picture. The viral basis of the disease can be confirmed by the finding of virally modified epithelial cells on cytologic smears of ruptured vesicular lesions.

Treatment

There is no specific treatment.

Herpes Zoster

Herpes zoster is an *inflammation of the posterior root ganglion of the spinal nerves* or an *extramedullary ganglion of a cranial nerve*. It is characterized by pain and burning and vesicle formation along the distribution of the involved nerve.

The etiologic agent is a filtrable virus closely related in morphology and physiology to the virus of herpes simplex and varicella. In some cases, trauma and leukemic infiltration may be predisposing factors. It occurs most frequently in the fifth and seventh decades, although occasionally the disease is found in children. As a general rule, the disease is more severe in older patients.

The herpetic eruption is usually preceded by pain or burning along the distribution of the involved nerve, which may last for 24 to 48 hours before the *typical vesicular eruption* appears. The vesicles, which are surrounded by a distinct *erythematous base*, appear in groups. They rupture and heal gradually in 5 to 10 days. The lesions are characteristically *unilateral*, although *bilateral* involvement has been reported.

Oral lesions

The *fifth cranial nerve* is involved in about 15 per cent of the cases. When the maxillary and mandibular divisions of the fifth cranial nerve are involved, lesions occur on the skin, oral mucosa, or both. The anterior portion of the tongue, soft palate, and cheek are the most frequent intra-oral sites. Burket[10] states that the oral lesions are of shorter duration than the dermal involvement.

Treatment

Besides palliative local treatment, the many different types of parenteral therapy include the use of posterior pituitary extract, dihydroergotamine, protamide, and convalescent serum. The large number of such agents and their wide differences of action are indications of their ineffectiveness. Antibiotics are used but their value is limited to controlling secondary infection.

Molluscum Contagiosum

Molluscum contagiosum is a virus disease of the epithelium that very rarely involves mucous membranes and is characterized by *small, nodular lesions,* which usually have *minute, rounded surface orifices.*

Oral lesions

The lesions may range from pin-head to pea size and develop slowly. At first they are *globular* in shape with broad bases, but as they enlarge they become *flattened* and *umbilicated.* They may be discrete or grouped. Their most common location in the oral cavity is on the dorsal surface of the *tongue,* although they have been reported on other areas, especially the lips.

Histopathology

Microscopically, molluscum contagiosum is characterized by the presence of "molluscum bodies," which are degenerating epithelial cells. The prickle cells increase in size as the surface of the lesion is approached, and inclusion bodies develop adjacent to the nuclei. Nearer the surface, the cells lose their nuclei but retain the inclusion bodies. At the surface, the inclusion bodies are no longer present and the cells appear as a homogeneous mass.

Treatment

The lesions are very amenable to local therapy. Piercing them with a sharp instrument usually stops their growth, and in a few days they deteriorate and drop off the surface. Electrodesiccation, cauterization, or "shelling out" with a blunt instrument may be employed in resistant cases.

Verruca Vulgaris

Oral lesions

Verruca vulgaris is a small lesion 2 to 6 mm. in size, commonly located on the *tongue, vestibule,* or *buccal mucosa.* It is usually grayish white in color and may bleed profusely if traumatized.

Histopathology

Microscopically, verruca vulgaris presents marked acanthosis and some hyperkeratosis of the epithelium. The lesion is confined to the epithelium without extending into the underlying tunica propria.

Treatment

Treatment consists of elimination by electrodesiccation or electrocautery. In addition, podophyllin in alcohol when applied topically to mucous membrane warts is an effective medication.

DRUG ERUPTIONS

An increase in the incidence of skin and oral manifestations of hypersensitivity to drugs has been noted since the advent of the sulfonamides, barbiturates, and the various antibiotics. The eruptive skin and oral lesions are attributed to the fact that the drug acts as an *allergen,* either alone or in combination, *sensitizing* the tissues and then causing the allergic reaction.

Eruptions in the oral cavity resulting from sensitivity to drugs that have been taken by mouth or parenterally are termed stomatitis medicamentosa. The local reaction from the use of a medicament in the oral cavity, such as a so-called "aspirin burn" and the stomatitis resulting from topical penicillin, is referred to as stomatitis venenata or contact stomatitis. Such changes may result from either the irritating local action of the drug or from drug sensitivity. In many cases skin eruptions may accompany the oral lesions.

In general, drug eruptions in the oral cavity are *multiform. Vesicular* and *bullous lesions* occur commonly, but *pigmented or nonpigmented macular lesions* are frequently observed. Erosions, often followed by deep ulceration with purpuric lesions, may also occur. The lesions are seen in different areas of the oral cavity, with the gingiva frequently being affected.

There are hundreds of drugs capable of producing skin eruptions with or without mouth lesions. Constitutional symptoms may be severe or entirely absent. Only a few of the important and most commonly used drugs that may be associated with skin and oral eruptions will be considered here.

Agranulocytosis characterized by *necrotic oral lesions, sore throat,* and *leukopenia* may follow the use of gold salts, arsphenamine, aminopyrine, phenacetin, sulfonamides, and antibiotics. The barbiturates[28] and salicylates[11] (Fig. 12–29) occasionally produce vesicular or bullous lesions followed by erosions in the oral cavity. Phenolphthalein, found in many proprietary laxatives, may produce bullous lesions followed by erosions (usually confined to a single lesion) on the skin and in the oral cavity (Fig. 12–30).

Iodides and bromides may give rise to bullous and hemorrhagic eruptions in the oral cavity and, on the skin, acne, urticaria, or suppurating and vegetating lesions. The sulfonamides are responsible for a variety of skin and oral lesions, including vesicles, bullae, and ulceration. Sulfonamide ointment has been a factor in producing sensitization in a large percentage of cases.[52] A so-called "fixed eruption" of mucous membrane and skin caused by sulfadiazine[12] has been reported. Atabrine (quinacrine hydrochloride), used in the prevention and treatment of malaria in World War II, produced a skin eruption called atypical lichenoid dermatitis characterized by lesions resembling lichen planus on the skin and oral mucosa.

Skin and oral eruptions and acute monilial infection have been associated with the widespread use of antibiotics (Fig. 12–31).

FUNGUS DISEASES OF THE ORAL CAVITY

Although fungus disease of the oral cavity is relatively uncommon, the following conditions are occasionally seen.

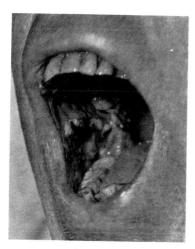

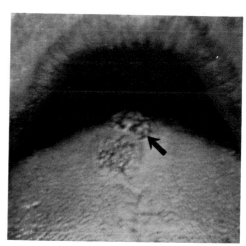

Fig. 12–29　　　　　　　　　　　Fig. 12–30

Figure 12–29　Stomatitis Medicamentosa resulting from bismuth salicylate showing necrosis of the buccal mucosa with pigmentation.

Figure 12–30　Fixed Eruption Due to Phenolphthalein. Note the bullous lesion on dorsum of tongue.

Acute Candidiasis (Moniliasis; Thrush)

Acute candidiasis is the most common mycotic infection of the oral mucosa. It is seen in three types of individuals—the debilitated or immunosuppressed adult, the young baby, and the adult who has been on antibiotic therapy for some period of time. The causative organism is *Candida albicans*, a common inhabitant of the mouth and normally nonpathogenic. In the severely debilitated adult, with significantly lowered tissue resistance, the organism may become invasive and destructive, penetrating the oral mucosa and producing necrosis of epithelium. Candidiasis is seen in immunosuppressed patients and is becoming increasingly frequent in cancer patients who have been treated with high dosages of radiation or chemotherapeutic drugs. The baby is born with a sterile mouth and the normal oral bacterial-mycotic flora gradually develops. During this early stage, while the flora is becoming established, the candidal organisms may proliferate and produce disease. *Candida albicans* may proliferate and invade the oral tissues if the normal bacterial components of the oral flora are removed by the use of antibiotics. However, the development of candidiasis as a complication of antibiotic therapy has been overemphasized. It usually requires the use of several different antibiotics over a period of several weeks or months, and these patients also tend to be debilitated by the conditions requiring the antibacterial therapy. An increased incidence of candidiasis is also seen in certain metabolic disorders such as diabetes and the hypothyroid–adrenocortical insufficiency syndrome. Women developing oral candidiasis may also develop vaginal candidiasis, since the organism is also a common inhabitant of the vaginal tract. Pregnancy and the use of contraceptive steroids tend to predispose the female to the development of both oral and vaginal candidiasis.

Microscopic examination of oral lesions of candidiasis reveal the invading mycelia of the organisms within epithelium that is undergoing necrosis. Biopsy is not necessary for diagnostic purposes, since a smear can adequately demonstrate the organisms. Culture of the organisms is unnecessary and misleading, since *Candida albicans* is usually present in normal mouths as part of the bacterial-mycotic flora. This disease is not contagious, since the organisms are normally present and require some predisposing loss of tissue resistance or depression of the immune response.

Oral lesions

The oral lesions may appear anywhere on the mucosal surface as a simple patch, but usually the lesions are multiple. The *characteristic lesions are creamy-white, simulating coagulated milk, adherent and, when forcibly removed, give rise to bleeding points* (Figs. 12–32 and 12–33). Intertriginous maceration at the labial commissures both in children and adults may reveal *C. albicans*.

Diagnosis

The diagnosis is based upon the history, clinical appearance of the lesions, and microscopic study of smears of scrapings from them. The smears are stained with gentian violet or methylene blue and will show spores and mycelia of *Candida albicans* (Fig. 12–34).

Swabs from the exudate on Sabouraud's culture medium at room temperature give rise to characteristic colonies of the fungus. The colonies grow in three to five days as creamy-white, medium-sized moist colonies with a definite odor of yeast.

Clinically, thrush may simulate *diphtheria, macerated epithelium* of the buccal mucosa from chronic irritation (biting habit), *leukoplakia*, and possibly *lichen planus*. These conditions are readily ruled out by smears of the necrotic white lesions.

Treatment

Current treatment of acute oral candidiasis favors the use of the antimycotic agent, nystatin, in a suspension or as a troche. A spoonful of the suspension (100,000 units/ml) is gently moved around in the mouth for about 1 minute and then swallowed. This is repeated four times daily for 7 to 10 days. Troches are more effective and are kept in the mouth until dissolved. This is repeated four times daily for 7 to 10 days. If oral troches or tablets are not available, vaginal tablets (100,000 units) are used as oral troches. Painting the lesions with 1 per cent gentian violet is an older but effective treatment if the clinician can paint all lesions every day for 7 days.

Fig. 12–31

Fig. 12–32

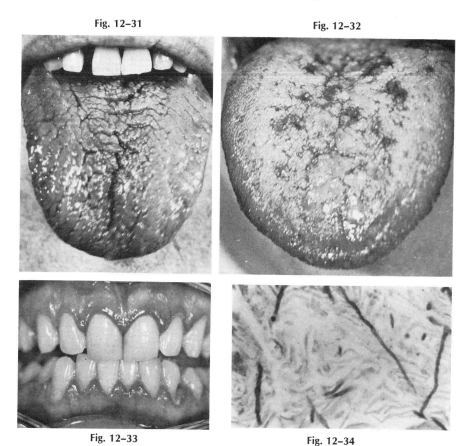

Fig. 12–33

Fig. 12–34

Figure 12–31   Prominent Papillae and Discoloration of the Tongue Associated With the Local Use of Penicillin.
Figure 12–32   Acute Moniliasis of the Tongue.
Figure 12–33   The Gingiva in Acute Moniliasis.
Figure 12–34   Smear from Lesion of Candidiasis showing Proliferating Mycelia of Candida albicans.

Chronic Candidiasis

This is a rare type of *C. albicans* infection resulting in a *granulomatous lesion* that begins in infancy or early childhood and may persist for several years.[29] The oral lesions are often accompanied by involvement of the nails and skin (Figs. 12–35 to 12–37). In contrast to the mild, superficial acute forms of monilial infection,

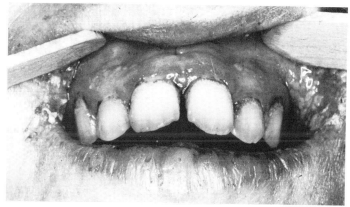

Figure 12–35   Chronic Candidiasis involving gingiva in 18-year-old female.

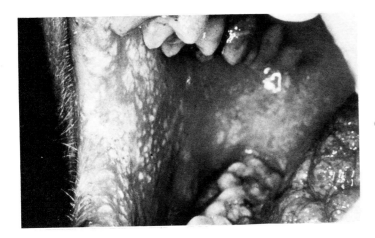

Figure 12–36 Lesions of **Chronic Candidiasis** on buccal mucosa.

monilial granuloma[19] manifests itself by a deep inflammatory reaction with the production of granulation tissue. Ultimate involvement of the lungs with multiple abscesses, often associated with kidney lesions, results in death in many cases.

Diagnosis

The diagnosis is confirmed by laboratory studies as for acute candidiasis.

Treatment

In chronic or systemic candidiasis, the treatment involves the systemic use of amphotericin B, a potent but relatively toxic antimycotic agent. Newer antimycotic agents for systemic use are currently being tested.

Actinomycosis

Actinomycosis, caused by Actinomyces, (A. bovis and A. israelii), is a disease that involves many parts of the body and is most frequently seen about the oral cavity. The Actinomyces are classified as an intermediate group between the fungi and bacteria, and may be considered as bacteria-like fungi. Actinomyces are common normal habitants of the oral cavity.

Approximately 90 per cent of the cases of actinomycosis are of the cervicofacial type, and a large percentage of these follow extraction of teeth. One of the characteristics of actinomycosis is the lack of immediate tissue reaction following invasion of the Actinomyces. Clinically, as described by Lamb et al.,[27] the cervicofacial type of actinomycosis presents the follow-

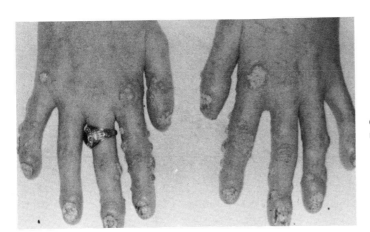

Figure 12–37 Lesions of **Chronic Candidiasis** on skin of hands and on fingernails.

ing features: dark-red discoloration of the skin, slate-blue elevated lesions, multiple nodules with formation of ridges and furrows in the creases of the skin and neck, distinct board-like induration and multiple sinuses with both macroscopic and microscopic granules in the purulent discharge. Pain is usually mild and sometimes absent.

The *tongue* or *buccal mucosa* is occasionally the primary site of the disease. It starts as a deep-seated, *painless nodule* that grows slowly and eventually breaks through the mucosa, discharging a *yellowish purulent material*. On the *gingiva*, the picture is somewhat similar. It takes about four to six weeks for an actinomycotic nodule to soften and discharge its contents.

Differential diagnosis

A large group of conditions may simulate actinomycosis. Among them are *tuberculosis, syphilitic gummas, blastomycosis, lymphogranuloma venereum or malignancy,* usually of the *lymphomatous type,* and *lupus vulgaris.*

Diagnosis

The purulent exudate from the lesions is collected from the draining sinuses and examined grossly for the yellow sulfur granules. **Microscopically, the granules appear as lobulated bodies composed of delicate branching, intertwined filaments. The organism can be grown anaerobically in thioglycollate medium.**

Treatment

Surgical drainage of the lesion is effective; filtered x-ray irradiation, systemic penicillin, amphotericin B, and other antibiotics and sulfa drugs are also used.

Histoplasmosis

Histoplasmosis, one of the rare fungus diseases of man, shows cutaneous or mucomembranous lesions in one half of the cases reported to date. Darling first reported cases in Panama and originally

named the causative agent *Histoplasma capsulatum.*[16] The method of transmission of this fungus to man is not definitely known; the dog may be the intermediate host, as *H. capsulatum* has been isolated from that animal.

Oral lesions occurred in 28 of 88 cases compiled by Miller.[37] The lesions may occur anywhere in the oral cavity, but the *tongue* is the most common site. The most common form is a *very indurated ulcer,* although *nodular lesions* are almost as common as ulcers. The lesion also presents as verrucous or granular masses.[6] Purpuric, macular areas may accompany the ulcerations.

The skin lesions may be multiform in character and include papules, ulcerations, purpuric lesions, impetiginous eruptions, and generalized scaling dermatosis. The disease presents systemic manifestations as well as cutaneous and oral lesions. The symptoms include elevated temperature, anemia, and leukopenia. Lymph node and pulmonary involvement resembling both lymphoblastoma and pulmonary tuberculosis occur in many cases.

Histopathology

Microscopically, histoplasmosis is classified among the chronic infectious granulomas and cannot be definitely differentiated on the basis of cellular changes from other members of the group. Multinucleated macrophages containing the yeast-like fungi are diagnostic. The fungi are seen in large mononuclear cells and appear as small oval bodies 1 to 4 microns in diameter surrounded by a nonstaining capsule. The organism has to be differentiated from the Leishmania protozoan parasites. Lymphocytic and plasma cell infiltration may be associated with focal areas of necrosis. Epithelial hyperplasia and fibrosis occur around the necrotic areas, and typical Langhans' giant cells are often present.

REFERENCES

1. Andreasen, J. O.: Oral lichen planus. I. A clinical evaluation of 115 cases. Oral Surg., 25:31, 1968.
2. Andreasen, J. O., and Poulsen, H. E.: Oral manifestations in discoid and systemic lupus erythematosus. 2. Histologic investigation. Acta Odontol. Scand., 22:389, 1964.

3. Baldridge, G. D., and Blank, H.: Effect of Aureomycin on the herpes simplex virus in embryonated eggs. Proc. Soc. Exp. Med. Biol., 72:506, 1949.

4. Barber, H. W.: Circumscribed scleroderma of the buccal mucosa. Proc. R. Soc. Med., 37:73, 1944.

5. Barcaglia, A.: Hemilateral scleroderma with hemiatrophy and vitiligo in a boy four years of age. Pediatria, 45:533, 1937.

6. Bennett, D. E.: Histoplasmosis of the oral cavity and larynx. Arch. Intern. Med. (Chicago), 120:417, 1967.

7. Beutner, E. H., et al.: The immunopathology of pemphigus and bullous pemphigoid. J. Invest. Derm., 51:63, 1968.

8. Brantzaeg, P.: Erytheme multiforme exudatium. Odont. T., 72:363, 1964.

9. Braun-Falco, O., and Vogell, W.: Elektronen-Mikroskopische Untersuchungen zur Dynamik der Akantholyse bei Pemphigus Vulgaris. II Mitteilung. Die Akantholytische Blase. Arch. Klin. Exp. Derm., 223:533, 1965.

10. Burket, L. W.: Oral Medicine. Philadelphia, J. B. Lippincott Co., 1946, p. 151.

11. Claman, H. N.: Mouth ulcers associated with prolonged chewing of gum containing aspirin. J.A.M.A., 202:651, 1967.

12. Cole, L. W.: Fixed eruption of mucous membrane and skin caused by sulfadiazine. Arch. Derm. Syph., 54:675, 1946.

13. Combes, F. L., and Canizares, O.: Pemphigus vulgaris, a clinicopathological study of one hundred cases. Arch. Derm. Syph., 62:786, 1950.

14. Cooke, B. E. D.: Diagnosing features of pemphigus affecting the oral mucosa. J. Dent. Res., 40:1281, 1961.

15. Coutts, W. E., and Banderas, B. T.: Lymphogranulomatosis venerea and its clinical syndromes. Urol. Cutan. Rev., 38:263, 1934.

16. Darling, S. T.: The morphology of the parasite (Histoplasma capsulatum) and lesions of histoplasmosis, a fatal disease of tropical America. J. Exp. Med., 11:515, 1909.

17. Foster, T. D., et al.: Dental involvement in scleroderma. Br. Dent. J., 124:353, 1968.

18. Frei, W.: On the skin test in lymphogranuloma inguinale. J. Invest. Derm., 1:367, 1938.

19. Gahan, E.: Lupus erythematosus. Clinical observations in 443 cases. Arch. Derm. Syph., 45:685, 1942.

20. Griffin, J. W.: Recurrent intraoral herpes simplex virus infection. Oral Surg., 19:209, 1965.

21. Hanser, P. V., and Rothman, S.: Monilial granuloma, report of case. Arch. Derm. Syph., 61:297, 1950.

22. Hashimoto, K., and Lever, W.: An electron-microscopic study of pemphigus vulgaris of the mouth and skin with special reference to the intercellular cement. J. Invest. Derm., 48:540, 1967.

23. Jandinski, J., and Shklar, G.: Lichen planus of the gingiva. J. Periodontol., 47:724, 1976.

24. Jansen, G. T., et al.: Generalized scleroderma. Treatment with immunosuppressive agents. Arch. Derm., 97:690, 1968.

25. Klemperer, P.: The concept of collagen diseases. Am. J. Pathol., 26:505, 1950.

26. Komori, A., Welton, N. A., and Kelln, E. E.: The behavior of the basement membrane of skin and oral lesions in patients with lichen planus, erythema multiforme, lupus erythematosus, pemphigus vulgaris, pemphigoid, and epidermolysis bullosa. Oral Surg., 22:752, 1966.

27. Lamb, J. H., Lain, E., and Jones, P.: Actinomycosis of face and neck. J.A.M.A., 134:351, 1947.

28. Lawson, B. F.: Severe stomatitis associated with barbiturate ingestion. J. Oral Med., 24:13, 1969.

29. Lehner, T.: Chronic candidiasis. Br. Dent. J., 116:539, 1964.

30. Lever, W. F.: Pemphigus. Medicine, 32:1, 1953.

31. Levy, B. P., Reeve, C. M., and Kierland, R. R.: The oral aspects of epidermolysis bullosa dystrophica: A case report. J. Periodontol., 40:431, 1970.

32. Magoffin, R. L., Jackson, E. W., and Lennette, E. H.: Vesicular stomatitis and exanthem: A syndrome associated with Coxsackie virus type A 16. J.A.M.A., 175:441, 1961.

33. McCarthy, F. P.: A clinical and pathologic study of oral disease based on 2300 consecutive cases. J.A.M.A., 116:16, 1941.

34. McCarthy, F. P.: Pyostomatitis vegetans. Arch. Derm. Syph., 60:750, 1949.

35. McCarthy, P. L., and Shklar, G.: Diseases of the Oral Mucosa. New York, McGraw Hill Book Company, 1964, p. 160.

36. Meyer, I., and Shklar, G.: The oral manifestations of acquired syphilis. Oral Surg., 23:45, 1967.

37. Miller, H. E., et al.: Histoplasmosis, cutaneous and mucomembranous lesions. Arch. Derm. Syph., 56:715, 1947.

38. Mitchell, D. F., and Chaudhry, A. P.: Roentgenographic manifestations of scleroderma. Oral Surg., 10:307, 1957.

39. Monash, S.: Oral lesions of lupus erythematosus. Dent. Cosmos, 73:511, 1931.

40. Montgomery, H.: Dermatopathology. New York, Harper and Row, 1967, p. 84.

41. O'Leary, P. A., and Nomland, R.: A clinical study of one hundred and three cases of scleroderma. Am. J. Med. Sci., 180:95, 1930.

42. Parsons, R. G., and Zarofonetis, C. J. D.: Histoplasmosis in man. Arch. Intern. Med., 75:1, 1945.

43. Pindborg, J. J.: Atlas of Diseases of the Oral Mucosa. Philadelphia, W. B. Saunders Company, 1973, p. 58.

44. Praetorius-Clausen, F.: Rare oral viral disorders. (Molluscum contagiosum, localized keratoacanthoma, verrucae, condyloma acuminatum and focal epithelial hyperplasia.) Oral Surg., 34:604, 1972.

45. Scópp, I. W., and Schlagel, E.: Scleroderma: Its orofacial manifestations. Oral Surg., 15:1510, 1962.

46. Shklar, G.: Oral lesions of erythema multiforme, histologic and histochemical observations. Arch. Derm., 92:495, 1965.

47. Shklar, G., et al.: Oral lesions in bullous pemphigoid. Arch. Derm., 99:663, 1970.
48. Shklar, G., and McCarthy, P. L.: The oral lesions of mucous membrane pemphigoid. A study of 85 cases. Arch. Otolaryngol., 93:83, 1971.
49. Shklar, G., and McCarthy, P. L.: The oral lesions of lichen planus. Oral Surg., 14:164, 1961.
50. Shklar, G., and McCarthy, P. L.: The Oral Manifestations of Systemic Disease. Boston, Butterworth's, 1976, p. 110.
51. Stafne, E. C., and Austin, L. T.: A characteristic dental finding in acrosclerosis and diffuse scleroderma. Am. J. Orthod., 30:25, 1944.
52. Sulzberger, M. B., Kanof, A., Baer, R. L., and Lowenberg, C.: Sensitization by topical application of sulfonamides. J. Allergy, 18:92, 1947.
53. Templeton, H. J.: Localized scleroderma with bullae. Arch. Derm. Syph., 43:360, 1941.
54. Weisberger, D.: Treatment of some diseases of the soft tissues of the mouth. Dent. Clin. North Am., March 1960, p. 215.
55. Whitten, J. B., Jr.: Intra-oral lichen planus simplex: An ultrastructure study. J. Periodontol., 41:261, 1970.
56. Wilgram, G. F., Caulfield, J. B., and Lever, W. F.: An electron microscopic study of acantholysis in pemphigus vulgaris. J. Invest. Derm., 36:373, 1961.
57. Zahorsky, J.: Herpetic sore throat. Southern Med. J., 13:871, 1920.

CHRONIC DESQUAMATIVE GINGIVITIS

Chronic desquamative gingivitis is a term that has been used in dental medicine for many years to describe a unique condition of the gingiva characterized by intense redness and desquamation of the surface epithelium. The cause of the condition was unknown and a variety of etiologic influences were suggested, particularly some endocrine imbalance, since most cases were described in postmenopausal females. McCarthy et al.[9] in 1960 reconsidered the literature on desquamative gingivitis and from a study of 40 cases concluded that desquamative gingivitis was not a specific disease entity, but rather a nonspecific gingival manifestation of a variety of systemic disturbances, some of which are better understood at present than others. A provisional classification can be suggested based on etiologic considerations.

1. Dermatoses
   a. Lichen planus
   b. Mucous membrane pemphigoid
   c. Bullous pemphigoid
   d. Pemphigus
2. Endocrine Imbalance
   a. Estrogen deficiency in females following hysterectomy with oophorectomy or menopause
   b. Testosterone deficiency in males
3. Aging (senile atrophic gingivitis)
4. Metabolic Disturbances
   a. Nutritional deficiency (gingivosis)
5. Abnormal Response to Irritation (modification of chronic marginal gingivitis)
6. Idiopathic
7. Chronic Infections
   a. Tuberculosis
   b. Chronic candidiasis
   c. Histoplasmosis

Since the large majority of cases of so-called chronic desquamative gingivitis are now understood to represent either lichen planus or mucous membrane pemphigoid, the topic is appropriately included in this chapter on the oral manifestations of dermatologic disease.

Prinz[12] first used the term "chronic diffuse desquamative gingivitis" in 1932 and described 12 cases with a chronic diffuse inflammation of the marginal gingiva characterized by desquamation of the epithelium of the papillae and adjacent gingiva. The denuded connective tissue bled upon the slightest irritation. The condition had been described earlier under other names by Tomes and Tomes[23] and by Goadby,[6] who thought that the disease was associated with an anemia. Merritt[10] and Sorrin[21] offered further descriptions, and Ziskin and Zegarelli[26] suggested that the condition resulted from a metabolic disorder such as estrogen deficiency or hypothyroidism, and they used estrogen ointment to treat the gingival erythema and desquamation. Ziskin and Zegarelli studied their cases histologically and found vesicle formation in almost half of them. Foss et al.[3] also suggested a disturbance of endocrine function and used topical cortisone to treat their cases. Glickman and Smulow[5] studied the histopathology of desquamative gingivitis and described two principal types—a bullous type characterized by edema and subepithelial vesiculation, and a lichenoid type characterized by a dense subepithelial band of chronic inflammatory cells, primarily lymphocytes. Histochemical[2, 20] and ultrastructural studies[1, 11, 24] have not contributed significant information. The electron microscopic changes described are extremely variable and resemble many of the changes described in lichen planus[8, 13] or mucous membrane pemphigoid.[22] Marked multiplication of basal lamina was noted by Nikai et al.[11] as well as interruptions of basal lamina and separation from basal cells. Similar basal lamina changes were described by Susi and Shklar[22] in mucous membrane pemphigoid, including thickening and irregularity. Separation of epithelium and connective tissue was seen to start with a separation of collagen fibrils and a decrease in the number of anchoring fibrils. Changes in oral lichen planus were described as a disruption of basement membrane and increased irregularity of nuclear membranes of epithelial cells with increased tonofibril thickness.[8, 13]

It is apparent that the microscopic changes described in so-called desquamative gingivitis are consistent with those of either lichen planus or mucous membrane pemphigoid. All cases of mucous membrane pemphigoid[19] and those cases of bullous pemphigoid with oral involvement[18] present a desquamative or erosive gingivitis. However, since mucous membrane pemphigoid is a relatively rare disease, it is probable that the majority of cases of so-called desquamative gingivitis are in fact lichen planus. A desquamative gingivitis is a rare manifestation of lichen planus (10 to 20 per cent of cases),[17, 25] but lichen planus is a relatively common disease of the mouth and the incidence of gingival lichen planus should be higher than that of mucous membrane pemphigoid. Careful examination of the mouth should reveal other manifestations of lichen planus in these cases, such as reticulate lesions of the buccal mucosa. However, some cases of lichen planus start with gingival involvement, and other lesions may appear as the disease progresses. Diagnosis may be possible by histologic studies. In mucous membrane pemphigoid, there may be conjunctival lesions as well as involvement of other mucous membrane sites such as nasal mucosa, vagina, rectum, and urethra. However, the involvement may be confined to gingiva in the early stages of the disease

and other oral lesions may follow. Biopsy studies may reveal the characteristic clean separation of epithelium from underlying connective tissue. In some cases of desquamative gingivitis, a severe nutritional deficiency background may be responsible, as suggested by Schour and Massler's observation[15] on "gingivosis" in Italian children of the immediate post-war era.

Clinical features

The clinical features of so-called desquamative gingivitis vary in severity, and mild, moderate, and severe forms have been described by Glickman and Smulow.[4]

MILD FORM. In its mildest form there is diffuse erythema of the marginal, interdental, and attached gingiva; the condition is usually painless and comes to the attention of the patient or dentist because of the over-all discoloration. The mild form occurs most frequently in young females between 17 and 23 years of age.

MODERATE FORM. This is a more advanced form. It presents a patchy distribution of bright red and gray areas involving the marginal and attached gingiva (Fig. 12–38A). The surface is smooth and shiny, and the normally resilient gingiva becomes soft. There is slight pitting upon pressure, and the epithelium is not firmly adherent to the underlying tissues. Massaging of the gingiva with the finger results in peeling of the epithelium and exposure of the underlying bleeding connective tissue surface.

The oral mucosa in the remainder of the mouth is extremely smooth and shiny. This condition is seen most frequently in persons between 30 and 40 years of age. Patients complain of a burning sensation and sensitivity to thermal changes. Inhalation of air is painful. The patient cannot tolerate condiments, and toothbrushing causes painful denudation of the gingival surface.

SEVERE FORM. In this and other forms of desquamative gingivitis the lingual surface is usually less severely involved than the labial (Fig. 12–38B) because the tongue and friction from food excursion reduce the accumulation of local irritants and limit the inflammation. This form is

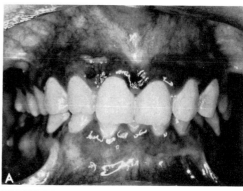

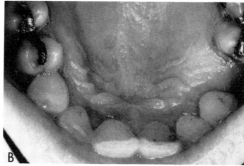

Figure 12–38 Chronic Desquamative Gingivitis of Varied Severity. *A,* Moderate. Generalized edema and erythema associated with inflammation and exposure of underlying connective tissue. *B,* Lingual view of patient shown in *A.* Aside from slight marginal erythema, there is little evidence of change in the gingiva and adjacent mucosa. *C,* Severe. Scattered, irregularly shaped denuded areas produce a mosaic appearance. Note the ulceration between the right maxillary lateral and canine. *D,* Severe. Complete denudation of the epithelium with exposure of underlying erythematous inflamed connective tissue.

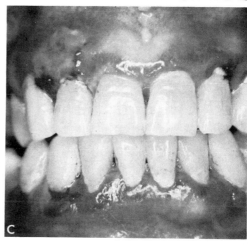

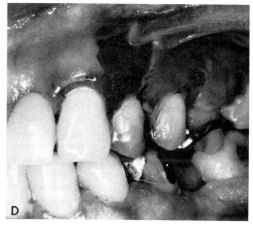

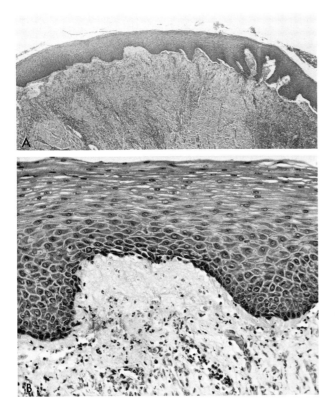

Figure 12–39 Chronic Desquamative Gingivitis—Bullous Type. *A,* There is massive replacement of the papillary and reticular connective tissue by inflammatory exudate, disruption of the epithelial–connective tissue junction, and the formation of large subepithelial bullae. *B,* Detailed view showing blunting of epithelial rete pegs and inflammatory exudate of edema, fibrin, and leukocytes which have replaced the connective tissue.

characterized by scattered, irregularly shaped areas in which the gingiva is denuded and strikingly red in appearance (Fig. 12–38*C*). Since the gingiva separating these areas is grayish blue, in over-all appearance the gingiva seems speckled. The surface epithelium is shredded and friable and can be peeled off in small patches (Fig. 12–38*D*).

There are occasionally surface vessels which rupture, releasing a thin, aqueous fluid and exposing an underlying surface that is red and raw. A blast of air directed at the gingiva causes elevation of the epithelium and the consequent formation of a bubble. The areas of involvement seem to shift to different locations on the gingiva. The mucous membrane other than the gingiva is smooth and shiny and may present a fissuring in the cheek adjacent to the line of occlusion.

The condition is extremely painful. The patient cannot tolerate coarse foods, condiments, or temperature changes. There is a constant, dry burning sensation throughout the oral cavity which is accentuated in the denuded gingival zones.

Histopathology

The microscopic appearance of so-called desquamative gingivitis often appears as a bullous type, resembling the histopathology of mucous membrane pemphigoid (Fig. 12–39), or as a lichenoid type with features similar to those of lichen planus (Fig. 12–40). Occasionally there will be a thin, atrophic epithelium with little or no keratin at the surface, and a dense, diffuse infiltration of chronic inflammatory cells in the underlying connective tissue. This tends to be the histopathologic picture in those rare cases of desquamative gingivitis due to menopausal alterations or the atrophic changes of aging.

Therapy

The therapy of so-called desquamative gingivitis must be based, if possible, on an

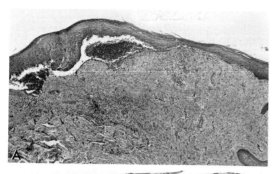

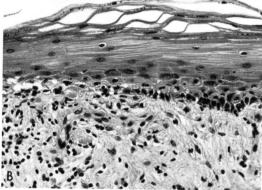

Figure 12–40 Chronic Desquamative Gingivitis—Lichenoid Type. A, The epithelium is atrophic, the connective tissue is inflamed, and the epithelium is separated from the connective tissue by a subepithelial vesicle. B, Detailed view, showing atrophic parakeratotic epithelium with vacuolization of the basal cells and microvesicle formation at the epithelium–connective tissue junction.

understanding of the basic disease process causing the gingival reaction.

1. A careful oral examination must be carried out so that other lesions may be discovered. In lichen planus the gingiva are rarely affected without other oral mucosal lesions being present.

2. A careful history should be taken for the possibility of co-existent extra-oral disease. A conjunctivitis and symptomatology of burning on urination or vaginal irritation may suggest multiple sites of mucosal disease and point to mucous membrane pemphigoid. The presence of papular skin lesions, particularly on sites such as wrists or ankles, would suggest lichen planus. Menopausal history or a history of hysterectomy would suggest a possible hormonal etiology.

3. Biopsy studies often point to the diagnosis of lichen planus or mucous membrane pemphigoid.

4. Local treatment is essential for all forms of desquamative gingivitis. The pa-

tient must be carefully instructed in plaque control, using a soft toothbrush, since the gingival surface is easily abraded with a hard brush. Oxidizing mouthwashes (hydrogen peroxide USP 3 per cent diluted to 1/3 peroxide:2/3 warm water) should be used twice daily. The reduction of gingival marginal inflammation also results in some reduction of the inflammation and desquamation of the attached gingiva. The use of topical corticosteroid ointments[7] and creams may be attempted, but their success has been limited. The gingival tissue is gently dried with a sterile sponge and an ointment or cream such as triamcinolone 0.1 per cent (Kenalog Aristocort) fluocinonide 0.05 per cent (Lidex), betamethasone 0.1 per cent (Valisone), or desonide 0.05 per cent (Tridesilon) is applied and gently rubbed into the gingiva several times daily.

5. Systemic therapy may be used in cases of severe gingival involvement. Systemic corticosteroid therapy is not to be considered lightly, since a variety of side effects is possible. The patient's general health should also be discussed with his physician prior to the use of systemic corticosteroids. If a diagnosis of mucous membrane pemphigoid is entertained, then moderate doses of corticosteroids are often helpful in alleviating discomfort and improving the tissue response. Prednisone can be used in a daily or every-second-day dose of 30 to 40 mg. and gradually reduced to a daily maintenance dose of 5 to 10 mg. Other steroids in comparable doses can be used. Systemic steroid therapy in lichen planus is helpful only in rare cases.

In a desquamative gingivitis due to a deficiency of estrogen or androgens, replacement therapy can be instituted, in consultation with the patient's physician. The estradiol or testosterone may stimulate growth of the atrophic gingival epithelium.

It must be emphasized that in many cases of desquamative gingivitis, it may not be possible to determine the basic etiology. However, local therapy together with diligence and patience will eventually improve the condition, and the etiologic background may be discovered by the eventual appearance of other lesions or symptoms. Particular care and patience is required in the atrophic gingivitis of aging, since there is no systemic therapy that has been found useful, other than nutritional supplements if the patient's nutritional status is deficient. Nutritional supplements[14] may be of value if the patient suffers from a true nutritional deficiency, such as vitamin B deficiency.

REFERENCES

1. Brusati, R., and Bracchetti, A.: Electron microscopic study of chronic desquamative gingivitis. J. Periodontol., 40:388–397, 1969.
2. Engel, M., Ray, H. G., and Orban, B.: The pathogenesis of desquamative gingivitis. J. Dent. Res., 29:410, 1950.
3. Foss, C. L., Grupe, H. E., and Orban, B.: Gingivosis. J. Periodontol., 24:207, 1953.
4. Glickman, I., and Smulow, J. B.: Chronic desquamative gingivitis: Its nature and treatment. J. Periodontol., 35:397, 1964.
5. Glickman, I., and Smulow, J. B.: Histopathology and histochemistry of chronic desquamative gingivitis. Oral Surg., 21:325, 1966.
6. Goadby, K.: Diseases of the gums and oral mucous membrane. London, Henry Froude and Hodder and Staughton, 1923, p. 22.
7. Goldman, H. M., and Ruben, M. P.: Desquamative gingivitis and its response to topical triamcinolone therapy. Oral Surg., 21:579, 1966.
8. Hashimoto, K., Dibella, R., Shklar, G., and Lever, W.: Electron microscopic studies of oral lichen planus. G. Ital. Dermatol., 107:765–788, 1966.
9. McCarthy, F. P., McCarthy, P. L., and Shklar, G.: Chronic desquamative gingivitis: A reconsideration. Oral Surg., 13:1300, 1960.
10. Merritt, A. H.: Chronic desquamative gingivitis. J. Periodontol., 4:30, 1933.
11. Nikai, H., Rose, G., and Cattoni, M.: Electron microscopic study of chronic desquamative gingivitis. J. Periodont. Res. (Suppl.), 6:1–30, 1971.
12. Prinz, H.: Chronic diffuse desquamative gingivitis. Dent. Cosmos, 74:331, 1932.
13. Pullon, P. A.: Ultrastructure of oral lichen planus. Oral Surg., 28:365–371, 1969.
14. Roth, H., and Ross, I. F.: The treatment of desquamative gingivitis. Oral Surg., 9:391, 1956.
15. Schour, I., and Massler, M.: Gingival disease in postwar Italy; gingivosis in hospitalized children in Naples. Am. J. Orthod., 33:756, 1947.
16. Shklar, G., and Mayer, I.: The histopathology and histochemistry of dermatologic lesions in the mouth. Oral Surg., 14:1069–1084, 1961.
17. Shklar, G.: Lichen planus as an oral ulcerative disease. Oral Surg., 33:376–388, 1972.
18. Shklar, C., Meyer, I., and Zacarian, S.: Oral lesions in bullous pemphigoid. Arch. Derm., 99:663–670, 1969.
19. Shklar, G., and McCarthy, P. L.: Oral lesions of mucous membrane pemphigoid. A study of 85 cases. Arch. Otolaryngol., 93:354–364, 1971.
20. Sognnaes, R. F., Weisberger, D., and Albright, J. T.: Pathologic desquamation of oral epithelium examined by electron microscopy and histochemistry. J. Natl. Cancer Inst., 17:329, 1956.
21. Sorrin, S.: Chronic desquamative gingivitis. J. Am. Dent. Assoc., 27:250, 1940.
22. Susi, F. R., and Shklar, G.: Histochemistry and fine structure of oral lesions of mucous membrane pemphigoid. Arch. Derm., 104:244–253, 1971.
23. Tomes, J., and Tomes, C.: Dental surgery. 4th ed. London, J. & A. Churchill, Ltd., 1894.
24. Whitten, J. B.: The fine structure of desquamative stomatitis. J. Periodontol., 39:75–80, 1968.
25. Ziskin, D., and Silvers, H. F.: Report of a case of desquamative gingivitis and lichen planus. J. Periodontol., 16:7, 1945.
26. Ziskin, D., and Zegarelli, E. V.: Chronic desquamative gingivitis. Am. J. Orthod., 33:756, 1947.

Part II

Periodontal Disease

Classification of Periodontal Disease

The term *chronic destructive periodontal disease* describes all forms of periodontal disease caused primarily by local factors (bacterial plaque and trauma from occlusion). It has been customary to classify chronic destructive periodontal disease into inflammatory, degenerative, and traumatic types. As useful background information some of the more relevant classifications proposed for the clinical management of periodontal disease are presented in Table 13–1.

CLASSIFICATION

The following classification includes all forms of chronic destructive periodontal disease in the light of recent investigations that have provided a different interpretation and categorization of laboratory and clinical findings. It attempts to provide a useful tool for the analysis and diagnosis of clinical cases:

Chronic destructive periodontal disease
  I. Periodontitis
    A. Simple
    B. Compound
    C. Juvenile form
      1. Generalized
      2. Localized (idiopathic juvenile periodontitis or periodontosis)
  II. Trauma from occlusion*
  III. Periodontal atrophy*

Review of other classifications

Because of varied interpretations of the nature of periodontal disease, its classification has been approached in many different ways. Representative classifications of periodontal disease are shown in Table 13–1.

PERIODONTITIS

Periodontitis† is the most common type of periodontal disease and results from the extension of the inflammatory process initiated in the gingiva to the supporting periodontal tissues (see Chapters 14 to 16).

---

*Both trauma from occlusion and periodontal atrophy, in their pure forms, are accommodation phenomena to changes in the environment. They are included under *diseases* for the sake of completeness and convenience for the clinician.

†Synonyms not in current usage include: schmutz-pyorrhea (Gottlieb), paradentitis (Weski-Becks), periodontoclasia, pericementitis, alveolar pyorrhea, alveoloclasia, Rigg's disease, and chronic suppurative periodontitis.

TABLE 13-1 REPRESENTATIVE CLASSIFICATIONS OF PERIODONTAL DISEASE

WESKI, 1937[21]

Paradentitis
(Gingivitis)
Hypertrophic
Simple
Ulcerative
Paradentosis
Partial atrophic (true form of paradentosis)
Total atrophic (alveolar atrophy?)
Diffuse atrophy
Paradentoma
Localized form
Epulis
Generalized form
Elephantiasis gingivae

KANTOROWICZ, 1924[13]

Inflammatory disease
Paradentitis
Dystrophic disease with little inflammation
Presenile atrophy
Dystrophy from occlusal trauma
Dystrophy from lack of occlusion
Diffuse atrophy

GOTTLIEB, 1928[7]

Inflammatory
Schmutzpyorrhea (poor oral hygiene)
Degenerative or atrophic
Diffuse alveolar atrophy (Systemic or metabolic causes)
Paradental pyorrhea

AMERICAN ACADEMY OF PERIODONTOLOGY, 1957[1]

Inflammation
Gingivitis
Periodontitis
Primary (simplex)
Secondary (complex)
Dystrophy
Occlusal traumatism
Periodontal disuse atrophy
Gingivosis
Periodontosis

JACCARD, 1930, 1933[11, 12]

Inflammatory complex
Pure gingivitis
Preparadontal gingivitis
Inflammatory paradentosis
Osteopathic dystrophic complex
Dystrophic paradentosis
Presenile atrophy
Senile atrophy

THOMA AND GOLDMAN, 1937[20]

Inflammatory conditions
Gingivitis (may be of local or systemic origin)
Marginal, Hypertrophic, Ulcerative
Marginal paradentitis (poor oral hygiene)
Degenerative conditions
Paradontosis (bone resorption, in turn affecting other periodontal structures)
Atrophy
Gingival recession (faulty toothbrushing)
Presenile atrophy (normal physiologic process, recession of gingivae, and resorption of alveolar crest)
Disuse atrophy
Decreased dental function or lack of function of jaws
Atrophy due to abnormal occlusal trauma
Syndrome of paradontitis and paradontosis

HÄUPL AND LANG, 1927[8]

Paradentitis
Marginal paradentitis
Etiology includes mechanical, thermal, chemical, infectious factors, as well as functional disturbances, tooth malformation, systemic disturbances, general resistance, etc.
Superficial marginal paradentitis
Epithelial changes
Regressive
Progressive
Formation of the pocket
Connective tissue changes
Subepithelial
Supra-alveolar
Changes in paradental bone
Marginal paradentitis profunda
Apical paradentitis

McPHEE AND COWLEY, 1969[15]

Gingivitis
Acute gingivitis
Acute specific
Ulceromembranous gingivitis
Herpetic gingivitis
Coccal gingivitis
Acute nonspecific
Acute gingivitis which does not present the features characteristic of ulceromembranous gingivitis; herpetic or coccal gingivitis.
Chronic gingivitis
Chronic nonspecific
Chronic edematous gingivitis
Chronic hyperplastic gingivitis
Chronic atrophic gingivitis
Periodontitis
Acute nonspecific
Periodontal abscess
Chronic nonspecific
Periodontitis simplex
Periodontitis complex

CARRANZA, 1959[3]

Inflammatory Periodontal Syndrome { Superficial / Deep
Traumatic Periodontal Syndrome { Compensated / Uncompensated
Combined Periodontal Syndrome { Compensated / Uncompensated

Table continued on the following page

TABLE 13–1 REPRESENTATIVE CLASSIFICATIONS OF PERIODONTAL DISEASE *(Continued)*

Box, McCall, 1940, 1925[2,14]	Fish, 1944[1]	Orban, 1949[17]	Hulin, 1949[10]
Gingivitis Acute Chronic **Periodontitis** Acute Chronic **Periodontitis simplex** (exogenous factors) **Periodontitis complex or rarefying pericementitis fibrosa** (endogenous factors)	**Gingivitis** Acute ulcerative Subacute marginal Chronic marginal Traumatic **Pyorrhea** Pyorrhea simplex (gradual deepening of sulcus) Pyorrhea profunda (deep pocket, pus formation, tooth mobility) Senile alveolar resorption **Neoplasia** Odontoclasma Cementoma Fibrous epulis	**Inflammatory conditions** **Gingivitis** Localized to free margin of gingiva Swelling, shallow pockets Acute or chronic according to duration Ulcerative, purulent, etc. according to symptoms Local or systemic according to etiology Local (extrinsic). Infectious. Physical. Chemical Systemic (intrinsic). Dietary deficiency. Endocrine disturbance **Periodontitis** Inflammation extends to deeper supporting tissues. May be deep pockets, suppuration, abscess formation. Varying degrees of alveolar resorption Simplex—following gingivitis Complex—following periodontosis **Degenerative conditions** **Gingivosis—systemic etiology** Degeneration of connective tissue **Periodontosis** Degeneration of collagenous fibers of the periodontal membrane Irregular bone resorption Primarily systemic etiology—inherited inferiority of dental organ Early—no inflammation Late—deep pockets with periodontitis **Atrophic conditions** Periodontal atrophy—bone recession Precocious aging. Aging. Disuse—loss of normal function. Trauma—toothbrush, orthodontia **Periodontal traumatism** Pressure necrosis and its consequences Primary—overstress, bruxism, etc. Secondary—loss of supporting tissue **Gingival hyperplasia** Overgrowth of gingiva in varying degrees Infections—pyogenic granuloma. Endocrine dysfunction—pregnancy. Drugs—Dilantin. Idiopathic.	**Inflammatory process** **Parodontitis** Exogenous gingivitis Tartar Bacteria Endogenous gingivitis Avitaminosis Intoxication **Degenerative processes** **Paradontosis** Precocious senile atrophy or Juvenile paradontosis Senile paradontosis Pyorrhetic paradontosis Traumatic paradontolysis **Paradontomes** Epulis Gingival elephantiasis

Held and Chaput, 1960[9]	Grant, Stern, and Everett, 1972[5]	Goldman and Cohen, 1972[6]	Prichard, 1972[18]	Schluger, Yuodelis and Page, 1977[19]
Parodontopathies Superficial 　Inflammatory — gingivitis 　Degenerative — gingivosis Deep 　Inflammatory — parodontitis 　Degenerative — parodontosis } parodontolysis Superficial and deep 　Neoplastic — parodontoma 　Reticular — parodontoreticulosis	Inflammatory 　Gingivitis 　Periodontitis Dystrophic 　Atrophic degenerative conditions 　　Recession 　　Disuse 　　Gingival hyperplasia 　Traumatic 　　Periodontal trauma 　　　Primary 　　　Secondary 　Unknown etiology 　　Periodontosis	I. Inflammation 　A. Gingivitis — with or without gingival enlargement (acute and chronic) 　B. Periodontitis 　　1. Secondary to long-standing gingivitis 　　2. Initial lesion 　　3. May occur in conjunction with occlusal traumatism 　　4. Secondary to periodontosis II. Dystrophy 　A. Occlusal traumatism 　B. Degenerative disease of attachment apparatus: periodontosis	Diseases affecting the surface or gingiva 　Inflammation without surface destruction 　　Marginal gingivitis 　　Generalized diffuse gingivitis 　　Gingival enlargement 　Inflammation with surface destruction 　　Necrotizing ulcerative gingivitis 　　Herpetic gingivostomatitis 　　Desquamative gingivitis 　　Oral ulcers Diseases that affect the deeper structures 　Chronic destructive periodontal disease or periodontitis 　Periodontal abscess 　Periodontal traumatism 　　Primary traumatism 　　Secondary traumatism	Gingivitis 　Plaque-associated gingivitis 　Acute ulcerative necrotizing gingivitis 　Hormonal gingivitis 　Drug-induced gingivitis Marginal periodontitis 　Adult type 　Juvenile type

REFERENCES TO TABLE 13–1

1. Bernier, J. L.: Report of the committee on classification and nomenclature. J. Periodontol., 28:56, 1957.
2. Box, H. K.: Periodontal studies. D. Items Int., 62:915, 1940.
3. Carranza, F. A., Sr., and Carranza, F. A., Jr.: A suggested classification of common periodontal disease. J. Periodontol., 30:140, 1959.
4. Fish, E. W.: Paradontal Disease. London, Eyre and Spottiswoode, 1944, p. 52.
5. Grant, D. A., Stern J., and Everett, F.: Orban's Periodontics, 4th ed. St. Louis, The C. V. Mosby Co., 1972.
6. Goldman, H. M., and Cohen, D. W.: Periodontal Therapy, 5th ed. St. Louis, The C. V. Mosby Co., 1972.
7. Gottlieb, B.: Parodontal pyorrhea and alveolar atrophy. J. Am. Dent. Assoc., 15:2196, 1928.
8. Häupl, K., and Lang, F. J.: Marginal Paradentitis. Berlin, H. Meusser, 1927.
9. Held, A.-J., and Chaput, A.: Les Parodontologies. J. Prelat, Paris, 1960.
10. Hulin, C.: Nomenclature and classification. Paradentologie, 3:82, 1949.
11. Jaccard, R.: Terminologie des Pyorrhees. Schwz. Mschr. Zahnhk., 40:661, 1930.
12. Jaccard, R.: Necessity of an international collaboration for paradentosis investigation. Schwz. Mschr. Zahnhk., 43:196, 1933.
13. Kantorowicz, A.: Two types of pyorrhea. Klin. Zahnheilk., 1924.
14. McCall, J. O., and Box, H. K.: Chronic periodontitis. J. Am. Dent. Assoc., 12:1300, 1925.
15. McPhee, T., and Cowley, G.: Essentials of Periodontology and Periodontitis. London, Blackwell Scientific Publications, 1969.
16. Orban, B.: Classification and nomenclature of periodontal diseases. J. Periodontol., 13:88, 1942.
17. Orban, B.: Classification of periodontal disease. Paradentologie, 3:159, 1949.
18. Prichard, J. F.: Advanced Periodontal Disease, 2nd ed. Philadelphia, W. B. Saunders Company, 1972.
19. Schluger, S., Yuodelis, R., and Page, R.: Periodontal Disease. Philadelphia, Lea & Febiger, 1977.
20. Thoma, K. H., and Goldman, H. M.: Classification and histopathology of parodontal disease. J. Am. Dent. Assoc., 24:1915, 1937.
21. Weski, O.: Paradentopathia and paradentosis. Paradentium, 8:169, 1937.

Lindhe et al.[13] have studied the sequential stages in the development of a periodontal lesion in dogs on the basis of clinical manifestations and measurements of gingival exudate. They describe the following stages:

1. *Phase of subclinical gingivitis*, characterized by rapidly increased gingival exudation and migration of crevicular leukocytes, i.e., signs of acute inflammation.

2. *Phase of clinical gingivitis*, characterized by changes in gingival color, texture, and bleeding tendency but only minor alterations in the number of migrating crevicular leukocytes.

3. *Phase of periodontal breakdown*, characterized by loss of fiber attachment; radiographic bone changes appear.

Periodontitis can be classified as *simple* or *marginal* periodontitis, in which the destruction of periodontal tissues is associated with inflammation alone; *compound* periodontitis, in which the tissue destruction resulting from inflammation is modified by trauma from occlusion; and *juvenile forms*, which constitute a special group of advanced lesions in children and adolescents.

Simple Periodontitis

CLINICAL FEATURES. Chronic inflammation of the gingiva, pocket formation, and bone loss usually accompany simple periodontitis. Tooth mobility and pathologic migration appear in advanced cases. This disease may be localized to a single tooth or group of teeth or generalized throughout the mouth, depending upon the distribution of the etiologic factors (Fig. 13–1).

Simple periodontitis progresses at a varied rate; its advanced stages are usually seen in the fifth and sixth decades of life. This contrasts with the juvenile form, which reaches advanced stages in the late teens and early adulthood.

Simple periodontitis is usually painless, but it may be accompanied by such symptoms as (1) sensitivity to thermal changes, food, and tactile stimulation associated with denudation of the roots; (2) dull deep radiating pain during and after chewing, caused by the forceful wedging of food into periodontal pockets; (3) acute symptoms such as throbbing pain and sensitivity to percussion from periodontal abscess formation or superimposed acute necrotizing ulcerative gingivitis; (4) pulpal symptoms such as sensitivity to sweets, thermal changes, or throbbing pain, which result from pulpitis associated with carious destruction of the root surfaces.

ETIOLOGY. Simple periodontitis is caused by dental plaque. The accumulation of plaque can be favored by a large variety of local irritants such as calculus, faulty restorations, food impaction.

Compound Periodontitis *

CLINICAL FEATURES. The clinical features are the same as those of simple periodontitis with the following exceptions: there is a higher incidence of infrabony pockets and angular rather than horizontal bone loss[6] (Fig. 13–2); widening of the periodontal ligament space is a more common finding; tooth mobility tends to occur earlier and to be more severe.

ETIOLOGY. Compound periodontitis is caused by the combined effect of bacterial plaque and the resultant inflammation, and trauma from occlusion.

On the basis of the rate of tissue destruction and some clinical features, simple and compound periodontitis can be subclassified in two groups. One is a *slow progressing lesion* associated with abundant plaque and calculus deposits. Obvious signs of gingival inflammation are found (changes in color, surface texture, abundant exudate, etc.). (See Chapters 7 to 11.)

The other type is a more *rapidly progressing lesion*, with less obvious signs of inflammation and associated with scantier amounts of plaque and calculus. Different composition and structure of bacterial plaque have been found in these two types of periodontitis.[22]

The clinical features of the slow and rapid

---

*Other terms used for this condition include occlusal periodontitis and traumatic periodontitis.

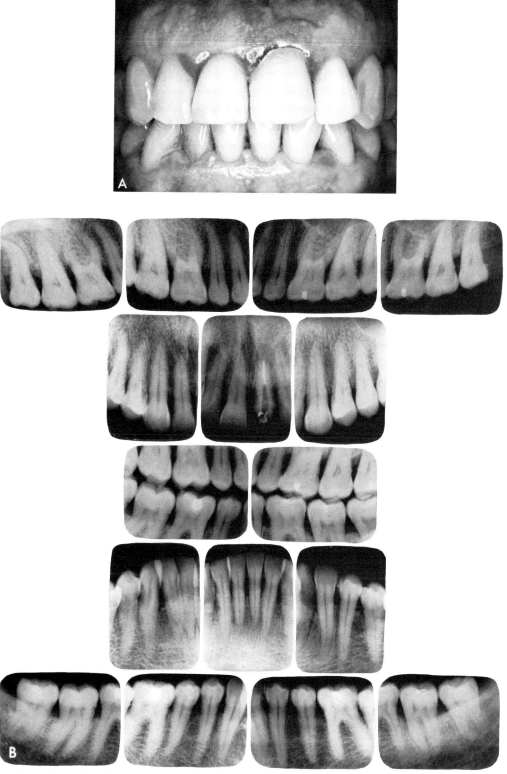

Figure 13–1 Simple Periodontitis in a 47-Year-Old Female. *A,* Clinical view showing generalized gingival inflammation and periodontal pocket formation. *B,* Radiographs showing generalized horizontal bone loss which varies in severity in different areas.

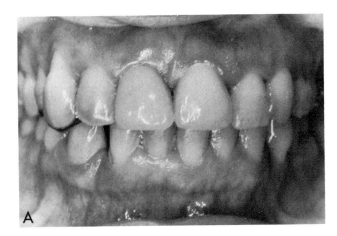

Figure 13–2 Compound Periodontitis in a 44-year-old Female. *A,* Generalized gingival inflammation with periodontal pocket formation. *B,* Generalized bone loss with angular destruction of the interdental septa caused by the combination of inflammation and trauma from occlusion.

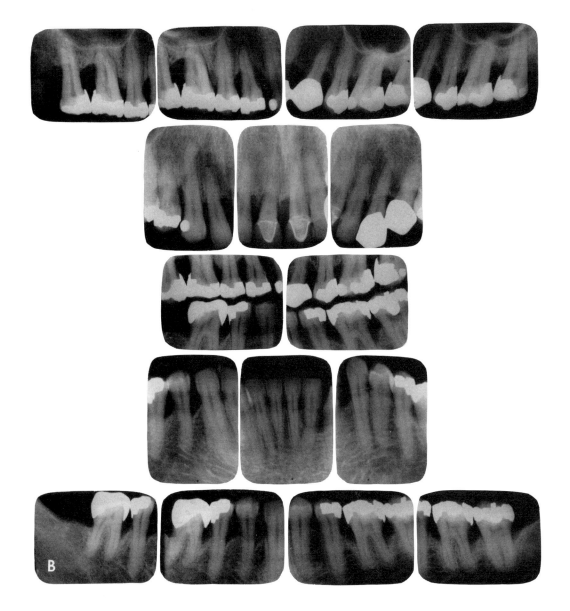

types of periodontitis are not yet clearly defined, and differential diagnosis is therefore difficult except on the basis of determining the rate of progression of periodontal destruction and its response to treatment. They may be compatible with the diagnosis of positive and negative bone factor as determined by Glickman.

Juvenile Form of Periodontitis

This form includes advanced destructive lesions in children and adolescents.* The distribution of lesions is the basis for its classification into generalized and localized forms. The generalized form involves the whole dentition while the localized form attacks first molars and incisors.

Generalized form

These are the diseases associated with systemic conditions such as Papillon-Lefèvre syndrome, hypophosphatasia, agranulocytosis, Down's syndrome, and others. They have different characteristics depending on the systemic condition and are dealt with in Chapter 21. Patients without underlying systemic predisposing factors have also been described.[1, 2]

Localized form

This includes the disease we now call "idiopathic juvenile periodontitis" or "periodontosis." It was first described by Gottlieb[9] in 1923 under the name "diffuse atrophy of the alveolar bone" in a fatal case of epidemic influenza. He described loss of collagen fibers in the periodontal ligament and its replacement by loose connective tissue and extensive bone resorption resulting in a widened periodontal ligament space. The gingiva was apparently not involved. In 1928 Gottlieb attributed this condition to the inhibition of continuous cementum formation, which he considered essential for maintenance of periodontal

---

*The terms precocious advanced alveolar atrophy,[16] juvenile atrophy, paradentose juvenile, and juvenile parodontopathia have been used to describe this condition.

ligament fibers; he termed it then "deep cementopathia." In an expansion of his theory Gottlieb felt that deep cementopathia was a "disease of eruption." Senescent cementum could act like a foreign body in an attempt by the host to exfoliate the tooth, resulting in bone resorption and pocket formation.[10]

In 1940 Thoma and Goldman[23] introduced the term "paradontosis" for this disease, the initial feature of which is located in the alveolar bone rather than in the cementum and which consists of vascular resorption and halisteresis rather than "lacunar resorption." In 1947 Goldman[8] described again these features in a spider monkey: a degenerative noninflammatory disease of the supporting structures.

In 1942 Orban and Weinmann[19] introduced the term "periodontosis" and on the basis of one autopsy case studied in detail described three stages in the development of the disease.

Stage 1, consisting of degeneration and desmolysis of the principal fibers of the periodontal ligament and probable cessation of cementum formation; there is simultaneous resorption of the alveolar bone owing to lack of functional stimulation from the tooth and increased tissue pressure caused by edema and capillary proliferation. In this stage tooth migration occurs as the earliest clinical sign and it occurs without detectable inflammatory involvement.

The *second stage* is characterized by the rapid proliferation of the junctional epithelium along the root and sometimes proliferation of the epithelial rests of Malassez. In this stage the earliest signs of inflammation appear. Clinically, both the first and second stage are of short duration and cannot be differentiated from each other.

The *third stage* is characterized by progressive inflammation and the development of deep periodontal pockets of the infrabony type. This is the stage most frequently seen.

All the above mentioned studies consider periodontosis a degenerative disease, caused by unknown systemic factors. Glickman in 1952[7] felt that these conditions did not represent a different type of periodontal disease but that they represented extreme variants of destructive processes

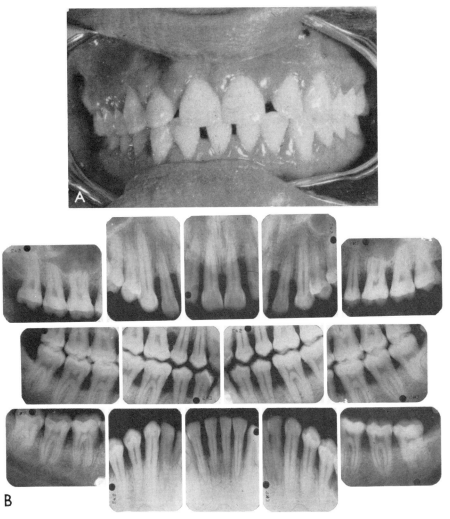

Figure 13–3 Idiopathic juvenile periodontitis ("periodontosis") in a 24-year-old Male. A, Pathologic migration of the maxillary and mandibular anterior teeth. B, Generalized bone loss accentuated in the maxillary and mandibular anterior areas.

common to all periodontal disease. Many authors have denied the existence of a degenerative type of periodontal disease and have attributed the changes to the effect of trauma from occlusion.[4, 11, 15, 20, 21] In 1966 the World Workshop in Periodontics[24] was of the opinion that the conventional concept of periodontosis as a degenerative entity was unsubstantiated and that the term should be eliminated from periodontal nomenclature. The committee did recognize that a clinical entity different from "adult" periodontitis may occur in adolescents and young adults.

Recent studies have revealed important differences between the "juvenile" and the "adult" types of periodontal destruction, particularly from the microbiological[17, 18]

and immunological[14] points of view. They are reviewed in detail in Chapter 25. They do not yet, however, give a clue to the reason for the peculiar distribution of the lesions in the mouth; they do point to a bacterial etiology particularly related to the presence of anaerobic microbes and to a possible immunologic predisposition.

CLINICAL FEATURES. Juvenile periodontitis affects both males and females and is seen most frequently in the period between puberty and the age of 25. In teenagers it is more prevalent in females.

The distribution in the mouth is characteristic and as yet unexplainable. The maxillary and mandibular incisors are affected earliest and most severely and usually bilaterally, but with time the involvement

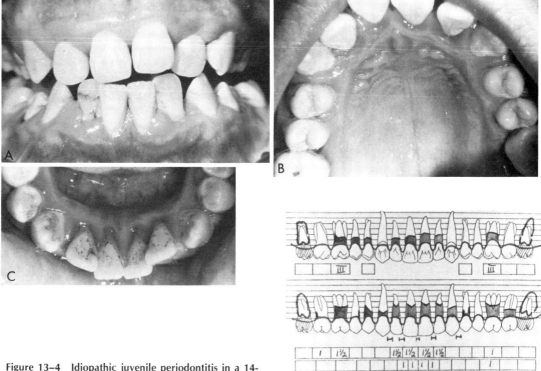

Figure 13–4   Idiopathic juvenile periodontitis in a 14-year-old male. *A, B, C,* Clinical picture showing gingival inflammation and migration of teeth with diastema formation. *D,* Diagram depicting pocket depth (shaded areas on teeth), tooth mobility (in boxes between upper and lower teeth) and furcation involvements (in boxes with Roman numerals adjacent to molars and first upper premolars). *E,* Radiographs demonstrating the typical molar-incision distribution of bone loss. Note the higher bone level in canines and premolars and in second molars.

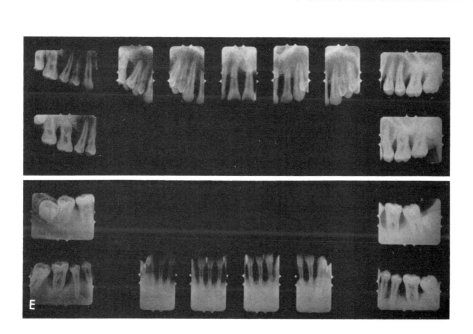

may become generalized. Least destruction occurs in the mandibular premolar area (Figs. 13–3 and 13–4).

The onset of osseous destruction is insidious, especially during the circumpubertal period from 11 to 13 years of age. The most striking feature of early juvenile periodontitis is the lack of clinical inflammation. Late in the incipient stages there is the beginning of deep pocket formation in the periodontium around these teeth, and, clinically, the most common presenting symptoms are mobility and migration of the incisors and first molars.

As the disease progresses, however, other symptomatology may arise. Denuded root surfaces become sensitive to thermal changes, foods, and tactile stimuli such as toothbrush bristles or curette blades. Deep, dull, radiating pain may be present upon mastication and is probably due to irritation of the supporting structures from mobile teeth and impacted food. Periodontal abscesses may form at this stage. Manson and Lehner[14] have reported a high incidence of regional lymph node enlargement in affected individuals.

Vertical loss of alveolar bone around the first molars and incisors in otherwise healthy individuals is taken to be a diagnostic sign of classical juvenile periodontitis. Roentgenographic findings include "an arc-shaped loss of alveolar bone extending from the distal surface of the second bicuspid to the mesial surface of the second molar."[16] Evidence indicates that bone loss is not from any developmental or congenital absence or defect. Alveolar bone in patients in this age group develops normally with tooth eruption and only subsequently does the alveolar bone undergo resorptive changes. Classically, one sees a distolabial migration of the maxillary incisors with diastemata formation. The lower incisors seem to have less of a propensity to migrate. Occlusal patterns and tongue pressures can vary the amount and type of migration noted. Along with anterior tooth migration, an apparent increase in size of the clinical crown, accumulation of plaque and calculus, and clinical inflammation appears. Kaslick and Chasens[12] reported that in many cases of periodontosis bilateral and symmetrical patterns of bone loss occur.

Juvenile periodontitis progresses rapidly. Evidence available indicates that the rate of bone loss is about three to four times faster than in typical periodontitis. In affected patients, bone resorption progresses until the teeth are either treated, exfoliated, or extracted. There is no consistent or reliable evidence to indicate that the disease process per se spreads to unaffected areas. However, it has been reported that in later stages of the disease other teeth are involved with a form of periodontitis accompanied by the usual inflammatory changes (Fig. 13–5).

Several authors have described a familial pattern of alveolar bone loss and have implicated (without substantial evidence) a genetic factor in periodontosis.[3, 5] Benjamin and Baer,[2] in the most comprehensive study on familial patterns, described the disease in identical twins, siblings, and first cousins, as well as in parents and offspring. Newman and Socransky[18] have also described a familial pattern and have suggested the possibility of a transmissible microbiologic component in the pathogenesis of the disease.

Baer has also considered a more generalized form of juvenile periodontitis. In this form the disease process may affect most of the dentition with the same initial signs and symptoms described for the localized or classical form of the disease. Recently, however, several investigators have suggested that the generalized form of the disease be separated from classical periodontosis. Until more substantial scientific and clinical data are presented, there will be continued confusion and disagreement, and at the present time, it is generally accepted that there are two forms of juvenile periodontitis, the localized or classical form and the generalized form.

The clinical course of juvenile periodontitis is rapid and fairly predictable. However, there is a phenomenon referred to as "burn out" that is seen in many cases. "Burn out" refers to a sudden and unexplainable decrease in the rate of bone destruction, and is almost always seen in the mid- and late twenties. In these cases, the onset of alveolar resorption apparently occurred in the mid- to late teens, rather than during the circumpubertal period.

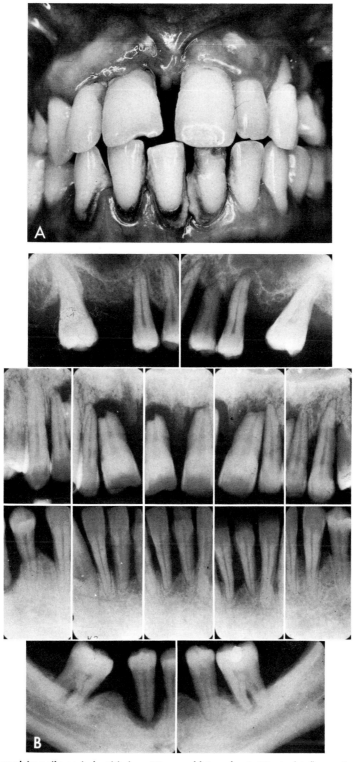

Figure 13–5   Advanced juvenile periodontitis in a 28-year-old Female. *A,* Gingival inflammation, heavy calculus deposits, anterior open bite with diastema formation associated with tongue thrusting habit. *B,* Severe generalized bone destruction obscures the limitation of bone loss to the anterior and molar regions seen in early periodontosis.

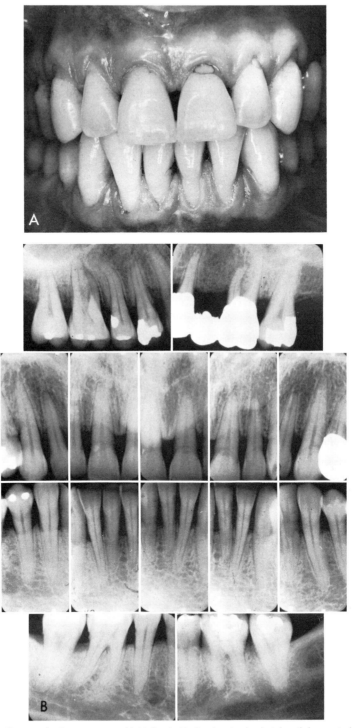

Figure 13–6   Presenile Atrophy in a 38-year-old Male. *A,* Reduction in the height of the periodontium and recession with slight gingival inflammation. *B,* Premature generalized bone loss.

Although many theories have been postulated regarding this phenomenon, none are based on scientific fact.

TRAUMA FROM OCCLUSION

Because gingival inflammation is so common, trauma from occlusion seldom occurs without it. When it is the sole pathological process it presents the following clinical features: tooth mobility, pronounced widening of the periodontal space in the gingival region of the root (with an associated angular destruction of bone) and thickening of the periodontal ligament at the apex. Isolated teeth and their antagonists are affected. It does not produce gingival inflammation or formation of periodontal pockets.

PERIODONTAL ATROPHY

Atrophy is a decrease in the size of the tissue or organ or of its cellular elements after it has attained its normal mature size. Generalized reduction in the height of the alveolar bone, accompanied by recession of the gingiva without overt inflammation or trauma from occlusion, occurs with increasing age and has been termed physiologic or senile atrophy. It is due not to aging but to the cumulative effect of repeated injuries to the periodontium.

Presenile Atrophy

Presenile atrophy is premature reduction in the height of the periodontium that is uniform throughout the mouth and without apparent local cause (Fig. 13–6).

Disuse Atrophy

Disuse atrophy results when the functional stimulation required for the maintenance of the periodontal tissues is markedly diminished or absent. Disuse atrophy is characterized by thinning of the periodontal ligament, thinning and reduction in the number of periodontal fibers and disruption

of the fiber bundle arrangement, thickened cementum and reduction in the height of the alveolar bone, and osteoporosis, which appears as a reduction in the number and thickness of the bone trabeculae.

REFERENCES

1. Baer, P. N.: The case for periodontosis as a clinical entity. J. Periodontol., *42*:516, 1971.
2. Benjamin, S. D., and Baer, P. N.: Familial patterns of advanced alveolar bone loss in adolescence (periodontosis). Periodontics, *5*:82, 1967.
3. Butler, J. H.: A familial pattern of juvenile periodontitis (periodontosis). J. Periodontol., *40*: 115, 1969.
4. Carranza, F. A., Sr., and Carranza, F. A., Jr.: A suggested classification of common periodontal disease. J. Periodontol., *30*:140, 1959.
5. Cohen, D. W., and Goldman, H. M.: Clinical observations on the modification of human oral tissue metabolism by local intraoral factors. Ann. N. Y. Acad. Sci., *85*:68, 1960.
6. Erausquin, R., and Carranza, F. A.: Primeros hallazgos paradentosicos. Rev. Odontol. (Buenos Aires), *27*:485, 1939.
7. Glickman, I.: Periodontosis: A critical evaluation. J. Am. Dent. Assoc., *44*:706, 1952.
8. Goldman, H. M.: Similar condition to periodontosis in two spider monkeys. Am. J. Orthod., *33*:749, 1947.
9. Gottlieb, B.: Die diffuse atrophy des alveolarknochens. Z. Stomatol., *21*:195, 1923.
10. Gottlieb, B.: The formation of the pocket: Diffuse atrophy of alveolar bone. J. A. Dent. Assoc., *15*:462, 1928.
11. Häupl, K., and Lang, F. J.: Marginal Paradentitis. Berlin, H. Meusser, 1927.
12. Kaslick, R. S., and Chasens, A. I.: Periodontosis with periodontitis: A study involving young adult males. Oral Surg., *25*:327, 1968.
13. Lindhe, J., Hamp, S. E., and Loe, H.: Experimental periodontitis in the Beagle dog. Intern. Dent. J., *23*:432, 1973.
14. Manson, J. D., and Lehner, T.: Clinical features of juvenile periodontitis (periodontosis) J. Periodontol., *45*:636, 1974.
15. Mezl, Z.: Contribution a l'histologie pathologique du paradentium. Paradentologie, *2*:60, 1948.
16. Miller, S. C.: Precocious advanced alveolar atrophy. J. Periodontol., *19*:146, 1948.
17. Newman, M. G.: Periodontosis. J. Western Soc. Periodont., *24*:5, 1976.
18. Newman, M. G., and Socransky, S. S.: Predominant cultivable microbiota in periodontosis. J. Periodont. Res., *12*:120, 1977.
19. Orban, B., and Weinmann, J. P.: Diffuse atrophy of alveolar bone. J. Periodontol., *13*:31, 1942.
20. Ramfjord, S. P.: Effect of acute febrile diseases with special reference to collagen fibers. J. Dent. Res., *31*:5, 1952.
21. Ramfjord, S. P.: Tuberculosis and periodontal

disease with special reference to collagen fibers. J. Dent. Res., *31*:5, 1952.

22. Socransky, S. S.: Personal communication.

23. Thoma, K. H., and Goldman, H. M.: Wandering and elongation of the teeth and pocket formation in paradontosis. J. Am. Dent. Assoc., *27*:335, 1940.

24. World Workshop in Periodontics. Ramfjord, S. P., Ash, M. M., and Kerr, D. A. (eds). University of Michigan, 1966.

The Periodontal Pocket

A periodontal pocket is a pathologically deepened gingival sulcus; it is one of the important clinical features of periodontal disease. Progressive pocket formation leads to destruction of the supporting periodontal tissues, and loosening and exfoliation of the teeth.

SIGNS AND SYMPTOMS

The only reliable method of locating periodontal pockets and determining their extent is careful probing of the gingival margin along each tooth surface.

The following clinical signs may indicate the presence of periodontal pockets:

1. Enlarged, bluish red marginal gingiva with a "rolled" edge separated from the tooth surface (Fig. 14–1).

2. A reddish blue vertical zone from the gingival margin to the attached gingiva and sometimes into the alveolar mucosa (Fig. 14–2).

3. A break in the faciolingual continuity of the interdental gingiva.

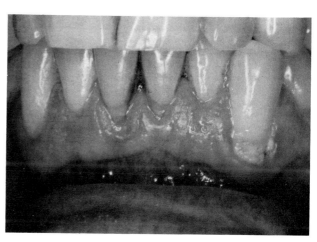

Figure 14–1 Periodontal Pockets around the central incisors and left canine, showing rolled margins and separation from the tooth surfaces. Note the materia alba on the canine.

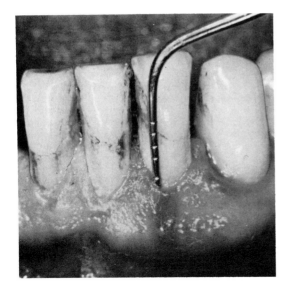

Figure 14-2 Periodontal Pocket with vertical discolored zone extending to the alveolar mucosa.

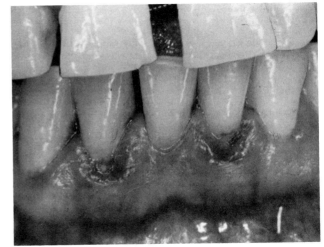

Figure 14-3 Periodontal Pockets with puffy discolored gingiva and exposed root surfaces.

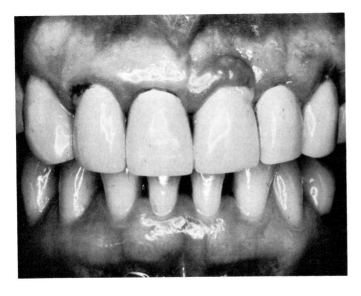

Figure 14-4 Purulent Exudate from periodontal pocket on the maxillary left central incisor.

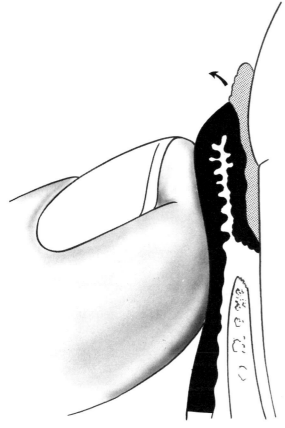

Figure 14–5 **Purulent Exudate Expressed from Periodontal Pocket by Digital Pressure.**

gin (Fig. 14–4), or its appearance in response to digital pressure on the lateral aspect of the gingival margin (Fig. 14–5).

7. Looseness, extrusion, and migration of teeth.

8. The development of diastemata where none had existed (Fig. 14–6).

Periodontal pockets are generally painless but may give rise to the following symptoms: localized pain or a sensation of pressure after eating, which gradually diminishes; a foul taste in localized areas; a tendency to suck material from the interproximal spaces; radiating pain "deep in the bone"; a "gnawing" feeling or feeling of itchiness in the gums; the urge to dig a pointed instrument into the gums with relief from the resultant bleeding; complaints that food "sticks between the teeth," the teeth "feel loose," or preference to "eat on the other side"; sensitivity to heat and cold; toothache in the absence of caries.

CLASSIFICATION

Periodontal pockets are classified according to morphology and their relationship to adjacent structures as follows:

Gingival pocket (relative or false)

A gingival pocket is formed by gingival enlargement without destruction of the underlying periodontal tissues. The sulcus is deepened because of the increased bulk of the gingiva (Fig. 14–7).

4. Shiny, discolored, and puffy gingiva associated with exposed root surfaces (Fig. 14–3).

5. Gingival bleeding.

6. Purulent exudate of the gingival mar-

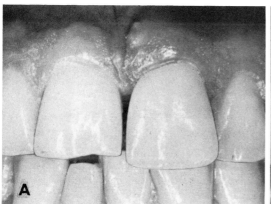
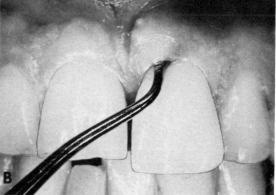

Figure 14–6 *A,* **Extrusion of Maxillary Left Incisor** and diastema associated with periodontal pocket. *B,* Entire length of periodontal probe inserted to the base of periodontal pocket on central incisor.

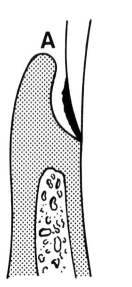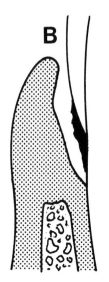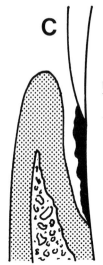

Figure 14–7 Different Types of Periodontal Pockets. *A,* Gingival pocket. There is no destruction of the supporting periodontal tissues. *B,* Suprabony pocket. The base of the pocket is coronal to the level of the underlying bone. Bone loss is horizontal. *C,* Infra-bony pocket. The base of the pocket is apical to the level of the adjacent bone. Bone loss is vertical.

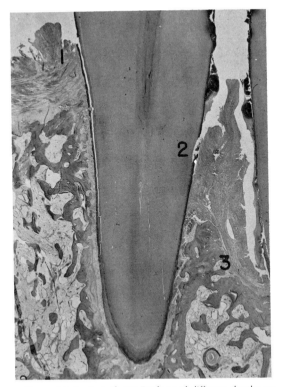

Figure 14–8 Suprabony Pockets of different depths on the distal (1) and mesial (2) surfaces of second premolar. Interdental space with suprabony pocket (2) and **Infrabony Pocket** (3) on the approximating tooth surfaces.

Periodontal pocket (absolute or true)

This is the type of pocket that occurs with destruction of the supporting periodontal tissues (Fig. 14–7). Absolute pockets are of two types: (1) *suprabony* (supracrestal), in which the bottom of the pocket is coronal to the underlying alveolar bone, and (2) *infrabony* (intrabony, subcrestal, or intra-alveolar), in which the bottom of the pocket is apical to the level of the adjacent alveolar bone. In this type the lateral pocket wall lies between the tooth surface and the alveolar bone (Fig. 14–7).

Pockets of different depths and types may occur on different surfaces of the same tooth and on approximating surfaces of the same interdental space (Fig. 14–8).

Pockets can also be classified according to the number of surfaces involved as follows:

SIMPLE. One tooth surface (Fig. 14–9).

COMPOUND. Two or more tooth surfaces. The base of the pockets is in direct communication with the gingival margin along each of the involved surfaces (Fig. 14–9).

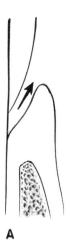
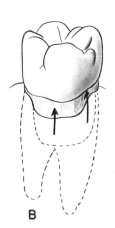
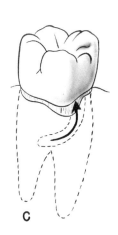

Figure 14–9 Classification of Pockets According to Involved Tooth Surfaces. *A,* Simple pocket. *B,* Compound pocket. *C,* Complex pocket.

A   **B**   **C**

COMPLEX. This is a spiral-type pocket that originates on one tooth surface and twists around the tooth to involve one or more additional surfaces (Figs. 14–9 and 14–10). The only communication with the gingival margin is at the surface where the pocket originates. To avoid missing the compound or complex types, all pockets should be probed laterally as well as vertically.

PATHOGENESIS

Periodontal pockets are caused by microorganisms and their products, which produce pathologic tissue changes and deepening of the gingival sulcus. **There are no systemic conditions which initiate periodontal pockets.** On the basis of depth alone, it is sometimes difficult to differentiate between a deep normal sulcus and a shallow periodontal pocket. In such borderline cases pathologic changes in the gingiva differentiate the two conditions.

Deepening of the gingival sulcus may occur by (1) movement of the gingival margin in the direction of the crown (this produces a "gingival" rather than a periodontal pocket; sulcus depth is increased by enlargement of the gingiva without destruction of supporting tissues); (2) migration of the junctional epithelium apically and its separation from the tooth surface; or (3) what is usually the case, a combination of both processes. In a sense, pocket formation may be likened to the stretching of an accordion, in that distance is increased by movement in opposite directions (Fig. 14–11).

The sequence of changes involved in transition from the normal gingival sulcus to the pathologic periodontal pocket is as follows:

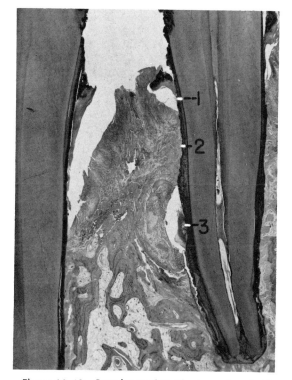

Figure 14–10 **Complex Pocket.** The base of pocket is shown at 3. The pocket then spirals around onto another surface of the tooth and communicates with the oral cavity at 1. In the area marked 2, the periodontal ligament is attached to the tooth.

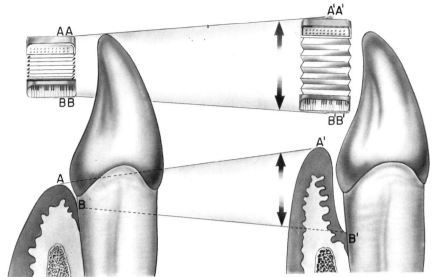

Figure 14–11 **Diagrammatic Representation of Pocket Formation** indicating expansion in two directions from the normal gingival sulcus *AB* to the periodontal pocket *A'B'*. Note comparison with expanding accordion *AA, BB,* to *A'A', B'B'*.

Pocket formation starts as an inflammatory change in the connective tissue wall of the gingival sulcus caused by bacterial plaque. The cellular and fluid inflammatory exudate causes degeneration of the surrounding connective tissue, including the gingival fibers. In association with the inflammation, the junctional epithelium proliferates along the root in the form of finger-like projections two or three cells in thickness. The coronal portion of the junctional epithelium detaches from the root as the apical portion migrates.

The coronal portion of the junctional epithelium is subject, as a result of inflammation, to an increased invasion by polymorphonuclear leukocytes, which are not joined to each other nor to the remaining epithelial cells by desmosomes. When the relative volume of polymorphonuclear leukocytes reaches approximately 60 per cent or more of the junctional epithelium tissue, this detaches from the tooth surface so that the sulcus bottom shifts apically and the oral sulcular epithelium occupies a gradually increasing portion of the sulcular lining.[42]

The degree of leukocyte infiltration of the junctional epithelium is independent of the volume of inflamed connective tissue so that the above mentioned steps may occur in a gingiva with a slight amount of clinical inflammation.[43]

With continued inflammation the gingiva increases in bulk and the crest of the gingival margin extends toward the crown. The junctional epithelium continues to migrate along the root and separate from it. The epithelium of the lateral wall of the pocket proliferates to form bulbous and cord-like extensions into the inflamed connective tissue. Leukocytes and edema from the inflamed connective tissue infiltrate the epithelium lining the pocket, resulting in varying degrees of degeneration and necrosis.

The transformation of a gingival sulcus into a periodontal pocket creates an area where plaque removal becomes impossible and therefore the following feedback mechanism is established:

Plaque → gingival inflammation → pocket formation → more plaque formation

The rationale for pocket elimination is based on the need to eliminate areas of plaque accumulation.

Page and Schroeder[36] have described the following stages in the pathogenesis of a periodontal lesion:

1. *The initial lesion,* characterized by "classic vasculitis of vessels subjacent to the junctional epithelium; exudation of fluid from the gingival sulcus; increased migration of leukocytes into the junctional epithelium and gingival sulcus; presence

of serum proteins, especially fibrin, extracellularly; alteration of the most coronal portion of the junctional epithelium; and loss of perivascular collagen."[36]

2. *The early lesion*, having the following features: "accentuation of the features described for the initial lesion; accumulation of lymphoid cells immediately subjacent to the junctional epithelium at the site of acute inflammation; cytopathic alterations in resident fibroblasts, possibly associated with interactions with lymphoid cells; further loss of the collagen fiber network supporting the marginal gingiva; beginning proliferation of the basal cells of the junctional epithelium."[36]

3. *The established lesion* with "persistence of the manifestations of acute inflammation; predominance of plasma cells but without appreciable bone loss; presence of immunoglobulins extravascularly in the connective tissues and in junctional epithelium; continuing loss of connective tissue; proliferation, apical migration, and lateral extension of the junctional epithelium; early pocket formation may or may not be present."[36]

4. *The advanced lesion*, distinguished by "persistence of features described for the established lesion; extension of the lesion into alveolar bone and periodontal ligament with significant bone loss; continued loss of collagen subjacent to the pocket epithelium with fibrosis at more distant sites; presence of cytopathically altered plasma cells in the absence of altered fibroblasts; formation of periodontal pockets; periods of quiescence and exacerbation; conversion of bone marrow distant from the lesion into fibrous connective tissue; widespread manifestations of inflammatory and immunopathologic tissue reactions."[36]

HISTOPATHOLOGY

The Suprabony Pocket

Once formed, the periodontal pocket is a chronic inflammatory lesion complicated by proliferative and degenerative changes. It presents the following microscopic features:

The soft tissue wall

The connective tissue is edematous and densely infiltrated with plasma cells (approximately 80 per cent[57]) and lymphocytes and a scattering of polymorphonuclear leukocytes. The blood vessels are increased in number, dilated, and engorged. The connective tissue presents varying degrees of degeneration. Single or multiple necrotic foci are occasionally present.[35] In addition to exudative and degen-

TABLE 14–1 CORRELATION OF CLINICAL AND HISTOPATHOLOGIC FEATURES OF THE PERIODONTAL POCKET

Clinical Features	Histopathologic Features
1. The gingival wall of the periodontal pocket presents varying degrees of bluish red discoloration, flaccidity, a smooth shiny surface, and pitting on pressure.	1. The discoloration is caused by circulatory stagnation; the flaccidity, by destruction of the gingival fibers and surrounding tissues; the smooth, shiny surface, by the atrophy of the epithelium and edema; the pitting on pressure, by edema and degeneration.
2. Less frequently the gingival wall may be pink and firm.	2. In such cases fibrotic changes predominate over exudation and degeneration, particularly in relation to the outer surface of the pocket wall. However, despite the external appearance of health, the inner wall of the pocket invariably presents some degeneration, and is often ulcerated (Fig. 14–16).
3. Bleeding is elicited by gently probing the soft tissue wall of the pocket.	3. Ease of bleeding results from increased vascularity, thinning and degeneration of the epithelium, and the proximity of the engorged vessels to the inner surface.
4. When explored with a probe the inner aspect of the periodontal pocket is generally painful.	4. Pain upon tactile stimulation is due to ulceration of the inner aspect of the pocket wall.
5. In many cases pus may be expressed by applying digital pressure.	5. This occurs in pockets with suppurative inflammation of the inner wall.

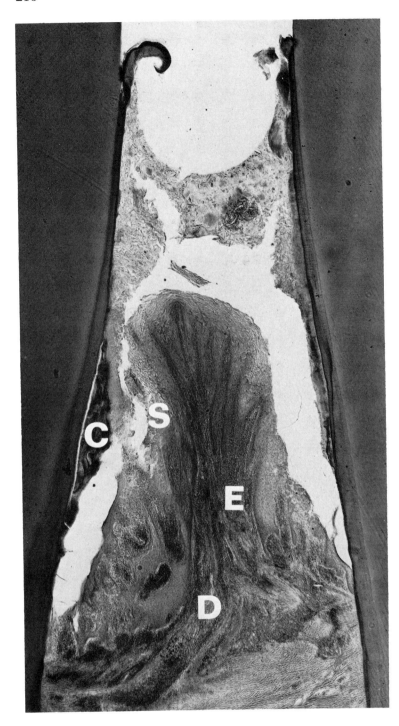

Figure 14–12 Interdental Papilla with Suprabony Pockets on Proximal Tooth Surfaces. *D,* Densely inflamed connective tissue; E, proliferating pocket epithelium; S, ulceration of lateral wall with pus exuding adjacent to calculus (C).

erative changes, the connective tissue presents proliferation of the endothelial cells with newly formed capillaries, fibroblasts, and collagen fibers (Fig. 14–12).

The junctional epithelium at the base of the pocket varies in the length, width, and condi-

tion of the epithelial cells. The variations range from the extremes of a long narrow band to a comparatively short wide clump of cells (Fig. 14–13). The cells may be well formed and in good condition or present slight to marked degeneration (Fig. 14–14).

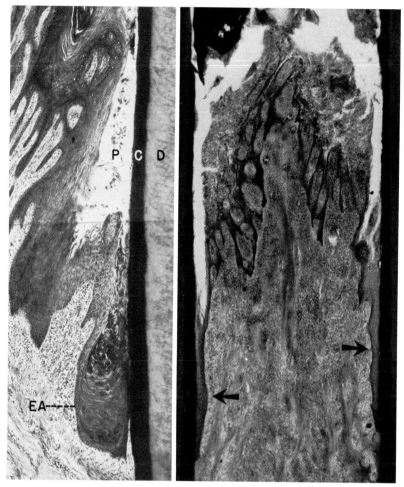

Figure 14–13 Varied Conformations of Junctional Epithelium. *Left,* Hyperkeratotic nodular junctional epithelium (EA) at the base of pocket (P), cementum (C), dentin (D). *Right,* Interdental papilla showing lengthy junctional epithelium (arrows) in two proximal pockets.

Special note should be made of the fact that extension of the junctional epithelium along the root requires the presence of healthy epithelial cells. Degeneration of the junctional epithelium would retard rather than accelerate pocket formation. Degenerative changes are seen in the junctional epithelium at the base of periodontal pockets, but they are usually less severe than those in the epithelium of the lateral pocket wall. Since migration of the junctional epithelium requires healthy viable cells, it is reasonable to assume that the degenerative changes seen in this area occurred after the junctional epithelium reached its position on the cementum.

The most severe degenerative changes in the periodontal pocket occur along the lateral wall. The epithelium of the lateral wall of the pocket presents striking proliferative and degenerative changes.[8] Epithelial buds or interlacing cords of epithelial cells project from the lateral wall into the adjacent inflamed connective tissue and frequently extend farther apically than the junctional epithelium. These epithelial projections, as well as the remainder of the lateral epithelium, are densely infiltrated by leukocytes and edema from the inflamed connective tissue. The cells undergo vacuolar degeneration and rupture to form vesicles. Progressive degeneration and necrosis of the

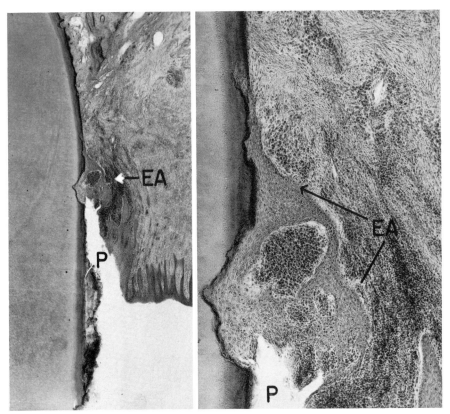

Figure 14–14   *A,* **Low-Power Section of Periodontal Pocket** (P). The location of the junctional epithelium is indicated by the arrow (*EA*). The lateral epithelial wall is ulcerated. *B,* **Detailed Study of Junctional Epithelium** (*EA*) at the base of the pocket (*P*). Note extension of well-formed epithelial cells (arrow) along the resorbed root surface. There is a dense accumulation of leukocytes enclosed within the epithelium.

epithelium leads to ulceration of the lateral wall, exposure of the underlying markedly inflamed connective tissue, and suppuration. In some cases acute inflammation is superimposed upon the underlying chronic changes.

The severity of the degenerative changes is not necessarily related to pocket depth. Ulceration of the lateral wall may occur in shallow pockets. Deep pockets are occasionally observed in which the lateral epithelium is intact and presents only slight degeneration (Fig. 14–15).

The epithelium at the crest of the periodontal pocket is generally intact and thickened, with prominent rete pegs. When acute inflammation occurs on the surface of the periodontal pocket, however, the crest of the gingiva undergoes degeneration and necrosis.

Periodontal pockets are healing lesions

Periodontal pockets are chronic inflammatory lesions, and as such are constantly undergoing repair.

The condition of the soft tissue wall of the periodontal pocket results from a balance between destructive and constructive tissue changes. The destructive changes consist of the fluid and cellular inflammatory exudate and the associated degenerative changes stimulated by the local irritation. The constructive changes consist of the formation of connective tissue cells, collagen fibers, and blood vessels in an effort to repair the tissue damage caused by inflammation.

Healing does not go to completion because of the persistence of local irritants. These irritants continue to stimulate fluid

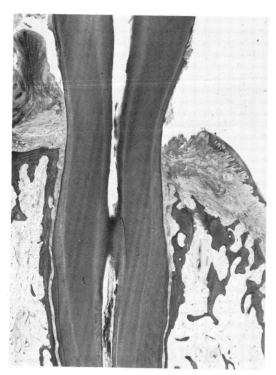

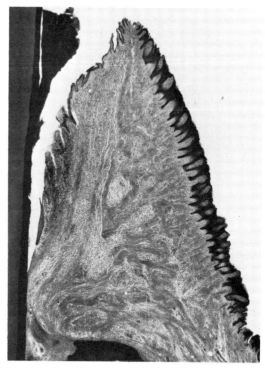

Figure 14–15   Shallow Ulcerated Pocket in Relation to One Surface of a Tooth (*right*) in contrast with intact deeper pocket in relation to other tooth surface (*left*).

Figure 14–16   Periodontal Pocket Wall. The inner half is inflamed and ulcerated, the outer half is densely collagenous.

and cellular exudate, which in turn causes degeneration of the new tissue elements formed in the continuous effort at repair.

The balance between exudative and constructive changes determines the color, consistency, and surface texture of the pocket wall. If the inflammatory fluid and cellular exudate predominate, the pocket wall is bluish red, soft, spongy, and friable, with a smooth, shiny surface. If there is a relative predominance of newly formed connective tissue cells and fibers, the pocket wall is firm and pink. At the clinical level the former is generally referred to as an edematous pocket, the latter as fibrotic (see Chapter 33).

Edematous and fibrotic pockets represent opposite extremes of the same pathologic process rather than different disease entities. They are subject to constant modification, depending upon the relative predominance of exudative and constructive changes.

The outer appearance of a periodontal pocket may be misleading because it is not necessarily a true indication of what is taking place throughout the pocket wall. The severest degenerative changes in periodontal pockets occur along the inner aspect. In some cases inflammation and ulceration on the inside of the pocket are walled off by fibrous tissue on the outer aspect (Fig. 14–16). Outwardly the pocket appears pink and fibrotic despite the degeneration taking place within.

The contents

Periodontal pockets contain debris which is principally microorganisms and their products (enzymes, endotoxins, and other metabolic products), dental plaque, gingival fluid, food remnants, salivary mucin, desquamated epithelial cells, and leukocytes. Plaque-covered calculus usually projects from the tooth surface (Fig. 14–17). If a purulent exudate is present, it consists of living, degenerated, and necrotic leukocytes (predominantly polymorphonuclear), living and dead bacteria,

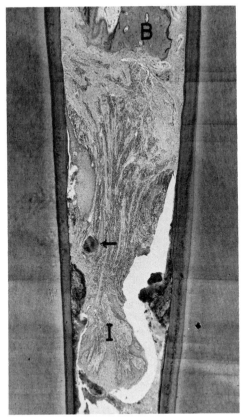

Figure 14–17 Interdental Papilla (I) with ulcerated suprabony periodontal pockets on its mesial and distal aspects. Calculus is present on the approximal tooth surfaces and within the gingiva (*arrow*). The bone is shown at *B*.

serum, and a scant amount of fibrin[32] (Fig. 14–18). The contents of periodontal pockets filtered free from organisms and debris have been demonstrated to be toxic when injected subcutaneously into experimental animals. [4]

The significance of pus formation

There is a tendency to overemphasize the importance of the purulent exudate and to equate it with the severity of periodontal disease. Because it is a dramatic clinical finding, early observers assumed it was responsible for the loosening and exfoliation of the teeth. *Pus is a common feature of periodontal disease, but it is only a secondary sign.* The presence of pus or the ease with which it can be expressed from the pocket merely reflects the nature of the inflammatory changes in the pocket wall. It is no indication of the depth of the pocket or the severity of destruction of the supporting tissues. Extensive pus formation may occur in shallow pockets, while deep pockets may present little or no pus.

The root surface wall

The root surface wall of periodontal pockets often undergoes changes that are

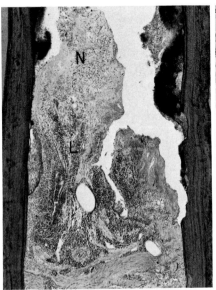

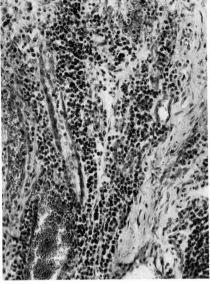

Figure 14–18 *Left,* **Pus Formation** (N) at the crest of a necrotic interdental papilla. There is a dense underlying leukocytic infiltration. *Right,* Detailed study of dense leukocytic infiltration and distended engorged capillaries.

significant because they may *cause pain and complicate periodontal treatment.* The following changes have been described in exposed cementum: (a) Presence of *pathologic granules,*[7, 10] which have been observed with optical and electron microscopy[4] and may represent areas of collagen degeneration or areas where collagen fibrils had not been initially fully mineralized.

(b) *Areas of increased mineralization,*[46] probably due to an exchange, upon exposure to the oral cavity, of minerals and organic components at the cementum-saliva interface. The hypermineralized zone is detectable by electron microscopy. Selvig[46] studied in detail these hypermineralized zones and found that the increased mineral content was associated with increased perfection of the crystal structure and organic changes suggestive of a subsurface cuticle.

These zones have also been seen in microradiographic studies[48] as a layer 10 to 20 microns thick, with areas as thick as 50 microns; no decrease in mineralization was found in deeper areas, indicating that increased mineralization does not come from adjacent areas.

Mineral content of exposed cementum is increased.[47] The following minerals are increased in diseased root surfaces: calcium,[48] magnesium,[33, 48] phosphorus,[33] and fluoride.[33] Microhardness, however, remains unchanged.[39, 55]

(c) *Areas of demineralization* which may be related to root caries.

Hatfield and Baumhammers[25] have demonstrated that roots of teeth with periodontal disease placed in a tissue culture induce irreversible morphologic changes in the cells of the culture; similar changes were not produced by unexposed roots. Aleo et al.[3] have found endotoxin in diseased roots that may be responsible for inducing changes in cultured cells. Endotoxin may come from plaque trapped in areas of decalcification or may become absorbed into the root surface.

The surface morphology of the tooth wall of a periodontal pocket has been studied by several authors.[6, 11, 27, 40, 41, 54] The following zones can be found in the bottom of a periodontal pocket:

1. Cementum covered by calculus, where all the changes described in previous paragraphs can be found.

2. Attached plaque which covers calculus and extends apically to it to a variable extension, probably 100 to 500 microns.

3. In extracted teeth a plaque-free zone has been described between the most apical level of attached plaque and the coronal border of the periodontal ligament fibers; it has been suggested that this area corresponds to the junctional epithelium. However, attached plaque is surrounded by unattached plaque[29] which extends apically; this unattached plaque is washed away in extracted teeth. It probably takes up most of this so-called plaque-free region. The plaque-free area would therefore be composed as follows: (a) a coronal portion of unattached plaque and (b) the area covered by the junctional epithelium.

The total width of the plaque-free zones varies according to the teeth (wider in molars than in incisors) and the depth of the pocket (narrower in deeper pockets).[41]

ROOT CARIES. Exposure to oral fluid and bacterial plaque results in proteolysis of the embedded remnants of Sharpey's fibers; the cementum may be softened and undergo fragmentation and cavitation.[26]

Involvement of the cementum is followed by bacterial penetration of the dentinal tubules, resulting in destruction of the dentin (Fig. 14–19). In severe cases, large sections of necrotic cementum become detached from the tooth and separated from it by masses of bacteria (Fig. 14–20).

The tooth may not be painful, but exploration of the root surface reveals the presence of a defect; penetration of the involved area with a probe elicits pain.

Caries of the root may lead to *pulpitis,* sensitivity to sweets and thermal changes, or severe pain. Pathologic exposure of the pulp occurs in severe cases. **It is well to bear in mind that root caries may be the cause of toothache in patients with periodontal disease without evidence of coronal decay.**

Caries of the cementum requires special attention when the pocket is treated. The necrotic cementum must be removed by scaling and root planing until firm tooth surface is reached, even if this entails extension into the dentin.

CELLULAR RESORPTION. Areas of cellular resorption of cementum and dentin are common in roots uninvolved with periodontal disease. These are of no particular significance because they are symp-

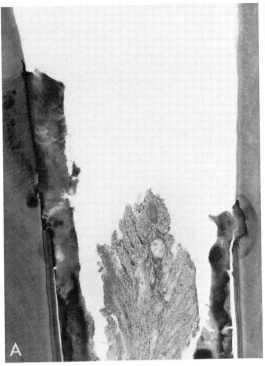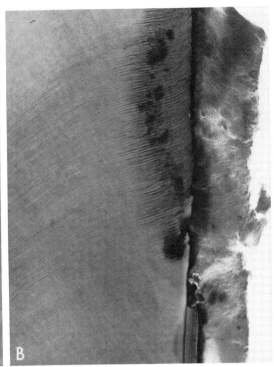

Figure 14–19   Caries on Root Surfaces Exposed by Periodontal Disease. *A,* Interdental space, showing inflamed gingiva and caries on proximal tooth surfaces. *B,* Caries of cementum and dentin, showing bacterial invasion of dentinal tubules. Note the filamentous structure of the dental plaque and darker staining of calculus adherent to the root.

tom-free, and so long as the root is covered by the periodontal ligament, they are apt to undergo repair. However, if the root is exposed by progressive pocket formation before repair of such areas occurs, they appear as isolated cavitations that penetrate into the dentin. These areas can be differentiated from caries of the cementum by their clear-cut outline and hard surface. Once exposed to the oral cavity, they may be sources of considerable pain and require restoration.

Pulp changes associated with periodontal pockets

Spread of infection from periodontal pockets may cause pathologic changes in the pulp.[45] *Such changes may give rise to painful symptoms or adversely affect the response of the pulp to restorative procedures.*

Involvement of the pulp in periodontal disease occurs through either the apical foramen or the lateral canals in the root after spread- **ing from the pocket through the periodontal ligament. Atrophy or hypertrophy of the odontoblastic layer, hyperemia, leukocytic infiltration, interstitial calcification, and fibrosis are the types of pulp changes that occur in such cases.**

The pulpal changes are correlated with the severity of periodontal involvement,[58] but not in all cases.[31] In experimental animals, artificially induced pulp inflammation spread to the furcation area (10 to 15 per cent), probably through lateral canals[44] and injury to the gingiva led to formation of secondary dentin.[50]

Gingival recession and pocket depth

Pocket formation causes recession of the gingiva and denudation of the root surface. The severity of recession is generally, but not always, correlated with the depth of the pocket. This is because the *degree of recession depends upon the location of*

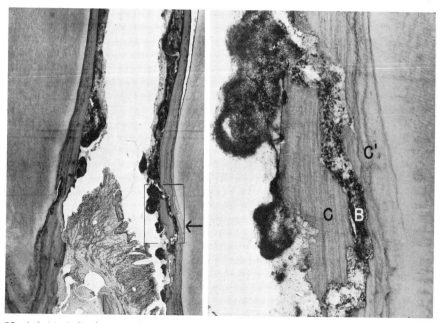

Figure 14–20   *Left,* Mesiodistal section through an interdental space in a patient with extensive periodontal destruction. An area of **Cementum Necrosis** is enclosed within the rectangle designated by the arrow.
   Right, Detailed section of area enclosed in the rectangle showing **Necrotic Fragment of Cementum** (C) separated from lamellated cementum (C′) by clumps of bacteria (*B*).

the base of the pocket on the root surface, whereas the depth is the distance between the base of the pocket and the crest of the gingiva. Pockets of the same depth may be associated with different degrees of recession (Fig. 14–21), and pockets of different depths may be associated with the same amount of recession (Fig. 14–22).

Exposure of the roots after pockets are eliminated depends upon the amount of recession before treatment is instituted. A realistic appraisal of recession associated with periodontal pockets will prevent the erroneous impression that it is caused by the treatment.

Relation of pocket depth to alveolar bone destruction

Severity of bone loss may generally be correlated with pocket depth—but not always. Extensive bone loss may be associated with shallow pockets, and slight loss with deep pockets. Destruction of alveolar bone may occur in the absence of

Figure 14–21   Same Pocket Depth—Different Amounts of Recession. *A,* Pocket depth (P), recession (R). *B,* Pocket depth (P) same as in *A,* more recession (R). *C,* Pocket depth (P) same as in *A,* still more recession (R).

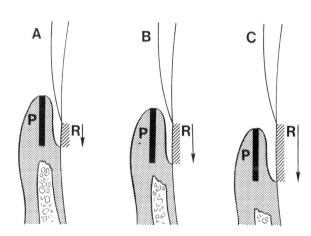

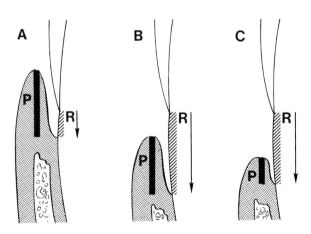

Figure 14–22 Difference Between Pocket Depth and Amount of Recession. *A,* Deep pocket (P), slight recession (R). *B,* Deep pocket (P), marked recession (R). *C,* Shallow pocket (P), marked recession (R).

periodontal pockets associated with trauma from occlusion and in cases of marked recession.

The area between the base of the pocket and the alveolar bone

Normally, the distance between the junctional epithelium and the alveolar bone is relatively constant. Stanley[51] measured histometrically in human specimens of periodontal pockets the distance between the bottom of the calculus and the alveolar crest and found it to be most constant, having a mean length of 1.97 mm. ± 33.16 per cent. This was confirmed by Wade.[53]

The Infrabony Pocket

In infrabony pockets the base is apical to the level of the alveolar bone, and the pocket wall lies between the tooth and bone. Infrabony pockets most often occur interproximally, but may be located on the facial and lingual tooth surfaces. Most often the pocket spreads from the surface on which it originates to one or more contiguous surfaces. Statistical information regarding the prevalence of infrabony pockets is not available. *The inflammatory, proliferative, and degenerative changes in infrabony and suprabony pockets are the same, and both lead to destruction of the supporting periodontal tissues.*

TABLE 14–2 DISTINGUISHING FEATURES OF SUPRABONY AND INFRABONY POCKETS

Suprabony Pocket	Infrabony Pocket
1. The base of the pocket is coronal to the level of the alveolar bone.	1. The base of the pocket is apical to the crest of the alveolar bone, so that the bone is adjacent to the soft tissue wall (Fig. 14–7).
2. The pattern of destruction of the underlying bone is horizontal.	2. The bone destructive pattern is vertically angular (Fig. 14–24).
3. Interproximally, the transseptal fibers that are restored during progressive periodontal disease are arranged horizontally in the space between the base of the pocket and the alveolar bone (Fig. 14–25).	3. Interproximally, the transseptal fibers are oblique rather than horizontal. They extend from the cementum beneath the base of the pocket along the bone, and over the crest to the cementum of the adjacent tooth (Fig. 14–26).
4. On the facial and lingual surfaces, the periodontal ligament fibers beneath the pocket follow their normal horizontal-oblique course between the tooth and the bone.	4. On the facial and lingual surfaces, the periodontal ligament fibers follow the angular pattern of the adjacent bone. They extend from the cementum beneath the base of the pocket along the bone and over the crest to join with the outer periosteum.

Differences between infrabony and suprabony pockets

The principal differences between infrabony and suprabony pockets are the relationship of the soft tissue wall of the pocket to the alveolar bone, the pattern of bone destruction, and the direction of the transseptal fibers of the periodontal ligament[13] (Fig. 14-23).

In a suprabony pocket the alveolar crest and the fibrous apparatus attached to it gradually attain a more apical position in relation to the tooth but retain their general morphology and architecture, while in infrabony pockets the morphology of the

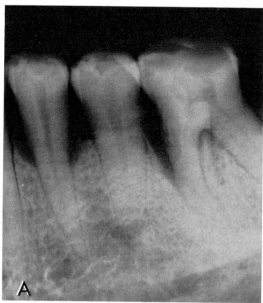

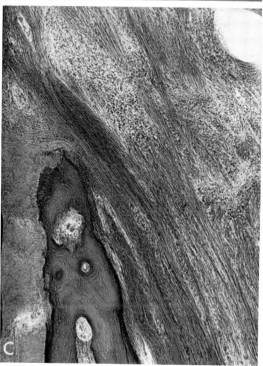

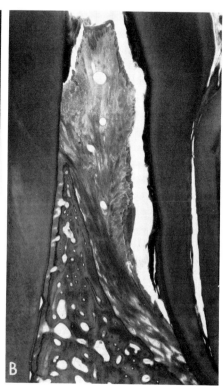

Figure 14-23 **Infrabony Pocket on Mesial Surface of Molar.** *A,* Radiograph showing deep angular defect on the mesial surface of the first molar. The bifurcation is also involved. There are shallower, broader defects on the first premolar. Note the calculus on the mesial surface of the molar. *B,* Interdental space between the second premolar with a suprabony pocket (*left*) and the first molar with an infrabony pocket. Note the following: the transseptal fibers which extend from the base of the infrabony pocket along the bone to the root of the premolar; the relationship of the epithelial lining of the pocket to the transseptal fibers; the calculus on the root. *C,* Transseptal fibers extending from the distal surface of the premolar over the crest of the bone into the infrabony pocket. Note the leukocytic infiltration of the transseptal fibers.

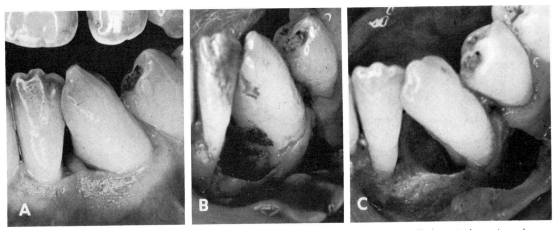

Figure 14–24   Infrabony Pocket on the Mesial Surface of the Mandibular Canine. *A,* Rolled gingival margin and space between gingiva and canine suggest presence of periodontal pocket. *B,* Flap reflected to show calculus on root and three wall bone defect. *C,* Bone defect, calculus removed.

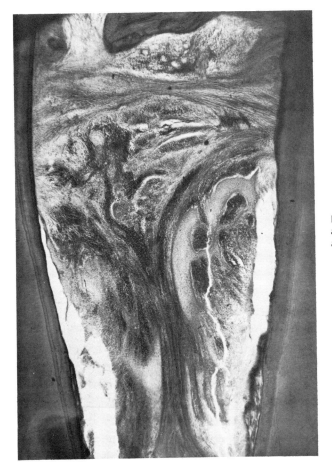

Figure 14–25 Two Suprabony Pockets in an Interdental Space between the maxillary cuspid and lateral incisor. Note the normal horizontal arrangement of the transseptal fibers.

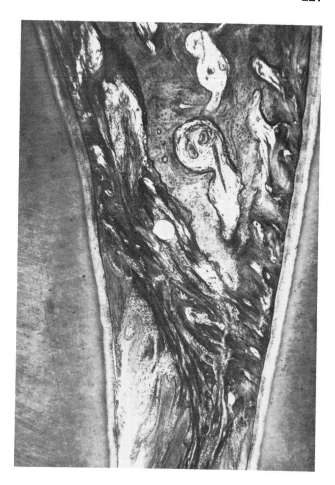

Figure 14–26 Vertical bone loss and suprabony pocket in maxillary incisor (*left*). Note the oblique arrangement of the transseptal fibers.

alveolar crest changes completely. This may have an effect on the function of the area.[12]

The distinguishing features of suprabony and infrabony pockets are summarized in Table 14–2. The morphologic features of the infrabony pocket are important because they necessitate modification in treatment techniques (see Chapter 51).

Classification of infrabony pockets

Infrabony pockets are classified in different ways; often used features are *the number of walls*[37] in the osseous defect (Fig. 14–27) and its *depth and width*, because they are important factors which influence the outcome of treatment. Infrabony defects may have one wall (Fig. 14–28), two walls, or three or four walls (Fig. 14–29). They are sometimes referred to as "**intrabony pockets**" when the os-

seous defect has three walls. When the number of walls in the apical portion of the defect is different from the number in the occlusal portion, the term *combined osseous defect* is used (Fig. 14–30).

Infrabony pockets are classified according to depth and width as follows:
Type 1. Shallow narrow
Type 2. Shallow wide (Fig. 14–31)
Type 3. Deep narrow (Fig. 14–32)
Type 4. Deep wide (Fig. 14–32)
Infrabony pockets generally occur in forms which represent gradients of the aforementioned types.

The etiology of infrabony pockets

Infrabony pockets are caused by the same local irritants as suprabony pockets. Trauma from occlusion may add to the effect of the inflammation by causing bone resorption lateral to the periodontal liga-

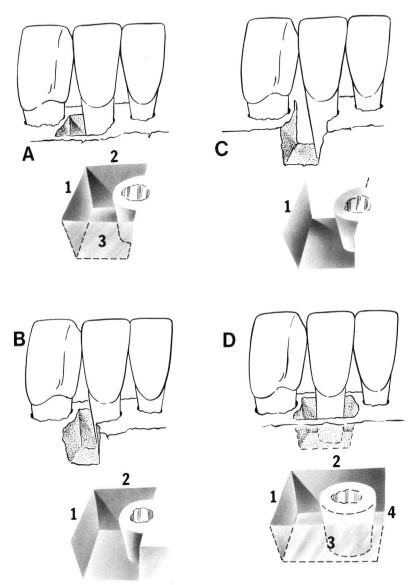

Figure 14–27   One-, Two-, Three-, and Four-Walled Infrabony Defects on right lateral incisor. *A,* Three bony walls: (1) distal, (2) lingual, and (3) facial wall. *B,* Two-wall defect: (1) distal and (2) lingual walls. *C,* One-wall defect: (1) distal wall only. *D,* Four-wall defect completely surrounds the root: (1) distal, (2) lingual, (3) facial, and (4) mesial walls.

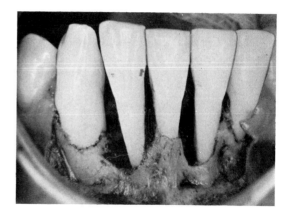

Figure 14-28 One-Wall Infrabony Defect on the mesial surface of the left lateral incisor and 1½-wall defect (distal wall and one half of the labial wall) on the distal surface of the right lateral.

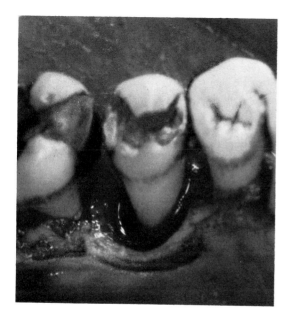

Figure 14-29 Four-Wall Infrabony Defect Viewed From the Lingual Surface, consisting of facial, lingual, mesial, and distal walls in relation to the second premolar. The facial bony wall is obscured by the tooth.

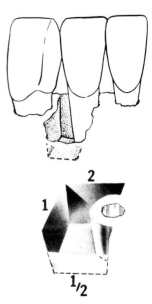

Figure 14-30 Combined Type of Osseous Defect. Because the facial wall is one half the height of the distal (1) and lingual (2) walls, this is an osseous defect with three walls in its apical half and two walls in the occlusal half.

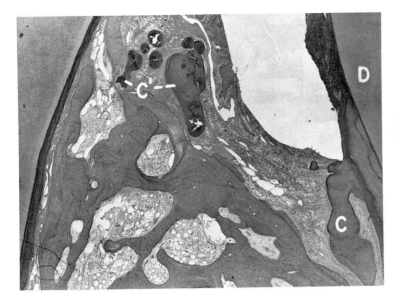

Figure 14–31 Shallow, Broad Infrabony Pocket. Cementicles in the pocket wall (C') represent an infrequent complication which may occur in any type of periodontal pocket. The epithelium at the base of the pocket is attached to a cementicle (C) which is adherent to the tooth (D).

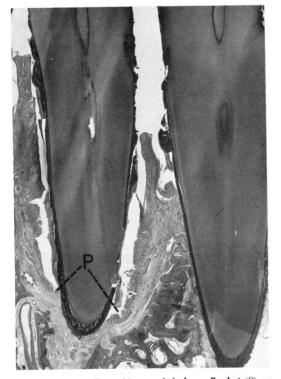

Figure 14–32 Deep Narrow Infrabony Pocket (P) on the mesial surface of the mandibular lateral incisor (*left*). Deep wide infrabony pocket (P) on the distal surface (*right*).

ment, worsening the bone loss caused by inflammation alone and leading to the creation of the osseous defect associated with infrabony pockets.*

Trauma may also add to the effect of inflammation in the following ways:[16, 17] (1) By altering the alignment of the transseptal periodontal fibers, it diverts the inflammation directly into the periodontal ligament space rather than into the interdental septum. (2) By injuring the periodontal ligament fibers, it aggravates the destruction produced by inflammation. This further reduces the obstruction to the proliferating pocket epithelium. Instead of remaining coronal to the bone, the epithelium extends between the root and the bone (Fig. 14–33), creating an infrabony pocket.

There are still other opinions regarding the etiology of infrabony pockets.[38] The causative role of inflammation combined with trauma from occlusion has been studied extensively, but other etiologic factors also play a role. Anatomic characteristics of the area such as wide bone margins may favor the production of angular lesions and

---

*This subject is discussed in detail in Chapter 19.

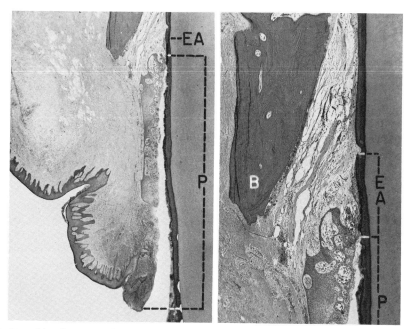

Figure 14–33   Transition from Suprabony Pocket to Infrabony Pocket. *Left,* Deep pocket (P) on the facial surface of a maxillary tooth. The junctional epithelium is shown at EA. *Right,* Base of the pocket. The junctional epithelium (EA) has migrated beyond the crest of the bone (B) and started to change the suprabony pocket to an infrabony pocket. At this early stage, the base of the pocket (P) is still coronal to the bone.

infrabony pockets. Food impaction and infrabony pockets often occur together,[37] but it has not been established whether the food impaction produces the pockets or aggravates infrabony pockets caused by other factors.

THEORIES ON THE PATHOGENESIS OF PERIODONTAL POCKETS

The histopathology of the periodontal pocket is well documented; however, it has been subjected to varied interpretations. The following theories regarding how periodontal pockets develop are presented as useful background information for the interpretation of current and future concepts.

I. Destruction of the Gingival Fibers is a Prerequisite for the Initiation of Pocket Formation.

This concept focuses attention upon the migration of gingival fibers. The conten-

tion is that proliferation of the junctional epithelium along the root can take place only if the underlying gingival fibers are destroyed.[15] These fibers are considered a barrier to the normal migratory tendency of the epithelium at the base of the sulcus,[18] and it is believed that their degeneration and necrosis occur secondary to gingival inflammation or the action of bacterial enzymes such as hyaluronidase.[2] As soon as the topmost fiber is digested and absorbed, the epithelium proliferates along the root until a healthy fiber is reached.

Gottlieb and Orban[23] have questioned this concept. They point to areas of repaired idiopathic tooth resorption immediately beneath the junctional epithelium, and note that since the resorption of the tooth entailed detachment of the gingival fibers, repair would not have been possible had the epithelium proliferated simply because the fibers had been destroyed. They also point out that when the junctional epithelium is attached to the enamel and is separated from the cementum by unattached connective tissue rather than fibers embedded in the tooth, pathologic migration of the epithelium does not occur.

II. The Initial Change in Pocket Formation Occurs in the Cementum.

In seeking an explanation for pocket formation, Gottlieb stresses the changes in tooth surface rather than in the gingiva. He envisions downgrowth of the junctional epithelium as a physiologic phenomenon that is part of the process of continuous eruption of teeth throughout life.[21, 22] Under physiologic conditions, the continuous deposition of new cementum acts as a barrier that prevents accelerated migration of the junctional epithelium. So long as continuous cementum deposition is not disturbed, migration of the junctional epithelium at a pathologic rate cannot occur.[19, 20] However, if the tooth surface is of low resistance, or if the normal deposition of cementum is impaired, inflammation or trauma can do additional harm by destroying either the cementum or the gingiva, or both. This dissolves the organic connection between the two, and the epithelium proliferates along the root until it meets undisturbed connective tissue fibers and cementum. Death of the cementum does not necessarily occur under such circumstances, as evidenced by the fact that epithelium attaches itself to cementum after its organic connection with the periodontal ligament fibers is destroyed.

III. Stimulation of the Junctional Epithelium by Inflammation Rather than Destruction of Gingival Fibers is the Prerequisite for the Initiation of the Periodontal Pocket.

Destruction of the underlying gingival fibers is not a prerequisite for epithelial migration.[1] Stimulated by inflammation, the epithelium migrates along the root without preceding destruction of the gingival fibers. In such instances the epithelial cells burrow between the intact gingival fibers and attach themselves farther apically on the cementum in bundle-free areas. The junctional epithelium may move between healthy connective tissue fibers, enmesh them in an epithelial network, and produce secondary fiber degeneration.

IV. Pathologic Destruction of the Junctional Epithelium due to Infection or Trauma is the Initial Histologic Change in Pocket Formation

According to Skillen,[49] the junctional epithelium has few protective qualities for safeguarding the underlying connective tissue against spread of infection. It is the normal downgrowth of the oral epithelium behind the junctional epithelium that protects the underlying connective tissue. The junctional epithelium is an area of low resistance subject to infection. In experimental animals, pocket formation occurs because of pathologic dissolution of the junctional epithelium due to infection or trauma, or both. Accumulation of debris in the pocket may be secondary—after the pocket is formed by dissolution of the junctional epithelium.

V. The Periodontal Pocket is Initiated by Invasion of Bacteria at the Base of the Sulcus or the Absorption of Bacterial Toxins Through the Epithelial Lining of the Sulcus.

According to Box,[10] either because of imperfect junction of the epithelial cells and the cementum or extreme thinness of the epithelium, the base of the sulcus offers a poor defense against bacteria. In the evolution of a pocket, initial invasion of bacteria at the base of the sulcus leads to the following changes: inflammation in the underlying connective tissue, ulceration at the base of the crevices, sloughing of the epithelium and loss of attachment to the cementum, progressive loss of connective tissue, and penetration of the pocket into the deeper tissues. Specific infective agents possibly related to *Leptothrix falciformis* are capable of deepening the periodontal pocket. Also Arnim and Holt[3] consider the epithelial lining of the sulcus a poor barrier against bacterial toxins, which initiate inflammatory changes leading to pocket formation.

VI. Pocket Formation is Initiated in a Defect in the Sulcus Wall.

According to Becks,[8] the formation and maintenance of the normal 1 mm.-deep sulcus results from the coordination of degeneration of the enamel epithelium, proliferation of the oral epithelium, and atrophy of the gingival papilla. Disturbance of this correlation, whether by inflammation or injury, leads to pathologic pocket formation.

Pocket formation occurs between the oral epithelium and the enamel epithelium, rather than by separation of enamel epithelium from the cuticle. If degeneration of the enamel epithelium takes place rapidly without being covered by the oral epithelium, a defect occurs in the lateral sulcus wall. This defect constitutes a "locus minoris resistentiae" which is a portal of entry for bacteria with resultant inflammation. This induces proliferation of the basal cells of the enamel epithelium and the oral epithelium, a protective mechanism for the connective tissue. Inflammation is a stimulant to oral epithelium proliferation, which shuts off nutrition from enamel epithelium, hastens its degeneration, and increases the pocket depth.

In some cases, pathologic pocket formation may be initiated without inflammation appearing to play a role. In such instances there is an accelerated degeneration of the enamel epithelium, possibly of systemic origin. This is followed by proliferation of the oral epithelium to cover the defect.

VII. Proliferation of the Epithelium of the Lateral Wall, Rather Than the Epithelium at the Base of the Sulcus, is the Initial Change in the Formation of the Periodontal Pocket.

Wilkinson[56] regards epithelial proliferation as the primary change in pocket formation. He describes the following sequence of changes: Proliferation and downgrowth of the oral epithelium or proliferation of the junctional epithelium result in a thickening of the epithelial lining of the sulcus. The cause of this proliferation is not known. Because of the increased thickness, the cells along the inner aspect of the sulcus are deprived of nutrition and undergo degeneration and necrosis. The degenerated and necrotic epithelial cells become calcified (serumal calculus). Separation of the calcified masses from the adjacent normal epithelium produces a pocket or trough. These changes are fol-

lowed by proliferation of the epithelium along the cementum, and detachment of its coronal portion from the root surface. The epithelial changes that initiate pocket formation are not caused by infection. Inflammatory changes in pocket formation are secondary to the epithelial changes. Wilkinson suggests that vitamin A deficiency may be an important factor in initiating pocket formation.

VIII. Two-stage Pocket Formation.

James and Counsel[28] disagree with the concept that proliferation of junctional epithelium followed by separation from cementum forms a pocket. Instead, they feel pocket formation occurs in two stages:

The first stage is proliferation of the subgingival epithelium (junctional epithelium). The second stage is loss of the superficial layers of the proliferated epithelium, which produces a space or pocket. The rate of proliferation of the epithelium at the base is such that it precedes the destruction of the superficial epithelium, and the pocket is therefore always lined with epithelium.

IX. Inflammation is the Initial Change in the Formation of the Periodontal Pocket.

According to this concept periodontal pockets start as inflammatory lesions.[34] The first reaction is a vascular change in the underlying connective tissue.

Inflammation in the connective tissue stimulates the following changes in the epithelial lining of the sulcus and in the junctional epithelium: increased mitotic activity in the basal epithelial layer, and sometimes in the prickle cell layer; increased production of keratin with desquamation. The cellular desquamation adjacent to the tooth surface tends to deepen the pocket.

The epithelial cells of the basal layer at the bottom of the sulcus and in the area of attachment proliferate into the underlying connective tissue and break up the gingival fibers. The dissolution of connective tissue results in the formation of what is described as an *open lesion*. It is the repair of the lesion in the absence of treatment that establishes the periodontal pocket. Granulation tissue fills in the defect created by the open lesion, and the epithelium proliferates inward. This forms a lining of the repaired open lesion to a point where the connective tissue is attached to the root. In pocket formation, the epithelium does not proliferate along the root; instead it proliferates from the gingival surface to cover the connective tissue lesion created by inflammation, and thereby forms the lining of the pocket.

X. Pathologic Epithelial Proliferation Occurs Secondary to Noninflammatory Degenerative Changes in the Periodontal Ligament.

Under the term "periodontosis" a condition has been described which is characterized by generalized noninflammatory degeneration of the collagen fibers embedded in the cementum. Under such condi-

tions, the normal barrier afforded by the gingival fibers is diminished. This facilitates the migration of the junctional epithelium along the root and pocket formation in the presence of local irritation.

Comment regarding pocket formation

The following salient facts regarding pocket formation are worthy of special note:

Local irritation is required for the initiation and progress of pocket formation.

Proliferation of the junctional epithelium along the root and degeneration of the underlying gingival fibers are primary changes in pocket formation.

Proliferation of the junctional epithelium is stimulated by local irritation. Inflammation caused by local irritation produces degeneration of the gingival fibers,

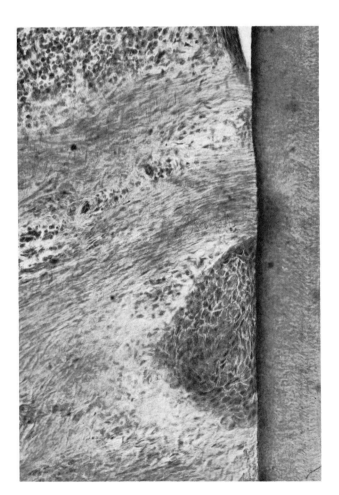

Figure 14–34 Section Showing Finger-Like Projection of Epithelium which has proliferated along the root surface into space created by destruction of gingival fibers. Some fibers still remain between the proliferated epithelium and the base of the pocket (*top*). Note inflammatory cells among the gingival fibers.

making it easier for the epithelium to move along the root (Fig. 14–34).

Systemic disorders do not initiate pocket formation, but they may affect pocket depth by causing degeneration of gingival and periodontal fibers.

REFERENCES

1. Aisenberg, M. S., and Aisenberg, A. D.: A new concept of pocket formation. Oral Surg., *1:* 1047, 1948.
2. Aisenberg, M. S., and Aisenberg, A. D.: Hyaluronidase in periodontal disease. Oral Surg., *4:*317, 1951.
3. Aleo, J. J., De Renzis, F. A., Farber, P. A., and Varboncoeur, A. P.: The presence and biologic activity of cementum bound endotoxin. J. Periodontol., *45:*672, 1974.
4. Armitage, G. C., and Christie, T. M.: Structural changes in exposed cementum. I. Light microscopic observations. J. Periodont. Res., 8: 343, 1973. II. Electron-microscopic observations. J. Periodont. Res., 8:356, 1973.
5. Arnim, S. S., and Holt, R. T.: The defense mechanism of the gingiva. J. Periodontol., 26:79, 1955.
6. Bass, C. C.: A demonstrable line on extracted teeth indicating the location of the outer border of the epithelial attachment. J. Dent. Res., 25:401, 1946.
7. Bass, C. C.: A previously undescribed demonstrable pathologic condition in exposed cementum and the underlying dentine. Oral Surg., 4:641, 1951.
8. Becks, H.: Normal and pathologic pocket formation. J. Am. Dent. Assoc., 16:2167, 1929.
9. Benson, L. A.: A study of a pathologic condition in exposed cementum. Oral Surg., 16:1137, 1963.
10. Box, H. K.: New aspects of periodontal research. J. Can. Dent. Assoc., 13:3, 1941.
11. Brady, J. M.: A plaque-free zone on human teeth – scanning and transmission electron microscopy. J. Periodontol., 44:416, 1973.
12. Carranza, F. A., and Carranza, F. A., Jr.: The management of alveolar bone in the treatment of the periodontal pocket. J. Periodontol., 27:29, 1956.
13. Carranza, F. A., Jr., and Glickman, I.: Some observations on the microscopic features of the infrabony pockets. J. Periodontol., 28:33, 1957.
14. Emslie, R. D., and Stack, M. V.: The micro hardness of roots of teeth with periodontal disease. Dent. Practit., 9:101, 1958.
15. Fish, E. W.: Surgical pathology of the mouth. London, Isaac Pitman and Sons, 1948, p. 316.
16. Glickman, I., and Smulow, J. B.: Alterations in the pathway of gingival inflammation into the underlying tissues induced by excessive occlusal forces. J. Periodontol., 33:7, 1962.
17. Glickman, I., and Smulow, J. B.: The combined effects of inflammation and trauma from occlusion in periodontitis. Intern. Dent. J., 19: 393, 1969.
18. Goldman, H. M.: The relationship of the epithelial attachment to the adjacent fibers of the periodontal membrane. J. Dent. Res., 23:177, 1944.
19. Gottlieb, B.: The formation of the pocket; diffuse alveolar atrophy. Proc. 7th Intern. Dent. Cong., 2:1631, 1926.
20. Gottlieb, B.: Tissue changes in pyorrhea. J. Am. Dent. Assoc., 14:2178, 1927.
21. Gottlieb, B.: Continuous deposition of cementum. J. Am. Dent. Assoc., 30:842, 1943.
22. Gottlieb, B.: The new concept of periodontoclasia. J. Periodontol., 17:7, 1946.
23. Gottlieb, B., and Orban, B.: Biology and pathology of the tooth. Trans. M. Diamond. New York, The Macmillan Co., 1938, p. 64.
24. Graham, J. W.: Toxicity of sterile filtrate from parodontal pockets. Proc. R. Soc. Med., 30: 1165, 1937.
25. Hatfield, C. G., and Baumhammers, A.: Cytotoxic effects of periodontally involved surfaces of human teeth. Arch. Oral Biol., 16:465, 1971.
26. Herting, H. C.: Electron microscope studies of the cementum surface structures of periodontally healthy and diseased teeth. J. Dent. Res., 46: [Suppl.]:1247, 1967.
27. Hoffman, I. D., and Gold, W.: Distances between plaque and remnants of attached periodontal tissues on extracted teeth. J. Periodontol., 42:29, 1971.
28. James, W., and Counsell, A.: A histological investigation into "so-called pyorrhea alveolaris." Br. Dent. J., 48:1237, 1927.
29. Listgarten, M.: Structure of the microbial flora associated with periodontal health and disease in man. J. Periodontol., 47:1, 1976.
30. Masi, P. L., and Benini, A.: Richerche su la microdurezza del dente umano parodontosico. Riv. Ital. Stomatol., 18:293, 1963.
31. Mazur, B., and Massler, M.: Influences of periodontal disease on the dental pulp. Oral Surg., 17:592, 1964.
32. McMillan, L., Burrill, D. Y., and Fosdick, L. S.: An electron microscope study of particulates in periodontal exudate. Abstract. Dent. Res., 37:51, 1958.
33. Nakata, T., Stepnick, R., and Zipkin, I.: Chemistry of human dental cementum. The effect of age and exposure on the concentration of F, Ca, P and Mg. J. Periodontol., 43:115, 1972.
34. Nuckolls, J., Dienstein, B., Bell, D. G., and Rule, R. W., Jr.: The periodontal lesions – The development of the lesion and the establishment and treatment of the periodontal pocket. J. Periodontol., 21:7, 44, 1950.
35. Orban, B., and Ray, A. G.: Deep necrotic foci in the gingiva. J. Periodontol., 19:91, 1948.
36. Page, R. C., and Schroeder, H. H.: Structure and pathogenesis. *In* Schluger, S., Yuodelis, R., and Page, R.: Periodontal disease. Philadelphia, Lea & Febiger, 1977.
37. Prichard, J.: A technique for treating infrabony pockets based on alveolar process morphology, Dent. Clin. North Am., March, 1960, p.85.
38. Proceedings, World Workshop in Periodontics. The University of Michigan, 1966, p.272.
39. Rautiola, C. A., and Craig, R. G.: The micro hardness of cementum and underlying dentin

of normal teeth and teeth exposed to periodontal disease. J. Periodontol., *32*:113, 1961.

40. Saglie, R., Johansen, J. R., and Tollefsen, T.:
Plaque-free zones on human teeth in periodontitis. J. Clin. Periodont., 2:190, 1975.

41. Saglie, R., Johansen, J. R., and Flotra, L.: The
zone of completely and partially destroyed
periodontal fibers in pathologic pockets. J.
Clin. Periodont., 2:198, 1975.

42. Schroeder, H. E., and Listgarten, M. A.: Fine
structure of the developing epithelial attachment of human teeth. Monographs in Developmental Biology. Vol. 2. Basel, S. Karger,
1971.

43. Schroeder, H. E.: Quantitative parameters of
early human gingival inflammation. Arch.
Oral Biol., *15*:383, 1970.

44. Seltzer, S., Bender, I., Nazimov, H., and Sinai, I.:
Pulpitis-induced interradicular periodontal
changes in experimental animals. J. Periodontol., 38:124, 1967.

45. Seltzer, S., Bender, I. B., and Ziontz, M.: The
interrelationship of pulp and periodontal disease. Oral Surg., *16*:1474, 1963.

46. Selvig, K. A.: Biological changes at the tooth-saliva interface in periodontal disease. J. Dent.
Res., *48* [Suppl.]:846, 1969.

47. Selvig, K. A.: Ultrastructural changes in cementum and adjacent connective tissue in periodontal disease. Acta Odontol. Scand., 24:459,
1966.

48. Selvig, K. A., and Zander, H. A.: Chemical analy-

sis and microradiography of cementum and
dentin from periodontally diseased human
teeth. J., Periodontol., *33*:303, 1962.

49. Skillen, W. G.: Normal characteristics of the gingiva and their relation to pathology. J. Am.
Dent. Assoc., *17*:1088, 1930.

50. Stahl, S. S.: Pulpal response to gingival injury in
adult rats. Oral Surg., *16*:1116, 1963.

51. Stanley, H. R.: The cyclic phenomenon of periodontitis. Oral Surg., 8:598, 1955.

52. Thilander, H.: Some structural changes in periodontal disease. Dent. Practit., *11*:191, 1961.

53. Wade, A. B.: The relation between the pocket
base, the epithelial attachment and the alveolar process. In "Les Parodontopathies"
16th A.R.P.A. Congress, Vienna, 1960.

54. Waerhaug, J.: The gingival pocket. Odont. Tidsk.,
60 [Suppl. 1], 1952.

55. Warren, E. B., Hansen, N. M., Swartz, M. L., and
Phillips, R. W.: Effects of periodontal disease
and of calculus solvents on microhardness of
cementum. J. Periodontol., 35:505, 1964.

56. Wilkinson, F. C.: A patho-histological study of
the tissue tooth attachment. Dent. Rec., 55:
105, 1935.

57. Wittwer, J. W., Dickler, E. H., and Toto, P. D.:
Comparative frequencies of plasma cells and
lymphocytes in gingivitis. J. Periodontol., *40*:
274, 1969.

58. Zilkens, K.: Some observations regarding the
pulp in periodontal disease. Fortschr. Zahnheilk., 3:289, 1927.

Chapter 15

Extension of Inflammation from the Gingiva to the Supporting Periodontal Tissues

The extension of inflammation from the marginal gingiva into the supporting periodontal tissues marks the transition from *gingivitis* to *periodontitis*. **Periodontitis is always preceded by gingivitis, but not all gingivitis proceeds to periodontitis.** Some cases will apparently never become periodontitis, and others will go through their "gingivitis phase" in a brief period of time. The factor or factors that are responsible for the extension of inflammation to the supporting structures and produce the conversion of a gingivitis to periodontitis are not known.

THE PATHWAYS OF GINGIVAL INFLAMMATION

For many years opinion differed regarding the pathway of gingival inflammation into the supporting tissues. Some considered it to be by way of the lymphatics of the periodontal ligament;[2, 6, 13] some felt that the inflammation extended along the fibers of the periodontal ligament or the outer periosteum of the alveolar bone;[5, 11] while others maintained that the inflam-

mation spread from the gingiva into the alveolar bone and that it rarely, if ever, extended directly into the periodontal ligament.[3, 9, 14] The findings of Weinmann[15] led to a general acceptance of the latter concept; namely, that gingival inflammation follows the course of the blood vessels through the loosely arranged tissues around them into the alveolar bone. **The pathway of the spread of inflammation is**

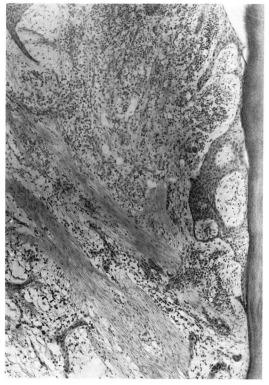

Figure 15–1 Destruction of Gingival Fibers associated with the extension of inflammation from the gingiva into the supporting periodontal tissues.

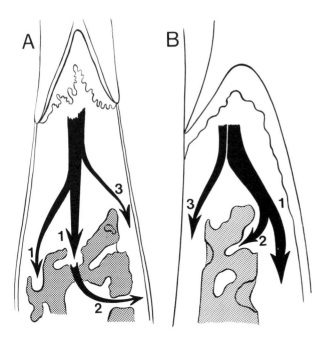

Figure 15–2 Pathways of Inflammation From the Gingiva into the Supporting Periodontal Tissues in Periodontitis. *A,* **Interproximally.** (1) From the gingiva into the bone, (2) from the bone into the periodontal ligament, (3) from the gingiva into the periodontal ligament. *B,* **Facially and Lingually.** (1) From the gingiva along the outer periosteum, (2) from the periosteum into the bone, (3) from the gingiva into the periodontal ligament.

critical, because it affects the pattern of bone destruction in periodontal disease.

Local irritation causes inflammation in the marginal gingiva and interdental papillae. The inflammation penetrates and destroys the gingival fibers, usually at a short distance from their attachment into the cementum (Fig. 15–1). It then spreads into the supporting tissues along the following pathways (Fig. 15–2):

Interproximal pathways

Interproximally, inflammation spreads in the loose connective tissue around the blood vessels through the transseptal fibers and then into the bone through vessel channels which perforate the crest of the interdental septum. **The location at which the inflammation enters the bone depends upon the location of the vessel channels.** It may enter the interdental septum at the center of the crest (Fig. 15–3), toward the side (Fig. 15–4) of the crest, or at the angle of the septum (Fig. 15–5), and it may enter the bone through more than one channel (Fig. 15–5). After reaching the marrow spaces, the inflammation may return from the bone into the periodontal ligament (Fig. 15–2). Less frequently, the inflammation spreads from the gingiva di-

rectly into the periodontal ligament and from there into the interdental septum (Fig. 15–2).[1]

Facial and lingual pathways

Facially and lingually, inflammation from the gingiva spreads **along the outer periosteal surface of the bone** (Fig. 15–2) and penetrates into the marrow spaces through **vessel channels in the outer cortex.**

Reestablishment of transseptal fibers

In its course from the gingiva to the bone, the inflammation destroys the transseptal fibers and reduces them to disorganized granular fragments interspersed among the inflammatory cells and edema (Figs. 15–6 and 15–4B). However, there is a continuous tendency to recreate transseptal fibers across the crest of the interdental septum further along the root as the bone destruction progresses. As a result, transseptal fibers are present even in cases of extreme periodontal bone loss (Fig. 15–7).

The dense transseptal fibers are of clinical significance when surgical procedures

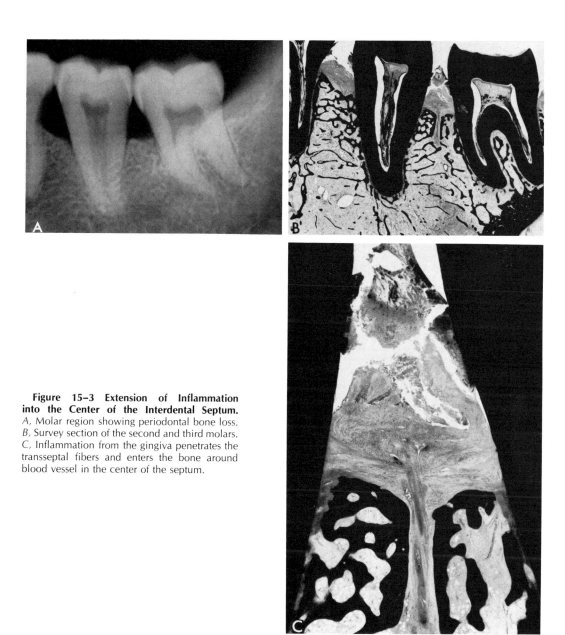

Figure 15-3 Extension of Inflammation into the Center of the Interdental Septum.
A, Molar region showing periodontal bone loss.
B, Survey section of the second and third molars.
C, Inflammation from the gingiva penetrates the transseptal fibers and enters the bone around blood vessel in the center of the septum.

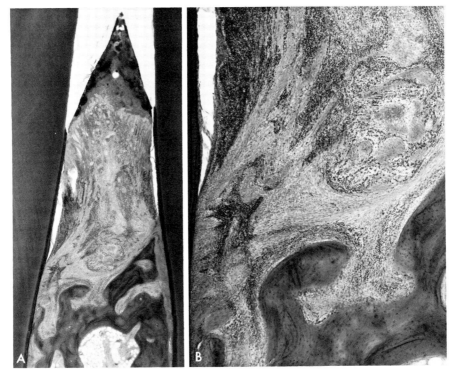

Figure 15–4   Inflammation Enters the Interdental Septum at the Center of the Crest and Near the Crestal Angle. *A,* Interdental periodontal pockets with inflammation extending into the bone. *B,* Inflammation enters the crest of the interdental bone at two areas. Note the granular necrosis of the collagen fibers in the inflamed area above the bone.

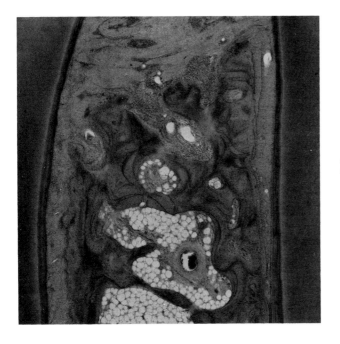

Figure 15–5   Inflammation Enters the Interdental Bone at the Angle of the Crest and in two other areas.

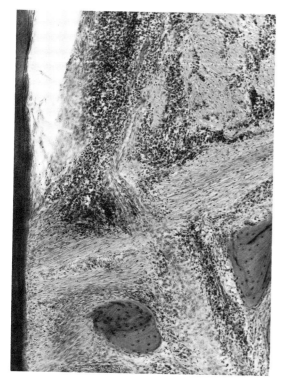

Figure 15–6 Penetration and Destruction of Transseptal Fibers as Inflammation Extends into the Bone.

are employed for the eradication of periodontal pockets. They form a firm covering over the bone, which is encountered after the superficial granulation tissue is removed.

The effect of trauma from occlusion

Considerable controversy has existed with reference to the possible changes in the pathway of gingival inflammation under the influence of trauma from occlusion. Excessive pressure affects the alignment of the transseptal fibers so that they become angular instead of horizontal; it also causes compression, degeneration, and realignment of periodontal ligament fibers so that they are more parallel than perpendicular to the tooth and bone. Glickman and Smulow[8] have described that instead of following its usual interdental course into the interdental bone, the inflammatory exudate is channeled between the transseptal fibers directly into the periodontal ligament (Fig. 15–8).

Other authors[4, 12] have been unable to arrive at similar conclusions. This change in the pathway of inflammation under the influence of trauma from occlusion would lead to vertical bone losses and infrabony pocket formation. Other mechanisms for this trauma-inflammation interaction have been suggested (see Chapter 19).

Excessive tension has also been described to affect the pathway of inflammation.[10] Tension causes stretching and unraveling of the principal fiber bundles of the periodontal ligament, reducing the barrier provided by the intact bundles and permitting the inflammation direct access to the periodontal ligament.

CLINICAL ASPECTS OF INFLAMMATION IN THE PERIODONTAL LIGAMENT

Regardless of whether it extends directly from the gingiva or indirectly through the alveolar bone, inflammation is often present in the periodontal ligament in periodontal disease, contributing to tooth mobility and pain.

Tooth mobility

Inflammation in the periodontal ligament is one of the factors responsible for pathologic tooth mobility, along with loss of alveolar bone and trauma from occlusion. The inflammatory exudate reduces tooth support by causing degeneration and destruction of the principal fibers and a break in the continuity between the root and the bone. The extent to which inflammation in the periodontal ligament contributes to tooth mobility is dramatically demonstrated when the inflammation is eliminated by treatment and the tooth becomes firm.

Pain

Inflammation in the periodontal ligament is usually chronic and asymptomatic. However, superimposed acute inflammation is frequently the cause of considerable pain. With the influx of the acute exudate, the tooth becomes elevated in its socket and there is a desire on the part of the patient to "grind" on it. Repeated con-

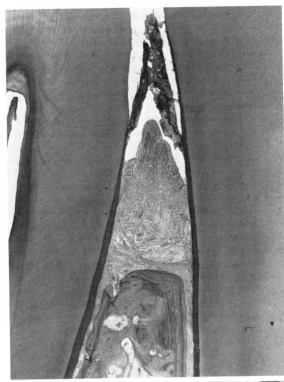

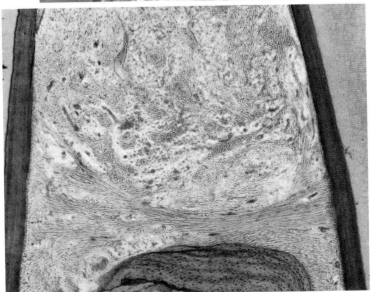

Figure 15–7 Reformation of the Transseptal Fibers in Periodontal Disease. *Top,* Mesiodistal section through the interdental septum showing gingival inflammation with pocket formation and bone loss. *Bottom,* Bone margin showing recreated transseptal fibers of the periodontal ligament just above the bone. Note pronounced degeneration of the connective tissue above the transseptal fibers.

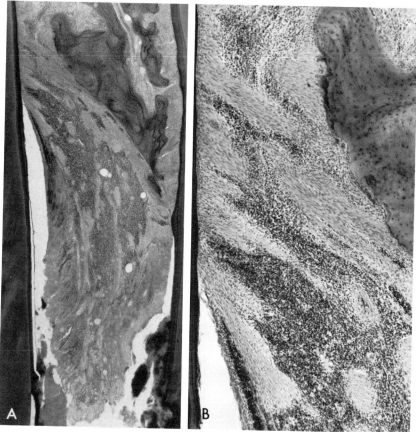

Figure 15–8   Inflammation Extends Directly into the Periodontal Ligament. *A,* Infrabony pocket on the mesial surface of maxillary premolar (*left*). *B,* Inflammation at the base of infrabony pocket extends directly into the periodontal ligament. Note the funnel-shaped widening of the periodontal ligament space and the osteoclastic resorption along the bone surface.

tact with the opposing teeth causes the tooth to become sensitive to percussion. The condition may develop into an acute periodontal abscess unless the irritating agents are removed.

REFERENCES

1. Akiyoshi, M., and Mori, K.: Marginal periodontitis: A histological study of the incipient stage. J. Periodontol. 38:45, 1967.
2. Black, G. V.: Operative Dentistry. Chicago, Medical-Dental Publishing Co., 1936, p. 165.
3. Box, H. K.: Twelve Periodontal Studies. Toronto, University of Toronto Press, 1940.
4. Comar, M. D., Kollar, J. D., and Gargiulo, A. W.: Local irritation and occlusal trauma as cofactors in the periodontal disease process. J. Periodontol., 40:193, 1969.
5. Coolidge, E. D.: Inflammatory changes in the gingival tissue due to local irritation. J. Am. Dent. Assoc., 18:2255, 1931.
6. Fish, E. W.: Bone infection. J. Am. Dent. Assoc., 26:691, 1939.
7. Fullmer, H. M.: A histochemical study of periodontal disease in the maxillary alveolar proc-

ess of 135 autopsies. J. Periodontol., 32:206, 1961.
8. Glickman, I., and Smulow, J. B.: Alterations in the pathway of gingival inflammation into the underlying tissues induced by excessive occlusal forces. J. Periodontol., 33:7, 1962.
9. Kronfeld, R.: Histopathology of the Teeth and Their Surrounding Structures. Philadelphia, Lea & Febiger, 1939, p. 315.
10. Macapanpan, L. C., and Weinmann, J. P.: The influence of injury to the periodontal membrane on the spread of gingival inflammation. J. Dent. Res., 33:263, 1954.
11. Noyes, F. B.: A review of the work on the lymphatics of dental origin. J. Am. Dent. Assoc., 14:714, 1927.
12. Stahl, S. S.: The response of the periodontium to combined gingival inflammation and occlusofunctional stresses in four surgical specimens. Periodontics, 6:14, 1968.
13. Talbot, E. S.: Interstitial gingivitis. Philadelphia, S. S. White Manufacturing Co., 1899.
14. Thoma, K. H., and Goldman, H. M.: The classification and histopathology of parodontal disease. J. Am. Dent. Assoc., 24:1915, 1937.
15. Weinmann, J. P.: Progress of gingival inflammation into the supporting structures of the teeth. J. Periodontol., 12:71, 1941.

Chapter 16

Bone Loss and Patterns of Bone Destruction in Periodontal Disease

The crux of the problem of chronic destructive periodontal disease lies in the changes that occur in the bone. Changes in the other tissues of the periodontium are important, but in the final analysis it is the destruction of bone that is responsible for loss of the teeth.

PHYSIOLOGIC ALVEOLAR BONE EQUILIBRIUM

The height of the alveolar bone is normally maintained by a constant equilibrium between bone formation and bone resorption,[1] which is regulated by local and systemic influences[5, 7] (Fig. 16–1). When resorption exceeds formation, bone height is reduced. It has been claimed[12] that a reduction in the height of the alveolar bone occurs physiologically with age and is termed *physiologic* or *senile atrophy*. This concept has been disputed by others.[24]

In bone destruction in periodontal disease the equilibrium is altered so that resorption exceeds formation. Any factor or combination of factors that changes the physiologic bone equilibrium so that resorption exceeds formation results in loss of alveolar bone.

Bone loss in periodontal disease may result from any of the following changes (Fig. 16–1):

1. Increased resorption in the presence of normal or increased formation.

2. Decreased formation in the presence of normal resorption.

3. Increased resorption combined with decreased formation.

BONE DESTRUCTION IN PERIODONTAL DISEASE

Bone destruction in periodontal disease is caused principally by local factors. It may also be caused by systemic factors, but their role has not been defined. Local factors responsible for bone destruction in periodontal disease fall into two groups: those that cause *gingival inflammation*, and those that cause *trauma from occlusion*. Acting singly or together, inflammation and trauma from occlusion are responsible for the locally caused bone destruction in periodontal disease and determine its severity and pattern.

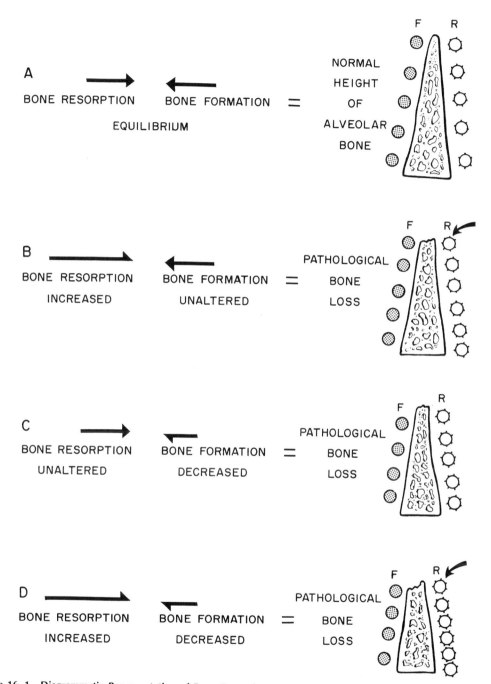

Figure 16–1   Diagrammatic Representation of Bone Formative – Bone Resorptive Relationships in Periodontal Health and Disease. *A,* Physiologic equilibrium between bone resorption (R) and bone formation (F) responsible for the maintenance of normal alveolar bone height. *B,* Pathological bone loss produced when bone resorption is increased (arrow). *C,* Pathological bone loss produced when bone formation is decreased. *D,* Pathological bone loss produced when bone resorption is increased (arrow) and bone formation decreased.

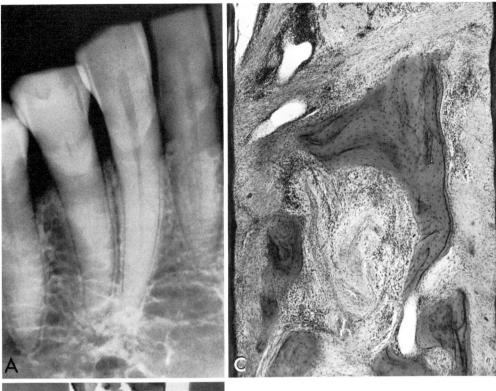

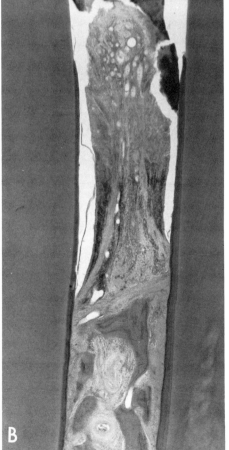

Figure 16–2 Early Periodontal Bone Destruction. *A,* Early periodontal bone loss in the canine and premolar areas. *B,* Interdental space between the canine and first premolar, showing calculus and periodontal pockets. *C,* Interdental septum beneath the periodontal pockets. The inflammation has invaded the marrow space, and there is lacunar resorption of the surrounding bone surface. Note the inflammation in the periodontal ligament on the right side.

Bone Destruction Caused by Chronic Inflammation

Chronic inflammation is the most common cause of bone destruction in periodontal disease.

Histopathology

Inflammation reaches the bone by extension from the gingiva (see Chapter 15). It spreads into the marrow spaces and replaces the marrow with a leukocytic and fluid exudate, new blood vessels, and proliferating fibroblasts (Fig. 16–2). Multinuclear osteoclasts and mononuclear phagocytes are increased in number,[7] and the bone surfaces are lined with cove-like resorption lacunae (Fig. 16–3). In the marrow spaces resorption proceeds from within, causing first a thinning of the surrounding bone trabeculae and enlargement of the marrow spaces, followed by destruction of the bone and reduction in bone height.

The inflammation also stimulates bone formation immediately adjacent to active bone resorption (Fig. 16–4) and along trabecular surfaces removed from the inflammation in an apparent effort to reinforce the remaining bone[2] (buttressing bone formation) (Fig. 16–5).

Mechanisms Whereby Inflammation and/or Plaque-Derived Products Destroy Bone in Periodontal Disease

The possible pathways by which plaque products could cause alveolar bone loss in periodontal disease have been listed by Hausmann[15] as follows:

1. Direct action of plaque products on bone progenitor cells induce their differentiation into osteoclasts.

2. Plaque products act directly on bone, destroying it through a noncellular mechanism.

3. Plaque products stimulate gingival cells, causing them to release mediators which in turn trigger bone progenitor cells to differentiate into osteoclasts.

4. Plaque products cause gingival cells to release agents that can act as cofactors in bone resorption.

5. Plaque products can cause gingival cells to release agents that destroy bone by direct chemical action without osteoclasts.

Goldhaber[10] has developed an in vitro method for the cultivation of rat calvaria in which he tested the influence of many factors on bone resorption. It was found that bone resorption is enhanced by parathyroid gland extract,[4] tumor fragments,[8] heparin,[9] and human gingiva.[10] The combination of heparin and gingival fragments increases bone resorption. Endotoxin from *Bacteroides melaninogenicus* stimulates osteoclastic bone resorption;[13, 30] lipoteichoic acid acts in a similar way.[15]

Prostaglandins are a group of naturally occurring lipids that participate in the inflammatory process and have hormone-like effects.[11] When injected intradermally they induce the vascular changes seen in in-

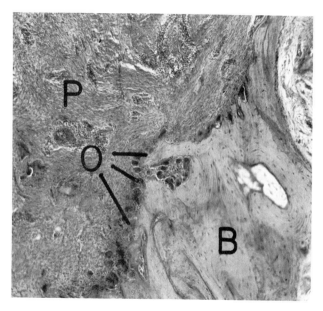

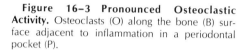

Figure 16–3 Pronounced Osteoclastic Activity. Osteoclasts (O) along the bone (B) surface adjacent to inflammation in a periodontal pocket (P).

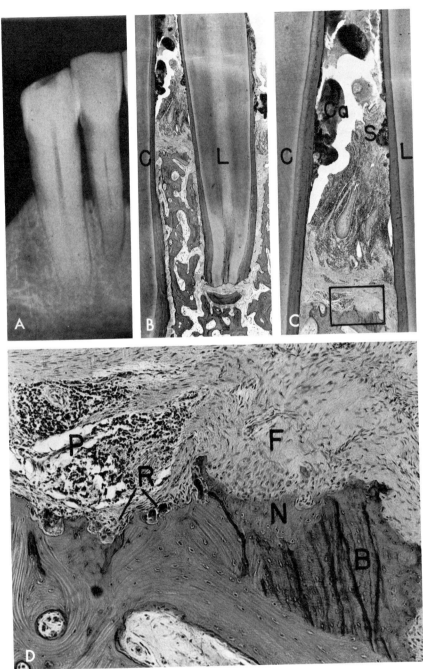

Figure 16–4 Bone Resorption and Formation in Active Periodontal Disease. *A,* Lateral incisor and canine with bone loss. *B,* Survey section of lateral (L) and canine (C). *C,* Interdental space between lateral (L) and canine (C), showing calculus (Ca) and periodontal pockets with suppuration (S). A detailed view of the bone margin within the rectangle is shown in C.

D, Bone margin beneath the periodontal pockets. Note the following: osteoclastic resorption (R) beneath the inflammation (P), and newly formed bone (N) with a thin surface layer of osteoid and osteoblasts adjacent to the resorption. The new bone is separated from the lamellanted bone (B) by an irregular resorption line. An area of fibrosis is shown at F.

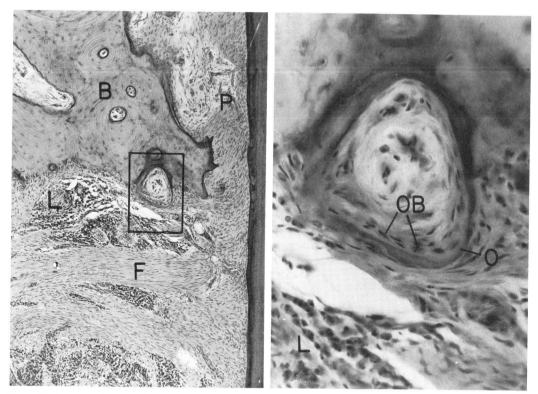

Figure 16–5 Central Buttressing Bone Formation in Chronic Periodontal Disease. *Left,* Survey section of crest of interdental bone (B) beneath inflamed connective tissue (L). The periodontal ligament is shown at P, the transseptal fibers at F. *Right,* High-power study of area in rectangle showing osteoblasts (OB) and layer of osteoid buttressing thinned remnant of resorbed bone (O). Leukocytic infiltration is shown at L.

flammation. When injected over a bone surface they induce bone resorption[19] in the absence of inflammatory cells and with scarce multinucleated osteoclasts.[11] Complement may enhance the synthesis of prostaglandins by the bone and therefore induce bone resorption.[29]

Bone resorption can also be induced by supernatants of leukocyte cultures stimulated by antigens from dental plaque.[16] Horton et al.[16] hypothesized that lymphocytes produce an **osteoclast-activating factor** (OAF) which induces osteoclast formation and activity.

Many investigations have been conducted and many explanations considered, but the mechanism or mechanisms of bone destruction in inflammatory periodontal disease have not as yet been determined.

Inflammation in periodontal disease is accompanied by an increase in osteoclasts and mononuclear phagocytes, both of which resorb bone by removing the min-

eral crystals and digesting the exposed collagen. The increased vascularity associated with inflammation may also cause bone resorption by stimulating an increase in osteoclasts and by elevating the local oxygen tension. The lowered pH of the inflammatory process may also affect bone resorption.[31]

Proteolytic enzymes in the periodontal tissues or produced by gingival bacteria may also participate in bone resorption.[17] Collagenase is present in the normal periodontium and increased in inflamed gingiva; it is also produced by oral bacteria. Collagenolytic activity is produced in resorbing bone in vitro, but the collagen content is not correlated with the severity of bone loss.[3] By breaking down the bone matrix ground substance, hyaluronidase produced by oral bacteria may influence the resorptive process.

Irving et al.,[17] in an experiment with gnotobiotic rats monoinfected with *Actin-*

omyces naeslundii, *Actinomyces viscosus,*
or *Streptococcus mutans,* and in another
experiment with conventional rats superin-
fected with *A. naeslundii,* found that bone
loss was not accompanied by osteoclasts
and seemed to be more a gradual cessation
of bone formation than active resorption.

**The bone destruction caused by inflam-
mation in periodontal disease is not a process of bone necrosis.**[7, 20] It entails the
activity of *living cells* along *viable bone.*
When tissue necrosis and pus are present in
periodontal disease, they occur in the soft
tissue walls of periodontal pockets, not
along the resorbing margin of the underlying bone. **The severity of bone loss is not
necessarily correlated with the depth of
periodontal pockets, the severity of ulceration of the pocket wall, or the presence or
absence of pus.**

Bone Formation in Periodontal Disease

It is significant that the response of alveolar bone to inflammation includes
bone formation as well as resorption. It
means that **bone loss in periodontal disease is not simply a destructive process
but results from the predominance of resorption over formation.** New bone formation retards the rate of bone loss, compen-
sating in some degree for the bone
destroyed by inflammation. Newly formed
osteoid is more resistant to resorption than
mature bone.[18] Because of the interaction
between bone resorption and bone formation, **bone loss in periodontal disease is
not necessarily continuous. It is a progressive process, but its rate cannot be predicted.**

Occasionally in autopsy specimens of
untreated disease, there are areas where
bone resorption has ceased and new bone
is being formed on the previously eroded
bone margin. **This indicates that bone resorption in periodontal disease may occur
as an intermittent process with periods of
remission and exacerbation.** This is consistent with the varied rates of progress observed clinically in untreated periodontal
disease.

The microscopic bone formation in response to inflammation varies in amount
and distribution. It is governed by the
severity and distribution of the inflammation and by systemic influences. In this
way systemic factors which affect the metabolic processes involved in bone formation influence the bone loss in periodontal
disease.[2]

**The presence of bone formation in re-
sponse to inflammation in active periodontal disease has a bearing on the outcome
of treatment.** Elimination of inflammation
to remove the stimulus to bone resorption
and the establishment of conditions conducive to healing are basic aims in periodontal treatment. Healing of the periodontium following treatment depends upon
the body's reparative processes, one of
which is the formation of new bone. An
active tendency toward bone formation in
untreated disease could benefit healing if
carried over into the post-treatment
period.

The radiograph is extremely useful in
diagnosis, but it does not detect microscopic resorptive and formative activities.
Sometimes, endosteal bone formation in
periodontal disease produces increased radiodensity (condensing osteitis) adjacent
to eroded bone margins. However, there
may be bone formation in periodontal disease without any radiographic suggestion
of its presence (Fig. 16–6).

Bone Destruction Caused by Trauma from Occlusion

Inflammation is the more common
cause of periodontal destruction, the other
being trauma from occlusion. Trauma from
occlusion can produce bone destruction in
the absence of inflammation or combined
with it.

Trauma in the absence of inflammation

In the absence of inflamation, the
changes in trauma from occlusion vary
from increased compression and tension of
the periodontal ligament and increased osteoclasis of alveolar bone[25] to necrosis of the
periodontal ligament and bone and resorption of bone and tooth structure. These
changes are reversible in that they are
repaired if the offending forces are re-

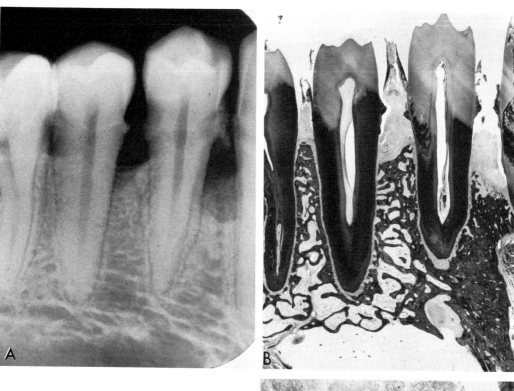

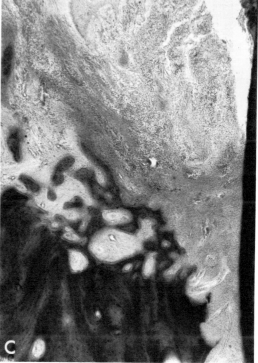

Figure 16–6 Bone Formation in Untreated Periodontal Disease. *A,* Radiograph showing bone destruction in the mandibular premolar areas. Note the heavy calculus deposits. *B,* Survey section of the distal surface of the canine (*right*), the first and second premolars and the mesial surface of the first molar, showing periodontal disease with bone loss. *C,* Interdental space between the canine and first premolar, showing inflammation and newly formed bone trabeculae on the previously resorbed bone margin.

moved. However, persistent trauma from occlusion causes funnel-shaped widening of the crestal portion of the periodontal ligament with resorption of the adjacent bone.[23] These changes, which may result in an angular shape of the bony crest, represent adaptation of the periodontal tissues to "cushion" increased occlusal force, but they produce defects in the bone which weaken tooth support and cause tooth mobility.

Trauma combined with inflammation

When combined with inflammation, trauma from occlusion acts as a codestructive factor in periodontal disease. It aggravates the bone destruction caused by the inflammation,[23] and causes bizarre bone patterns.

Bone Destruction Caused by Systemic Disorders

Local and systemic factors regulate the physiologic equilibrium of bone.[5] When there is a generalized tendency toward bone resorption, bone loss initiated by local inflammatory processes may be magnified. This systemic influence upon the response of alveolar bone loss has been termed the *"bone factor"* in periodontal disease.[5]

The "Bone Factor" Concept

The individual bone factor affects the severity of bone loss associated with local destructive factors in periodontal disease. The destructive effect of inflammation and trauma from occlusion varies with the status of the individual "bone factor." It is less severe in a healthy individual in the presence of a positive "bone factor" than when superimposed upon a systemically induced bone-destructive tendency (negative "bone factor"). In the presence of a negative "bone factor" the normal adaptive capacity of alveolar bone to occlusal forces is altered so that a normal functional relationship may become a local destructive force.

The bone factor concept, developed by Irving Glickman,[5] differs from the traditional division of periodontal disease into "local" and "systemic" types. It envisions a systemic component in all cases of periodontal disease.

In addition to the amount and virulence of plaque bacteria, it is the nature of the systemic component and not its presence or absence that influences the severity of periodontal destruction. For the application of the bone factor concept to diagnosis and prognosis, see Chapters 32 and 33.

Periodontal bone loss may also occur in generalized skeletal disturbances such as hyperparathyroidism, leukemia, Hand-Schüller-Christian disease, etc., by mechanisms totally unrelated to the usual periodontal problem.

BONE LOSS AND TOOTH MOBILITY

Loss of alveolar bone in periodontal disease is an important cause of tooth mobility, but other factors are involved. As a result, the degree of tooth mobility in periodontal disease is not necessarily correlated with the amount of bone loss (see Chapter 20).

FACTORS DETERMINING BONE MORPHOLOGY IN PERIODONTAL DISEASE

Normal Variation in the Morphology of Alveolar Bone

There is considerable normal variation in the morphology of alveolar bone (see Chapter 4), and it affects the osseous contours produced by periodontal disease. The bone features that significantly affect the bone destructive pattern in periodontal disease are the *thickness, width,* and *crestal angulation of the interdental septa, the thickness of the facial and lingual alveolar plates, the presence of fenestrations and dehiscences on the root surfaces, thickening of the alveolar bone margins to accommodate functional demands, and the alignment of the teeth.*

For example, angular osseous defects cannot form in thin facial or lingual alveolar plates, which have little or no cancellous bone between the outer and inner cortical layers. In such instances, the entire crest of the plate is destroyed and the height of the bone is reduced.

Exostoses

Exostoses are outgrowths of bone of varied size and shape. They occur more often on the facial surface than on the lingual, and apparently serve no useful purpose. The cervical margin of the alveolar bone is often thickened in response to increased functional demands so that it is sometimes difficult to differentiate between linear exostoses and functional adaptaton.

The Pathway of Inflammation

Because chronic inflammation is an important cause of bone destruction, its path-

way in the supporting tissues is a significant determinant of the bone morphology produced by periodontal disease.

Traumatic Forces

Trauma from occlusion is a critical factor in determining the dimension and shape of bone deformities. This may be due to a change in the initial morphology of the bone (angular defects, buttressing bone — see below) upon which inflammatory changes will later be superimposed, or as a codestructive factor that changes the bone destructive pattern of inflammation.

Buttressing Bone Formation (Lipping)

Bone formation sometimes occurs in an attempt to buttress bone trabeculae weak-

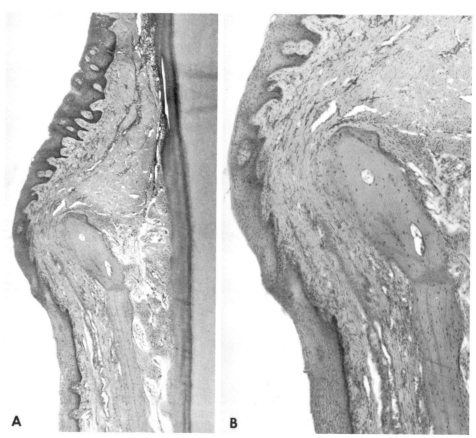

A **B**

Figure 16–7 Lipping of Facial Bone. *A,* Peripheral buttressing bone formation along the external surface of facial bony plate and at the crest. Note the deformity in the bone produced by the buttressing bone formation and the bulging of the mucosa. *B,* Detailed view showing "lipping" and deformity produced by buttressing bone formation.

ened by resorption. When it occurs within the jaw it is termed *central buttressing bone formation.*[6] When it occurs on the external surface it is referred to as *peripheral buttressing bone.* The latter may cause bulging of the bone contour, termed *lipping,* which sometimes accompanies the formation of osseous craters and infrabony defects (Fig. 16–7).

Food Impaction

Interdental bone defects often occur where the proximal contact is abnormal or absent. Pressure and irritation from food impaction contribute to the inverted bone architecture. In some instances the poor proximal relationship may be the result of a shift in tooth position because of extensive bone destruction that preceded food impaction. In such cases food impaction is a complicating factor, rather than the initial cause of the bone defect.

Juvenile Periodontitis (Periodontosis)

Vertical or angular destruction of alveolar bone is found in juvenile periodontitis.

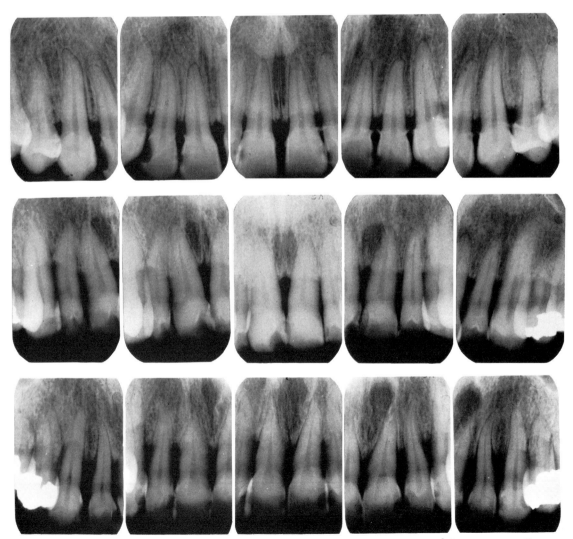

Figure 16–8   Horizontal Bone Loss. Three patients with different degrees of destruction in the anterior maxilla.

The cause for the bone destructive pattern in this type of periodontal disease is unknown.

BONE DESTRUCTIVE PATTERNS IN PERIODONTAL DISEASE

In addition to reducing bone height, periodontal disease alters the morphology of the bone. An understanding of the nature and pathogenesis of these alterations is essential for effective diagnosis and treatment.

Horizontal Bone Loss

This is the most common pattern of bone loss in periodontal disease. The bone is reduced in height and the bone margin is horizontal or slightly angulated. Interdental septa and the facial and lingual plates are affected, but not necessarily to an equal degree around the same tooth (Fig. 16–8).

Bone Deformities (Osseous Defects)

The following are types of bone deformities produced by periodontal disease.[20] They usually occur in adults but have been reported in human skulls with deciduous dentitions.[22] Their presence may be sug-

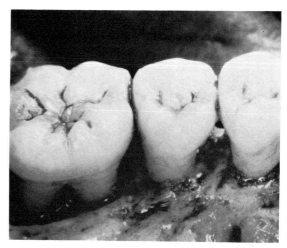

Figure 16–10 **Osseous Crater** and furcation involvement around mandibular first molar.

gested by the radiograph, but **careful probing and surgical exposure of the area are required to determine their conformation and dimensions.**

OSSEOUS CRATERS. These are concavities in the crest of the interdental bone confined within facial and lingual walls (Fig. 16–9), and less frequently between the tooth surface and facial or lingual bony plate (Fig. 16–10). Craters have been found to represent about one third of all defects (35.2 per cent) and about two thirds (62.0 per cent) of all mandibular defects.[26] Manson[26] lists the following factors as responsible for the frequent occurrence of interdental craters:

(1) The interdental area collects plaque and is difficult to clean.

(2) The normal flat or even concave buccolingual shape of the interdental septum in lower molars; the lack of cortical bone in the crest.

(3) Inflammation travels on vascular pathways and therefore more rapidly through vascular cancellous trabeculation.

(4) Cancellous trabeculation has a more rapid turnover than cortical bone.

VERTICAL (ANGULAR) DEFECTS. Such defects are hollowed-out troughs in the bone alongside one or more denuded root surfaces enclosed within one, two, or three bony walls (Fig. 16–11). The base of the

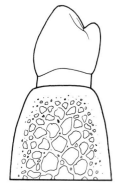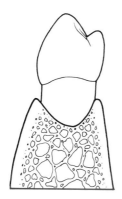

Figure **16–9** Diagrammatic representation of an osseous crater in a facio-lingual section between two lower premolars. Left, Normal bone contour. Right, Osseous crater.

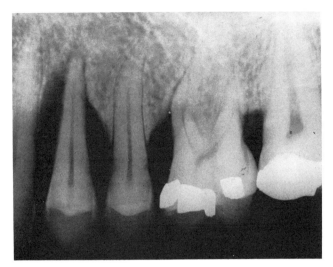

Figure 16–11   Angular (Vertical) Defects of different depths.

defect is located apical to the surrounding bone (see Chapter 14).

In human skulls it was observed that angular defects are most common on the mesial surface of the maxillary and mandibular second and third molars; that they are present in an increasing percentage of individuals from age 2 to 44, when the maximum is reached; and that the number of defects per individual is greatest after age 60.[21] In another study[26] angular defects were found to predominate in the maxilla rather than in the mandible.

BULBOUS BONE CONTOURS.   These are bony enlargements caused by exostoses, adaptation to function, or buttressing bone formation (Fig. 16–12). They are found much more frequently in the maxilla.[26]

HEMISEPTA.   The remaining portion of an interdental septum after the mesial or distal portion has been entirely destroyed by disease is termed a hemiseptum (Fig.

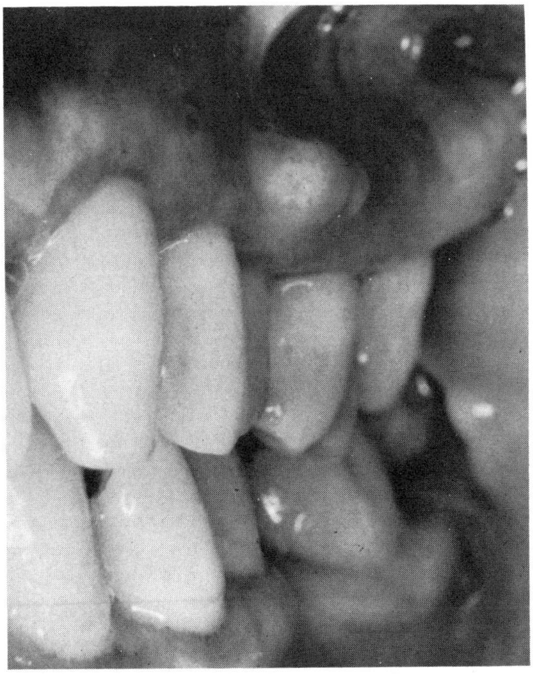

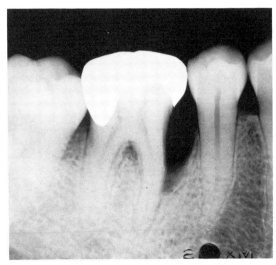

Figure 16–12   Exostoses.

Figure 16–13   Angular Defect on the Mesial Surface of the First Molar. Note also the furcation involvement.

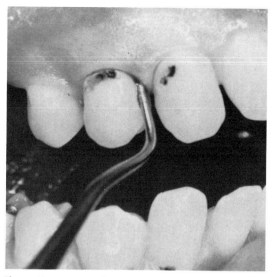
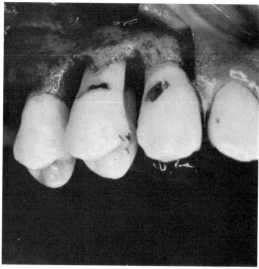

Figure 16–14   Irregular Bone Margin. *Left,* Probe in deep infrabony pocket on the mesial surface of maxillary premolar. *Right,* Elevated flap shows irregular bone margin with notching of interdental bone.

16–13). This term is synonymous with one wall vertical or angular bone loss.

INCONSISTENT MARGINS. These are angular or U-shaped defects produced by resorption of the facial or lingual alveolar plate or abrupt differences between the height of the facial or lingual margins and the height of the interdental septa (Fig. 16–14). These defects have also been termed *reversed architecture.* They are more frequent in the maxilla.[26]

LEDGES. Ledges are plateau-like bone margins caused by resorption of thickened bony plates (Fig. 16–15).

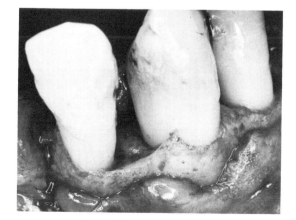

Figure 16–15   Labial Ledge produced by interproximal resorption.

REFERENCES

1. Carranza, F. A., Jr., and Cabrini, R. L.: Histometric studies of periodontal tissues. Periodontics, 5:308, 1967.
2. Carranza, F. A., Jr., Simes, R. J., Mayo, J., and Cabrini, R. L.: Histometric evaluation of periodontal bone loss in rats. J. Periodont. Res., 6: 65, 1971.
3. Fullmer, H. M., et al.: Collagenase and gingival disease. Proceedings, First Pan-Pacific Congress of Dental Research, 1970, pp. 167–171.
4. Gaillard, P. J.: Parathyroid gland tissue and bone in-vitro. Exp. Cell Res., 3:154, 1955.
5. Glickman, I.: The experimental basis for the "bone factor" concept in periodontal disease. J. Periodontol., 20:7, 1951.
6. Glickman, I., and Smulow, J.: Buttressing bone formation in the periodontium. J. Periodontol., 36:365, 1965.
7. Glickman, I., and Wood, H.: Bone histology in periodontal disease. J. Dent. Res., 21:35, 1942.
8. Goldhaber, P.: Enhancement of bone resorption in tissue culture by mouse fibrosarcoma. Proc. Am. Assoc. Cancer Res., 24:254, 1960.
9. Goldhaber, P.: Bone resorption factors, co-factors and giant vacuole osteoclasts in tissue culture. *In* Gaillard, P. J., et al.: The Parathyroid Glands: Ultrastructure, Secretion and Function. Chicago, University of Chicago Press, 1965, p. 153.
10. Goldhaber, P.: Tissue culture studies of bone as a model system for periodontal research. J. Dent. Res., 50:279, 1971.
11. Goodson, J. M., McClatchy, K., and Revell, C.: Prostaglandin-induced resorption of the adult calvarium. J. Dent. Res., 53:670, 1974.
12. Gottlieb, B., and Orban, B. J.: Biology and Pathology of the Tooth and its Supporting Mechanism. New York, Macmillan, Inc., 1938.

13. Hausmann, E., Raisz, L. G., and Miller, W. A.: Endotoxin: Stimulation of bone resorption in tissue culture. Science, 168:862, 1970.

14. Hausmann, E., Genco, R., Weinfeld, N., and Sacco, R.: Effects of sera on bone resorption in tissue culture. Calc. Tiss. Res., 13:311, 1973.

15. Hausmann, E.: Potential pathways for bone resorption in human periodontal disease. J. Periodontol., 45:338, 1974.

16. Horton, J. E., Raisz, L. G., Simmons, H. A., Oppenheim, J. J., and Mergenhagen, S. E.: Bone resorbing activity in supernatant fluid from cultured human peripheral blood leukocytes. Science, 177:793, 1972.

17. Irving, J. T.: Factors concerning bone loss associated with periodontal disease. J. Dent. Res., 49:262, 1970.

18. Irving, J. T., and Heeley, J. D.: Tissue reaction to the implantation of labeled isogenous bone. Abstract. I.A.D.R. Program and Abstracts of Papers, 1969, p. 224.

19. Klein, D. C., and Raisz, L. G.: Prostaglandins: Stimulation of bone resorption in tissue culture. Endocrinology, 86:1436, 1970.

20. Kronfeld, R.: Condition of alveolar bone underlying periodontal pockets. J. Periodontol., 6:22, 1935.

21. Larato, D. C.: Intrabony defects in the dry human skull. J. Periodontol., 41:496, 1970.

22. Larato, D. C.: Periodontal bone defects in the juvenile skull. J. Periodontol., 41:473, 1970.

23. Lindhe, J., and Svanberg, G.: Influence of trauma from occlusion on progression of experimental periodontitis in beagle dogs. J. Clin. Periodont., 1:3, 1974.

24. Loe, H.: The Structure and Physiology of the Dentogingival Junction. In Miles, A. E. W. (ed.): Structural and Chemical Organization of Teeth. Academic Press, 1967.

25. Lopez-Otero, R., et al.: Histologic and histometric study of bone resorption after tooth movement in rats. J. Periodont. Res., 8:327, 1973.

26. Manson, J. D.: Bone morphology and bone loss in periodontal disease. J. Clin. Periodont., 3:14, 1976.

27. Melcher, A. H., and Eastoe, J. E.: Biology of the Periodontium. New York, Academic Press, 1969, pp. 315–319.

28. Prichard, J. F.: Periodontal Surgery, Practical Dental Monographs. Chicago, Year Book Medical Publishers, Inc., Nov., 1961, pp. 16–19.

29. Raisz, L. G., Sandberg, A. L., Goodson, J. M., Simmons, H. A., and Mergenhagen, S. E.: Complement-dependent stimulation of prostaglandin synthesis and bone resorption. Science, 185:789, 1974.

30. Rizzo, A. A., and Mergenhagen, S. E.: Histopathologic effects of endotoxin injected into rabbit oral mucosa. Arch. Oral Biol., 9:659, 1964.

31. Swenson, O., and Claff, L. C.: Changes in the hydrogen ion concentration of healing fractures. Proc. Soc. Exp. Biol. Med., 61:151, 1946.

Furcation Involvement

The term *furcation involvement* refers to commonly occurring conditions in which the bifurcation and trifurcation of multi-rooted teeth are denuded by periodontal disease.[1, 2] The mandibular first molars are the most common sites, and the maxillary premolars the least common; the number of furcation involvements increases with age.[4]

CLINICAL FEATURES

The denuded bifurcation or trifurcation may be visible or obscured by the inflamed wall of a periodontal pocket. The extent of involvement is determined by exploration with a blunt probe, with a simultaneous blast of warm air to facilitate visualization. The tooth may or may not be mobile and is usually symptom-free, but there may be painful complications. These include **sensitivity to thermal changes** caused by caries or lacunar resorption of the root in the furcation area, **recurrent or constant throbbing pain** caused by pulp changes, and **sensitivity to percussion** from acute inflammatory involvement of the periodontal ligament. Furcation involvement may result in acute periodontal or periapical abscess formation, with all the symptoms that accompany such lesions (Figs. 17–1 and 17–2).

MICROSCOPIC FEATURES

Microscopically, furcation involvement presents no unique pathologic features. It is simply a phase in the rootward extension of the periodontal pocket. In its early stages, it presents widening of the periodontal space with cellular and fluid inflammatory exudation (Fig. 17–3), followed by epithelial proliferation into the bifurcation area from an adjoining periodontal pocket (Fig. 17–4). Extension of the inflammation into the bone leads to resorption and reduction in bone height (Fig. 17–5). Bone formation is often present adjacent to areas of resorption and along adjoining medullary spaces (Fig. 17–6). The bone destructive pattern may be horizontal or may produce angular osseous defects associated with infrabony pockets (Fig. 17–7). Plaque, calculus, and bacterial debris occupy the de-

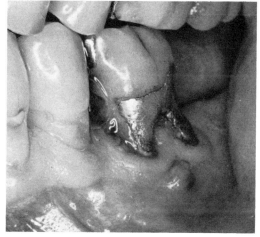

Figure 17–1 Bifurcation Involvement Complicated by Periodontal Abscess.

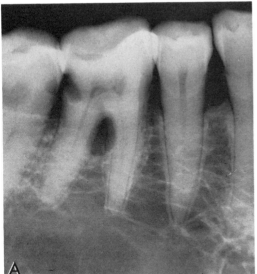

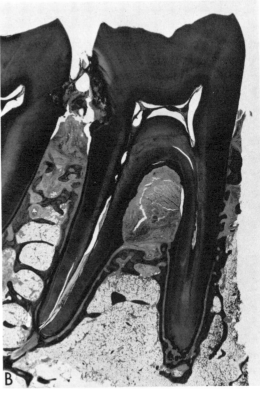

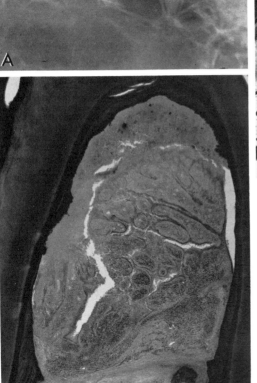

Figure 17–2 Furcation Involvement Complicated by Abscess Formation. *A,* Bifurcation involvement of mandibular first molar. Also note caries. *B,* Section through mandibular first molar showing periodontal disease with bifurcation involvement. Note the caries. *C,* Abscess in the bifurcation. Note extension of the inflammation into the bone and thickened blood vessel.

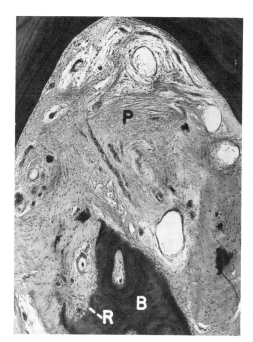

Fig. 17-3

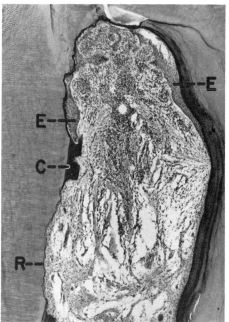

Fig. 17-4

Figure 17-3   Bifurcation Area in a Mandibular Molar. The periodontal space is widened. There is edema, degeneration, and slight leukocytic infiltration of the periodontal ligament, and an area of resorption (R) at the margin of the bone (B).

Figure 17-4   Bifurcation Area showing proliferation of epithelium (E), edema and degeneration of connective tissue, bone loss, and destruction of cementum (C) and dentin with irregularly hollowed-out lacunae along the dentinal surface (R).

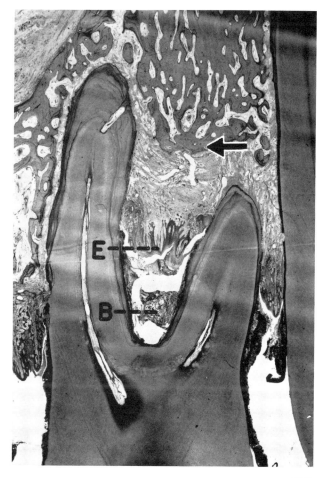

Figure 17-5   Trifurcation Involvement. Maxillary first molar showing pronounced bone loss, inflammation, and epithelial proliferation (E). Bacterial debris is shown at B. The area indicated by the arrow is shown in Figure 17-6.

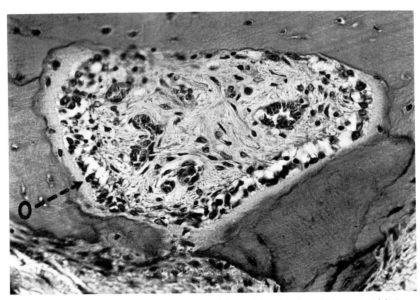

Figure 17–6 Detail of Figure 17–5 (*arrow*) showing osteoblasts (O) and pale staining osteoid lining medullary space adjoining bone margin undergoing resorption.

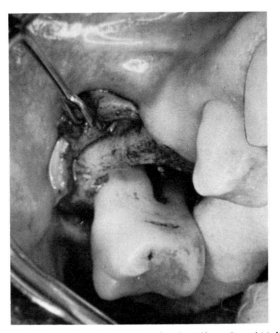

Figure 17–7 Crater-like Osseous Defect in Trifurcation of Molar.

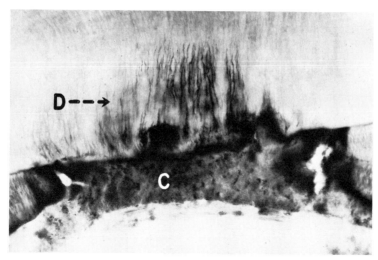

Figure 17–8   Trifurcation Showing Destruction of Cementum (C) and Caries of Dentin (D).

nuded furcation space. Findings that complicate furcation involvement and account for painful symptoms include caries of cementum and dentin with involvement of the dentinal tubules (Fig. 17–8); idiopathic tooth resorption in which cementum is absent and the dentin presents a clear-cut, irregular margin with hollowed-out lacunae (Fig. 17–4); and abscess formation in the furcation area.

ETIOLOGY

Bifurcation and trifurcation involvement are stages of progressive periodontal disease and have the same etiology. However, of all areas of the periodontium, the bifurcation and trifurcation are the most sensitive to injury from excessive occlusal forces.[3] Trauma from occlusion should be particularly suspect as a contributing etiologic factor in cases of furcation involvement with crater-like or angular deformities in the bone, especially when bone destruction is localized to one of the roots.

RADIOGRAPHIC FEATURES

Definitive diagnosis of furcation involvement is made by clinical examination which includes careful probing. Radiographs are helpful but present artefacts which make it possible for furcation involvement to be present without detectable radiographic changes.

For example, in Figure 17–9, the trifurcation of the maxillary first molar appears involved, whereas that of the second molar does not. Microscopic sections of the au-

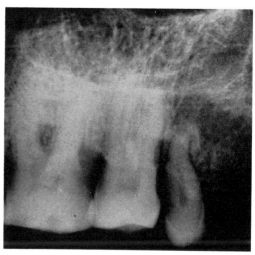

Figure 17–9 Radiograph Showing Trifurcation Involvement of the Maxillary First Molar. Compare with Figures 17–10 and 17–11.

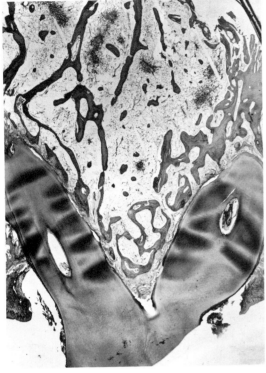

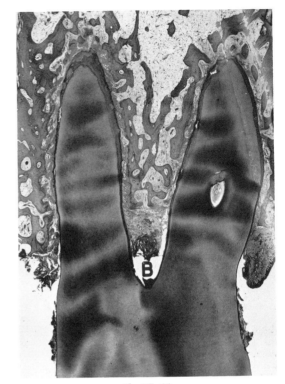

Fig. 17–10

Fig. 17–11

Figure 17–10 Buccopalatal section through the **Maxillary First Molar** shown in Figure 17–9. The trifurcation is involved and there are periodontal pockets on the buccal (*left*) and palatal roots (*right*).

Figure 17–11 Buccopalatal section through the **Maxillary Second Molar** shown in Figure 17–9. There is involvement of the trifurcation at B, which is clearly detectable in the radiograph.

topsied jaw indicate that both the first (Fig. 17–10) and second (Fig. 17–11) molars are involved. The opaque palatal root of the second molar hides the bone loss in the trifurcation.

Variations in radiographic technique may obscure the presence and extent of furcation involvement. A tooth may present marked bifurcation involvement in one film (Fig. 17–12A), but appear uninvolved in another (Fig. 17–12B). Films should be taken at different angles to reduce the risk of missing furcation involvement.

Aids in radiographic interpretation

The recognition of large, clearly defined radiolucency in the furcation area presents no problem (Fig. 17–12A), but less clearly defined radiographic changes produced by furcation involvement are often overlooked. To assist in the radiographic detection of furcation involvement the following criteria are suggested:

1. The slightest radiographic change in the furcation area should be investigated clinically, especially if there is bone loss on adjacent roots (Fig. 17–13).

2. Diminished radiodensity in the furcation area in which outlines of bone trabeculae are visible (Fig. 17–14).

3. Whenever there is marked bone loss in relation to a single molar root, it may be assumed that the furcation is also involved (Figs. 17–15) and 17–16). This is an extremely important rule. Treatment limited to the root with extensive bone loss may

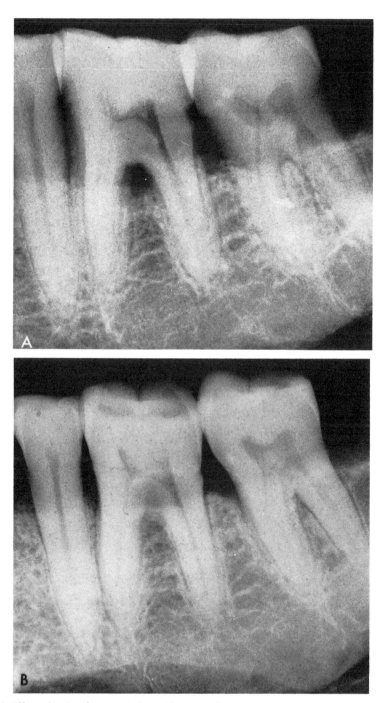

Figure 17–12 *A,* **Bifurcation Involvement** indicated by triangular radiolucence in bifurcation area of mandibular first molar. The second molar presents only a slight thickening of the periodontal space in the bifurcation area. *B,* Same area, different angulation. The triangular radiolucence in the bifurcation of the first molar is obliterated and involvement of the second molar bifurcation is apparent.

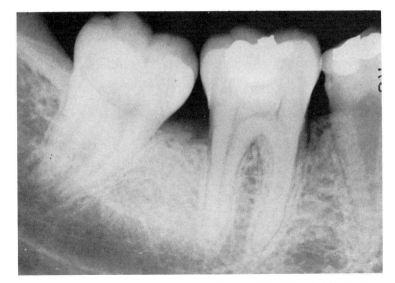

Figure 17–13 Early Furcation Involvement suggested by fuzziness in the bifurcation of the mandibular first molar, particularly when associated with bone loss on the roots.

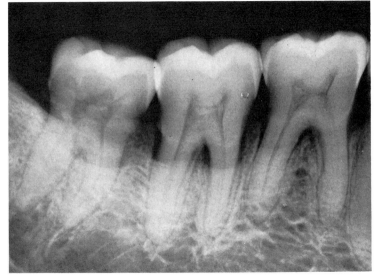

Figure 17–14 Bifurcation Involvement of Mandibular First and Second Molars Indicated by Thickening of Periodontal Space in Bifurcation Area. The bifurcation of the third molar is also involved but the thickening of the periodontal space is partially obscured by the external oblique line.

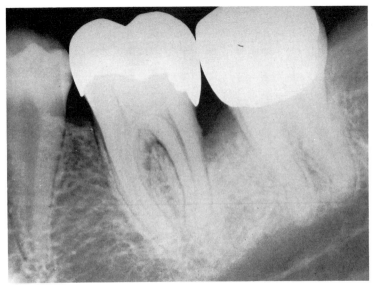

Figure 17–15 Bifurcation Involvement of first molar, associated with bone loss on the distal root.

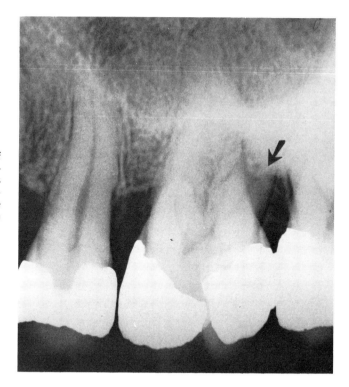

Figure 17–16 Trifurcation Involvement of the First Molar Partially Obscured by the Radiopaque Lingual Root. The horizontal line across the distobuccal root demarcates the apical portion (arrow) which is covered by bone, from the remainder of the root where the bone has been destroyed.

seal the infected bifurcation or trifurcation, prevent drainage, and lead to formation of a periodontal abscess.

REFERENCES

1. Easley, J. R., and Drennan, G. A.: Morphological classification of the furca. J. Can. Dent. Assoc., 35:104, 1969.

2. Glickman, I.: Bifurcation involvement in periodontal disease. J. Am. Dent. Assoc., 40:528, 1950.

3. Glickman, I., Stein, R. S., and Smulow, J. B.: The effects of increased functional forces upon the periodontium of splinted and non-splinted teeth. J. Periodontol., 32:290, 1961.

4. Larato, D. C.: Furcation involvements: incidence of distribution. J. Periodontol., 41:499, 1970.

The Periodontal Abscess

A *periodontal abscess is a localized purulent inflammation in the periodontal tissues*. It is also known as a *lateral* or *parietal abscess*. Periodontal abscess formation may occur as follows:

1. Deep extension of infection from a periodontal pocket into the supporting periodontal tissues, and localization of the suppurative inflammatory process along the lateral aspect of the root.

2. Lateral extension of inflammation from the inner surface of a periodontal pocket into the connective tissue of the pocket wall. Localization of the abscess results when drainage into the pocket space is impaired (Fig. 18–1).

3. In a pocket that describes a tortuous course around the root (complex pocket), a periodontal abscess may form in the cul-de-sac, the deep end of which is shut off from the surface.

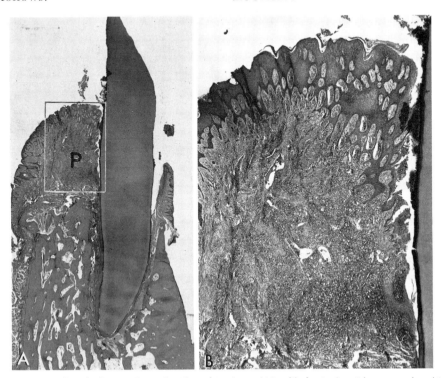

Figure 18–1 *A*, **Periodontal Abscess (P) on the Lingual Surface of Mandibular Incisor** (abscess enclosed in rectangle). *B*, Detailed view of periodontal abscess showing dense leukocytic infiltration and suppuration.

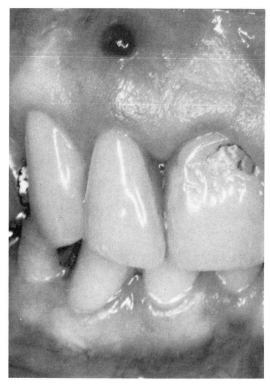

Figure 18–2 **Periodontal Abscess** deep in the periodontium showing hemorrhagic tissue at the sinus orifice.

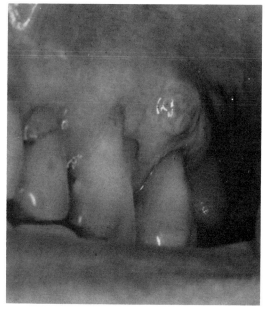

Figure 18–4 **Periodontal Abscess on Maxillary Second Molar.**

4. Incomplete removal of calculus during treatment of a periodontal pocket. In this instance, the gingival wall shrinks, occluding the pocket orifice, and a periodontal abscess occurs in the sealed-off portion of the pocket.

5. A periodontal abscess may occur in the absence of periodontal disease, following trauma to the tooth or perforation of the lateral wall of the root in endodontic therapy.

Classification

Periodontal abscesses are classified according to location as follows:

1. *Abscess in the supporting periodontal tissues* along the lateral aspect of the root. In this condition, there is generally a sinus in the bone, which extends laterally from the abscess to the external surface (Fig. 18–2).

Figure 18–3 **Chronic Periodontal Abscess in the Wall of a Deep Pocket.**

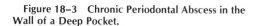

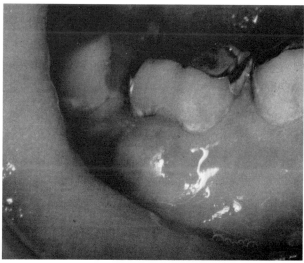

2. *Abscess in the soft tissue wall of a deep periodontal pocket* (Figs. 18–3 and 18–4).

Clinical features

Periodontal abscess may be *acute* or *chronic.* Acute lesions often subside but persist in the chronic state, whereas chronic lesions may exist without having been acute. Chronic lesions frequently undergo acute exacerbations.

ACUTE ABSCESS. The acute periodontal abscess is accompanied by symptoms such as **throbbing radiating pain, exquisite tenderness of the gingiva to palpation, sensitivity of the tooth to percussion, tooth mobility, lymphadenitis, and systemic effects such as fever, leukocytosis, and malaise.**

The acute periodontal abscess appears as an ovoid elevation of the gingiva along the lateral aspect of the root (Figs. 18–5 and 18–6). The gingiva is edematous and red, with a smooth, shiny surface. The shape and consistency of the elevated area vary. It may be dome-like and relatively firm, or pointed and soft. In most instances, pus may be expressed from the gingival margin by gentle digital pressure. Occasionally, the patient may present symptoms of an acute

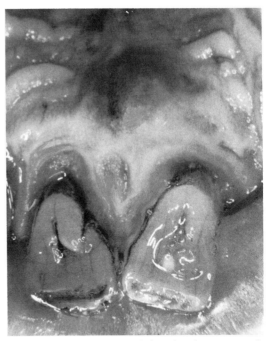

Figure 18–6 Acute Periodontal Abscess on the Lingual Surface.

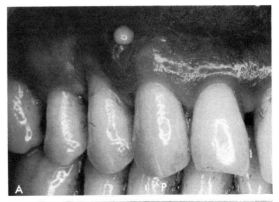

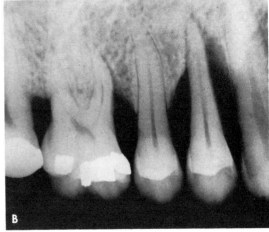

Figure 18–7 Suppuration from a Chronic Periodontal Abscess. *A,* Suppurative draining sinus between the canine and first premolar. *B,* Radiograph showing extensive bone destruction in the area of the draining sinus.

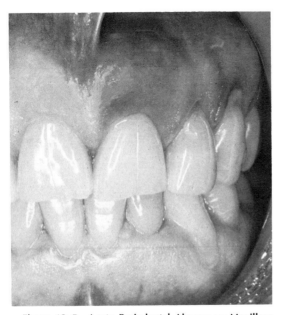

Figure 18–5 Acute Periodontal Abscess on Maxillary Left Central Incisor.

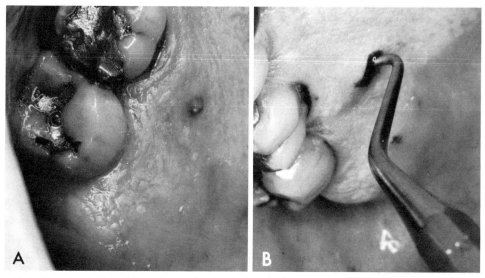

Figure 18–8 Pinpoint Orifice of Sinus from Palatal Periodontal Abscess. *A,* Pinpoint orifice on the palate indicative of sinus from periodontal abscess. *B,* Probe extends into abscess deep in the periodontium.

periodontal abscess *without any notable clinical lesion or radiographic changes.*

CHRONIC ABSCESS. The chronic periodontal abscess usually presents a sinus that opens onto the gingival mucosa somewhere along the length of the root. There may be a history of intermittent exudation (Fig. 18–7). The orifice of the sinus may appear as a difficult-to-detect pinpoint opening, which when probed reveals a sinus tract deep in the periodontium (Fig. 18–8). The sinus may be covered by a small, pink, beadlike mass of granulation tissue (Fig. 18–9).

The chronic periodontal abscess is usually asymptomatic. The patient may report episodes characterized by **dull gnawing pain, slight elevation of the tooth, and a desire to bite down and grind the tooth.** The chronic periodontal abscess

often undergoes acute exacerbations with all the associated symptoms.

Radiographic appearance

The typical radiographic appearance of the periodontal abscess is that of a discrete area of radiolucence along the lateral aspect of the root (Figs. 18–10 and 18–11). However, the radiographic picture is not always typical (Fig. 18–12) because of many variables such as:

1. The stage of the lesion. In the early stages the acute periodontal abscess is extremely painful but presents no radiographic changes.

2. The extent of bone destruction and the morphology of the bone.

3. The location of the abscess.

Figure 18–9 Granulation Tissue at the orifice of sinus from periodontal abscess.

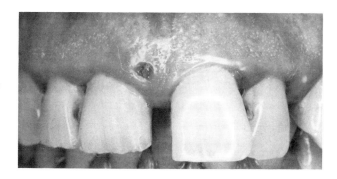

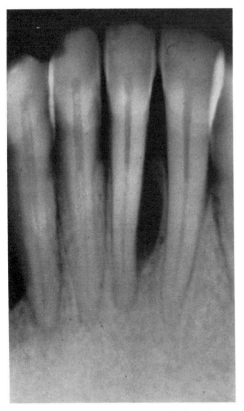

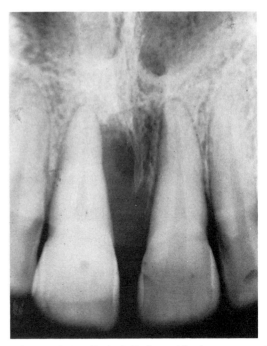

Figure 18–11 Typical Radiographic Appearance of Periodontal Abscess on Right Central Incisor.

Figure 18–10   Radiolucent Area on the lateral aspect of root with chronic periodontal abscess.

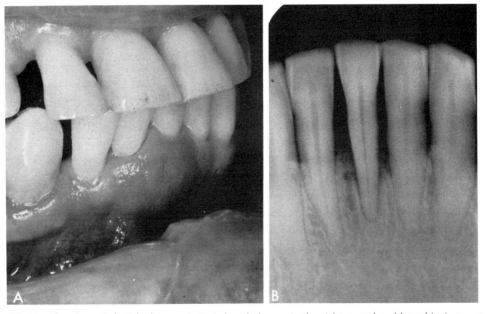

Figure 18–12   Chronic Periodontal Abscess. *A,* Periodontal abscess in the right central and lateral incisor area. *B,* Extensive bone destruction and thickening of the periodontal ligament space around the right central incisor.

Lesions in the soft tissue wall of a periodontal pocket are less likely to produce radiographic changes than those deep in the supporting tissues.

Abscesses on the facial or lingual surface are obscured by the radiopacity of the root; interproximal lesions are more likely to be visualized radiographically.

The radiograph alone cannot be relied upon for the diagnosis of a periodontal abscess.

Diagnosis

Diagnosis of the periodontal abscess requires correlation of the history and clinical and radiographic findings. **Continuity of the lesion with the gingival margin is clinical evidence of the presence of a periodontal abscess.** The suspected area should be probed carefully along the gingival margin in relation to each tooth surface for the presence of a channel from the marginal area to the deeper periodontal tissues. **The abscess is not necessarily located on the same surface of the root as the pocket from which it is formed.** A pocket on the facial or lingual surface may give rise to a periodontal abscess interproximally. It is common for a periodontal abscess to be localized on a root surface other than that along which the pocket originated because impairment of drainage is more likely to occur when a pocket follows a tortuous course.

Differential diagnosis between a periodontal and periapical abscess

The following are useful guides in the differential diagnosis between a *periodontal* and *periapical* abscess:

If the tooth is nonvital, the lesion is most likely periapical. In severe cases a periodontal abscess may extend to the apex and cause pulp involvement and necrosis. Except in such cases, however, periodontal abscesses do not cause devitalization of teeth.

An apical abscess may spread along the lateral aspect of the root to the gingival margin, but when the apex and lateral surface of a root are involved by a single lesion that can be probed directly from the gingival margin, it is more likely to have originated as a periodontal abscess.

Radiographic findings are helpful in differentiating between a periodontal and periapical lesion, but their usefulness is limited. Early acute periodontal and periapical abscesses present no radiographic changes. Ordinarily an area of radiolucence along the lateral surface of the root suggests the presence of a periodontal abscess, whereas apical rarefaction suggests a periapical abscess. **However, acute periodontal abscesses that show no radiographic changes frequently cause symptoms in teeth with long-standing radiographically detectable periapical lesions that are not contributing to the patient's complaint.** Clinical findings such as the presence of extensive caries, pocket formation, tooth vitality, and the existence of a continuity between the gingival margin and the abscess area, often prove to be of greater diagnostic value than radiographs.

A draining sinus on the lateral aspect of the root suggests periodontal rather than apical involvement, whereas a sinus from a periapical lesion is more likely to be located further apically. However, sinus location is not conclusive. In many instances, particularly in children, the sinus from a periapical lesion drains on the side of the root rather than at the apex.

The periodontal abscess and the gingival abscess

The principal differences between the periodontal abscess and the gingival abscess are location and history. (Described under Acute Inflammatory Gingival Enlargement, Chapter 10.) The gingival abscess is confined to the marginal gingiva, and it often occurs in previously disease-free areas. It is usually an acute inflammatory response to foreign material forced into the gingiva. In rare instances it results from infection of an epithelial-lined gingival cyst.[2] The periodontal abscess involves the supporting periodontal tissues and generally occurs in the course of chronic destructive periodontal disease.

The periodontal cyst

This is an uncommon lesion which produces localized destruction of the periodontal tissues along a lateral root surface, most often in the mandibular canine–

premolar area.[3] It is believed to be an odontogenic cyst caused by proliferation of the epithelial rests of Malassez, but the stimulus initiating the cellular activity is not understood. Other theories regarding its origin suggest that (a) it may be a lateral dentigerous cyst retained in the jaw after the tooth erupted, that (b) it may be caused by traumatic implantation of oral epithelium, or that (c) it may result from stimulation of the epithelial rests of the periodontal ligament by infection from a periodontal abscess or from the pulp through an accessory root canal. A periodontal cyst is usually asymptomatic and without grossly detectable changes, or it may present a localized tender swelling. Radiographically, when located interproximally it appears on the side of the root as a radiolucent area bordered by a radiopaque line, which cannot be differentiated from the radiographic appearance of a periodontal abscess.

REFERENCES

1. Cross, W. G.: Lateral periodontal cyst: Report of a case. J. Periodontol., 25:287, 1954.
2. Ritchey, B., and Orban, B.: Cysts of the gingiva. Oral Surg., 6:765, 1952.
3. Standish, S. N., and Shafer, W. G.: The lateral periodontal cyst. J. Periodontol., 29:27, 1958.

Chapter 19

Trauma from Occlusion

THE FUNCTIONAL COMPONENT IN PERIODONTAL HEALTH

Periodontal health depends upon a balance between an internal systemically controlled milieu that governs tissue metabolism and the external environment of the tooth, of which occlusion is an important component. To remain structurally and metabolically sound, the periodontal ligament and alveolar bone require the mechanical stimulation of occlusal forces.

The relationship of occlusion to periodontal health starts with the development of the tooth. When the crown of the tooth is completed, it is contained within a bony crypt in the jaw, protected from external environmental factors. As the tooth erupts into the oral cavity, it becomes confronted with an entirely new world. Pressure from the lips and the tongue, the cheeks, the child's fingers, the pacifier, and food is thrust upon it. To enable the crown to withstand such forces the root is built as the tooth erupts and the periodontium develops around the root to hold it in the jaw. **The periodontium is custom built to meet the functional demands of the tooth; support of the tooth is the only reason for its existence.**

Just as the tooth depends upon the periodontal tissues to keep it in the jaw, so do the periodontal tissues depend upon the functional activity of the tooth to remain healthy. When there is insufficient functional stimulation the periodontal tissues atrophy; when the tooth is extracted the periodontium disappears. **Occlusion is the lifeline of the periodontium.** In periodontal health, it provides the mechanical stimulation which marshals the complex biologic mechanisms responsible for the well-being of the periodontium.

PHYSIOLOGIC ADAPTIVE CAPACITY OF THE PERIODONTIUM TO OCCLUSAL FORCES

When there is an increased functional demand upon it, the periodontium tries to accommodate to the demand. The adaptive capacity varies in different persons and in the same person at different times. The effect of occlusal forces upon the periodontium is influenced by their **magnitude, direction, frequency, and duration.**

When the **magnitude of occlusal forces** is increased, the periodontium responds by a thickening and increase in the fibers in the periodontal ligament and increase in the density of alveolar bone.

Changing the **direction of occlusal forces** causes a reorientation of the stresses and strains within the periodontium.[23] The principal fibers of the periodontal ligament are arranged so that they can best accommodate occlusal forces in the long axis of the tooth. When *axial forces* are increased there is viscoelastic distortion of the periodontal ligament and ultimate compression of the periodontal fibers and resorption of bone in the apical areas. The fibers in relation to the remainder of the root are placed under tension, and new bone is formed.[63] **In designing dental restorations and prostheses, every effort is made to direct occlusal forces axially in order to benefit from the greater tolerance of the periodontium to forces in this direction.**[38]

Lateral or horizontal forces are ordinarily accommodated by bone resorption in areas of pressure and bone formation in areas of tension (Fig. 19–1). The most advantageous point of application of a lateral force is near the cervical line. As the point of application is moved coronally, the distance from the center of rotation or lever arms is lengthened and the force upon the periodontal ligament increases.[76]

Torques or rotational forces cause both tension and pressure which, under physiologic conditions, result in bone formation and bone resorption respectively.[64] Torques are the type of force most likely to injure the periodontium.

Duration and frequency affect the response of alveolar bone to occlusal forces.[46] Constant pressure on bone causes resorption, whereas intermittent force favors bone formation. The time lapse between pressure applications apparently influences the bone response. Recurrent forces over short intervals of time have essentially the same resorbing effect as constant pressure.

An inherent "margin of safety" common to all tissues permits some variation in occlusion without the periodontium being adversely affected. However, when occlusal forces exceed the adaptive capacity of the tissues, they are injured.[1, 7, 8, 14, 27, 35–37, 49, 51] **The injury is called trauma from occlusion.**

TRAUMA FROM OCCLUSION

Periodontal tissue injury caused by occlusal forces is called trauma from occlu-

sion.* **Trauma from occlusion is the tissue injury—not the occlusal force.** An occlusion which produces such injury is called a traumatic occlusion.[4] Excessive occlusal forces may also disrupt the function of the masticatory musculature and *cause painful spasms, injure the temporomandibular joints,* or *produce excessive tooth wear,* but the term "trauma from occlusion" is generally used in connection with injury in the periodontium.

Trauma from occlusion may be *acute* or *chronic. Acute trauma* from occlusion results from an abrupt change in occlusal force such as that produced by a restoration or prosthetic appliances which interfere with the occlusion or alter the direction of occlusal forces on the teeth. The results are pain, sensitivity to percussion, and increased tooth mobility. If the force is dissipated by a shift in the position of the tooth or by wearing away or correction of the restoration, the injury heals and the symptoms subside. Otherwise, periodontal injury may worsen and develop into necrosis with periodontal abscess formation, or it may persist as a chronic condition. Acute trauma can also produce cemental tears (see Chapter 3).

Chronic trauma from occlusion is more common than the acute form and is of greater clinical significance. It most often develops from gradual changes in the occlusion produced by tooth wear, drifting, and extrusion of teeth, combined with parafunctional habits such as bruxism and clenching, rather than as a sequel to acute periodontal trauma. The features of chronic trauma from occlusion and their significance are discussed below.

The causes of trauma from occlusion

Trauma from occlusion may be caused by (1) alterations in occlusal forces, (2) reduced capacity of the periodontium to withstand occlusal forces, or a combination of both.

The criterion which determines whether

---

*This term is used throughout the text to designate periodontal tissue injury produced by occlusal forces. It is also known as "traumatism" and "occlusal trauma."

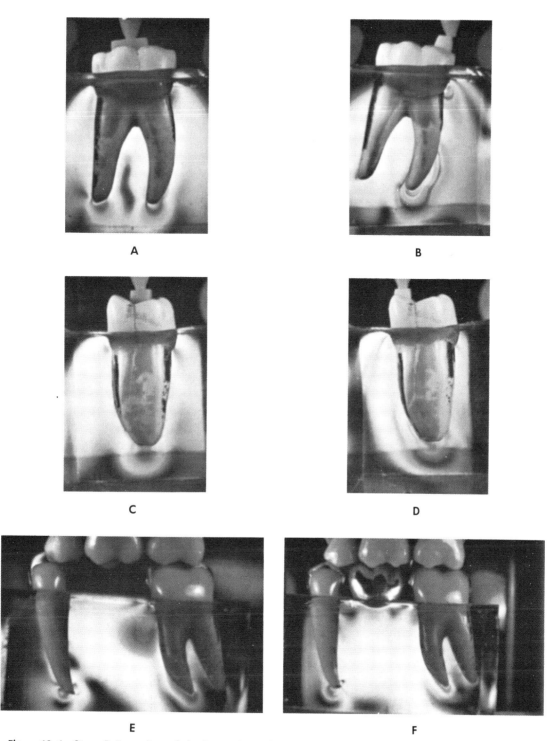

Figure 19–1 **Stress Patterns Around the Roots Changed by Shifting the Direction of Occlusal Forces (Experimental Model Using Photoelastic Analysis).** *A,* Buccal view of ivorine molar subjected to an **axial force.** The shaded fringes indicate that the internal stresses are at the root apices. *B,* Buccal view of ivorine molar subjected to a **mesial tilting force.** The shaded fringes indicate that the internal stresses are along the mesial surface and at the apex of the mesial root. *C,* Ivorine molar subjected to **axial force** viewed from the mesial proximal surface. The shaded fringes indicate that the stresses are concentrated at the apex. *D,* Ivorine molar subjected to **lingual tilting force** viewed from the mesial proximal surface. The shaded fringes indicate that the internal stresses are along the lingual surface and at the apex. *E,* **Stress patterns around the roots of teeth adjacent to an edentulous space.** Note particularly the stress fringes in the mesial cervical region of the molar. *F,* **Changes in stress patterns produced by inserting a fixed bridge.** Note the disappearance of the fringes in the cervical region of the molar (compare with *E.*)

277

an occlusion is traumatic is whether it produces injury, rather than how the teeth occlude. Any occlusion which produces periodontal injury is traumatic. Malocclusion is not necessary to produce trauma; it may occur when the occlusion appears "normal."[47] The dentition may be anatomically and esthetically acceptable, but functionally injurious. Conversely, not all malocclusions are necessarily injurious to the periodontium. Occlusal relationships which are traumatic are referred to by such terms as "occlusal disharmony," "functional imbalance," or "occlusal dystrophy." This is because of their effect upon the periodontium, not because of the position of the teeth. Since trauma from occlusion refers to the tissue injury rather than to the occlusion, an increased occlusal force is not traumatic if the periodontium can accommodate it.

Trauma from occlusion is sometimes described as being a *primary* or *secondary* factor in the etiology of periodontal destruction. Periodontal inflammation and trauma from occlusion so often occur together that it is difficult to determine which came first.

PRIMARY TRAUMA FROM OCCLUSION. Trauma from occlusion may be considered the primary etiologic factor in periodontal destruction if the only local alteration to which a tooth is subjected is one of occlusion. Examples are periodontal injury produced around teeth with a *previously healthy periodontium* (1) following insertion of a "high filling," (2) following insertion of a prosthetic replacement which creates excessive forces on abutment and antagonistic teeth, (3) following the drifting or extrusion of teeth into spaces created by unreplaced missing teeth, and (4) following the orthodontic movement of teeth into functionally unacceptable positions. Most of the studies made on experimental animals on the effect of trauma from occlusion have been on this primary type of trauma.

SECONDARY TRAUMA FROM OCCLUSION. Trauma from occlusion is considered a secondary cause of periodontal destruction when the adaptive capacity of the tissues to withstand occlusal forces is impaired. The periodontium becomes vulnerable to injury and previously well-tolerated occlusal forces become traumatic.

The following factors impair the capability of the periodontium to withstand occlusal forces: (1) Bone loss due to marginal inflammation. This will reduce the periodontal attachment area, increasing the burden upon the remaining tissues because there is less tissue to support the forces and because the leverage upon the remaining tissues is modified. This is the most common cause of secondary trauma and may be very difficult to solve. (2) Systemic disorders which inhibit the anabolic activity or induce degenerative changes in the peridontium.[29, 68]

Three stages of trauma from occlusion

Trauma from occlusion occurs in three stages.[12, 17] The first is injury, the second is repair, and the third is a change in the morphology of the periodontium. Tissue injury is produced by excessive occlusal forces. Nature attempts to repair the injury and restore the periodontium. This can occur if the force is diminished or the tooth drifts away from it. If, however, the offending force is chronic, the periodontium is remodeled to cushion its impact. The ligament is widened at the expense of the bone, angular bone defects occur without periodontal pockets, and the tooth becomes loose.

Stage I: Injury. The severity, location, and pattern of the tissue damage depend upon the severity, frequency, and direction of the injurious forces. *Slightly excessive pressure* stimulates resorption of the alveolar bone, with a resultant widening of the periodontal ligament space. *Slightly excessive tension* causes elongation of the periodontal ligament fibers and opposition of alveolar bone. In areas of increased pressure the blood vessels are numerous and reduced in size; in areas of increased tension they are enlarged.[81]

Greater pressure produces a gradation of changes in the periodontal ligament, starting with compression of the fibers, which produces areas of hyalinization,[57, 58] and subsequent injury to the fibroblasts and other connective tissue cells leading to necrosis of areas of the ligament.[60, 61] Vascular changes are also produced: within 30 minutes, retardation and stasis of blood

Figure 19–2   Periodontal Accommodation to Lateral Forces. *A,* Mandibular premolar. *B,* Lingual surface, showing new bone formation in response to tension on the periodontal ligament. Note the pale-staining osteoid bordered by osteoblasts and the incremental lines indicative of previous additions to the bone. *C,* Facial surface shows compression of the periodontal ligament and osteoclastic resorption of the bony plate. Note the new bone formed on the external surface. This is **Peripheral Buttressing Bone,** which reinforces the resorbing facial plate. Note, too, that the buttressing bone has produced a bulge in the bony contour.

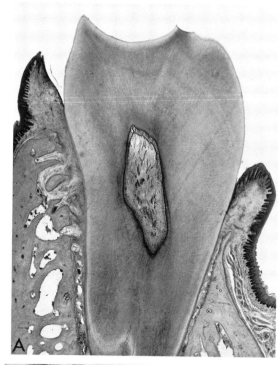

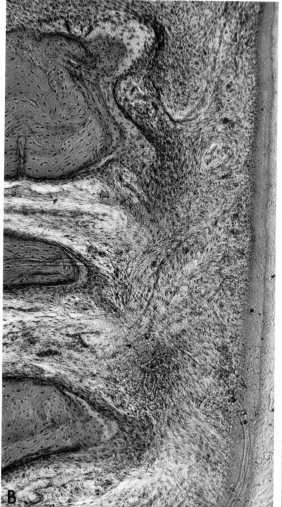

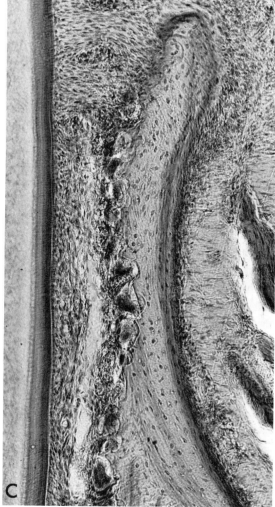

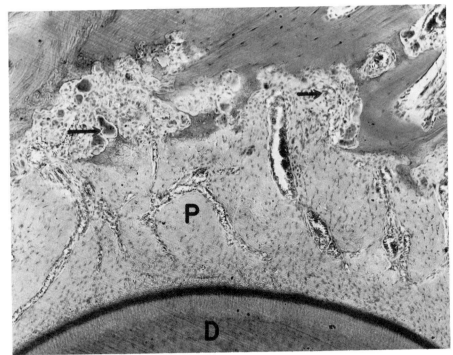

Figure 19–3 Trauma from Occlusion at Root Apex. Note bone resorption with prominent osteoclasts (*arrow*). The periodontal ligament (P) is widened as the result of bone resorption, and the blood vessels are engorged. The root is shown at D.

flow; at 2 to 3 hours, blood vessels appear packed with erythrocytes, which start to fragment; and between 1 and 7 days there is disintegration of the blood vessel walls and release of its contents into the surrounding tissue.[59] There is also excessive resorption of alveolar bone and, frequently, resorption of tooth surface[36, 41] (Fig. 19–2 and 19–3).

Severe tension causes widening of the periodontal ligament, thrombosis, hemorrhage, tearing of the periodontal ligament, and resorption of alveolar bone.

Pressure severe enough to force the root against bone causes necrosis of the periodontal ligament and bone. The bone is resorbed from viable periodontal ligament adjacent to the necrotic area and from the marrow spaces, a process called "undermining resorption."[33, 49]

The bifurcation and trifurcation are the areas of the periodontium most susceptible to injury from excessive occlusal forces.[30]

With injury to the periodontium there is a temporary depression in mitotic activity and in the rate of proliferation and differentiation of fibroblasts,[51] collagen, and bone formation,[36, 65, 70] which return to normal following dissipation of the force.

Stage II: Repair. Repair is constantly going on in the normal periodontium. In trauma from occlusion the injured tissues stimulate increased reparative activity. The damaged tissues are removed, and new connective tissue cells and fibers, bone, and cementum are formed in an attempt to restore the injured periodontium (Figs. 19–4 and 19–5). A force remains traumatic only so long as the damage it produces exceeds the reparative capacity of the tissues. Cartilage-like material sometimes develops in the periodontal ligament spaces as an aftermath of the trauma.[20] Formation of crystals from erythrocytes has also been shown.[62]

BUTTRESSING BONE FORMATION. When bone is resorbed by excessive occlusal forces, nature attempts to reinforce the thinned bone trabeculae with new bone (Fig. 19–6). This attempt to compensate for lost bone is called buttressing bone formation and is an important feature of

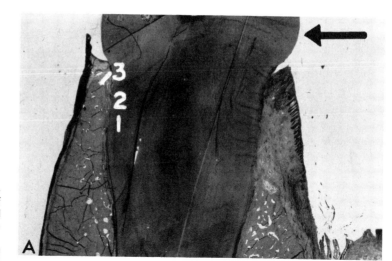

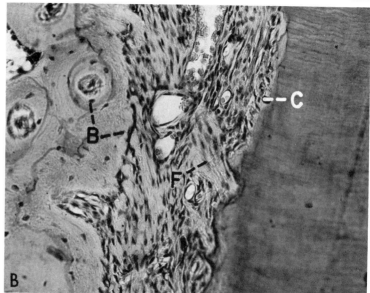

Figure 19–4 *A,* Faciolingual survey section of mandibular tooth of dog, subjected to **Excessive Lateral Force** *(arrow)* that injured periodontium in area marked 1,2,3.

B, **Reversibility of Trauma from Occlusion.** Healing in area marked 1,2,3, one month after cessation of force. There is new bone formation (B) in relation to the periodontal ligament and endosteal bone margins. Cementum (C) is being deposited along the eroded dentinal surface. Note the fibroblasts with collagen fibers (F) being embedded in the cementum and extending into the newly formed bone.

the reparative process associated with trauma from occlusion.[26] It also occurs when bone is destroyed by inflammation or osteolytic tumors.

Buttressing bone formation occurs within the jaw (central) and on the bone surface (peripheral). In central buttressing bone formation the endosteal cells deposit new bone, which restores the bone trabeculae and reduces the size of the marrow spaces (Fig. 19–6). Peripheral buttressing bone formation occurs on the facial and lingual surfaces of the alveolar plate. Depending upon its severity, it may produce a shelf-like thickening of the alveolar margin referred to as lipping (Figs. 19–2, 19–6, and 19–7) or a pronounced bulge in the contour of the facial and lingual bone[17, 26] (see Chapter 16).

Stage III: Adaptive Remodeling of the Periodontium. If the repair cannot keep pace with the destruction caused by the occlusion, the periodontium is remodeled in an effort to create a structural relationship in which the forces are no longer injurious to the tissues. To cushion the impact of the offending forces, the periodontal ligament is widened and the adjacent bone loss is absorbed.[24] The involved teeth become loose.[80] The results are a

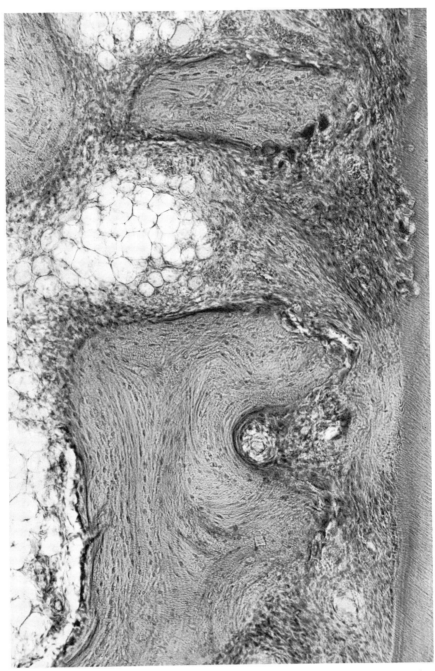

Figure 19–5 Trauma from Occlusion. Injury more severe than in Figure 19–3. The cementum (*right*) is undergoing resorption, the periodontal ligament is compressed and necrotic, and the bone is undergoing resorption. Note the osteoblasts and new bone (central buttressing bone formation) on the trabecular margins adjacent to the marrow.

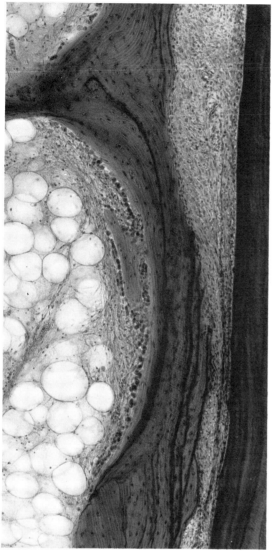

Figure 19–6 Central Buttressing Bone. New bone formation on the marrow side of alveolar bone which is undergoing resorption on the side of the periodontal ligament.

thickened periodontal ligament, funnel-shaped at the crest, and angular defects in the bone with no pocket formation. An increased vascularization has also been reported.[18]

The three stages described in the evolution of traumatic lesions have been shown histometrically by means of the relative amounts of periodontal bone surface undergoing resorption or formation.[11, 17] (Fig. 19–8). The injury phase shows an increase in areas of resorption and a decrease in

bone formation, while the repair phase demonstrates increased formation and decreased resorption. After adaptive remodelling of the periodontium, resorption and formation return to normal (Fig. 19–8).

Effects of insufficient occlusal force

Insufficient occlusal force may also be injurious to the supporting periodontal tissues.[13] Insufficient stimulation causes degeneration of the periodontium manifested by thinning of the periodontal ligament, atrophy of the fibers, osteoporosis of the alveolar bone, and reduction in bone height. Hypofunction results from an open bite relationship, absence of functional antagonists, or unilateral chewing habits that neglect one side of the mouth.

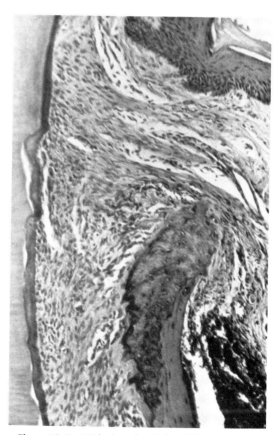

Figure 19–7 Widening of periodontal ligament space in cervical area and change in shape of margin alveolar bone as a result of chronic prolonged trauma from occlusion in rats.

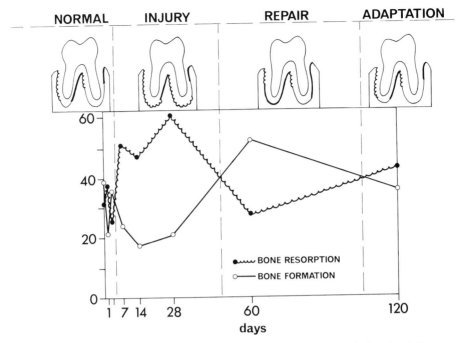

Figure 19–8 Evolution of traumatic lesions as depicted experimentally in rats by variations in relative amounts of areas of bone formation and bone resorption in periodontal bone surfaces. Horizontal axis: days after initiation of traumatic interference. Vertical axis: percentage of bone surface undergoing resorption or formation. The stages in the evolution of the lesions are represented in the top drawings, which show the average amount of bone activity for each group. See reference 17.

Trauma from occlusion is reversible

Trauma from occlusion is reversible. When trauma is artificially induced in experimental animals, the teeth move away or are intruded into the jaw. The impact of the artificially created force is relieved and the tissues undergo repair. The fact that trauma from occlusion is reversible under such conditions does not mean that it always corrects itself and therefore is temporary and of limited clinical significance. The injurious force must be relieved in order for repair to occur.[30, 54] If conditions in humans do not permit the teeth to escape from or adapt to excessive occlusal force, periodontal damage persists[14] until the excessive forces are corrected by the clinician. Traumatic forces that affect the teeth in balancing positions, i.e., nonaxial, often are such that severe lesions result because there is a tendency for teeth to be maintained in the position dictated by axial forces, i.e., intercuspal position. Axial forces are most important in determining tooth position.

The presence of inflammation in the area due to plaque accumulation may, however, impair the reversibility of traumatic lesions.[39, 54]

The effects of excessive occlusal forces on the dental pulp

The effects of excessive occlusal forces upon the dental pulp have not been established. Some clinicians report the disappearance of pulp symptoms following correction of occlusal forces. Pulp reactions have been noted in animals subjected to increased occlusal forces,[16, 78] but not when the forces were light and over short periods.[42]

THE ROLE OF TRAUMA FROM OCCLUSION IN THE ETIOLOGY OF PERIODONTAL DISEASE

Just as the occlusion is a critical environmental factor in the life of the healthy

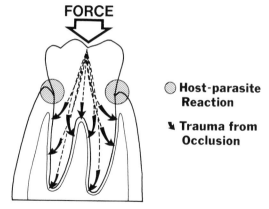

Figure 19–9   The reaction between dental plaque and the host takes place in the gingival sulcus region. Trauma from occlusion appears in the supporting tissues of the tooth.

The role of trauma from occlusion in gingivitis and periodontitis is best understood if the periodontium is considered as consisting of two zones (Figs. 19–9 and 19–10): the *zone of irritation* and the *zone of co-destruction.*

The zone of irritation

The zone of irritation consists of the marginal and interdental gingiva with its boundary formed by the gingival fibers (Fig. 19–10). This is where gingivitis and periodontal pockets start. They are caused by local irritation from plaque, bacteria, calculus, and food impaction. With few exceptions,[5, 74] researchers agree that trauma from occlusion does not cause gingivitis or periodontal pockets.[4, 31, 36, 55, 78, 80, 82]

The local irritants which start gingivitis and periodontal pockets affect the marginal gingiva, but trauma from occlusion occurs in the supporting tissues and does not affect the gingiva. The marginal gingiva is unaffected by trauma from occlusion because its blood supply is sufficient to maintain it even when the vessels of the periodontal ligament are obliterated by excessive occlusal forces.[32]

periodontium, its influence continues in periodontal disease. Inflammation in the periodontium cannot separate it from the influence of occlusion. Because occlusion is the constant monitor of the condition of the periodontium, it affects the response of the periodontium to inflammation and becomes a factor in all cases of periodontal disease.

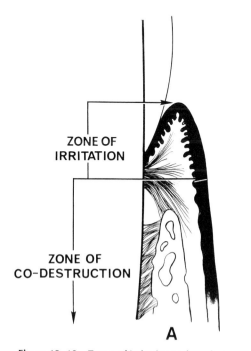

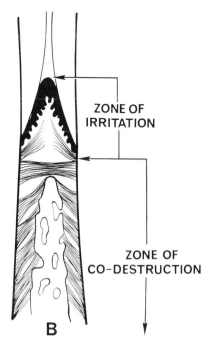

Figure 19–10   **Zones of Irritation and Co-destruction in Periodontal Disease.** *A,* Facial or lingual surface. *B,* Interproximal area.

So long as inflammation is confined to the gingiva it is not affected by occlusal forces.[40] When it extends from the gingiva into the supporting periodontal tissues (that is, when gingivitis becomes periodontitis), plaque-induced inflammation enters the zone of co-destruction.

The zone of co-destruction

The zone of co-destruction begins with the transseptal fibers interproximally and the alveolar crest fibers facially and lingually (Fig. 19–10). It consists of the supporting periodontal tissues, the periodontal ligament, alveolar bone, and cementum. When inflammation reaches the supporting periodontal tissues, the destruction it causes comes under the influence of the occlusion.

If occlusion is unfavorable, that is, if it is excessive or inadequate, it alters the environment of inflammation, produces periodontal injury, and becomes a co-destructive factor which affects the pattern and severity of tissue destruction in periodontal disease.[24]

Trauma from occlusion does not alter the inflammatory process but changes the tissue environment around the inflammatory exudate, leading to angular osseous defects and infrabony pocket formation.[3, 19, 27, 28, 43, 79] The mechanisms for this interaction of trauma and inflammation are as yet unclear, but the following have been proposed:

1. An alteration in the pathway of extension of gingival inflammation to the underlying tissue under the influence of trauma directing it to the periodontal ligament rather than to the bone. As a consequence, bone loss would be angular and the pocket could become infrabony[3, 22, 25, 27, 45] This explanation has been extensively investigated by Glickman and co-workers[22, 25, 27] but is disputed by others.[15, 52, 67, 69]

2. Excessive occlusal forces alter the alignment of the transseptal and alveolar crest fibers[3, 10] and the shape of the crestal bone.[17, 24, 52] These changes favor an angular type of bone loss.

3. Excessive occlusal forces produce periodontal ligament damage and bone resorption which aggravate tissue destruc-

tion caused by inflammation.[43] Fusion of plaque-induced inflammation with a traumatized periodontal ligament region may facilitate infrabony pocket development and increased rate of destruction.

4. Trauma-induced areas of root resorption uncovered by apical migration of the inflamed gingival attachment may offer a more favorable environment for the formation and attachment of uncalcified and calcified deposits and may be responsible for deeper lesions.[66]

There is considerable variability in the response of the periodontium to the combination of inflammation and trauma from occlusion. Inflammation from the gingiva may reach the periodontal ligament through vessel channels in the bone in the absence of trauma from occlusion;[2] the combination of tilting or excessive occlusal forces and inflammation does not necessarily lead to infrabony pockets,[15, 21, 67] and angular bone destruction may occur beneath suprabony pockets.[28]

The existence of a co-destructive relationship between inflammation and trauma from occlusion does not rule out the possibility that both may be present without the production of infrabony pockets and angular defects. The inflammation or the trauma may not be severe enough, or the anatomy of the tooth or bone may not be conducive to their formation. For example, if the facial or lingual bone is very thin, it may undergo resorption before an angular defect can develop. For similar reasons the absence of infrabony pockets and osseous defects does not rule out the presence of trauma from occlusion. Such periodontal lesions may be produced by etiologic factors other than the combination of inflammation and trauma from occlusion. In summary, not every infrabony pocket is due to a combination of trauma and inflammation, but this combination apparently increases the likelihood of a periodontal pocket becoming infrabony.

Changes produced by trauma from occlusion alone

In the absence of local irritants severe enough to produce periodontal pockets, trauma from occlusion may cause excessive loosening of teeth, widening of the periodontal ligament, and angular (vertical) defects in the alveolar bone without pockets.[17, 44]

The most common sign of trauma to the periodontium is *increased tooth mobility.* Tooth mobility produced by trauma occurs in two phases: the *initial phase* is due to alveolar bone resorption increasing the width of the periodontal ligament and reducing the number of periodontal fibers. The *second phase* occurs after repair of the traumatic lesion and adaptation to the increased forces resulting in permanent widening of the periodontal ligament space. See Chapter 20 for a more detailed description of tooth mobility.

Radiographic signs of trauma from occlusion

The radiographic signs of trauma from occlusion are shown in Figures 19–11 and 19–12. They include (1) widening of the periodontal space, often with thickening of the lamina dura in the following areas: along the lateral aspect of the root, in the apical region, and in bifurcation areas; (2) "vertical" rather than "horizontal" destruction of the interdental septum, with the formation of infrabony defects; (3) radiolucence and condensation of the alveolar bone; and (4) root resorption.

It should be understood that widening of the periodontal space and thickening of the lamina dura do not necessarily indicate destructive changes. They may result from thickening and strengthening of the periodontal ligament and alveolar bone, which constitute a favorable response to increased occlusal forces (Fig. 19–13) (see Chapter 32).

Other clinical changes attributed to trauma from occlusion

A wide variety of clinical changes has been attributed to trauma from occlusion,[48, 66, 72, 73] *based upon clinical impressions rather than substantiated evidence.* These are summarized as a matter of interest: Food impaction. Abnormal habits. Obscure facial pain. Erosion. Recession. Gingival bleeding. Cheek biting. Sensitivity of the occlusal and incisal surfaces. Chronic necrotizing ulcerative gingivitis. Hyperplasia of the gingiva. Pericementitis. Bruxism. Unilateral mastication. Limited excursion of the mandible (insufficient wear). Unlimited excursion of the mandible (excessive wear). Interproximal caries. Formation of subgingival calculus and gingivitis. Tendency toward epulis formation. Blanching of the gingiva upon the application of occlusal force. In the pulp: hyperemia resulting in hypersensitivity to cold; pulpitis; pulp necrosis; pulp stones.

Box[6] and Stillman[71] considered trauma to be the causative factor for the following incipient signs of periodontal disease:

Traumatic crescent, a crescent-shaped, bluish red zone of gingiva confined to about one sixth of the circumference of the root.

Congestion, ischemia, or hyperemia of the marginal gingiva.

Recession of the gingiva, which may be asymmetrical, associated with resorption of the alveolar crest.

Stillman's clefts, indentations in the gingival margin, generally on one side of the tooth. Two clefts frequently occur on the same tooth. Intermittent compressions of the periodontal ligament followed by abnormal flushing of the gingival capillaries and enlargment and engorgement of the gingival vessels were considered to be the mechanism responsible for the cleft.

McCall's festoons, discrete semilunar enlargement of the marginal gingiva.

Absence of stippling, interpreted as evidence of edema secondary to trauma.

Injection of the blood vessels in the marginal gingiva.

Sharply demarcated linear depressions in the alveolar mucosa, parallel to the long axis of the root and overlying the septal bone.

Distended veins in the oral mucosa.

It bears emphasis, however, that none of these changes has been conclusively shown to be associated with trauma to the periodontium.

SUMMARY

Trauma from occlusion is an important factor in periodontal disease. It is an integral part of the destructive process in

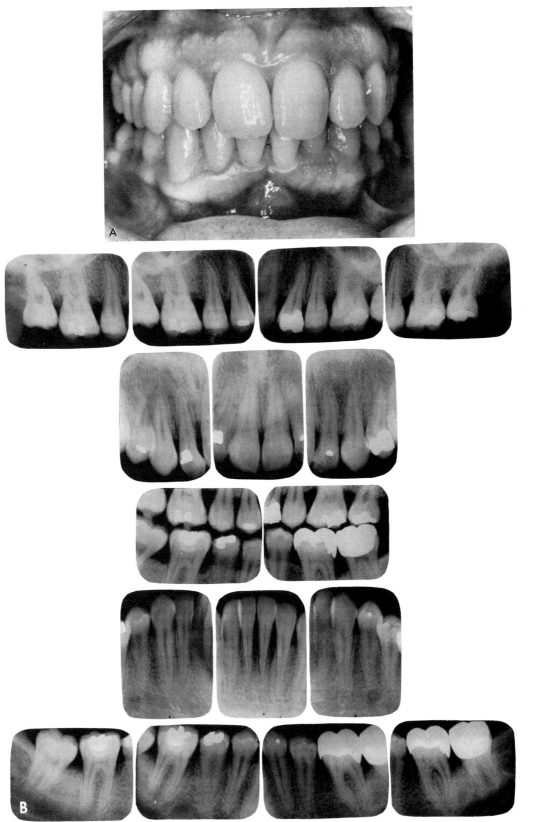

Figure 19–11   Radiographic Signs of Trauma from Occlusion. *A,* Twenty-seven year old female with only slight clinical evidence of periodontal disease. Little suggestion of the bone destruction shown radiographically. *B,* Radiographs show typical signs of trauma from occlusion: widening of the periodontal space in the mandibular anterior region, early angular bone destruction, and furcation involvement in the molar areas.

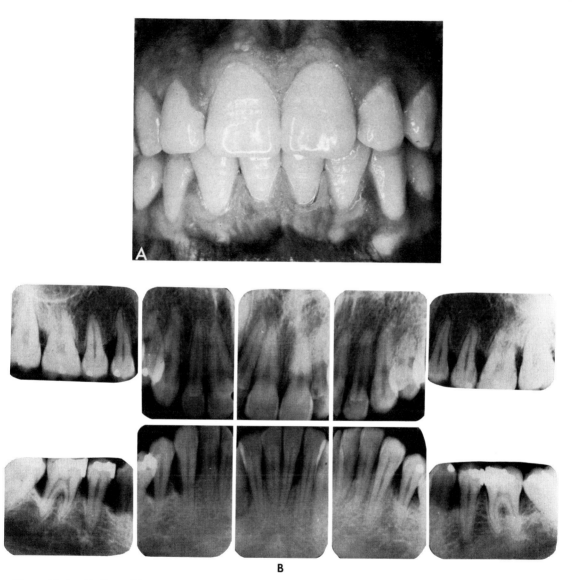

Figure 19–12 Radiographic Signs of Trauma from Occlusion. *A,* Thirty year old female with slight gingival disease. *B,* Radiographs show typical signs of trauma from occlusion: thickening of lamina dura, varied degrees of angular bone destruction, and furcation involvement.

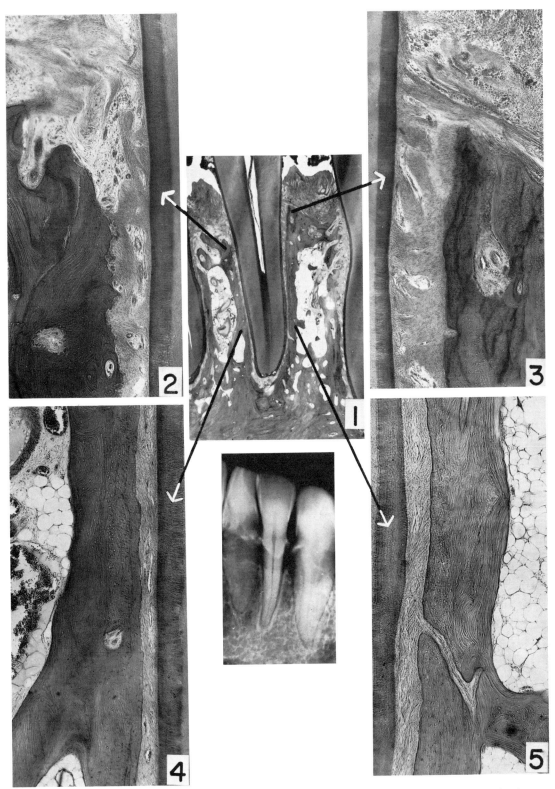

Figure 19–13   Widened Periodontal Space Produced by Two Types of Tissue Response to Increased Occlusal Forces. Radiograph shows thickening of periodontal space and lamina dura around the lateral incisor. *1,* Survey microscopic section of lateral incisor. *2,* Mesial surface-widening of the periodontal space has resulted from resorption of alveolar bone associated with pressure. *3,* Distal surface-widening of the periodontal space has resulted from thickening of the periodontal ligament which is a favorable response to increased tension. *4 and 5,* Thinned periodontal ligament at axis of rotation, one-third the distance from the apex.

periodontal disease. It does not start gingivitis or periodontal pockets, but it affects the progress and severity of periodontal pockets started by local irritation. Understanding its effect upon the periodontium is useful in the clinical management of periodontal problems.

REFERENCES

1. Adrion, W.: Structural changes in the paradontium in traumatic influence. Dtsch. Monatsschr. Stomatol., 3:97, 1933.
2. Akiyoshi, M., and Mori, K.: Marginal periodontitis: A histologic study of the incipient stage. J. Periodontol., 38:45, 1967.
3. Balbe, R., Carranza, F. A., and Erausquin, R.: Los paradencios del caso ocho. Rev. Odont. (Buenos Aires), 26:606, 1938.
4. Bhaskar, S. N., and Orban, B.: Experimental occlusal trauma. J. Periodontol., 26:270, 1955.
5. Box, H. K.: Experimental traumatogenic occlusion in sheep. Oral Health, 25:9, 1935.
6. Box, H. K.: Signs of incipient periodontal disease. J. Am. Dent. Assoc., 12:1150, 1925.
7. Box, H. K.: Traumatic occlusion and traumagenic occlusion. Oral Health, 20:642, 1930.
8. Box, H. K.: Twelve Periodontal Studies. Toronto, University of Toronto Press, 1940, p. 55.
9. Breitner, C.: Tissue changes caused by so-called bite-raising acting on the front teeth. Z. Stomatol., 30:1185, 1932.
10. Carranza, F. A., Jr., and Glickman, I.: Some observations on the microscopic features of the infrabony pocket. J. Periodontol., 28:33, 1957.
11. Carranza, F. A., Jr., and Cabrini, R. L.: Histometric studies of periodontal tissues. Periodontics, 5:308, 1967.
12. Carranza, F. A., Jr.: Histometric evaluation of periodontal pathology. J. Periodontol., 38:741, 1970.
13. Cohn, S. A.: Disuse atrophy of the periodontium in molar teeth of mice. J. Dent. Res., 40:707, 1961.
14. Coolidge, E. D.: Traumatic and functional injuries occurring in the supporting tissues on human teeth. J. Am. Dent. Assoc., 25:343, 1938.
15. Comar, M. D., Kollar, J. A., and Gargiulo, A. W.: Local irritation and occlusal trauma as co-factors in the periodontal disease process. J. Periodontol., 40:193, 1969.
16. Cooper, M. B., Landay, M. A., and Seltzer, S.: The effects of excessive occlusal forces on the Pulp. II. Heavier and longer term forces. J. Periodontol., 42:353, 1971.
17. Dotto, C. A., Carranza, F. A., Jr., and Itoiz, M. E.: Effectos mediatos del trauma experimental en ratas. Rev. Asoc. Odont. Argent., 54:48, 1966.
18. Dotto, C. A., Carranza, F. A., Jr., Cabrini, R. L., and Itoiz, M. E.: Vascular changes in experimental trauma from occlusion. J. Periodontol., 38:183, 1967.

19. Erausquin, R., and Carranza, F. A.: Primeros hallazgos paradentosicos. Rev. Odont. (Buenos Aires), 27:486, 1939.
20. Everett, F. G., and Bruckner, R. J.: Cartilage in the periodontal ligament space. J. Periodontol., 41:165, 1970.
21. Ewen, S. J., and Stahl, S. S.: The response of the periodontium to chronic gingival irritation and long term tilting forces in adult dogs. Oral Surg., 15:1426, 1962.
22. Glickman, I.: Occlusion and the periodontium. J. Dent. Res., 46 (Supplement 53), 1967.
23. Glickman, I., Roeber, F., Brion, M., and Pameijer, J.: Photoelastic analysis of internal stresses in the periodontium created by occlusal forces. J. Periodontol., 41:30, 1970.
24. Glickman, I., and Smulow, J. B.: Adaptive alterations in the periodontium of the Rhesus monkey in chronic trauma from occlusion. J. Periodontol., 39:101, 1968.
25. Glickman, I., and Smulow, J. B.: Alterations in the pathway of gingival inflammation into the underlying tissues induced by excessive occlusal forces. J. Periodontol., 33:7, 1962.
26. Glickman, I., and Smulow, J. B.: Buttressing bone formation in the periodontium. J. Periodontol., 36:365, 1965.
27. Glickman, I., and Smulow, J. B.: Effect of excessive occlusal forces upon the pathway of gingival inflammation in humans. J. Periodontol., 36:141, 1965.
28. Glickman, I., and Smulow, J. B.: The combined effects of inflammation and trauma from occlusion to periodontitis. Intern. Dent. J., 19:393, 1969.
29. Glickman, I., Smulow, J. B., and Moreau, J.: Effect of alloxan diabetes upon the periodontal response to excessive occlusal forces. J. Periodontol., 37:146, 1966.
30. Glickman, I., Stein, R. S., and Smulow, J. B.: The effects of increased functional forces upon the periodontium of splinted and nonsplinted teeth. J. Periodontol., 32:290, 1961.
31. Glickman, I., and Weiss, L.: Role of trauma from occlusion in initiation of periodontal pocket formation in experimental animals. J. Periodontol., 26:14, 1955.
32. Goldman, H.: Gingival vascular supply in induced occlusal traumatism. Oral Surg., 9:939, 1956.
33. Gottlieb, B., and Orban, B.: Changes in the Tissue Due to Excessive Force Upon the Teeth. Leipzig, G. Thieme, 1931.
34. Gottlieb, B., and Orban, B.: Tissue changes in experimental traumatic occlusion with special reference to age and constitution. J. Dent. Res., 11:505, 1931.
35. Grohs, R.: Changes in the human periodontal membrane due to overstress. Z. Stomatol., 29:386, 1931.
36. Itoiz, M. E., Carranza, F. A., Jr., and Cabrini, R. L.: Histologic and histometric study of experimental occlusal trauma in rats. J. Periodontol., 34:305, 1963.
37. Karolyi, M.: Beobachtungen uber Pyorrhea Alveolaris. Oest. Viertel Ischr. Z., 17:279, 1901.
38. Kemper, W. W., Johnson, J. F., and Van Huysen, G.: Periodontal tissue changes in response to

high artificial crowns. J. Pros. Dent., *20*:160, 1968.

39. Kantor, M., Polson, A. N., and Zander, H. A.: Alveolar bone regeneration after removal of inflammatory and traumatic factors. J. Periodontol., *46*:687, 1976.

40. Kenney, E. B.: A histopathologic study of incisal dysfunction and gingival inflammation in the Rhesus monkey. J. Periodontol., *42*:3, 1971.

41. Kvam, E.: Scanning electron microscopy of tissue changes on the pressure surface of human premolars following tooth movement. Scand. J. Dent. Res., *80*:357, 1972.

42. Landay, M. A., Nazimov, H., and Seltzer, S.: The effects of excessive occlusal forces on the pulp. J. Periodontol., *41*:3, 1970.

43. Lindhe, J., and Svanberg, G.: Influence of trauma from occlusion on progression of experimental periodontitis in the Beagle dog. J. Clin. Periodont., *1*:3, 1974.

44. Lindhe, J., and Ericsson, I.: The influence of trauma from occlusion on reduced but healthy periodontal tissues in dogs. J. Clin. Periodont., *3*:110, 1976.

45. Macapanpan, L. C., and Weinmann, J. P.: The influence of injury to the periodontal membrane on the spread of gingival inflammation. J. Dent. Res., *33*:263, 1954.

46. Mazzoni, J., Gonzales, V., Haskel, E., and Sales, G.: Effect of traumatic forces applied on the molars of the rat. Odont. Uruguaya, *20*:5, 1964.

47. McCall, J. O.: Traumatic occlusion. J. Am. Dent. Assoc., *26*:519, 1939.

48. Miller, S. C.: Textbook of Periodontia. 3rd ed. Philadelphia, Blakiston Co., 1950, p. 350.

49. Orban, B.: Tissue changes in traumatic occlusion. J. Am. Dent. Assoc., *15*:2090, 1928.

50. Orban, B.: Classification of periodontal diseases. Paradentologie, *3*:159, 1949.

51. Orban, B., and Weinmann, J.: Signs of traumatic occlusion in average human jaws. J. Dent. Res., *13*:216, 1933.

52. Polson, A. M.: Trauma and progression of marginal periodontitis in squirrel monkeys. II. Co-destructive factors of periodontitis and mechanically-produced injury. J. Periodontol. Res., *9*:108, 1974.

53. Polson, A. M., Meitner, S. W., and Zander, H. A.: Trauma and progression of marginal periodontitis in squirrel monkeys. III. Adaption of interproximal alveolar bone to repetitive injury. J. Periodont. Res., *11*:279, 1976.

54. Polson, A. M., Meitner, S. W., and Zander, H. A.: Trauma and progression of marginal periodontitis in squirrel monkeys. IV. Reversibility of bone loss due to trauma alone and trauma superimposed upon periodontitis. J. Periodontal Res., *11*:290, 1976.

55. Ramfjord, S. P., and Kohler, C. A.: Periodontal reaction to functional occlusal stress. J. Periodont., *30*:95, 1959.

56. Rothblatt, J. M., and Waldo, C. M.: Tissue response to tooth movement in normal and abnormal metabolic states. J. Dent. Res., *32*:678, 1953.

57. Rygh, P.: Ultrastructural changes in pressure zones of human periodontium incident to orthodontic tooth movement. Acta Odont. Scand., *31*:109, 1973.

58. Rygh, P.: Ultrastructural changes of the periodontal fibers and their attachment in rat molar periodontium incident to orthodontic tooth movement. Scand. J. Dent. Res., *81*:467, 1973.

59. Rygh, P.: Ultrastructural vascular changes in pressure zones of rat molar periodontium incident to orthodontic movement. Scand. J. Dent. Res., *80*:307, 1972.

60. Rygh, P.: Elimination of hyalinized periodontal tissues associated with orthodontic tooth movement. Scand. J. Dent. Res., *82*:57, 1974.

61. Rygh, P.: Ultrastructural cellular reactions in pressure zones of rat molar periodontium incident to orthodontic movement. Acta Odont. Scand., *30*:575, 1972.

62. Rygh, P., and Selvig, K. A.: Erythrocytic crystallization in rat molar periodontium incident to tooth movement. Scand. J. Dent. Res., *81*:62, 1973.

63. Schwarz, A. M.: Movement of teeth under traumatic stress. D. Items Intern., *52*:96, 1930.

64. Skillen, W. C., and Reitan, K.: Tissue changes following rotation of teeth in the dog. Angle Ortho., *10*:140, 1940.

65. Solt, C. W., and Glickman, I.: A histologic and radioautographic study of healing following wedging interdental injury in mice. J. Periodontol., *39*:249, 1968.

66. Sottosanti, J. S.: A possible relationship between occlusion, root resorption and the progression of periodontal disease. J. Western Soc. Periodont., *25*:69, 1977.

67. Stahl, S. S.: The responses of the periodontium to combined gingival inflammation and occluso-functional stresses in four human surgical specimens. Periodontics, *6*:14, 1968.

68. Stahl, S. S., Miller, S. C., and Goldsmith, E. D.: The effects of vertical occlusal trauma on the periodontium of protein deprived young adult rats. J. Periodontol., *28*:87, 1957.

69. Stahl, S. S.: Accomodation of the periodontium to occlusal trauma and inflammatory periodontal disease. Dent. Clin. North Am., *19*:531, 1975.

70. Stallard, R. E.: The effect of occlusal alterations on collagen formation within the periodontium. Periodontics, *2*:49, 1964.

71. Stillman, P. R.: Differential diagnosis of early periodontal lesions. Bull. Ont. Dent. Assoc., 1925.

72. Stillman, P. R.: Early clinical evidences of disease in the gingiva and periodontium. J. Dent. Res., *3*:25, 1921.

73. Stillman, P. R., and McCall, J. O.: Textbook of Clinical Periodontia. New York, Macmillan, Inc., 1937, p. 116.

74. Stones, H. H.: An experimental investigation into the association of traumatic occlusion with paradontal disease. Proc. Soc. Med., *31*:479, 1938.

75. Svanberg, G., and Lindhe, J.: Vascular reactions to the periodontal ligament incident to trauma from occlusion. J. Clin. Periodont., *1*:58, 1974.

76. Thurow, R. C.: The periodontal membrane in function. Angle Orthod., *15*:8, 1945.

77. Ubios, A. M.: Estudio Autorradiografico de la Reabsorcion Osea en los Movimientos Orto-doncicos de los Molares de Rata. Thesis, University of Buenos Aires, 1972.

78. Waerhaug, J.: Pathogenesis of pocket formation in traumatic occlusion. J. Periodontol., *26*: 107, 1955.

79. Waerhaug, J., and Hansen, E. R.: Periodontal changes incidental to prolonged occlusal overload in monkeys. Acta Odont. Scand., *24*:91, 1966.

80. Wentz, F. M., Jarabak, J., and Orban, B.: Experimental occlusal trauma imitating cuspal interferences. J. Periodontol., *29*:117, 1958.

81. Zaki, A. E., and Van Huysen, G.: Histology of the periodontium following tooth movement. J. Dent. Res., *42*:1373, 1963.

82. Zander, H. A., and Muhlemann, H. R.: The effect of stresses on the periodontal structures. Oral Surg., *9*:380, 1956.

Chapter 20

Pathologic Migration; Tooth Mobility

PATHOLOGIC MIGRATION

Pathologic migration refers to tooth movement that results when the balance among the factors which maintain physiologic tooth position is disturbed by periodontal disease. Pathologic migration is relatively common and may be an early sign of disease, or it may occur associated with gingival inflammation and pocket formation as the disease progresses.

Pathologic migration occurs most frequently in the anterior region, but posterior teeth may also be affected. The teeth move in any direction, usually accompanied by mobility and rotation. Pathologic migration in the occlusal or incisal direction is termed extrusion or elongation, the former term being preferred. All degrees of pathologic migration are encountered, and one or more teeth may be affected (Fig. 20–1). It is important to detect it in its early stages (Fig. 20–2) and to prevent

more serious involvement by eliminating the causative factors. Even in the early stage, some degree of bone loss has occurred.

Pathogenesis

Pathologic migration represents the cumulative effect of a combination of factors. The normal position of the teeth in the arch is maintained by an equilibrium between many factors, such as the health of the periodontal tissues, the forces of occlusion, presence of a full complement of teeth, tooth morphology and cuspal inclination, pressure from the lips, cheeks and tongue, the physiologic tendency toward mesial migration, the nature and location of contact point relationships, approximal, incisal and occlusal attrition, and the axial inclination of the teeth. Alterations in any of these factors start an interrelated sequence of changes in the environment of a single tooth or group of teeth that results in pathologic migration.

Pathologic migration occurs under the following conditions:

Inflammatory periodontal disease (periodontitis)

Pathologic migration consists of two components: (1) *destruction of tooth-supporting tissues by periodontal disease and* (2) *a force to move the weakened tooth.* Destruction of the periodontal tissues creates an imbalance between the tooth and the occlusal and muscular forces it is ordinarily called upon to bear. The weakened tooth is unable to maintain its normal position in the arch and moves away

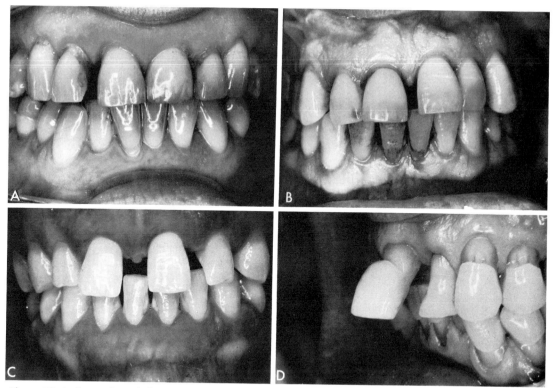

Figure 20–1 Stages in Pathologic Migration. *A,* Migration of right maxillary lateral incisor. *B,* Labial migration of maxillary central incisors and left canine, and mesial migration of right lateral. *C,* Migration and extrusion of maxillary and mandibular incisors. *D,* Severe migration of maxillary central incisor.

from the force, unless it is restrained by proximal contact. The force that moves the weakened tooth may be created by a variety of factors such as occlusal contacts, the tongue, or the food bolus.

It is important to understand that **the abnormality in pathologic migration rests with the weakened periodontium.** The force itself need not be abnormal. Forces that are acceptable to the intact periodon-

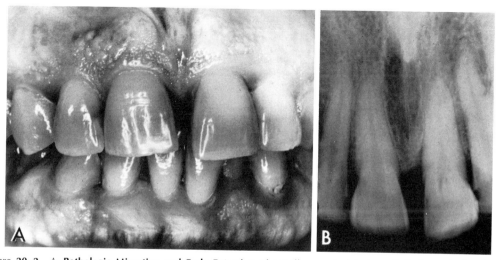

Figure 20–2 *A,* **Pathologic Migration and Early Extrusion** of maxillary central incisor. *B,* Radiograph showing bone loss on extruded central incisor.

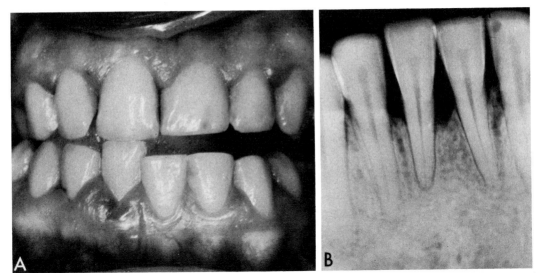

Figure 20–3 Pathologic Migration Aggravated by Excessive Occlusal Force. A, Mandibular central incisor extruded beyond the line of occlusion. Note that the maxillary central incisor is also extruded. B, Thickening of the periodontal ligament space around the central incisor, and angular bone destruction pattern typical of injury produced by excessive occlusal forces.

tium become injurious when periodontal support is reduced. An example of this is the tooth with abnormal proximal contacts. Abnormally located proximal contacts convert the normal anterior component of force to a wedging force, which forces the tooth occlusally or incisally. The wedging force, withstood by the intact periodontium, causes the tooth to extrude when the periodontal support is weakened by disease. **As its position changes, the tooth is subjected to abnormal occlusal forces which aggravate the destruction and the migration (Fig. 20–3).**

Pathologic migration may continue after a tooth no longer contacts its antagonist (Fig. 20–4). Pressure from the tongue, from the food bolus in mastication, and from proliferating granulation tissue provides the force.

Drifting following failure to replace missing teeth

Drifting of teeth often occurs into the spaces created by unreplaced missing teeth. **Drifting differs from pathologic migration in that it does not result from de-**

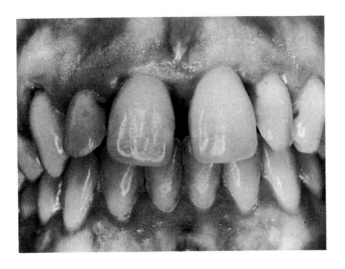

Figure 20–4 Pathologic migration continues despite absence of contact between mandibular and maxillary incisors.

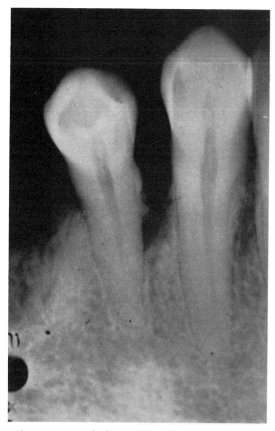

Figure 20–5 Calculus and Bone Loss on mesial surface of canine that has drifted distally.

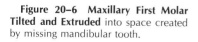

struction of the periodontal tissues. However, drifting usually creates conditions that lead to periodontal disease, so that the initial tooth movement becomes aggra-

vated by loss of periodontal support (Fig. 20–5).

Drifting generally occurs in a mesial direction, combined with tilting or extrusion beyond the occlusal plane. The premolars frequently drift distally (Figs. 20–6 and 20–7). Although drifting is a common sequel of unreplaced missing teeth, it does not always occur (Fig. 20–8).

FAILURE TO REPLACE FIRST MOLARS *The pattern of changes that may follow failure to replace missing first molars is characteristic.* In extreme cases it consists of the following:

1. Tilting of the second and third molars, resulting in a decrease in vertical dimension (Fig. 20–9).

2. The premolars move distally and the mandibular incisors tilt or drift lingually. The mandibular premolars, while drifting distally, lose their intercuspating relationship with the maxillary teeth and may tilt distally.

3. Anterior overbite is increased. The mandibular incisors strike the maxillary incisors near the gingiva or traumatize the gingiva.

4. The maxillary incisors are pushed labially and laterally (Fig. 20–10).

5. The anterior teeth extrude because the incisal apposition has largely disappeared.

6. Diastemata are created by the separation of the anterior teeth (Fig. 20–9).

The disturbed proximal contact relationships lead to food impaction, gingival inflammation, and pocket formation, fol-

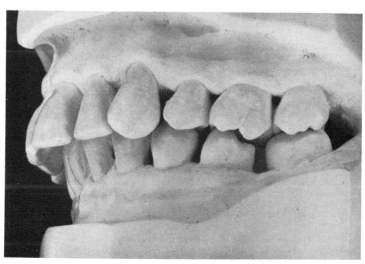

Figure 20–6 Maxillary First Molar Tilted and Extruded into space created by missing mandibular tooth.

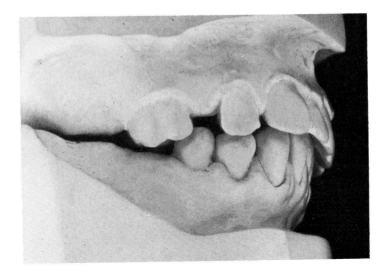

Figure 20–7   Distal Drifting of Maxillary and Mandibular Premolars. The maxillary molar is extruded and tilted.

lowed by bone loss and tooth mobility. Occlusal disharmonies created by the altered tooth positions traumatize the supporting tissues of the periodontium and aggravate the destruction caused by the inflammation. Reduction in periodontal support leads to further migration of the teeth and mutilation of the occlusion.

Idiopathic juvenile periodontitis (periodontosis)

Pathologic migration is an early sign of idiopathic juvenile periodontitis. The teeth are weakened by loss of periodontal support. The maxillary and mandibular anterior incisors drift labially, rotate and extrude, and create diastemata between the teeth (Fig. 20–11).

Trauma from occlusion

Trauma from occlusion may cause a shift in tooth position either by itself, or combined with inflammatory periodontal disease. The direction of movement depends upon the occlusal force.

Tongue pressure

Pressure from the tongue may cause drifting of the teeth in the absence of periodontal disease or contribute to patho-

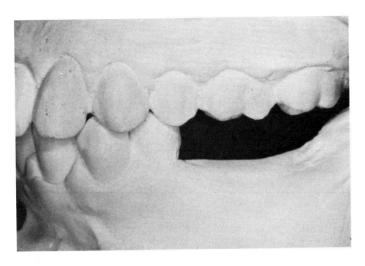

Figure 20–8   No Drifting or Extrusion despite four years' absence of mandibular teeth.

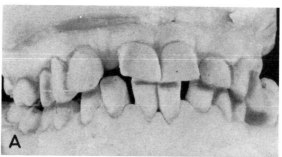

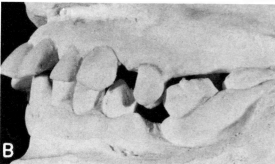
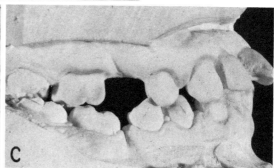

Figure 20–9 Mutilation of Occlusion Associated with Unreplaced Missing Teeth. Note pronounced pathologic migration, disturbed proximal contacts, and functional relationships with "closing of the bite."

logic migration of teeth with reduced periodontal support (Fig. 20–12).

Pressure from Chronic Inflammatory Granulation Tissue

In teeth weakened by periodontal destruction, pressure from the granulation tissue of periodontal pockets may contribute to pathologic migration. The teeth may return to their original positions after the pockets are eliminated, but, if there has been more destruction on one side of a tooth than the other, the healing tissues tend to pull in the direction of the lesser destruction.

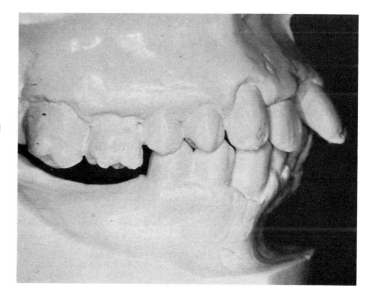

Figure 20–10 Maxillary Incisors Pushed Labially in Patient with bilateral unreplaced mandibular molars. Note extrusion of the maxillary molars.

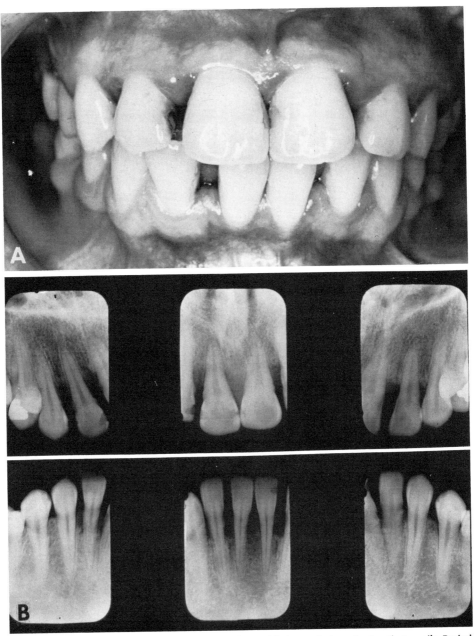

Figure 20–11 *A,* **Pathologic Migration** of maxillary and mandibular teeth in patient with **Juvenile Periodontitis.** *B,* Radiographs showing bone loss around the anterior teeth.

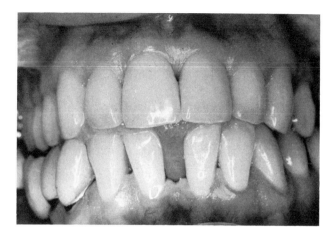

Figure 20–12 Pathologic Migration associated with tongue pressure.

Disturbance in the synchronism between active and passive eruption

Gottlieb[1] considered pathologic migration to be caused by a disturbance in the balance between active and passive eruption. It is produced when the teeth do not erupt at an even rate and some are worn down more by attrition than others. Teeth with least attrition must bear the entire biting force and are most susceptible to pathologic migration.

TOOTH MOBILITY

Normal Mobility

Teeth normally have a certain range of mobility,* single rooted teeth more than multirooted, and the incisors have the most. The mobility is principally in a horizontal direction; it also occurs axially but to a much lesser degree.[7] The range of physiologic tooth mobility varies among individuals and from hour to hour in individual teeth in the same person. It is highest upon arising, possibly because of slight extrusion in the absence of function during the night, and diminishes during the day, possibly from intrusion by pressure from chewing and swallowing. The 24-hour variations in tooth mobility are less in patients with a healthy periodontium and greater in patients with periodontal disease or occlusal habits such as bruxism and clenching.

Tooth mobility occurs in two stages: (1) **The initial or intrasocket stage,** in which the tooth moves within the confines of the periodontal ligament. This is associated with viscoelastic distortion of the ligament and redistribution of periodontal fluids, interbundle content, and fibers.[3] (2) **The secondary stage,** which occurs gradually and entails elastic deformation of the alveolar bone in response to increased horizontal forces.[5] The tooth itself is also deformed by the impact of a force applied to the crown, but not to a clinically significant degree.

Elastic recoil, slow recovery, and periodontal pulse[4]

When a force such as that normally applied to teeth in occlusion is discontinued, the teeth return to their original position in two stages; the first is an *immediate spring-like elastic recoil;* the second is a slow *asymptomatic recovery movement.* The recovery movement is pulsating and apparently associated with the normal pulsation of the periodontal vessels which occurs in synchrony with the cardiac cycle.

Abnormal (Pathologic) Mobility

Mobility beyond the physiologic range is termed abnormal or pathologic. It is

---

*For a comprehensive review of the subject of mobility, including an excellent bibliography, the reader is referred to the articles by H. R. Mühlemann[4] and by T. J. O'Leary.[6]

pathologic in the sense that it exceeds the limits of normal mobility values, rather than that the periodontium is necessarily diseased at the time of examination. Pathologic mobility is caused by one or more of the following factors:

1. **Loss of tooth support (bone loss).** The amount of mobility depends upon the severity and distribution of the tissue loss on individual root surfaces, the length and shape of the roots, and the root size compared to the crown. A tooth with short tapered roots is more likely to loosen than one with normal-sized or bulbous roots with the same amount of bone loss. Because bone loss is not the sole cause of tooth mobility and tooth mobility usually results from a combination of factors, the severity of tooth mobility does not necessarily correspond to the amount of bone loss.

2. **Trauma from occlusion.** Injury produced by excessive occlusal forces and incurred during abnormal occlusal habits such as bruxism and clenching which are aggravated by emotional stress is a common cause of tooth mobility. Mobility is also increased by hypofunction. Mobility produced by trauma from occlusion occurs initially as a result of resorption of the cortical layer of bone and later as an adaptation phenomenon resulting in a widened periodontal space.

3. **The extension of inflammation from the gingiva into the periodontal ligament results in degenerative changes which increase mobility.** The changes usually occur in periodontal disease which has advanced beyond the early stages, but tooth mobility is sometimes observed in severe gingivitis. The spread of inflammation from an acute periapical abscess produces a temporary increase in tooth mobility in the absence of periodontal disease.

Mobility is also temporarily increased for a short period after periodontal surgery.

4. **Tooth mobility is increased in pregnancy, and sometimes associated with the menstrual cycle or the use of hormonal contraceptives.** It occurs in patients with or without periodontal disease, presumably because of physicochemical changes in the periodontal tissues.

Mobility can also result from jaw processes that destroy the alveolar bone and/or the roots of the teeth. Osteomyelitis and tumors of the jaws belong in this category.

REFERENCES

1. Gottlieb, B.: Formation of the pocket; Diffuse atrophy of alveolar bone. J. Am. Dent. Assoc., *15*:462, 1928.
2. Hirschfeld, I.: The dynamic relationship between pathologically migrating teeth and inflammatory tissue in periodontal pockets: A clinical study. J. Periodontol., *4*:35, 1933.
3. Kurashima, K.: Viscoelastic properties of periodontal tissue. Bull. Tokyo Med. Dent. Univ., *12*: 240, 1965.
4. Mühlemann, H. R.: Tooth mobility: A review of clinical aspects and research findings. J. Periodontol., *38*:686, 1967.
5. Mühlemann, H. R., Savdir, S., and Rateitschak, K. H.: Tooth mobility—Its causes and significance. J. Periodontol., *36*:148, 1965.
6. O'Leary, T. J.: Tooth mobility. Dent. Clin. North Am., *13*:567, 1969.
7. Parfitt, G. J.: Measurement of the physiologic mobility of individual teeth in an axial direction. J. Dent. Res., *39*:608, 1960.

Chapter 21

Gingival and Periodontal Disease in Childhood

The terminal effects of periodontal disease observed in adults have their inception earlier in life. Gingival disease in childhood may progress to jeopardize the periodontium of the adult. The increasing awareness of the prevalence of gingival and periodontal disease in children,[56] coupled with the need for more information regarding the early stages of periodontal disease, have focused attention upon the periodontium in childhood.[8, 10, 56]

The developing dentition and certain systemic metabolic patterns are peculiar to childhood. There are also gingival and periodontal disturbances that occur more frequently in childhood and are, therefore, identified with this period. Consequently, some degree of coherence is provided by grouping the facts regarding gingival and periodontal problems in childhood in a separate chapter.

THE PERIODONTIUM OF THE DECIDUOUS DENTITION

The *gingiva* in the deciduous dentition is pale pink, firm, and either smooth or stippled (in 35 per cent of children in the 5-to-13 age group[51]) (Fig. 21–1). The interdental gingiva is broad faciolingually and tends to be relatively narrow mesiodistally in conformity with the contour of the approximal tooth surfaces. It is comparable to that of the adult in that it consists of a facial and lingual papilla with an intervening depression or *col*. The mean gingival sulcus depth for the primary dentition is 2.1 mm. ± 0.2 mm.[46]

Microscopically, the stratified squamous epithelium of the gingiva presents well-differentiated rete pegs with a parakeratinized (Fig. 21–2) or keratinized surface, the latter correlated with stippling. The connective tissue is predominantly fibrillar and is differentiated into papillary and reticular layers. The well-differentiated collagen bundles seen in the adult are not present in childhood.

The epithelium initially covering the col is a

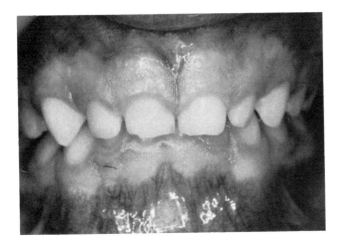

Figure 21-1 Deciduous Dentition with Stippled Gingiva.

few cells thick and nonkeratinized. The *periodontal ligament* of the deciduous teeth is wider than that of the permanent dentition. During eruption the principal fibers are parallel to the long axis of the teeth; the bundle arrangement seen in the adult dentition occurs when the teeth encounter their functional antagonists.

The *alveolar bone* in relation to the deciduous dentition shows a prominent lamina dura radiographically, in the crypt stage and during eruption. The trabeculae of the alveolar bone are fewer but thicker, and the marrow spaces tend to be larger than in the adult. The crests of the interdental septa are flat.[10]

PHYSIOLOGIC GINGIVAL CHANGES ASSOCIATED WITH TOOTH ERUPTION

During the transitional period in the development of the dentition, changes occur

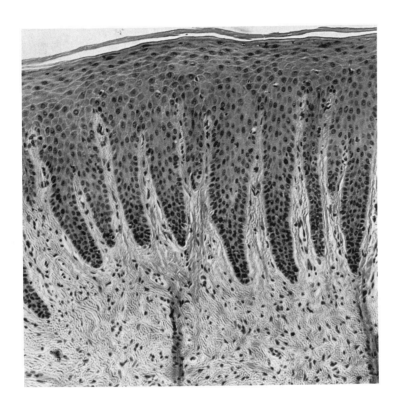

Figure 21-2 Normal Gingiva in a Four-Year-Old Patient Showing Stratified Squamous Epithelium with Rete Pegs and Surface Keratinization. The papillary arrangement of the underlying connective tissue can also be seen.

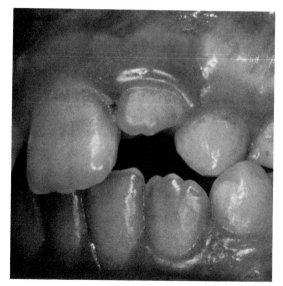

Figure 21–3   Gingivitis Associated with Tooth Eruption. Prominent rolled gingival margin which is slightly inflamed and edematous around erupting maxillary lateral incisor.

in the gingiva associated with eruption of the permanent teeth. It is important to recognize these physiologic changes and to differentiate them from gingival disease that often accompanies tooth eruption. The following are physiologic changes in the gingiva associated with tooth eruption:

Pre-eruption bulge

Before the crown appears in the oral cavity, the gingiva presents a bulge which is firm, may be slightly blanched, and conforms to the contour of the underlying crown.

Formation of the gingival margin

The marginal gingiva and sulcus develop as the crown penetrates the oral mucosa. In the course of eruption the gingival margin is usually edematous, rounded, and slightly reddened (Fig. 21–3).

Normal prominence of the gingival margin

During the period of the mixed dentition it is normal for the marginal gingiva around the permanent teeth to be quite prominent, particularly in the maxillary anterior region. At this stage in tooth eruption the gingiva is still attached to the crown, and it appears prominent when superimposed upon the bulk of the underlying enamel (Fig. 21–4).

GINGIVAL DISEASE

Chronic Marginal Gingivitis

This is the most prevalent type of gingival change in childhood. The gingiva presents all the changes in color, size, consistency, and surface texture characteristic of chronic inflammation. Fiery red surface discoloration is often superimposed upon underlying chronic changes.

ETIOLOGY.   In   children, as in adults, the most common cause of gingivitis is local irritation, as well as local conditions which lead to the accumulation of local

Figure 21–4   Prominent Marginal Gingiva on the cervical third of partially erupted maxillary anterior teeth.

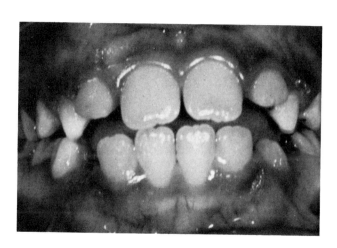

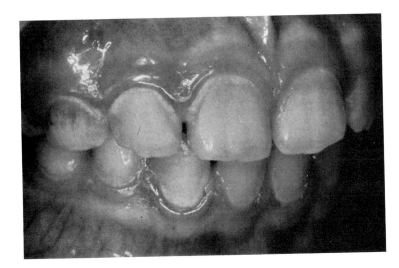

Figure 21–5 Chronic Marginal Gingivitis associated with plaque and materia alba.

irritants. In a study in preschool children the gingival response to bacterial plaque was found to be reduced.[33] Most gingivitis in children is caused by *poor oral hygiene, dental plaque,* and *materia alba* (Fig. 21–5). Dental plaque appears to form more rapidly in children (aged 8. to 12) than in adults.

Calculus. Calculus is uncommon in infants,[9] occurs in approximately 9 per cent of children between the ages of 4 and 6, 18 per cent at ages 7 to 9, and 33 to 43 per cent at ages 10 to 15.[21] In children with *cystic fibrosis,* calculus formation is more common (77 per cent at ages 7 to 9, 90 per cent at ages 10 to 15) and more severe, probably related to increased concentrations of phosphate, calcium, and protein in the saliva.[40]

Gingivitis Associated with Tooth Eruption. The frequency with which gingivitis occurs around erupting teeth has given rise to the term *eruption gingivitis.* However, tooth eruption per se does not cause gingivitis. The inflammation results from plaque accumulation around erupting teeth. The inflammatory changes accentuate the normal prominence of the gingival margin and create the impression of a marked gingival enlargement (Fig. 21–6).

Loose and Carious Teeth. Partially exfoliated loose deciduous teeth frequently cause gingivitis. The eroded margin of partially resorbed teeth favors plaque accumulation that causes gingival changes varying from slight discoloration and edema to abscess formation with suppuration. Other

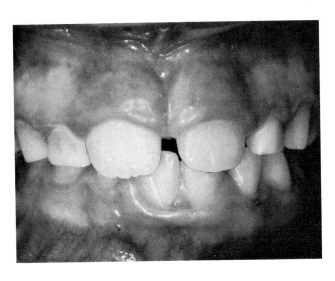

Figure 21–6 Developmental Gingival Enlargement caused by inflammation superimposed upon the normal prominence of the gingiva at this stage of tooth eruption.

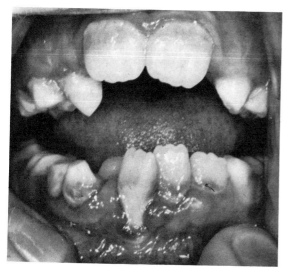

Figure 21–7   **Severe Gingivitis** associated with accumulation of plaque around malposed teeth.

ment, bluish red discoloration, ulceration (Fig. 21–7), and the formation of deep pockets from which pus can be expressed. Gingival health and contour are restored by correction of the malposition (Figs. 21–8 and 21–9), elimination of local irritants, and, when necessary, surgical removal of the enlarged gingiva.

Gingivitis is increased in children with *excessive overbite* and *overjet*, with *nasal obstruction*, and with *mouth breathing*.[50] *Pyogenic granulomas* and *peripheral giant cell reparative granulomas* occasionally occur in the gingiva.[5] (For a description of these lesions, see Chapter 10.)

Localized Gingival Recession

Gingival recession around individual teeth or groups of teeth is a common source of concern. The gingiva may be inflamed or free of disease, depending upon the presence or absence of local irritants. There are many causes of gingival recession (see Chapter 9), but in children the *position of the tooth in the arch* is the most important.[44] Gingival recession occurs on teeth in labial version (Fig. 21–10) or on those which are tilted or rotated so that the roots project labially. The recession may be a transitional phase in tooth eruption and may correct itself when the teeth attain proper alignment, or it may be necessary to realign the teeth orthodontically.

factors favoring plaque are food impaction and materia alba accumulation around teeth partially destroyed by caries. Children frequently develop *unilateral chewing habits* to avoid loose or carious teeth, aggravating the accumulation of plaque on the nonchewing side.

Malposed Teeth and Malocclusion. Gingivitis occurs more frequently and with greater severity around malposed teeth because of the increased tendency toward accumulation of plaque and materia alba. Severe changes include gingival enlarge-

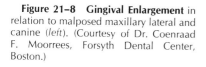

Figure 21–8   **Gingival Enlargement** in relation to malposed maxillary lateral and canine (*left*). (Courtesy of Dr. Coenraad F. Moorrees, Forsyth Dental Center, Boston.)

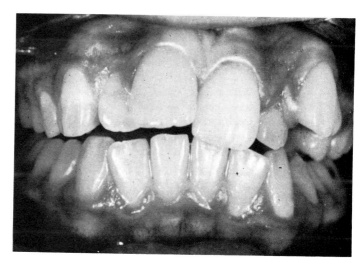

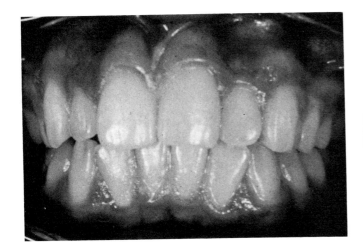

Figure 21–9 Disappearance of gingival enlargement shown in Figure 21–8 following orthodontic correction of the malposed teeth. (Courtesy of Dr. Coenraad F. Moorrees.)

Acute Gingival Infections

ACUTE HERPETIC GINGIVOSTOMATITIS. This is the most common type of acute gingival infection in childhood. It often occurs as a sequel to upper respiratory tract infection. (For a full discussion, see Chapter 11.)

CANDIDIASIS. This is a mycotic infection of the oral cavity caused by the fungus *Candida albicans,* and is most often *acute* (Fig. 21–11) but may be *chronic.* (For a full discussion, see Chapter 12.)

ACUTE NECROTIZING ULCERATIVE GINGIVITIS. The incidence of acute necrotizing ulcerative gingivitis in childhood is low. (For a full discussion, see Chapter 11.) In areas of chronic malnutrition and in children with Down's syndrome, the incidence and severity of acute necrotizing ulcerative gingivitis seems to increase.[28, 45] Acute herpetic gingivostomatitis, which is more common in childhood, is occasionally erroneously diagnosed as acute necrotizing ulcerative gingivitis.

TRAUMATIC CHANGES IN THE PERIODONTIUM

Traumatic changes may occur in the periodontal tissues of deciduous teeth under several conditions. In shedding deciduous teeth, resorption of teeth and bone weakens the periodontal support so that the existing functional forces are injurious to the remaining supporting tissues.[5] Excessive occlusal forces may be produced by malalignment, mutilation,

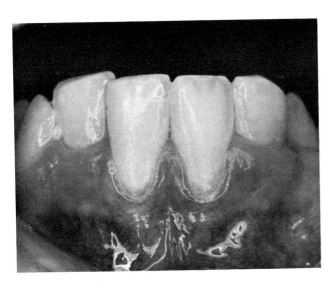

Figure 21–10 **Gingival Recession** on labially positioned mandibular central incisors.

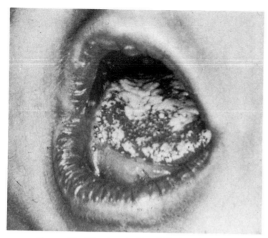

Figure 21–11   Acute Candidiasis (Thrush).

loss or extractions of teeth, or dental restorations. In the mixed dentition, the periodontium of the permanent teeth may be traumatized because they bear an increased occlusal load when the adjacent deciduous teeth are shed. The periodontal ligament of an erupting permanent tooth may be injured by occlusal forces transmitted through the deciduous tooth it is replacing.[25]

Microscopically,[2, 31, 41, 42] **the least severe traumatic changes consist of compression, ischemia, and hyalinization of the periodontal ligament. With severe injury there is crushing and necrosis of the periodontal ligament (See Chapter 19).**

In most instances the injuries are repaired and tooth loss does not result. However, such traumatized teeth may be sore or loose. Repair may result in *ankylosis* of the tooth to the bone, fixing the tooth in situ. When the permanent dentition erupts, ankylosed deciduous teeth appear to be *submerged.*

PERIODONTAL DISEASE

Periodontitis occurs occasionally in the deciduous dentition[26] and in 5 per cent of teenagers. There are also situations of severe rapid periodontal destruction and premature tooth loss in children and teenagers, the etiology of which is not well understood. These are infrequent; they are referred to as *juvenile periodontitis* and can

be classified as generalized or localized (idiopathic juvenile periodontitis or periodontosis).

Juvenile Periodontitis (Generalized Form)

This type of juvenile periodontitis attacks the whole dentition or a large part of it and is usually associated to systemic disturbances such as Papillon-Lefèvre syndrome, Down's syndrome, etc. In very rare cases it is unrelated to any detectable systemic disturbances. The latter cases have been considered a generalized form of periodontosis.[1] They present a severe periodontal destruction with some teeth completely denuded of bone (Figs. 21–12 and 21–13), accompanied by tooth mobility and pathologic migration. There is also generalized severe gingival inflammation with gingival enlargement and purulent pocket exudate. Medical history, examination, and laboratory tests are essentially negative, with no notable changes in other bones.

Other types of generalized juvenile periodontitis include the following:

Papillon-Lefèvre Syndrome. This is a syndrome characterized by hyperkeratotic skin lesions, severe destruction of the periodontium, and, in some cases, calcification of the dura.[1, 14, 23, 34, 43] The skin and periodontal changes usually appear together before the age of four. The skin lesions consist of

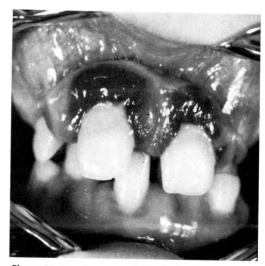

Figure 21–12   Pronounced Gingival Inflammation and pathologic migration in an eight-year-old patient. (Courtesy of Drs. P. Losch and C. Boyes, Children's Hospital, Boston.)

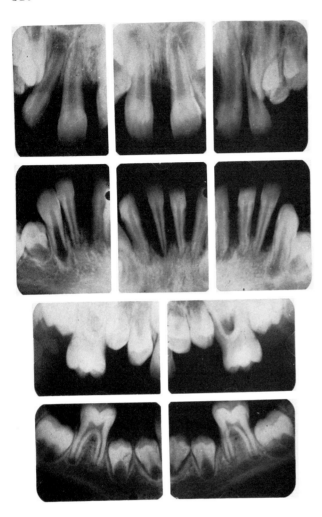

Figure 21–13 Radiographs of patient shown in Figure 21–12 showing pronounced generalized bone loss.

hyperkeratosis and ichthyosis of localized areas in palms, soles, knees, and elbows (Figs. 21–14 and 21–15).

Periodontal lesions consist of early inflammatory involvement leading to bone loss and exfoliation of teeth. Primary teeth are lost by five or six years of age. The permanent dentition then erupts normally, but within a few years the teeth are exfoliated due to destructive periodontal disease. By the age of 15 patients are usually edentulous except for the third molars. These are also lost a few years after they erupt.

The microscopic changes observed in one case[34] include marked chronic inflammation of the lateral wall of the pocket with active osteoclastic activity and apparent lack of osteoblastic activity; in the tooth studied, cementum was very thin or almost non-existent

except in the apical area where a comparatively wide area of cellular cementum was seen. Bacterial studies of plaque in a case of Papillon-Lefèvre syndrome revealed a flora

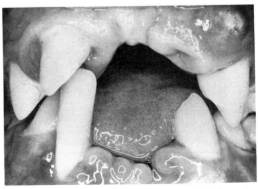

Figure 21–14 Dentition of a 17-year-old male patient with **Papillon-Lefèvre syndrome.** The missing teeth were exfoliated.

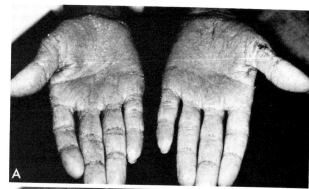

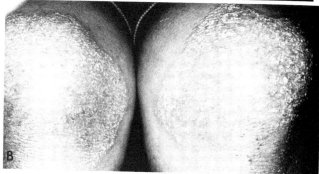

Figure 21–15   *A,* Palms and (*B*) knees of the same patient in Figure 21–14. Note the hyperkeratotic scaly lesions.

similar to that of periodontitis and not of periodontosis.[39]

The syndrome is inherited and appears to follow an autosomal recessive pattern.[24] Parents are not affected and both must carry the autosomal genes for the syndrome to appear in the offspring. It may occur in siblings; males and females are equally affected. The estimated frequency is one to four per million.[24]

Patients with skin lesions similar to those of Papillon-Lefèvre syndrome but no periodontal destruction are diagnosed as having Meleda's disease.[43]

Down's Syndrome* (synonyms: mongolism, trisomy 21). This is a congenital disease caused by a chromosomal abnormality and characterized by mental deficiency and growth retardation. The prevalence of periodontal disease in Down's syndrome is high, and although plaque, calculus, and periodontal pockets are present, the severity of periodontal destruction exceeds that explainable by local factors alone.[17, 29, 54]

Periodontal disease in Down's syndrome

---

*An excellent review on this subject has been done by Baer and Benjamin.[1]

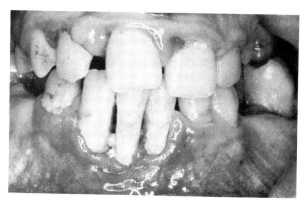

Figure 21–16   Down's syndrome patient, 14 years old, with severe periodontal destruction.

is characterized by formation of deep periodontal pockets associated with high plaque score and moderate gingivitis (Fig. 21–16). These findings are usually generalized, although they tend to be more severe in the lower anterior region; marked recession is sometimes also seen in this region, apparently associated with high frenum attachment. Acute necrotizing lesions are also a frequent finding.

No valid explanation has been offered for the increased prevalence and severity of periodontal destruction in children with Down's syndrome. The following have been mentioned: general physical deterioration of these patients at an early age,[3] reduced resistance to infections due to poor circulation especially in areas of terminal vascularization such as the gingival tissues,[19] or neurodystrophic processes.[17] Increased numbers of *Bacteroides melaninogenicus* have been reported in these children's mouths.[32]

Neutropenias. See Chapter 30.

Hypophosphatasia. This is a rare familial skeletal disease which in some cases results in loss of primary teeth, particularly the incisors. An association with abnormal alkaline phosphatase activity has been suggested but not proved.[1]

Eosinophilic Granuloma and Related Syndromes. This is a group of diseases characterized by proliferation of eosinophils and mononuclear cells that infiltrate the bone marrow and other tissues. Three entities are usually included in this group: (1) *Eosinophilic granuloma*, which is the most benign and presents unifocal bone lesions;[13, 49] (2) *Hand-Schüller-Christian disease*, which shows multifocal bone lesions and occurs mostly in young children; and (3) *Letterer-Siwe disease*, which is widespread to all major organs and occurs in babies and young children.

One of the initial manifestations, particularly of Hand-Schüller-Christian disease but also of the others, may be radiolucent lesions in the jaws and severe gingival inflammation with loss of bone leading to looseness and exfoliation of teeth.[12, 13, 48]

Congenital Heart Disease. Gingival disease and other oral symptoms may occur in children with congenital heart disease.[6, 30] In cases of *tetralogy of Fallot*, which is characterized by pulmonary stenosis, right ventricular enlargement, a defect in the interventricular septum, and malposition of the aorta to the right, the oral changes include purplish red discoloration of the lips and severe marginal gingivitis and periodontal destruction (Figs. 21–17 and 21–18). The tongue is coated, fissured, and edematous, and there is extreme reddening of the fungiform and filiform papillae. There is an increased number of subepithelial capillaries, which returns nearly to normal following cardiac surgery.[22]

In cases of *tetralogy of Eisenmenger* there is pulmonary insufficiency and a diastolic murmur; the lips, cheeks, and buccal mucous membranes are cyanotic but less markedly so than in the tetralogy of Fallot. Severe generalized marginal gingivitis is a common finding. In cases where there is *transposition of the aorta and superior vena cava vessels*, cyanotic discoloration and marginal gingivitis of a lesser degree are noted. In *coarctation of the aorta* there is a narrowing of the vessel in the region where it is joined by the ductus arteriosus. These

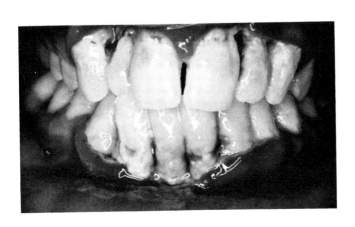

Figure 21–17 Extensive marginal inflammation with ulceronecrotic lesions and periodontal destruction in an adolescent with tetralogy of Fallot.

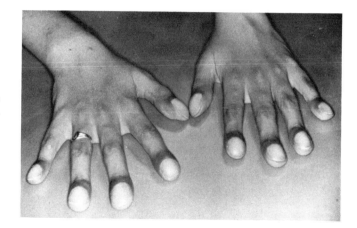

Figure 21–18 Characteristic clubbing of the fingers in the patient shown in Figure 21–17.

cases show marked inflammation of the gingiva in the anterior part of the mouth.

Diabetes. In childhood, uncontrolled diabetes may be accompanied by marked destruction of alveolar bone.[47] Although gingival inflammation is a frequent finding in such cases, the extent of alveolar bone loss is in excess of that generally seen in children with comparable gingival involvement.

Cerebral Palsy. Hypoplasia, attrition, malocclusion, and temporomandibular dysfunction are increased in cerebral palsy.[53] Because oral hygiene is a problem, the prevalence of periodontal disorders and caries may be high.

Erythroblastic Anemia (Cooley's Anemia). This is an inherited disorder characterized by a hemolytic anemia, spleno-

megaly, nucleated red blood cells in the peripheral blood, and generalized skeletal lesions.[16] Skeletal changes are absent or minimal during the first year of life. The osteoporosis characteristic of the disease occurs during early childhood and is followed by sclerosis. The most characteristic bony changes are noted in the metacarpals and femurs. Pneumatization of the paranasal sinuses is retarded.

Oral changes[16] include pallor and cyanosis of the mucous membrane and marked malocclusion owing to overgrowth of the alveolar ridge of the maxilla (Fig. 21–19). There is an associated spreading of the teeth with creation of large interproximal spaces. Radiographic examination reveals generalized rarefaction of the bones of the jaw with an alteration in trabecular pattern characterized by an irregularly arranged heterogenous lattice, with obliteration of the lamina dura in some areas (Fig. 21–20).

Acute and Subacute Leukemia. These diseases in children are accompanied by gingival changes (Fig. 21–21) (see Chapter 30).

Nutritional Deficiencies. Oral changes associated with deficiencies in components of the vitamin B complex and vitamin C (Fig. 21–22) sometimes occur secondary to gastrointestinal disorders. (Oral changes in vitamin deficiencies are described in Chapter 28.)

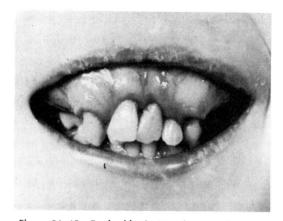

Figure 21–19 Erythroblastic Anemia. Note the prominence of the maxilla and pallor of the gingival mucosa. (Courtesy of Dr. M. M. Cohen and Dr. J. M. Baty, Floating Hospital, Boston.)

Localized form of juvenile periodontitis

This disease attacks only the first molar-incisor regions and is called idiopathic ju-

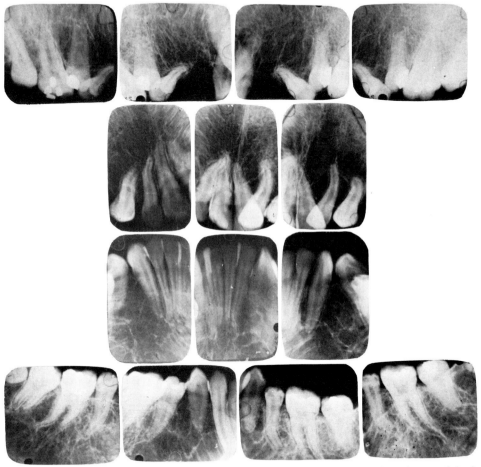

Figure 21–20   Radiographs of Patient with Erythroblastic Anemia. There is generalized rarefaction of the bone and enlarged irregularly arranged medullary spaces. (Courtesy Dr. M. M. Cohen and Dr. J. M. Baty.)

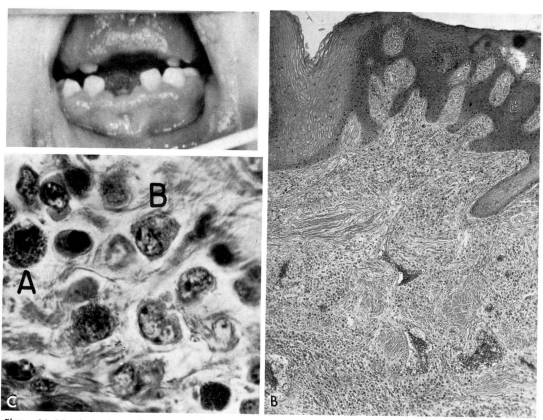

Figure 21–21 *A,* **Acute Myelogenous Leukemia,** showing diffuse gingival enlargement. *B* Section of gingival biopsy, showing dense leukocytic infiltration. *C,* Detailed study of myeloid cells in gingival biopsy. Myelocytes are shown at A and B.

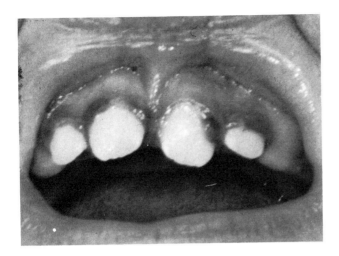

Figure 21–22 **Scorbutic Child** with discoloration and enlargement of the gingiva.

venile periodontitis or periodontosis. It is described in detail in Chapter 13.

THE ORAL MUCOUS MEMBRANE IN CHILDHOOD DISEASES

Certain childhood diseases present specific alterations in the oral cavity.[7, 27] Among these are the communicable diseases.

CHICKENPOX (VARICELLA). Successive papillary eruptions and vesicles appear on the buccal mucosa as well as on the face and remainder of the cutaneous body sur-

face (Fig. 21–23). On the buccal mucosa the vesicles break down to become small ulcerated craters with surrounding erythema resembling the lesions of acute herpetic stomatitis. Comparable but more extensive oral lesions are seen in *smallpox* (variola).

MEASLES (RUBEOLA). Koplik spots are pathognomonic of measles and are found in 97 per cent of patients. They are seen two to three days before the rash appears. They occur most often on the buccal mucosa opposite the first molars or on the inner aspect of the lower lip, and appear as bluish white specks — pinpoint in

Figure 21–23 **Chickenpox (Varicella).** *A,* Skin lesions. *B,* Vesicles on gingiva.

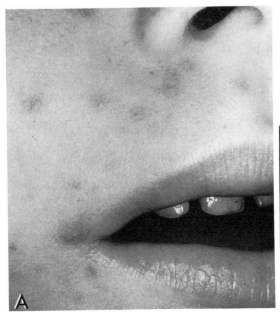

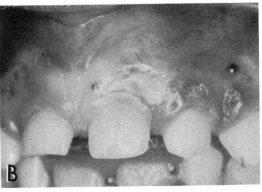

size—surrounded by a bright red areola. They are best seen in daylight. At first only a few are present, but later they become numerous and coalesce. In addition to these specific lesions, measles may also be accompanied by erythema and edema of the gingiva and remainder of the oral mucosa, and discrete bluish red discolored areas on the soft palate.

SCARLET FEVER (SCARLATINA). Diffuse fiery red discoloration of the oral mucosa occurs in scarlet fever. Characteristic tongue changes include (1) "raspberry tongue," a bright red, shiny discoloration with prominent papillae, and (2) "strawberry tongue," a coated surface covering an underlying bright red discoloration with prominent papillae.

DIPHTHERIA. Diphtheria is characterized by pseudomembrane formation in the oropharynx that appears as a gray, friable, curtain-like extension in the area of the anterior faucial pillars. Diffuse erythema of the oral mucous membrane with vesicle formation is also commonly seen in this condition.

REFERENCES

1. Baer, P. N., and Benjamin, S. D.: Periodontal disease in children and adolescents. Philadelphia, J. B. Lippincott Co., 1974.
2. Bauer, W.: Ueber traumatische Schadigungen des Zementmantels der Zahne mit einem Beitrag zu Biologie des Zementes. Dtsch. Monatschr. Zahnhk., 45:769, 1927.
3. Benda, C. E.: Mongolismo y cretinismo. 2nd. ed. Barcelona, Cientifica Medica, 1954.
4. Benjamin, S. D., and Baer, P. N.: Familial patterns of advanced alveolar bone loss in adolescence (periodontosis). Periodontics, 5:82, 1967.
5. Bernick, S., and Freedman, N.: Microscopic studies of the periodontium of the primary dentitions of monkeys. II. Posterior teeth during the mixed dentitional period. Oral Surg., 7:322, 1954.
6. Blitzer, B., Sznajder, N., and Carranza, F. A., Jr.: Hallazgos clinicos periodontales en niños con cardiopatias congenitas. Rev. Asoc. Odont. Argent., 63:169, 1975.
7. Blackstone, C. H.: A clinical and roentgenographic study of periodontic problems in children with systemic disease. J. Am. Dent. Assoc., 29:1664, 1942.
8. Bradley, R. E.: Periodontal lesions of children—Their recognition and treatment. D. Clin. North Am., Nov., 1961, p. 671.
9. Brauer, J. C.: Periodontal problems in the child patient. J. Periodontol., 11:7, 1940.
10. Brauer, J. C., Highley, L. B., Massler, M., and Schour, I.: Dentistry for children. 2nd ed. Philadelphia, The Blakiston Company, 1947.
11. Butler, J.: A familial pattern of juvenile periodontitis (periodontosis). J. Periodontol., 40:115, 1969.
12. Carraro, J. J., Sereday, M., and Sznajder, N.: Oral manifestations of histiocytosis X. J. Periodontol., 38:521, 1967.
13. Carraro, J. J., Sznajder, N., Barros R., and Martinez Lalis, R.: Periodontal involvement in eosinophilic granuloma. J. Periodontol., 43:427, 1972.
14. Carvel, R. I.: Palmar-plantar hyperkeratosis and premature periodontal destruction. J. Oral Med., 24:73, 1969.
15. Cohen, D. W., and Goldman, H. M.: Periodontal disease in children. P.D.M., July, 1962, p. 3.
16. Cohen, M. M., and Baty, J. M.: Oral manifestations of erythroblastic anemia. J. Am. Dent. Assoc., 32:1396, 1945.
17. Cohen, M. M., Winer, R. A., Schwartz, S., and Shklar, G.: Oral aspects of mongolism. Part I. Periodontal disease in mongolism. Oral Surg., 14:92, 1961.
18. Cooley, T. B., Witwer, E. R., and Lee, P.: Anemia in children with splenomegaly and peculiar changes in bones. Am. J. Dis. Child., 34:347, 1927.
19. Dow, R. S.: Preliminary study of periodontoclasia in mongolian children at Polk State School. Am. J. Ment. Defic., 55:535, 1951.
20. Eichel, R. A.: A Clinical Television Evaluation of Plaque Formation in Children. Internat. Assn. for Dent. Res. Program and Abstracts, 48th General Meeting, 1970, p. 171.
21. Everett, F. G., Tuchler, H., and Lu, K. H.: Occurrence of calculus in grade school children in Portland, Oregon. J. Periodontol., 34:54, 1963.
22. Forsslund, G.: Occurrence of subepithelial gingival blood vessels in patients with morbus caeruleus (tetralogy of Fallot). Acta Odont. Scand., 20:301, 1962.
23. Galanter, D. R., and Bradford, S.: Hyperkeratosis palmoplantaris and periodontosis: The Papillon-Lefèvre syndrome. J. Periodontol., 40:40, 1969.
24. Gorlin, R. J., Sedano, H., and Anderson, V. E.: The syndrome of palmar-plantar hyperkeratosis and premature periodontal destruction of the teeth. J. Pediatr., 65:895, 1964.
25. Grimmer, E. A.: Trauma in an erupting premolar. J. Dent. Res., 18:267, 1939.
26. Harndt, E.: Marginal periodontal disease in the deciduous dentition. A.R.P.A. Internat., 13:1, 1955.
27. Jacobs, M. H.: Oral lesions in childhood. Oral Surg., 9:871, 1956.
28. Jimenez, M., Ramos, J., Garrington, G., and Baer, P. N.: The familial occurrence of acute necrotizing gingivitis in Colombia. J. Periodontol., 40:414, 1969.
29. Johnson, N. P., and Young, M. A.: Periodontal disease in Mongols. J. Periodontol., 34:41, 1963.

30. Kaner, A., Losch, P., and Green, H.: Oral manifestations of congenital heart disease. J. Pediatr., 29:269, 1946.
31. Kronfeld, R., and Weinmann, J.: Traumatic changes in the periodontal tissues of deciduous teeth. J. Dent. Res., 19:441, 1940.
32. Loesche, W. J., Hockett, R. N., and Syed, S. A.: The predominant cultivable flora of tooth surface plaque removed from institutionalized subjects. Arch. Oral Biol., 17:1311, 1972.
33. Mackler, S. B., and Crawford, J. J.: Plaque development in the primary dentition. J. Periodontol., 44:18, 1973.
34. Martinez Lalis, R. R., Lopez Otero, R., and Carranza, F. A., Jr.: A case of Papillon-Lefèvre syndrome. Periodontics, 3:292, 1965.
35. McCombie, F., and Stothard, D.: Relationships between gingivitis and other dental conditions. J. Can. Dent. Assoc., 30:506, 1964.
36. McIntosh, W. G.: Gingival and periodontal disease in children. J. Can. Dent. Assoc., 20:12, 1954.
37. Miller, S. C., Wolf, A., and Seidler, B. B.: Generalized rapid alveolar atrophy. J. Dent. Res., 19:306, 1940.
38. Newman, M. G.: Periodontosis. J. Western Soc. Periodont./Periodont. Abs., 24:5, 1976.
39. Newman, M. G., Angel, I., Karge, H., Weiner, M., Grinenko, V., and Schusterman, L.: Bacterial studies of the Papillon-Lefèvre syndrome. J. Dent. Res., 56:545, 1977.
40. Notman, S., Mandel, I. D., and Mercadante, J.: Calculus in Normal Children and Children with Cystic Fibrosis. Intern. Assoc. for Dent. Res. Program and Abstracts, 48th General Meeting, 1970, p. 64.
41. Oppenheim, A.: Histologische Befunde beim Zahnwechsel. Z. Stomatol., 20:543, 1922.
42. Orban, B., and Weinmann, J.: Signs of traumatic occlusion in average human jaws. J. Dent. Res., 13:216, 1933.
43. Papillon, M. M., and Lefèvre, P.: Deux Cas de Keratodermie Palmaire et Plantaire Syme-trique Familiale (Maladie de Meleda) chez le Frere et la Soeur. Coexistance dans les Deux Cas d'Alterations Dentaires Graves. Soc. Franc. Derm. Syph., 31:82, 1924.
44. Parfitt, G. J., and Mjor, I. A.: A clinical evaluation of local gingival recession in children. J. Dent. Child., 31:257, 1964.
45. Pindborg, J. J., Bhat, M., Devanath, K. R., Narayana, H. R., and Ramachandra, S.: Occurrence of acute necrotizing gingivitis in South India children. J. Periodontol., 37:14, 1966.
46. Rosenblum, F. N.: Clinical study of the depth of the gingival sulcus in the primary dentition. J. Dent. Child., 5:289, 1966.
47. Rutledge, C. E.: Oral and roentgenographic aspects of the teeth and jaws of juvenile diabetics. J. Am. Dent. Assoc., 27:1740, 1940.
48. Sedano, H., Cernea, P., Hosxe, G., and Gorlin, R. J.: Histiocytosis X. Oral Surg., 27:760, 1969.
49. Shklar, G., Taylor, R., and Schwartz, S.: Oral lesions of eosinophilic granuloma. Oral Surg., 19:613, 1965.
50. Somjen, I.: Seltene Falle von Gingivitis. Korrespond. Zahnaerzt., 57:122, 1933.
51. Soni, N. N., Silberkweit, M., and Hayes, R. L.: Histological characteristics of stippling in children. J. Periodontol., 34:31, 1963.
52. Standish, S. M., and Shafer, W. G.: Gingival reparative granulomas in children. J. Oral Surg., 19:367, 1961.
53. Sznajder, N.: Oral diseases in cerebral palsy children. Rev. Asoc. Odont. Argent., 52:96, 1964.
54. Sznajder, N., Carraro, J. J., Otero, E., and Carranza, F. A., Jr.: Clinical periodontal findings in trisomy 21 (mongolism). J. Periodont. Res., 3:1, 1968.
55. Teuscher, G. W.: Systemic disease in children of interest to the dentist. D. Clin. North Am., July, 1958, p. 481.
56. Thomas, B. O. A.: The child patient as a future periodontal problem. J. Am. Dent. Assoc., 35:763, 1947.

Chapter 22

The Epidemiology of Gingival and Periodontal Disease

Epidemiologic surveys conducted throughout the world point to the universal distribution of gingival and periodontal disease.[31, 126, 128] From the earliest times, disease of the supporting structures of the teeth has been recognized in almost every culture. Paleontologic studies indicate that periodontal disease existed in early man as far back as 2000 B.C.[123, 166]

Progress in the study of the periodontal diseases has been retarded by several important features that do not exist in the study of dental caries. The pathology of dental caries involves hard calcified tis-sues, whereas periodontal disease involves both soft and hard tissues. Unlike dental caries, which has its greatest attack rate from the time the permanent teeth erupt in the mouth through and including the middle twenties, the greatest incidence and prevalence,* of destructive periodontal disease does not occur until later, at approximately 35 years of age. Periodontal disease does not lend itself easily to objective measurement because the signs of periodontal pathology involve color changes in the soft tissues, swelling, bleeding, and bone changes that are reflected in sulcus depth changes or pathologic pocket formation and loss of tooth function due to mobility. Therefore, the signs of dental caries lend themselves better to objective assessment than the pathologic parameters used to define periodontal disease.[39]

Dental epidemiology, by definition, is the study of the **pattern (distribution)** and **dynamics** of dental diseases in a population of people. **Pattern** implies that certain people are selected for attack by a disease and that the association between a disease and a people can be described by variables such as age, sex, racial-ethnic groups, occupation, social characteristics, place of residence, susceptibility, and exposure to specific agents. The term **dynamics** refers to a temporal pattern (distribution) and is concerned with trends, cyclic patterns, and the time that elapses between the exposure to inciting factors and the onset of the specific disease.[139] Russell's definition of

---

*Incidence is defined as the rate of occurrence of new disease in a population during a given period of time. Prevalence is the proportion of persons affected by a disease at a specific point in time, such as a cross-sectional survey.

dental epidemiology may provide a better overview: ". . . (It) is not so much the study of disease as a process as it is a study of the condition of the people in whom disease occurs."[124]

The **purposes or objectives** of epidemiology are to increase the understanding of the disease process, thereby leading to methods of control and prevention. In addition, it attempts to discover populations at high and low risk and to define the specific problem under investigation. The design, conduct, and interpretation of clinical trials of preventive and curative measures are also considered in its purview.[139] One of the most valuable techniques employed in dental epidemiology is the epidemiologic index.

Epidemiologic indices attempt to quantitate clinical conditions on a graduated scale, thereby permitting and facilitating comparison with other populations examined by the same criteria and methods. Unlike the absolute or definitive diagnosis it is possible to make on an individual patient, an epidemiologic index (i.e., numerical value) will estimate only the **relative** prevalence or occurrence of the clinical condition. In general, indices are actually *underestimates* of the true clinical condition. The **criteria** of a good epidemiologic index are that it must be easy to use, permit the examination of many people in a short period of time, define clinical conditions objectively, be highly reproducible in assessing a clinical condition when used by one or many examiners, be amenable to statistical analysis, and be strongly related numerically to the clinical stages of the specific disease under investigation. Calibration or standardization of the examiner(s) in reference to the use of the indices' criteria is imperative to ensure the reliability of the data.[124]

In general, there are two types of dental indices. The first type of index measures the **number or proportion** of people in a population with and without a specific condition at a specific point in time or interval of time. The second type of dental index measures the **number** of people affected **and the severity** of the specific condition at a specific time or interval of time.[124] More explicitly, this type of index

will not only help to identify the person in the population affected with a specific condition, but will also assess the condition under study on a graduated scale. Owing to the almost universal distribution of gingival or periodontal disease, those of the latter type can provide more meaningful information.

INDICES USED TO STUDY PERIODONTAL PROBLEMS

Although there are many indices for recording and quantitating the many entities included under the term periodontal disease, space limitations permit only the inclusion of indices that historically contributed to our understanding of periodontal diseases or those indices that are currently in frequent use. An excellent comprehensive review of indices not covered in this chapter is available in two symposia publications.[23, 25]

The indices that will be discussed in this chapter can, for the purpose of convenience and reason, be divided into those that evaluate:

a. The degree of inflammation of the gingival tissues.

b. The degree of periodontal destruction.

c. The amount of plaque accumulated.

d. The amount of calculus present.

Indices Used to Assess Gingival Inflammation

P.M.A. index (Schour and Massler[142])

Originally the P.M.A. Index consisted of counting the number of gingival units affected with gingivitis.[141, 142] This approach was predicated on the belief that the number of units affected would convey the degree or severity of gingival inflammation. The facial surface of gingiva around a tooth was divided into three gingival scoring units: the mesial dental papilla (P), the gingival margin (M), and the attached gingiva (A). The presence or absence of inflammation on each gingival unit was recorded as

1 or 0, respectively. The P, M, and A numerical values are totaled separately, added together, and expressed numerically as the P.M.A. Index **score per person.** Although all of the facial tissues surrounding all of the teeth could be assessed in this manner, usually only the maxillary and mandibular incisors, canines, and premolars were examined. The developers of this index eventually added a severity component in assessing gingivitis so that the papillary units (P) were scored on a scale of 0 to 5 and the marginal (M) and attached gingiva (A) were scored on a scale of 0 to 3.[81] The value of this index lies in its broad application to epidemiologic surveys and clinical trials as well as to individual patients. The criteria and approach for assessing gingival inflammation developed by Schour and Massler[142] has served as the basis for many of the indices to be discussed.

Some indices that are based on modifications of the P.M.A. Index were developed by Mühlemann and Mazor,[97] Lobene,[73] and Suomi and Barbano.[155] Mühlemann et al.[97] assessed the prevalence and severity of gingivitis on only the gingival and papillary units surrounding each tooth. The areas were scored on a scale of 0 to 4, using light probing to determine the extent of bleeding.

Examining only the papilla and gingival margin of the facial and lingual surfaces surrounding each tooth (i.e., six scoring units per tooth), Lobene [73] assessed the presence of gingivitis on a scale 0 to 3. Suomi et al.[155] assessed the presence and severity of gingivitis on each papilla and gingival margin of all the teeth on a scale of 0 to 2. When this criterion was applied only to the entire facial and lingual surface of eight selected teeth (teeth numbered 3, 8, 12, 14, 19, 24, 28, and 30), it became known as the Dental Health Center Index (DHCI)[152] after the center where it was developed.

Periodontal index (Russell[134])

The Periodontal Index (PI) was intended to estimate deeper periodontal disease than the P.M.A. Index by measuring the presence or absence of gingival inflammation, its severity, pocket formation, and loss of masticatory function. The criteria appearing in Table 22–1 are used to examine all of the gingival tissues surrounding each tooth (i.e., all of the tissue surrounding a tooth is considered a scoring or gingival unit). Because it measures both reversible and irreversible aspects of periodontal disease, it illustrates an epidemiologic index with a true biologic gradient.[124] A PI **score per individual** is determined by summing all of the tooth scores and dividing by the number of teeth examined.

Since only a mouth mirror and no calibrated probe or radiographs are used when performing the Periodontal Index examination, the results tend to underestimate the true level of periodontal disease in a population. The index was developed for use in epidemiologic surveys, but with care it may be used in clinical trials. The abstractness of the numerical score, an often-stated criticism concerning epidemiologic indices, is minimized in the PI because group scores may be associated with clinical conditions of periodontal disease (Table 22–1).[130]

The significance of the Periodontal Index lies in the fact that more data have been assembled using this index than any other index of periodontal disease. As a result, much of what we know about the distribution of periodontal disease in the United States and throughout the world resulted from using this index. It is also used in the National Health Survey,[63] the largest ongoing health survey in the United States.

Gingivitis component of the periodontal disease index (Ramfjord[119])

The Periodontal Disease Index (PDI) is used to measure the presence and severity of periodontal disease. It does so by combining the assessments of gingivitis and gingival sulcus depth, on six selected teeth (Nos. 3, 9, 12, 19, 25, and 28). Calculus and plaque are also examined to assist in formulating a more comprehensive assessment of periodontal status. Only gingivitis will be discussed in this section. Other components will be described in following sections of this chapter.

The tissue circumscribing each of the six

TABLE 22-1 THE PERIODONTAL INDEX (RUSSELL)[134]

Score	Criteria and Scoring for Field Studies	Additional X-ray Criteria Followed in the Clinical Test
0	NEGATIVE. There is neither overt inflammation in the investing tissues nor loss of function due to destruction of supporting tissues.	Radiographic appearance is essentially normal.
1	MILD GINGIVITIS. There is an overt area of inflammation in the free gingivae, but this area does not circumscribe the tooth.	
2	GINGIVITIS. Inflammation completely circumscribes the tooth, but there is no apparent break in the epithelial attachment.	
4	(Used when radiographs are available.)	There is early, notchlike resorption of the alveolar crest.
6	GINGIVITIS WITH POCKET FORMATION. The epithelial attachment has been broken and there is a pocket (not merely a deepened gingival crevice due to swelling in free gingivae). There is no interference with normal masticatory function, the tooth is firm and has not drifted.	There is horizontal bone loss involving the entire alveolar crest, up to half of the length of the tooth root.
8	ADVANCED DESTRUCTION WITH LOSS of MASTICATORY FUNCTION. The tooth may be loose; may have drifted; may sound dull on percussion with a metallic instrument; may be depressible in its socket.	There is advanced bone loss, involving more than one-half of the length of the tooth root, or a definite infrabony pocket with widening of the periodontal ligament. There may be root resorption, or rarefaction at the apex.

RULE: When in doubt, assign the lesser scores.

$$\text{Periodontal Index Score per Person} = \frac{\text{Sum of individual scores}}{\text{Number of teeth present}}$$

Clinical Condition	Group PI Scores*	Stage of Disease
Clinically normal supportive tissues	0 to 0.2	
Simple gingivitis	0.3 to 0.9	Reversible
Beginning destructive periodontal disease	0.7 to 1.9	
Established destructive periodontal disease	1.6 to 5.0	Irreversible
Terminal disease	3.8 to 8.0	

*130

selected teeth is assessed using the criteria described in Table 22–2. The six index teeth have been tested as reliable indicators of the various regions of the mouth. A numerical score for the **gingival status** of the PDI is obtained by summing all of the gingival units and dividing by the number of teeth present (i.e., Gingivitis Index score per person).[120] The Index has been used in epidemiologic surveys, longitudinal studies of periodontal disease, and clinical trials of therapeutic or preventive procedures. It is considered to be the gingival index of choice in longitudinal studies of periodontal disease.[49]

Gingival index (Löe and Silness[75])

The Gingival Index (GI) was developed solely for the purpose of assessing the severity of gingivitis and its location in four possible areas. The tissues surrounding each tooth are divided into four gingival scoring units: distal-facial papilla, facial margin, mesial-facial papilla, and the entire lingual gingival margin. Unlike the facial surfaces, the lingual surface is not subdivided in an effort to minimize examiner variability in scoring, since it will most likely be viewed indirectly with a

TABLE 22–2 CRITERIA FOR SEVERAL COMPONENTS OF THE PERIODONTAL DISEASE INDEX (RAMFJORD)[119]

Gingival Status (Gingivitis Index)
0 = Absence of signs of inflammation.
1 = Mild to moderate inflammatory gingival changes, not extending around the tooth.
2 = Mild to moderately severe gingivitis extending all around the tooth.
3 = Severe gingivitis characterized by marked redness, swelling, tendency to bleed, and ulceration.[120]

Sulcular Measurements
A. If the gingival margin is on enamel, measure from gum margin to cemento-enamel junction and record the measurement. If the epithelial attachment is on the crown and the cemento-enamel junction cannot be felt by the probe, record the depth of the gingival crevice on the crown. Then record the distance from the gingival margin to the bottom of the pocket if the probe can be moved apically to the cemento-enamel junction without resistance or pain. The distance from the cemento-enamel junction to the bottom of the pocket can then be found by subtracting the first from the second measurement.
B. If the gingival margin is on cementum, record the distance from the cemento-enamel junction to the gingival margin as a minus value. Then record the distance from the cemento-enamel junction to the bottom of the gingival sulcus as a plus value. Both loss of attachment and actual sulcus depth can easily be assessed from the scores.[120]

Periodontal Disease Index Criteria for Surveys (PDI)
If the gingival sulcus in none of the measured areas extended apically to the cemento-enamel junction, the recorded score for gingivitis is the PDI score for that tooth. If the gingival sulcus in any of the two measured areas extended apically to the cemento-enamel junction but not more than 3 mm. (including 3 mm. in any area), the tooth is assigned a PDI score of 4. The score for gingivitis then is disregarded in the PDI score for that tooth. If the gingival sulcus in any of the two recorded areas of the tooth extends apically to from 3 to 6 mm. (including 6 mm.) in relation to the cemento-enamel junction, the tooth is assigned the PDI score of 5 (again the gingivitis score is disregarded). Whenever the gingival sulcus extends more than 6 mm. apically to the cemento-enamel junction in any of the measured areas of the tooth, the score of 6 is assigned as the PDI score for that tooth (again disregarding the gingivitis score).[120]

Shick-Ash Modification[150] of Plaque Criteria
0 = Absence of dental plaque.
1 = Dental plaque in the interproximal or at the gingival margin covering less than one third of the gingival half of the facial or lingual surface.
2 = Dental plaque covering more than one third but less than two thirds of the gingival half of the facial or lingual surface.
3 = Dental plaque covering two thirds or more of the gingival half of the facial or gingival surface of the tooth.[150]

Calculus Criteria
0 = Absence of calculus.
1 = Supragingival calculus extending only slightly below the free gingival margin (not more than 1 mm.).
2 = Moderate amount of supra- and subgingival calculus or subgingival calculus alone.
3 = An abundance of supra- and subgingival calculus.[120]

mouth mirror. A blunt instrument, such as a periodontal pocket probe, is used to assess the bleeding potential of the tissues. Hence, each of the four gingival units is assessed according to the criteria appearing in Table 22–3.

Totaling the scores around each tooth yields the Gingival Index for the **area.** If the scores around each tooth are totaled and divided by four, the GI score for the **tooth** is obtained. Totaling all of the indices per tooth and dividing by the number of teeth examined provides the GI **score per person.** The Gingival Index may be obtained for a segment of the mouth or group of teeth in the same way.[74]

Except for the consideration of bleeding, the criteria used in the GI index are similar to those used by Lobene.[73] The numerical scores of the GI may be associated with varying degrees of gingivitis clinically as follows:

TABLE 22–3 CRITERIA FOR THE GINGIVAL INDEX (LÖE AND SILNESS)[75] AND THE PLAQUE INDEX (SILNESS AND LÖE)[151]

Gingival Index (GI)
0 = Normal gingiva.
1 = Mild inflammation, slight change in color, slight edema; *no bleeding on probing.*
2 = Moderate inflammation; redness, edema, and glazing; *bleeding on probing.*
3 = Severe inflammation, marked redness and edema; ulcerations; *tendency to spontaneous bleeding.*[74]

Plaque Index (PlI)
0 = No plaque in the gingival area.
1 = A film of plaque adhering to the free gingival margin and adjacent area of the tooth. The plaque may be recognized only by running a probe across the tooth surface.
2 = Moderate accumulation of soft deposits within the gingival pocket, on the gingival margin, and/or adjacent tooth surface, which can be seen with the naked eye.
3 = Abundance of soft matter within the gingival pocket and/or the gingival margin and adjacent tooth surface.[74]

Gingival Scores	Condition
0.1–1.0	Mild gingivitis
1.1–2.0	Moderate gingivitis
2.1–3.0	Severe gingivitis

The index is used in determining the prevalence and severity of gingivitis in epidemiologic surveys as well as in the individual dentitions. This latter attribute has contributed to making the GI Index the index of choice in controlled clinical trials of preventive or therapeutic agents.[49]

Gingival periodontal index (O'Leary et al.[107])

The Gingival Periodontal Index (GPI) is a modification of the Periodontal Disease Index (PDI, Ramfjord) for the purpose of screening individuals to determine who is in need of periodontal treatment. The GPI assesses three components of periodontal disease: gingival status; periodontal status (sulcus depth); and, collectively, materia alba, calculus, and overhanging restorations. The latter triad is independently called the *Irritation Index*. Only the criteria for the gingival status will be described in this section.

The maxillary and mandibular arches are each divided into three segments: the six anterior teeth, the left posterior teeth, and the right posterior teeth. The primary objective in using the index is to determine the tooth, or its surrounding tissues, with the severest condition within each segment. Hence, each segment is assessed for each of the three components of periodontal disease described above. The specific criteria for the gingival status of the GPI are as follows:

0 = Tissue tightly adapted to the teeth, firm consistency with physiologic architecture.

1 = Slight to moderate inflammation as indicated by changes in color and consistency, involving one or more teeth in the same segment but not completely surrounding any one tooth.

2 = The above changes singularly or combined completely encircle one or more teeth in a segment.

3 = Marked inflammation as indicated by loss of surface continuity (ulceration), spontaneous hemorrhage, loss of faciolingual continuity or any interdental papilla, marked deviation from normal contour, such as gross thickening or enlargement covering more than one third of the anatomic crown, recession, and clefts.

The area with the highest score gives the gingival score for the entire segment, and the **gingival status** for the mouth is obtained by dividing the sum of the gingival scores by the number of segments.

The index has been used extensively in military populations. Unlike the traditional

TABLE 22–4 CRITERIA FOR THE PERIODONTAL TREATMENT NEED SYSTEM (PTNS) CLASSIFICATION*

PTNS classi-fication	Unit	Plaque	Calculus and/or overhangs	Inflam-mation	Pocket depth
Class 0	mouth	no	no	no	not considered
Class A	mouth	yes	no	yes	≤ 5 mm.
Class B	quadrant	yes	yes	yes	≤ 5 mm.
Class C	quadrant	yes	yes	yes	> 5 mm.

* After Bellini.[10a]

indices used in epidemiology (i.e., traditional indices attempt only to assess the status of a specific disease condition with only the crudest suggestion of determining treatment needs), the GPI was developed for the specific purpose of detecting periodontal disease early so that treatment may be instituted promptly.[105]

A recently developed index, the **Periodontal Treatment Need System (P.T.N.S.)**,[49] has been used in Oslo with interesting results. It attempts to classify individuals into one of four categories based on treatment procedures required as follows:

Class O: No treatment needed.

Class A: Motivation and oral hygiene instruction

Class B: Scaling and removal of overhangs.

Class C Surgery.

It considers the presence or absence of gingivitis and plaque, and the presence of 5 mm. or greater pockets in each quadrant of the mouth, as shown in Table 22–4.

Indices Used to Measure Periodontal Destruction

In 1973 Ramfjord summarized the state of the art in measuring periodontal destruction by saying "categorically . . . none of the present periodontal indices provide data with adequate details for studies and clinical trials involving loss or gain of periodontium."[118] Although little has changed since this statement was made, it is possible and necessary to make the most of what is known and to describe the epidemiologic indices and techniques that have made it possible to quantitate the irreversible loss of alveolar bone. Some of the approaches that will be discussed in this section include gingival sulcus measurements, radiographic evaluations of bone loss, gingival recession, and tooth mobility.

Gingival sulcus measurement component of the periodontal disease index (Ramfjord[120])

The technique developed by Ramfjord for measuring gingival sulcus depth with a calibrated periodontal probe approaches the most quantitative method currently available for assessing the status of periodontal support. It consists of measuring the distance from the cemento-enamel junction to the free gingival margin and the distance from the free gingival margin to the bottom of the gingival crevice or pocket. The difference between the two measurements yields the gingival **sulcus depth**, which translates into epithelial attachment level. This is considered to be the most important clinical measurement in determining the status of the periodontium. It is considered useful in epidemiologic surveys, longitudinal studies of periodontal disease, and clinical trials of preventive and therapeutic agents.[118]

The first measurement in this two-step process may be used in assessing **gingival loss (recession) or gain**. It is considered more accurate and reliable in clinical trials than the Gingival Recession Index used in epidemiologic surveys.[118]

The probe used for the sulcus depth measurements is graduated in 3-mm. increments. All measurements are rounded to the nearest millimeter. Anything close to 0.5 mm. is rounded to the lower whole number. This "underscoring" has increased the reproducibility of the measurements using the above criteria. The placement of the periodontal probe in a standardized position relative to the tooth and gingival sulcus is also crucial. Measurements are made on the facial surface equidistant between the mesial and distal surfaces; the mesial-facial line angle at the interproximal contact area; the lingual surface, equidistant between the mesial and distal surfaces; and the distal-lingual line angle at the interproximal contact area. In making the facial-mesial and distal-lingual measurements, the probe is in contact with the adjacent tooth.[120] Measurements at the distal-lingual line angle are considered optional because their omission does not significantly decrease the accuracy of sulcus measurements per person on Periodontal Disease Index (PDI) score.[118] The criteria developed by Ramfjord for making sulcular determinations appear in Table 22–2.

When the measurements are rounded to the nearest millimeter, as described above, the Ramfjord criteria are most applicable to longitudinal studies of periodontal disease and clinical trials of preventive or therapeutic agents. Either the six teeth

(teeth numbered 3, 9, 12, 19, 25, and 28) used by Ramfjord or whatever teeth are appropriate to the objective of the study may be assessed.

In an epidemiologic survey (i.e., cross-sectional survey) in which the purpose is to determine the prevalence of total periodontal disease (PDI), only the six index teeth should be used. The criterion for a cross-sectional survey is called the **Periodontal Disease Index (PDI)** and appears in Table 22–2. By strict definition, the PDI includes only the assessment of the gingival tissues and the gingival sulci. The Periodontal Disease Index **score for the individual** is obtained by totaling the scores of the teeth and dividing by the number of teeth examined (a maximum of 6).[120]

Radiographic approaches to measuring bone loss

In general, the use of radiographs in the study of the epidemiology of periodontal disease would appear to overcome some of the criticisms of the more subjective clinical measurements. They present a permanent objective record of interdental bone levels; in longitudinal studies they may present less variability than poorly standardized dental examiners; they present the only method available for making crown and root measurements. Their disadvantages are that they are not useful in the buccal or lingual assessment of bone level;

they do not provide adequate information on soft tissue attachment; and their value may be lost if improper angulation is used[43] (see Chap. 32).

There are several indices that have been specifically designed to evaluate the radiographic assessment of periodontal disease, and techniques for making reasonably accurate measurements from radiographs have been developed.

GINGIVAL-BONE COUNT (DUNNING AND LEACH[40]). The Gingival-Bone Count (GB) Index records the gingival condition and the level of condition of the crest of the alveolar bone. The bone level is assessed by clinical examination, but radiographs are recommended for greater accuracy. The ·Gingival-Bone Count is scored as shown in Table 22–5. The average Gingival score per person is added to the average Bone score per person to yield the Gingival-Bone Count per person.

Sheiham and Striffler[149] developed an index similar to the bone count component of the GB Count Index. The criteria for evaluating radiographs is as follows:

0 = Normal.

4 = Lack of continuity of cortical plate at the crest of the interdental bone with possible widening of periodontal ligament.

5 = Up to one third of supporting bone lost.

6 = More than one third and up to two thirds of supporting bone lost.

TABLE 22–5   THE GINGIVAL-BONE COUNT (DUNNING AND LEACH)[40]

Gingival score (One score is assigned to each tooth studied. A mean is then computed for the whole mouth.)

Negative	0
Mild gingivitis involving the free gingiva (margin, papilla or both)	1
Moderate gingivitis involving both free and attached gingivia	2
Severe gingivitis with enlargement and easy hemorrhage	3

Bone score (One score is assigned to each tooth studied. A mean is then computed for the whole mouth.)

No bone loss	0
Incipient bone loss or notching of the alveolar crest	1
Bone loss approximating one fourth of root length or pocket formation one side not over one half root length	2
Bone loss approximating one half of root length or pocket formation one side not over three fourths root length; mobility slight°	3
Bone loss approximating three fourths of root length or pocket formation one side to apex; mobility moderate°	4
Bone loss complete; mobility marked°	5
Maximum possible GB count per person	8

°If mobility or impairment of masticatory function varies considerably from that to be expected with bone loss seen, the score may be altered up or down one point.

7=More than two thirds of supporting bone lost.[43]

The strength of each of the above indices is in epidemiologic surveys in which evaluation time is limited because of large study populations.

TECHNIQUES USED TO OBTAIN MORE ACCURATE MEASUREMENTS OF RADIOGRAPHS. Miller and Seidler[91, 92] used a scale of 0 to 5 to assess tooth-to-marginal bone level ratios from radiographs. A percentage value was used as the index of periodontal disease. Schei et al.[140] introduced a graded scale to estimate bone loss using the cemento-enamel junction as a point of reference. Bjorn et al.[14, 15] developed a method involving the projection of radiographs at a fixed distance onto a screen with a graded scale of 20 divisions. The number of divisions between the most coronal level of bone and the apical base of the bone were counted.

One additional technique that offers great practicality is the use of wire grids (with 1 mm. squares) embedded in thin plastic which are attached to the radiograph before exposure.[47, 157] Either direct observation or projection of the radiographs permits measurements relative to the cemento-enamel junction rounded to the nearest 0.5 mm.

The time restraints of epidemiologic surveys limit the use of radiographic assessment of periodontal support to longitudinal studies of periodontal disease, whether descriptive or experimental.

Techniques used to measure horizontal tooth mobility*

The most subjective method used to assess horizontal tooth mobility was described by Miller[90] and consists of assessing the mobility of a tooth on a scale from 0 to 3 when the tooth is held between two instruments. The numerical values correspond to movement in 1 mm. increments. Although this approach is useful in clinical diagnosis and treatment planning, it is of little value in longitudinal or clinical studies.

Parfitt[109, 111] used an electronic instru-

ment to measure tooth movement with an accuracy of 0.001 mm. ± 7 per cent. Picton[114, 115] developed a method that used resistance-wire strain gauges where any movement relative to the adjacent tooth was measured. A system using electronic transducers was developed by Korber and Korber.[69–71] All of these devices are complex, and the time required to use them is prohibitive for epidemiologic surveys or large clinical trials.

Mühlemann[94, 96] has developed two instruments for measuring tooth mobility: the macroperiodontometer and the microperiodontometer. Although many studies have been completed using the first device, its value is limited to specific areas of the mouth.[95] The latter device is more difficult to master and its results are less reproducible.[104]

The Periodontometer (USAFSAM) developed by O'Leary and Rudd[106] has been used more extensively than any device to measure tooth mobility. It measures the facial or palatal deflection of a tooth in increments of 0.0001 inch when 500 grams of force are applied. It requires two investigators, extensive training in its use, and a minimum of 8 to 10 minutes per quadrant. Therefore, its use could be considered only in clinical trials.[104]

Indices Used to Measure Plaque Accumulation

In general, most of the indices used to measure plaque accumulation assess on a numerical scale the extent of the surface area of a tooth covered by plaque. For our purposes, plaque will be defined as a nonmineralized soft tooth deposit including debris and materia alba. No attempt will be made to present the various indices according to the subtle differences that exist in definitions of plaque, debris, and materia alba (e.g., the terms *plaque* and *debris* will be used interchangeably unless otherwise stated) (see Chap. 24 and 25).

Plaque component of periodontal disease index (Ramfjord[120])

The first index that attempted to assess on a numerical scale the extent of plaque

---

*The reader is referred to an excellent review on this subject by Timothy O'Leary.[104]

covering the surface area of a tooth was developed by Ramfjord. The plaque component of the Periodontal Disease Index (PDI) is used on the six teeth selected by Ramfjord (teeth numbered 3, 9, 12, 19, 25, and 28) after staining with Bismarck brown solution. The criteria measure the presence and extent of plaque on a scale of 0 to 3, looking specifically at all interproximal facial and lingual surfaces of the index teeth. The criteria are suitable for longitudinal studies of periodontal disease.[120] Even though the plaque component is not a part of the PDI score, it is helpful in a total assessment of periodontal status.

Shick and Ash[150] modified the original criteria of Ramfjord by excluding consideration of the interproximal areas of the teeth and "restricting the scoring of plaque to the gingival half"[118] of the facial and lingual surfaces of the index teeth. The criteria for the Shick-Ash modification of the Ramfjord plaque criteria appear in Table 22–2.

The plaque **score per person** is obtained by totaling all of the individual tooth scores and dividing by the number of teeth examined. The modified plaque criteria are suitable for clinical trials of preventive or therapeutic agents.

Simplified oral hygiene index (Greene and Vermillion[56])

In the early development of the indices used to measure gingivitis and periodontal disease, it became apparent that the data lacked meaning or significance unless the level of oral hygiene or cleanliness was evaluated as a separate component. The lack of a simple, objective set of criteria that minimized examiner variability prompted Greene and Vermillion to develop the Oral Hygiene Index (OHI).[55] Their goal was to develop a measuring technique that could be used in "studying the epidemiology of periodontal disease and oral calculus, when assessing toothbrushing efficiency, and when evaluating the dental health practices of a community and the immediate as well as the long-term effects of dental health education"[53] programs. Realizing that it was not necessary or practical to assess all of the teeth to determine a person's level of oral cleanliness, Greene and Vermillion selected six index tooth surfaces that were representative of all anterior and posterior segments of the mouth based on whole mouth examinations. This modification of the OHI was called the Simplified Oral Hygiene Index (OHI-S).[56] The OHI-S measures the surface area of the tooth covered by debris and calculus. The imprecise term *debris* was used because it was not practical to observe the soft deposits microscopically and to make the subtle distinction that exists between plaque, debris, and materia alba. In addition, the practicality of determining the weight and thickness of the soft deposits prompted the assumption that the dirtier the mouth, the greater the tooth surface area covered by debris. This assumption also implied a time factor, because the longer oral hygiene practices are neglected, the greater the surface area of the tooth that will be covered by debris.

The OHI-S consists of two components: a Debris Index (DI-S) and a Calculus Index (CI-S). Each component is assessed on a scale of 0 to 3. Only a mouth mirror and shepherd's crook or sickle-type dental explorer, and no disclosing agent, are used for the examination. The six tooth surfaces examined in the OHI-S are the facial surfaces of the teeth numbered 3, 8, 14, and 24 and the lingual surfaces of the teeth numbered 19 and 30. Each tooth surface is divided horizontally into gingival, middle, and incisal thirds.

For the Debris Index (DI-S) a dental

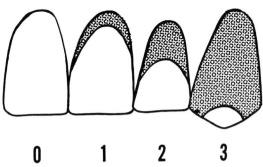

0   1   2   3

Figure 22–1   Criteria for Scoring Oral Debris (DI-S) Component of OHI-S.[56]

0 — No debris or stain present.

1 — Soft debris covering not more than one third of the tooth surface, or the presence of extrinsic stains without other debris regardless of surface area covered.

2 — Soft debris covering more than one third but not more than two thirds of the exposed tooth surface.

3 — Soft debris covering more than two thirds of the exposed tooth surface.

explorer is placed on the incisal third of the tooth and moved toward the gingival third according to the criteria illustrated in Figure 22–1. The Debris Index **score per person** is obtained by totaling the debris score per tooth surface and dividing by the number of surfaces examined.

The Calculus Index (CI-S) is performed by gently placing a dental explorer into the distal gingival crevice and drawing it subgingivally from the distal contact area to the mesial contact area (i.e., one half of a tooth's circumference is considered a scoring unit). The criteria for scoring the calculus component of the OHI-S appear in Figure 22–2. The Calculus Index **score per person** is obtained by totaling the calculus score per tooth surface and dividing by the number of surfaces examined. The **OHI-S score per person** is the total of the DI-S and CI-S scores per person.

The clinical levels of oral cleanliness for debris that can be associated with group Simplified Debris Index scores are as follows:[53]

Good	0.3 to 0.6
Fair	0.7 to 1.8
Poor	1.9 to 3.0

The clinical levels of oral hygiene that can be associated with group OHI-S scores are as follows:[53]

Good	0.0 to 1.2
Fair	1.3 to 3.0
Poor	3.1 to 6.0

The significance of the OHI-S is that, like Russell's Periodontal Index, it has been used extensively throughout the world and has contributed greatly to our understanding of periodontal disease. It is also used in the National Health Survey.[64] The high degree of correlation ($r = 0.82$)[144] between the OHI-S and PI makes it possible, knowing one of the two scores, to calculate the other score using regression analysis.[52] The major strength of the OHI-S is its use in epidemiologic surveys[80] and in evaluating dental health education programs (longitudinal). It can also be used to evaluate an individual's level of oral cleanliness and, to a more limited extent, can be used in clinical trials. The index is easy to use because the criteria are objective, the examination may be performed quickly, and a high level of reproducibility is possible with a minimum of training sessions.[53]

Turesky modification[161] of the Quigley-Hein[117] plaque index

In 1962, Quigley and Hein[117] presented the results of a plaque index that focused attention on the gingival third of the tooth surface. They examined only the facial surfaces of the anterior teeth, after disclosing the subject with a basic fuchsin

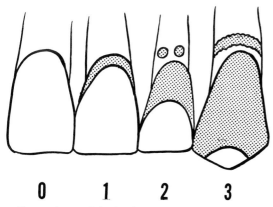

0   1   2   3

Figure 22–2 Criteria for Scoring Calculus (CI-S) Component of OHI-S.[56]

0 — No calculus present.

1 — Supragingival calculus covering not more than one third of the exposed tooth surface.

2 — Supragingival calculus covering more than one third but not more than two thirds of the exposed tooth surface or the presence of individual flecks of subgingival calculus around the cervical portion of the tooth or both.

3 — Supragingival calculus covering more than two thirds of the exposed tooth surface or a continuous heavy band of subgingival calculus around the cervical portion of tooth or both.

TABLE 22–6 TURESKY-GILMORE-GLICKMAN MODIFICATION[161] OF THE QUIGLEY-HEIN PLAQUE INDEX[117]

0 = No plaque.

1 = Separate flecks of plaque at the cervical margin of the tooth.

2 = A thin continuous band of plaque (up to 1 mm.) at the cervical margin.

3 = A band of plaque wider than 1 mm. but covering less than one third of the crown.

4 = Plaque covering at least one third but less than two thirds of the crown.

5 = Plaque covering two thirds or more of the crown.[79]

mouthwash, using a numerical scoring system of 0 to 5.

Turesky et al.[161] strengthened the objectivity of the Quigley-Hein criteria by redefining the scores of the gingival third area. The Turesky modification of the Quigley-Hein criteria appears in Table 22–6. They assessed plaque on the facial and lingual surfaces of all of the teeth after using a disclosing agent. A plaque **score per person** was obtained by totaling all of the plaque scores and dividing by the number of surfaces examined. This system of scoring plaque is relatively easy to use because of th objective definitions of each numeri score. The strength of this plaque index is its application to longitudinal studies and clinical trials of preventive and therapeutic agents. Mandel has suggested that if the Turesky modification of the Quigley-Hein criteria were applied to the distal, middle, and mesial thirds of the facial and lingual surfaces of the teeth, it would be the plaque index of choice in clinical trials.[80]

Glass criteria for scoring debris[50]

The only other index that assesses the presence and extent of debris accumulation is a system developed by Glass[50] for assessing toothbrushing efficacy. All of the teeth are scored, and the facial and lingual surfaces are scored as a scoring unit. In addition to assessing debris, Glass also developed criteria for measuring gingival changes, tooth stain, and calculus accumulation. However, only the debris criteria will be described. The system for scoring debris according to the Glass criteria is as follows:

0 = No visible debris.
1 = Debris visible at gingival margin, but discontinuous — less than 1 mm. in height.
2 = Debris continuous at gingival margin — greater than 1 mm. in height.
3 = Debris involving entire gingival third of tooth.
4 = Debris generally scattered over tooth surface.

The debris index **score per person** is obtained by totaling all of the debris scores per tooth and dividing by the number of teeth examined. Because it places more emphasis on the gingival third of the tooth than does the OHI-S, its strength lies in clinical trials of preventive or therapeutic agents.[79]

Patient hygiene performance index (Podshadley and Haley[116])

The Patient Hygiene Performance Index (PHP)[116] is the only index developed for the sole purpose of assessing an individual's performance in removing debris after toothbrushing instruction (i.e., patient education). It assesses the presence or absence of debris as a 1 or 0, respectively, using the six OHI-S teeth (six surfaces). The PHP Index is relatively more sensitive than the OHI-S because it divides each tooth surface into five areas: three longitudinal thirds — distal, middle, and mesial; the middle third is subdivided horizontally into incisal, middle, and gingival thirds. The scoring is preceded by the use of a disclosing agent. The PHP **score per person** is obtained by totaling the five subdivision scores per tooth surface and dividing by the number of tooth surfaces examined. This index is easy to use because of its dichotomous criteria and can be performed quickly. Although it can be used in group studies of health education, its value lies in its application to individual patient education (i.e., an education aid).

Plaque index (Silness and Löe[151])

The Plaque Index (PlI) is unique among the indices described so far because it ignores the coronal extent of plaque on the tooth surface area and concentrates on assessing only the **thickness** of plaque at the gingival area of the tooth. Since it was developed as a component to parallel the Gingival Index (Löe and Silness[75]), it examines the same scoring units of the teeth: distal-facial, facial, mesial-facial, and lingual surfaces. A mouth mirror, dental explorer, and air drying of the teeth are used in assessing plaque in the Plaque Index. Unlike most indices, it does not exclude or substitute for teeth with gingival restorations or crowns. Either all or only selected teeth may be used in the P1I. The criteria for the Plaque Index of Silness and Löe appear in Table 22–3.

The P1I score for the **area** is obtained by totaling the four plaque scores per tooth. If the sum of the plaque scores per tooth is divided by four, the P1I score for the **tooth** is obtained. The P1I **score for the person** is obtained by summing the P1I scores per tooth and dividing by the number of teeth examined. The P1I may be obtained for a segment of the mouth or group of teeth in a similar manner.

The strength of the P1I is in its application to longitudinal studies and clinical trials. In spite of the studies that have been conducted to insure the reliability of the P1I data, the subjectiveness of plaque thickness requires highly trained and experienced examiners to insure valid data.[79]

Modified Navy plaque index[42]

This index was developed for the purpose of evaluating oral hygiene performance in Navy personnel. It records the presence or absence of plaque, by a score of 1 or 0, respectively, on nine areas of each tooth surface of the six index teeth used by Ramfjord. Each tooth surface is divided horizontally into gingival, middle, and incisal thirds. The gingival third is further divided in half horizontally, following the scallop shape of the gingiva. The lower half is immediately adjacent to the gingiva and does not exceed 1 mm. in width. Both of the gingival halves are divided longitudinally into distal, middle, and mesial thirds. The middle third (horizontally) of the tooth surface is divided into distal and mesial halves, and the incisal third is coronal to the contact area and is not subdivided. This approach emphasizes the gingival two-thirds of the tooth with the gingival one-third weighted twice as heavily (i.e., the plaque in closest proximity to the gingival tissues is weighted more heavily because of its importance). A Modified Navy Plaque Index **score per person** is obtained by totaling all nine of the subdivision scores per tooth surface and dividing by the number of tooth surfaces examined. Like the PHP Index of Podshadley and Haley, the Modified Navy Plaque Index is of value in assessing health education programs as well as the ability of individuals to perform oral hygiene practices.

Other plaque indices

Plaque is one of the two factors measured in the Irritants Index,[105, 107] which is a component of the Gingival Periodontal Index (GPI) of O'Leary et al. The presence and coronal extent of plaque is scored on a scale of 0 to 3. Other factors that contribute to the Irritants Index are supra- and subgingival calculus and subgingival irritants, such as overhanging or deficient restorations.

Bjorby and Löe[13] developed a Retention Index that not only examined supra- and subgingival calculus, but grossly assessed dental caries and the quality of the margins of restorations. Collectively, all of these parameters were scored on a numerical scale of 0 to 3.[74]

Indices Used to Measure Calculus

In general, the choice of indices used to assess calculus may be conveniently divided into those that are most appropriate to epidemiologic surveys; those that are appropriate to longitudinal studies, with an examination every three to six months; and those that are used in short-term clinical studies, usually no longer than six weeks.

Simplified oral hygiene index (Greene and Vermillion[56])

The Simplified Calculus Index (CI-S component of the OHI-S) was presented in detail under *Indices Used to Measure Plaque Accumulation,* because it is less separable from its scoring system than any of the other indices that combine several component measures. The value of the CI-S component is its application to epidemiologic surveys and longitudinal studies of periodontal disease.[53] Figure 22–2 illustrates the specific criteria of the OHI-S used to assess calculus.

Calculus component of the periodontal disease index (Ramfjord[119])

The calculus component of the PDI assesses the presence and extent of calculus on six index teeth (i.e., the facial and lingual surfaces of teeth numbered 3, 9, 12, 19, 25, and 28) on a numerical scale of 0 to 3. A mouth mirror and a dental explorer and/or periodontal probe are used in the examination. The criteria for assigning a score to each tooth surface for the calculus component of the PDI appears in Table 22–2. Like the plaque component of the PDI, calculus is not included in the PDI score, but it is considered useful in a total assessment of periodontal status.

The calculus scores per tooth are totaled and then divided by the number of teeth examined to yield the calculus **score per person**. Like the Simplified Calculus Index of the OHI-S, the calculus component of the PDI has a high degree of examiner reproducibility, can be performed quickly, and has its best application in epidemiologic surveys and longitudinal studies.[120]

Probe method of calculus assessment (Volpe and Manhold[163])

The Probe Method of Calculus Assessment was developed to assess the quantity of supragingival calculus formed in longitudinal studies. A periodontal probe graduated in millimeter divisions is used to measure the deposits of calculus on the lingual surfaces of the lower six anterior teeth. The smallest unit used to record the presence of calculus is 0.5 mm. A mouth mirror and air are used to dry the teeth prior to examination. Measurements are made in three planes: gingival, distal, and mesial. The gingival measurement is made with the probe held parallel to the long axis of the tooth and equidistant between the mesial and distal surfaces. The probe should be simultaneously in contact with the calculus and the incisal edge of the tooth. The distal measurement is made by holding the probe diagonally so that the tip is in contact with the distal aspect of the tooth and the opposite end (i.e., the portion toward the shank of the probe) is bisecting the mesial-incisal line angle of the tooth. The opposite

is true for the mesial measurement. The measurement may be calculated and expressed in three different ways: per measurement score, per tooth score, and per subject score. The **measurement score** is simply the total of all the scores divided by the number of measurements made. The **tooth score** is the total of all of the scores divided by the number of teeth scored. The **subject score** is simply the total of all of the scores (subjects with less than six teeth are excluded).[162]

The Probe Method of Calculus Assessment has been shown to possess a high degree of inter- and intraexaminer reproducibility. It requires extensive training under an experienced investigator in order to master it.

Calculus surface index (Ennever et al.[46])

The Calculus Surface Index (CSI) is one of two indices that are used in short-term (i.e., less than six weeks) clinical trials of calculus inhibitory agents. The object of this type of study is to determine rapidly whether or not a specific agent has any effect on reducing or preventing supra- or subgingival calculus. The CSI assesses the presence or absence of supra- and/or subgingival calculus on the four mandibular incisors. The index has also been applied to the six mandibular anterior teeth. The category of presence and absence is determined by visual or tactile examination using a mouth mirror and sickle type dental explorer. Each incisor is divided into four scoring units. The facial (or labial) surface is considered one surface and the lingual surface is divided longitudinally into three subdivisions: the distal-lingual third, the lingual third, and the mesial-lingual third. The total number of surfaces with calculus is considered the Calculus Surface Index score per person. The index has been shown to have good intraexaminer reproducibility, and scoring can be performed in a relatively short period of time. Hence, using a 1 to indicate the presence of calculus (and a 0 the absence of calculus), the maximum number of surfaces (scoring mandibular incisors) per person that could have calculus is 16.[162]

A companion index to the Calculus Surface Index (CSI) is the Calculus Surface

Severity Index (CSSI).[46] The CSSI measures the quantity of calculus present, on a scale of 0 to 3, on each of the surfaces examined in the CSI examination. The criteria[26] for the Calculus Surface Severity Index are as follows:

0 = No calculus present.

1 = Calculus observable, but less than 0.5 mm. in width and/or thickness.

2 = Calculus not exceeding 1.0 mm. in width and/or thickness.

3 = Calculus exceeding 1.0 mm. in width and/or thickness.

Marginal line calculus index (Mühlemann and Villa[98])

The second index that is frequently used in short-term (i.e., less than six weeks) clinical trials of anticalculus agents is the Marginal Line Calculus Index (MLCI). This index was developed to assess the accumulation of supragingival calculus on the gingival third of the tooth, or more specifically supragingival calculus along the margin of the gingiva.

Using a mouth mirror and air to dry the surfaces under examination, only the cervical areas on the lingual surfaces of the four mandibular incisors are examined. The cervical third of each lingual surface is divided into distal and mesial halves. Each half is examined for the extent of calculus covering the surface and a score on a scale of percentages is assigned as follows: 0, 12.5, 25, 50, 75, and 100 per cent. The MLCI **score per tooth** is determined by averaging the two half units per each tooth. The MLCI **score per person** is determined by totaling the scores per tooth and dividing by the number of teeth examined. Like the Calculus Surface Index, the Marginal Line Calculus Index has shown good reproducibility.[162]

DESCRIPTIVE EPIDEMIOLOGY OF GINGIVAL AND PERIODONTAL DISEASE

Prevalence of Gingivitis

Gingivitis has been observed in children less than five years of age.[85, 159] In general the prevalence and severity of gingivitis increases with increasing age,[1] beginning at approximately five years of age and reaching its highest point in puberty and then very gradually decreasing[110] but remaining relatively high throughout life (Fig. 22–3). The rapid increase in the incidence of gingivitis prior to 10 years of age is asso-

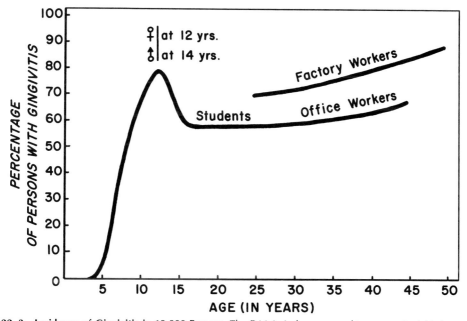

Figure 22–3 **Incidence of Gingivitis in 10,000 Persons.** The P.M.A. Index was used to assess gingivitis in persons 2 to 60 years of age. (Courtesy of Dr. Maury Massler.[82])

TABLE 22-7　PREVALENCE OF GINGIVITIS IN CHILDREN AND YOUNG ADULTS

Investigators	Year	Group Studied	No. Children in Group	Age Group	Percentage of Persons Affected with Gingivitis
Ainsworth and Young[1]	1925	School children in England and Wales	4063	2–14 yrs.	40
McCall[85]	1933	New York	4600	1–14 yrs.	98
Messner et al.[87]	1938	Children in twenty-six states of U.S.	1,438,318	6–14 yrs.	3.5–8.6
Marshall-Day and Tandan[37]	1940	Middle class children in Lahore, India	756	approx. 13 yrs.	68
Marshall-Day[28]	1940	Fluoride endemic area in Northern India	203	5–18 yrs.	59.6
King[66]	1940	Isle of Lewis	2280	6–15 yrs.	90
Campbell and Cook[22]	1942	Dundee Hospital in Scotland	1924		2.2
Marshall-Day[30]	1944	Boys in Kangra district of India (poor nutrition)	200	approx. 13 yrs.	81
Marshall-Day and Shourie[34]	1944	Low-middle class school children	613	5–15 yrs.	80
King, Franklyn and Allen[68]	1944	English boys	403	11–14 yrs. Group A Group B	77.4 87.6
	1944	Gibraltar evacuees in England	135	10–14 yrs.	85.2
King[67]	1945	Primary school children in Dundee, Scotland	103	12–14 yrs.	90
	1945	Harpenden Institution, England	170	11–14 yrs.	Groups vary 56.4–97.5
Marshall-Day and Shourie[33]	1947	Low to middle class male school children in Lahore, India	1054	9–17 yrs.	99.4
Marshall-Day and Shourie[33]	1947	Girls of high socio-economic level at Lahore, India	179	9–17 yrs.	73.3
Schour and Massler[141]	1947	Four communities in Italy suffering from malnutrition	682 721	6–10 yrs. 11–20 yrs.	40.3 55.3
Marshall-Day et al.[32]	1948	Puerto Rico	1648	6–18 yrs.	60–79
Massler, Schour, and Chopra[84]	1950	Suburban Chicago school children	804	5–14 yrs.	64.3
Marshall-Day and Shourie[32]	1950	Virgin Island (91% Negro population)	823 860	6–18 yrs. 5–13 yrs.	57.0 26.9
Stahl and Goldman[153]	1953	School children in Massachusetts	1300	13–17 yrs.	29.0
Russell[133]	1957	Urban United States White { Negro {	6682 15,922 4031 37 494	5–9 yrs. 10–14 yrs. 15–19 yrs. 5–9 yrs. 10–19 yrs.	10.8 25.5 37.3 8.1 28.7
Greene[54]	1960	School boys in low socio-economic area of India	1613	11–17 yrs.	96.9
		School boys in low socio-economic area of Atlanta, Georgia	577	11–17 yrs.	92.0
Zimmerman and Baker[167]	1960	White children from Maryland	529	6–12 yrs.	35
		Negro children from Texas	442	6–12 yrs.	67
		White children from Texas	435	6–12 yrs.	79
Jamison[59]	1963	Tecumseh, Michigan (deciduous teeth only)	159	5–14 yrs.	99.4
McHugh et al.[86]	1964	Dundee, Scotland, boys and girls	2905	13 yrs.	99.4
Dutta[41]	1965	Calcutta, India, boys and girls	1424	6–12 yrs.	89.8
Wade[164]	1966	Iraq	200	13–15 yrs.	97.0
		London	222	13–15 yrs.	
Sheiham[147]	1968	Nigeria	1620	10 yrs. and older	99+
Sheiham[148]	1969	Surrey	756	11–17 yrs.	99.7

TABLE 22–7 PREVALENCE OF GINGIVITIS IN CHILDREN AND YOUNG ADULTS (*Continued*)

Investigators	Year	Group Studied	No. Children In Group	Age Group	Percentage of Persons Affected with Gingivitis
Murray[100]	1969	West Hartlepool, 1.5–2.0 ppm. fluoride			
		Boys	211	15 yrs.	94.8
		Girls	175	15 yrs.	86.3
		York, 0.2 ppm. fluoride			
		Boys	202	15 yrs.	95.5
		Girls	179	15 yrs.	85.5
Downer[38]	1970	Secondary school children in London, England	373	11–14 yrs.	79.0
Murray[99]	1972	West Hartlepool, 1.5–2.0 ppm. fluoride			
		Boys	141	15–19 yrs.	90.1
		Girls	449	15–19 yrs.	88.4
		York, 0.2 ppm. fluoride			
		Boys	61	15–19 yrs.	86.9
		Girls	102	15–19 yrs.	84.3
Jorkjend and Birkeland[61]	1973	Primary school children in Porsgrunn, Norway	154	11–13 yrs.	99.0
Bowden et al.[18]	1973	Cheshire, England	622	15 yrs.	81.2
Murray[101]	1974	West Hartlepool, 1.5–2.0 ppm. fluoride			
		Boys	1470	8–18 yrs.	92.9
		Girls	1406	8–18 yrs.	91.1

ciated with the eruption of the permanent dentition.[84] Surveys of the prevalence and severity of gingivitis are summarized in Table 22–7. Data from the National Health Survey (NHS, Fig. 22–4) show that for children 6 to 11 years of age[62] the prevalence of gingivitis (i.e., periodontal disease with no pockets) is approximately 38 per cent; for adolescents 12 to 17 years of age[138] the prevalence of gingivitis is 62 per cent; for young adults 18 to 24 years of age[63] the prevalence is 57 per cent. Thereafter, the prevalence of gingivitis continues gradually to decrease with increasing age. Hence, the

Figure 22–4 Prevalence of Periodontal Disease by Age. Data are from the National Health Survey (NHS) and covers the periods of 1963-1965 (children, 6-11 years), 1966-1970 (youths, 12-17 years), and 1960-1962 (adults, 18-79 years). The per cent distribution is by mild to moderate gingivitis (no pockets) and periodontal disease with one or more pockets; it is based on Periodontal Index (PI) scores. Males and females were combined. Adapted from Kelly and Sanchez,[62] Sanchez,[138] and Kelly and Van Kirk.[63]

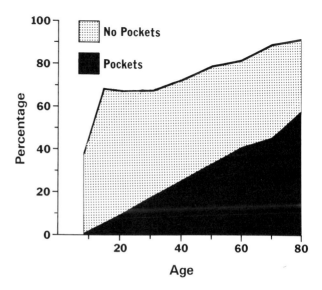

highest prevalence of gingivitis occurs during puberty.

Prevalence of Periodontal Disease

On a worldwide basis the United States ranks relatively low in the magnitude and prevalence of periodontal disease. Table 22–8 shows mean Periodontal Index scores by various population groups throughout the world. Compared with South America and the Asian countries, the severity of periodontal disease in groups in the United States is relatively low.[126]

Although there is no precise method of determining the absolute magnitude of periodontal disease in the United States, sufficient data do exist to arrive at a relatively accurate estimate of the prevalence. In adults 18 to 79 years of age, for example, three out of four adults (75 per cent) have some form of periodontal disease, and one out of four (25 per cent) has destructive periodontal disease.[63] Hence, 50 per cent of these adults have mild to severe gin-

givitis. Out of the 11.2 per cent of the adult population that is completely edentulous,[21] it is reasonable to assume that a substantial number of people lost their teeth because of periodontal disease. Also, adults who have teeth in only ,one arch have more severe periodontal disease than people with some teeth in both arches.[63] All adults will at some time during their lifetime experience some deterioration of their periodontal structures. Collectively, all of these observations lead to the conclusion that periodontal disease has a more deleterious effect on dental health than the percentage values indicate. As more people retain their teeth throughout their lifetime and as the proportion of older people increases, more teeth would be at risk to periodontal disease. Hence, the prevalence of periodontal disease will likely increase in the future!

Prevalence of Juvenile Periodontitis

It is difficult to arrive at a statement of prevalence for juvenile periodontitis because of the lack of uniform criteria for recognizing and classifying juvenile periodontitis and the small sample sizes of the groups studied. A review of the literature will reveal a range of prevalence values from 0.1 to 15 per cent.[8, 36, 88, 102, 108, 122, 131, 133] The age group that appears to be most affected by juvenile periodontitis is the interval from puberty to approximately 30 years of age.[36, 88, 131] Most investigators agree on this generalization. An examination of the per cent distribution of periodontal disease for persons in the United States (see Fig. 22–4) shows that the prevalence of destructive periodontal disease (i.e., disease with pockets) is 5.8 per cent for adolescents 12 to 17 years of age,[138] 10 per cent for young adults 18 to 24 years of age, and approximately 17 per cent for adults 30 to 34 years of age.[63] Assuming that approximately half of these individuals had juvenile periodontitis, it would be reasonable to expect that the true prevalence of juvenile periodontitis would be some value less than 8 per cent, and even this may be a high estimate. Some investigators[8, 122] believe that females are affected more frequently than males, but this has not been clearly established.[102] Intraorally, the teeth that are most severely affected are the maxillary and mandibular

TABLE 22–8 AVERAGE PERIODONTAL INDEX IN CIVILIANS (BOTH SEXES), AGED 40–49 YEARS, SURVEYED BY EXAMINERS OF THE NATIONAL INSTITUTE OF DENTAL RESEARCH, UNITED STATES*

Population Group	Average Periodontal Index
Baltimore, Maryland (white)	1.03
Colorado Springs, Colorado	1.04†
Alaska; primitive Eskimos	1.17‡
Ecuador	1.85
Ethiopia	1.86
Baltimore, Maryland (Negro)	1.99
Uganda[99]	2.50§
Vietnam; Vietnamese	2.18
Colombia	2.21
Alaska; urban Eskimos	2.31‡
Chile	2.74
Lebanon; Lebanese	2.98
Thailand	3.30
Lebanon; Palestinian refugees	3.52
Burma	3.58
Jordan; Jordanian civilians	3.96
Vietnam; Hill Tribesmen	3.97
Trinidad	4.21
Jordan; Palestinian refugees	4.41

*Modified from Russell, A. L.[126]
†Ages 40–44 only.
‡Males only.
§Age over 40.

incisors and the first molars; the least affected teeth are the mandibular premolars.[8, 89] When greater agreement among investigators is reached relative to the parameters used to describe juvenile periodontitis, a more accurate estimate of its prevalence will be possible.

FACTORS AFFECTING THE PREVALENCE AND SEVERITY OF GINGIVITIS AND PERIODONTAL DISEASE

Age

The prevalence of periodontal disease increases directly with increasing age.[126] Figure 22–4 shows the distribution of periodontal disease, with and without pockets.[62, 63, 138] The prevalence of periodontal disease is approximately 45 per cent at 10 years of age, 67 per cent at 20 years, 70 per cent at 35 years, and approximately 80 per cent at 50 years of age. This gradual increase in the prevalence of periodontal disease supports the statement that virtually no one escapes the ravages of periodontal disease. The distribution of periodontal disease with pockets is approximately 1 per cent at 10 years of age, approximately 10 per cent at 20 years of age, slightly over 20 per cent at 35 years of age, and almost 40 per cent at 50 years of age. There is a dramatic fivefold increase in the prevalence of destructive disease with pockets between 20 and 75 years of age. This pattern of disease with pockets closely parallels the reduction in bone height that occurs with increasing age.[31, 35] Although destructive periodontal disease is primarily a disease of adults, its onset during puberty has been observed with greater frequency in other countries[131] than in the United States.[138]

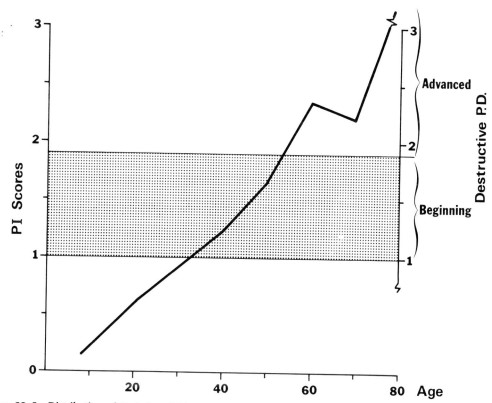

Figure 22–5 **Distribution of Periodontal Disease Severity by Age.** Data are from the NHS and combines whites and blacks together. Severity is indicated by mean Periodontal Index (PI) scores. The subdivisions of destructive periodontal disease approximate the group PI scores that correspond to the various clinical conditions (Table 22–1). Adapted from Kelly,[62] Sanchez,[138] and Kelly.[63]

The severity of periodontal disease as indicated by mean Periodontal Index Scores **increases directly with age** (Fig. 22–5). At approximately 35 years of age, the average adult enters the beginning phase of destructive periodontal disease. It then takes approximately 20 more years before the average adult (55 years of age) enters the advanced phase of destructive periodontal disease.[63]

Sex

In general, **males consistently have a higher prevalence and severity of periodontal disease than females** (Fig. 22–6). Before 20 years of age the differences between males and females are very slight.[62, 133, 138] At 20 years of age males have only a 25 per cent higher Periodontal Index score than females.[60, 63] Starting at 35 years of age and continuing through age 60, however, males have 50 per cent more severe periodontal disease than females.

The differences in severity between males and females increase to 66 per cent after 60 years of age. It is also interesting to note that as a group males enter the beginning phase of destructive periodontal disease at approximately 35 years of age, compared with females, who enter the beginning phase at approximately 45 years of age; that males enter the advanced stage of periodontal disease at approximately 55 years of age, compared with females, who enter the advanced stage at approximately 75 years of age.

Race

Figure 22–7 compares the severity of periodontal disease by racial-ethnic group for the National Health Survey (NHS)[62, 63, 138] and the Ten-State Nutrition Survey (10-SNS or National Nutrition Survey).[159] When whites and blacks from the National Health Survey are compared, blacks appear consistently to have more severe periodontal

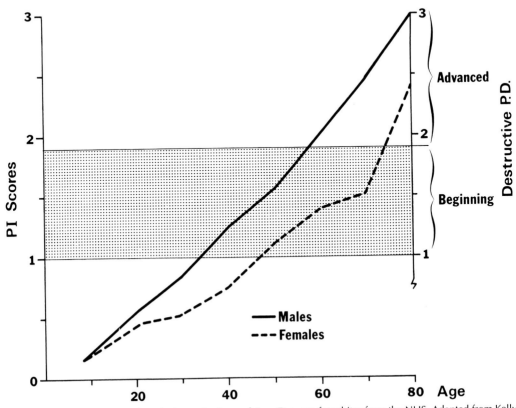

Figure 22–6   Severity of Periodontal Disease by Sex and Age. Data are for whites from the NHS. Adapted from Kelly[62, 63] and Sanchez.[138]

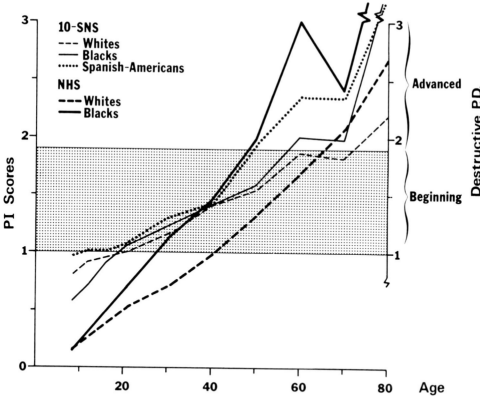

Figure 22–7   Severity of Periodontal Disease by Racial-Ethnic Group and Age. Data are from the NHS and the Ten-State Nutrition Survey (10-SNS or National Nutrition Survey, 1968-1970), high income ratio states. Adapted from Kelly,[62] Sanchez,[138] Kelly,[63] and Ten-State Nutrition Survey, 1968-1970.[159]

disease than whites.[63] After 20 years of age, blacks average 50 per cent more severe periodontal disease than whites.[133] Even though the differences that exist between whites and blacks are not as great in the data from the Ten-State Nutrition Survey, the same general trend still holds (i.e., blacks have more periodontal disease than whites).

Education

Figure 22–8[63] illustrates two important associations relative to periodontal disease. First, **periodontal disease is inversely related to increasing levels of education.**[57, 132, 135] In whites, the decrease in periodontal disease severity is 63 per cent and in blacks the decrease is 47 per cent. Second, **the apparent differences that** were observed between whites and blacks with periodontal disease (see Fig. 22–7) may be explained by differences in education, since no significant differences exist between whites and blacks of similar education. It is not surprising that occupation, which is so closely tied to education in the United States, shows a relationship to periodontal disease that is similar to that of education. For example, the prevalence and severity of periodontal disease is lower in office personnel than in factory workers and also lower in occupations that require more educational background.[5, 82]

Income

The association between periodontal disease and income is similar to the association observed between periodontal disease and education. **Periodontal disease is inversely**

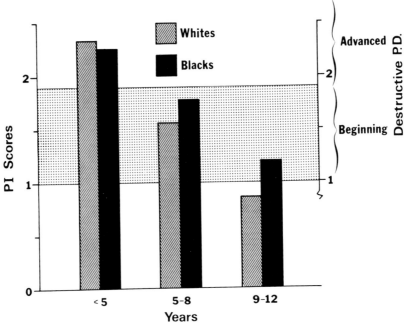

Figure 22–8 Comparison of Periodontal Disease Severity by Education and Racial-Ethnic Groups. Data are for adults from the NHS by the number of years or the highest grade of elementary or high school completed. Adapted from Kelly and Van Kirk.[63]

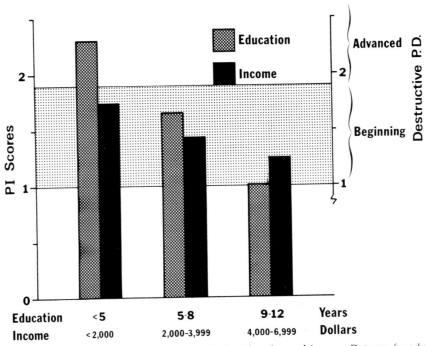

Figure 22–9 Comparison of Periodontal Disease Severity by Education and Income. Data are for adults, whites and blacks combined, from the NHS. Adapted from Kelly and Van Kirk.[63]

related to increasing levels of income. Data from the NHS show that the decrease in the severity of periodontal disease that occurs with increasing income is 38 per cent for whites and 20 per cent for blacks.[63] The differences that were observed between whites and blacks in Figure 22–7 are not influenced as strongly by income as they are by education.

The stronger influence of education over income relative to periodontal disease is more vividly illustrated in Figure 22–9.[63] When the Periodontal Index scores of whites and blacks are combined by education and income, the decrease due to education is 55 per cent, whereas the decrease due to income is only 28 per cent.

Residence

In general, the prevalence and severity of periodontal disease is slightly higher in rural areas than it is in urban areas.[11, 63]

Geographic Area

Within the United States some investigators have shown geographic differences in the prevalence and severity of periodontal disease,[83, 167] but no significant differences were observed for adults (6672 persons, 18 to 79 years of age) in the NHS.[63] Children (7119; 6 to 11 years)[62] and youths (6768; 12 to 17 years)[138] living in the South, however, did have slightly higher PI scores than their counterparts living in the Midwest and West.

ETIOLOGIC FACTORS OF GINGIVAL AND PERIODONTAL DISEASE

Oral Hygiene

The strong positive association that exists between poor oral hygiene and gingival and periodontal disease[6, 52, 54, 56, 64, 77, 121, 135, 148] makes it a primary etiologic agent. Based on observations of periodontal disease in the United States and throughout the world, Russell states that "active (gingival and periodontal) disease is rarely found in the absence of oral debris (plaque) or calculus."[125] One vivid example that puts a perspective on the importance of oral hy-

giene relative to the other demographic variables, described under the descriptive epidemiology of periodontal disease, is a multiple correlation analysis of the combined effects of age, sex, and oral hygiene (OHI-S scores) to Periodontal Index scores in 752 South Vietnamese over 15 years of age.[136] The coefficient of multiple correlation was r = 0.82, which under the above conditions, means that statistically 67 per cent of the variance was attributed to oral hygiene and approximately 31 per cent was attributed to age. In the National Health Survey, a comparison of the partial correlation coefficients of oral hygiene (OHI-S), age, education of the head of the household, and family income to Periodontal Index scores showed that oral hygiene was the best predictor of the prevalence and severity of periodontal disease.[137, 138] Hence, **statistically as well as clinically, plaque is a primary etiologic factor of periodontal disease.**

Nutrition

The nutrients that have been specifically associated with the periodontal tissues are vitamins A, B complex, C, and D, and the elements calcium and phosphorus (see Chap. 28). Deficiencies in each of these nutrients and their effects on the periodontium have all been clearly demonstrated in appropriately designed animal studies. The evidence for deficiencies in these nutrients being associated with periodontal disease in humans, however, has been less than convincing.[145] In a series of nutrition surveys (conducted under the auspices of the Interdepartmental Committee on Nutrition for National Defense, ICNND),[129] designed specifically to determine associations between nutrient levels and disease, the strongest residual associations between periodontal disease and nutritional deficiencies were expressed in partial correlations (holding the effects of age, debris, and calculus constant) of minus 0.11 for vitamin A and minus 0.19 for hematocrit levels.[126] The partial correlation coefficient (minus 0.11) for the vitamin A deficiency accounts for approximately 1 per cent of the variance in the Periodontal Index scores; the strongest partial correlation coefficient (minus 0.19) accounts for less than 4 per cent of the variance in the Periodontal Index scores. Little or no effect could be attributed to serum ascorbic acid, serum carotene, and total serum protein; urinary thiamine, riboflavin and N'methylnicotinamide and hemoglobin. The vitamin A deficiency and a subnormal hematocrit level were found in a South Vietnam population, but neither of these deficiencies was found to be associated with periodontal disease in subsequent ICNND surveys. In the Ten-State Nutrition Survey,[159] the simple correlation coefficient (−0.03) for PI scores and plasma vitamin A deficiency accounted for 0.1 per cent of the variance in the Periodontal Index scores. All of these correlation coefficients are at best weak associations. The ICNND nutrition surveys found no consistent correlation between nutrition and periodontal disease. They also concluded, however, that "despite the independence of the nutritive state of the individual adult and his periodontal condition," there is a trend toward a higher prevalence and severity of periodontal disease in adults in areas[66] where protein calorie malnutrition or vitamin A deficiency are common in children."[126]

Nutrition is, therefore, a secondary factor in the etiology of periodontal disease.

Fluorides

No definitive statement can be made concerning the prevalence and severity of gingival or periodontal disease in cities with optimal or high levels of fluoride in the drinking water. Some investigators have reported that optimal levels of fluoride did not have any effect on the gingival tissues,[45, 58, 93, 100] and others have reported a lower prevalence and severity of gingivitis and periodontal disease in optimally fluoridated areas.[7, 44, 127]

Adverse Habits

Tobacco smoking[4, 5, 154] and betel nut chewing[9] have been associated with increased periodontal disease.[27] Although this association is not unequivocal, it seems reasonable that any habit that increases irritation to the gingival tissues or lowers the resistance of the tissues would be a predisposing or secondary factor in initiating periodontal disease (see Chap. 26).

PROFESSIONAL DENTAL CARE

The incidence and severity of periodontal disorders are lower in individuals under regular dental care.[19, 78, 135, 156, 165] The prevalence and severity of disease increases with neglect (see Chap. 58).

DISTRIBUTION OF DISEASE IN DIFFERENT AREAS OF THE MOUTH

The strong association that was previously described between plaque and calculus and periodontal disease may in its initial stages be explained by the dynamics of plaque and gingivitis formation over

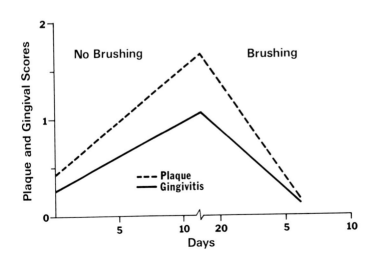

Figure 22–10 Rate of Plaque and Gingivitis Formation. Data are for 12 young Scandinavian adults, averaging 23 years of age. The Gingival Index (GI) and Plaque Index (PlI) were used for the clinical assessments. Adapted from Löe, Theilade, and Jensen.[76]

TABLE 22–9 SEVERITY OF GINGIVITIS FOR THREE DIFFERENT AREAS BY ARCH*

Areas	Arch	Mean GI
Interproximal	Upper > Lower	1.44 > 1.20
Facial	Upper > Lower	1.23 > 1.13
Lingual	Lower > Upper	0.89 > 0.46

*Adapted from Löe et al.[76]

time. Figure 22–10 shows the rate of plaque and gingivitis formation that Löe et al.[76] observed in their classic study of experimental gingivitis. It shows that, when brushing is withheld from oral hygiene cleansing procedures, the formation of plaque and gingivitis closely parallel each other and both increase with time, reaching a maximum between 15 and 21 days, when all subjects experienced a maximum of gingivitis. Reinstituting toothbrushing not only illustrated the reversible nature of gingival inflammation, but also showed a concomitant decrease in the plaque-gingivitis association.

Dividing the mouth into interproximal, facial, and lingual areas by upper and lower arches (Table 22–9), Löe showed that the area most severely affected by gingivitis was the interproximal followed by the facial and lingual surfaces. Dividing each of the areas into upper and lower arches revealed that gingivitis was more severe in the upper arch than it was in the lower arch for the interproximal and facial areas, and in the lingual area it was more severe in the lower arch than in the upper arch.[76] Suomi and Barbano[155] examined the severity of gingivitis by facial and lingual surfaces for three areas of the mouth (Fig. 22–11) and found the same general pattern observed by Löe. For facial surfaces, the areas most severely affected by gingivitis, in descending order, were the upper first and second molars, lower anteriors, upper anteriors, upper premolars, lower first and second molars, and the lower premolars. For lingual surfaces, the areas most severely affected by gingivitis, in descending order, were the lower first and second molars, lower premolars, lower anteriors, upper first and second molars, upper premolars, and upper anteriors. This intraoral pattern of gingivitis was similar to that observed by Marshall-Day,[29] with the exception of the facial surfaces of the upper anteriors, which he found to be the most severely affected by gingivitis. Several investigators[12, 155] have observed a slightly higher trend of gingivitis on the right half of the arch when compared with the left half. This may be due to the difficulty that right-handed people have in brushing the right half of the mouth.

The thorough and conscientious removal of plaque will not only prevent gingivitis from occurring but will also prevent or at least retard the calcification of plaque, which results in calculus. Histologically, the calcification of plaque has been observed as early as 4 to 8 hours. Clinically, the calcification of plaque has been observed as early as 48 hours.[160] The dynamics of calculus formation in heavy calculus formers are illustrated in Figure 22–12.[26] Following a thorough prophylaxis, calculus was clinically detected in measurable

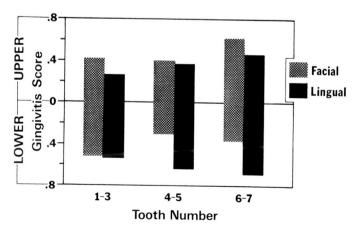

Figure 22–11 **Intraoral Distribution of Gingivitis Severity by Tooth Surface and Area of Mouth.** Data are for 400 males, 15–34 years of age. The Dental Health Center Index (DHCI) was used to assess gingivitis by marginal and papillary units for all teeth. Tooth numbers are defined as follows: 1 = central incisor, 2 = lateral incisor, 3 = canine, 4 = first premolar, 5 = second premolar, 6 = first molar, 7 = second molar. Adapted from Suomi and Barbano.[155]

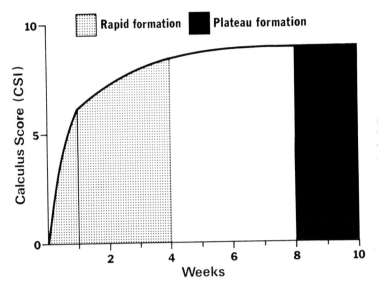

Figure 22–12 **Rate of Calculus Formation.** Data are for 39 subjects who were heavy calculus formers. The Calculus Surface Index (CSI) was used to assess calculus on the four mandibular incisors. Adapted from Conroy and Sturzenberger.[26]

quantities by the end of the first week, the most rapid period of formation. The rapid formation of calculus continued until the fourth week and then the rate started to diminish until it reached a plateau at eight weeks. Hence, the significance of this study is that it provides an upper limit on the rate of calculus formation that may be expected in some people.

The intraoral pattern of supra- and subgingival calculus by individual teeth appears in Figure 22–13.[143] For supragingival calculus, the upper first molars followed by the lower centrals and laterals had the most calculus and the upper anteriors (centrals, laterals, and canines) had the least calculus. For subgingival calculus, the lower centrals and laterals followed by the upper first molars had the most calculus; the upper anteriors (centrals, laterals, and canines)

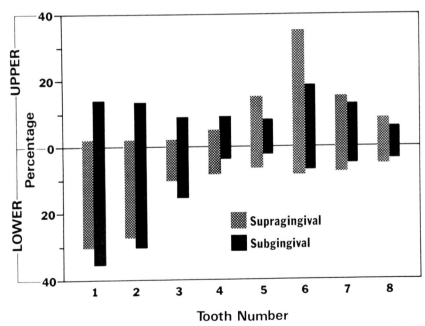

Figure 22–13 **Intraoral Prevalence of Calculus by Individual Teeth.** The percentage of supra and subgingival calculus is presented by tooth and arch. Tooth numbers are defined in Figure 22–11. Adapted from Schroeder.[143]

and upper second molars had intermediate percentages of calculus; the lower first and second premolars and the lower third molars had the least calculus. Combining both supra- and subgingival calculus, the lower centrals and laterals and the upper first molars had the most calculus; the upper second premolars and the upper second molars had intermediate percentages of calculus; the lower second premolars and the lower third molars had the least calculus.[112, 143]

In general, the severity of bone loss follows the intraoral pattern of gingivitis and the intraoral pattern of calculus when supra- and subgingival calculus were combined. The incisors and molar areas are more severely involved than are the canine and premolars areas.[35, 48, 92, 140, 158] with the least bone loss occurring in the lower canine and premolar regions. Bone loss in the maxilla is generally more severe than in the mandible,[10] except for the anterior region, where the situation is reversed.[35, 165] Also, the severity of bone loss is greater interproximally than it is facially and lingually.

The upper and lower limits of the various patterns of plaque, gingivitis, calculus, and bone loss all converge to produce the intraoral pattern of periodontal disease by individual teeth in Figure 22–14.[17] The end result of all of the above parameters shows that the *teeth that are the most severely affected* by periodontal disease are the lower centrals and laterals and upper molars (first, second, and third). The *teeth that are moderately affected* by periodontal disease are the lower molars (first, second, and third), the upper centrals, laterals, and premolars (first and second), and the lower canine; the *teeth that are the least affected* are the lower premolars (first and second) and the upper canines.

THE RELATIONSHIP BETWEEN PERIODONTAL DISEASE AND DENTAL CARIES

Even though numerous investigators have attempted to determine a relationship between the occurrence of periodontal disease and dental caries, no clear-cut positive or negative relationship between the two has been established.[24, 51, 65, 72] Some investigators consider them antagonistic processes with the presence of one precluding the occurrence of the other.[20, 51, 65] Several statistical studies suggest a positive correlation between caries and gingival disease,[16, 146] but this has not been substantiated.[30, 67, 165] Although both diseases share

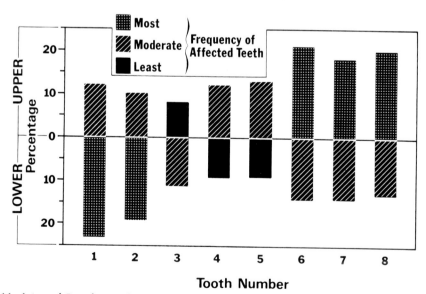

Figure 22–14 Intraoral Prevalence of Periodontal Disease by Individual Teeth. The percentages of teeth affected by periodontal disease are classified as most, moderate, and least. Data are for industrial workers 40–44 years of age, with males and females combined. Tooth numbers are defined in previous figures. Adapted from Bossert and Marks.[17]

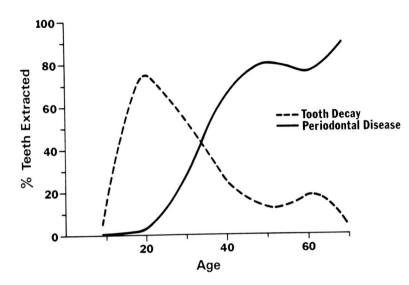

Figure 22–15 **Tooth Extractions Due to Dental Caries and Periodontal Disease.** A comparison of the percentage of teeth indicated for extraction due to caries and periodontal disease by age was determined from almost 225,000 dental records of the U.S. Public Health Service facilities from 1948 through 1952. Adapted from Pelton, Pennell, and Druzina.[113]

dental plaque as their etiology, caries and periodontal disease appear to be two independent processes.[91, 165]

The terminal result of either dental caries or periodontal disease is the loss of teeth. Hence, comparing the percentages of teeth extracted because of caries and periodontal disease will provide a common denominator for describing the relationship between the two processes. Figure 22–15[113] shows that extractions due to caries start shortly after the teeth erupt in the mouth and reaches its greatest prevalence at approximately 20 years of age and gradually decreases in a skewed pattern. The greatest incidence of tooth extraction due to periodontal disease occurs between 20 and 50 years of age, and **after 35 years of age more teeth are lost because of periodontal disease than dental caries.**[2, 3]

It has been shown that periodontal disease is responsible for approximately **50 per cent** of the total tooth loss after age **15**, and caries for approximately **38 per cent**, with the remainder of teeth lost by other causes such as accidents, impactions, orthodontic or prosthetic reasons.[113]

REFERENCES

1. Ainsworth, N. J., and Young, M.: The incidence of dental disease in children. Med. Res. Council, Special Report Series No. 97. London, His Majesty's Stationery Office, 1925.
2. Allen, E. F.: Statistical study of the primary causes of extraction. J. Dent. Res., 23:453, 1944.
3. Andrews, G., and Krogh, H. W.: Permanent tooth mortality. Dent. Progress, 1:130, 1961.
4. Arno, A., Schei, O., Lovdal, A., and Waerhaug, J.: Alveolar bone loss as a function of tobacco consumption. Acta Odont. Scand., 17:3, 1959.
5. Arno, A., Waerhaug, J., Lovdal, A., and Schei, O.: Incidence of gingivitis as related to sex, occupation, tobacco consumption, toothbrushing and age. Oral Surg., 11:587, 1958.
6. Ash, M. M., Gitlin, B. N., and Smith, W. A.: Correlation between plaque and gingivitis. J. Periodontol., 35:424, 1964.
7. Ast, D. B., and Schlesinger, E. R.: The conclusion of a ten-year study of fluoridation. Am. J. Pub. Health, 46:265, 1956.
8. Baer, P. N., and Benjamin, S. D.: Periodontal Disease in Children and Adolescents. Philadelphia, J.B. Lippincott Co., 1974, pp. 139–181.
9. Balendra, W.: The effect of betel chewing on the dental and oral tissues and its possible relationship to buccal carcinoma. Br. Dent. J., 87:83, 1949.
10. Beagrie, G. S., and James, G. A.: The association of posterior tooth irregularity and periodontal disease. Br. Dent. J., 113:239, 1962.
10a. Bellini, H. T.: A system to determine the periodontal therapeutic needs of a population. Universitetsforlagets trykningssentral, Oslo, 1973.
11. Benjamin, E. M., Russell, A. L., and Smiley, R. D.: Periodontal disease in rural children of 25 Indian countries. J. Periodontol., 28:294, 1957.
12. Beube, F. E., Schwartz, M., and Thompson, R. H.: A comparison of effectiveness in plaque removal of an electric toothbrush and a conventional hand toothbrush. Periodontics, 2:71, 1964.
13. Bjorby, A., and Löe, H.: The relative significance

of different local factors in the initiation and development of periodontal inflammation. J. Periodont. Res., 2:76 (Abstract), 1967.

14. Bjorn, H., Halling, A., and Thyberg, H.: Radiographic assessment of marginal bone loss. Odont. Revy, 20:165, 1969.

15. Bjorn, H., and Holmberg, K.: Radiographic determination of periodontal bone destruction in epidemiological research. Odont. Revy, 17:232, 1966.

16. Black, G. V.: Something of the etiology and early pathology of the diseases of the periodontal membrane with suggestions as to treatment. Dent. Cosmos, 55:1219, 1913.

17. Bossert, W. A., and Marks, H. H.: Prevalence and characteristics of periodontal disease of 12,800 persons under periodic dental observation. J. Am. Dent. Assoc., 52:429, 1956.

18. Bowden, D. E. J., Davies, R. M., Holloway, P. J., Lennon, M. A., and Rugg-Gunn, A. J.: A treatment need survey of a 15-year old population. Br. Dent. J., 134:375, 1973.

19. Brandtzaeg, P., and Jamison, H. C.: The effect of controlled cleansing of the teeth on periodontal health and oral hygiene in Norwegian Army Recruits. J. Periodontol., 35:308, 1964.

20. Broderick, F. W.: Antagonism between dental caries and pyorrhea. Am. Dent. Surg., 49:103, 1929.

21. Burnham, C. E.: Edentulous Persons, United States 1971. Washington, D.C., U.S.P.H.S., U.S. Department of Health, Education and Welfare, National Center for Health Statistics, Publication No. (HRA) 74–1516. Series 10, No. 89, 1974.

22. Campbell, H. G., and Cook, R. P.: Incidence of gingivitis at Dundee Dental Hospital. Year Book of Dentistry. Chicago, Year Book Publishers, 1942.

23. Chilton, N. W. (ed.): International conference on clinical trials of agents used in the prevention/treatment of periodontal diseases. J. Periodont. Res., 9:7–211 (Suppl. 14), 1974.

24. Citron, J.: About the question of the internal etiology of paradentosis. Zahnärztl. Rdsch., 37:1319, 1928.

25. Cohen, D. W., and Ship, I. I. (eds.): Clinical methods in periodontal diseases based on a conference held on May 20-23, 1967. J. Periodontol., 38:580-795, 1967.

26. Conroy, C. W., and Sturzenberger, O. P.: The rate of calculus formation in adults. J. Periodontol., 39:142, 1968.

27. Davies, G. N.: Social customs and habits and their effect on oral disease. J. Dent. Res., 42:209, 1963.

28. Day, C. D. Marshall-: Chronic endemic fluorosis in Northern India. Br. Dent. J., 68:409, 1940.

29. Day, C. D. Marshall-: The epidemiology of periodontal disease. J. Periodontol., 22:13, 1951.

30. Day, C. D. Marshall-: Nutritional deficiencies and dental caries in northern India. Br. Dent. J., 76:115, 143, 1944.

31. Day, C. D. Marshall-: Periodontal disease: Present status and interpretation of epidemio-

logical research. In Muhler, J. C., and Hine, M. K.: A Symposium on Preventive Dentistry. St. Louis, The C.V. Mosby Co., 1956, p. 174.

32. Day, C. D. Marshall-, and Shourie, K. L.: Gingival disease in the Virgin Islands, J. Am. Dent. Assoc., 40:175, 1950.

33. Day, C. D. Marshall-, and Shourie, K. L.: Hypertrophic gingivitis in Indian children and adolescents. Ind. J Med. Res., 35:261, 1947.

34. Day, C. D. Marshall- and Shourie, K. L.: The incidence of periodontal disease in the Punjab. Ind. J. Med. Res., 32:47, 1944.

35. Day, C. D. Marshall-, and Shourie, K. L.: A roentgenographic study of periodontal disease in India. J. Am. Dent. Assoc., 39:572, 1949.

36. Day, C. D. Marshall-, Stephens, R. G., and Quigley, L. F.: Periodontal disease: Prevalence and incidence. J. Periodontol., 26:185, 1955.

37. Day, C. D. Marshall-, and Tandan, G. C.: The incidence of dental caries in the Punjab. Br. Dent. J., 69:389, 1940.

38. Downer, M. C.: Dental caries and periodontal disease in girls of different ethnic groups: A comparison in a London secondary school. Br. Dent J., 128:379, 1970.

39. Dunning, J. M.: Principles of Dental Public Health. 2nd ed., Cambridge, Harvard University Press, 1970, pp. 68–69, 161–162.

40. Dunning, J. M., and Leach, L. B.: Gingival-bone count: A method for epidemiological study of periodontal disease. J. Dent. Res., 39:506, 1960.

41. Dutta, A.: A study on prevalence of periodontal disease and dental caries amongst the school-going children in Calcutta. J. All Ind. Dent. Assn., 37:367, 1965.

42. Elliot, J. R., Bowers, G. M., Clemmen, B. A., and Rovelstad, G. H.: Evaluation of an oral physiotherapy center in the reduction of bacterial plaque and periodontal disease. J. Periodontol., 43:221, 1972.

43. Emslie, R. D.: Formal discussion. In Ramfjord, S. P.: Design of studies or clinical trials to evaluate the effectiveness of agents or procedures for the prevention, or treatment, of loss of the periodontium. J. Periodont. Res., 9:78 (Suppl. 14), 1974.

44. Englander, H. R., Kesel, R. G., and Gupta, O. P.: Effect of natural fluoride on the periodontal health of adults. Am. J. Publ. Health, 53:1233, 1963.

45. Englander, H. R., and White, C. L.: Periodontal and oral hygiene status of teenagers in optimum and fluoride-deficient cities. J. Am. Dent. Assoc., 68:173, 1964.

46. Ennever, J., Sturzenberger, O. P., and Radike, A. W.: Calculus surface index for scoring clinical calculus studies. J. Periodontol., 32:54, 1961.

47. Everett, F. G., and Fixott, H. C.: Use of an incorporated grid in the diagnosis of oral roentgenograms. Oral Surg., 16:1061, 1963.

48. Fleming, W. C.: Localization of pyorrhea involvement. Dent. Cosmos, 54:538, 1926.

49. Gjermo, P.: Formal discussion. *In* Hazen, S. P.: Indices for the measurement of gingival inflammation in clinical studies of oral hygiene and periodontal disease. J. Periodont. Res., 9:61 (Suppl. 14), 1974.

50. Glass, R. L.: Hand and electric toothbrushing. J. Periodontol., 36:323, 1965.

51. Gottlieb, B.: Zur Aetiologie und Therapie der Alveolarpyorrhoe. Z. Stomatol., 18:59, 1920.

52. Greene, J. C.: Oral hygiene and periodontal disease. Am. J. Publ. Health, 53:913, 1963.

53. Greene, J. C.: The oral hygiene index—Development and uses. Part II. J. Periodontol., 38:625, 1967.

54. Greene, J. C.: Periodontal disease in India: Report of an epidemiological study. J. Dent. Res., 39:302, 1960.

55. Greene, J. C., and Vermillion, J. R.: Oral hygiene index: A method for classifying oral hygiene status. J. Am. Dent. Assoc., 61:172, 1960.

56. Greene, J. C., and Vermillion, J. R.: The simplified oral hygiene index. J. Am. Dent. Assoc., 68:7, 1964.

57. Horton, J. E., and Sumnicht, R. W.: Relationships of educational levels to periodontal disease and oral hygiene with variables of age and geographic regions. J. Periodontol., 38:335, 1967.

58. James, P. M. C., et al.: Gingival health and dental cleanliness in English school children. Arch. Oral Biol., 3:57, 1960.

59. Jamison, H. C.: Prevalence of periodontal disease of the deciduous teeth. J. Am. Dent. Assoc., 66:207, 1963.

60. Johnson, E. S., Kelly, J. E., and VanKirk, L. E.: Selected Dental Findings in Adults by Age, Race and Sex, United States 1960–1962. Washington, D.C., U.S. Department of Health, Education and Welfare, National Center for Health Statistics, Publication No. 1000, Series 11, No. 7, 1965.

61. Jorkjend, L., and Birkeland, J. M.: Plaque and gingivitis among Norwegian children participating in a dental health program. Community Dent. Oral Epidemiol., 1:41, 1973.

62. Kelly, J. E., and Sanchez, M. J.: Periodontal Disease and Oral Hygiene Among Children, United States. Washington, D.C., U.S.P.H.S., U.S. Department of Health, Education and Welfare, National Center for Health Statistics, Publication No. (HSM) 72–1060, Series 11, No. 117, 1972.

63. Kelly, J. E., and Van Kirk, L. E.: Periodontal Disease in Adults, United States 1960–1962. Washington, D.C., U.S.P.H.S., U.S. Department of Health, Education and Welfare, National Center for Health Statistics, Publication No. 1000, Series 11, No. 12, 1966.

64. Kelly, J. E., Van Kirk, L. E., and Garst, C. C.: Oral Hygiene in Adults, United States 1960–1962. Washington, D.C., U.S.P.H.S., U.S. Department of Health, Education and Welfare, National Center for Health Statistics, Publication No. 1000, Series 11, No. 16, 1966.

65. Kesel, R. G.: Are dental caries and periodontal disease incompatible? J. Periodontol. 21:30, 1950.

66. King, J. D.: Dental disease in the Isle of Lewis. Medical Research Council, Special Report Series, No. 241. London, His Majesty's Stationery Office, 1940.

67. King, J. D.: Gingival disease in Dundee, Dent. Record, 65:9, 32, 55, 1945.

68. King, J. D., Franklyn, A. B., and Allen, I.: Gingival disease in Gibraltar evacuee children. Lancet, 1:495, 1944.

69. Körber, K. H.: Electronic registration of tooth movements. Int. Dent. J., 21:466, 1971.

70. Körber, K. H.: Periodontal pulsation. J. Periodontol., 41:382, 1970.

71. Körber, K. H., and Körber, E.: Untersuchungen Zur Biophysik des Parodontiums. Dtsch. Zahnärztl. Z., 17:1585, 1962.

72. Landgraph, E., und Banhigyi, S.: Untersuchungen über den Cholesterin-, Bilirubin- und Reservealkaligehalte des Blutes bei Paradentosekranken. Z. Stomatol., 29:11, 1931.

73. Lobene, R. R.: The effect of an automatic toothbrush on gingival health. J. Periodontol., 35:137, 1964.

74. Löe, H.: The gingival index, the plaque index and the retention index systems. Part II. J. Periodontol., 38:610, 1967.

75. Löe, H., and Silness, J.: Periodontal disease in pregnancy. Acta Odontol. Scand., 21:533, 1963.

76. Löe, H., Theilade, E., and Jensen, S. B.: Experimental gingivitis in man. J. Periodontol., 36:177, 1965.

77. Lovdal, A., Arno, A., and Waerhaug, J.: Incidence of clinical manifestations of periodontal disease in light of oral hygiene and calculus formation. J. Am. Dent Assoc., 56:21, 1958.

78. Lovdal, A., Arno, A., Schei, O., and Waerhaug, J.: Combined effect of subgingival scaling and controlled oral hygiene on the incidence of gingivitis. Acta Odontol. Scand., 19:537, 1961.

79. Mandel, I. D.: Indices for measurement of soft accumulations in clinical studies of oral hygiene and periodontal disease. J. Periodont. Res., 9:7 (Suppl. 14), 1974.

80. Mandel, I. D.: Indices for measurement of soft accumulations in clinical studies of oral hygiene and periodontal disease (Continued). J. Periodont. Res., 9:106 (Suppl. 14), 1974.

Marshall-Day, C. D. See Day.

81. Massler, M.: The P-M-A index for the assessment of gingivitis. Part II. J. Periodontol., 38:592, 1967.

82. Massler, M., and Schour, I.: The P-M-A-index of gingivitis. J. Dent. Res., 28:634 (Abstract), 1949.

83. Massler, M., Cohen, A., and Schour, I.: Epidemiology of gingivitis in children. J. Am. Dent. Assoc., 45:319, 1952.

84. Massler, M., Schour, I., and Chopra, B.: Occurrence of gingivitis in suburban Chicago school children. J. Periodontol., 21:146, 1950.

85. McCall, J. O.: The periodontist looks at children's dentistry. J. Am. Dent. Assoc., 20:1518, 1933.

86. McHugh, W. D., McEven, J. D., and Hitchin, A. D.: Dental disease and related factors in

13-year-old children in Dundee. Brit. Dent. J., *117*:246, 1964.

87. Messner, C. T., Gafaver, W. M., Cady, F. C., and Dean, H. T.: Dental Survey of School Children Ages 6 to 14 Years Made in 1933–1934 in 26 states. Public Health Bulletin 226. Washington, D.C., U.S. Government Printing Office, 1938.

88. Miglani, D.C.: Incidence of acute necrotizing ulcerative gingivitis and periodontosis among cases seen at the government hospital, Madras. J. All India Dent. A., 37:183, 1965.

89. Miller, S. C.: Precocious advanced alveolar atrophy. J. Periodontol., 19:146, 1948.

90. Miller, S. C.: Textbook of Periodontia, 3rd ed., Philadelphia, Blakiston, 1950.

91. Miller, S. C., and Seidler, B. B.: A correlation between periodontal disease and caries. J. Dent Res., 19:549, 1940.

92. Miller, S. C., and Seidler, B. B.: Relative alveoloclastic experience of the various teeth. J. Dent. Res., 21:365, 1942.

93. Moore, R. M., Muhler, J. C., and McDonald, R. E.: A study of the effect of water fluoride content and socio-economic status on the occurrence of gingivitis in school children. J. Dent. Res., 43:782, 1964.

94. Mühlemann, H. R.: Periodontometry, a method for measuring tooth mobility. Oral Surg., 4:1220, 1951.

95. Mühlemann, H. R.: 10 years of tooth-mobility measurements. J. Periodontol., 31:110, 1960.

96. Mühlemann, H. R.: Tooth mobility: I. The measuring method—Initial and secondary tooth mobility. J. Periodontol., 25:125, 1954.

97. Mühlemann, H. R., and Mazor, Z. S.: Gingivitis in Zurich school children. Helv. Odontol. Acta, 2:3, 1958.

98. Mühlemann, H. R., and Villa, P.: The marginal line calculus index. Helv. Odontol. Acta, 11:175, 1967.

99. Murray, J. J.: Gingivitis and gingival recession in adults from high-fluoride and low-fluoride areas. Arch. Oral. Biol., 17:1269, 1972.

100. Murray, J. J.: Gingivitis in 15-year old children from high fluoride and low fluoride areas. Arch. Oral Biol., 14:951, 1969.

101. Murray, J. J.: The prevalence of gingivitis in children continuously resident in a high fluoride area. J. Dent. Child., 41:133, 1974.

102. Newman, M. G.: Periodontosis. J. West. Soc. Periodontol., 24:5, 1976.

103. Nizel, A. E.: The Science of Nutrition and Its Application in Clinical Dentistry, 2nd ed. Philadelphia, W. B. Saunders Company, 1966, pp. 408–420.

104. O'Leary, T. J.: Indices for measurement of tooth mobility in clinical studies. J. Periodont. Res., 9:94 (Suppl. 14), 1974.

105. O'Leary, T. J.: The periodontal screening examination. J. Periodontol., 38:617, 1967.

106. O'Leary, T. J., and Rudd, K. D.: An instrument for measuring horizontal tooth mobility. USAF School of Aerospace Medicine TDR 63–58, August 1963. Periodontics, 1:249, 1963.

107. O'Leary, T., Gibson, W. A., Shannon, I. L., Schuessler, C. F., and Nabers, C. L.: A screening examination for detection of gingival and periodontal breakdown and local irritants. Periodontics, 1:167, 1963.

108. Orban, B.: Classification of periodontal disease. Parodontologie, 4:159, 1949.

109. Parfitt, G. J.: Development of an instrument to measure tooth mobility, J. Dent Res., 37:64 (Abstract), 1958.

110. Parfitt, G. J.: A five year longitudinal study of the gingival condition of a group of children in England. J. Periodontol., 28:26, 1957.

111. Parfitt, G. J.: Measurement of the physiological mobility of individual teeth in an axial direction. J. Dent. Res., 39:608, 1960.

112. Parfitt, G. J.: A survey of the oral health of Navajo Indian children. Arch. Oral Biol., 1:193, 1959.

113. Pelton, W. J., Pennell, E. H., and Druzina, A.: Tooth morbidity experience of adults. J. Am. Dent. Assoc., 49:439, 1954.

114. Picton, D. C. A.: A method of measuring physiological tooth movements in man. J. Dent. Res., 36:814, 1957.

115. Picton, D. C. A.: A study of normal tooth mobility and the changes with periodontal disease. Dent. Pract., 12:167, 1962.

116. Podshadley, A. G., and Haley, J. V.: A method for evaluating patient hygiene performance by observation of selected tooth surfaces. Publ. Health Rep., 83:259, 1968.

117. Quigley, G., and Hein, J.: Comparative cleansing efficiency of manual and power brushing. J. Am. Dent. Assoc., 65:26, 1962.

118. Ramfjord, S. P.: Design of studies or clinical trials to evaluate the effectiveness of agents or procedures for the prevention, or treatment, of loss of the periodontium. J. Periodont. Res., 9:78, (Suppl. 14), 1974.

119. Ramfjord, S. P.: Indices for prevalence and incidence of periodontal disease. J. Periodontol., 30:51, 1959.

120. Ramfjord, S. P.: The periodontal index (PDI). J. Periodontol., 38:602, 1967.

121. Ramfjord, S. P.: The periodontal status of boys 11 to 17 years old in Bombay, India. J. Periodontol., 32:237, 1961.

122. Rao, S. S., and Tewani, S. V.: Prevalence of periodontosis among Indians. J. Periodontol., 37:27, 1968.

123. Ruffer, M. A.: Studies in the Palaeopathology of Ancient Egypt. Chicago, University of Chicago Press, 1921.

124. Russell, A. L.: Epidemiology and the rational bases of dental public health and dental practice. In Young, W. O., and Striffler, D. F.: The Dentist, His Practice, and His Community, 2nd ed. Philadelphia, W. B. Saunders Company, 1969, pp. 35–57.

125. Russell, A. L.: The epidemiology of dental caries and periodontal diseases. In Young, W. O., and Striffler, D. F.: The Dentist, His Practice, and His Community, 2nd ed. Philadelphia, W.B. Saunders Company, 1969, pp. 73–86.

126. Russell, A. L.: Epidemiology of periodontal disease. Int. Dent. J., 17:282, 1967.

127. Russell, A. L.: Fluoride, domestic water and periodontal disease. Am. J. Publ. Health, 47:688, 1957.

128. Russell, A. L.: The Geographical Distribution and

Epidemiology of Periodontal Disease. World Health Organization Expert Committee on Dental Health (Periodontal Disease). WHO/DH/34. Geneva, 1960.

129. Russell, A. L.: International nutrition surveys: A summary of preliminary dental findings. J. Dent. Res., 42:233, 1963.

130. Russell, A. L.: The periodontal index. J. Periodontol., 38:585, 1967.

131. Russell, A. L.: The prevalence of periodontal disease in different populations during the circumpubertal period. J. Periodontol., 42:508, 1971.

132. Russell, A. L.: A social factor associated with the severity of periodontal disease. J. Dent. Res., 36:922, 1957.

133. Russell, A. L.: Some epidemiological characteristics of periodontal disease in a series of urban populations. J. Periodontol., 28:286, 1957.

134. Russell, A. L.: A system of classification and scoring for prevalence surveys of periodontal disease. J. Dent Res., 35:350, 1956.

135. Russell, A. L., and Ayers, P.: Periodontal disease and socio-economic status in Birmingham, Ala. Am. J. Publ. Health, 50:206, 1960.

136. Russell, A. L., Leatherwood, E. C., Consolazio, C. F., and Van Reen, R.: Periodontal disease and nutrition in South Vietnam. J. Dent. Res., 44:775, 1965.

137. Sanchez, M. J.: Oral Hygiene Among Youths 12–17 Years, United States. Washington, D.C., U.S.P.H.S., U.S. Department of Health, Education and Welfare, National Center for Health Statistics, Publication No. (HRA) 76–1633, Series 11, No. 151, 1975.

138. Sanchez, M. J.: Periodontal Disease Among Youths 12–17 Years, United States. Washington, D.C., U.S.P.H.S., U.S. Department of Health, Education and Welfare, National Center for Health Statistics, Publication No. (HRA) 74–1623, Series 11, No. 141, 1974.

139. Sartwell, P. E. (ed.): Maxcy-Rosenau Preventive Medicine and Public Health, 10th ed., New York, Appleton-Century-Crofts, 1973, pp. 1–58.

140. Schei, O., Waerhaug, J., Lovdal, A., and Arno, A.: Alveolar bone loss as related to oral hygiene and age. J. Periodontol., 30:7, 1959.

141. Schour, I., and Massler, M.: Gingival disease in postwar Italy (1945). I. Prevalence of gingivitis in various age groups. J. Am. Dent. Assoc., 35:475, 1947.

142. Schour, I., and Massler, M.: Survey of gingival disease using the PMA index. J. Dent. Res., 27:733, 1948.

143. Schroeder, H. E.: Formation and Inhibition of Dental Calculus. Berne, H. Huber Publishers, 1969, pp. 66–68.

144. Shapiro, S., Pollack, B. R., and Gallant, D.: A special population available for periodontal research. Part II. A correlation and association analysis between oral hygiene and periodontal disease. J. Periodontol., 42:161, 1971.

145. Shaw, J. H., and Sweeney, E. A.: Nutrition in relation to dental medicine. In Goodhart, R. S., and Shils, M. E. (eds.): Modern Nutrition in Health and Disease: Dietotherapy, 5th ed. Philadelphia, Lea and Febiger, 1973, pp. 756–764.

146. Shay, H., and Smart, G. A.: The association of local factors with gingivitis. Br. Dent. J., 78:135, 1945.

147. Sheiham, A.: The epidemiology of chronic periodontal disease in Western Nigerian children. J. Periodont. Res., 3:257, 1968.

148. Sheiham, A.: The prevalence and severity of periodontal disease in Surrey school children. Dent. Pract., 19:232, 1969.

149. Sheiham, A., and Striffler, D. F.: A comparison of four epidemiological methods of assessing periodontal disease. J. Periodont. Res., 5:148, 1970.

150. Shick, R. A., and Ash, M. M.: Evaluation of the vertical method of toothbrushing. J. Periodontol., 32:346, 1961.

151. Silness, P., and Löe, J.: Periodontal disease in pregnancy. Acta Odontol. Scand., 22:121, 1964.

152. Smith, L. W., Suomi, J. D., Greene, J. C., and Barbano, J. P.: A study of intraexaminer variation in scoring oral hygiene status, gingival inflammation and epithelial attachment level. J. Periodontol., 41:671, 1970.

153. Stahl, D. G., and Goldman, H. M.: Incidence of gingivitis among a sample of Massachusetts school children. Oral Surg., 6:707, 1953.

154. Summers, C., and Oberman, A.: Association of oral disease with twelve selected variables. I. Periodontal disease. J. Dent. Res., 47:457, 1968.

155. Suomi, J. D., and Barbano, J. P.: Patterns of gingivitis. J. Periodontol., 39:71, 1968.

156. Suomi, J. D., Greene, J. C., Vermillion, J. R., Doyle, J., Chang, J. J., and Leatherwood, E. C.: The effect of controlled oral hygiene procedures on the progression of periodontal disease in adults: Results after third and final year. J. Periodontol., 42:152, 1971.

157. Suomi, J. D., Plumbo, J., and Barbano, J. P.: A comparative study of radiographs and pocket measurements in periodontal disease evaluation. J. Periodontol., 39:311, 1968.

158. Tenenbaum, B., Karshan, M., Ziskin, D., and Nahoun, K. I.: Clinical and microscopic study of the gingivae in periodontosis. J. Am. Dent. Assoc., 40:302, 1950.

159. Ten-State Nutrition Survey 1968–1970, by Health Services and Mental Health Administration, U.S. Department of Health, Education and Welfare. Atlanta Center for Disease Control. Atlanta, Publication No. (HSM) 72–8131, 1972, volume III, pp. 126–131.

160. Tibbetts, L. S., and Kashiwa, H. K.: A histochemical study of early plaque mineralization. In I.A.D.R. Program and Abstracts of Papers, Abstract No. 616, p. 202, 1970.

161. Turesky, S., Gilmore, N. D., and Glickman, I.: Reduced plaque formation by the chloromethyl analogue of victamine C. J. Periodontol., 41:41, 1970.

162. Volpe, A. R.: Indices for the measurement of hard deposits in clinical studies of oral hygiene and periodontal disease. J. Periodont. Res., 9:31 (Suppl. 14), 1974.

163. Volpe, A. R., Manhold, J. H., and Hazen, S. P.: In

vivo calculus assessment: A method and its reproducibility. J. Periodontol., *36*:292, 1965

164. Wade, A. B.: Validity of anterior segment gingival scores in epidemiologic studies. J. Periodontol., *37*:55, 1966.

165. White, C. L., and Russell, A. L.: Some relations between dental caries experience and active periodontal disease in two thousand adults. N.Y. J. Dent., *32*:211, 1962.

166. Wilkinson, F. C., Adamson, K. T., and Knight, F.: A study of the incidence of dental disease in the aborigines, from the examination of 65 in the collection found in the Melbourne University. Austr. J. Dent., *33*:109, 1929.

167. Zimmerman, E. R., and Baker, W. A.: Effect of geographic location and race on gingival disease in children. J. Am. Dent. Assoc., *61*: 542, 1960.

Interaction of Etiologic Factors in Periodontal Disease

Etiologic factors of periodontal disease have customarily been classified into local and systemic, although their effects are interrelated. *Local factors* are those in the immediate environment of the periodontium, while *systemic factors* result from the general condition of the patient.

Local factors cause inflammation, which is the principal pathologic process in periodontal disease; systemic factors monitor the tissue response to local factors, so that the effect of local irritants may be dramatically aggravated by unfavorable systemic conditions. The following diagram, modified from that developed by A. Bahn[1], shows in schematic form the role of the different factors:

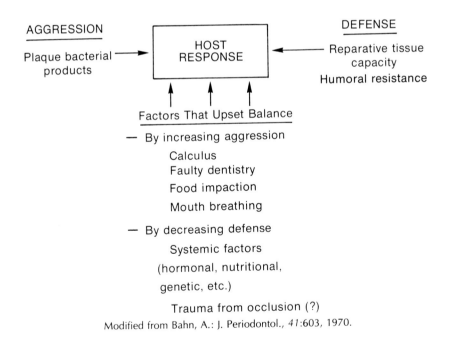

AGGRESSION

Plaque bacterial products

HOST RESPONSE

DEFENSE

Reparative tissue capacity

Humoral resistance

Factors That Upset Balance

— By increasing aggression

 Calculus

 Faulty dentistry

 Food impaction

 Mouth breathing

— By decreasing defense

 Systemic factors

 (hormonal, nutritional,

 genetic, etc.)

Trauma from occlusion (?)

Modified from Bahn, A.: J. Periodontol., *41*:603, 1970.

Plaque is necessary to initiate the disease. A small but variable amount of plaque can, however, be controlled by the body defense mechanisms, resulting in an equilibrium between aggression and defense. This equilibrium can be broken either by increasing the amount and/or the virulence of the bacteria, or by reducing the defensive capacity of the tissues. The following factors favor the accumulation of plaque: calculus, inadequate restorations, food impaction, and mouth breathing.

Factors that reduce the defensive capacity of the tissues include all the systemic conditions that may disturb the tissue response to irritation. Their exact mechanism of action is in most cases obscure. The possibility that in some cases they may act by producing changes in the oral flora has not been adequately explored.

It should also be clearly understood that other diseases besides periodontal disease can attack the periodontal tissues. These other diseases may result from a variety of causes, by direct extension from the oral mucosa or the jaw bones or owing to a systemic involvement. Within this group of diseases which we shall term "periodontal manifestations of other diseases," the following can be found: herpetic gingivostomatitis, tuberculous, syphilitic and other bacterial infections, monilial infections and other mycoses, different dermatoses such as lichen planus, pemphigus, erythema multiforme, blood diseases such as acute leukemia, and various benign and malignant tumors.

Systemic factors can therefore act either by reducing tissue resistance to plaque or by producing changes *per se*. In the former case the resulting disease will be periodontal disease; in the latter it will be a periodontal manifestation of the systemic disease.

REFERENCE

1. Bahn, A.: Microbial potential in the etiology of periodontal disease. J. Periodontol., *41*:603, 1970.

The Host Response in Periodontal Disease

The state of periodontal health or disease depends upon the interaction between the resident microbiota and the host response.

Emphasis in periodontal disease research has been focused on understanding the immunopathologic mechanisms which may operate in the development and maintenance of periodontal inflammatory changes. This chapter will briefly review the basis of the immunologic and inflammatory responses as they may relate to the etiology and pathogenesis of periodontal diseases.

Previous investigators have considered periodontal disease to be one disease process in which the nature and severity differed according to the individual's host resistance and the specific etiologic and predisposing factors present.[91] Recent evidence suggests that the term "periodontal disease" may represent different diseases of the periodontium, each demonstrating unique clinical, bacterial, pathologic, biochemical, and immunologic patterns.[140, 142, 165] In most individuals, the host response mechanisms depend on the presence of specific microorganisms and their particular toxic and/or antigenic products.[13, 111, 126, 147, 171] The nature and severity of periodontal pathology are modified by factors such as leukocytic defects,[19, 22] mechanical and traumatic forces, drug ingestion, nutritional deficiencies, systemic disease, and age.

The histopathology of gingivitis and periodontitis suggests that an immunologic response occurs in the pathogenesis of these diseases (Fig. 23–1). Inflammation in the periodontal tissues is triggered by the continuous presence of antigenic and non-antigenic bacterial products from the dental plaque microorganisms. The gingival tissues are infiltrated with plasma cells, which produce immunoglobulins potentially active in immediate hypersensitivity and immune complex disease. Lymphocytes, which are active in cell-mediated reactions, as well as mast cells, polymorphonuclear leukocytes, and macrophages, are found in these tissues. Although inflammation is a defense mechanism by which the body localizes and destroys foreign materials, the host's own tissues may be destroyed in the process.[140] Thus,

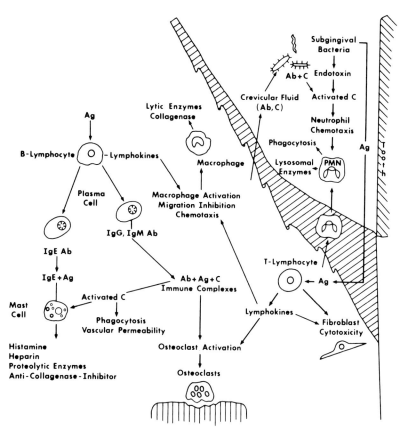

Figure 23–1   Immunologic Responses in Gingivitis and Periodontitis. Potential immunopathologic processes which may occur in the course of human gingivitis and periodontitis. (From Nisengard, R. J.: J. Periodontol., 48:505, 1977.)

inflammation may account for part of the tissue loss seen in the course of human periodontal disease.

INITIAL HOST RESPONSE

As a consequence of bacteria or their products in the gingival sulcus, an initial vascular response occurs. This consists of increased blood flow and permeability of the small vessels of the gingiva.[34, 35] Serum components, fibrin, erythrocytes, and granulocytes accumulate and form an inflammatory exudate. Clinically, this type of response can occur in two to four days of plaque accumulation and is characterized as acute gingivitis.[126] The events which take place as a result of the host's response may be protective or destructive.

The nature and character of the host response determines whether this initial lesion resolves rapidly, with the tissue restored to normal, or evolves into a chronic inflammatory lesion. If the latter occurs, an infiltrate of macrophages and lymphoid cells appears in a few days.[126]

The acute inflammatory exudate and the changes in the microcirculation are induced by chemical substances released in the gingiva. Increased vascular permeability is due to release of histamine, 5-hydroxytryptamine, kinins, complement components, and prostaglandins. Histamine is released from mast cells, platelets, and endothelial cells. Mast cell degranulation occurs by interaction with bacteria, endotoxins, IgE, immune complexes, complement components, mechanical trauma, basic peptides, and proteolytic enzymes.[70, 140]

The   increased   permeability   which

occurs in the gingival microvasculature increases the cells and chemical constituents which have the potential to cause tissue damage. The resulting edema, together with leakage of the junctional epithelium, allows the flow of gingival fluid into the gingival sulcus. Because of its cellular and chemical, constituents, the fluid could serve to neutralize bacteria and their products, and/or furnish essential nutrients to potentially pathogenic organisms located deep in periodontal pockets.[110] The presence of the protein-rich gingival fluid is a very important ecologic factor favoring the accumulation and growth of the protein- and amino acid–requiring gram-negative rods and spirochetes. These organisms increase in number during the development of gingivitis and in periodontitis (see Chap. 24).

INFLAMMATORY CELL RESPONSE

In response to specific biochemical stimuli, inflammatory cells migrate (chemotaxis) and concentrate in localized areas where they phagocytize bacteria or their components (Fig. 23–1). Some of these cells increase in number (blastogenesis), release vasoactive products, and may produce substances that cause the lysis of other host cells or the destruction of alveolar bone.[140] The cells involved are mast cells, polymorphonuclear leukocytes (PMN's or neutrophils), macrophages, and lymphocytes.

Mast Cells

Mast cells may play a role in the pathogenesis of gingivitis and periodontitis, since their numbers are inversely related to the degree of gingival inflammation.[17, 27, 32, 143, 156, 157, 188] Normal gingiva contains more mast cells per area than does moderately inflamed tissue. Severely inflamed gingiva contains the fewest mast cells.[17] This has suggested that degranulation occurs during the development of periodontal disease. Mast cell counts decrease during periodontitis and increase following successful periodontal therapy.[111] During periods of decrease, mast cell granules are seen in tissue spaces.[4, 5, 6]

Mast cells are important because the granules they release (subsequent to binding by cytophilic IgE antibody) could in turn release histamine and other factors into the gingival tissues.[8, 57, 75, 178] These reactions form the basis of anaphylaxis. In addition, a mast cell "factor" has recently been shown to enhance collagenase activity,[173] and heparin (contained in other granules)[85] may enhance bone resorption[51] by potentiating the effect of parathyroid hormone (Fig. 23–1).

Neutrophils (PMN's)

Neutrophils are important in the host's defense against injury and infection. These cells are found in all inflammatory lesions, where they concentrate at sites of injury and engulf, kill, and digest microorganisms and neutralize other noxious substances (Fig. 23–1). In periodontal diseases, neutrophils apparently play both a protective and a destructive role.[2, 84, 111, 126, 140, 152, 174] When these cells are depressed in number, as in cyclic neutropenia,[22] or in function, as in idiopathic juvenile periodontitis (periodontosis),[10] periodontal destruction is more severe.

In idiopathic juvenile periodontitis (periodontosis),[18, 19, 77] there is a reduction in phagocytosis and a decreased response of neutrophils to chemotactic stimuli. Healthy siblings of patients with this disease may also have a chemotactic defect. These alterations may impair host defenses against implicated gram-negative bacteria. A similar severe alveolar bone loss occurs in other disorders in which there is neutrophil dysfunction: cyclic neutropenia,[22] agranulocytosis,[7] and Chédiak-Higashi disease.[76, 175] Neutrophil defects have been described in patients with chronic infections[160, 183] and chronic candidiasis[56] and are thought to be responsible for increased incidence of bacterial infections in cirrhosis[92] and rheumatoid arthritis.[104]

PMN's may also cause tissue destruction. Their granules contain substances capable of killing, digesting, and neutralizing microorganisms and/or their products, and they also contain a specific collagenase.[40, 54, 65, 94, 170, 172] The actual evidence that they play a destructive role remains circumstantial. It is important to note that the localized tissue damage seen in the Arthus reaction (see below) depends upon the presence of neutrophils.

Macrophages

Macrophages have direct and important functions in cell-mediated immunity (see below). These large, highly phagocytic cells are part of the scavenger reticuloendothelial system.[31] They participate with T-lymphocytes in aiding the response of B-lymphocytes to many immunogens.[16, 37, 74, 109] This helper function stems from observations which demonstrate that trace amounts of antigen bound to the macrophage surface are far more potent immunogenically than the same amount of free, unbound antigen.[98, 122] In inflammatory lesions, macrophages arise by differentiation of monocytes carried to the lesion by the blood. These cells act nonspecifically with antigens, which provide them with the capability of destroying a diverse, antigenically unrelated group of bacteria.[166]

Macrophages and monocytes are not the most common cell types found in periodontal lesions, but they may play an important role in the pathogenesis of this disease.[127] Mononuclear cells are attracted to sites of inflammation by lymphokines (substances released by lymphocytes) and complement factors, and once present they are retained at these sites by other lymphokines (Fig. 23–1). The ability of the macrophages to ingest, kill, and digest microorganisms is dependent upon interaction with other leukocytes, the immune system in general, and complement. Prior interaction of specific antigens with antibody and complement enhances the ability of macrophages to phagocytize.

Macrophages also appear to produce prostaglandins,[102] cyclic AMP, and collagenase[43, 78, 99, 128-130, 179, 180] in response to stimulation by bacterial endotoxin, immune complexes, or lymphokines. Macrophage collagenase may play a significant role in collagen destruction in the diseased periodontal tissues.

ANTIBODY

The host can respond to the presence of oral bacteria and their products by the production of antibodies, primarily by mature plasma cells. The possible role antibodies may play in periodontal and gingival disease is summarized in Table 23–1.

These proteins, derived from the blood and functioning as antibodies, are the effectors of humoral immunity.[31] They are referred to as immunoglobulins or Ig. All Ig's have a similar structural organization but differ according to their antigenic properties and amino acid sequences. Every antibody molecule has a specific group of antigens with which it can react.

Human Ig's are divided into five classes on the basis of chemical differences and by their biological effects subsequent to antigen binding (Table 23–2). The five classes are called IgG, IgM, IgA, IgE, and IgD. Four subclasses of IgG have been identified (IgG_1, IgG_2, IgG_3, and IgG_4), two subclasses of IgA (IgA_1 and IgA_2), and two subclasses of IgM (IgM_1 and IgM_2). Ig

TABLE 23–1 POSSIBLE ROLE OF ANTIBODIES IN PERIODONTAL AND GINGIVAL DISEASE*

Reaction or Process	Effects
Activation of C' by Ag-Ab complexes	Protective early changes in inflammation
Phagocytosis of Ag-Ab complexes by PMN's with release of lysosomes	Destructive
Enhanced lymphocyte stimulation by Ag-Ab complexes	Release of lymphokines with protective and destructive effects
Blocking of lymphocytes by free antibody or by Ag-Ab complexes	Suppression of cell-mediated immune reactions
Neutralization of bacterial allergins, toxins, or histolytic enzymes	Protective
Enhanced opsonization or bacteriolysis of plaque bacteria	Protective

*Modified from Genco, R., et al.: J. Periodontol., 45:336, 1974.

TABLE 23–2   PROPERTIES OF IMMUNOGLOBULINS*

	IgG				IgA	IgM	IgD	IgE
	1	2	3	4				
Serum concentration (mg./ml.)	total IgG: 12				2	1.2	0.03	0.00004
Complement fixation								
Classic pathway	+	±	+		−	+	−	−
Alternate pathway	+	+	+	?	+	+	−	+
Placental transfer	+	+	+	+	−	−	−	+
Reaginic activity	−	−	−	−	−	−	?	?
Antibacterial lysis	+	+	+	+	+	+	?	?

*From Nisengard, R. J.: J. Periodontol., 48:505, 1977.

molecules are made up of small (light) and enlarged (heavy) polypeptide chains. Each of the five classes of Ig's has similar sets of light chains but antigenically distinct sets of heavy chains. Any particular Ig molecule has identical heavy chains and identical light chains.[31, 36]

A variety of studies have suggested that IgG molecules are Y-shaped. The tail of the Y is made up of a set of heavy chains, the end of which is referred to as the FC fragment. It is in this region that complement binding takes place. The "V" area of the Y-shaped molecule is made up of heavy and light chains and is the FAb or antibody-binding site. The number of these binding sites is called valence.

Biological Properties of Immunoglobulins

IGG. IgG is the most abundant of the serum immunoglobulins and is distributed equally between the blood and the extravascular fluids. Its major role is to neutralize bacterial toxins by binding to organisms enhancing their phagocytosis. Although IgG concentration in serum is very high, its concentration in secretions is low. IgG constitutes 80 per cent of the total serum immunoglobulins, passes the placenta, and provides newborns with the humoral immunity of the mother.[31]

IGM. Antibodies of the IgM class, in contrast to those of the IgG class, are the first to be formed in the immune response and nearly always at low levels. The levels of IgM during the course of an infection become negligible in comparison with those of IgG. However, IgM molecules are composed of five basic immunoglobulin structural units with a correspondingly larger number of sites for interaction with antigen. This early synthesis suggests an important role for IgM in the early stages of infection. IgM is also the most efficient activator of the complement system.[63]

IGE. IgE (reaginic antibody) is present in human sera at about 125,000th the level of IgG. Despite the low concentration, this class of antibody is responsible for severe, acute allergic reactions and may be important in acute phases of periodontal disease. The cells that produce IgE are abundant in mucosa of the respiratory and intestinal tracts, and IgE is also found in exocrine secretion. Higher concentrations of these antibodies are found in patients with asthma, hay fever, and drug and food allergies. This class of antibodies has an affinity for cell surfaces, mediated by an attachment site on their FC fragment. In man the cells to which IgE attach are mast cells and basophilic leukocytes. Thus, when antigens bind with IgE antibodies already attached to mast cells, the antigen-antibody reaction causes histamine and other pharmacologically active substances to be released.[154]

IGD. IgD is an immunoglobulin which is found at extremely low levels in serum, although its role in the immune system is not clear. Recent evidence suggests that it is the antigen receptor on the surface of lymphocytes. It may serve in the important role of triggering lymphocyte stimulation by antigen, thus initiating the immune response.[63]

IGA. IgA occurs in a variety of polymeric forms of the basic IgG molecule from monomer to trimer and even higher forms. IgA is the principal Ig in exocrine secretions (milk, respiratory secretions, intestinal mucin, saliva (see Chap. 25), and tears). It is present at one fifth the concentration of IgG in human serum. The cells that produce IgA are concentrated in the subepithelial tissue of exocrine glands and apparently respond to antigens that are present locally. Serum IgA is mostly monomer, while exocrine IgA is a dimer.

Properties of secretory IgA antibodies make them unique and influence the way in which they function on mucosal surfaces.[156] Secretory IgA is more resistant to digestion with proteolytic enzymes than are other immunoglobulins. It has been suggested that the secretory component of a polypeptide chain which is attached to the FC portion of secretory IgA stabilizes this portion of the molecule, facilitating transport across the glandular epithelium. It is also possible that the J chain, the fourth type of polypeptide chain found associated with secretory IgA, may function in making secretory IgA more resistant to proteolysis. The valance of secretory IgA molecules generally found in saliva is four.[98]

Recently, there has been a wide range of interest regarding the possible protective effects of secretory antibodies against bacterial diseases on mucosal surfaces. Serum IgA, unlike serum IgG and serum IgM, does not have the ability to fix the first component of complement. Recently, an alternative pathway of immunologic activation of the complement system has been described which involves utilization of the latter complement components, C3 through C9, but not C1, C4, or C2 (see section on complement).

Prevention of adhesion of bacteria to tissue surfaces by secretory antibodies may be important.[48a] This mechanism of protection may be active in bacterial diseases such as cholera, dental caries, and in the early phase of periodontal disease, in which bacterial adhesion and colonization of mucosal or dental tissues is a necessary step in pathogenesis[100] (see Chap. 24). The antibacterial role of IgA in established periodontal lesions is unclear, since saliva probably does not penetrate into the depths of the lesion.

Antibody and Periodontal Disease

The presence of IgG, IgM, IgE, and (serum derived) IgA in the gingival sulcus of clinically healthy individuals suggests that these immunoglobulins gain access to the gingival sulcus.[141] These immunoglobulins are detected in higher concentrations in sulcular fluid of individuals with periodontal disease.[15, 44, 111, 114, 134] The local synthesis of these antibodies and the demonstration of immunoglobulin-coated bacteria in subgingival plaque indicate that some of these immunoglobulins possess specificity for oral microorganisms.[9, 58]

The *in vivo* coating of subgingival bacteria with immunoglobulins and complement may directly influence the numbers and types of subgingival bacteria.[1, 117, 150] Reactions with gram-negative bacteria could promote lysis and with gram-positive bacteria could promote phagocytosis. *In vivo* coating could also affect the growth characteristics of the bacteria by limiting their numbers.[14, 53]

Antibody titers to oral bacteria may also have a protective effect. Frequently, but not always, titers increase with increased severity of disease.[38, 50, 113, 124, 151, 169] Localized antibody production also occurs in gingival tissues.[111] Antibodies to bacilli,[97] spirochetes,[119, 167–169] cocci and filamentous bacteria,[41, 50] and specifically to *Fusobacterium, Leptotrichia*,[97] and *Veillonella*[15] have been identified. These antibodies could aid in phagocytosis and removal of bacterial products from the tissues through complement activation by immune complexes.

Serum antibody and complement titers to plaque flora and to organisms isolated in and lesions of idiopathic juvenile periodontitis (IJP) have been assayed.[120] Significant elevated titers occurred to *Bacteroides* species. For some of the other juvenile periodontitis–associated organisms, titers were significantly greater in patients with this disease than in older healthy patients, individuals with periodontitis, and siblings of patients with IJP.

The general concept that develops from studies of antibody titers to oral bacteria is that most humans with clinically healthy periodontal tissues have a spectrum of antibodies to plaque organisms. In periodontitis, antibody titers vary in concentration depending on the specific organism for which antibodies have been detected. Further work must be done to elucidate the significance of these antibody responses in the pathogenesis of periodontal diseases.

COMPLEMENT

An important and potentially harmful biological consequence of antigen-antibody interaction is the activation of complement (Fig. 23–2). Complement consists of at least 11 proteins that make up approximately 10 per cent of the globulins in normal serum of man and other vertebrates.[31, 48, 49, 95, 105] These proteins are not immunoglobulins, and they are not increased in concentration by immunization. These substances may be synthesized in the liver, small intestine, macrophage, and other mononuclear cells.[96, 140] They react with a wide variety of antibody-antigen complexes and exert their primary biological effects on cell membranes, causing lysis and functional alteration. Of primary importance is their effect on mast cells. In these cells degranulation by complement causes the release of histamine and other biologically active substances which increase permeability of small blood vessels. Migration of polymorphonuclear leukocytes, increased phagocytic activity by leukocytes and macrophages, hemolysis, and bacteriolysis also take place. Red blood cell lysis (hemolysis) as a consequence of complement activation has been analyzed in greatest detail because it is simple to measure. This provides the basis for the complement fixation assay, an important laboratory procedure for detecting and measuring many different kinds of antigens and antibodies and their effects on the complement system.

The reaction sequence in the activation of the complement system is similar in nature to the cascading pathway in the blood coagulation system (Fig. 23–3). After one component of the complement system is bound by antibody-antigen complexes, the other components of the complement system react in an ordered sequence. In general, an activated protein cleaves the next reacting member of the series into fragments, and so on until the cascade has been completed. Some of the smaller fragments during cleavage have phlogistic activity; that is, they cause inflammatory tissue changes[98] (Table 23–3). These include increased vascular permeability and attraction of polymorphonuclear leukocytes. Other biological activities of complement fixation are also shown in Table 23–4. The "classic" pathway is activated by antigen reacting with IgG or IgM antibodies and by aggregated immunoglobulins. The sequence is C1, C4, C2, C3, C5, C6, C7, C8, C9. C3 is cleaved by C42 into C3b, which binds to the cell membrane, and C3a, which has biological activity (see Fig. 23–2).

An alternate pathway for complement

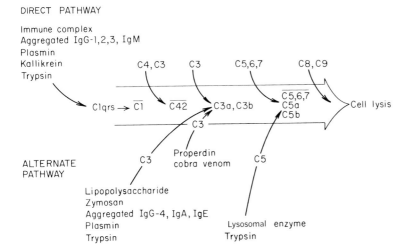

DIRECT PATHWAY

Immune complex
Aggregated IgG-1,2,3, IgM
Plasmin
Kallikrein
Trypsin

ALTERNATE PATHWAY

Lipopolysaccharide
Zymosan
Aggregated IgG-4, IgA, IgE
Plasmin
Trypsin

Figure 23–2 Schematic diagram of the complement sequence. Direct (classical) and alternate pathways in the activation of complement components. See Table 23–4. (From Page, R. *In* Schluger, S., Yuodelis, R. A., and Page, R. C.: Periodontal Disease. Philadelphia, Lea and Febiger, 1977.

TABLE 23–3 BIOLOGICAL EFFECTS OF COMPLEMENT*

Activity	Complement Components
Cytolytic and cytotoxic damage to cells	C1-9
Chemotactic activity for leukocytes	C3a, C5a, C567
Histamine release from mast cells	C3a, C5a
Increased vascular permeability	C3a, C5a
Kinen activity	C2, C3a
Lysosomal enzyme release from leukocytes	C5a
Promotion of phagocytosis	C3, C5
Enhancement of blood clotting	C6
Promotion of clot lysis	C3, C4
Inactivation of bacterial lipopolysaccharides from endotoxin	C5, C6

*From Nisengard, R. J.: J. Periodontol., 48:505, 1977.

activation also exists.[125, 161] Antibodies of the IgG, IgA, and IgE class can initiate the complement sequence by activating the third component of complement (C3) without triggering the sequence of complement activation at the beginning of the "cascade" or C1 component. The alternate pathway begins with cleavage of C3 after conversion of C3 proactivator. The sequence after C3 activation is identical to that of the "classic" pathway: C5, C6, C7, C8, C9.

Recent studies have demonstrated that the alternate pathway of complement activation occurs in most periodontal pockets, and that the classic pathway is activated only occasionally.[111, 140] Bacterial antigens such as endotoxins and polysaccharides such as dextran are activators of the alternate pathway.[159] Upon activation of complement by endotoxin, biologically active fragmentation products are released. Complement components that are present in the gingival sulcular fluid have been shown to be activated by some plaque bacteria and bacterial proteases.[1, 16, 149, 158] The resultant effect of complement activation by these various pathways could result in mechanisms which destroy the periodontal tissues.[135]

Although cell lysis has dominated the study of complement activation, the main physiological effects of activated complement are related to cellular and tissue changes associated with inflammation.

When the C3a and C5a components of the complement system are liberated, they cause the release of histamine from mast cells, which in turn causes a marked increase in capillary permeability. Injection of C3a into human skin elicits a wheal, and the effect can be specifically blocked by antihistamine drugs.

Chemotaxis of polymorphonuclear leukocytes is brought about by the activation of the C5a component of the complement system.[162-164] There is some speculation that the C3a component is also involved in this activity. Chemotaxis is neither stimulated by histamine nor blocked by antihistamine drugs.

In addition to chemotactic factors derived from complement, certain species of bacteria produce low molecular weight peptides that are directly chemotactic and do not require complement for activity.[140] These products could contribute to the accumulation of inflammatory cells in the periodontal lesion.

An important reaction involved with complement activation occurs against gram-negative bacteria coated with specific antibody. These bacteria can by lysed by complement acting through the same reaction sequence as occurs in the lysis of red blood cells. It appears that gram-positive bacteria are not susceptible to this lytic action of complement. The overall effect of complement activation in the course of periodontal disease may be increased permeability of gingival tissues, allowing a greater penetration of toxic products from plaque, and may in turn initiate a vicious cycle in the destruction of the periodontal tissues (see Fig. 23–1).

The necessary prerequisites for complement activation via either pathway or by direct enzymatic cleavage are present in the periodontal lesion. Endotoxin from gram-negative bacteria can activate the alternative pathway, immune complexes can activate the classic pathway, and bacterial and host tissue proteases can cleave complement components directly.

Several complement components (C3, C4, and Factor B) have been identified in sulcular fluid and in the gingival connective tissue of normal individuals as well as those with clinical symptoms of periodontal disease.[140, 176] Immunofluorescent staining of

C3 demonstrates a more intense fluorescent pattern in inflamed gingiva than in nondiseased tissue. As indicated earlier, the findings of a conversion product of C3 and reduced C4 levels in sulcular fluid from inflamed gingiva strongly suggest local complement activation.[1, 149, 150]

Complement studies of sulcular fluid from patients with ideopathic juvenile periodontitis (IJP) suggest that complement is activated by the alternate pathway.[148] This activation may be induced by endotoxins from the predominantly gram-negative flora in the periodontal lesion.

IMMUNE MECHANISMS

Immune mechanisms are usually protective responses of the host to the presence of foreign substances such as bacteria and viruses, but they may also cause local tissue destruction by triggering several types of overreactions or *hypersensitivity.* Tissue damage (immunopathology) may occur in a sensitized host upon subsequent exposure to the sensitizing antigen. There are four types of hypersensitivity reaction described by Gell and Coombs;[11, 41, 42] they are designated as types I, II, III, and IV (Fig. 23–3).

There are three *antibody*-mediated responses of importance to periodontal disease which are classified as *hypersensitivity reactions.*[138] They are anaphylaxis (Type I), cytotoxic reactions (Type II), and immune complex or Arthus reactions (Type III). In addition, reactions to transfused blood are involved with immediate hypersensitivity reactions. Another type of hypersensitivity which depends upon the interaction of immunocompetent *cells* is called delayed or cell-mediated (Type IV).

Anaphylaxis (Type I)

Two types of anaphylactic hypersensitivity are differentiated by the route of administration of the antigen. If the antigen is injected locally into the skin, it is called *cutaneous anaphylaxis.* If the antigen is injected intravenously, it is called *systemic* or *generalized. anaphylaxis.* The basic mechanisms in both types of immediate hypersensitivity are the same.

In anaphylaxis, both IgG and IgE are involved; however, only IgE is capable of sensitizing the skin. This sensitizing capability is referred to as *reaginic* and the IgE antibody as *reagin.* IgG antibody combines with antigen and prevents "sensitization." These antibodies are referred to as *blocking* antibodies. There are several major features which distinguish these types of blocking antibodies from reaginic or sensitizing antibodies.

IgE antibodies involved in anaphylactic reactions combine strongly at the Fc portion of the antibody to perivascular mast cells and to basophilic leukocytes primarily in the skin and other connective tissues such as the gingiva. These sensitizing IgE antibodies are called monocytotrophic antibodies because they bind only to human mast cells. In contrast, IgG blocking antibodies bind to mast cells of other phylogenetically distinct species and are termed heterocytotrophic antibodies. A very important component in anaphylactic hypersensitivity is the fact that IgE antibodies normally do not fix (activate) complement.

Since plasma cells are known to produce immunoglobulins, the finding of IgE-containing cells in the periodontal and other tissues is thought to represent localized synthesis of IgE antibodies.[111, 114] These IgE-forming cells are found primarily in respiratory and gastrointestinal mucosa and in regional lymph nodes. It has been suggested that IgE formed locally in tissue may then participate in local disease processes.

MECHANISMS OF ANAPHYLACTIC HYPERSENSITIVITY

Antigen capable of inducing anaphylaxis binds to sensitizing antibody fixed to mast cells at the Fab portion of the antibody. This antibody-antigen reaction causes the release of pharmacologically active substances from the sensitized cell (Table 23–4). It is these substances that cause the response and have the potential to induce tissue damage in periodontal disease.[112, 133]

Of the several active pharmacologic substances released during anaphylaxis, histamine pre-exists in the cells and is promptly released by antibody-antigen

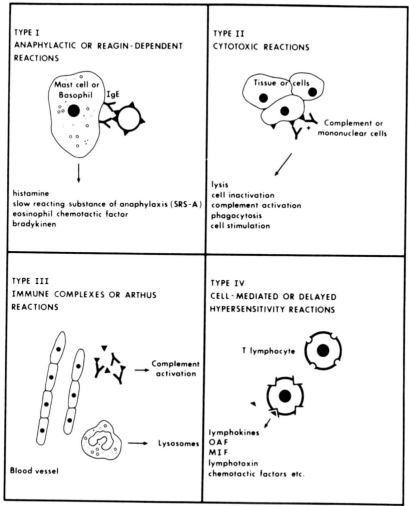

TYPE I
ANAPHYLACTIC OR REAGIN-DEPENDENT
REACTIONS

Mast cell or
Basophil   IgE

histamine
slow reacting substance of anaphylaxis (SRS-A)
eosinophil chemotactic factor
bradykinen

TYPE II
CYTOTOXIC REACTIONS

Tissue or cells

Complement or
mononuclear cells

lysis
cell inactivation
complement activation
phagocytosis
cell stimulation

TYPE III
IMMUNE COMPLEXES OR ARTHUS
REACTIONS

Complement
activation

Lysosomes

Blood vessel

TYPE IV
CELL-MEDIATED OR DELAYED
HYPERSENSITIVITY REACTIONS

T lymphocyte

lymphokines
OAF
MIF
lymphotoxin
chemotactic factors etc.

Figure 23–3   Immunologic Mechanisms of Tissue Damage. The four types of hypersensitivity reactions described by Gell and Coombs and depicted by Nisengard. (From Nisengard, R. J.: J. Periodontol., *48*:505, 1977.)

complexes. Other pharmacologically active substances, the kinins and "SRS-A" (slow-reacting substance of anaphylaxis), are produced only *after* the antigen-antibody complexes are formed.

An α_2-macroglobulin which blocks the normally found inhibitor for collagenase is released from sensitized cells, as are prostaglandins and an eosinophil chemotactic factor.

Histamine has been the most extensively studied chemical mediator of immediate hypersensitivity. As mentioned previously, it is widely found in mammalian tissues. Mast cells, platelets, and basophilic leuko-

cytes contain this substance. Histamine levels in chronically inflamed gingiva are significantly higher than levels in normal gingiva.[36] Some of the pharmacologic actions of histamine include increased capillary permeability, smooth muscle contraction, stimulation of exocrine glands, and dilatation and increased venule permeability. The biological effects of histamine can be blocked with antihistamine drugs, but no apparent change in the course of periodontal disease has been demonstrated with these drugs.

Slow-reacting substances of anaphylaxis (SRS-A) are acidic lipids which cause a sus-

TABLE 23–4 PHARMACOLOGICALLY ACTIVE MEDIATORS RELEASED BY HUMAN MAST CELLS*

Mediator	Pharmacologic Action
Histamine	Increased capillary permeability Smooth muscle contraction Stimulation of exocrine glands Dilation and increased venule permeability Skin response: wheal and erythema Bone resorption?
SRS-A	Smooth muscle contraction Increased vascular permeability
Bradykinin	Smooth muscle contraction Vasodilation Increased capillary permeability Migration of leukocytes Stimulation of pain fibers
Alpha$_2$-macro-globulin	Colagenase activation

*Modified from Nisengard, R.: J. Periodontol., 45: 345, 1972.

tained slow contraction of the guinea-pig ileum. This contraction is not inhibited by antihistamines. In addition to causing constriction of smooth muscle, SRS-A has some permeability-enhancing activity.

Bradykinin, a peptide formed by the enzymatic action of kallikrein on an alpha$_2$-globulin of plasma, has a number of pharmacologic activities and is considered to be a major pharmacologic mediator of anaphylactic hypersensitivity. These biological activities include smooth muscle contraction, vasodilation, increased capillary permeability, migration of leukocytes, and stimulation of pain fiber. The action of bradykinin is not inhibited by antihistamine drugs.

Anaphylactic-type reactions to oral bacteria have been demonstrated to correlate with severity of periodontal disease in humans.[69, 111, 115] Skin test reagents prepared from an extract of *Actinomyces* and other oral bacteria by Nisengard[52] have provided an *in vitro* test demonstrating that humans have immediate (anaphylactic) and delayed reactions to these oral filamentous bacteria.[118] A statistically significant correlation was found between the incidence of immediate hypersensitivity and the severity of periodontal disease.

The greatest incidence of hypersensitivity was in periodontitis. In patients with generalized gingivitis, the incidence of immediate hypersensitivity was significantly depressed compared with patients with normal gingiva, localized gingivitis, and periodontitis.[111]

Cytotoxic Reactions (Type II)

In these types of reactions, Type II (Fig. 23–2) antibodies react directly with antigens tightly bound to cells. These antigens may be natural components of the cell such as the cell membrane polysaccharide antigens of red blood cells. A cytotoxic reaction in which these cells are involved may result in hemolysis. Cytotoxic antibodies may also react with antigens that have become associated with tissue cells. These cell-associated antigens include those derived from bacteria, drugs, or altered tissue components. Cytotoxic antibodies are of the IgG or IgM class. These antibodies have the ability to fix complement, although complement fixation is not required for all types of cytotoxic antibody reactions. In addition to inducing cell lysis, cytotoxic antibody may cause tissue damage by increasing the synthesis and release of lysosomal enzymes by cells (PMN's) coated with antigen. The tissues exposed to these enzymes may then be damaged. Hemolytic transfusion reactions, hemolytic disease of newborn, and autoallergic hemolytic anemia are examples of cytotoxic reactions induced by these antibody-antigen reactions.[31] Cytotoxic reactions are seen in autoimmune disease in which antibodies react with a patient's own tissue components.[116, 144] This occurs, for example, in pemphigus, in which antibodies react with cell membranes, and in pemphigoid, in which antibodies react with the epithelial basement membrane.[10, 57, 61, 111, 144] To date there is no evidence which suggests an important role of cytotoxic reactions in gingivitis and periodontitis.[15]

Arthus Reactions (Type III)

When high levels of antigen (capable of antibody reaction) are present, antigen-antibody complexes precipitate in and around small blood vessels, causing tissue damage at the site of the local reaction[20, 21, 33, 55, 83, 139, 177] (Fig. 23–2). Inflammation, hemorrhage, and necrosis may occur. Tissue damage appears to be due to the release of lysosomal enzymes from polymorphonuclear leukocytes (PMN's). This reaction is referred to as Arthus reaction and is usually mediated by IgM or IgG type antibodies. These antibodies have the ability to fix complement, which is partially responsible for the chemotactic attraction of the polymorphonuclear leukocytes crucial to the Arthus reaction (Fig. 23–1).

The presence of antibodies to many oral bacteria, together with the recognition of continual antigen penetration of the gingiva, provides the basis for immune complex or Arthus reaction.[24–26, 106, 186] Experimental gingival Arthus reactions have a histopathology similar to that of human gingivitis and periodontitis.[136–138, 141] In vitro studies have also demonstrated that immune complexes with complement activation induce osteoclastic activity,[42, 111] possibly by prostaglandin E synthesis.[135]

A reduction in antibodies, which are necessary for immune complex disease, has little or no effect on gingivitis or periodontitis. Gingivitis can be seen in hypogammaglobulinemia.[111] Immunosuppression with azathioprine in combination with prednisone may also influence periodontal disease.[153] When these drugs are employed after organ (usually kidney) transplants, the correlation between severity of periodontal disease and plaque has not been demonstrated. Whether this lack of relationship results from suppressed humoral immunity, cell-mediated immunity, or a direct effect of the prednisone on inflammation by stabilization of lysosomal membranes is not known.[111] It is also possible that these drugs may affect the plaque bacteria directly.

Cell-mediated Immunity – Delayed Hypersensitivity (Type IV)

The phenomenon of delayed hypersensitivity belongs to the class of immune responses known as cell-mediated immunity. These reactions are referred to as Type IV (Fig. 23–2). Lymphocytes sensitized to plaque antigens undergo morphologic and functional transformation (in vitro), which results in a chronic infiltration with lymphocytes and macrophages and the formation of biologically active substances.

Another important type of reaction is seen when the lymphocytes are transferred from an immunologically competent donor to an allogenically incompetent recipient. These reactions have increasing clinical importance because of therapeutic attempts to transfer normal thymus or bone marrow cells to immunodeficient humans. These transplantation techniques are becoming increasingly common and have been used in patients with genetic defects and in patients with leukemia treated with cytotoxic drugs and whole body irradiation.[153] Often such patients have concomittant periodontal manifestations of their primary systemic disease (see Chap. 29).

Cellular immunity does not involve circulating antibodies but is based on the interaction of antigens with the surface of lymphocytes. There are two populations of lymphocytes involved with cellular immunity (Fig. 23–4). Antibody-producing lymphocytes are designated as "B" cells because they were found to proliferate in the bursa of Fabricius in birds and in the bone marrow of mammals. These cells circulate from the blood or thoracic duct to lymphatic tissues, where they predominate in the cortical germinal centers of lymph nodes and red pulp of the spleen and differentiate into plasma cells.[98] These differentiated cells are then induced to produce antibody. Recently B-lymphocytes have been shown to produce biologically active lymphokines[89, 90, 181] (see below).

In contrast, the "T" cells migrate to the thymus from the bone marrow, where they divide and become immunocompetent (Fig. 23–4). From the thymus they migrate to the paracortical areas of lymph nodes and the white pulp of the spleen.[98] The relationship between T- and B-lymphocytes and cellular and humoral immunity is not as simple as previously thought, since interactions frequently occur between these cells.[111]

T-lymphocytes sensitized to react to an immunizing antigen can be stimulated to

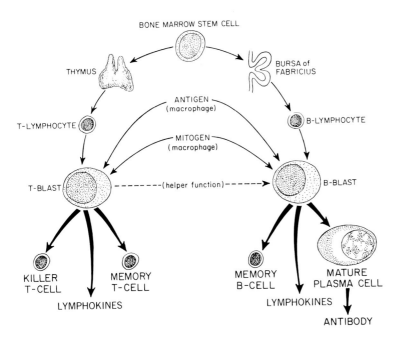

Figure 23–4 Schematic diagram illustrating the derivation and response of B- and T-lymphocytes. Antigen- and mitogen-induced responses resulting from the presence of macrophages. From Page, R.: *In* Schluger, S., Yuodelis, R. A., and Page, R. C.: Periodontal Disease. Philadelphia, Lea and Febiger, 1977.

undergo "blastogenesis" or transformation *in vitro* and presumably *in vivo*. This consists of morphological enlargement, synthesis of proteins RNA and DNA, and ultimately mitotic division. This increases the number of immunocompetent lymphoid cells which are specific for a particular antigen.

Lymphokines

In the process of blastogenesis a variety of soluble biologically active substances (mediators) are made by the cultured T-lymphocytes. B-lymphocytes can presumably produce lymphokines without prior blastogenesis. These mediators, called lymphokines, appear in the supernatant of lymphocyte cultures.[28] The accumulation of plasma cells and lymphocytes in the periodontal tissues suggests that lymphokines participate in periodontal pathology. Since the number of currently identified lymphokines is extensive[140] (Table 23–5), only the major ones will be discussed. These are macrophage migration inhibitory factor (MIF), lymphotoxin (LT), osteoclast activating factor (OAF), and leukocyte derived chemotactic factor (CTX).

MACROPHAGE ACTIVATING FACTOR (MAF)

It is postulated that in periodontitis macrophages are attracted to the periodontal tissues by chemotactic factor (CTX), retained there by MIF, and activated by the lymphokine, macrophage activating factor (MAF).[101, 107, 108, 148] MAF stimulates the macrophages to secrete collagenase.[129]

MACROPHAGE MIGRATION INHIBITORY FACTOR (MIF)

The lymphokine responsible for the inhibition of macrophage migration from an area in which the lymphokines have been released by activated lymphocytes is called macrophage migration inhibitory factor (MIF).[8, 30, 73, 93, 155] *In vivo* this mediator may concentrate macrophages at the local inflammatory site, where they function to phagocytize and digest antigen.

LEUKOCYTE DERIVED CHEMOTACTIC FACTOR (CTX)

The inflammatory lesion in periodontal disease is characterized by polymorphonuclear and mononuclear leukocytes. It is suggested that this is due to the production of chemotactic factors.[182, 184] These may be

TABLE 23–5 LYMPHOKINES: BIOLOGICAL ACTIVITY OF MEDIATORS OF CELL-MEDIATED IMMUNITY

Biological Activity	Lymphokine (or Mediator)
Effects on Macrophages	
Chemotaxis	Chemotactic factor (CTX)
Inhibition of migration	Migration inhibition factor (MIF)
Activation	Activation factor (MAF)
Effects on Other Cells	
Inhibition of leukocyte migration	Inhibition factors
Chemotaxis of neutrophils, basophils, and eosinophils	Chemotactic factors
	Eosinophil chemotactic factor (ECF)
Blast formation of lymphocytes	Mitogenic factor
Cytotoxicity (fibroblasts and other cells)	Lymphotoxin (LT)
Activation of osteoclasts	Osteoclast activating factor (OAF)
Other effects	
Transfer of cell-mediated immunity	Transfer factors
Inhibition of virus replication	Interferon
Inhibition of yeasts *(in vitro)*	Antifungal factors

from the complement system, plaque bacteria, and host lymphocytes which produce a leukocyte chemotactic factor (CTX). T- or B-lymphocytes can be stimulated *in vitro* by endotoxins and other antigens to produce this lymphokine.

LYMPHOTOXIN (LT)

In vitro experiments have demonstrated that lymphotoxin may be cytotoxic for cultures of human gingival fibroblasts.[27, 61, 72, 145, 146, 185] A correlation exists between the degree of periodontal disease of the lymphocyte donor and the amount of lymphotoxin elaborated by the cells in response to plaque antigens. Thus, there may be some *in vivo* correlation with the *in vitro* experiments.

Cytotoxicity of tissue cells may also be affected through a direct lymphocyte interaction with target cells containing a specific stimulating antigen on their surface.[98, 176] Although antigen recognition by sensitized lymphocytes is generally quite specific, the cytotoxic effect produced by lymphocyte host cell interaction is generally nonspecific. These lymphocyte interactions suggest that the persistent deposition of plaque antigen into the gingival tissue could favor the generation of lymphotoxin-producing cells and/or direct lymphocytotoxicity, resulting in tissue damage seen in periodontal diseases.[111]

OSTEOCLAST ACTIVATING FACTOR (OAF)

Osteoclast activating factor (OAF) induces osteoclastic resorption of bone in organ cultures.[59, 60, 62, 99] Histologically, the resorption is characteristically associated with the appearance of increased numbers of osteoclasts and the loss of bony matrix. Osteoclast activating factor can be distinguished from other bone resorbing substances such as parathormone, active metabolites of vitamin D, and prostaglandins.

Assays

The assays for lymphocyte transformation are *in vitro*. Small lymphocytes harvested from peripheral blood or lymphoid organs can be transformed (induced) to larger lymphocytes (blastogenesis). During the process of transformation, the cells synthesize DNA, RNA, and proteins. By labeling or incorporating radioactive precursor substances of the DNA, the transformation reaction can be quantitated.[31, 123] Radioisotopes such as tritiated thymidine are incorporated into DNA and subsequently quantitated. The degree of transformation is compared with that of control substances capable of stimulating a majority of lymphocytes. These stimulants are nonspecific and are called mitogens. Mitogens include phytohemaglutinin (PHA), antilymphocyte serum (ALS), and mercuric chloride.[12, 39, 47]

Cellular Immunity in Periodontal Disease

Delayed hypersensitivity reactions as measured by lymphocyte transformation suggests that this type of response may play an important role in the pathogenesis of periodontal disease[51, 66-68, 79-81, 103] (see Fig. 23–1). Peripheral blood lymphocytes from patients with moderate periodontal disease react to a greater degree than those from patients with mild disease, and patients with more severe or extensive periodontal destruction manifest a diminished reaction to the particular stimulant. This phenomenon may occur because patients with extensive periodontal destruction have blocking factors which could limit the disease process in severe periodontal destruction. This assumption is made if one considers that this immunopathologic reaction actually occurs *in vivo*.

A similar correlation of cell-mediated immunity and periodontal disease has been observed with sonicated plaque antigens.[43, 44] A diminished response to plaque, however, was not observed in severe periodontitis. Cell-mediated immunity to other microorganisms, including *Actinomyces israelii, A. naeslundii, Arachnia proprionica, Proprionibacterium acnes, Leptotrichia buccalis* and an anaerobic gram-negative rod (24N),[64, 110] from IJP also correlated with disease state.[73, 74]

Cell-mediated immunity to some bacteria is frequently long lasting. Patients edentulous for at least five years respond to *A. viscosus, A. naeslundii,* and homologous dental plaque to the same degree as do patients with gingivitis and periodontitis.[47, 121, 131, 187] This suggests that lymphocyte stimulation is from a source other than the periodontium. These edentulous subjects did not respond to *Veillonella alcalescens, Leptotrichia buccalis,* and *Bacteroides melaninogenicus*. Thus, cell-mediated immunity to gram-negative bacteria may relate more directly to periodontitis.

Cell-mediated immune responses in idiopathic juvenile periodontitis (IJP) are dependent on the type of antigen. No statistically significant stimulation was observed to *Veillonella, Bacteroides, Fusobacterium,* *Actinomyces,* and plaque,[82] while gram-negative bacteria isolated from lesions of patients with this disease did elicit a significant response.[3]

Clinical periodontal therapy consisting of scaling and root planing in patients with advanced periodontitis does not result in reduction of cell-mediated immunity to *A. viscosus* or *A. naeslundii*.[45]

REFERENCES

1. Attström, R., Laurel, A., Larsson, U., and Sjöholm, A.: Complement factors in gingival crevice material from healthy and inflamed gingiva in humans. J. Peridont. Res., *10*:19, 1974.
2. Attström, R.: Studies on neutrophil polymorphonuclear leukocytes at the dento-gingival junction in gingival health and disease. J. Periodont. Res., 8 (Suppl):1, 1971.
3. Baker, J. J., Chan, S. P., Socransky, S. S., Oppenheim, J. J., and Mergenhagen, S. E.: Importance of *Actinomyces* and certain gram-negative anaerobic organisms in the transformation of lymphocytes from patients with periodontal disease. Infect. Immun., *13*:1363, 1976.
4. Barnett, M. L.: The fine structure of human epithelial mast cells in periodontal disease. J. Periodont. Res., 8:371, 1973.
5. Barnett, M. L.: Mast cells in the epithelial layer of human gingiva. J. Ultrastruct. Res., *43*:247, 1973.
6. Barnett, M. L.: The fine structure of human connective tissue mast cells in periodontal disease. J. Periodont. Res., 9:84, 1974.
7. Bauer, W. H.: The supporting tissues of the tooth in acute secondary agranulocytosis (arsphenamin neutrophenia). J. Dent. Res., 25:501, 1946.
8. Benditt, E. P., and Lagunoff, D.: The mast cell: Its structure and function. Prog. Allergy, 8:195, 1964.
9. Berglund, S. E.: Immunoglobulins in human gingiva with specificity for oral bacteria. J. Periodontol., 42:546, 1971.
10. Beutner, E. H., Chorzelski, T. P., and Jordan, R. E.: Autosensitization in pemphigus and bullous pemphigoid. Springfield, Ill., Charles C Thomas, Publisher, 1970.
11. Bickley, H. C.: A concept of allergy with reference to oral disease. J. Periodontol., 41:302, 1970.
12. Bourne, H. R., Epstein, L. B., and Melmon, L. L.: Lymphocyte cyclic adenosine monophosphate (AMP) synthesis and inhibition of phytohemagglutinin-induced transformation. J. Clin. Invest., 50:10a, 1971.
13. Brandtzaeg, P.: Immunology of inflammatory periodontal lesions. Int. Dental J., 23:438, 1973.
14. Brandtzaeg, P., Fjellanger, I., and Gjeruldsen S. T.: Adsorption of immunoglobulin A onto oral bacteria in vivo. J. Bacteriol., 96:242, 1968.

15. Brandtzaeg. P., and Kraus, F. W.: Autoimmunity and periodontal disease. Odont. Tids., 73: 282, 1965.

16. Cardella, C. J., Davies, P., and Allison, A. C.: Immune complexes induce selective release of lysosomal hydrolases from macrophages. Nature, 247:46, 1974.

17. Carranza, F. A., Jr., and Cabrini, R. L.: Mast cells in human gingiva. Oral Surg., 8:1093, 1955.

18. Cianciola, L., Genco, R., Patters, M., and McKenna, J.: A family study of neutrophil chemotaxis in idiopathic juvenile periodontitis (periodontosis). AADR Abstract, p. B90, 1977.

19. Cianciola, L. J., Genco, R. J., Patters, M. R., McKenna, J., and van Oss, C. J.: Defective polymorphonuclear leukocyte functions in a human periodontal disease. Nature, 265:445, 1977.

20. Cochrane, C. G.: The Arthus phenomenon, a mechanism of tissue damage. Arthritis Rheum., 10:392, 1967.

21. Cochrane, C. G.: Mechanisms involved in the deposition of immune complexes in tissues. J. Exp. Med., 134:75, 1971.

22. Cohen, M. M., and Morris, A. L.: Periodontal manifestations of cyclic neutropenia. J. Periodontol., 32:159, 1961.

23. Cohen, S., and Winkler, S.: Cellular immunity and the inflammatory response. J. Periodontol., 45:348, 1974.

24. Colbe, H. M.: Transitory bacteremia. Oral Surg., 7:609, 1954.

25. Corner, H. D., Hamberman, S., Collings, C. K., and Winford, T. E.: Bacteremias following periodontal scaling in patients with healthy appearing gingiva. J. Periodontol., 38:466, 1967.

26. Courant, P. R., and Bader, H.: *Bacteroides melaninogenicus* and its product in the gingiva of man. Periodontics, 4:131, 1966.

27. Coyne, J., et al.: Guinea pig lymphotoxin (LT). J. Immunol., 110:1630, 1973.

28. David, J. R.: Delayed hypersensitivity in vitro: Its mediation by cell-free substances formed by lymphoid cell-antigen interaction. Proc. Natl. Acad. Sci. U.S.A., 56:72, 1966.

29. David, J. R.: Lymphocyte mediators and cellular hypersensitivity. N. Engl. J. Med., 288:143, 1973.

30. David, J. R., and David, R.: Assay for inhibition macrophage migration. *In* Bloom, B. R., and Glade, P. R. (eds.): In Vitro Methods in Cell Mediated Immunity. New York, Academic Press, Inc., 1971, p. 249.

31. Davis, B. D. et al.: Microbiology. 2nd ed. New York, Harper & Row, Publishers, Inc., 1973.

32. Dienstein, B., Ratcliff, P. A., and Williams, R. K.: Mast cell density and distribution in gingival biopsies: Quantitative study. J. Periodontol., 38:198, 1967.

33. Dixon, F. J.: Antigen-antibody complexes and autoimmunity. Ann. N.Y. Acad. Sci., 124:162, 1965.

34. Egelberg, J.: Permeability of the dento-gingival blood vessels. II. Clinically healthy gingivae. J. Periodont. Res., 1:276, 1966.

35. Egelberg, J.: Permeability of the dento-gingival blood vessels. III. Chronically inflamed gingivae. J. Periodont. Res., 1:287, 1966.

36. Eisen, H. N.: Immunology. An Introduction to Molecular and Cellular Principles of the Immune Responses. New York, Harper & Row, 1974.

37. Erb, P., and Feldman, M.: Role of macrophages in in vitro induction of T-helper cells. Nature, 254:352, 1975.

38. Evans, R. T., Spaeth, S., and Mergenhagen, S. E.: Bactericidal antibody in mammalian serum to obligatorily anaerobic gram-negative bacteria. J. Immunol., 97:112, 1966.

39. Ferraris, V. A., and DeRubertis, F. R.: Release of prostaglandin by mitogen and antigen-stimulated leukocytes in culture. J. Clin. Invest., 54:378, 1974.

40. Freedman, H. L., Taichman, N. S., and Keystone, J.: Inflammation and tissue injury. II. Local release of lysosomal enzymes during mixed bacterial infection in the skin of rabbits. Proc. Soc. Exp. Biol. Med., 125:1209, 1967.

41. Gell, P. G. H., and Coombs, R. R. A. (eds.): Clinical Aspects of Immunology. Philadelphia, F. A. Davis Co., 1968.

42. Gell, P. G. H., Coombs, R. R. A., and Lachman, P. J.: Clinical Aspects of Immunology, 3rd ed. Oxford, Blackwell Scientific Publications, 1975.

43. Gemsa, D., et al.: Release of cyclic AMP from macrophages by stimulation with prostaglandins. J. Immunol., 144:1422, 1975.

44. Genco, R. J., and Krygier, G.: Localization of immunoglobulins, immune cells and complement in human gingiva. J. Periodont. Res., 10 (Suppl.):30, 1972.

45. Genco, R. J., Krygier, G., Singh, S., Patters, M., and Ellison, S. A.: Immune responses of patients with advanced periodontitis during initial periodontal therapy. IADR Abstract, p. B207, 1976.

46. Genco, R. J., Mashimo, P. A., Krygier, G., and Ellison, S. A.: Antibody-mediated effects on the periodontium. J. Periodontol., 45:330, 1974.

47. Gery, I., and Waksman, B. H.: Potentiation of the T-lymphocyte response to mitogens. J. Exp. Med., 136:143, 1972.

48. Gewurz, H.: The immunologic role of complement. Hosp. Pract., 2:45, 1967.

48a. Gibbons, R. J., and Van Houte, J.: Selective bacterial adherence to oral epithelial surfaces and its role as an ecological determinant. Infect. Immun., 3:567, 1971.

49. Gigli, I.: Immunochemistry and immunobiology of the complement system. J. Invest. Dermatol., 67:346, 1976.

50. Gilmour, M. N., and Nisengard, R. J.: Interactions between serum titers to filamentous bacteria and their relationship to human periodontal disease. Arch. Oral Biol., 19:959, 1974.

51. Goldhaber, P.: Heparin enhancement of factors stimulating bone resorption in tissue culture. Science, 147:407, 1965.

52. Granger, G. A.,: Lymphokines – the mediators of cellular immunity. Ser. Haematol., 4:8, 1972.

53. Green, L. H., and Kass, E. H.: Quantitative determination of antibacterial activity of the rabbit gingival sulcus. Arch. Oral Biol., 15: 491, 1970.

54. Hawkins, D.: Neutrophilic leukocytes in immu-

nologic reactions: Evidence for the selective release of lysosomal constituents. J. Immunol., 108:310, 1972.

55. Henson, P. M.: Interaction of cells with immune complexes: Adherence, release of constituents, and tissue injury. J. Exp. Med., 134:114, 1971.

56. Hill, H. R., Estensen, R. D., Hogan, N. A., and Quie, P. G.: Severe staphylococcal disease associated with allergic manifestations, hyperimmunoglobulinemia E, and defective neutrophil chemotaxis. J. Lab. Clin. Med., 88:796, 1976.

57. Hook, W. A., Snyderman, R., and Mergenhagen, S. E.: Further characterization of a factor from endotoxin-treated serum which releases histamine and heparin from mast cells. Infect. Immun., 5:909, 1972.

58. Horton, J. E., Leiken, S., and Oppenheim, J. J.: Human lymphoproliferative reaction to saliva and dental plaque deposits: An *in vitro* correlation with periodontal disease. J. Periodontol., 43:522, 1972.

59. Horton, J. E., et al.: Macrophage-lymphocyte synergy in the production of osteoclast activating factor. J. Immunol., 113(4):1278–1287, 1974.

60. Horton, J. E., Oppenheim, J. J., and Mergenhagen, S. E.: A role for cell mediated immunity in the pathogenesis of periodontal disease. J. Periodontol., 45:351, 1974.

61. Horton, J. E., Oppenheim, J. J., and Mergenhagen, S. E.: Elaboration of lymphotoxin by cultured human peripheral blood leukocytes stimulated with dental-plaque deposits. Clin. Exp. Immunol., 13:383, 1973.

62. Horton, J. E., Raisz, L. G., Simmons, H. A., Oppenheim, J. J., and Mergenhagen, S. E.: Bone resorbing activity in supernatant fluid from cultured human peripheral blood leukocytes. Science, 177:793, 1972.

63. Iacono, V.: Defense Mechanisms. *In* Baer, P., and Morris, M. (eds.): Textbook of Periodontics. Philadelphia, J. B. Lippincott, 1977.

64. Irving, J. T., Newman, M. G., Socransky, S. S., and Heeley, J. O.: Histologic changes in experimental periodontal disease in rats monoinfected with a gram-negative organism. Arch. Oral Biol., 20:219, 1975.

65. Ishikawa, I., Cimasoni, G., and Ahmad-Zadeh, C.: Possible role of lysosomal enzymes in the pathogenesis of periodontitis. A study on cathepsin D in human gingival fluid. Arch. Oral Biol., 17:111, 1972.

66. Ivanyi, L., and Lehner, T.: Stimulation of lymphocyte transformation by bacterial antigens in patients with periodontal disease. Arch. Oral Biol., 15:1089, 1970.

67. Ivanyi, L., Wilton, J. M. A., and Lehner, T.: Cell-mediated immunity in periodontal disease; cytotoxicity, migration inhibition and lymphocyte transformation studies. Immunology, 22:141, 1972.

68. Ivanyi, L., and Lehner, T.: The significance of serum factors in stimulation of lymphocytes from patients with periodontal disease by *Veillonellia alcalescens*. Int. Arch. Allergy Appl. Immunol., 41:620, 1971.

69. Jayawardine, A., and Goldner, M.: Reagin-like activity of serum in human periodontal disease. Infect. Immun., 15:665, 1977.

70. Kaliner, M., and Austen, K. F.: Immunologic release of chemical mediators from human tissues. Elliott, H. W., George, R., and Okum, R. (eds.), Annual Review of Pharmacology.

71. Kiger, R. D., Wright, W. H., and Creamer, H. R.: The significance of lymphocyte transformation responses to various microbial stimulants. J. Periodontol., 45:780, 1974.

72. Kolb, W. P., and Granger, G. A.: Lymphocyte in vitro cytotoxicity: Characterization of human lymphotoxin. Proc. Natl. Acad. Sci. U.S.A., 61:1250, 1968.

73. Koopman, W., Gillis, M. H., and David, J. R.: Prevention of MIF activity by agents known to increase cellular cyclic AMP. J. Immunol., 110:1609, 1973.

74. Krahenbuhl, J. L., Rosenberg, L. T., and Remington, J. S.: The role of thymus derived lymphocytes in the in vitro activation of macrophages to kill Lysteria monocytogenes. J. Immunol., 111:992, 1973.

75. Lagunoff, D.: The properties of mast cell proteases. Biochem. Pharmacol. (Suppl.), 221–227, 1968.

76. Lavine, W. S., Page, R. C., and Padgett, G. A.: Host response in chronic periodontal disease. V. The dental and periodontal status of mink and mice affected by Chediak-Higashi Syndrome. J. Periodontol., 47:621, 1976.

77. Lavine, N., Stolman, J., Maderazo, E., Ward, P., and Cozen, R.: Defective neutrophil chemotaxis in patients with early onset periodontitis. IADR Abstract, 1976.

78. Lazarus, G. S., et al.: Human granulocyte collagenase. Science, 159:1483, 1968.

79. Lehner, T.: Cell-mediated immune responses in oral disease: A review. J. Oral Pathol., 1:39, 1972.

80. Lehner, T., et al.: Sequential cell-mediated immunoresponse in experimental gingivitis in man. Clin. Exp. Immunol., 16:481, 1974.

81. Lehner, T., Challacombe, S. J., Wilton, J. M. A., and Ivanyi, L.: Immunopotentiation by dental microbial plaque and its relationship to oral disease in man. Arch. Oral Biol., 21:749, 1976.

82. Lehner, T., Wilton, J. M. A., Ivanyi, L., and Manson, J. D.: Immunologic aspects of juvenile periodontitis (periodontosis). J. Periodont. Res., 9:261, 1974.

83. Lerner, C.: Arthus reaction in the oral cavity of laboratory animals. J. Periodontol 3:18, 1965.

84. Lindhe, J., and Hellden, L.: Neutrophilic chemotactic activity elaborated by dental plaque. J. Periodont. Res., 7:297, 1972.

85. Lucas, O. N., and Wright, W. H.: Heparin in normal and inflamed gingival tissue. J. Dent. Res., Suppl. 55, Abstr. No. 793, 1976.

86. Mackaness, G. B.: The immunological basis of acquired cellular resistance. J. Exp. Med., 120:105, 1964.

87. Mackaness, G. B.: The relationship of delayed hypersensitivity to acquired cellular resistance. Br. Med. Bull., 23:52, 1967.

88. Mackler, B. F., Frostad, K. B., Robertson, P. B., and Levy, B. M.: Immunoglobulin bearing lymphocytes and plasma cells in human periodontal disease. J. Periodont. Res., *12*: 37, 1977.

89. Mackler, B. F., et al.: Induction of lymphokine production by EAC and of blastogenesis by soluble mitogens during human B cell activation. Nature, *249*:834, 1974.

90. Mackler, B. F., et al.: Blastogenesis and lymphokine synthesis by T and B lymphocytes from patients with periodontal disease. Infec. Immun., *10*:844, 1974.

91. MacPhee, T. (ed.): Host Resistance to Commensal Bacteria: The Response to Dental Plaque. Edinburgh, Churchill, Livingstone, 1972.

92. Maderazo, E. G., Ward, P. A., and Quintiliani, R.: Defective regulation of chemotaxis in cirrhosis. J. Lab. Clin. Med., *85*:621, 1975.

93. Manheimer, S., and Pick, E.: The mechanism of action of soluble lymphocyte mediators. I. A pulse exposure test for the measurement of macrophage migration inhibitory factor. Immunology, *24*:1027, 1973.

94. May, C. D., Levine, B. E., and Weissmann, G.: Effects of compounds which inhibit antigenic release of histamine and phagocytic release of lysosomal enzyme on glucose utilization by leukocytes in humans. Proc. Soc. Exp. Biol. Med., *133*:758, 1970.

95. Mayer, M. M.: The complement system. Sci. Am., *229*:54, 1973.

96. Mergenhagen, S. E.: Complement as a mediator of the inflammatory response: Interaction of complement with mammalian and bacterial enzymes. J. Dent. Res., *51* (Suppl. 2):251, 1972.

97. Mergenhagen, S. E., DeAraujo, W. C., and Varah, E.: Antibody to Leptotrichia buccalis in human sera. Arch. Oral Biol., *10*:29, 1965.

98. Mergenhagen, S. E., and Scherp, H. W. (eds.): Comparative Immunology of the Oral Cavity. DHEW Publ. No. 73–438, 1973.

99. Mergenhagen, S. E., Wahl, S. M., Wahl, L. M., Horton, J. E., and Raisz, L. G.: The role of lymphocytes and macrophages in the destruction of bone and collagen. Ann. N.Y. Acad. Sci., *256*:132, 1975.

100. Michalek, S. M., et al.: Ingestion of *Streptococcus mutans* induces secretory immunoglobulin A and caries immunity. Science, *192*:1238–40, 1976.

101. Mooney, J. J., and Waksman, B. H.: Activation of normal rabbit macrophages by supernatants of antigen-stimulated lymphocytes. J. Immunol., *105*:1138, 1970.

102. Morley, H.: Prostaglandins and lymphokines in arthritis. Prostaglandins, 8:315, 1974.

103. Movius, D. L., Rogers, R. S., and Reeve, C. M.: Lymphocyte-mediated cellular immunity and the pathogenesis of periodontal disease. Program and Abstracts, 52nd Gen. Mtg. IADR, Abs. No. 498, 1974.

104. Mowat, A. G., and Baum, J.: Chemotaxis of polymorphonuclear leukocytes from patients with rheumatoid arthritis. J. Clin. Invest., *50*:2541, 1971.

105. Müller-Eberhard, H. J.: Complement. Ann. Rev. Biochem., *44*:697, 1975.

106. Murray, M., and Moosnick, F.: Incidence of bacteremia in patients with dental disease. J. Lab. Clin. Med., *26*:801, 1941.

107. Nath, I., Poulter, L. W., and Turk, J. L.: Effect of lymphocyte mediators on macrophages in vitro. A correlation of morphological and cytochemical changes. Clin. Exp. Immunol., *13*:455, 1973.

108. Nathan, C. F.., Karnovsky, M. L., and David, J. R.: Alterations of macrophage functions by mediators from lympocytes. J. Exp. Med., *133*: 1356, 1971.

109. Nelson, D. S.: Production by stimulated macrophages of factors depressing lymphocyte transformation. Nature, *246*:306, 1973.

110. Newman, M. G., Socransky, S., Savitt, E. D., Propas, E. D., and Crawford, A.: Studies of the microbiology of periodontosis. J. Periodontol., *47*:373, 1976.

111. Nisengard, R. J.: The role of immunology in periodontal disease. J. Periodontol., *48*:505, 1977.

112. Nisengard, R. J., and Beutner, E. H.: Relation of immediate hypersensitivity to periodontitis in animals and man. J. Periodontol., *41*:223, 1970.

113. Nisengard, R. J., and Beutner, E. H.: Immunologic studies of periodontal disease. V. IgG type antibodies and skin test responses to *Actinomyces* and mixed oral flora. J. Periodontol., *41*:149, 1970.

114. Nisengard, R. J., Beutner, E. H., and Gauto, M. S.: Immunofluorescent studies of IgE in periodontal disease. Ann. N.Y. Acad. Sci., *177*:39, 1971.

115. Nisengard, R. J., Beutner, E. H., and Hazen, S. P.: Immunologic studies of periodontal disease. III. Bacterial hypersensitivity and periodontal disease. J. Periodontol., *39*:329, 1968.

116. Nisengard, R. J., Jablonska, S., Beutner, E. H., Shu, S., Chorzelski, T. P., Jarzabek, M., Blaszczyk, M., and Pzesa, G.: Diagnostic importance of immunofluorescence in oral bullous diseases and lupus erythematosus. Oral. Surg., *40*:365, 1975.

117. Nisengard, R., and Jarrett, C.: Coating of subgingival bacteria with immunoglobulin and complement. J. Periodontol., *47*:518, 1976.

118. Nisengard, R. J., and Jarrett, C.: Hypersensitivity reactions to four oral microorganisms. IADR Abstract, March, 1974, p. 137.

119. Nisengard, R. J., Myers, D., Fischman, S., and Socransky, S.: Immunologic studies of acute necrotizing ulcerative gingivitis. IADR Abstract, p. B206, 1976.

120. Nisengard, R. J., Myers, D., and Newman, M. G.: Human antibody titers to periodontosis—associated microbiota. IADR Abstract, p. A23, 1977.

121. Nobreus, N., Attström, R., and Egelberg, J.: Effect of antithymocyte serum on chronic gingival inflammation in dogs. J. Periodont. Res., 9:236, 1974.

122. Opitz, H. G., et al.: Inhibition of H-thymidine incorporation of lymphocytes by a soluble factor from macrophages. Cell. Immunol., *16*:379, 1975.

123. Oppenheim, J. J.: Relationships of *in vitro* lymphocyte transformation to delayed hyper-

sensitivity in guinea pig and man. Fed. Proc., 27:21, 1968.

124. Orstavik, D., and Brandtzaeg, P.: Serum antibodies to plaque bacteria in subjects with dental caries and gingivitis. Scand. J. Dent. Res., 85:106, 1977.

125. Osler, A. G., and Sandberg, A. L.: Alternate complement pathways. Prog. Allergy, 17:51, 1973.

126. Page, R. C.: Pathogenic mechanisms. In Schluger, S., Yudalis, R., and Page, R. C.: Periodontal Disease: Basic Phenomena, Clinical Management and Restorative Interrelationships. Philadelphia, Lea & Febiger, 1977.

127. Page, R. C., Davies, P., and Allison, A. C.: Effects of dental plaque on the production and release of lysosomal hydrolases by macrophages in culture. Arch. Oral Biol., 18:1481, 1973.

128. Pantalone, R. M., and Page, R. C.: Lymphokine induced production and release of lysosomal enzymes by macrophages. Proc. Natl. Acad. Sci. U.S.A., 72:2091, 1975.

129. Pantalone, R. M., and Page, R. C.: The production and secretion of collagenase and lysosomal hydrolases by macrophages activated with lymphokines. Unpublished paper.

130. Parakkal, P. F.: Involvement of macrophages in collagen resorption. J. Cell. Biol., 41:345, 1969.

131. Patters, M. R., Genco, R. J., Reed, M. J., and Mashimo, P. A.: Blastogenic response of human lymphocytes to oral bacterial antigens: Comparison of individuals with periodontal disease to normal and edentulous subjects. Infect. Immun., 14:1213, 1976.

132. Pick, E., and Turk, J. L.: The biological activities of soluble lymphocyte products. Clin. Exp. Immunol., 10:1, 1972.

133. Piper, P. J., and Vane, J. R.: Release of additional factors in anaphylaxis and its antagonism by anti-inflammatory drugs. Nature, 223:29, 1971.

134. Platt, D., Crosby, R. G., and Dalbow, N. H.: Evidence for the presence of immunoglobulins and antibodies in inflamed periodontal tissues. J. Periodontol., 41:215, 1970.

135. Raisz, L. G., et al.: Complement-dependent stimulation of prostaglandin synthesis and bone resorption. Science, 185:789, 1974.

136. Ranney, R. R., and Zander, H. A.: Allergic periodontal disease in sensitized squirrel monkeys. J. Periodontol., 41:12, 1970.

137. Rizzo, A. A.: Histologic and immunologic evaluation of antigen penetration into oral tissues after topical application. J. Periodontol., 41:210, 1970.

138. Rizzo, A. A., and Mergenhagen, S. E.: Studies on the significance of local hypersensitivity in periodontal disease. Periodontics, 3:271, 1965.

139. Rizzo, A. A., and Mergenhagen, S. E.: Local Shwartzman reaction in rabbit oral mucosa with endotoxin from oral bacteria. Proc. Soc. Exp. Biol. Med., 104:580, 1968.

140. Rizzo, A. A., and Mergenhagen, S. E.: Host responses in periodontal disease. Proceedings of the International Conference on Research on the Biology of Periodontal Disease. Chicago, Ill., 1977.

141. Rizzo, A. A., and Mitchell, C. T.: Chronic allergic inflammation induced by repeated deposition of antigen in rabbit gingival pockets. Periodontics, 4:5, 1966.

142. Robertson, P. B., Grupe, Jr., H. E., Taylor, R. E., Shyu, K. W., and Fullmer, H. M.: The effect of collagenase-inhibitor complexes on collagenolytic activity of normal and inflamed gingival tissue. J. Oral Pathol., 2:28, 1973.

143. Robinson, L. P., and DeMarco, T. J.: Alteration of mast cell densities in experimentally inflamed human gingiva. J. Periodontol., 43:614, 1972.

144. Rogers, R. S., Sheridan, P. J., and Jordan, R. E.: Desquamative gingivitis. Oral Surg., 42:316, 1976.

145. Rosenberg, S. A., et al.: Guinea pig lymphotoxin (LT). I. In vitro studies of LT produced in response to antigen stimulation of lymphocytes. J. Immunol., 110:1623, 1973.

146. Russell, S. W., et al.: Purification of human lymphotoxin. J. Immunol., 109:784, 1972.

147. Sandberg, A. L., and Mergenhagen, S. E.: Periodontal disease: Potential role of immunologic mechanisms of tissue injury. In Textbook of Dental Microbiology. New York, Harper and Row, Publishers, 1977.

148. Schenkein, H., Cianciola, L., and Genco, R.: Complement activation in gingival pocket fluid from patients with periodontosis and severe periodontitis. IADR Abstract, 1976.

149. Schenkein, H. A., and Genco, R. J.: Gingival fluid and serum in periodontal diseases. I. Quantitative study of immunoglobulins, complement components and other plasma proteins. J. Periodontol., 48:772, 1977.

150. Schenkein, H. A., and Genco, R. J.: Gingival fluid and serum in periodontal diseases. II. Evidence for cleavage of complement components C3, C3 proactivator (factor B) and C4 in gingival fluid. J. Periodontol., 48:778, 1977.

151. Schneider, T. F., et al.: Specific bacterial antibodies in the inflamed human gingiva. Periodontics, 4:53, 1966.

152. Schroeder, H. E.: Transmigration and infiltration of leucocytes in human junctional epithelium. Helv. Odont. Acta, 17:6, 1973.

153. Schuller, P. D., Freedman, H. L., and Lewis, D. W.: Periodontal status of renal transplant patients receiving immunosuppressive therapy. J. Periodontol., 44:167, 1973.

154. Schwartz, J., and Dibblee, M.: The role of IgE in the release of histamine from gingival mast cells. J. Periodontol., 46:171, 1975.

155. Seravalli, E., and Taranta, A.: Release of macrophage migration inhibitory factor(s) from lymphocytes stimulated by streptococcal preparations. Cell. Immunol., 8:40, 1973.

156. Shapiro, S., Ulmansky, M., and Scheuer, M.: Mast cell population in gingiva affected by chronic destructive periodontal disease. J. Periodontol., 40:276, 1969.

157. Shelton, L. E., and Hall, W. B.: Human gingival mast cells. Effects of chronic inflammation. J. Periodont. Res., 3:214, 1968.

158. Shillitoe, E. J., and Lehner, T.: Immunoglobulins and complement in crevicular fluid, serum and saliva in man. Arch. Oral Biol., 17:241, 1972.

159. Snyderman, R.: Role for endotoxin and complement in periodontal tissue destruction. J. Dent. Res., 51 (Suppl. 2):356, 1972.

160. Snyderman, R., Altman, L. C., Frankel, A., and Blaese, R. M.: Defective mononuclear leukocyte chemotaxis: A previously unrecognized immune dysfunction. Studies in a patient with chronic mucocutaneous candidiasis. Ann. Intern. Med., 78:509, 1973.

161. Snyderman, R., Gewurz, H., and Mergenhagen, S. E.: Interactions of the complement system with endotoxic lipopolysaccharide. J. Exp. Med., 128:259, 1968.

162. Snyderman, R., Phillips, J. K., and Mergenhagen, S. E.: Biological activity of complement in vivo: Role of C5 in the accumulation of polymorphonuclear leukocytes in inflammatory exudates. J. Exp. Med., 134:1131, 1971.

163. Snyderman, R., Shin, H. S., and Dannenberg, A. M.: Macrophage proteinase and inflammation. Production of chemotactic activity from the fifth component of complement by macrophage proteinase. J. Immunol., 109:896, 1972.

164. Snyderman, R. H., Shin, H. W., and Hausmann, M. H.: A chemotactic factor from mononuclear phagocytes. Proc. Soc. Exp. Biol. Med., 138:378, 1971.

165. Socransky, S. S.: Microbiology of periodontal disease. Present status and future considerations. J. Periodontol., 48:497, 1977.

166. Spector, W. G.: The macrophage in inflammation. Ser. Haematol., 3:132, 1970.

167. Steinberg, A. I.: Evidence for the presence of circulating antibodies to an oral spirochete in the sera of clinic patients. J. Periodontol., 41:213, 1970.

168. Steinberg, A. I., and Gershoff, S.: Quantitative differences in spirochetal antibody observed in periodontal disease. J. Periodontol., 39:286, 1968.

169. Steinberg, A. I., Socransky, S. S., Gershoff, S. N., and Weinstock, A.: Use of tanned-cell hemagglutination to demonstrate circulating antibody against an oral spirochete. J. Bacteriol., 91:2114, 1966.

170. Taichman, N. S., Freedman, H. L., and Uriuhara, T.: Inflammation and tissue injury. I. The response to intradermal injections of human dentogingival plaque in normal and leukopenic rabbits. Arch. Oral Biol., 11:1385, 1966.

171. Taichman, N. S., and McArthur, W. P.: Current concepts in periodontal disease. In Annual Reports in Medicinal Chemistry, vol. 10. New York, Academic Press, Inc., 1975.

172. Taichman, N. S., Pruzanski, W., and Ranadive, N. S.: Release of intracellular constituents from rabbit polymorphonuclear leukocytes ex-

posed to soluble and insoluble immune complexes. Int. Arch. Allergy Appl. Immunol., 43:182, 1972.

173. Taylor, A. C.: Collagenolysis in cultured tissue: II. Role of mast cells. J. Dent. Res., 50:1301, 1971.

174. Tempel, T. R., et al.: Factors from saliva and oral bacteria, chemotactic for polymorphonuclear leukocytes. Their possible role in gingival inflammation. J. Periodontol., 41:71, 1970.

175. Temple, T. R., Kimball, H. R., Kakehashi, S., and Amen, C. R.: Host factors in periodontal disease: Periodontal minfestations of Chédiak-Higashi Syndrome. J. Periodont. Res. (Suppl.), 10:26, 1973.

176. Tempel, T. R., Snyderman, R., Jordan, H. V., and Mergenhagen, S. E.: Factors from saliva and oral bacteria, chemotactic for polymorphonuclear leukocytes: Their possible role in gingival inflammation. J. Periodontol., 41:71, 1970.

177. Terner, C.: Arthus reaction in the oral cavity of laboratory animals. Periodontics, 3:18, 1965.

178. Terner, V. K., Muszbek, L., and Csaba, B.: Der histamingehalt bei verschiedenen erkrankungen des zahnfleisches. Stoma (Heidelbr), February, 100, 1969.

179. Wahl, L. M., et al.: Collagenase production by endotoxin-activated macrophages. Proc. Natl. Acad. Sci. U.S.A., 71:598, 1974.

180. Wahl, L. M., et al.: Collagenase production by lymphokine-activated macrophages. Science, 187:261, 1975.

181. Wahl, S. M., Iverson, G. M., and Oppenheim, J. J.: Induction of guinea pig B-cell lymphokine synthesis by mitogenic and nonmitogenic signals to Fc, Ig and C3 receptors. J. Exp. Med., 140:1631, 1974.

182. Ward, P. A., Remold, H. G., and David, J. R.: The production of antigen-stimulated lymphocytes of a leukotactic factor distinct from migration inhibitory factor. Cell Immunol., 1:162, 1970.

183. Ward, P. A., and Schlegel, R. J.: Impaired leukotactic responsiveness in a child with recurrent infections. Lancet, 2:344, 1969.

184. Ward, P. W., Remold, H. G., and David, J. R.: Leukotactic factor produced by sensitized lymphocytes. Science, 163:1079, 1967.

185. Williams, T. W., and Granger, G. A.: Lymphocyte in vitro cytotoxicity: Lymphotoxins of several mammalian species. Nature, 219:1076, 1968.

186. Winford, T. E., and Haberman, S.: Isolation of aerobic Gram-positive filamentous rods from diseased gingivae. J. Dent. Res., 45:1159, 1956.

187. Wright, W. E., Oppenheim, J. J., Baker, J. J., and Chan, S. P.: Effect of clinical therapy on lymphocyte transformation in severe periodontitis. IADR Abstract, p. B206, 1976.

188. Zachrisson, B. U.: Mast cells of the human gingiva. J. Periodont. Res., 2:87, 1967.

Chapter 24

The Role of Microorganisms in the Etiology of Gingival and Periodontal Disease

The major change in our concepts regarding the etiology and progression of periodontal diseases is based on a better understanding of the structure and composition of the bacterial plaque associated with the gingival and periodontal tissues.

A number of reviews have documented the evidence that bacterial plaque is the major etiologic agent in most forms of periodontal disease (i.e., gingivitis, acute

necrotizing ulcerative gingivitis, periodontitis) and bacteria have been implicated in juvenile periodontitis (periodontosis).[*] The exact nature of the microbiota associated with periodontal disease and health is of great concern to the dentist.

Earlier theories regarding the role of dental plaque suggested that it was composed of a complex and homogeneous bacterial mass which would lead to disease where allowed to overgrow.[13, 14, 37, 39] Recent studies have revealed that the bacterial composition of plaque associated with healthy sites is different from that of the plaque associated with disease. Even more important has been the observation that characteristic microbial floras may be associated with clinically different periodontal diseases.[†]

The advances in the last decade have permitted a more realistic view of dental plaque. Previous difficulties encountered were more technical in nature and included problems in the dispersion of plaque samples[93, 158] (while maintaining cell viability) and in the recovery of microorganisms which were often oxygen sensitive or fastidious in their growth requirements. Newer procedures include the use of anaerobic techniques, better methods of sampling and dispersion of plaque, as well as improvements in culture media and methods of identification of the isolated organisms. Microbiologic sampling from discrete sites and microscopy of sections of

---

[*]See references 9, 26, 30, 38, 44, 45, 53, 61, 73, 86, 91, 105, 116, 137, 149, 190, 203, and 206.

[†]See references 19, 23, 46, 115, 140, 162, 182–184, 201, and 218.

human plaque *in situ* have permitted a clearer understanding of the localization of colonization of possible subgingival pathogens.† Much of this work is relatively recent and technically difficult to carry out. Thus information is limited. A brief synthesis of existing information is discussed below to aid in understanding the microbiologic approaches taken in studying periodontal diseases. Gaps in present knowledge may alter some but certainly not all of the viewpoints expressed.[196]

PLAQUE

General Characteristics

Many types of deposits exist on the tooth surface. In the past they were designated by a variety of terms, often with the same term applied to different deposits (Table 24–1). More recently there has been interest in identifying distinguishing features and disease-producing potential of the deposits based on their origin and nature.

Small amounts of plaque are not clinically visible unless they are discolored by pigments from within the oral cavity or stained by disclosing solutions or wafers (Plate III). As plaque accumulates it becomes a visible globular mass with a pin-point nodular surface that varies from gray to yellowish gray to yellow in color.

Plaque occurs supragingivally, mostly on the gingival third of the teeth, and subgingivally, with a predilection for surface cracks, defects, and roughness and overhanging margins of dental restorations.

Supragingival plaque formation begins by the adhesion of bacteria on the acquired pellicle or tooth surface (Fig. 24–1). Plaque mass grows by (1) the addition of new bacteria, (2) the multiplication of bacteria, and (3) the accumulation of bacterial products.

Measurable amounts of supragingival plaque may form within one hour after teeth are thoroughly cleaned,[207] with maximum accumulation reached in approximately 30 days or less. The rate of formation and the location vary among indi-

†See references 1a, 12, 21, 56, 91a, 105, 117, 132, 137, 140, 164, 168, 182–184, and 203.

TABLE 24–1 HISTORICAL REVIEW OF TERMINOLOGY USED FOR SOFT ORAL DEPOSITS°

1897	J. C. Williams	A thick felt-like mass of acid-forming microorganism
1897	G. V. Black	Gelatinous layers of microorganisms
1898	G. V. Black	Gelatinous microbial plaque
1898	J. C. Williams	Microbic plaques
1899	G. V. Black	Gelatinous microbic plaque—transparent gelatin layers produced by microbes
1902	W. D. Miller	Bacterial plaque
1941	W. Wild	Plaque—adheres to the surface in the habitually unclean spaces of the dentition, and is composed of finely distributed food debris (carbohydrate, protein, fat) saliva (mucin, desquamated epithelial cells) and various bacteria
1953	R. M. Stephan	Plaque—the sum total of all soft, exogenous material which adheres to dental surfaces
1961	World Health Organization	Plaque—primarily microorganisms; materia alba—oral debris, microorganisms, epithelial and blood cells and little food debris
1963	C. Dawes, G. N. Jenkins, C. H. Tongue	Dental plaque—all soft deposits, exclusive of food debris
1969	R. S. Schwartz, M. Massler[155]	Classified soft deposits as follows: 1. Acquired pellicle—a noncellular thin film 2. Dental plaque—an organized transparent deposit which is primarily composed of bacteria and their products 3. Materia alba—soft, whitish deposit, with no specific architecture, which can be removed with water spray 4. Food debris—retained food, which is usually removed by saliva and oral muscular action
1976	M. Listgarten	Classified surface coatings on teeth based on origin and nature: 1. Coatings of developmental origin—reduced enamel epithelium, coronal cementum, the dental cuticle, subsurface enamel matrix 2. Acquired coatings—salivary, bacterial, calculus, surface stains, subsurface pellicle, complex coatings

°Abstracted from Schroeder, H. E.[151] with additions.

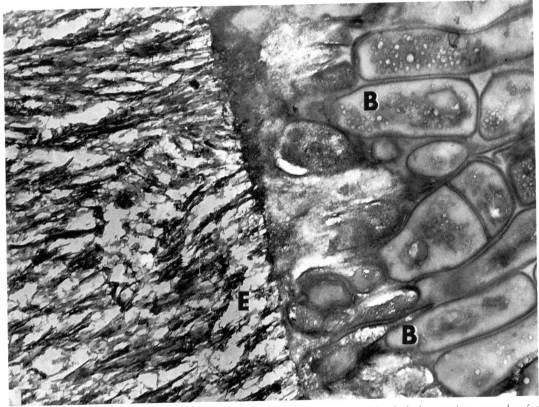

Figure 24–1   Plaque Formed Directly on Enamel Surface. Electromicrograph of decalcified noncarious enamel surface, showing remnants of enamel matrix (E) and bacteria in attached plaque (B). (Courtesy of Frank, R. M., and Brendel, A.)

viduals, on different teeth in the same mouth, and on different areas of individual teeth.

Composition of Supragingival Dental Plaque

Supragingival plaque consists principally of proliferating microorganisms (see below) and a scattering of epithelial cells, leukocytes, and macrophages in an adherent intercellular matrix (Fig. 24–2). Organic and inorganic solids form about 20 per cent of the plaque; the remainder is water. Bacteria constitute approximately 70 to 80 per cent of the solid material, and the rest is intercellular matrix.[40, 187] Supragingival plaque stains positive with periodic acid-Schiff (PAS) stain and orthochromatic with toluidine blue.

Supragingival plaque matrix

ORGANIC CONTENT.   The organic matrix consists of a polysaccharide-protein complex of which the principal components are carbohydrates and proteins, approximately 30 per cent each, and lipids, approximately 15 per cent, with the nature of the remainder unclear. These components represent extracellular products of plaque bacteria, their cytoplasmic and cell membrane remnants, ingested foodstuff, and derivatives of salivary glycoproteins. The carbohydrate present in greatest amount in the matrix of supragingival plaque is dextran, a bacteria-produced polysaccharide which forms approximately 9.5 per cent of the total plaque solid (Table 24–2). Other matrix carbohydrates are levan, another polysaccharide bacterial product, galactose, and methylpentose in the form of rhamnose.

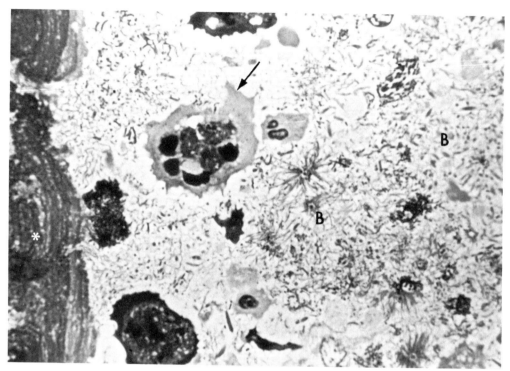

Figure 24–2 Histologic section of plaque showing nonbacterial components such as white blood cells (arrow), and epithelial cells (asterisk) interspersed among bacteria (B). (Courtesy of Dr. Max Listgarten.)

Bacterial remnants provide muramic acid, lipids, and some matrix protein, for which salivary glycoproteins are the principal source.

INORGANIC CONTENT. The principal inorganic components of supragingival plaque matrix are calcium and phosphorus, with small amounts of magnesium, potassium, and sodium. They are bound to the organic components of the matrix. The inorganic content is higher on the mandibular an-

terior teeth than in the remainder of the mouth and is also generally higher on lingual surfaces. The total inorganic content of early supragingival plaque is small, with the greatest increase occurring in plaque which is transformed to calculus (see chap. 25). Fluoride topically applied to the teeth and in drinking water becomes incorporated in the plaque.

Diet and Supragingival Plaque Formation

Dental plaque is not a food residue. Supragingival plaque forms more rapidly during sleep, when no food is ingested, than following meals. This may be because the mechanical action of food and the increased salivary flow during mastication may deter plaque formation. The consistency of the diet also affects the rate of plaque formation. Supragingival plaque forms rapidly on soft diets, whereas hard chewy foods retard it. (For additional discussion of food consistency and plaque formation, see Chapter 28.)

In man and in some laboratory animals, dietary supplements of sucrose increase

TABLE 24–2 CARBOHYDRATE CONTENT OF PLAQUE MATRIX°

	Percentage of Lyophilized Matrix Weight	
	Mean	Range
Dextran (polymer of glucose)	9.5%	8–10%
Hexosamine	4%	3–6%
Methylpentose	3.1%	2–4%
Galactose	2.6%	1.7–4.4%
Levan (polymer of fructose)	0.4%	0.1–0.7%

°Modified from Mandel, I. D.[110]

supragingival plaque formation[45, 46] and affect its bacterial compositon. This is attributed to extracellular polysaccharides produced by bacteria; glucose supplements do not have a similar effect. Plaque formation occurs on high-protein low-fat diets and on carbohydrate-free diets, but in small amounts.

DIFFICULTIES IN STUDYING PERIODONTAL DISEASE

Disease Activity

The clinical characteristics of periodontal disease present several problems in the search for its etiology (Table 24–3). One of the most important considerations is the chronic nature of periodontal disease. It is not clear whether periodontal destruction occurs in a chronic steady state or whether there are periods of exacerbation and remission which result in the loss of the periodontal tissues. This rate of periodontal destruction or *periodontal disease activity* is very difficult to assess. Any analysis of the microbiota (or potential immunopathologic process) associated with a particular periodontal lesion or healthy area must take into account the nature of disease activity. It is possible that certain bacteria will be associated with periods of destruction while other groups of bacteria may be associated with remission or quiescent periods.[196]

Host Resistance

Host resistance is another factor which can lead to erroneous conceptions regarding the role of microorganisms in periodontal diseases (Table 24–3). The balance between host resistance and bacterial virulence will determine the state of periodontal health or disease. Thus it is important to consider the nature of the host's defensive (and potentially destructive) relationship with the bacteria colonizing the periodontal tissues. The complexity of the host response has been discussed in detail in Chapter 23.)

Animal Models

In the study of periodontal disease, *animal models* are often used. These models are associated with conceptual and technical problems.[190, 191] First, all animals thus far tested have a distinctly different microbiota from that of man.[28, 57, 80–82, 88, 90] Therefore, results from experiments using animal models are not *directly* transferable in the consideration of human periodontal diseases. In addition, investigators have found great difficulty in establishing human organisms in the mouths of many animals.[20, 75, 76, 190]

Complexity of Bacteria

The bacteria which are associated with the periodontium exist in an extremely complex arrangement. Our understanding regarding the nature of the microbiota associated with periodontal disease or health has been very limited even though this area of investigation is very important. Earlier studies of the bacterial etiology revealed problems in sampling the resident microorganisms, cultivation, and the description of the isolated bacteria (Table 24–3).[29, 40, 41, 76, 112, 187] For example, the use of pooled plaque samples described in earlier studies tended to obscure actual differences in bacterial distribution from site to site. Often bacteria from periodontally involved sites were mixed with bacteria from normal sites. Thus, any differences which may have existed could not be detected. The inability adequately to cultivate oxygen-sensitive microorganisms found in the gingival crevice has led to further problems.

Recent evidence suggests the possibility

TABLE 24–3 DIFFICULTIES IN STUDYING THE MICROBIOLOGY OF PERIODONTAL DISEASE

Disease Characteristic	Problems Encountered
Disease activity	Periods of exacerbation and remission
Host resistance	Variable, difficult to measure
Animal models	Different bacteria
Bacterial complexity	Cultivation, enumeration, sampling

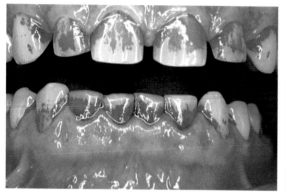

A

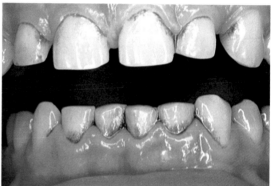

B

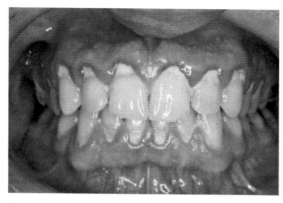

C

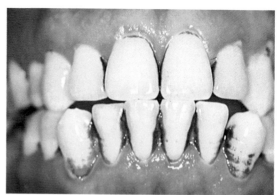

D

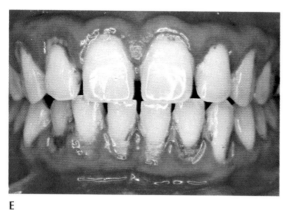

E

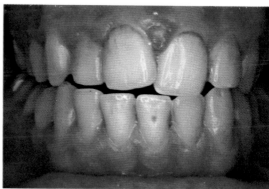

F

Plate III

A, Disclosed supragingival plaque covering one half to two thirds of clinical crowns (courtesy of Dr. S. Socransky, Boston).

B, The same patient as in *A,* disclosed with an oxidation-reduction dye indicating reduced (anaerobic) areas of plaque. The supragingival anaerobic areas (purple stain) are located interproximally and along the gingival margin (courtesy of Dr. S. Socransky, Boston).

C, Materia alba generalized throughout the mouth with heaviest accumulation near the gingiva. Note the gingivitis present.

D, Teeth stained by several weeks of mouth rinses with alexidine. This stain can be easily removed.

E, Supragingival calculus in a patient with gingival inflammation.

F, Green stain on anterior teeth. Note inflamed, enlarged interdental papilla between maxillary central incisors.

that different forms of periodontal disease may have specific microbial etiologies. Examination of the microbiota associated with periodontal health and with different forms of disease revealed previously unsuspected differences in microbial composition. The once prevalent view that dental plaque composition was reasonably consistent from individual to individual and site to site is clearly not valid.[196] The feeling that plaques were similar in composition was derived in part from studies of the infectious potential of plaque by subcutaneous injection into experimental animals[20, 24, 119, 161, 180] and partly from studies of the microbial composition of pooled dental plaque. Since supragingival plaque is usually more abundant (and more easily removed) than subgingival plaque, the samples often reflected the organisms dominant in the supragingival sites.

Despite these problems, several major advances occurred which allowed investigators to analyze more completely the resident microbiota (Table 24–4). In 1970, Sigmund Socransky et al. working at the Forsyth Dental Center in Boston, began developing methods which allowed investigators to sample and cultivate approximately 70 per cent of the bacteria from human oral ecologic sites.* Of primary concern was the recognition that a majority of the subgingival plaque bacteria were anaerobic in nature.[66, 114, 200] Thus, the newer methods of analysis include strict anaerobic techniques. Conceptual changes regarding the nature of plaque also began

to appear around the same time. The primary change was the knowledge that **plaque is not homogeneous in its qualitative and quantitative bacterial composition.**

CRITERIA FOR THE BACTERIAL ETIOLOGY OF PERIODONTAL DISEASE

Classically the criteria for the bacterial etiology in human infectious disease are known as *Koch's postulates.* These postulates, formulated by Robert Koch in the late 1800's, provide a theoretical basis by which a specific bacterial agent may be defined as a causative agent.[25] When these concepts are modified as criteria for periodontal disease etiology,[194] they state that: (1) a suspected organism or group of organisms must be present in the periodontal tissues, (2) the organism or organisms must be able to induce a similar (to human) disease in an animal model system, and (3) the organism or organisms must be shown to have an effect on the periodontal tissues in the course of human disease. Although these criteria appear to be straightforward, they are extremely difficult to fulfill.[190] A major problem is the attempt to establish the etiologic significance of an organism or group of organisms in the presence of a complex and heterogenous microbiota. The bulk of periodontal microbiology research has been directed toward fulfilling the third criterion. The evidence below summarizes the current knowledge, which has resulted in the present-day concept of a **primary bacterial etiology in periodontal disease.**

*See references 20, 21, 23, 125, 126, 132, 133, 135, 136, 139, 168, 195, and 197.

TABLE 24–4 MAJOR CONCEPTUAL AND TECHNICAL CHANGES IN PERIODONTAL DISEASE ETIOLOGY

Conceptual
Anaerobic nature of flora
Bacterial specificity
Architectural arrangement of plaque
Unique bacterial types

Technical
Anaerobic techniques
Sampling refinements
Plaque dispersion
Development of taxonomy schemes

EVIDENCE FOR A PRIMARY BACTERIAL ETIOLOGY IN PERIODONTAL DISEASE

There is growing evidence that bacteria are the etiologic agents of different clinical forms of periodontal disease (Table 24–5), but the major question facing both the researcher and the clinician is whether or not there are specific agents causing periodontal destruction.

The effective treatment of acute necrotizing ulcerative gingivitis (ANUG) with the systemic administration of antibiotics provides a clear and direct example of a

TABLE 24–5 EVIDENCE FOR A PRIMARY BACTERIAL ETIOLOGY IN PERIODONTAL DISEASE

Effectiveness of antibiotics in ANUG
Plaque accumulation and development of gingivitis
Experimental gingivitis eliminated with oral hygiene
Use of antimicrobial agents reduces gingivitis
Epidemiology of periodontal diseases associated with plaque
Histologic evidence of plaque associated with disease
Oral hygiene status
Germ-free animal studies
Efficacy of periodontal therapy

bacterial etiology in this form of periodontal disease.[54, 131, 171] These bacteria have been shown to be large spirochetes possessing up to 20 or more axial fibrils and fusiforms. These spirochetes are not observed in normal, healthy gingiva or in bacterial plaque deposits when disease is absent[100–102] (see Chapter 11.)

The correlation of bacterial accumulation with gingivitis serves as an additional example of the association between bacteria and disease.[1, 2, 147] Löe et al.[95, 150] have demonstrated that gingivitis develops within 10 to 21 days following elimination of oral hygiene procedures (Fig. 24–3). If oral hygiene procedures are then initiated, the gingiva returns to a healthy condition. The association of bacterial plaque deposits and gingival inflammation can also be demonstrated by the elimination of gingivitis with the topical administration of antibiotics and antimicrobial substances.*

---
*See references 24, 49, 78, 108–110, 124, 141, 146, 153, 154, and 210.

Epidemiologic studies have demonstrated the correlation between bacterial accumulation and bone loss in many studies, and there is substantial histologic evidence which demonstrates an association between bacterial accumulations and bone loss in both animals and humans.[4, 118, 169] Thus, the individual state of oral hygiene correlates well with the degree of alveolar bone loss.[16, 199]

Studies with germ-free animals have also suggested a central role for bacteria in the etiology of periodontal disease. From these experiments, it has been demonstrated that mechanical irritation (such as calculus) alone does not cause alveolar bone loss.[34, 163]

The efficacy of periodontal therapy in humans suggests that bacteria are the primary etiologic agents in the destruction of the periodontium. The efficacy of periodontal therapy is primarily based on reducing bacterial plaque accumulations, either directly by improving oral hygiene or indirectly by eliminating gingival and periodontal pockets. The removal of bacteria-laden calculus deposits (see Fig. 24–11) and the design of adequate restorations is also necessary.[211–215]

Human bacterial plaque has the pathogenic potential and the requisite armamentarium to lead to the destruction of the periodontium.[5, 18, 85] Plaque microorganisms are capable of causing destructive abscesses in humans[36, 127] or experimental animals.[37, 181] A number of toxic products can be detected in dental plaque, including endotoxins,[68, 69, 128, 129, 186] cell wall mucopeptides,[176] fatty and organic acids,[111, 113, 189, 216]

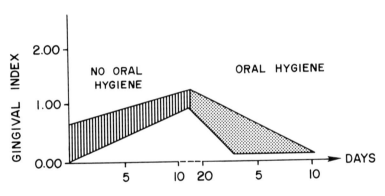

Figure 24–3 Accumulation of Plaque and Development of Gingivitis within 10 to 21 days after cessation of oral hygiene procedures (left side), followed by disappearance of plaque and gingivitis after oral hygiene procedures are reinstated (right side). (Löe, H., Theilade, E., and Jensen, S. B.[107])

hydrogen sulfide,[121, 157] ammonia,[122, 156] indole,[121] amines,[188] etc.[70, 72, 77, 143, 204] In addition, enzymes have been shown to be produced by whole plaque or individual microorganisms from plaque which can be demonstrated to hydrolyze a wide variety of tissue constituents.* Finally, the bacterial masses which accumulate at or in the gingival sulcus possess an array of antigens capable of triggering the host-mediated events that have been postulated as mechanisms of tissue destruction.

POTENTIAL MECHANISMS OF BACTERIA-MEDIATED DESTRUCTION

Periodontal health is maintained as long as the balance between host resistance and bacterial virulence is in favor of the host. It is clear from histologic studies that **bacteria do not invade the periodontal tissues in periodontitis or gingivitis.** Because of the nature of the inflammatory tissue reaction to resident bacteria, the presence of bacterial substances which stimulate host-mediated responses must penetrate the periodontal connective tissue. The presence of bacteria or bacterial products in the periodontal tissues can *indirectly* stimulate the host by triggering potential immunopathologic processes. This area of interest has been an important research endeavor in the last decade. The specific potential immunopathologic mechanisms are discussed in Chapter 23.

The bacteria which colonize the periodontal tissues may also cause tissue destruction by *direct* means. Considerable attention has been focused on characterizing the organisms which produce lytic enzymes or toxic products which could be responsible for destroying the periodontium. This attention was primarily due to the fact that, in earlier cultural studies, samples of pooled gingival material (bacteria) of either healthy or diseased individuals suggested that specific groups of bacteria were not associated with clinical disease. It was, therefore, hypothesized that periodontitis was bacteriologically nonspecific and that certain bacterial me-

tabolites such as lytic enzymes were probably responsible for the tissue destruction.[27, 121] Analysis of whole plaque demonstrated a variety of enzymes capable of destroying the major components of the gingival connective tissue.[16] Furthermore, specific gingival bacteria were also found to produce a variety of substances. In addition to lytic enzymes, there is a wide variety of other potentially toxic products elaborated by gingival bacteria. These factors can be divided into three major areas (Table 24–6): (a) factors that affect intercellular matrix, (b) direct cellular toxicity factors, and (c) inflammatory stimulants.[172–175, 198]

The pathogenic potential of organisms isolated in periodontal lesions has been demonstrated in other ways. For example, bacteria colonizing the mouth of humans can initiate dangerous infections in other parts of the body. Infections initiated by oral organisms can occur accidentally through skin punctures with dental probes or from human bite wounds[36, 127] (Fig. 24–4). Organisms associated with periodontal disease have also been associated with infected surgical wounds and in pleuropulmonary abscesses due to aspiration.[33] Bacterial endocarditis due to bacteria associated with periodontal disease has also increased in occurrence.[33]

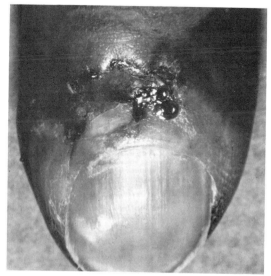

Figure 24–4 Infected finger from accidental puncture with periodontal curette (Courtesy of Dr. R. Barbanell, Long Beach, Cal.)

*See references 27, 39, 59, 133, 145, 146, 169, 174, and 207.

TABLE 24–6 FACTORS INVOLVED IN
BACTERIA-MEDIATED DESTRUCTION

INTRACELLULAR MATRIX

Bacteria	*Substance Elaborated*
Staphylococci	Hyaluronidase
Streptococci	β-glucuronidase
Diphtheroids	Chondroitin sulfatase
Bacteroides	Collagenase

CYTOTOXIC SUBSTANCES

Bacteria	*Substance Elaborated*
Many plaque bacteria	Ammonia, proteases
Many plaque bacteria	Hydrogen sulfide
Many plaque bacteria	Indole, toxic amines
Many plaque bacteria	Organic acids

INFLAMMATORY STIMULANTS

Bacteria	*Substance Elaborated*
Gram-negative organisms	Endotoxin
Gram-positive organisms	Peptidoglycans

Studies in Experimental Animals

The periodontopathic potential of organisms isolated from human periodontal disease can be demonstrated in experimental animals. Ideally animals in which these experiments are carried out should have conditions similar to those which occur in man. Unfortunately, there has been the lack of a good animal model system which develops periodontal pathology comparable to that of humans. Recently, however, great interest has been generated regarding the Beagle dog animal model system.[17, 98] These animals will develop gingivitis and subsequent loss of supporting bone similar to human disease when maintained on soft diets for long periods of time (Fig. 24–5).[165] There are many similarities in the oral flora in the animals, but it is quite clear that these dogs have a characteristic indigenous microbiota different from that of man.[87, 89, 138] Consequently, direct extrapolation of bacteriologic findings from animals to humans should be done with great caution.

Bacteriologic studies have been carried out in other animal model systems.[21] The subcutaneous injection of gingival plaque into Guinea pigs, mice, and rabbits results in the formation of large purulent abscesses which contain a complex array of bacteria similar to those present in the original inoculum. In addition, the lesions

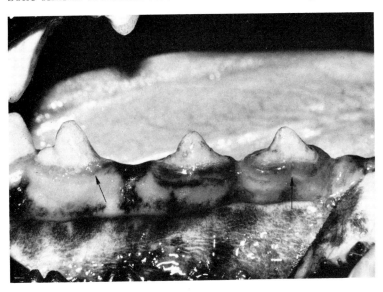

Figure 24–5 Beagle dog demonstrating classic signs of inflammatory periodontal disease. Note inflamed gingival margins (arrow) adjacent to plaque-laden teeth.

are transmissible because exudate obtained from the produced lesions will cause abscesses in other animals. Purification of individual bacterial species from this plaque demonstrated that the transmissible mixed infections could not be initiated with pure cultures of a variety of species within the complex mixture.[20, 35, 119, 120, 161, 180] These types of infections are referred to as **mixed anaerobic infections,** and they represent an example of bacterial synergism in the production of disease[123] (Fig. 24–6). Earlier investigators described these types of infections as "fuso-spirochetal" infections, because fusiform bacteria and spirochetes were usually found to be the predominant organism in exudates.[62, 119] In a series of studies by Macdonald and co-workers, the exact nature of the microorganisms necessary for the induction of mixed anaerobic infections was elucidated.[119, 120] Macdonald clearly demonstrated that *Bacteroides melaninogenicus* was always required in the induction of an infection.[120] Subsequent studies on *B. melaninogenicus* demonstrated that this organism has the biochemical potential to be an overt pathogen. In addition, it has been isolated from a wide variety of human infections, including appendicitis, abscesses of the lung, brain, skin, peritoneal cavity, and other infected wounds.[33] Other studies have demonstrated that *B. melaninogenicus* produces a wide variety of toxic substances and lytic enzymes such as collagenases, deoxyribonuclease, hydrogen sulfide, ammonia, and endotoxin. However, its *direct* role in human periodontal disease has not been elucidated.

Shortly after Keyes demonstrated the transmissible nature of dental caries, observations were made in hamsters regarding periodontal disease.[88] Jordan and Keyes also demonstrated the transmissible nature of a periodontal syndrome between golden hamsters and albino hamsters.[80, 82] Analysis of the plaque demonstrated large numbers of gram-positive filamentous organisms. Pure cultures of these bacteria were effective in initiating periodontal disease when implanted intraorally in susceptible animals. These organisms were identified as *Actinomyces viscosus.* Other investigators demonstrated that the periodontal syndrome in strains of the rice rat were transmissible and that similar gram-positive filamentous bacteria were involved.[28, 177, 179] Thus, for the first time, these studies demonstrated that there is a high degree of *bacterial specificity* in periodontal disease in these animal model systems.

Germ-free animal experiments

A substantial body of knowledge regarding the pathogenic potential of many bacterial isolates from human periodontal disease has been gained using the gnotobiotic rat and pathogen-free hamster.

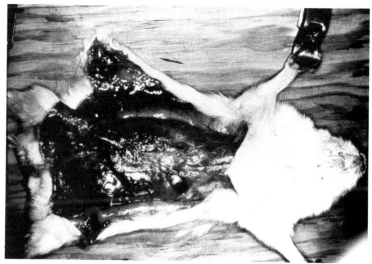

Figure 24–6 Transmissible mixed infection caused by bacteria isolated from human periodontal lesion. (Courtesy of Dr. S. S. Socransky.)

In an important series of experiments, it was demonstrated that the presence of mechanical irritation alone does not cause gingival inflammation or induce alveolar bone loss.[34, 58, 163] Other studies of periodontal disease in these animals suggest that there is specificity in the nature of organisms which cause periodontal destruction, since many species of conventional animals do not demonstrate periodontal destruction even though they harbor a reasonably complex microbiota.

Some gram-positive organisms from the human oral cavity can initiate periodontal destruction in gnotobiotic rats. These include strains of *Streptococcus mutans*, *S. salivarius*, *Actinomyces naeslundii*, *A. viscosus*, *Bacillus* species, and *Nocardia* species.* More recently, certain gram-negative isolates have been shown to be periodontopathic as monocontaminants in gnotobiotic rats. These include strains of *Bacteroides* and *Capnocytophaga*† isolated from idiopathic juvenile periodontitis (periodontosis), *Capnocytophaga*, *Eikenella corrodens*, *Bacteroides melaninogenicus*, *Fusobacterium nucleatum*, and *Selenomonas sputigena*[20, 75, 76] isolated from periodontitis.

The clinical and histologic features of the gram-positive and the gram-negative infections differ (Fig. 24–7). In the gram-positive infections there is generally massive subgingival plaque formation, root caries, and loss of alveolar bone. The mechanism of bone loss in this infection is not clear. Irving and co-workers[74] suggest that bone loss may be associated with an inhibition of osteoblastic activity diminishing bone formation in the animal. Garant,[37] in light and electron microscopic studies of *Actinomyces naeslundii* infection in rats, suggests that brief flare-ups of osteoclastic activity may account for the observed loss of bone. In animals monocontaminated with gram-negative organisms there is little plaque formation and no root caries but massive loss of alveolar bone associated with the presence of large numbers of os-

teoclasts,[75, 76] It is clear that the gram-negative organisms tested were more pathogenic on a per cell basis than the tested gram-positive organisms, since approximately equal destruction was caused in a given period of time by the two types of organisms. However, the numbers of gram-positive organisms were approximately 1000 times higher than gram-negative organisms. This difference in pathogenic potential is of interest because these gram-negative forms have been found in higher numbers in destructive periodontal diseases. It is important to stress that not all oral bacterial isolates cause periodontal destruction in these animal model systems. Specific strains which have failed to cause destruction include strains of *Streptococcus mutans*, *S. sanguis*, *S. mitis*, *S. salivarius*, *Actinomyces naeslundii*, *A. viscosus*, *A. odontolyticus*, *Rothia dentocariosa*, *Escherichia coli*, *Veillonella alcalescens*, *V. parvula*, *Fusobacterium polymorphym*, *F. nucleatum*, *Treponema denticola*, *T. macrodentium*, *Bacillus cereus*, *Arachnia proprionicus*, *Bacterionema matruchotic*, and *Leptotrichia buccalis*.[20]

STRUCTURE AND ORGANIZATION OF SUBGINGIVAL PLAQUE

The gingival sulcus and periodontal pocket harbor a diverse collection of bacteria. The nature of the organisms which colonize these retentive sites differs dramatically from that of the organisms found in supragingival plaque. The morphology of the gingival sulcus makes it less subject to the cleansing activities of the mouth. Thus, these retentive areas form a relatively stagnant environment where organisms which cannot readily adhere to a tooth surface may colonize. Therefore, it is not surprising to find that the majority of the motile bacteria in the mouth colonize these sites. These organisms may also adhere to other bacteria and/or the subgingival epithelium. In addition, organisms within these retentive sites have direct access to nutrients present in sulcular fluid. The oxidation-reduction potential (anaerobic nature) of the gingival sulcus and periodontal pocket has been demonstrated to be very low. Thus, organisms which can exist

---

*See references 42, 43, 74, 82, 83, 85, 86, 115-117, 191, and 192.

†Tentative classification for gram-negative capnophilic fusiform rods which exhibit surface translocation. Possible synonym: *Bacteroides ochreacius*.

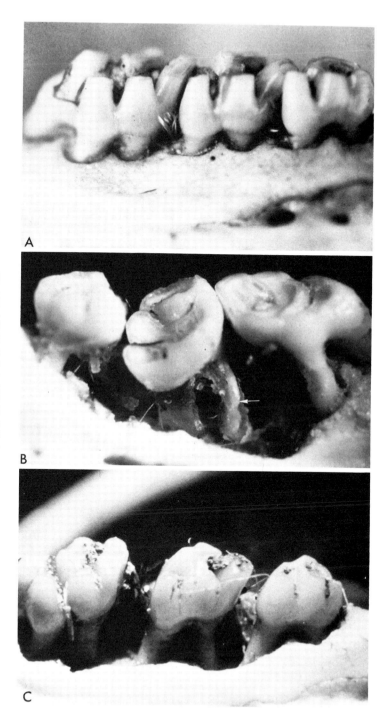

Figure 24–7 *A,* Skull of noninfected control germ-free rat 90 days old. *B,* Massive alveolar bone destruction and root caries (arrow) caused by monoinfection with a periodontopathic strain of *Actinomyces naeslundii* in 90-day-old gnotobiotic rat. Organism isolated from a patient with periodontitis. *C,* Extreme alveolar bone loss caused by monoinfection with a periodontopathic strain of *Capnocytophaga* in a 90-day-old gnotobiotic rat. Organism was isolated from lesion in patient with juvenile periodontitis (periodontosis). Note that these organisms did not cause root surface caries.

TABLE 24–7 MORPHOLOGIC
CHARACTERISTICS OF SUBGINGIVAL PLAQUE

ATTACHED ZONE
Gram-positive bacteria predominate
Does not extend to junctional epithelium
Periodontopathic organisms isolated
Associated with calculus formation
Associated with root caries
May be continuous with supragingival plaque

UNATTACHED ZONE
Gram-negative bacteria predominate
In contact with sulcular and junctional epithelium
Periodontopathic organisms isolated
Increases in size in rapid and juvenile periodontitis
May be "advancing front" of periodontal lesion

only in areas of low oxygen concentration can survive in the gingival sulcus area.

Of major importance in understanding the colonization of microorganisms in oral ecologic sites has been the morphologic description of plaque and plaque development. Light and electron microscopic observation of extracted teeth and adjacent tissues from human patients has been of paramount importance.[104, 105, 170] These studies have demonstrated that the subgingival microbiota exist in at least two components (Table 24–7). These components are differentiated on the basis of their anatomical relation to the tooth surface.

Attached Subgingival Plaque

In the gingival sulcus and periodontal pocket, there is a zone of plaque bacteria which is *attached* to the tooth surface (Table 24–7; Fig. 24–8). These organisms are usually gram-positive rods and cocci such as *Streptococcus mitis, S. sanguis, Actinomyces viscosus, A. naeslundii,* and *Propionibacterium.*[103, 141, 197] In addition, some gram-negative cocci and rods can be found in this attached component. The attached component is apparently continuous with the supragingival plaque and usually extends near the apex of the gingival sulcus or periodontal pocket in chronic periodontitis. Microorganisms of

the attached component have not been demonstrated to be in direct contact with the junctional epithelium.

The attached component of subgingival plaque is associated with the deposition of mineral salts, the formation of calculus, and probably with root caries and root resorption areas. (Fig. 24–9). However, it is not clear whether this attached component develops before other bacteria are found in the gingival sulcus area.

Adjacent to the predominately gram-positive attached component of subgingival plaque is an intermediate zone which separates the attached from the unattached component. There are no clear-cut delineations which demarcate one zone from another.

Unattached Subgingival Plaque

Another discernible area within the subgingival plaque is not directly attached to the tooth surface. It contains motile and gram-negative organisms (Table 24–7; Fig. 24–8). The *unattached* component of the subgingival plaque in chronic periodontitis extends from the gingival margin to the junctional epithelium. Organisms within this zone are in direct contact with the epithelium of the gingival sulcus or periodontal pocket; however, penetration or invasion of bacteria has never been demonstrated. Recent cultural (taxonomy) studies employing techniques which permit more precise localization of the bacterial plaque samples have confirmed the histologic observations of a predominately gram-negative unattached zone.[23, 28, 136] The conceptualization of an unattached zone of plaque at the apical extent of the periodontal pocket or gingival sulcus challenges earlier concepts of a "plaque-free" zone (see Chap. 14). It can readily be seen that removal of teeth for study would disrupt and eliminate the unattached component, leaving a zone immediately coronal to the junctional epithelium devoid of plaque bacteria.

The proportion of the unattached to the attached component of the subgingival plaque varies. The relative size of each

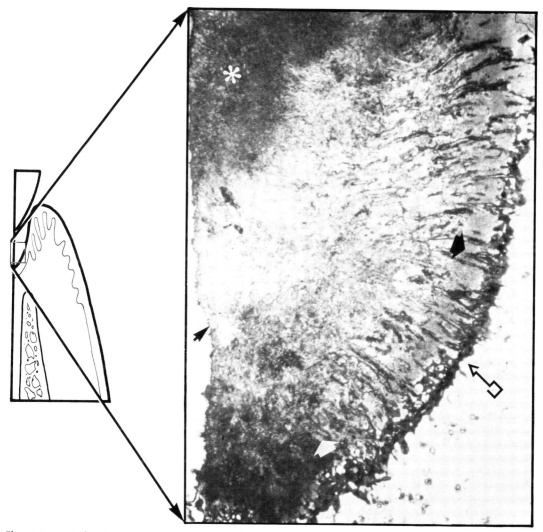

Figure 24–8   *Left,* Diagrammatic representation of the histologic structure of subgingival plaque. *Right,* Histologic section of subgingival plaque. *Arrow with box,* Sulcular epithelium. *White arrow,* Predominantly gram-negative unattached zone. *Black arrow,* Tooth surface. *Asterisk,* Predominantly gram-positive attached zone. (From Listgarten, M.: J. Periodontol., 46:10, 1975.)

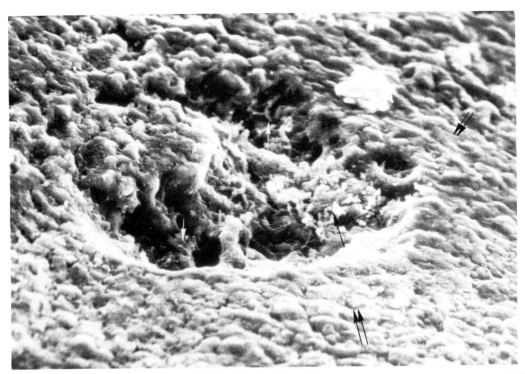

Figure 24–9   Minute lesion on surface of root (resorption concavity) previously covered by plaque. Note microorganisms (single arrow) within lesion. Cemental mounds can easily be identified (double arrows). (Courtesy Dr. J. Sottosanti.)

zone appears to be related to the nature of disease which is present. In rapidly advancing lesions such as idiopathic juvenile periodontitis the attached component of the subgingival plaque appears to be minimal. Instead, the periodontal pocket contains loosely adherent gram-negative rods and spirochetes which make-up the subgingival plaque (Fig. 24–10). Listgarten has also reported a similar pattern of subgingival colonization in patients with a rapid form of periodontitis.[105] In addition, several investigators have suggested that the unattached component adjacent to the sulcular and junctional epithelium may be the "advancing front" of the periodontal lesion.[133, 194] Organisms isolated from both the attached and the unattached components have been shown to be periodontopathic in germ-free animals.

Further examination of the structure of the subgingival plaque reveals characteristics of each component which are important in understanding the relationship of certain groups of microorganisms to disease. It is clear from clinical examination that cal-

culus is attached to the tooth surface and not to the epithelium.[1] Thus, the attached zone of subgingival plaque is most important in calculus formation. In addition, root caries undoubtedly result from a subgingival plaque which is also in contact with the root surface (Fig. 24–9). Bacteriologic information (see next section) confirms that a gram-positive flora typical of the attached plaque is associated with calculus formation and root caries. **Calculus is always covered by adherent plaque** (Fig. 24–11).

MICROBIOLOGY

Historical Background Regarding the Etiologic Role of Oral Microorganisms

One of the earliest complete studies of the bacterial flora associated with periodontal disease was performed by Goadby.[52] He found various streptococci, *"Bacillus fusiformis"* and spirochetes, and a great number of other organisms. His conclusion was that lowered resistance re-

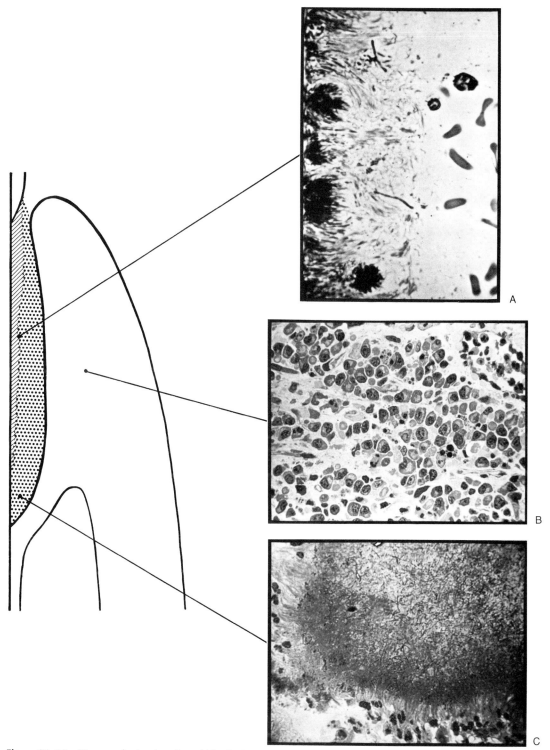

Figure 24–10   Diagram depicts location of histologic sections A, B, and C, from a case of juvenile periodontitis (periodontosis) *A,* Sparsely colonized root surface (R). *B,* Biopsy of adjacent connective tissue showing plasma cells (P) and lymphocytes (L). *C,* Unattached plaque surrounded by PMN's from adjacent connective tissue. (Histologic sections courtesy of Dr. Max Listgarten.)

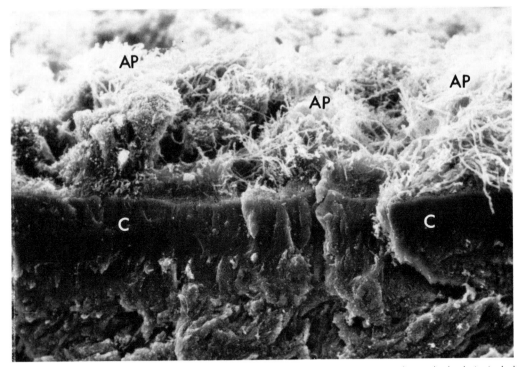

Figure 24–11   Scanning electron photomicrograph of cross-section of cementum (C) with attached subgingival plaque (AP). Area shown is within a periodontal pocket. (Courtesy of Dr. J. Sottosanti.)

sulting from insufficient production of substances immune to the oral flora was the primary factor in the etiology of the disease. He was interested in autogenous vaccines made from the organisms of the periodontal lesions to assist in curing the disease. Glynn[51] considered the nonhemolytic streptococci to be the chief pathogenic aerobic organisms in periodontal infections. According to Hartzell,[63, 64] the leading role in the etiology of periodontal disease was played by the streptococci, which were thought to be the first to penetrate the tissues and create the initial lesion, and prepared the way for other organisms.

Noguchi[144] isolated in pure culture the particular spirochete, which he called *Treponema mucosum*, from the exudate in the periodontal pockets. The organisms apparently thrived on injured or impaired tissue but did not grow on healthy or intact tissue. He also recognized the presence in chronic periodontal disease of streptococci, staphylococci, and pneumococci, but believed that specific oral spiro-

chetes were directly responsible for the disease. He also noted the presence of other spiral forms, as well as the fusiform bacillus. Since Noguchi was one of the first bacteriologists to perfect techniques for the cultivation of spirochetes, he tended to place much emphasis upon their presence. Actually, Leeuwenhoek,[92] in the late seventeenth century, was the first to record the existence of oral spirochetes. The discovery of the oral spirochetes was the initial step in the development of the field of general bacteriology.

Kritchevsky and Sèguin[92] recovered spirochetal forms of bacteria from every case of chronic destructive periodontal disease that they studied. Considering the bacteria a possible cause, they treated their cases with intravenous salvarsan, but obtained only temporary results unless careful scaling of the teeth was included in the treatment. They assumed that the spirochetes were secondary invaders because they flourished in the debris and microaerophilic environment of the periodontal pocket. Hemmens and Harrison[65] found little difference between the bacterial flora of normal gingiva and of suppurative lesions. They believed bacteria in periodontal disease to be secondary invaders, possibly responsible for the suppurative phase. Smith,[185] however, concluded that *Treponema microdentium* and the fusiform bacillus, as well as anaerobic streptococcus and a vibrio, could cause suppurative periodontal disease in the absence of any other factors. Tunnicliff et al.[208] found that a combination of fusiform bacilli and spirilla became pathogenic when the vitality of the tissue was impaired. Gins[44] believed that all gingival disease was caused by spirilla and should therefore be designated "spirillosis."

At one time there was considerable interest in the amebae as causative factors in periodontal disease. Barrett[6] and Bass[7] considered *Entamoeba gingivalis* and *E. buccalis* of such etiologic significance that they recommended the amebicide emetine for the treatment of periodontal disease. Glynn[51] found the ameba *E. buccalis* abundant in mouths with poor oral hygiene. It was present in periodontal pockets, but not consistently so. It was not found in healthy periodontal tissues, and emetine had no effect upon it. Hartzell also studied the use of emetine in the treatment of periodontal disease and became convinced of its uselessness. Keilty[84] found *E. gingivalis* present in direct smears in 95.5 per cent of 201 cases of destructive periodontal disease, and absent in control cases. He concluded that it is a harmless parasite.

Conant and Rosebury[15] discussed the presence of *Actinomycetes* in the oral cavity, and Rosebury[160] reviewed the subject in considerable detail. These are a varied group of filamentous microorganisms with characteristics between bacteria and molds. They are found in the normal gingival sulcus and in calculus. *Actinomyces* is a true parasite of mucous membrane and occurs in the presence of low-grade, nonspecific, inflammatory processes in the gingiva. The accepted concept is that it may produce disease as an endogenous infection, comparable to *Streptococcus viridans* in endocarditis or *Escherichia coli* in cystitis. The disease, however, is not periodontal disease but actinomycosis.

In the past decade there have been a number of changes in our concepts of the etiology of periodontal disease. In the 1960's it was generally accepted that dental plaque was in some way associated with human periodontal destruction. It was felt that the presence of plaque initiated a series of as-yet-undefined events which led to the destruction of the periodontium. The composition of plaque was thought to be relatively similar from patient to patient and site to site within patients. Variability was recognized, but the true extent of differences in bacterial composition was not appreciated. It was thought that the major event triggering destructive periodontal disease was an increase in mass of bacterial plaque, possibly accompanied by a diminution of host resistance. Indeed, in the mid 1960's the classic studies of Löe and co-workers[101, 205] convincingly deonstrated that plaque accumulation directly preceded and initiated gingivitis. It was also felt by many investigators that gingivitis was harmful, leading eventually to the destruction of the periodontal tissues, probably by host-mediated events.

Certain observations troubled clinicians and research workers. For example, the localized nature of destruction occurring in individual mouths was of considerable concern. If all plaques were alike and the host responded consistently to a constant challenge, then why was destruction taking place adjacent to one tooth but not another? Another troublesome observation was the presence of large accumulations of plaque and severe gingivitis in individuals for years without destruction of the supporting structures. In contrast, individuals were observed with little detectable plaque or clinical inflammation and yet dramatic loss of the periodontium. If host-mediated changes associated with inflammation were the main mechanisms of destruction, why were so many teeth retained in the presence of continual gingivitis? One explanation could be the additional effect of local factors such as trauma from occlusion, overhanging fillings, etc.

Other explanations can be derived from studies of the microbiology of periodontal disease. The major changes in concept of the etiology of periodontal disease are based largely on the concepts and work of Socransky.[190, 193, 196] Through his pioneering efforts in the technical aspects of plaque analysis, a better understanding of the structure and composition of the bacterial plaque associated with gingival and periodontal tissues has been obtained. This work has set the stage for future studies.

Oral Flora

The oral cavity is sterile at birth, but a simple, primarily aerobic flora becomes established within six to ten hours.[193] Anaerobes appear in *some* mouths within the first 10 days, and are present in *most* by five months of age, before the teeth erupt, and in 100 per cent of mouths when the incisors appear. The anaerobes increase with age, but the facultative types remain numerically predominant. Microscopic counts in saliva range from 43 million to 5.5 billion organisms per milliliter, with an average of 750 million.[13] A representative census of the salivary bacterial population is shown in Table 24–8. Also present are fungi, including *Candida*, *Cryptococcus*, and *Saccharomyces* and protozoa such as *Entamoeba gingivalis* and *Trichomonas tenax*.[13] In some instances viruses can be found in the oral cavity.

Most of the salivary bacteria are derived from the dorsum of the tongue, from which they are detached by mechanical action; lesser amounts come from the remainder of the oral mucous membrane. The number of microorganisms increases temporarily during sleep, and decreases after eating or toothbrushing.

Supragingivally, bacteria associated with periodontal health can accumulate up to approximately 12 cells thick on the tooth surface consisting of mainly gram-positive coccal and rod-shaped bacteria (Fig.24–12).

These organisms initiate plaque growth by their ability to adhere to the tooth surface (pellicle) and then proliferate in that particular ecological niche. The colonization of the tooth surface by supragingival plaque bacteria appears to be quite specific and apparently depends upon the interaction of the bacterial surface with the salivary glycoprotein of the pellicle. *Streptococcus sanguis* and gram-positive rods have been shown to be the major groups of bacteria which initiate supragingival plaque.[46]

Once supragingival plaque growth is initiated, secondary growth and maturation take place. During this phase bacterial population shifts occur. Filamentous organisms and gram-negative bacteria increase in proportion. In general this plaque appears more compact (Figs. 24–12 and 24–13). Bacterial cohesive interactions are also more evident (Figs. 24–13 and 24–14).

The microorganisms commonly encountered in such sites in adults include *Strep-*

TABLE 24–8   INDIGENOUS FLORA OF HUMAN SALIVA*

Bacterial Group	Predominant Isolates of the Group	Percentage
Gram-positive facultative cocci	Streptococci represent 41 per cent of all isolates and are composed of S. salivarius, S. mitis, and small numbers of enterococci; the remainder are staphylococci	46.2
Gram-negative anaerobic cocci	Veillonella	15.9
Gram-positive anaerobic cocci	Peptostreptococcus or Peptococcus	13.0
Gram-positive facultative rods	Diphtheroids, Actinomyces,	11.8
Gram-negative anaerobic rods	Campylobacter sputorum, Bacteroides, Fusobacterium	4.8
Gram-positive anaerobic rods	Propionibacterium, Actinomyces	4.8
Gram-negative facultative rods	Unidentified	2.3
Gram-negative facultative cocci	Unidentified	1.2

*Modified from Gordon, D. F., Jr., and Jong, B. B.: Appl. Microbiol., *16*:428, 1968.

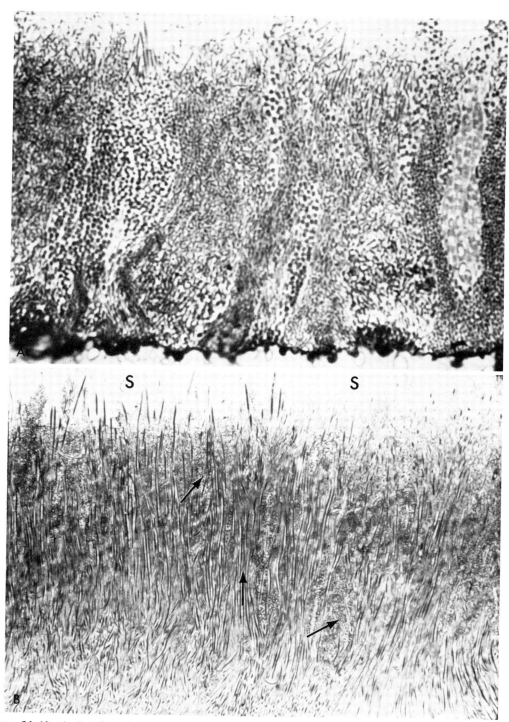

Figure 24–12 *A,* One-day-old plaque. Microcolonies of plaque bacteria extend perpendicularly away from tooth surfaces. (From Dr. Max Listgarten. J. Periodontol., *46:10, 1975*). *B,* Developed supragingival plaque showing overall filamentous nature and microcolonies (arrows) extending perpendicularly away from tooth surface. Saliva-plaque interface shown (S). (Courtesy of Dr. Max Listgarten.)

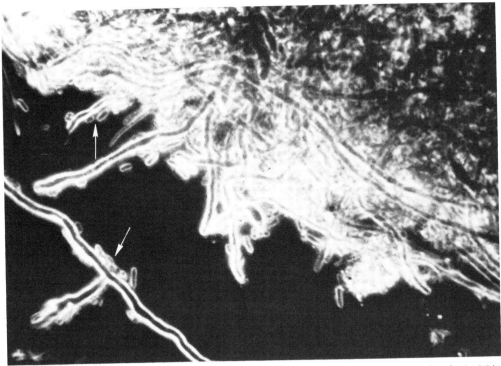

Figure 24–13   Darkfield photomicrograph demonstrates filamentous nature of plaque associated with gingivitis. Note attachment of smaller bacteria to filaments. (arrows).

tococcus mitis, S. sanguis, Staphylococcus epidermidis, Rothia dentocariosa, Actinomyces viscosus, A. naeslundii, and occasionally species of *Neisseria* and *Veillonella.*[41, 136, 197, 209] This list is not meant to exclude other forms which can frequently be detected, but to indicate the organisms most likely to be encountered.

Gingivitis

The development of gingivitis is thought to be a major consequence of the bacteria associated with an increase in supragingival plaque formation. The gram-positive filamentous rods, mainly *Actinomyces,* appear to be of major significance in this

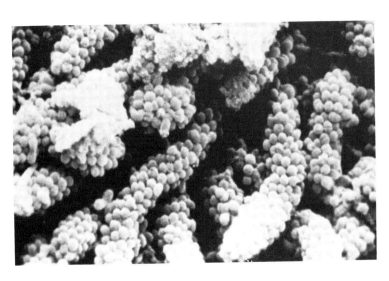

Figure 24–14   Longstanding supragingival plaque near the gingival margin demonstrates "corn cob" arrangement. Central gram-negative filamentous core (*Leptotrichia buccalis*). Coccal forms held in position by firm intercellular attachment (cohesion). (Courtesy of Dr. Z. Skobe, 1975).

clinical condition.[115, 202] The sequence of development of supragingival plaque (discussed in an earlier section) is associated with an increase in absolute numbers and percentages of *Actinomyces* species. The appearance of gram-negative forms, such as spirochetes, *Bacteroides, Leptotrichia*, vibrios, and other motile forms in the late stages of the development of gingival redness clearly indicate a sequential process in the development of gingivitis, since these organisms are associated with subgingival plaque. However, the initial insult to the periodontal structures in gingivitis may be associated with noxious elements of large masses of the gram-positive bacteria associated with this supragingival plaque. It is suggested that the increased numbers of bacteria would subject the gingival tissues to larger quantities of potentially destructive substances. Thus, as bacterial plaque accumulates in the gingival sulcus area, clinically detectable gingivitis will invariably but not always develop. An interesting arrangement of bacteria often observed at the external surface of supragingival plaque near the gingival margin is the "corn cob" arrangement[79] (Fig. 24–14). This usually consists of a central gram-negative filament, *Leptotrichia buccalis*, which is covered by coccal forms of a second species. The significance of these in gingivitis is not clear.

It has been suggested by many investigators that repeated episodes of gingivitis can lead to periodontal bone loss (periodontitis). This fact is a general clinical observation. It stems from many epidemiologic studies which have demonstrated that the continued presence of bacterial plaque is associated with alveolar bone loss. However, it is quite clear that some individuals may have recurrent episodes of gingivitis without periodontitis developing. It is not clear whether the microbiota in these individuals is different from that of those who develop gingivitis and, subsequently, periodontitis.

The microbiota associated with **pregnancy gingivitis** has recently been described. *B. melaninogenicus* and *Capnocytophaga* were found in high concentrations. Their proliferation may be due to a direct stimulating effect of increased levels of hormone in saliva and sulcular fluid.[1a, 91a]

The microbiota associated with A.N.U.G. has been described in Chapter 11.

Gingival Sulcus

To date there have been few technically acceptable studies which have specifically documented the nature of the *sulcular* microbial flora associated with periodontal health. In general terms the healthy periodontal tissues of humans appear to be associated with a minimal microbial flora both supragingivally and subgingivally. Depending on the methods used for sampling and cultivating these flora, certain patterns have emerged.[148, 164, 166]

Subgingivally the nature of the microbiota apparently conforms to the architectural arrangement previously described. Gram-positive organisms[183] and gram-negative organisms such as *Capnocytophaga, Bacteriodes* species, *Campylobacter,* and *Fusobacterium* can be isolated. These organisms are found in the apparently sparse unattached zone of the subgingival plaque.[140]

Periodontitis

There are limited data which suggest that specific organisms, or groups of organisms, are associated with different forms of human periodontal diseases. This is especially true when one considers the microbiota associated with periodontitis. However, there are important observations which demonstrate that trends or patterns of bacterial colonization in periodontal pockets actually exist. The exact nature of this microbiota depends on the state of periodontal destruction, disease activity, and host resistance. Whether the lesion is associated with chronic disease or whether it is associated with a more rapid form of periodontal destruction is an important consideration.

In the chronic forms of periodontitis (most common), there is a large component of attached subgingival plaque. Filamentous organisms such as *Actinomyces israelii, A. naeslundii*, and *A. viscosus* are numerous[23, 218] (Fig. 24–15). These organisms may constitute 30 to 40 per cent of the bacteria present. In almost all cases this attached plaque is associated with varying degrees of calculus formation. *A. naeslundii* and *A. israelii* demonstrate a characteristic pathogenicity when implanted as monocontaminants in germ-free

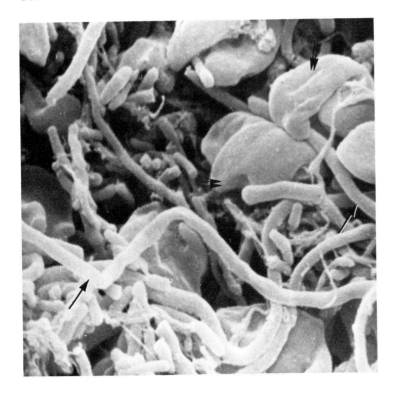

Figure 24–15 Scanning electron photomicrograph of attached subgingival plaque from chronic periodontitis. Filamentous organism (single arrows) and red blood cells (double arrows) can be seen.

rats[20, 74, 191, 192] (see Fig. 24–7). These organisms form large accumulations of bacterial plaque and cause root caries. Alveolar bone loss appears to be associated with a suppression of osteoblasts.

The unattached component of the subgingival plaque in chronic periodontitis has not been adequately studied. However, electron microscopic observations suggest that this zone contains numerous gram-negative rods and spirochetes. Limited information from cultural studies also suggests that *Bacteroides melaninogenicus, Fusobacterium, Capnocytophaga, Campylobacter,* and *Selenomonas* species vary in concentration.

In rapid destructive forms of periodontitis, the unattached component of the pocket flora predominates at the apical portion of the periodontal pocket[105, 201] (Fig. 24–16). The microbiota associated with this rapid periodontitis is characterized by the presence of large numbers of gram-negative microorganisms, including *Fusobacterium nucleatum, Bacteroides melaninogenicus ss assacharolyticus,Eikenella corrodens, B. fragilis,* and anaerobic vibrios. In addition, *Capnocytophaga* organisms and *Selenonomas sputigena* are found in periodontitis lesions. When organisms from this zone of the subgingival microbiota are implanted into germ-free animals as monocontaminants, they are extremely periodontopathic. However, the resultant destruction in these animals differs markedly from that observed when gram-positive organisms are established. Infection with these gram-negative organisms results in rapid alveolar bone destruction, a lack of large bacterial masses, no root caries,and a stimulation of osteoclastic activity (see Fig. 24–7). Thus, it appears that the virulence of these organisms in experimental animals appears to be of a higher order than that of the gram-positive organisms associated with the attached component of subgingival plaque from *chronic* periodontitis. Gibbons suggests that if infection with gram-negative organisms is superimposed upon that produced by gram-positive organisms, the rate of tissue destruction is accelerated.[41] The findings of higher proportions of gram-negative anaerobic organisms in the depths of rapid periodontitis pockets substantiate this suggestion. These organisms may accelerate the rate of destruction because of their elaboration of endotoxins.

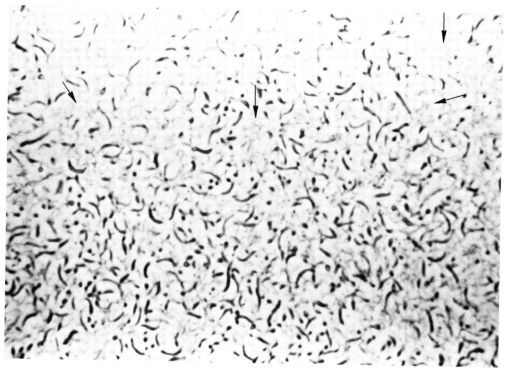

Figure 24–16 Histologic section of unattached plaque from a patient with a rapidly destructive form of periodontitis. Arrows indicate spirochetes forming a light-staining background. Vibrio and spiral-shaped organisms (*Selenomonas*) predominate. (From Listgarten, M., et al.: J. Periodontol., *47*:1, 1976.)

Idiopathic Juvenile Periodontitis (Periodontosis)

Recent evidence has suggested that gram-negative rods predominate in the molar-incisor lesions of patients diagnosed as having juvenile periodontitis (periodontosis).[133–137, 139, 182, 203] These patients exhibit minimal plaque accumulation and calculus and minimal clinically evident gingivitis and root caries. Almost all of the bacteria located in these periodontal pockets are unattached to the tooth surface, and they are saccharolytic[105, 133] (see Fig. 24–10). The subgingival bacteria are often seen surrounded by polymorphonuclear leukocytes. The connective tissue adjacent to the lesions demonstrates a histologic picture similar to chronic periodontitis (see Fig. 24–10).

Many of the organisms isolated from young patients with the molar-incisor lesions differ from those found in chronic periodontitis. The isolates from localized sites do not fall into easily recognizable species. One group frequently detected in most patients are the gram-negative surface translocating fusiform organisms *Capnocytophaga*. Another group of bacteria commonly found in large numbers in subgingival sites include members of the genus *Bacteroides*. Other gram-negative isolates have been frequently but not consistently encountered. In contrast, bacteria from healthy sites in some of the same patients make up a gram-positive microbiota typical of that seen in mixed plaque from subgingival sites in other healthy individuals.

The pathogenic potential of the gram-negative organisms isolated from juvenile periodontitis lesions has been demonstrated in germ-free rats[20, 75, 136, 195, 196] (see Fig. 24–7). The destruction caused by monoinfection with individual organisms isolated from juvenile periodontitis lesions results in minimal plaque formation, no root caries, extensive loss of alveolar bone, and a marked osteoclastic response.

The circumstantial evidence of isolating groups of bacteria at the site of rapid

TABLE 24–9 GENERAL DISTRIBUTION OF MICROORGANISMS ISOLATED FROM HEALTHY AND DISEASED PERIODONTIUMS

A Subgingival
B Marginal
C Supragingival
* Comparison with subgingival healthy site

	HEALTH		GINGIVITIS		PERIODONTITIS										
	AGED	HEALTHY	GINGIVITIS	ANUG	INCIPIENT		ADVANCED		RAPID		ABSCESS			JUVENILE		CHILDREN	
	A	C	A	B	C	A	B	C	A	A	*	A	*	A	*	A	B	*	A	*	A	*

| GRAM POSITIVE |
| STREPTOCOCCUS |
| STAPHYLOCOCCUS |
| ACTINOMYCES |
| ROTHIA, ARACHNIA |
| PEPTOCOCCUS |
| PEPTOSTREPTOCOCCUS |
| PROPIONIBACTERIUM |
| OTHER |
| GRAM NEGATIVE |
| VEILLONELLA |
| EIKENELLA |
| CAPNOCYTOPHAGA |
| BACTEROIDES MELANINOGENICUS |
| BACTEROIDES |
| FUSOBACTERIUM |
| LEPTOTRICHIA |
| SELENOMONAS |
| CAMPYLOBACTER |
| "VIBRIO–CORRODING" |
| UNIDENTIFIED |
| SPIROCHETES |

periodontal breakdown, and their pathogenicity in animal model systems suggests that bacteria may be of major significance in this form of human periodontal disease.

The Concept of Specificity

The concept of bacterial specificity suggests that periodontal disease may be a group of diseases with different etiologies and clinical course, but with similar clinical symptomatology. With the recognition of a diverse group of etiologic agents, more accurate clinical and laboratory diagnosis could be made.[136, 196] Our inabilities to separate clinically such disease entities at the present time reflects a lack of diagnostic acumen, as well as insufficient basic understanding of periodontal disease pathogenesis. Accurate identification of organisms is a prerequisite to this understanding.

Specific disease entities may be due to the interaction of bacteria with host-derived products such as hormones.[91a, 141] Table 24–9 is a compilation of the current information regarding the general distribution of microorganisms isolated from healthy and diseased periodontiums.

REFERENCES

1. Arno, A., Waerhaug, J., Lovdahl, A., and Schei, O.: Incidence of gingivitis as related to sex, occupation, tobacco consumption, toothbrushing and age. Oral Surg., 11:587, 1958.
1a. Angel, J., Newman, M. G., and Carranza, F. A., Jr.: Unpublished observations, 1978.
2. Ash, M. M., Jr., Gitlin, B. N., and Smith, W. A.: Correlation between plaque and gingivitis. J. Periodontol., 35:424, 1964.
3. Axelsson, P., and Lindhe, J.: The effect of a preventive programme on dental plaque, gingivitis and caries in school children. Results after one and two years. J. Clin. Periodont., 1:126, 1974.

4. Baer, P. N., Keyes, P. H., and White, C. L.: Studies on experimental calculus formation in the rat. XII. On the transmissibility of factors affecting dental calculus. J. Periodontol., 39:86, 1968.

5. Bahn, A. N.: Microbial potential in the etiology of periodontal disease. J. Periodontol., 41:603, 1970.

6. Barrett, M. T.: Clinical Report upon amoebic pyorrhea. Dent. Cosmos., 56:1345, 1914.

7. Bass, C. C., and Johns, M.: Pyorrhea dentalis and alveolaris-specific cause and treatment. J.A.M.A., 64:553, 1915.

8. Bergey's Manual of Determinative Bacteriology. 8th ed. Baltimore, The Williams & Wilkins Company, 1974.

9. Bowen, W.: Nature of plaque. Oral Sci. Rev., 9:3, 1976.

10. Boyden, S.: The chemotactic effect of mixtures of antibody and antigen on polymorphonuclear leukocytes. J. Exp. Med., 115:453, 1962.

11. Brandtzaeg, P., and Kraus F.: Autoimmunity and periodontal disease. Odont. Tidskrift, 73:285, 1965.

12. Bricknell, K., Grinenko, V., Carlton, D., and Newman, M.G.: GLC rapid analysis of bacteria in dental plaque. IADR Abs., 1978.

13. Burnett, G. W., and Scherp, H. W.: Oral Microbiology and Infectious Diseases. 3rd Ed. Baltimore, The Williams & Wilkins Company, 1968.

14. Burnett, H., et al.: Microbiology of dental infection. Dent. Clin. North Am., 14:681, 1970.

15. Conant, N. F., and Rosebury, T.: The Actinomycetes. In Dubois, R.: Bacterial and Mycotic Infections of Man: Philadelphia, J. B. Lippincott Company, 1974.

16. Courant, P. R., Paunio, I., and Gibbons, R. J.: Infectivity and hyaluronidase activity of debris from healthy and diseased gingiva. Arch. Oral Biol., 10:119, 1965.

17. Courant, P. R., Saxe, S. R., Nash, L., and Roddy S.: Sulcular bacteria in the Beagle dog. Periodontics, 6:250, 1968.

18. Cowley, G.: Effect of plaque on gingival epithelium. Oral Sci. Rev., 1:103, 1972.

19. Crawford, A., Socransky, S. S., and Bratthall, G.: Predominant cultivable microbiota of advanced periodontitis. J. Dent. Res., 54:209, 1975.

20. Crawford, A., Socransky, S., Smith, E., and Philips, R.: Pathogenicity testing of oral isolates in gnotobiotic rats. J. Dent. Res., 568:275, 1977.

21. Darwish, S., Hyppa, T., Manganiello, A., and Socransky, S. S.: Predominant cultivable microorganisms in periodontitis and periodontosis. II. Early periodontitis. J. Dent. Res., 52:289, 1973.

22. Darwish, S., and Socransky, S. S.: Personal communication, 1975.

23. Darwish, S., Hyppa, T., and Socransky, S. S.: Studies of the predominant cultivable microbiota of early periodontitis. J. Periodont. Res., 1976, in press.

24. Davies, R. M., Jensen, S. B., Schiott, C. R., and Loe, H.: The effect of topical application of chlorhexidine on the bacterial colonization of the teeth and gingiva. J. Periodont. Res., 5:96, 1970.

25. Davis, B. D., Dulbecco, R., Eisen, H. N., Ginsberg, H. S., Wood, W. B., and McCarty, M.,: Microbiology. 2nd ed. Hagerston, Md., Harper and Row, Publishers, Inc., 1973.

26. de Araujo, W. C., and MacDonald, J. B.: Gingival crevice microbiota of pre-school children. Arch. Oral Biol., 9:227, 1964.

27. Dewar, M. R.: Bacterial enzymes and periodontal disease. J. Dent. Res., 37:100, 1958.

28. Dick, D. S., and Shaw, J. H.: The infectious and transmissible nature of the periodontal syndrome of the rice rat. Arch. Oral Biol., 11:1095, 1966.

29. Dwyer, D. M., and Socransky, S. S.: Predominant cultivable micro-organisms inhabiting periodontal pockets. Br. Dent. J., 124:560, 1968.

30. Ellison, S. A.: Oral bacteria and periodontal disease. J. Dent. Res., 49:198, 1970.

31. Engee, M.: Mycoplasma salivarium in human gingival sulcus. J. Periodont. Res., 5:163, 1970.

32. Evans, R. T., Spaeth, S., and Mergenhagen, S. E.: Bacteriocidal antibody in mammalian serum to obligatory anaerobic gram-negative bacteria. J. Immunol., 97:112, 1966.

33. Finegold, S.: Anaerobic Bacteria in Human Disease. New York, Academic Press, Inc., 1977.

34. Fitzgerald, R. J., and McDaniel, E. G.: Dental calculus in germfree rats. Arch. Oral Biol., 2:239, 1960.

35. Foley, G., and Rosebury, T.: Comparative infectivity for Guinea pigs of fusospirochetal exudates from different disease. J. Dent. Res., 21:375, 1942.

36. Fritzell, K. E.: Infections of hand due to human mouth organisms. Lancet, 60:135, 1940.

37. Garant, P. R.: An electron microscopic study of the periodontal tissues of germfree rats and rats monoinfected with Actinomyces naeslundii. J. Periodont. Res., Suppl., 15:1, 1976.

38. Genco, R. J., Evans, R. T., and Ellison, S. A.: Dental research in microbiology with emphasis on periodontal disease. J. Am. Dent. Assoc., 78:1016, 1969.

39. Gibbons, R. J., and Macdonald, J. B.: Degradation of collagenous substrates by Bacteroides melaninogenicus. J. Bacteriol., 81:614, 1961.

40. Gibbons, R. J., Socransky, S. S.: Sawyers, S., Kapsimalis, B., and Macdonald, J. B.: The microbiota of the gingival crevice area of man-II. Arch. Oral Biol., 8:281, 1963.

41. Gibbons, R. J., et al.: Studies of the predominant cultivable microbiota of dental plaque. Arch. Oral Biol., 8:281, 1963.

42. Gibbons, R. J., Berman, K. S., Knoettner, P., and Kapsimalis, B.: Dental caries and alveolar bone loss in gnotobiotic rats infected with capsule forming streptococci of human origin. Arch. Oral Biol., 11:549, 1966.

43. Gibbons, R. J., and Banghart, S.: Induction of dental caries in gnotobiotic rats with a levan-forming streptococcus and a streptococcous isolated from subacute bacterial endocarditis. Arch. Oral Biol., 13:297, 1968.

44. Gibbons, R. J.: Bacterial plaque as common denominator in dental caries and periodontal

disease. Am. Inst. Oral Biol. Ann. Meeting, 1969, pp. 39–46.

45. Gibbons, R. J.: Microbiological model and dental disease. Va. Dent. J., 49:7, 1972.

46. Gibbons, R., and Van Houte, J.: On the formation of dental plaque. J. Periodontol., 44:347, 1973.

47. Gibbons, R. J., and Van Houte, J.: Microbiology of Periodontal Disease. In Textbook of Oral Biology. Philadelphia, W. B. Saunders Company, in press.

48. Gins, H. A.: The significance of spirillosis for the pathogenesis of the periodontal disturbances. Dtsch. Zahnarzt. Z., 2:282, 1947.

49. Gjermo, P., Baastad, K. L., and Rolla, G.: The plaque inhibiting capacity of 11 antibacterial compounds. J. Periodont. Res., 5:102, 1970.

50. Glickman, I.: Periodontal disease. N. Engl. J. Med., 284:1071, 1971.

51. Glynn, E. E.: The organisms found in periodontal infections and their relations to the toxemia. Br. Dent. J., 44:601, 1923.

52. Goadby, K.: Diseases of the Gums and Oral Mucous Membrane. New York, Oxford University Press, 1928.

53. Gold, R.: Dental caries and periodontal disease considered as infectious diseases. Adv. Appl. Microbiol., 11:135, 1969.

54. Goldhaber, P., and Giddon, D. B.: Present concepts concerning the etiology and treatment of acute necrotizing ulcerative gingivitis. Int. Dent. J., 14:468, 1964.

55. Gottlieb, B., Entamoeba gingivitis in periodontal disease. J. Periodont., 42:412, 1970.

56. Grinenko, V., Weiner, M., Karge, H., Angel, I., Newman, M., and Sims, T.: The predominant cultivable microbiota of periodontal abscesses. J. Dent. Res., 56B:278, 1977.

57. Gupta, O. R., Auskaps, A. M., and Shaw, J. H.: Periodontal disease in the rice rat. IV. The effects of antibiotics on the incidence of periodontal lesions. Oral Surg., 10:1169, 1957.

58. Gustafsson, B. E., and Krasse, B.: Dental calculus in germfree rats. Acta Odont. Scand., 20:135, 1962.

59. Hampp, E. G., Mergenhagen, S. E., and Omata, R. R.: Studies of mucopolysaccharase activity on oral spirochetes. J. Dent. Res., 38:979, 1959.

60. Handleman, S. L., and Hess, C.: Bacterial populations of selected tooth surface sites. J. Dent. Res., 48:67, 1969.

61. Hardie, J.: Normal microbial flora of mouth. Soc. Appl. Bact. Symp. Ser., 3:47, 1974.

62. Hari, T.: Fusiforms in gingival material. Br. Dent. J., 126:82, 1969.

63. Hartzell, T. B.: The use of emetine in the treatment of periodontal disease. J. All. Dent. Soc., 2:143, 1915.

64. Hartzell, T. B.: Etiology of pyorrhea alveolaris with simplified treatment. J. Am. Dent. Assoc., 12:1452, 1925.

65. Hemmens, E. S., and Harrison, R. W.: Studies on the anaerobic bacterial flora of suppurative periodontitis. J. Infect. Dis., 70:131, 1942.

66. Holdeman, L. V., and Moore, W. E. C.: Polytechnical Institute and State University Anaerobe Laboratory Manual. Virginia University, 1972.

67. Holt, S. C., Simpson, J. L., and Leadbetter, E. R.: Some characteristics of "gliding" bacteria isolated from human dental plaque. J. Dent. Res., 54:L208, 1975.

68. Hook, W. A., Snyderman, R., and Mergenhagen, S. E.: Histamine releasing factor generated by the interaction of endotoxin with hamster serum. Infect. Immun., 2:462, 1970.

69. Hook, W. A., Snyderman, R., and Mergenhagen, S. E.: Further characterization of a factor from endotoxin-treated serum which releases histamine and heparin from mast cells. Infect. Immun., 5:909, 1972.

70. Horton, J. E., Leikin, S., and Oppenheim, J. J.: Human lymphoproliferative reaction to saliva and dental plaque-deposits: An in vitro correlation with periodontal disease. J. Periodontol., 43:522, 1972.

71. Horton, J. E., Raisz, L. G., Simmons, H. A., Oppenheim, J. J., and Mergenhagen, S. E.: Bone resorbing activity in supernatant fluid from cultured human peripheral blood leukocytes. Science, 177:793, 1972.

72. Horton, J. E., Oppenheim, J. J., and Mergenhagen, S. E.: Elaboration of lymphotoxin by cultured human peripheral blood leukocytes stimulated with dental plaque deposits. Clin. Exp. Immunol., 13:383, 1973.

73. Hutchins, A.: Study of plaque distribution in gingival crevice. Oral Surg., 35:585, 1973.

74. Irving J. T., Socransky, S. S., and Heeley, J. D.: Histological changes in experimental periodontal disease in gnotobiotic rats and conventional hamsters. J. Periodont. Res., 9:73, 1974.

75. Irving, J. T., Newman, M. G., Socransky, S. S., and Heeley, J. D.: Histological changes in experimental periodontal disease in rats monoinfected with gram negative organism. Arch. Oral Biol., 20:219, 1975.

76. Irving, J. T., Socransky, S. S., Newman, M. G., and Savitt, E. Periodontal destruction induced by Capnocytophaga in gnotobiotic rats. IADR Abstract #783, 1976.

77. Ivanyi, L., and Lehner, T. Stimulation of lymphocyte transformation by bacterial antigen in patients with periodontal disease. Arch. Oral Biol., 15:1089, 1970.

78. Johnson, N. W., and Kenney, E. B.: Effects of topical application of chlorhexidine on plaque and gingivitis in monkeys. J. Periodont. Res., 7:180, 1972.

79. Jones, S.,: A special relationship between spherical and filamentous microorganisms in mature human dental plaque. Arch. Oral Biol., 17:613, 1972.

80. Jordan, H. V., and Keyes, P. H.: Aerobic, gram-positive, filamentous bacteria as etiologic agents of experimental periodontal disease in hamsters. Arch. Oral Biol., 9:401, 1964.

81. Jordan, H. V.: Periodontal lesions in hamsters and gnotobiotic rats injected with Actinomyces of human origin. J. Periodont. Res., 7:21, 1972.

82. Jordan, H. V., Keyes, P. H., and Bellack, S.: Periodontal lesions in hamsters and gno-

tobiotic rats infected with *Actinomyces* of human origin. Arch. Oral Biol., *17*:175, 1972.

83. Kaslick, R. S., West, T. L., Chasens, A. I., Terasaki, P. I., Lazzara, R., and Weinberg, S.: Association between HL-A2 antigen and various periodontal diseases in young adults. J. Dent. Res., *54*:424, 1975.

84. Keilty, R. A.: Focal infection. A bacteriological study of the gums in 200 cases. J. Med. Res., *43*:377, 1922.

85. Kelstrup, J., and Gibbons, R. J.: Induction of dental caries and alveolar bone loss by a human isolate resembling *Streptococcus Salivarius*. Caries Res., *4*:360, 1970.

86. Kelstrup, J., and Thailade, E.: Microbes and periodontal disease. J. Clin. Periodont., *1*:15, 1974.

87. Keyes, P. H., Fitzgerald, R. J., Jordan, H. V., and White, C. L.: The effects of various drugs on caries and periodontal disease in albino hamsters. Proc. 9th ORCA Cong., 1963.

88. Keyes, P. H., and Jordan, H. V.: Periodontal lesions in the Syrian hamster. III. Findings related to an infectious and transmissible component. Arch. Oral Biol., 9:377, 1964.

89. Keyes, P. H., Rowberry, S. A., Englander, H. R., and Fitzgerald, R. J.: Bi-assays of medicaments for the control of dento-bacterial plaque, dental caries, and periodontal lesions in Syrian hamster. J. Oral Ther., 3:157, 1966.

90. Keyes, P. H., Baer, P. N., and Socransky, S. S.: Induction of periodontal lesions in hamsters and rats. IADR Abstract #292, 1969.

91. Keyes, P. H.: Are periodontal pathoses caused by bacterial infections on cervicoradicular surfaces of teeth? J. Dent. Res., 49:223, 1970.

91a. Kornman, K., and Roesche, W.: Personal communication, 1977.

92. Kritchevsky, B., and Seguin, P.: The unity of spirochetes of the mouth. D. Cosmos, 66:511, 1924.

93. Leadbetter, E. R., and Holt, S. A.: Influence of sonication on cultivable microbiota of dental plaque. J. Dent. Res., 53:208, 1974.

94. Lehner, T., and Clarry, E. D.: Acute ulcerative gingivitis, an immunofluorescent investigation. Br. Dent. J., 120:366, 1966.

95. Lehner, T.,: Stimulation of lymphocyte transformation by tissue homogenates in recurrent oral ulceration. Immunology, 13:159, 1967.

96. Lehner, T., Wilton, M. A., Ivanyi, L., and Manson, J. D.: Immunological aspects of juvenile periodontitis (periodontosis). J. Periodont. Res., 9:261–272, 1974.

97. Lightner, L. M., O'Leary, T. J., Drake, R. B., Crump, P. P., and Allen, M. F.: Preventive periodontic treatment procedures: Results over 46 months. J. Periodontol., *42*:555, 1971.

98. Lindhe, J. G., Hampp, E., Loe, H., and Schiott, C. R.: Influence of topical application of chlorhexidine on chronic gingivitis and gingival wound healing in the dog. Scand. J. Dent. Res., 78:471, 1970.

99. Lindhe, J., and Nyman, S.: The effect of plaque control and surgical pocket elimination on the establishment and maintenance of periodontal health. A longitudinal study of periodontal therapy in cases of advanced periodontitis. J. Clin. Periodont., 2:67, 1975.

100. Listgarten, M. A.: Electron microscopic observation on the bacterial flora of acute necrotizing ulcerative gingivitis. J. Periodont., 36:328, 1965.

101. Listgarten, M. A., and Socransky, S. S.: Electron microscopy as an aid in the taxonomic differentiation of oral spirochetes. Arch. Oral Biol., 10:127, 1965.

102. Listgarten, M. A., and Lewis, D. W.: The distribution of spirochetes in the lesion of acute necrotizing ulcerative gingivitis: An electron microscopic and statistical survey. J. Periodontol., 38:379, 1967.

103. Listgarten, M. A.: Personal communication, 1975.

104. Listgarten, M. A., Mayo, H. E., and Tremblay, R.: Development of dental plaque on epoxy resin crowns in man. A light and electron microscopic study. J. Periodont., *46*:10, 1975.

105. Listgarten, M. A.: Structure of the microbial flora associated with periodontal disease and health in man. A light and electron microscopic study. J. Periodontol., 47:1, 1976.

106. Listgarten, M. A.: Structure of surface coatings on teeth. A review. J. Periodontol., 47:139, 1976.

107. Löe, H. E., Theilade, E., and Jensen, S. B.: Experimental gingivitis in man. J. Periodontol., 36:177, 1965.

108. Löe, H., Theilade, E., Jensen, S. B., and Schiott, C.: Experimental gingivitis in man. III. The influence of antibiotics on gingival plaque development. J. Periodont. Res., 2:282, 1967.

109. Löe, H., and Schiott, C. R.: The effect of mouth rinses and topical application of chlorhexidine on the development of dental plaque and gingivitis in man. J. Periodont. Res., 5:79, 1970.

110. Löe, H., Schiott, C. R., Glavind, L., and Karring, T.: Two years of oral use of chlorhexidine in man. I. General design and clinical effects. J. Periodont. Res., *11*:135, 1976.

111. Loesche, W. J., Socransky, S. S., and Gibbons, R. J.: *Bacteroides oralis:* Proposed new species isolated from the oral cavity of man. J. Bacteriol., 88:1329, 1964.

112. Loesche, W. J., and Gibbons, R. J.: A practical scheme for identification of the most numerous oral gram negative anaerobic rods. Arch. Oral Biol., 10:723, 1965.

113. Loesche, W. J., and Gibbons, R. J.: Amino acid fermentation by *Fusobacterium nucleatum*. Arch. Oral Biol., 13:191, 1968.

114. Loesche, W.: Oxygen sensitivity of various anaerobic bacteria. Appl. Microbiol., *18*:723, 1969.

115. Loesche, W. J., and Syed, S. A.: Bacteriology of dental plaque in experimental gingivitis. I. Relationship between gingivitis and flora. A.A.D.R. Abstract #108, 1975.

116. Loesche, W.: Chemotherapy of dental plaque infections. Oral Sci. Rev., 9:65, 1976.

117. Loesche, W.; Personal communication, 1977.

118. Lovdahl, A., Schei, O., Waerhaug, J., and Arno, A.: Tooth mobility and alveolar bone loss as related to oral hygiene and age. Acta Odont. Scand., 17:61, 1959.

119. Macdonald, J. B., Sutton, R. M., and Knoll, M. L.: The production of fusospirochetal infections in Guinea pigs with recombined pure cultures. J. Infect. Dis., 95:275, 1954.

120. Macdonald, J. B., Sutton, R. M., Knowll, M. L., Madlener, E . M., and Graisner, R. M.: The pathogenic components of an experimental fusospirochetal infection. J. Infect. Dis., 98:15, 1956.

121. Macdonald, J. B., Gibbons, R. J., and Socransky, S. S.: Bacterial mechanisms in periodontal disease. Ann. N.Y. Acad. Sci., 85:467, 1960.

122. Macdonald, J. B., and Gibbons, R. J.: The relationship of indigenous bacteria to periodontal disease. J. Dent. Res., 41:320, 1962.

123. Macdonald, J. B., Socransky, S. S., and Gibbons, R. J.: Aspects of the pathogenesis of mixed anaerobic infections of mucous membranes. J. Dent. Res., 42:529, 1963.

124. Mackenzie, I. C., Nuki, K., Loe, H., and Schiott, C. R.: Two years of oral use of chlorhexidine in man. V. Effects on stratum corneum of oral mucosa. J. Periodont. Res., 11:165, 1976.

125. Manganiello, A. D.: Thesis, Northeastern University, 1973.

126. Manganiello, A. D., Socransky, S. S., Propas, D., Oram, V., and Dogon, I. L.: Attempts to increase viable count recovery of human dental plaque. J. Periodont., in press.

127. McMaster, P. E.: Human bite infection. Am. J. Surg., 45:60, 1939.

128. Mergenhagen, S. E.: Endotoxic properties of oral bacteria as revealed by the local Schwartzman reaction. J. Dent. Res., 39:267, 1960.

129. Mergenhagen, S. E., Hampp, E. G., and Scherp, H. W.: Preparation and biological activities of endotoxins from oral bacteria. J. Infect. Dis., 108:304, 1961.

130. Mitchell, D. F., and Johnson, M.: The nature of the gingival plaque in the hamster. Production, prevention and removal. J. Dent. Res., 35:651, 1956.

131. Mitchell, D. F., and Baker, B. R.: Topical antibiotic control of necrotizing ulcerative gingivitis. J. Periodontol., 39:81, 1968.

132. Morgan, B., Socransky, S. S., and Schilder, H.: Predominant cultivable microbiota of necrotic root canals with periapical radiolucencies. J. Dent. Res., 53:68, 1974.

133. Newman, M. G., Socransky, S. S., and Listgarten, M. A.: Relationship of microorganisms to the etiology of periodontosis. J. Dent. Res., 53: 290, 1974.

134. Newman, M. G., Socransky, S. S., Savitt, E., Krichevsky, M., Listgarten, M., and Lai, W.: Characterization of bacteria isolated from periodontosis. J. Dent. Res., 53:325, 1974.

135. Newman, M. G., Williams, R. C., and Crawford, A.: Predominant cultivable microbiota of periodontosis, III. J. Dent. Res., 54:211, 1975.

136. Newman, M. G., Socransky, S. S., Savitt, E. D., Propas, D. A., and Crawford, A.: Studies of the microbiology of periodontosis. J. Periodontol., 47:373, 1976.

137. Newman, M. G., Sandler, M., Ormerod, W., Angel, L., and Goldhaber, P.: The effect of dietary cantrisin supplements on the flora of periodontal pockets in four Beagle dogs. J. Periodont. Res., 12:129, 1977.

138. Newman, M. G.: Periodontosis. J. West. Soc. Periodont., 24:5, 1976.

139. Newman, M. G., and Socransky, S. S.: Predominant cultivable microbiota in periodontosis. J. Periodont. Res., 12:120, 1977.

140. Newman, M. G., Weiner, M. S., Angel, I., Grinenko, V., and Karge, H. J.: Predominant cultivable microbiota of the gingival crevice in "supernormal" patients. J. Dent. Res., 56:277, 1977.

141. Newman, M. G., Angel, J., Karge, H., Weiner, M., Grinenko, V., and Schusterman, L.: Bacterial studies of Papillon-Lefèvre syndrome. J. Dent. Res., 56:220, 1977.

142. Nisengard, R., Beutner, E. H., and Hazen, S. P.: Immunologic studies of periodontal diseases. IV. Bacterial hypersensitivity and periodontal disease. J. Periodontol., 39:329, 1968.

143. Nisengard, R. J., and Beutner, E. H.: Immunologic studies of periodontal disease. V. IgG type antibodies and skin test responses to Actinomyces and mixed oral flora. J. Periodontol., 41:149, 1970.

144. Noguchi, H.: Treponema mucosum (new species): A mucous producing spirochete from pyorrhea alveolaris, grown in pure culture. J. Exp. Med., 16:194, 1912.

145. Nord, C. E., Frostell, G., and Soder, P. O.: A comparison between proteolytic enzymes in dental plaque material from children and adults. Svensk. Kem. T., 62:3, 1969.

146. Nuki, K., Schlenker, R., Loe, H., and Schiott, C. R.: Two years of oral use of chlorhexidine in man. VI. Effects on oxidative enzymes in oral epithelia. J. Periodont. Res., 11:172, 1976.

147. O'Leary, T. J., Shannon, I. L., and Prigmore, J. R.: Clinical correlations and systemic status in periodontal disease. S. Cal. Dent. J., 30:47, 1962.

148. Osterberg, S. K. A., Sudo, S. Z., and Folke, L. E. A.: Microbial succession in subgingival plaque of man. J. Periodont. Res., 11:243, 1976.

149. Page, R. C.: Dental deposits. In Schluger, S., Yuodelis, R., and Page, R.: Periodontal Disease. Philadelphia, Lea and Febiger, 1977.

150. Paul, W. E.: Functional specificity of antigen-binding receptors of lymphocytes. Transplant Rev., 5:130, 1970.

151. Poole, A. E., and Gilmour, M. N.: The variability of unstandardized plaques obtained from single or multiple subjects. Arch. Oral Biol., 16:681, 1971.

152. Rindom, K. A., Schiott, C., Briner, W. W., Kirkland, J. J., and Löe, H.: Two years of oral use of chlorhexidine in man. III. Changes in sensitivity of the salivary flora. J. Periodont. Res., 11:153, 1976.

153. Rindom, K. A., Schiott, C., Briner, W. W., and Löe, H.: Two years oral use of chlorhexidine in man. II. The effect on the salivary bacterial flora. J. Periodont. Res., 11:145, 1976.

154. Rindom, K. A., Schiott, C., Löe, H., and Briner, W. W.: Two years of oral use of chlorhexidine in man. IV. Effect on various medical parameters. J. Periodont. Res., *11*:158, 1976.

155. Ritz, H. L.: Microbial population shifts in developing human dental plaque. Arch. Oral Biol., *12*:1561, 1967.

156. Rizzo, A. A.: Rabbit corneal irrigation as a model system for studies on the relative toxicity of bacterial products implicated in periodontal disease. The toxicity of neutralized ammonia solutions. J. Periodontol., 38:491, 1967.

157. Rizzo, A. A.: The possible role of hydrogen sulfide in human periodontal disease. I. Hydrogen sulfide production in periodontal pockets. Periodontics, 5:233, 1967.

158. Robrish, S. A., Grove, S. B., Bernstein, R., and Amdur, B.: Differential breakage plaque dispersion. J. Dent. Res., 54:236, 1975.

159. Rosan, B., and Williams, N. B.: Hyaluronidase production by oral enterococci. Arch. Oral Biol., 9:291, 1964.

160. Rosebury, T.: The parasitic actinomycetes and other filamentous micro-organisms of the mouth. A review. Bacteriol. Rev., 8:189, 1944.

161. Rosebury, T., MacDonald, J. B., and Clark, A. R.: A bacteriologic survey of gingival scrapings from periodontal infections by direct examination, Guinea pig innoculations and anaerobic cultivation. J. Dent. Res., 29:718, 1950.

162. Ross, T.: Quantitative studies on saliva flora. J. Clin. Pathol., 24:717, 1971.

163. Rovin, S., Costich, E. R., and Gordon, H. A.: The influence of bacteria and irritation in the initiation of periodontal disease in germfree and conventional rats. J. Periodont. Res., 1:193, 1966.

164. Saviston, U.: Anaerobic bacteria from advanced periodontal lesions. J. Periodont., 43:199, 1972.

165. Sage, S. R., Green, J. C., Bonanhan, H. M., and Vermillion, S. R.: Oral debris, calculus and periodontal disease in the Beagle dog. Periodontics, 5:217, 1967.

166. Salkind, A., Oshrain, H. I., and Mandel, I. D.: Bacterial aspects of developing supragingival and subgingival plaque. J. Periodontol., 42:706, 1971.

167. Sasaki, S., Socransky, S., Lescord, M., and Sweeney, E.: Destructive periodontal disease in children. II. Microbiological and immunological findings. J. Dent. Res., 56B:422, 1977.

168. Savitt, E. D., Socransky, S. S., Hammond, B. F., and Newman, M. G.: Characterization of fusiform organisms isolated from periodontosis. J. Dent. Res., 54:208, 1975.

169. Schei, O., Waerhaug, J., Lovdahl, A., and Arno, A.: Alveolar bone loss as related to oral hygiene and age. J. Periodontol., 30:7, 1959.

170. Schroeder, H. E., and De Boever, J.: The structure of microbial dental plaque. *In* McHugh, W. D. (ed.): Dental Plaque. Edinburg, E. & S. Livingston, 1970.

171. Schuessler, C. F., Fairchild, J. M., and Stransky, I. M.: Penicillin in the treatment of Vincent's infection. J. Am. Dent. Assoc., 32:551, 1945.

172. Schultz-Haudt, S., Bibby, B. G., and Bruce, M. A.: Tissue destructive products of gingival bacteria from non-specific gingivitis. J. Dent. Res., 33:624, 1954.

173. Schultz-Haudt, S., and Scherp, H. W.: Lysis of collagen by human gingival bacteria. Proc. Soc. Exp. Biol. Med., 89:697, 1955.

174. Schultz-Haudt, S., and Scherp, H. W.: Production of hyaluronidase by viridans streptococci isolated from gingival crevices. J. Dent. Res., 34:924, 1955.

175. Schultz-Haudt, S., and Scherp, H. W.: Production of chondrosulfatase by microorganisms isolated from human gingival crevices. J. Dent. Res., 35:299, 1956.

176. Schuster, G. S., Hayashi, J. A., and Bahn, A. N.: Toxic properties of the cell wall of gram positive bacteria. J. Bacteriol., 93:47, 1967.

177. Shapiro, L., et al.: Endotoxin determinations in gingival inflammation. J. Periodontol., 43:591, 1972.

178. Shaw, J. H., Griffiths, D., and Auskaps, A. M.: The influence of antibiotics on the periodontal syndrome in the rice rat. J. Dent. Res., 40:511, 1961.

179. Shaw, J. H.: Further studies on the sensitivity of the periodontal syndrome in the rice rat to dietary antibiotics. J. Dent. Res., 44:431, 1965.

180. Shpuntoff, H., and Rosebury, T.: Infectivity of fusospirochetal exudate for Guinea pigs, hamsters, mice and chick embryos by several routes of inoculation. J. Dent. Res., 28:7, 1949.

181. Skobe, Z.: Personal observations. Forsyth Dental Center, 1976.

182. Slots, J.: The predominant cultivable organisms in juvenile periodontitis. Scand. J. Dent. Res., 84:1, 1976.

183. Slots, J.: The microflora in the healthy gingival sulcus in man. Scand. J. Dent. Res., 85:247, 1977.

184. Slots, J.: The predominant cultivable microflora of advanced periodontitis. Scand. J. Dent. Res., 85:114, 1977.

185. Smith, D. T.: Spirochetes and related organisms in fuso-spirochetal disease. Baltimore, The Williams & Wilkins Company, 1932.

186. Snyderman, R.: Role for endotoxin and C' in periodontal tissue destruction. J. Dent. Res., 51:356, 1972.

187. Socransky, S. S., Gibbons, R. J., Dale, A. C., Bortnick, L., Rosenthal, E., and Macdonald, J.: The microbiota of the gingival crevice area of man. I. Total microscopic and viable count of specific organisms. Arch. Oral Biol., 8:275, 1963.

188. Socransky, S. S., Loesche, W. J., Hubersak, C., and Macdonald, J. B.: Dependency of *Treponema microdentium* on other oral organisms for isobutyrate, polyamines, and a controlled oxidation-reduction potential. J. Bacteriol., 88:200, 1964.

189. Socransky, S. S., Listgarten, M. A., Hubersak, C., Cotmore, J., and Clark, A.: Morphological and biochemical differentiation of three types of small oral spirochetes. J. Bacteriol., 98:878, 1969.

190. Socransky, S. S.: The relationship of bacteria to the etiology of periodontal disease. J. Dent. Res., 49:2, 203, 1970.

191. Socransky, S. S., Hubersak, C., and Propas, D.: Induction of periodontal destruction in gnotobiotic rats by a human oral strain of *Actinomyces naeslundii.* Arch Oral Biol., 15:993, 1970.

192. Socransky, S. S., Hubersak, C., Propas, D., and Rozanis, J.: "Pathogenic potential" of human gram positive rods for oral tissues. IADR Abstract #151, 1970.

193. Socransky, S. S., and Manganiello, A. D.: The oral microbiota of man from birth to senility. J. Periodont., 42:485, 1971.

194. Socransky, S. S.: Personal communication, 1975.

195. Socransky, S. S.: Personal communication. 1977.

196. Socransky, S. S.: Microbiology of periodontal disease. Present status and future considerations. J. Periodontol., 48:497, 1977.

197. Socransky, S. S., Manganiello, A. D., Oram V., and Van Houte, J. Bacteriological studies of developing supragingival dental plaque. Periodont. Res., 12:90, 1977.

198. Soder, P. O., and Frostell, G.: Proteolytic activity of dental plaque material on azocoll, casein and gelatin. Acta Odont. Scand., 24:501, 1966.

199. Suomi, J. D., Greene, J. C., Vermillion, J. R., Doyle, J., Chang, J., and Leatherwood, E. C.: The effect of controlled oral hygiene procedures on the progression of periodontal disease in adults: Results after third and final year. J. Periodontol., 42:152, 1971.

200. Sutter, V. L., Attebery, H. R., Rosenblatt, J. E., Bricknell, K. S., and Finegold, S. M.: Anaerobic Bacteriology Manual. UCLA, 1972.

201. Sweeney, E., Stossel, T., Sesaki, S., and Socransky, S.: Destructive periodontal disease of children. Oral and septemic findings in 6 patients. J. Dent. Res., 56B:421, 1977.

202. Syed, S. A., Loesche, W. J., and Löe, H.: Bacteriology of dental plaque in experimental gingivitis. 2. Relationship between time, plaque score and flora. AADR Abstract #109, 1975.

203. Tanzer, J.: Microbiology section summary. Proceedings of the International Workshop in the Biology of Periodontal Disease, 1977. In press.

204. Tempel, T. R., Snyderman, R., Jordan, H. V., and Mergenhagen, S. E.: Factors from saliva and oral bacteria, chemotactic for polymorphonuclear leukocytes: Their possible role in gingival inflammation. J. Periodontol., 41:71, 1970.

205. Theilade, E., Wright, W. H., Jensen, S. B., and Loe, H.: Experimental gingivitis in man. II. A longitudinal, clinical and bacteriological investigation. J. Periodont. Res., 1:1, 1966.

206. Theilade, E., and Theilade, J.: Role of plaque in the etiology of periodontal disease and caries. Oral Sci. Rev., 9:23, 1976.

207. Thonard, J. C., Hefflin, C. M., and Steinberg, A. I.: Neurominidase activity in mixed culture supernatant fluids of human oral bacteria. J. Bacteriol., 89:924, 1965.

208. Tunnicliff, R., et al.: Fusiform bacilli and spirilla in gingival tissue. J. Am. Dent. Assoc., 23:1959, 1936.

209. Van Palestein-Halderman, W. H.: Total viable count and differential count of vibrio (Campylobacter) sputorum, fusobacterium nucleatum, selenomonas sputigena, Bacteriodes ochraceous and Veillonella in the inflamed and non-inflamed human gingival crevice J. Periodont. Res., 10:294, 1976.

210. Volpe, A. R., Kupczak, L. J., Brant, J. H., King, W. J., Kestenbaum, R. C., and Schlissel, H. J.: Antimicrobial control of bacterial plaque and calculus and the effects of these agents on oral flora. J. Dent. Res., 48:832, 1969.

211. Waerhaug, J.: Observations on replanted teeth plated with gold foil. Oral Surg., 9:780, 1956.

212. Waerhaug, J.: Effect of rough surfaces upon gingival tissue. J. Dent. Res., 35:323, 1956.

213. Waerhaug, J.: Effect of zinc phosphate cement fillings on gingival tissues. J. Periodontol., 27:284, 1956.

214. Waerhaug, J.: Tissue reaction to metal wires in healthy gingival pockets. J. Periodontol., 28:239, 1957.

215. Waerhaug, J.: Histological considerations which govern where the margins of restorations should be located in relation to the gingiva. Dent. Clin. North Am., 1960, p. 161.

216. Wahren, A., and Gibbons, R. J.: Amino acid fermentation by *Bacteroides melaninogenicus.* Antonie van Leuwenhoek, 36:149, 1970.

217. Watanabe, S.: Possible role of mycoplasmas in periodontal disease. Bull. Tokyo Med. Dent. Univ., 19:93, 1972.

218. Williams, B. L., Pantalone, R. M., and Sherris, J. C.: Subgingival micro-flora and periodontitis. J. Periodont. Res., 11:1, 1976.

Chapter 25

Saliva, Acquired Pellicle, Calculus, Materia Alba, Food Debris, and Dental Stains

SALIVA

Salivary secretions are protective in nature because they maintain the oral tissues

in a physiologic state (Table 25–1). In addition, saliva exerts a major influence on plaque initiation, maturation, and metabolism. Calculus formation and dental caries and some periodontal diseases are also influenced by salivary flow and composition.

The fluids secreted by the various salivary glands differ in composition from each other and are affected by (1) the type, intensity, and duration of stimulation, (2) diet, (3) sex, (4) age, (5) disease state, (6) time of day, and (7) drugs. Therefore, studies which control for these variables such as standardized stimulation, similar time of day, and the distinction between whole saliva and glandular secretion will provide more accurate information.[141]

The fluids secreted by the parotid, submaxillary, sublingual, and minor salivary glands mix together with bacterial, cellular, and food debris to form *whole saliva.* Whole saliva is the fluid collected by expectoration. In a 24-hour period the total salivary flow is approximately 1250 ml.[76] The secretions of the parotid and submaxillary glands make up 90 per cent of the total volume (each contributing half). During noneating periods, salivary flow is minimal. During masticatory or gustatory stimulation the flow rate of saliva is approximately 10 times that of a resting state. Therefore these activities account for the major salivary volume.

An increase in inflammatory gingival diseases, dental caries, and rapid tooth destruction associated with cervical or cemental caries is partially a consequence of decreased salivary gland secretion (xerostomia). Xerostomia may be a consequence of a variety of different factors, including sialolithiasis, sarcoidosis, Sjögren's syn-

405

TABLE 25–1   ROLE OF SALIVA IN ORAL HEALTH

Function	Salivary Components	Probable Mechanism
Lubrication	Glycoproteins, Mucoids	Coating similar to gastric mucin
Physical protection	Glycoproteins, Mucoids	Coating similar to gastric mucin
Cleansing	Physical flow	Clearance of debris and bacteria
Buffering	Bicarbonate and phosphate	Antacids
Tooth integrity	Minerals	Maturation, remineralization
	Glycoprotein pellicle	Mechanical protection
Antibacterial	IgA	Control of bacterial colonization
	Lysozyme	Breaks bacterial cell walls
	Lactoperoxidase	Oxidation of susceptible bacteria

drome, drugs, Mikulicz's disease, irradiation, surgical removal of salivary glands, diabetes mellitus, menopause, Parkinson's disease, anxiety, mental stress, and iatrogenic causes.

Salivary secretions are controlled by unconditioned reflex stimulation of the superior and inferior salivary nuclei located in the medulla. Taste bud stimulation (gustatory), stimulation of periodontal ligament propriocepters, and mastication (masticatory) provide the major source of saliva. Olfactory stimulation, oral pain, and irritation can also induce salivary stimulation.

Salivary Contents

Saliva is 99 per cent water and 1 per cent organic and inorganic substances. Its pH ranges from slightly acidic (pH 6.2) prior to secretion in the oral cavity to slightly alkaline (pH 7.4) upon excretion from the gland. Bicarbonate concentration increases at elevated flow rates, causing a rise in pH and an increase in buffering capacity.

In general the concentration of most substances is higher in the parotid than in the submaxillary glands; the exception being calcium, which has a submaxillary concentration approximately twice that of the parotid.

The protein concentration of saliva is very low compared to that of blood. The enzymes normally found in the saliva[18] (Table 25–2) are derived from the salivary glands, bacteria, leukocytes, oral tissue, and ingested substances; the major enzyme is parotid amylase. Certain salivary enzymes have been reported to increase in periodontal disease; they are hyaluronidase and lipase,[32] B-glucoronidase and chondroitin sulfatase,[42] amino acid decarboxylases,[57] catalase, peroxidase, and collagenase.[86, 101]

A mixture of glycoprotein components of saliva appear to make up salivary mucin. Mucin concentration is primarily responsible for the control of salivary viscosity. The glycoproteins are produced by the mucous cells of all salivary glands; however, some are produced exclusively by individual glands.

The high molecular weight mucinous glycoproteins in saliva bind specifically to many plaque-forming bacteria. The glycoprotein-bacterial interactions facilitate bacterial accumulation on the exposed tooth surface.[52, 67-69, 234]

The specificity of these interactions has been demonstrated. The interbacterial matrix of human plaque appears to contain polymers similar to salivary glycoproteins which may aid in maintaining the integrity of plaque. In addition, these glycoproteins selectively adsorb to the hydroxyapatite to make up part of the acquired pellicle (see section on Acquired Pellicle). Other salivary glycoproteins inhibit the sorption of some bacteria to the tooth surface and to oral mucosa epithelial cells.[67] This activity appears to be associated with the glycoproteins which possess blood group reactivity.[1, 52, 67, 68, 234] Glycoproteins and a glycolipid present on mammalian cell surfaces, appear to serve as receptors for the attachment of some viruses and bacteria. Thus the close similarity between the glycoproteins of salivary secretions and the components of the epithelial cell surface suggests that the secretions can competitively inhibit antigen sorption and thus may limit pathologic alterations.

Saliva exerts a major influence on plaque

TABLE 25–2 SOURCE OF ENZYMES FOUND IN SALIVA*

Enzyme	Source Indicated by X		
	Glands	Microorganisms	Leukocytes
Carbohydrases			
Amylase	X	—	—
Maltase	—	X	X
Invertase	—	X	—
Beta-glucuronidase	X	X	X
Beta-D-galactosidase	—	X	X
Beta-D-glucosidase	—	X	—
Lysozyme	X	—	X
Hyaluronidase	—	X	—
Mucinase	—	X	—
Esterases			
Acid phosphatase	X	X	X
Alkaline phosphatase	X	X	X
Hexosediphosphatase	—	X	—
Aliesterase	X	X	X
Lipase	X	X	X
Acetylcholinesterase	X	—	X
Pseudo-cholinesterase	X	X	X
Chondrosulfatase	—	X	—
Arylsulfatase	—	X	—
Transferring enzymes			
Catalase	—	X	—
Peroxidase	X	—	X
Phenyloxidase	—	X	—
Succinic dehydrogenase	X	X	X
Hexokinase	—	X	X
Proteolytic enzymes			
Proteinase	—	X	X
Peptidase	—	X	X
Urease	—	X	—
Other enzymes			
Carbonic anhydrase	X	—	—
Pyrophosphatase	—	X	—
Aldolase	X	X	X

*From Chauncey, H. H.: J.A.D.A., 63:360, 1961.

by mechanically cleansing the exposed oral surfaces, controlling acids produced by bacteria through its buffering capacity and by its antibacterial activities. Systemically administered antibiotics may also be secreted into the saliva.[108]

Salivary Antibodies

Saliva as well as sulcular fluid contains antibodies reactive with oral indigenous bacterial species. Although IgG and IgM are present, the predominant immunoglobulin found in saliva is IgA, whereas IgG predominates in sulcular fluid.[131, 157, 216, 217]

The IgA antibodies found in saliva differ from those found in serum and in tissues. It is composed of two "monomer" IgA molecules joined by a polypeptide chain called the secretory components,[21, 157] and an additional polypeptide called J chain.[95, 96, 200] J chain is depicted as being involved in maintaining the integrity of the secretory IgA dimer. Currently it is suggested that the secretory component is a product of gland ductile epithelium. Its postulated roles are that it (a) acts as a receptor on secretory epithelial cells facilitating the transfer of IgA from the gland cells to the duct lumen; (b) may be a molecule which "recognizes" and "attracts" plasma cell precursors to the glandular tissue; and (c) may protect the IgA molecule from proteolysis in secretions *in vivo.*

IgA lymphoid cells have been found in the bronchial and nasal mucosae and associated with exocrine glandular epithelium along submaxillary, parotid, lacrimal, and mammary gland ducts.[29, 85, 176, 180, 217] Salivary antibodies appear to be synthesized locally, for they will react with strains of bacteria indigenous to the mouth but not with organisms characteristic of the intestinal canal.[67, 68] Many bacteria found in saliva have been shown to be coated with IgA, and the bacterial deposits on teeth contain both IgA and IgG in quantities greater than 1 per cent of their dry weight.[69] It has been shown that IgA antibodies present in parotid saliva can inhibit the attachment of oral *Streptococcus* species to epithelial cells.[52, 234]

Gibbons suggests that antibodies in secretions may react with bacteria while they are proliferating on the surfaces of mucosal epithelial cells;[67-69] hence, when the organisms become dislodged, they would have an impaired ability to reattach. It is possible that this mechanism may play a major role in determining the bacterial diseases such as cholera, dental caries,[28, 88, 116, 131] and periodontal disease where bacterial adhesion and colonization of mucosal or dental tissues may be a necessary step in pathogenesis (Fig. 25-1). Inhibition of bacterial adherence has not been found to require accessory factors such as complement in the systems so far studied. Secretory IgA has a valence of

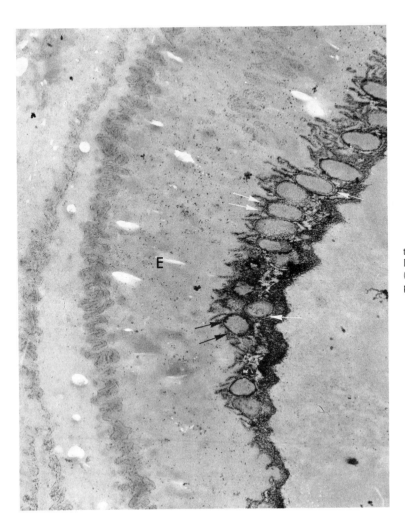

Figure 25-1 Attachment of bacteria (single arrows) to oral epithelial cell (E) surface (double arrows) (Barkin, M. and Newman, M. unpublished observations.)

four, which may lead to multivalent binding to cell surfaces, thereby increasing the efficiency of secretory IgA antibodies.

The antibacterial activities of secretory IgA antibodies are not very well understood. There is conflicting evidence regarding the ability of secretory IgA antibodies to function in bacterial opsonization and bactericidal activities. These conflicting results may be resolved by further studies defining the assay systems and accessory factors in more detail.

Salivary Buffers

The maintenance of physiologic hydrogen ion concentration (pH) at the mucosal epithelial cell and tooth surface is an important function of salivary buffers. Its primary effect has been studied in relationship to dental caries.

In saliva the most important salivary buffer is the bicarbonate-carbonic acid system.[76, 141] Bicarbonate concentration increases with increased flow rate, providing greater salivary buffering capacity. The system acts by the loss of carbon dioxide, which tends to raise the pH. In addition its pK = 6.1, which is similar to that in whole plaque and therefore would be more effective in maintaining physiologic pH. Urea and phosphate buffers also occur in saliva and contribute to the maintenance of a physiologic pH.

Lysozyme

Lysozyme is a hydrolytic enzyme which cleaves the linkage between structural components of the glycopeptide muramic acid–containing region of the cell wall of certain bacteria *in vitro*. The concentration of lysozyme appears to be higher in sublingual and submandibular saliva than in parotid saliva. The antibacterial effect in vivo is poorly understood and probably plays a minor role in controlling bacterial colonization in dental plaque or on mucosal surfaces.

Lactoperoxidase

The lactoperoxidase-thiocyanate system in saliva has been shown to be antibac-

terial to certain strains of *Lactobacillus* and *Streptococcus*.[152, 175] It is present in submandibular and parotid saliva. The system prevents the accumulation of lysine and glutamic acid by susceptible bacteria, both essential for bacterial growth.

Coagulation Factors

Several factors (VIII, IX, X, PTA, and the Hageman factor) that hasten blood coagulation and protect wounds from bacterial invasion have been identified in saliva,[121] and the presence of an active fibrinolytic enzyme has been suggested.[133]

Vitamins

Thiamine, riboflavin, niacin, pyridoxine, pantothenic acid, biotin, folic acid, and vitamin B_{12} are the principal vitamins found in saliva;[144] vitamin C and vitamin K have also been reported.[153] Suggested sources of the vitamins are microbial synthesis and secretion by salivary glands, food debris, degenerating leukocytes, and exfoliated epithelial cells.

Leukocytes

In addition to desquamated epithelial cells, the saliva contains all forms of leukocytes, of which the principal cells are the polymorphonuclear leukocytes. The number of leukocytes varies from person to person and at different times of the day, and is increased in gingivitis. Leukocytes reach the oral cavity by migrating through the lining of the gingival sulcus. Living polymorphonuclear leukocytes in saliva are sometimes referred to as *orogranulocytes* (OGC's), and their rate of migration into the oral cavity as the *orogranulocytic migratory rate* (OMR). Some feel that the rate of migration is correlated with the severity of gingival inflammation and is therefore a reliable index for assessing gingivitis;[166] others disagree.[178]

ACQUIRED PELLICLE

Acquired pellicle is a thin, amorphous coating primarily of salivary origin which forms on teeth as well as other solid surfaces exposed to saliva. When stained with disclosing agents, pellicle appears as a thin, pale-staining surface. In general, the staining properties of pellicle are quite similar to those of dried salivary films. It stains positively for sugars and proteins, but does not bind dyes that are specific for collagen or keratin. It does not contain heme or melanin, but may become brownish in color from the presence of tannins (see section on stains). When viewed with the electron microscope, the acquired pellicle is an acellular, afibrillar, faintly granular homogeneous material of variable thickness in intimate contact with its supporting surface (Fig. 25–2).

The age and method of preparation of pellicle appear to affect the observed morphology. Material forming for short time periods on previously polished tooth surfaces or on intraoral plastic strips exhibits a smooth, even surface. Coccal bacteria deposit first in the depressions of these surface irregularities, but initial deposition appears to be independent of actual bacterial growth. Armstrong[2, 3] and Schrieder[189] showed in cross-sectional views that pellicle has a scalloped border on the edge away from the surface of the cementum. Arm-

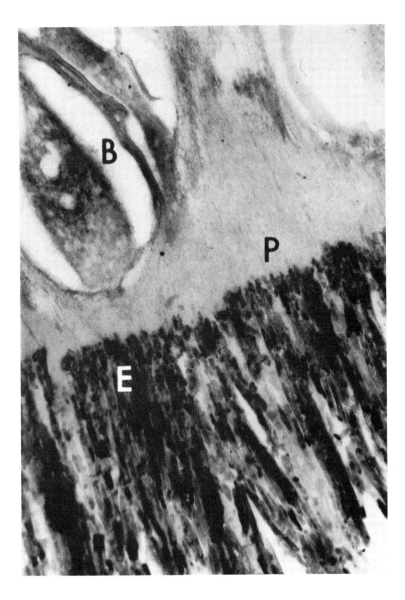

Figure 25–2 Dental Plaque Formed on Pellicle. Electronmicrograph of undecalcified incisor, showing bacterial plaque (B) and acquired pellicle (P) on enamel surface (E). ×36,000. (Courtesy of Leach, S. A., and Saxton, C. A.[115])

strong presented the possibility that salivary mucoproteins precipitate onto the tooth surface. Microorganisms then settle on the material. These same bacteria subsequently produce enzymes which bring about further deposition of salivary material. This additional material is seen as an elevation on a scalloped border in a cross-sectional view with the transmission electron microscope. Sottosanti[204] showed surface views of this attachment pellicle and revealed a strikingly symmetrical honeycombed effect (Fig. 25-2). These depressions very often harbor one bacterial organism or its cell remnants.

Formation

Pumice-containing polishing compounds remove the acquired pellicle as well as other uncalcified coatings. Within minutes after exposure of the cleaned tooth surface to saliva, a film free of microorganisms covers the tooth surface and fills in minor surface defects. Within hours a fully established pellicle, usually less than a micron thick, is formed. It appears likely that the acquired pellicle is formed primarily by the selective adsorption of salivary glycoproteins to the hydroxyapatite enamel surface.[87]

In addition to salivary glycoproteins, there may be variable amounts of microbiological products in the pellicle. Most of these observed products are cell wall constituents that can also be found in the saliva. After several days the acquired pellicle constituents become highly insoluble, because of the intermolecular interactions which "mature" the pellicle or by partial bacterial degradation.[201, 202]

Classification and Function

Three types of acquired pellicle are recognized. A *subsurface* or *"dentritic"* pellicle is most intimately associated with the enamel surface. It is characterized by processes which can extend 1 to 3 microns into microscopic defects present in the enamel surface. *Surface* pellicle covers most of the tooth surface and when it occurs on the lingual and palatal surfaces it usually appears to be calcified. *Stained* pellicle is usually thicker than other types of acquired pellicle, being approximately 1 to 10 microns in thickness. This type of pellicle may absorb chromogenic substances from a variety of sources and become visible to the naked eye (see section on Stains).

There appear to be three major "functions" of the acquired pellicle. The first and most studied is its role in the formation of supragingival bacterial plaque (Fig. 25-3). The sorption of bacteria from saliva to the surface of the acquired pellicle is highly selective and a primary step in supragingival plaque formation. The second and less understood function of the acquired pellicle appears to be protective. Enamel coated with pellicle is more resistant to acid decalcification than non-pellicle-covered enamel. The third function is postulated to be a repair function. It is suggested that the acquired pellicle may participate in the repair of early carious lesions by filling in surface defects.

CALCULUS

Although acquired bacterial coatings (plaque and materia alba) have been demonstrated to be the major factors in the initiation of periodontal diseases, the presence of calculus is of great concern to the clinician. Calculus is always covered by plaque, so its significance is primarily due to its relationship to the bacteria in plaque and their products (Figs. 25-3 to 25-7). The mechanical irritation attributed to calculus has long been considered of primary importance. However, experiments with germ-free animals (see Chapter 24) have demonstrated that the direct physical effect of calculus is secondary to the primary etiologic role of plaque bacteria. Therefore, these calcified deposits play a role in maintaining and accentuating periodontal disease. Consequently, when calculus is present the gingival tissues are inflamed and when it is present in deep subgingival lesions the potential for repair and reattachment is virtually nonexistent. Therefore, the clinician must be extremely competent in

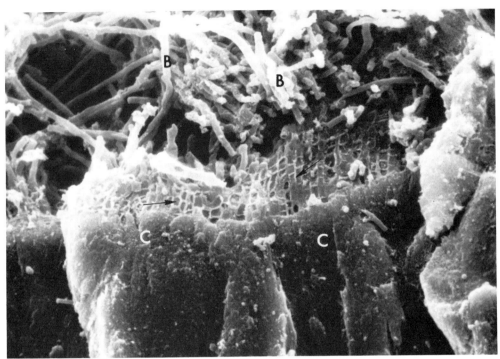

Figure 25–3   Attachment "spaces" (arrows) for subgingival bacteria (B) in pellicle-like substance on surface of cementum (C). (Courtesy of Dr. John Sottosanti.)

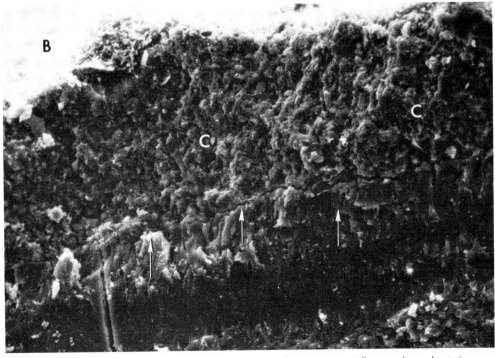

Figure 25–4   Subgingival calculus (C) attached to cementum surface (arrows). Adherent plaque bacteria on calculus surface (B). (Courtesy of Dr. John Sottosanti.)

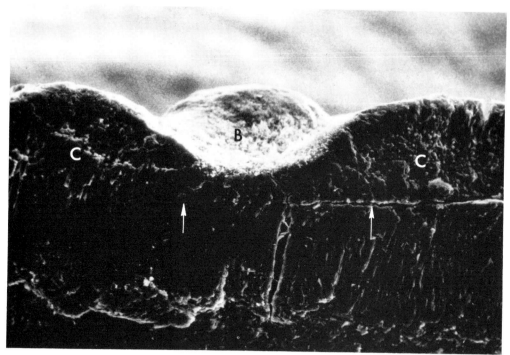

Figure 25–5 Subgingival calculus (C) attached to cementum surface (arrows). Adherent plaque bacteria (B) attached in depression on calculus surface. (Courtesy of Dr. John Sottosanti.)

Figure 25–6 Detailed Examination of Calculus showing an inner structure (C), filamentous organisms (F), other bacteria (B), and desquamated epithelial cells (E).

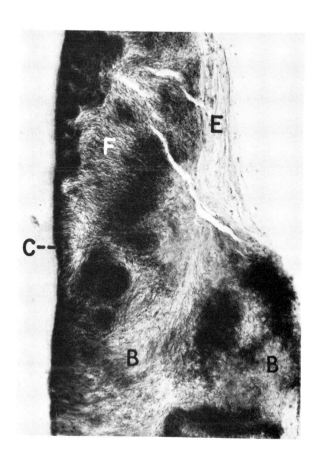

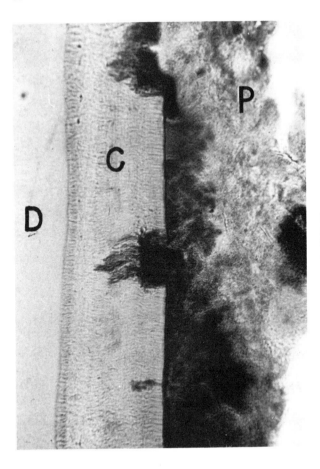

Figure 25–7 Calculus on Tooth Surface Embedded within the Cementum (C). Note the early stage of penetration shown in the lower portion of the illustration. The dentin is at D. (P) Plaque attached to calculus.

his/her ability to remove calculus and the necrotic cementum to which it attaches.

An excellent review regarding the structure and composition of calculus has been done by Schroeder.[186]

History

Calculus was recognized as a clinical entity in some way related to periodontal disease as far back as the tenth century. Albucasis of Cordova,[232] an Arabian physician, designed a set of scaling instruments for removing calculus in patients afflicted with periodontal disease. Fauchard, in 1728, termed it tartar or slime and referred to it as "a substance which accumulates on the surface of the teeth and which becomes, when left there, a stony crust of more or less considerable volume. The most common cause of the loss of teeth is the negligence of these people who do not clean their teeth when they might, and that they perceive the lodgment of this foreign substance which produces diseases of the gums."

Supragingival and Subgingival Calculus

Calculus is an adherent, calcified or calcifying mass that forms on the surface of natural teeth and dental prostheses. Ordinarily calculus consists of mineralized bacterial plaque. It is classified according to its relation to the gingival margin as follows:

Supragingival calculus (visible calculus) refers to calculus coronal to the crest of the gingival margin and visible in the oral cavity (Fig. 25–8). Supragingival calculus is usually white or white-yellow, of hard, claylike consistency, and easily detached from the tooth surface. Its recurrence after removal may be rapid, especially in the lingual of the mandibular incisors. The color is affected by such factors as tobacco

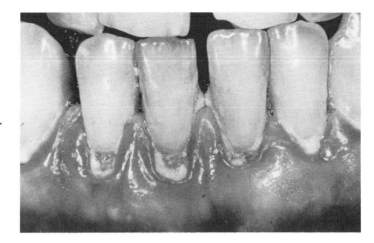

Figure 25–8   Supragingival Calculus.

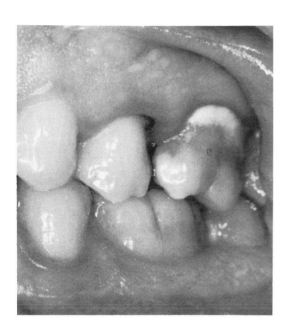

Figure 25–9   Calculus on Molar Opposite Stensen's Duct.

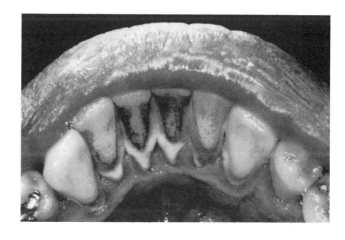

Figure 25–10   Calculus and Stain on lingual surface in relation to orifice of submaxillary and sublingual glands.

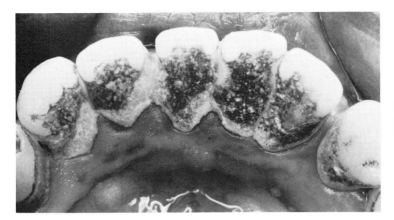

Figure 25–11 **Calculus** forming a bridge-like structure on the lingual surface of the mandibular anterior teeth.

or food pigment. It may localize on a single tooth or a group of teeth, or be generalized throughout the mouth. Supragingival calculus occurs most frequently and in greatest quantity on the buccal surfaces of the maxillary molars opposite Stensen's duct (Fig. 25–9), the lingual surfaces of the mandibular anterior teeth opposite Wharton's duct, and more on the central incisors than on the laterals (Fig. 25–10).[219] In extreme cases calculus may form a bridge-like structure along adjacent teeth (Fig. 25–11) or cover the occlusal surface of teeth without functional antagonists (Fig. 25–12).

Subgingival calculus refers to calculus below the crest of the marginal gingiva, usually in periodontal pockets, and is not visible upon usual oral examination. Determination of the location and extent of subgingival calculus requires careful detection with an explorer (Fig. 25–13). It is

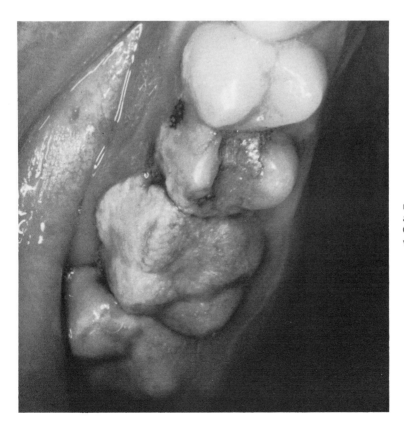

Figure 25–12 **Calculus** covering nonfunctioning maxillary molars and part of the second premolar. Compare with the first premolar, which has functional antagonists.

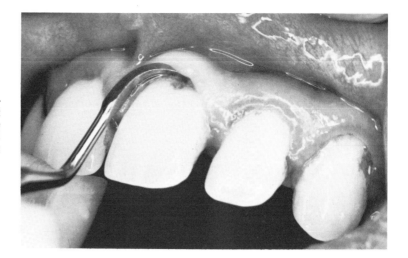

Figure 25–13   Subgingival Calculus revealed by deflecting the pocket wall. Note the inflammation of the marginal gingiva on adjacent lateral incisor and canine associated with supra- and subgingival calculus.

usually dense and hard, dark brown or green-black, flintlike in consistency, and firmly attached to the tooth surface (Figs. 25–14 and 25–15). Supragingival and subgingival calculus generally occur together, but one may be present without the other. Microscopic studies demonstrate that the deposits usually extend near but do not reach the base of periodontal pockets in chronic periodontal lesions.

Supragingival calculus has also been referred to as *salivary*, and subgingival calculus as *serumal*—predicated on the assumption that the former is derived from the saliva and the latter from the blood serum. This concept, overshadowed for a long time by the feeling that saliva was the sole source of all calculus, has been revised. It is the current consensus that the minerals for the formation of supragin-

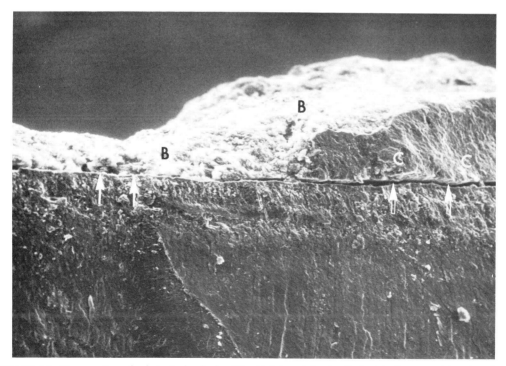

Figure 25–14   Cross-section of subgingival calculus (C) which is not firmly attached to the cemental surface (arrows). Note bacteria (B) attached to calculus and cemental surface. (Courtesy of Dr. John Sottosanti.)

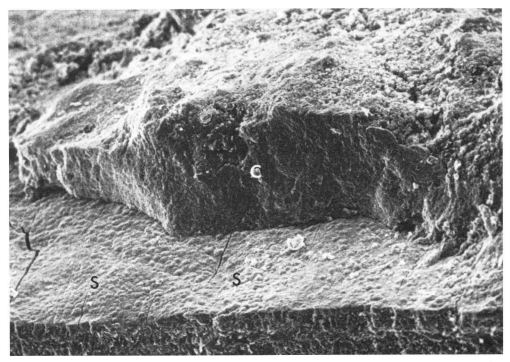

Figure 25–15   Cross-sectional view of subgingival calculus (C) attached to the cementum surface. (Courtesy of Dr. John Sottosanti.)

gival calculus come from the saliva, whereas the gingival fluid which resembles serum is the main mineral source for subgingival calculus.[99, 207]

When the gingival tissues become atrophic (recede) subgingival calculus becomes exposed and is classified as supragingival. Thus, supragingival calculus can be composed of both the supragingival and subgingival type.

Supra- and subgingival calculus usually appears in the early teens and increases with age.[78, 122, 169] The supragingival type is more common; subgingival calculus is uncommon in children, and supragingival calculus is uncommon up to the age of nine. The reported prevalence of both types of calculus at different ages varies considerably, according to the examination criteria of different investigators and in different population groups. Between the ages of 9 and 15, supragingival calculus has been reported in from 37[55] to 70 per cent[118] of the individuals studied; in the 16 to 21 age group it ranges from 44[190] to 88 per cent, and in 86[13] to 100 per cent after age 40.[128] The prevalence of subgingival calculus is generally slightly lower than that of the supragingival type, but it approaches a range of 47 to 100 per cent of individuals after the age of 40.

Supra- and subgingival calculus is often seen in roentgenograms (see Chapter 32). Supragingivally, well-calcified deposits are readily detectible, forming irregular contours of the roentgenographic crown. Interproximal calculus, both supra- and subgingival, is much more detectible, since these deposits form irregularly shaped projections into the interdental space. Normally the location does not indicate the depth of the periodontal pocket, since the most apical plaque is not calcified enough to be roentgenographic.

Composition of Calculus

Inorganic content

Supragingival calculus consists of inorganic (70 to 90 per cent)[73] and organic components. The inorganic portion consists of 75.9 per cent calcium phosphate, $Ca_3(PO_4)_2$; 3.1 per cent calcium carbonate, $CaCO_3$; and traces of magnesium phosphate, $Mg_3(PO_4)_2$, and other metals. The percentage of inorganic constituents of calculus is similar to that of other calcified tissues of the body. The principal inorganic components are calcium, 39 per cent; phosphorous, 19 per cent; magnesium, 0.8 per cent; carbon dioxide, 1.9 per cent; and trace amounts of sodium, zinc, strontium, bromine, copper, manganese, tungsten, gold, aluminum, silicon, iron, and fluorine.[155] At least two thirds of the inorganic component is crystalline in structure.[121] The four main crystal forms and their percentages are hydroxyapatite, $Ca_{10}(PO_4)_6(OH)_2$, approximately 58 per cent; brushite, $CaHOP_4 \cdot 2H_2O$, approximately 9 per cent; and magnesium whitlockite, $Ca_9(PO_4)_6$ X $PO_7 \cdot (X = Mg_{11} \cdot F_{11})$ and octacalcium phosphate $Ca_4H(PO_4)_3 \cdot 2H_2O$, approximately 21 per cent each.[177] Generally two or more crystal forms occur in a calculus sample, with hydroxyapatite and octacalcium phosphate being the most common (in 97 to 100 per cent of all supragingival calculus) and in the greatest amounts. Brushite is more common in the mandibular anterior region and whitlockite in the posterior areas. The incidence of the four crystal forms varies with the age of the deposit.[188]

Organic content

The organic component of calculus consists of a mixture of protein-polysaccharide complexes, desquamated epithelial cells, leukocytes, and various types of microorganisms (Fig. 25–6);[86, 137] 1.9 to 9.1 per cent of the organic component is carbohydrate, which consists of galactose, glucose, rhamnose, mannose, glucuronic acid, galactosamine, and sometimes arabinose, galacturonic acid, and glucosamine, all of which are present in salivary glycoprotein, except arabinose and rhamnose.[125, 205] Protein derived from the saliva accounts for 5.9 to 8.2 per cent, and includes most of the amino acids.[125, 137, 205] Lipids account for 0.2 per cent of the organic content in the forms of neutral fats, free fatty acids, cholesterol, cholesterol esters, and phospholipids.[126]

The composition of subgingival calculus is similar to supragingival, with some differences. It has the same hydroxyapatite content,[214] more magnesium and whitlockite, and less brushite and octacalcium phosphate.[177] The ratio of calcium to phosphate is higher subgingivally, and the sodium content increases with the depth of periodontal pockets.[127] Salivary proteins present in supragingival calculus are not found subgingivally.[15] Dental calculus, salivary duct calculus, and calcified dental tissues are similar in inorganic composition.

Attachment of Calculus to the Tooth Surface

Differences in the manner in which calculus is attached to the tooth surface affect the relative ease or difficulty encountered in its removal. The frequency of various modes of attachment was first described by Zander.[238] Subsequent articles by others presented further information.[110, 140, 184, 192, 203, 204] Calculus, particularly on enamel, can be attached by means of an organic pellicle. It can also be attached by mechanical locking into surface irregularities such as unrepaired cemental and dentinal resorptions (see Fig. 25–17) and by interlocking of inorganic crystals of calculus with those of the tooth structure. Selvig, using the transmission electron microscope, observed that the surface of cementum subsequent to chipping of the overlying calculus had crystals remaining that were previously attached to the calcified intermicrobial matrix or pellicle.[192] He concluded that the intercrystalline forces of the inorganic components may represent a significant contributing factor in the attachment of calculus to cementum (Fig. 25–16).

Sottosanti,[203, 204] using the scanning electron microscope, showed that most root surfaces were relatively smooth and retention of calculus depended on the close adaptation of its undersurface depressions to the gentle sloping mounds on the unaltered surface of cementum (Fig. 25–17 and 25–18).

Calculus Formation

Calculus is attached dental plaque which has undergone mineralization. The soft plaque is hardened by precipitation of mineral salts, which usually starts between

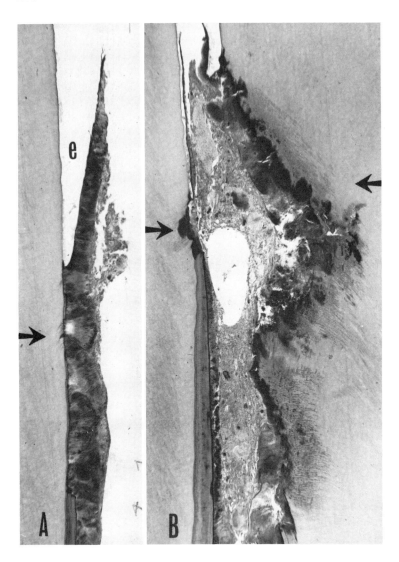

Figure 25–16 Calculus. A, Calculus attached to pellicle on enamel surface (e). The enamel was removed in preparation of the specimen. Also note calculus attached to dentin and associated penetration of dental tubules (arrow). B, Interproximal area with early and advanced root caries of adjacent teeth and with calculus attached to carious surfaces (arrows).

the first and the fourteenth day of plaque formation, but calcification has been reported as early as four to eight hours.[215] Calcifying plaques may become 50 per cent mineralized in two days and 60 to 90 per cent in 12 days.[152, 187, 193]

All plaque does not necessarily undergo calcification. Early plaque contains a small amount of inorganic material, which increases as plaque develops into calculus. Plaque which does not develop into calculus reaches a plateau of maximum mineral content by two days.[152, 187, 193] Microorganisms are not always essential in calculus formation, since it occurs readily in germ-free rodents.[72, 83]

Saliva is the mineral source for supragingival calculus, and the gingival fluid or exudate furnishes the minerals for subgingival calculus. Plaque has the ability to concentrate calcium to 2 to 20 times its level in saliva.[41] Early plaque of heavy calculus formers contains more calcium, three times more phosphorus, and less potassium than that of nonformers, suggesting that phosphorus may be more critical than calcium in plaque mineralization.[134]

Calcification entails binding of calcium ions to the carbohydrate-protein complexes of the organic matrix,[135] and the precipitation of crystalline calcium phosphate salts. Crystals initially form in the intercellular

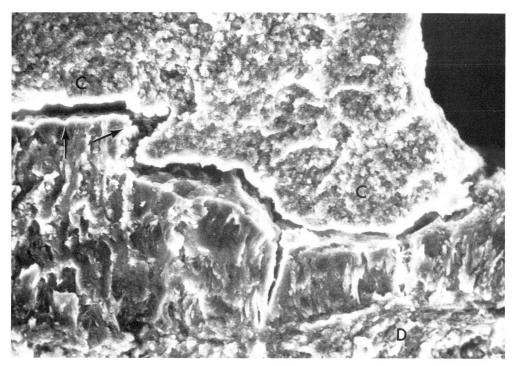

Figure 25–17   Subgingival calculus (C) embedded beneath the cementum surface (arrow) and penetrating to the dentin (D), making removal difficult. (Courtesy of Dr. John Sottosanti.)

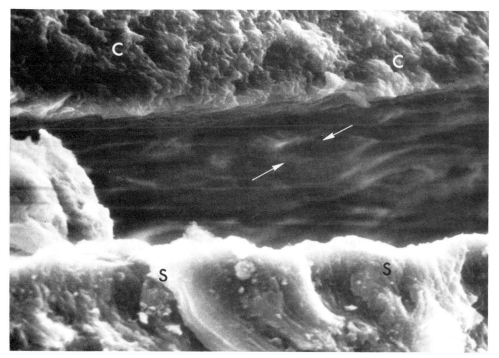

Figure 25–18   Under surface of subgingival calculus (C) previously attached to cementum surface (S). Note impression of cementum mounds in calculus (arrows). (Courtesy of Dr. John Sottosanti.)

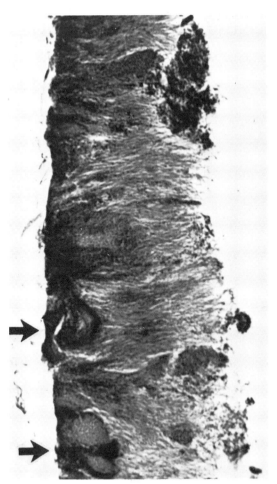

Figure 25–19 Five-Day Plaque, showing spherical calcification foci (*arrows*), and perpendicular alignment of filamentous organisms along the inner surface and colonies of cocci on the outer surface. (From Turesky, S., Renstrup, G., and Glickman, I.[221])

matrix and on the bacterial surfaces, and finally within the bacteria.[75, 239]

Calcification begins along the inner surface of the supragingival plaque (and in the attached component of subgingival plaque) adjacent to the tooth in separate foci that increase in size and coalesce to form solid masses of calculus (Fig. 25–19). It may be accompanied by alterations in the bacterial content and staining qualities of the plaque. With the occurrence of calcification, filamentous bacteria increase in number. In the calcification foci there is a change from basophilia to eosinophilia; the staining intensity of periodic acid–Schiff positive groups and sulfydryl and amino groups is reduced; and staining with toluidine blue,

initially orthochromatic, becomes metachromatic and disappears.[229] Calculus is formed in layers, often separated by a thin cuticle which becomes embedded in it as calcification progresses.[151]

Rate of formation and accumulation

The starting time and rate of calcification and accumulation of calculus vary from person to person, in different teeth, and at different times in the same person.[154, 218] Based on these differences, individuals may be classified as heavy, moderate, or slight calculus formers, or as nonformers. The average daily increment in calculus formers is from 0.10 to 0.15 per cent of dry weight.[193, 217]

Calculus formation continues until it reaches a maximum, from which it may be reduced in amount. The time required to reach the maximum level has been reported as ten weeks,[37] 18 weeks,[144] and six months.[225] The decline from maximum accumulation (reversal phenomenon)[153, 225] may be explained by the vulnerability of bulky calculus to mechanical wear from food and from the cheeks, lips, and tongue.

Theories regarding the mineralization of calculus

Theories regarding the mechanisms whereby plaque is mineralized to form calculus fit into two principal concepts:[155]

According to the first concept, mineral precipitation results from a local rise in the degree of saturation of calcium and phosphate ions, which may be brought about in several ways: (1) A rise in pH of the saliva causes precipitation of calcium phosphate salts by lowering the precipitation constant. The pH may be elevated by the loss of carbon dioxide and by the formation of ammonia by dental plaque bacteria, or by protein degradation during stagnation.[19, 92, 156] (2) Colloidal proteins in saliva bind calcium and phosphate ions and maintain a supersaturated solution with respect to calcium phosphate salts. With stagnation of saliva, colloids settle out; the supersaturated state is no longer maintained, leading to precipitation of calcium phosphate salts.[86, 168] (3) Phosphatase liberated from dental plaque, desquamated epithelial cells, or bacteria is believed to play a role in the precipitation of calcium phosphate by hydrolyzing organic phosphates in saliva and thus increasing the concentration of free phosphate ions:[36, 233] Another enzyme, esterase, present in the cocci, filamentous organisms, leukocytes, macrophages, and desquamated epithelial cells of dental plaque, may initiate calcification by hydrolyzing fatty esters into free fatty acids.[8] The fatty acids form soaps with calcium and magnesium that are converted later into the less soluble calcium phosphate salts.

According to the second concept, seeding agents induce small foci of calcification, which enlarge and coalesce to form a calcified mass.[158] This concept has been referred to as the epitactic concept. The seeding agents in calculus formation are not known, but it is suspected that the intercellular matrix of plaque plays an active role.[140, 152, 239] The carbohydrate-protein complexes may initiate calcification by removing calcium from the saliva (chelation) and binding with it to form nuclei that induce subsequent deposition of minerals.[135, 226] Plaque bacteria have also been implicated as possible seeding agents (discussed in the following section).

Role of microorganisms in the mineralization of calculus

Mineralization of plaque may start extracellularly around both gram-positive and gram-negative organisms,[115] but may start intracellularly. Filamentous organisms, diptheroids, and *Bacterionema* and *Veillonella* species have the ability to form intracellular apatite crystals. Calculus formation spreads until the matrix and bacteria are calcified.[75, 172, 239] Some feel that plaque bacteria actively participate in the mineralization of calculus by forming phosphatases, changing the plaque pH, or inducing mineralization,[53, 135] but the prevalent opinion is that they are only passively involved[75, 171, 231] and are simply calcified along with other plaque components. The occurrence of calculus-like deposits in germ-free animals encourages this opinion.[72, 83] However, other experiments suggest that transmissible factors are involved in calculus formation, and that penicillin in the diet of some of these animals reduces calculus formation.[9]

It is difficult to separate the effects of calculus and plaque upon the gingiva, because calculus is always covered with a nonmineralized layer of plaque.[185] There is a positive correlation between calculus and the prevalence of gingivitis,[169] but it is not as high as between plaque and gingivitis.[77] In young individuals the periodontal condition is more closely related to plaque accumulation than to calculus, but the situation is reversed with age.[77, 122]

Calculus, gingivitis, and periodontal disease increase with age. It is extremely rare to find a periodontal pocket in adults without subgingival calculus, although in some cases it may be of microscopic proportions (Fig. 25-20).

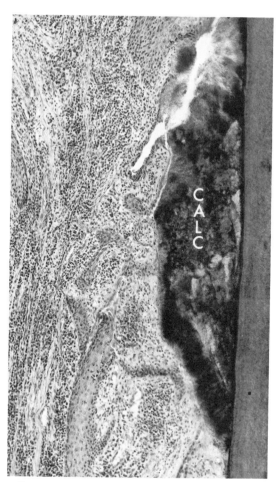

Figure 25-20 Suppurative Inflammation in periodontal pocket wall adjacent to uncalcified plaque on calculus surface (CALC).

The nonmineralized plaque on the calculus surface is the principal irritant,[203, 204] but the underlying calcified portion may be a significant contributing factor. It does not irritate the gingiva directly, but it provides a fixed nidus for the continued accumulation of irritating surface plaque and holds the plaque against the gingiva.

Subgingival calculus may be the product rather than the cause of periodontal pockets. Plaque initiates the gingival inflammation which starts pocket formation, and the pocket provides a sheltered area for plaque and bacterial accumulation. Increased flow of gingival fluid associated with gingival inflammation provides the minerals which convert the continually accumulating plaque into subgingival calculus.

Regardless of its primary or secondary relationship in pocket formation, and although the principal irritating feature of calculus is surface plaque rather than its calcified interior, calculus is a significant pathogenic factor in periodontal disease.

MATERIA ALBA

Materia alba* is primarily an acquired bacterial coating which is a yellow or gray-white, soft, sticky deposit somewhat less adherent than dental plaque.[186] Materia alba is clearly visible without using disclosing solutions and forms on tooth surfaces, restorations, calculus, and gingiva.[136, 152] It tends to accumulate on the gingival third of the teeth and on malposed teeth. It can form on previously cleaned teeth within a few hours, and during periods when no food is ingested.[166] Materia alba can be flushed away with a water spray, but mechanical cleansing is required to assure complete removal.

Long considered to consist of stagnant food debris, materia alba is now recognized to be a concentration of microorganisms, desquamated epithelial cells, leukocytes, and a mixture of salivary proteins and lipids,[136, 186, 236] with few or no food

---

*Materia alba is a traditional clinical term for a material which is essentially a heavy accumulation of plaque.

particles.[166] It lacks a regular internal pattern such as is observed in plaque. The irritating effect of materia alba upon the gingiva is most likely caused by bacteria and their products. Materia alba has also been demonstrated to be toxic when injected into experimental animals after the bacterial component has been destroyed by heat.[18]

FOOD DEBRIS

Most food debris is rapidly liquefied by bacterial enzymes and cleared from the oral cavity within five minutes after eating, but some remains on the teeth and mucosa.[20, 166] Salivary flow, mechanical action of the tongue, cheeks, and lips, and form and alignment of the teeth and jaws affect the rate of food clearance, which is accelerated by increased chewing and low viscosity of saliva.[112] Although it contains bacteria, food debris is different from the bacterial coatings (plaque and materia alba). Dental plaque is not a derivative of food debris, nor is food debris an important cause of gingivitis.[50] Food debris should be differentiated from fibrous strands trapped interproximally in areas of food impaction.*

The rate of clearance from the oral cavity varies with the type of food and the individual. Liquids are cleared more readily than solids. For example, traces of sugar ingested in aqueous solution remain in the saliva for approximately 15 minutes, whereas sugar consumed in solid form is present as long as 30 minutes after ingestion.[223] Sticky foods, such as figs, bread, toffee, and caramel, may adhere to tooth surfaces for over an hour, whereas coarse foods and raw carrots and apples are quickly cleared. Plain bread is cleared faster than bread with butter,[20, 79] brown rye bread faster than white,[112] and cold foods slightly faster than hot. The chewing of apples and other fibrous foods can effectively remove most of the food debris from the oral cavity, although it has no significant effect on reduction of plaque.[22, 123]

---

*Food impaction is discussed in Chapter 26.

DENTAL STAINS

Pigmented deposits on the tooth surface are called *stains*. They are primarily esthetic problems. Stains result from the pigmentation of ordinarily colorless developmental and acquired dental coatings by chromogenic bacteria, foods, and chemicals. They vary in color and composition and in the firmness with which they adhere to the tooth surface.

BROWN STAIN. This is a thin, translucent, acquired, usually bacteria-free, pigmented pellicle.[142, 222] It occurs in individuals who do not brush sufficiently or who use a dentifrice with inadequate cleansing action. It is found most commonly on the buccal surface of the maxillary molars and on the lingual surface of the mandibular incisors. The brown color is usually due to the presence of tanning.

TOBACCO STAINS. Tobacco produces dark brown or black tenacious surface deposits and brown discoloration of tooth substance. Staining results from coal tar combustion products and penetration of pits and fissures, enamel, and dentin by tobacco juices. Staining is not necessarily proportional to the tobacco consumed, but depends to a considerable degree upon pre-existent acquired coatings which attach the tobacco products to the tooth surface.

BLACK STAIN. This usually occurs as a thin black line on the teeth facially and lingually near the gingival margin, and as a diffuse patch on the proximal surfaces. It is firmly attached, tends to recur after removal, is more common in women, and may occur in mouths with excellent hygiene. The black stain that occurs on human primary teeth is typically associated with low incidence of caries in affected children.[199, 209] Chromogenic bacteria have been implicated. The microflora of black stain is dominated by gram-positive rods, primarily *Actinomyces* species, and evidence implicates these bacteria as a probable cause. Isolated *Actinomyces* species can produce black pigmentation, and other *in vitro* investigations have demonstrated black pigment formation caused by *Actinomyces* in the dentin.[6, 162, 199] The chromogenic bacteria, *Bacteroides melaninogenicus*, accounts for less than 1 per cent of isolated bacteria and is not considered important for the color of black stain.[199]

GREEN STAIN. This is a green or green-yellow stain, sometimes of considerable thickness, which is common in children (see Color Plate 3). It is considered to be the stained remnants of the enamel cuticle but this has not been substantiated.[5] The discoloration has been attributed to fluorescent bacteria and fungi such as *Penicillium* and *Aspergillus*.[6] Green stain usually occurs on the facial surface of the maxillary anterior teeth, in the gingival half, more often in boys (65 per cent) than in girls (43 per cent).[119] A high incidence has been reported in children with tuberculosis of cervical lymph nodes and other tuberculous lesions.

ORANGE STAINS. Orange stain is less common than green or brown stains. It may occur on both the facial and lingual surfaces of anterior teeth. *Serratia marcescens* and *Flavobacterium lutescens* have been suggested as the responsible chromogenic organisms.[14]

METALLIC STAINS. Metals and metallic salts may be introduced into the oral cavity in metal-containing dust inhaled by industrial workers, or through orally administered drugs. The metals combine with acquired dental coatings (usually pellicle), producing a surface stain, or penetrate the tooth substance and cause permanent discoloration. Copper dust produces a green stain and iron dust a brown stain. Iron-containing medicines cause a black iron sulfite deposit. Other occasionally seen metallic stains are manganese (black), mercury (green-black), nickel (green), and silver (black).

CHLORHEXIDINE STAIN. Chlorhexidine was introduced as a general disinfectant with a broad antibacterial action against gram-positive and gram-negative bacteria and yeast[71, 130] (Fig. 25–5). It has been observed clinically that the continued use of chlorhexidine solution may promote discoloration in the mouth.[70, 71, 130, 160] In vivo experiments using radioactive carbon–labelled chlorhexidine have shown retention of chlorhexidine in the human oral cavity.[24, 70, 71] The retention is attributed to its affinity for sulfate and acidic groups such as those found in plaque constituents, carious lesions, pellicle, and bacterial cell walls.[24, 71, 90, 160] The retention of chlorhexidine is concentration- and time-dependent. It is not influenced by the temperature or pH of the rinsing solution.[24]

Chlorhexidine stain imparts a yellowbrown to brownish color to the tissues of the oral cavity.[54, 70, 71] The staining appears in the cervical and interproximal regions of the teeth, on restorations, in plaque, and on the surface of the tongue.[70, 71, 90, 130, 160] It appears that the presence of aldehydes and ketones, which are normally intermediates of both mammalian and microbial metabolism, are essential for formation of discoloration by chlorhexidine.[160] No permanent staining of the enamel or dentine is observed clinically, since toothbrushing with dentifrice or professional prophylaxis can remove the stain accumulating on the teeth.[130] A similar stain occurs with the use of alexidine.

REFERENCES

1. Adinolfi, M., Mollison, P. L., Polley, M. J., and Rose, J. M.: A blood group antibodies. J. Exp. Med., 123:951–967, 1966.
2. Armstrong, W. G.: Origin and nature of the acquired pellicle. Proc. R. Soc. Med., 61:923, 1968.
3. Armstrong, W. G., and Hayward, A. F.: Acquired organic integuments of human enamel: A comparison of analytical studies with optical, phase-contrast and electron microscope examinations. Caries Res., 2:294, 1968.
4. Ash, M. M., Gitlin, B. N., and Smith, W. A.: Correlation between plaque and gingivitis. J. Periodontol., 35:424, 1964.
5. Ayers, P.: Green stains. J. Am. Dent. Assoc., 26:3, 1939.
6. Badanes, B. B.: The role of fungi in deposits upon the teeth. Dent. Cosmos, 75:1154, 1933.
7. Badanes, B. B., and Parodneck, C. B.: The influence of emotional states upon tartar formation. J. Am. Dent. Assoc., 24:1421, 1937.
8. Baer, P. N., and Burstone, M. S.: Esterase activity associated with formation of deposits on teeth. Oral Surg., 12:1147, 1959.
9. Baer, P. N., Keyes, P. H., and White, C. L.: Studies on experimental calculus formation in the rat. XII. On the transmissibility of factors affecting dental calculus. J. Periodontol., 39:86, 1968.
10. Baer, P. N., Stephan, R. M., and White, C. L.: Studies on experimental calculus formation in the rat. I. Effect of age, sex, strain, high carbohydrate, high protein diets. J. Periodontol., 32:190, 1961.
11. Baer, P. N., and White, C. L.: Studies on experimental calculus formation in the rat. IX. The effect of varying the protein and fat content of the diet on calculus deposition and alveolar bone loss. J. Periodontol., 37:113, 1966.
12. Barkin, M., and Bernard, G.: Ultrastructural cytochemical localization of polysaccharides in dental plaque. J. Dent. Res., 49:979, 1970.
13. Barros, L., and Witkop, C. P.: Oral and genetic study of chileans, 1960. III. Periodontal disease and nutritional factors. Arch. Oral Biol., 8:195, 1963.
14. Bartels, H. A.: A note on chromogenic micro-organisms from an organic colored deposit of the teeth. Intern. J. Orthod., 25:795, 1939.
15. Baumhammers, A., and Stallard, R. E.: A method for the labeling of certain constituents in the organic matrix of dental calculus. J. Dent. Res., 45:1568, 1966.
16. Beck, D. J., et al.: A simple method for public health dental survey in developing countries. New Zealand Dent. J., 60:274, 1964.
17. Becks, H., Wainwright, W. W., and Morgan, A. F.: Comparative study of oral changes in dogs due to deficiencies of pantothenic acid, nicotinic acid and vitamin B complex. Am. J. Orthod., 29:183, 1943.
18. Beckwith, T. D., and Williams, A.: Materia alba as toxic material. Am. Dent. Surg., 49:73, 1929.
19. Bibby, B. G.: The formation of salivary calculus. Dent. Cosmos, 77:668, 1935.
20. Bibby, B. G., Goldberg, H. J. V., and Chen, E.: Evaluation of caries-producing potentialities of various foodstuffs. J. Am. Dent. Assoc., 42:491, 1951.
21. Bienenstock, J.: Immunoglobulins of the hamster. II. Characterization of the gamma A and other immunoglobulins in serum and secretions. J. Immunol., 104:1228, 1970.
22. Birkeland, J., and Jorkjend, L.: The effect of chewing apples on dental plaque and food debris. Community Dent. Oral Epidemiol., 2:161–162, 1974.
23. Björn, H., and Carlsson, J.: Observations on a dental plaque morphogenesis. Odont. Rev., 15:23, 1964.
24. Bonesvell, D., Lokken, P., and Rolla, G.: Influence of concentration, time, temperature and pH on the retention of chlorhexidine in the human oral cavity after mouth rinses. Arch. Oral Biol., 19:1025–1029, 1974.
25. Bowen, W. H., and Cornick, D.: Effects of carbohydrate restriction in monkeys (Mirus) with active caries. Helv. Odont. Acta, 11:27, 1967.
26. Bowen, W. H., and Gilmour, M. N.: Actinomyces and calculus formation (Abst.). J. Dent. Res., 38:709, 1959.
27. Brandtzaeg, P., and Jamison, H.: A study of periodontal health and oral hygiene in Norwegian army recruits. J. Periodontol., 35:302, 1964.
28. Brandtzaeg, P., Tjellanger, I., and Gjeruldsen, S. I.: Human secretory immunoglobulins. I. Salivary secretions from individuals with normal or low levels of serum immunoglobu-

lins. Scand. J. Haemat. [Suppl.], *12*:1–83, 1970.

29. Brandtzaeg, P., Tjellanger, J., and Gjeruldsen, S. J.: Localization of immunoglobulins in human mucosa. Immunochemistry, *4*:57–60, 1967.

30. Carlsson, J.: Presence of various types of nonhemolytic streptococci in dental plaque and in other sites of the oral cavity of man. Odont. Revy, *18*:55, 1967.

31. Carlsson, J., and Egelberg, J.: Effect of diet on early plaque formation in man. Odont. Revy, *16*:112, 1965.

32. Carlsson, J., and Egelberg, J.: Local effect of diet on plaque formation and development of gingivitis in dogs. II. Effect of high carbohydrate versus high protein-fat diets. Odont. Revy, *16*:42, 1965.

33. Chauncey, H. H.: Salivary enzymes. J. Am. Dent. Assoc., *63*:360, 1961.

34. Chawla, T. N., Nanda, R. S., and Mathur, M. N.: Bacterial plaque and its relation to periodontal disease. All-India Dent. Assoc. J., *31*:121, 1959.

35. Ciba Foundation Symposium: Caries Resistant Teeth. Boston, Little, Brown and Company, 1965, pp. 292–296.

36. Citron, S.: The role of actinomyces israeli in salivary calculus formation. J. Dent. Res., *24*:87, 1945.

37. Conroy, C., and Sturzenberger, O.: The rate of calculus formation in adults. J. Periodontol., *39*:142, 1968.

38. Critchley, P., Wood, J. M., Saxton, C. A., and Leach, S. A.: The polymerisation of dietary sugars by dental plaque. Caries Res., *1*:112, 1967.

39. da Costa, T., and Gibbons, R. J.: Hydrolysis of levan by human plaque streptococci. Arch. Oral Biol., *13*:609, 1968.

40. Dawes, C., et al.: The relation between the fluoride concentrations in the dental plaque and in drinking water. Br. Dent. J., *119*:164, 1965.

41. Dawes, C., and Jenkins, G. N.: Some inorganic constituents of dental plaque and their relationship to early calculus formation and caries. Arch. Oral Biol., *7*:161, 1962.

42. Dawes, C., Jenkins, G. N., and Tonge, C. H.: The nomenclature of the integuments of the enamel surface of teeth. Br. Dent. J., *115*:65, 1963.

43. De Stopelaar, J. D., Van Houte, J., and De Moor, C. E.: The presence of dextran forming bacteria identified as *Streptococcus bovis* and *Streptococcus sanguis* in human dental plaque. Arch. Oral Biol., *12*:1199, 1967.

44. Dewar, M. R.: Bacterial enzymes and periodontal disease. J. Dent. Res., *37*:100, 1958.

45. Doku, H. C., and Taylor, R. G.: Thromboplastin generation by saliva. Oral Surg., *15*:1295, 1962.

46. Dornan, D. C.: Dental plaque: Its inflammatory potential. Periodont. Abstr., *16*:138, 1968.

47. Dreizen, S., and Hampton, J. K., Jr.: Radioisotopic studies of the glandular contribution of selected B vitamins in saliva. J. Dent. Res., *48*:579, 1969.

48. Eastcott, A., and Stallaad, R.: Sequential changes in developing human dental plaque as visualized by scanning electron microscopy. J. Periodontol., *44*:218, 1973.

49. Egelberg, J.: Local effect of diet on plaque formation and development of gingivitis in dogs. Part I. Effect of hard and soft diets. Odont. Revy, *16*:31, 1965.

50. Egelberg, J.: Local effect of diet on plaque formation and development of gingivitis in dogs. III. Effect of frequency of meals and tube feeding. Odont. Revy, *16*:50, 1965.

51. Eichel, R. A.: A clinical television evaluation of plaque formation in children. I.A.D.R. Abstracts, 1970, No. 491, p. 171.

52. Ellen, R. P., and Gibbons, R. J.: M-Protein associated adherence of streptococcus pyogenes to epithelial surfaces: Prerequisite for virulence. Infect. Immun., *5*:826, 1972.

53. Ennever, J.: Microbiologic mineralization: A calcifiable cell-free extract from a calcifiable microorganism. J. Dent. Res., *41*:1383, 1962.

54. Eriksen, H., and Gjermo, P.: Incidence of stained tooth surfaces in students using chlorhexidine-containing dentifrices. Scand. J. Dent. Res., *81*:533–537, 1973.

55. Everett, F. G., Tuchler, H., and Lu, K. H.: Occurrence of calculus in grade school children in Portland, Oregon, J. Periodontol., *34*:54, 1963.

56. Fitzgerald, R. J.: Plaque microbiology and caries. Ala. J. Med. Sci., *5*:239, 1968.

57. Fitzgerald, R. J., and Jordan, H. V.: Polysaccharide producing bacteria and dental caries. *In* Harris, R. S. (Ed.): The Art and Science of Dental Caries Research. New York, Academic Press, Inc., 1968.

59. Vogel, J. J., and Amdur, B. H.: Inorganic pyrophosphate in parotid saliva and its relation to calculus formation. Arch. Oral Biol., *12*:159, 1967.

60. Frank, R. M., and Brendel, A.: Ultrastructure of the approximal dental plaque and the underlying normal and carious enamel. Arch. Oral Biol., *11*:883, 1966.

61. Fundak, C. P., and Ash, M.: Correlation between supragingival plaque, subgingival plaque and gingival crevice depth. I.A.D.R. Abstracts, 1969, No. 349, p. 128.

62. Gibbons, R. J.: Dental Plaque. Edited by W. D. McHugh. London, E. & S. Livingstone Co., 1970, p. 207.

63. Gibbons, R. J., and Banghart, S. B.: Induction of dental caries in gnotobiotic rats with a levan forming streptococcus and a streptococcus isolated from subacute bacterial endocarditis. Arch. Oral Biol., *13*:297, 1968.

64. Gibbons, R. J. and Banghart, S. B.: Synthesis of extracellular dextran by cariogenic bacteria and its presence in human dental plaque. Arch. Oral Biol., *12*:11, 1967.

65. Gibbons, R. J., Kapsimalis, B., and Socransky, S. S.: The source of salivary bacteria. Arch. Oral Biol., *9*:101, 1964.

66. Gibbons, R. J., Socransky, S. S., De Araugo, W. C., et al.: Studies of the predominant cutivable microbiota of dental plaque. Arch. Oral Biol., *9*:365, 1964.

67. Gibbons, R. J., and van Houte, J.: Selective bacterial adherence to oral epithelial surfaces and its role as an ecological determinant. Infect. Immun., 3:567, 1971.

68. Gibbons, R. J., van Houte, J., and Liljemark, W. F.: Some parameters effecting the adherence of S. salivarius to oral epithelial surfaces. J. Dent. Res., 51:424, 1972.

69. Gibbons, R. J., and van Houte, J.: On the formation of dental plaques. J. Periodontol., 44:347, 1973.

70. Gjermo, P., Basstad, K., and Rolla, G.: The plaque-inhibiting capacity of 11 antibacterial compounds. J. Periodont. Res., 5:102–109, 1970.

71. Gjermo, P.: Chlorhexidine in dental practice. J. Clin. Periodontol., 1:143–152, 1974.

72. Glas, J. E., and Krasse, B.: Biophysical studies on dental calculus from germ free and conventional rats. Acta. Odont. Scand., 20:127, 1962.

73. Glock, G. E., and Murray, M. M.: Chemical investigation of salivary calculus. J. Dent. Res., 17:257, 1938.

74. Gochman, N., Meyer, R. K., Blackwell, R. Q., and Fosdick, L. S.: The amino acid decarboxylase of salivary sediment. J. Dent. Res., 38:998, 1959.

75. Gonzales, F., and Sognnaes, R. F.: Electromicroscopy of dental calculus. Science, 131:156, 1960.

76. Grant, D., Stern, I., and Everett, F.: Orban's Periodontics. 4th ed., The C. V. Mosby Co., St. Louis, 1972.

77. Greene, J. C.: Oral hygiene and periodontal disease. Am. J. Public Health, 53:913, 1963.

78. Greene, J. C., and Vermillion, J. R.: The oral hygiene index. J. Am. Dent. Assoc., 68:7, 1964.

79. Grenby, T.: The influence of sticky foods of high sugar content on dental caries in the rat. Arch. Oral Biol., 14:1259–1265, 1969.

80. Gressly, F.: Experimental calculus formation. Periodontics, 1:53, 1963.

81. Grøn, P., Yao, K., and Spinelli, M.: A study of inorganic constituents in dental plaque. J. Dent. Res., 48:799, 1969.

82. Grossman, L. I.: Effect of chemical agents on a calculus substitute. Oral Surg., 7:484, 1954.

83. Gustafsson, B. E., and Krasse, B.: Dental calculus in germ free rats. Acta Odont. Scand., 20:135, 1962.

84. Haber, G. G.: The effect of the differences in the quality of bread upon nutrition and the development of dental caries and tartar in Germany and Switzerland, 1932–1937. Brit. Dent. J., 68:142, 1940.

85. Hachwald, G. M., Jacobson, E. B., and Thorbecke, G. J.: C14 amino acid incorporation into transferrin and B. 2-A-globulin by ectodermal glands in vitro. (Absts.) Fed. Proc., 23:557, 1964.

86. Hampar, B., Mandel, I. D., and Ellison, S. A.: The carbohydrate components of supragingival calculus. (Absts.) J. Dent. Res., 40:752, 1961.

87. Hay, D. I.: The adsorption of salivary proteins by hydroxyapatite and enamel. Arch. Oral Biol., 12:937, 1967.

88. Heremans, J. E., and Crabbe, P. A.: IgA deficiency: General considerations and relation to human diseases. In Immunologic Deficiency Diseases in Man, Birth Defects Original Article Series, Vol. 4, New York: The National Foundation—March of Dimes, 1968, p. 298.

89. Herrenknecht, W., and Becks, H.: Oral hygiene. Fortschr. Zahnhk., 4:736, 1928.

90. Heyden, G.: Relation between locally high concentration of chlorhexidine and staining as seen in the clinic. J. Periodont. Res., 8 [Suppl.]:12:76–80, 1973.

91. Heylings, R. T.: Study of the prevalence and severity of gingivitis in undergraduates at Leeds University (1960). Dent. Practit., 12:129, 1961.

92. Hodge, H. C., and Leung, S. W.: Calculus formation. J. Periodontol., 21:211, 1950.

93. Hoover, D. R., and Robinson, H. B. G.: Effect of automatic and hand toothbrushing on gingivitis. J. Am. Dent. Assoc., 65:361, 1962.

94. Howell, A., Rizzo, A., and Paul, F.: Cultivable bacteria in developing and mature human dental calculus. Arch. Oral Biol., 10:307, 1965.

95. Hurlimann, J., and Zuber, C.: In vitro protein synthesis by human salivary gland. I. Synthesis of salivary IgA and serum proteins. Immunology, 14:809–817, 1968.

96. Hurlimann, J., and Zuber, C.: In vitro protein synthesis by human salivary glands. II. Synthesis of proteins specific to saliva and other secretions. Immunology, 14:819–824, 1968.

97. James, P.M.C., et al.: Gingival health and dental cleanliness in English schoolchildren. Arch. Oral Biol., 3:57, 1960.

98. Jenkins, G. N.: The chemistry of plaque. Ann. N. Y. Acad. Sci., 131:786, 1965.

99. Jenkins, G. N.: The Physiology of the Mouth. Oxford, Blackwell Scientific Publications, 1966, p. 495.

100. Jenkins, G. N., Ferguson, D. B., and Edgar, W. M.: Fluoride and the metabolism of salivary bacteria. Helv. Odont. Acta, 11:2, 1967.

101. Jensen, A. T., and Danø, M.: Crystallography of dental calculus and precipitation of certain calcium phosphates. J. Dent. Res., 33:741, 1954.

102. Kakehashi, S., Baer, P. N., White, C., and Gluck, G.: Studies on experimental calculus formation in the rat. VI. Effect of diet intubation, meal feeding and nibbling. J. Periodontol., 34:513, 1963.

103. King, J. D.: Experimental investigation of periodontal disease in the ferret and in man, with special reference to calculus formation. Dent. Practit., 4:157, 1954.

104. Kinoshita, S., and Mühlemann, H. R.: Effect of sodium ortho- and pyrophosphate on supragingival calculus. Helv. Odont. Acta, 10:46, 1966.

105. Kinoshita, S., Schait, A., Brebou, M., and Mühlemann, H. R.: Effect of sucrose on early dental calculus and plaque. Helv. Odont. Acta, 10:134, 1966.

106. Kleinberg, I. and Jenkins, G. N.: The pH of dental plaques in different areas of the mouth before and after meals and their relationship to the

pH and rate of flow of resting saliva. Arch. Oral Biol., 9:493, 1964.

107. Klinkhamer, J. M.: Saliva. *In* Lazzari, E.: Dental Biochemistry. Philadelphia, Lea and Febiger, 1968.

108. Krasse, B.: Human streptococci and experimental caries in hamsters. Arch. Oral Biol., 11:429, 1966.

109. Kraus, F. W., Perry, W. I., and Nickerson, J. F.: Salivary catalase and peroxidase values in normal subjects and in persons with periodontal disease. Oral Surg., 11:95, 1958.

110. Kupczyk, L., and Conroy, M.: The attachment of calculus to root planed surfaces. Periodontics, 6:78–83, 1968.

111. Kupczak, L. J., Volpe, A. R., and King, W. J.: Dental plaque: Relationship between accumulation patterns in human adult dentition and clinical investigations. I.A.D.R. Abstracts, 1969, No. 642, p. 201.

112. Lanke, L. S.: Influence on salivary sugar of certain properties of foodstuffs and individual oral conditions. Acta Odont. Scand., 15:3, [Suppl. 23.] 1957.

113. Leach, S. A.: Plaque chemistry and caries. Ala. J. Med. Sci., 5:247, 1968.

114. Leach, S. A., Critchley, P., Kolendo, A. B., and Saxton, C. A.: Salivary glycoproteins as components of the enamel integuments. Caries Res., 1:104, 1967.

115. Leach, S. A., and Saxton, C. A.: An electron microscopic study of the acquired pellicle and plaque formed on the enamel of human incisors. Arch. Oral Biol., 11:1081, 1966.

116. Lehner, J., Cardwell, J. E., and Clarry, E. D.: Immunoglobulins in saliva and serum in dental caries. Lancet, 2:1294–1297, 1967.

117. Lenz, H., and Mühlemann, H. R.: Repair of etched enamel exposed to the oral environment. Helv. Odont. Acta, 7:47, 1963.

118. Leung, S. W.: Role of calculus deposits in periodontal disease. *In* A Symposium on Preventive Dentistry. St. Louis, The C. V. Mosby Company, 1956, p. 206.

119. Leung, S. W.: Naturally occurring stains on the teeth of children. J. Am. Dent. Assoc., 41:191, 1950.

120. Leung, S. W.: The uneven distribution of calculus in the mouth. J. Periodontol., 22:7, 1951.

121. Leung, S. W., and Jensen, A. T.: Factors controlling the deposition of calculus. Intern. Dent. J., 8:613, 1958.

122. Lilienthal, B., Amerena, V., and Gregory, G.: An epidemiological study of chronic periodontal disease. Arch. Oral Biol., 10:553, 1965.

123. Lindhe, J., and Wicen, P.: The effects on the gingivae of chewing fibrous foods. J. Periodont. Res., 4:193–201, 1969.

124. Lisanti, V. F.: Hydrolytic enzymes in periodontal tissues. Ann. N.Y. Acad. Sci., 85:461, 1960.

125. Little, M. F., Bowman, L., Casciani, C. A., and Rowley, J.: The composition of dental calculus. III. Supragingival calculus—the amino acid and saccharide component. Arch. Oral Biol., 11:385, 1966.

126. Little, M. F., Bowman, L. M., and Dirksen, T. R.: The lipids of supragingival calculus. J. Dent. Res., 43:836, 1964.

127. Little, M. F., and Hazen, S. P.: Dental calculus composition. 2. Subgingival calculus: Ash, calcium, phosphorus and sodium. J. Dent. Res., 43:645, 1964.

128. Littleton, N. W.: Dental caries and periodontal disease among Ethiopian civilians. Public Health Rep., 78:631, 1963.

129. Littleton, N. W., Carter, C. H., and Kelly, R. T.: Studies of oral health in persons nourished by stomach tube. J. Am. Dent. Assoc., 74:119, 1967.

130. Löe, H., and Schiott, C.: The effect of mouth rinses and topical application of chlorhexidine on the development of dental plaque and gingivitis in man. J. Periodont. Res., 5:79–83, 1970.

131. Lo Grippo, G. A., Hayashi, H., and Perry, M.: Immunoglobulins in serum and saliva in health and diseases. Fed. Proc., 28:553, 1969.

132. Lovdal, A., Arno, A., Schei, O., and Waerhaug, J.: Combined effect of subgingival scaling and controlled oral hygiene on the incidence of gingivitis. Acta Odont. Scand., 19:537, 1961.

133. Lovdal, A., Arno, A., and Waerhaug, J.: Incidence of clinical manifestations of periodontal disease in light of oral hygiene and calculus formation. J. Am. Dent. Assoc., 56:21, 1958.

134. Mandel, I. D.: Biochemical aspects of calculus formation. J. Periodont. Res., 4:(Suppl. 4)7, 1969.

135. Mandel, I. D.: Calculus formation. The role of bacteria and mucoprotein. Dent. Clin. North Am., 1960, p. 731.

136. Mandel, I. D.: Dental plaque: Nature, formation, and effects. J. Periodontol., 37:357, 1966.

137. Mandel, I. D.: Histochemical and biochemical aspects of calculus formation. Periodontics, 1:43, 1963.

138. Mandel, I. D.: Plaque and calculus. Ala. J. Med. Sci., 5:313, 1968.

139. Mandel, I. D.: Plaque and calculus measurements—Rate of formation and pathologic potential. J. Periodontol., 38:721, 1967.

140. Mandel, I. D., Levy, B. M., and Wasserman, B. H.: Histochemistry of calculus formation. J. Periodontol., 28:132, 1957.

141. Mandel, I.: Relation of saliva and plaque to caries. J. Dent. Res. [Suppl.], 53:246–266, 1974.

142. Manly, R. S.: A structureless recurrent deposit on teeth. J. Dent. Res., 22:479, 1943.

143. Marshall-Day, C. D., and Shourie, K. L.: Gingival disease in the Virgin Islands. J. Am. Dent. Assoc., 40:175, 1950.

144. Matt, M. M., Stout, F. W., and Swancar, J. R.: Deposition curves of in vivo calculus formation. I.A.D.R. Abstracts, 1970, No. 705, p. 225.

145. McCombie, F., and Stothard, D.: Relationship between gingivitis and other dental conditions. J. Can. Dent. Assoc., 30:506, 1964.

146. McDougall, W. A.: Studies on the dental plaque. I. The histology of the dental plaque and its attachment. Australian Dent. J., 8:261, 1963.

147. McDougall, W. A.: Studies on the dental plaque. IV. Levans and the dental plaque. Australian Dent. J., 9:1, 1964.

148. McHugh, W. D., McEwen, J. D., and Hitchin, A.

D.: Dental disease and related factors in 13-year-old children in Dundee. Br. Dent. J., *117*:246, 1964.

149. Meckel, A. H.: The formation and properties of organic films on teeth. Arch. Oral Biol., *10*:585, 1965.

150. Morrison, M., and Steele, W.: Lactoperoxidase, the peroxidase in the salivary gland. *In* Person, P. (ed.): Biology of the Mouth. Washington, D.C. AAAS, 1968.

151. Moskow, B. S.: Calculus attachment in cemental separations. J. Periodontol., *40*:125, 1969.

152. Mühlemann, H. R., and Schroeder, H.: Dynamics of supragingival calculus formation. Adv. Oral Biol., *1*:175, 1964.

153. Mühlemann, H. R., and Villa, P. R.: The marginal line calculus index. Helv. Odont. Acta, *11*: 175, 1967.

154. Muhler, J. C., and Ennever, J.: Occurence of calculus through several successive periods in a selected group of subjects. J. Periodontol., *33*:22, 1962.

155. Mukherjee, S.: Formation and prevention of supragingival calculus. J. Periodont. Res., Suppl. 2, 1968.

156. Naeslund, C.: A comparative study of the formation of concretions in the oral cavity and in the salivary glands and ducts. Dent. Cosmos, *68*:1137, 1926.

157. Nash, D. R., Vaerman, J. P., Bazin, H., and Heremans, J. F.: Comparative molecular size of mouse IgA in different body fluids. Int. Arch. Allergy, *37*:167–174, 1970.

158. Neuman, W. F., and Neuman, M. W.: The Chemical Dynamics of Bone Mineral. Chicago, University of Chicago Press, 1958, p. 209.

159. Niles, E. S.: Odontolithus influenced by calcic and phosphatic diathesis (salivary calculus). D. Cosmos, *23*:203, 242, 502, 1881.

160. Nordbo, H.: Discoloration of human teeth by a combination of chlorhexidine and aldehydes or ketones in vitro. Scand. J. Dent. Res., *79*:356–361, 1971.

161. O'Leary, T. J., Shannon, I. L., and Prigmore, J. R.: Clinical correlation and systemic status in periodontal disease. J. Periodontol., *33*:243, 1962.

162. Onisi, M., and Nuckolls, J.: Description of actinomycetes and other pleomorphic organisms recovered from pigmented carious lesions of the dentine of human teeth. Oral Surg., *11*:910–930, 1958.

163. O'Rourke, J. T.: The relation of the physical character of the diet to the health of the periodontal tissues. Am. J. Orthod., *33*:687, 1947.

164. Oshrain, H. I., Salkind, A., and Mandel, I. D.: Studies of the histology and bacteriology of subgingival plaque and calculus. J. Periodont. Res., Suppl. 4, 1969, p. 9.

165. Parfitt, G. J.: A survey of the oral health of Navajo Indian children. Arch. Oral Biol., *1*:193, 1959.

166. Parfitt, G. J.: Summary of the problem of the prevention of periodontal disease. Ala. J. Med. Sci., *5*:395, 1968.

167. Perlitsh, M. J., and Glickman, I.: Salivary neuraminidase. III. Its relation to oral disease. J. Periodontol., *38*:189, 1967.

168. Prinz, H.: The origin of salivary calculus. Dent. Cosmos, *63*:231, 369, 503, 619, 1921.

169. Ramfjord, S. P.: The periodontal status of boys 11 to 17 years old in Bombay, India. J. Periodontol., *32*:237, 1961.

170. Ritz, H. L.: Microbial population shifts in developing human dental plaque. Arch. Oral Biol., *12*:1561, 1967.

171. Rizzo, A. A., Martin, G. R., Scott, D. B., and Mergenhagen, E. E.: Mineralization of bacteria. Science, *135*:439, 1962.

172. Rizzo, A. A., Scott, D. B., and Bladen, H. A.: Calcification of oral bacteria. Ann. N.Y. Acad. Sci., *109*:14, 1963.

173. Rogon, I., and Amdur, B.: Further characterization of an antibacterial factor in human parotid secretions active against lactobacillus casei. Arch. Oral Biol., *10*:605, 1965.

174. Rolla, G., Kornstad, L., Mathiesen, P., and Povatong, L.: Selective adsorption of an acidic glycoprotein from human saliva to tooth surfaces. J. Periodont. Res., Suppl. 4, Inter. Conf. Periodont. Res., 8, 1969.

175. Rosebury, T., and Karshan, M.: Salivary Calculus. Dental Science and Dental Art. Philadelphia, Lea & Febiger, 1938.

176. Rossen, R. D., Morgan, C., Hsu, K. C., Butler, W. J., and Rose, H. M.: Localization of its external secretory IgA by immunofluorescence in tissues lining the oral and respiratory passages in man. J. Immunol., *100*:706–717, 1968.

177. Rowles, S. L.: The inorganic composition of dental calculus. *In* Blackwood, H. J. J. (ed.): Bone and Tooth. Oxford, Pergamon Press, 1964, pp. 175–183.

178. Russell, A. L.: International nutrition surveys: A summary of preliminary dental findings. J. Dent. Res., *42*:233, 1963.

179. Russell, A. L., Leatherwood, E. C., Consolazio, C. F., and Van Reen, R.: Periodontal disease and nutrition in South Vietnam. J. Dent. Res., *44*:775, 1965.

180. Salmon, S. E., Markey, G., and Fudenberg, H. H.: "Sandwich" solid phase radio immunoassay for the quantitative determination of human immunoglobulins. J. Immunol., *103*:129–137, 1969.

181. Sandham, H. J., Lopez, H., Zuniga, M. A., and Koulourides, T.: Relation between location, composition and demineralizing potential of dental plaque. I.A.D.R. Abstracts, 1970, No. 614, p. 202.

182. Schie, O., Waerhaug, J., Lovdal, A., and Arno, A.: Alveolar bone loss as related to oral hygiene and age. J. Periodontol., *30*:7, 1959.

183. Schiott, C. R., and Löe, H.: The origin and variation in the number of leukocytes in the human saliva. J. Periodont. Res. [Suppl.] *4*: 24, 1969.

184. Schoff, F. R.: Periodontia: An observation on the attachment of calculus. Oral Surg., *8*:154–160, 1955.

185. Schroeder, H. E.: Crystal morphology and gross

structures of mineralizing plaque and of calculus. Helv. Odont. Acta, 9:73, 1965.

186. Schroeder, H. E.: Formation and Inhibition of Dental Calculus. Berne, Stuttgart and Vienna, Hans Huber Publ., 1969, pp. 12–15.

187. Schroeder, H. E.: Inorganic content and histology of early dental calculus in man. Helv. Odont. Acta, 7:17, 1963.

188. Schroeder, H. E., and Bambauer, H. U.: Stages of calcium phosphate crystallization during calculus formation. Arch. Oral Biol., 11:1, 1966.

189. Schroeder, H. E., and De Boever, J.:The structure of microbial dental plaque. In McHugh, W. D. (ed.): Dental Plaque. Edinburgh, E. & S. Livingstone, Ltd., 1970, pp. 49–74.

190. Schroeder, H. E., and Marthaler, T.: In Schroeder, H. E.: Formation and Inhibition of Dental· Calculus. Berne, Stuttgart, and Vienna, Hans Huber Publ., 1969, p. 22.

191. Selvig, K. A.: The formation of plaque and calculus on recently exposed tooth surfaces. J. Periodont. Res. [Suppl. 4] 4:10, 1969.

192. Selvig, J.: Attachment of plaque and calculus to tooth surfaces. Periodont. Res., 5:8, 1970.

193. Sharawy, A., Sabharwal, K., Socransky, S., and Lobene, R.: A quantitative study of plaque and calculus formation in normal and periodontally involved mouths. J. Periodontol., 37:495, 1966.

194. Silness, J., and Löe, H.: Periodontal disease in pregnancy. Acta Odont. Scand., 22:121, 1964.

195. Silverman, G., Kay, M., and Kleinberg, I.: Chemical binding between the macromolecular constituents of dental plaque. I.A.D.R. Abstracts 1965, p. 136.

196. Silverman, G., and Kleinberg, I.: Fractionation of human dental plaque and the characterization of its cellular and acellular components. Arch. Oral Biol., 12:1387, 1967.

197. Simaan, C., and Skach, M.: Clinical and histological evaluation of gingival massage in the treatment of chronic gingivitis. J. Periodontol., 37:383, 1966.

198. Skongaard, M. R., Bay, I., and Klinkhamer, J. M.: Correlation between gingivitis and orogranulocytic migratory rate. J. Dent. Res., 48:716, 1969.

199. Slots, J.: The microflora of black stain on human primary teeth. Scand. J. Dent. Res., 82:484–490, 1974.

200. Smith, R. S., Sherman, N. A., and Newcomb, R. W.: Synthesis and secretion of immunoglobulin, including IgA, by human tonsil and adenoid tissue cultured in vitro. Intern. Arch. Allergy, 46:785–801, 1974.

201. Sonju, T., and Rolla, G.: Chemical analysis of pellicle formed in two hours on cleaned human teeth in vivo. Rate of formation and amino acid analysis. Caries Res., 7:30, 1972.

202. Sonju, T., and Rolla, G.: Chemical analysis of acquired pellicle formed in two hours on cleaned human teeth in vitro. Caries Res., 7:30, 1973.

203. Sottosanti, J. S.: A possible relationship between occlusion, root resorption, and the progres-

sion of periodontal disease. J. Western Soc. Periodont., 25:69, 1977.

204. Sottosanti, J. S.: Relationship of calculus to root surfaces. J. Periodontol., in press.

205. Standford, J. W.: Analysis of the organic portion of dental calculus. J. Dent. Res., 45:128, 1966.

206. Stanton, G.: The relation of diet to salivary calculus formation. J. Periodontol., 40:167, 1969.

207. Stewart, R. T., and Ratcliff, P. A.: The source of components of subgingival plaque and calculus. Periodont. Abstr., 14:102, 1966.

208. Stewart, W. H., and Burnett, G. W.: The relationship of certain dietary factors to calculus-like formation in albino rats. J. Periodontol., 31:7, 1960.

209. Sutcliffe, P.: Extrinsic tooth stains in children. Dent. Practit., 17:175–179, 1967.

210. Taylor, R. G., Doku, H. C., and Romero, J.: Direct determination of fibrinolytic activity of human saliva. J. Dent. Res., 43:86, 1964.

211. Theilade, E., Wright, W. H., Jensen, S. B., and Löe, H.: Experimental gingivitis in man. II. A longitudinal clinical and bacteriological investigation. J. Periodont. Res., 1:1, 1966.

212. Theilade, J.: Electron microscopic study of calculus attachment to smooth surfaces. Acta Odont. Scand., 22:379, 1964.

213. Theilade, J., and Fitzgerald, R. J.: Dental calculus in the rat: Effect of diet and erythromycin. Acta Odont. Scand., 21:571, 1963.

214. Theilade, J., and Schroeder, H. E.: Recent results in dental calculus research. Inter. Dent. J., 16:205, 1966.

215. Tibbetts, L. S., and Kashiwa, H. K.: A histochemical study of early plaque mineralization. I.A.D.R. Abst. 1970, No. 616, p. 202.

216. Tomasi, T. B., and Bienenstock, J.: Secretory immunoglobulins. Adv. Immunol., 9:1–96, 1968.

217. Tomasi, J. B., Jr., and Zigelbaum, S.: The excretion of gamma globulin in human saliva, colostrum, and urine. Arthritis Rheum., 5:662, 1962.

218. Turesky, S., et al.: Effects of changing the salivary environment on progress of calculus formation. J. Periodontol., 33:45, 1962.

219. Turesky, S., Gilmore, N. D., and Glickman, I.: Calculus inhibition by topical application of the chloromethyl analogue of victamine C. J. Periodontol., 38:142, 1967.

220. Turesky, S., Gilmore, N. D., and Glickman, I.: Reduced plaque formation by the chloromethyl analogue of Victamine C. J. Periodontol., 41:41, 1970.

221. Turesky, S., Renstrup, G., and Glickman, L.: Histologic and histochemical observations regarding early calculus formation in children and adults. J. Periodontol., 32:7, 1961.

222. Vallotton, C. F.: An acquired pigmented pellicle of the enamel surface. J. Dent. Res., 24:161, 171, 183, 1945.

223. Volker, J. F., and Pinkerton, D. M.: Acid production in saliva-carbohydrates. J. Dent. Res., 26:229, 1947.

224. Volpe, A. R., Kupczak, L. J., and King, W. J.: In vivo calculus assessment: Part III. Scoring

techniques, rate of calculus formation, partial mouth exams vs. full mouth exams and intra-examiner reproducibility. Periodontics, 5: 184, 1967.

225. Volpe, A. R., Kupczak, L. J., King, W. J., Goldman, H., and Schulmann, S.M.: In vivo calculus assessment. Part IV. Parameters of human clinical studies. J. Periodontol., 40:76, 1969.

226. Von der Fehr, F., and Brudevold, F.: In vitro calculus formation. J. Dent. Res., 39:1041, 1960.

227. Voreadis, E. G., and Zander, H. A.: Cuticular calculus attachment. Oral Surg., 11:1120, 1958.

228. Waerhaug, J.: Effect of rough surfaces upon gingival tissue. J. Dent. Res., 35:323, 1956.

229. Waerhaug, J.: The source of mineral salts in subgingival calculus. J. Dent. Res., 34:563, 1955.

230. Wallace, J. S.: The newer knowledge of hygiene in diet. J. Am. Dent. Assoc., 18:1322, 1931.

231. Wasserman, B. H., Mandel, J. D., and Levy, B. M.: In vitro calcification of calculus. J. Periodontol., 29:145, 1958.

232. Weinberger, B. W.: An Introduction to the History of Dentistry. St. Louis, The C. V. Mosby Co., 1948, p. 203.

233. Wilkinson, F. C.: A patho-histological study of the tissue of tooth attachment. Dent. Record, 55:105, 1935.

234. Williams, R. W., and Gibbons, R. J.: Inhibition of bacterial adherence by secretory immuno-globulin A: A mechanism of antigen disposal. Science, 177:697, 1972.

235. Wood, J. M., and Critchley, P.: The extracellular polysaccharide produced from sucrose by a cariogenic streptococcus. Arch. Oral Biol., 11:1039, 1966.

236. World Health Organization: Periodontal disease: Report of an expert committee on dental health. Intern. Dent. J., 11:544, 1961.

237. Yardeni, J.: Dental calculus. J. Dent. Res., 27:532, 1948.

238. Zander, H. A.: The attachment of calculus to root surfaces. J. Periodontol., 24:16, 1953.

239. Zander, H. A., Hazen, S. P., and Scott, D. B.: Mineralization of dental calculus. Proc. Soc. Exper. Biol. Med., 103:257, 1960.

Chapter 26

Faulty Dentistry, Food Impaction, and Other Local Factors in the Etiology of Periodontal Disease

The cause of gingival inflammation is bacterial plaque (see Chap. 24). Several factors previously considered to be of direct etiologic significance in periodontal disease now are known to act only by favoring plaque accumulation. They include calculus (described in Chap. 25), faulty restorations and partial removable prostheses, food impaction, and others presented in this chapter.

This chapter also includes other factors (habits, toothbrush trauma, chemical irritation, and radiation) that will produce gingival inflammation and/or periodontal destruction by different mechanisms. It should be understood that they do not produce periodontal pockets and therefore the so-called "periodontitis" unless they become complicated by bacterial plaque.

FAULTY DENTISTRY

Faulty dental restorations and prostheses are common causes of gingival inflammation and periodontal destruction. Inadequate dental procedures may also injure the periodontal tissues. The following characteristics of restorations and partial dentures are of importance from a periodontal viewpoint: margin, contour, occlusion, materials, and design of removable partial dentures. They will be described in this chapter, as they play a role in the etiology of periodontal lesions; a more comprehensive review with special emphasis on the recommended approach to this procedure will be presented in Chapter 56.

MARGINS OF RESTORATIONS. Overhanging margins provide ideal locations for the accumulation of plaque and the multiplication of bacteria (Figs. 26–1 and 26–2). A study has shown that 75 per cent of the restorations show marginal defects and that 55 per cent of the defects equal or surpass 0.2 mm. A highly significant statistical relationship was found between marginal defects and reduced bone height.[10]

Numerous studies have shown positive correlation between subgingival margins and gingival inflammation.[26, 32, 36, 64] It has also been shown that even high quality restorations, if placed subgingivally, will

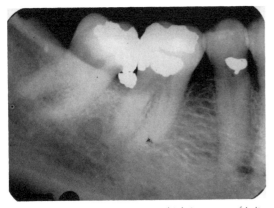

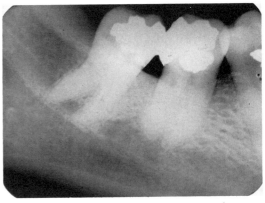

Figure 26–1   Amalgam Excess which is source of irritation to the gingiva.

Figure 26–2   Amalgam Excess Removed.

increase plaque accumulation, gingival inflammation[65] and the rate of gingival fluid flow.[55]

CONTOURS. In recent years the relationship between crown contour and gingival health has been clarified. It has been shown that overcontoured crowns and restorations tend to accumulate plaque and possibly prevent the self-cleaning mechanisms of the adjacent cheek, lips, and tongue[3, 41, 50, 89]   (Fig. 26–3). Previous claims that undercontouring of crowns may also have a deleterious effect owing to lack of protection of the gingival margin during mastication have not been proved.[89]

Inadequate or improperly located proximal contacts, and failure to reproduce the normal protective anatomy of the occlusal marginal ridges and developmental grooves, lead to food impaction. Failure to reestablish adequate interproximal embrasures fosters the accumulation of irritants.

OCCLUSION. Restorations that do not conform to the occlusal patterns of the mouth cause occlusal disharmonies that may be injurious to the supporting periodontal tissues.

MATERIALS. Restorative materials are not injurious by themselves to the periodontal tissues. [3, 37] One exception to this may be self-curing acrylics.[86]

Restorative materials differ in relation to their capacity to retain plaque,[87] but all can be adequately cleaned if they are polished[54, 70] and accessible to brushing. The composition of plaque formed on restora-

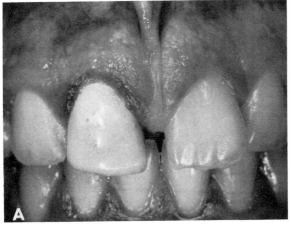

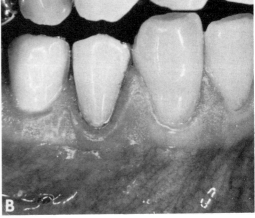

Figure 26–3 *A,* **Gingival inflammation and Recession** associated with accumulated irritants on rough margin of crown. *B,* **Inadequate Mesioproximal Contour on First Premolar Restoration** leads to accumulation of irritants and gingival inflammation.

tive materials is similar, with the exception of that formed on silicate.[54] Plaque formed at the margins of various restorations is similar to that formed on adjacent tooth surfaces.

REMOVABLE PARTIAL DENTURES. Several investigations have shown that after the insertion of partial dentures there is an increase in mobility of the abutment teeth, gingival inflammation, and periodontal pocket formation.[9, 16, 73] Other studies that emphasized regular check-ups and reinforced oral hygiene instructions periodically did not find the same periodontal changes.[8]

DENTAL PROCEDURES. The use of rubber dam clamps, copper bands, matrix bands, and disks in such a manner as to lacerate the gingiva results in varying degrees of inflammation. Although for the most part such transient injuries undergo repair, they are needless sources of discomfort to the patient. Injudicious tooth separation and excessively vigorous condensing of gold foil restorations are sources of injury to the supporting tissues of the periodontium, which may be attended by acute symptoms such as pain and sensitivity to percussion.

FOOD IMPACTION

Food impaction is the forceful wedging of food into the periodontium by occlusal forces. It may occur interproximally or in relation to the facial or lingual tooth surfaces. Food impaction is a very common cause of gingival and periodontal disease. Far too frequently, failure to recognize and eliminate food impaction is responsible for the unsuccessful outcome of an otherwise thoroughly treated case of periodontal disease.

The Mechanism of Food Impaction

The forceful wedging of food normally is prevented by the integrity and location of the proximal contact, the contour of the marginal ridges and developmental grooves, and the contour of the facial and lingual surfaces. An intact, firm proximal contact relationship prevents the forceful wedging of food interproximally. The location of the contact is also important in protecting the tissues against food impaction. The optimal cervico-occlusal location of the contact is at the longest mesiodistal diameter of the tooth, close to the crest of the marginal ridge. The proximity of the contact point to the occlusal plane reduces the tendency toward food impaction in the smaller occlusal embrasure. The absence of contact or the presence of an unsatisfactory proximal relationship is conducive to food impaction (Fig. 26–4).

The contour of the occlusal surface established by the marginal ridges and related developmental grooves normally

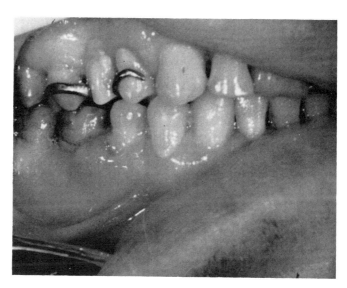

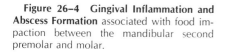

Figure 26–4 Gingival Inflammation and Abscess Formation associated with food impaction between the mandibular second premolar and molar.

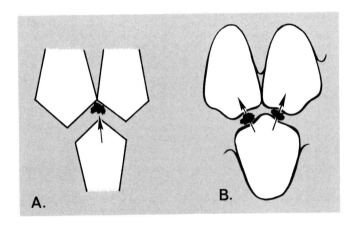

Figure 26-5   Food Impaction. *A,* Wedging effect upon food bolus *(arrow)* which results from wearing away of normal occlusal convexities and protective marginal ridges (after Hirschfeld). *B,* Food impaction corrected by restoring occlusal convex surfaces and marginal ridges and directing food onto the occlusal surface *(arrows).*

serves to deflect food away from the interproximal spaces (Fig. 26–5). As the teeth wear down and flattened surfaces replace the normal convexities, the wedging effect of the opposing cusp into the interproximal space is exaggerated (Fig. 26–5), and food impaction results. Cusps that tend to forcibly wedge food interproximally are known as *plunger cusps*. The plunger cusp effect may occur with wear as indicated above, or may be the result of a shift in tooth position following the failure to replace missing teeth.

Excessive anterior overbite is a common cause of food impaction. The forceful wedging of food into the gingiva on the facial surfaces of the mandibular anterior teeth and the lingual surfaces of the maxillary teeth produces varying degrees of periodontal involvement. Gingival changes in the mandibular anterior region, associated with excessive anterior overbite, are

easily detectable (Fig. 26–6). Unless they are severe, however, the effects of food impaction on the lingual surface of the maxilla are often overlooked. It should be stressed that inflammation caused by lingual food impaction may spread to the contiguous facial gingival margin. The possibility that lingual food impaction may be a contributory factor should always be explored when the etiology of gingival disease in the anterior maxilla is being considered.

In a classic dissertation on the subject, Hirschfeld[29] presented the following classification of factors causing food impaction:

Class I. Occlusal wear

Type A. Wedging action produced by the transformation of occlusal convexities into oblique facets (Fig. 26–7).

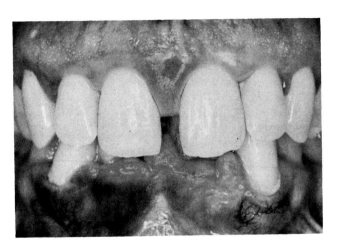

Figure 26-6   Inflammatory Gingival Enlargement in the mandibular anterior region associated with overbite and food impaction.

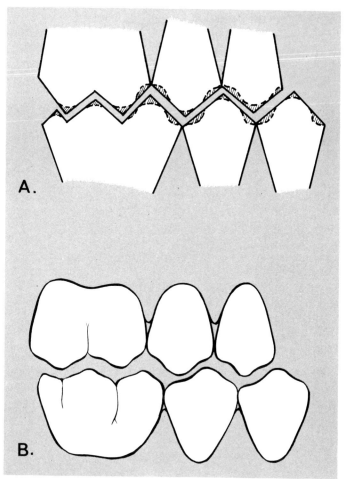

Figure 26–7   Correction of Food Impaction in Worn Dentition. *A,* Flattened occlusal surfaces result in food impaction. Dotted lines show recontouring of occlusal surfaces necessary to correct food impaction. *B,* Recontoured occlusal surfaces.

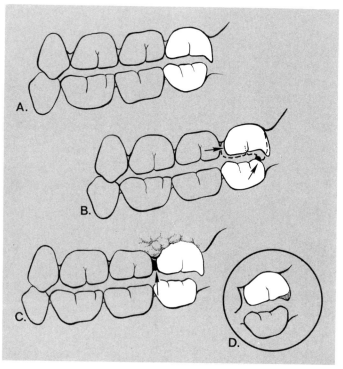

Figure 26–8   Distal Overhang on Worn Tooth Results in Food Impaction. *A,* Occlusal surface of the maxillary third molar is worn so as to produce a distal projection overhanging the mandibular molar. *B,* The maxillary molar is forced distally (*arrow*) by bolus of food during mastication (*arrow*). *C,* Food impaction (*arrow*) on the mesial surface of the maxillary molar. *D,* Occlusal surface is recontoured as initial step in correcting food impaction.

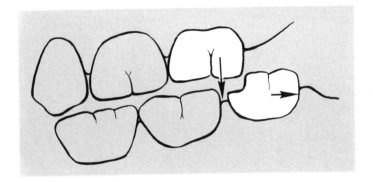

Figure 26–9 Food Impaction. Mandibular third molar forced distally (*arrow*) because of notch created by attrition. Food impaction (*arrow*) on the mesial surface is the result.

Type B. Remaining obliquely worn cusp of a maxillary tooth overhanging the distal surface of its functional antagonist (Fig. 26–8).

Type C. Obliquely worn mandibular tooth overlapping the distal surface of its functional antagonist (Fig. 26–9).

Class II. Loss of proximal support

Type A. Loss of distal support through the removal of a distally adjacent tooth (Fig. 26–10).

Type B. Loss of mesial support due to extraction.

Type C. Oblique drifting due to nonreplacement of a missing tooth.

Type D. Permanent occlusal openings to interdental spaces.

1. Drifting after extraction.
2. Habits forcing teeth out of position.
3. Periodontal disease.
4. Caries (Fig. 26–11).

Class III. Extrusion beyond the occlusal plane

Type A. Extrusion of a tooth retaining contiguity with the adjacent mesial and distal members.

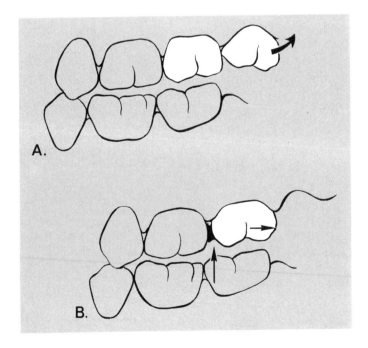

Figure 26–10 Food Impaction. *A*, Removal of maxillary third molar (*arrow*) permits second molar to be forced distally when teeth contact in occlusion. *B*, Bolus of food forced interproximally (*arrow*) as maxillary second molar is wedged distally (*arrow*).

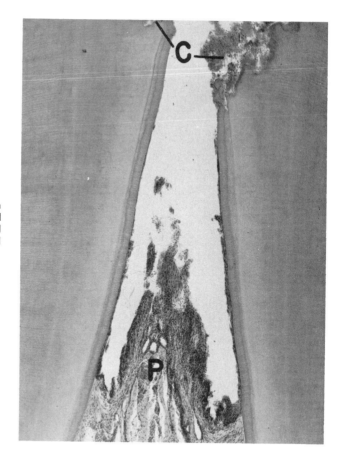

Figure 26–11 Mesiodistal section through mandibular premolars showing loss of proximal contact because of caries (C), which results in food impaction and inflammation of the interdental gingiva (P).

Class IV. Congenital morphologic abnormalities

Type A. Position of a tooth in torsion (Figs. 26–12 and 26–13).

Type B. Emphasized embrasures between thick-necked teeth.

Type C. Faciolingual tilting.

Type D. Lingual or facial position of a tooth (Fig. 26–14).

Class V. Improperly constructed restorations

Type A. Omission of contact points (Fig. 26–15).

Type B. Improper location of contact points.

Type C. Improper occlusal contour.

Type D. Improperly constructed cantilever restorations.

Type E. Scalloped cervical bevels on the tissue-borne areas of prosthetic restorations.

It should, however, be understood that the presence of the above-mentioned abnormalities does not necessarily lead to food impaction and periodontal disease. A study of interproximal contacts and marginal ridge relationships in three groups of periodontally healthy males revealed that from 61.7 to 76 per cent of the proximal contacts were defective and 33.5 per cent of adjacent marginal ridges were uneven.[56]

Lateral food impaction

In addition to food impaction by occlusal forces, lateral pressure from the lips, cheeks, and tongue may force food interproximally. This is more likely to occur when the gingival embrasure is enlarged by tissue destruction in periodontal disease or by recession. Impaction results when food forced into such an embrasure during mastication is retained instead of passing through.

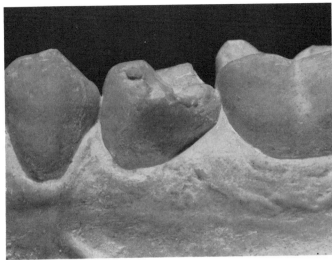
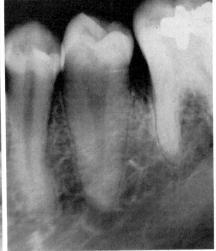

Fig. 26–12   Fig. 26–13

Figure 26–12 Improper Proximal Contact Relationship Associated with Malposed Premolar. Note inclined "plateau" which directs food from occlusal surface of the premolar into the distal interdental space.

Figure 26–13 Bone Loss in area of food impaction associated with improper contact between mandibular second premolar and molar.

Sequelae of Food Impaction

Food impaction serves to initiate gingival and periodontal disease and aggravates the severity of pre-existent pathologic changes. The following signs and symptoms occur associated with food impaction:

1. Feeling of pressure and the urge to dig the material from between the teeth.

2. Vague pain, which radiates deep in the jaws.

3. Gingival inflammation with bleeding and a foul taste in the involved area.

4. Gingival recession.

5. Periodontal abscess formation.

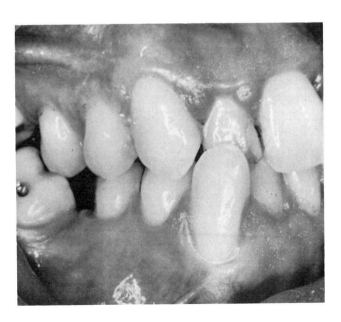

Figure 26–14 **Malposed Teeth** with food impaction and gingival inflammation.

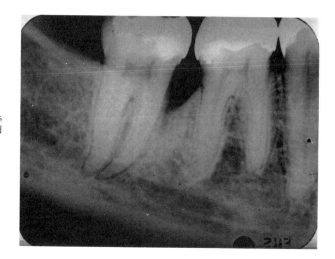

Figure 26–15 **Food Impaction** and bone loss associated with restorations that fail to restore and maintain proximal contact.

6. Varying degrees of inflammatory involvement of the periodontal ligament with an associated elevation of the tooth in its socket, prematurity in functional contact, and sensitivity to percussion.

7. Destruction of alveolar bone.

8. Caries of the root.

UNREPLACED MISSING TEETH

Failure to replace extracted teeth initiates a series of changes producing varying degrees of periodontal disease.[18, 30] In isolated cases, spaces created by tooth extraction may not cause undesirable sequelae. However, the frequency with which periodontal disease results from the failure to replace one or more missing teeth points to the advisability and prophylactic value of early prosthesis.

The ramifications of the failure to replace the first molar are sufficiently consistent to be recognized as a clinical entity. When the mandibular first molar is missing, the initial change is a mesial drifting and tilting of the mandibular second and third molars and extrusion of the maxillary molar. The distal cusps of the mandibular second molar are elevated and act as plungers impacting food into the interproximal space between the extruded maxillary first molar and the maxillary second molar (Fig. 26–16). If there is no maxillary

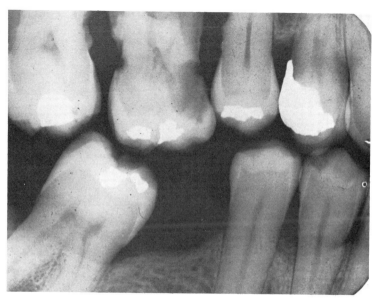

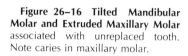

Figure 26–16 **Tilted Mandibular Molar and Extruded Maxillary Molar** associated with unreplaced tooth. Note caries in maxillary molar.

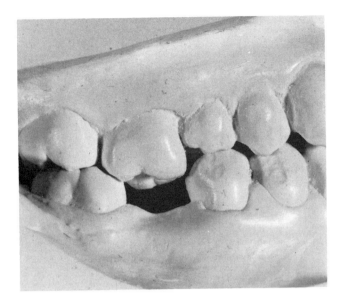

Figure 26–17 **Extrusion of Maxillary First Molar** into space created by unreplaced mandibular molar.

third molar, the distal cusps of the mandibular second molar act as a wedge which breaks the contact between the maxillary first and second molars and deflects the maxillary second molar distally. This results in food impaction, gingival inflammation, and bone loss in the interproximal area between the maxillary first and second molars. Tilting of the mandibular molars and extrusion of the maxillary molars alter the respective contact relationships of these teeth, thereby favoring

food impaction. Bone loss and pocket formation are commonly seen in relation to the extruded and tilted teeth (Figs. 26–17 to 26–19).

Tilting of the posterior teeth also results in reduction in the vertical dimension and accentuation of the anterior overbite. The mandibular anterior teeth slide gingivally along the palatal surfaces of the maxillary anterior teeth, resulting in a distal shift in the position of the mandible. In addition, there is food impaction and pocket forma-

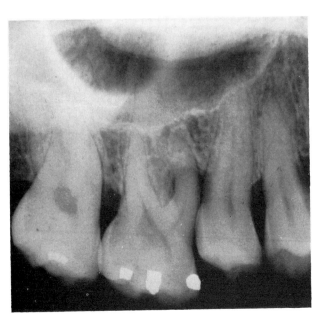

Figure 26–18 **Extruded Maxillary First Molar with Trifurcation Involvement.**

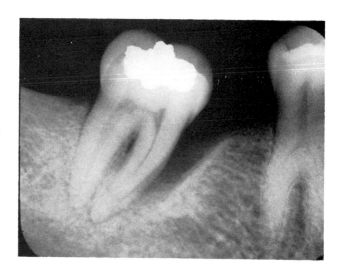

Figure 26–19 Angular Bone Loss on the Mesial Surface of Tilted Molar.

tion in relation to the anterior teeth and a tendency toward labial migration and diastema formation in the maxilla. Distal drifting of the second premolar with food impaction and pocket formation in relation to the opened interproximal space between the premolars may be further complications. The aforementioned changes are accompanied by alterations in the functional relationships of the inclined cusps, with resultant occlusal disharmonies injurious to the periodontium.

The combination of changes associated with the unreplaced mandibular first molar does not occur in all cases, nor are all the

changes identified with failure to replace other teeth in the arch. In general, however, drifting and tilting of the teeth, with alterations in proximal contact, result from failure to replace teeth that have been extracted. These changes are common factors in the etiology of periodontal disease.

MALOCCLUSION

Depending upon its nature, malocclusion exerts a varied effect in the etiology of gingivitis and periodontal disease.[49, 61, 67] Irregular alignment of teeth will make

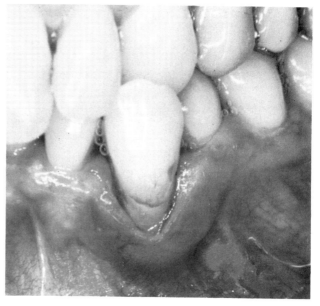

Figure 26–20 Gingival Recession and Inflammation on Malposed Canine.

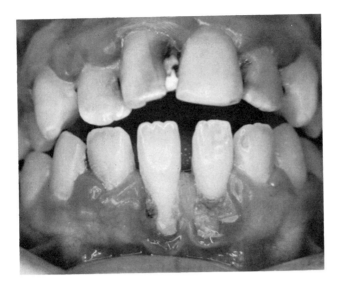

Figure 26–21 **Chronic Gingivitis** associated with "open bite" and accumulation of plaque and food debris.

plaque control difficult or even impossible. Several authors have found a positive correlation between crowding and periodontal disease;[13, 58, 81] others, however, have found no correlation.[25]

Gingival recession is associated with facially displaced teeth (Fig. 26–20). Occlusal disharmony associated with malocclusion results in injury to the periodontium.[51, 57] The incisal edges of the anterior teeth often cause irritation to the gingiva in the opposing jaw in patients with severe overbite. Open bite relationships lead to unfavorable periodontal changes caused by accumulation of plaque and an absence or diminution in function (Fig. 26–21).[14, 39] The prevalence and severity of periodontal

disease are increased in children with bimaxillary protrusions.[31]

MOUTH BREATHING

Gingivitis is often seen associated with mouth breathing.[45] The gingival changes include erythema, edema, enlargement, and a diffuse surface shininess in the exposed areas. The maxillary anterior region is the common site of such involvement. In many cases the altered gingiva is clearly demarcated from the adjacent unexposed normal mucosa (Fig. 26–22). The exact manner in which mouth breathing affects gingival changes has not been dem-

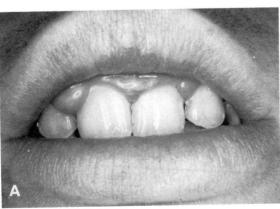
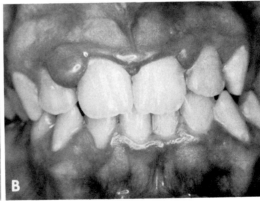

Figure 26–22 **Gingivitis in Mouth Breather.** A, High lip line in mouth breather. B, Gingivitis and inflammatory gingival enlargement in exposed area of gingiva.

onstrated. Its harmful effect is generally attributed to irritation from surface dehydration. However, comparable changes could not be produced by "air drying" the gingiva of experimental animals.[40]

Several recent studies have shown conflicting evidence with respect to the association of mouth breathing and gingivitis. The following has been reported: mouth breathing has no effect on prevalence or extent of gingivitis except in patients with considerable calculus;[1] mouth breathers have more severe gingivitis than non-mouth breathers with similar plaque scores;[34] there is no relationship between mouth breathing and prevalence of gingivitis except a slight increase in severity;[81] crowding of teeth is associated with gingivitis only in mouth breathers.[35]

HABIT

Habit is an important factor in the initiation and progress of periodontal disease. Frequently the presence of an unsuspected habit is revealed in cases that have failed to respond to periodontal therapy. Habits of significance in the etiology of periodontal disease have been classified as follows by Sorrin:[77]

1. *Neuroses*, such as lip biting and cheek biting, which lead to extrafunctional positioning of the mandible, toothpick biting and wedging between the teeth, "tongue-thrusting," fingernail biting, pencil and fountain pen biting, and occlusal neuroses.

2. *Occupational habit*, such as the holding of nails in the mouth as practiced by cobblers, upholsterers, or carpenters, thread biting, and pressure of a reed during the playing of certain musical instruments.

3. *Miscellaneous*, such as pipe (Fig. 26–23) or cigarette smoking, tobacco chewing, incorrect methods of toothbrushing, mouth breathing, and thumb sucking.

Tongue-Thrusting

Special mention should be made of "tongue-thrusting" because it is so frequently undetected. It entails persistent forceful wedging of the tongue against the teeth, particularly in the anterior region. Instead of placing the dorsum of the tongue against the palate with the tip behind the maxillary teeth during swallowing, the tongue is thrust forward against the mandibular anterior teeth which tilt and also spread laterally (Fig. 26–24).

Ray and Santos[63] divide patients with tongue-thrusting into two groups: (1) those in whom tongue-thrusting is part of a syndrome including a *hyposensitive palate and macroglossia*, and (2) those in whom the tongue-thrusting is a habit acquired in childhood or adult life. Tongue-thrusting is generally associated with abnormal swallowing habits (reverse swallow). These habits usually develop in infancy, and some[2, 80] suspect that they arise from bottle feeding with improperly designed nipples. Nasopharyngeal disease and allergy have also been implicated as possible causes of tongue-thrusting.

Tongue-thrusting causes excessive lateral pressure, which may be traumatic to the periodontium.[17, 19, 74] It also causes spreading and tilting of the anterior teeth, with an open bite anteriorly, posteriorly or in the premolar area (Fig. 26–24).

Numerous secondary sequelae may develop from tongue-thrusting. The altered inclination of the maxillary anterior teeth results in a change in the direction of the functional forces so that lateral pressure against the crowns is increased. This aggravates the labial drift and undesirable labiolingual rotational forces.The antagonism between forces that direct the tooth labially, and inward pressure from the lip, may lead to tooth mobility. The altered inclination of the teeth also interferes with food excursion and favors the accumulation of food debris at the gingival margin. The loss of proximal contact leads to food impaction. Tongue-thrusting is an important contributing factor responsible for pathologic migration.[17, 18]

Bruxism, Clenching, and Tapping

Bruxism consists of aggressive, repetitive or continuous grinding or gritting of the teeth during the day or night[66] or both—most frequently by adults but also by children. *Clenching* is continuous or

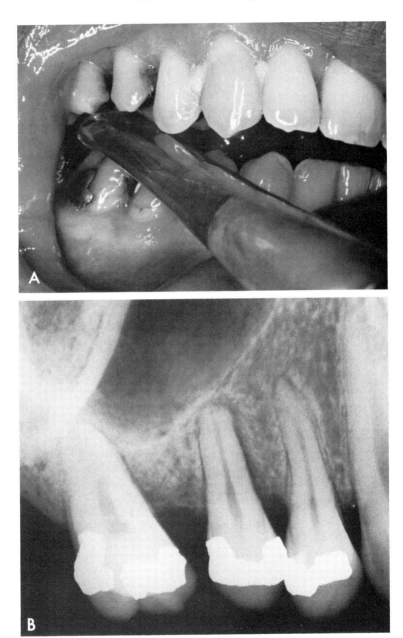

Figure 26–23   Trauma Associated with Holding Pipe in Fixed Position. *A,* Pipe held by maxillary first and second premolars and molar. Note the intruded second premolar and tilted molar. *B,* Radiograph showing intruded second premolar with apical resorption and widened periodontal ligament and angular bone destruction on the mesial surface. Note the widened periodontal ligament on the first premolar and the tilted molar.

intermittent closure of the jaws under pressure, and *tapping* is repetitive tooth contacts made on isolated prominent tooth surfaces or dental restorations. Bruxism, clenching, and tapping are different occlusal habits which should be considered to-

gether because their etiology is the same and they may produce comparable symptoms.

Patients are usually unaware of the habit, but may complain of pain or a tired feeling in the jaws or muscles, particularly

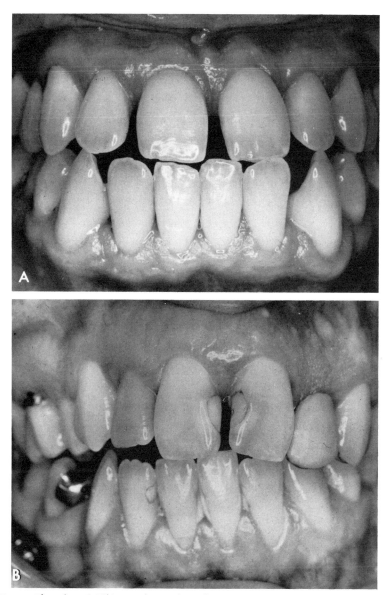

Figure 26–24 Tongue-Thrusting. A, Tilting and spreading of anterior teeth associated with tongue thrusting. B, Hypo-occlusion of lateral incisor, canine, and premolar associated with tongue-thrusting.

upon arising in the morning, which may radiate to the head and neck, a burning sensation in the muscles,[68] or headache.[52]

The aforementioned habits represent perversions of occlusion that are potentially injurious to the periodontal tissues, the masticatory muscles, and the temporomandibular joint. They are referred to by the term *parafunction*, which designates tooth contacts in other than chewing and swallowing.[20]

The etiology of bruxism and related occlusal habits is not known, but they are usually attributed to occlusal abnormalities and/or emotional tension.[44, 53] It is felt that the habits are triggered by occlusal disharmonies such as occlusal prematurities, and represent struggling movements of the mandible in an attempt to wear away or push aside the offensive tooth surfaces.[22] This opinion is supported by the finding that bruxism is accompanied by abnormal muscle activity, and both disappear when occlusal disharmonies are corrected.[62] There is also evidence that emotional tension, anxiety, and deep-seated aggression could cause or aggravate bruxism, clenching, and tapping.[82-84]

The relative significance of occlusal disharmonies and emotional factors in the etiology of bruxing, clenching, and tapping is not clear. Almost everybody has some form of occlusal disharmony, but there is no indication of how severe it must be to trigger an occlusal habit. People differ in their reaction to occlusal disharmonies. This is where the emotional factors enter the picture. Emotional tension may alter the individual threshold to tolerate the annoyance caused by an occlusal disharmony. A bruxing habit would be the result. Comparable occlusal disharmonies may trigger occlusal habits in some patients and not in others, and the response of a given individual to an occlusal disharmony may vary according to his emotional status.

The effects of bruxism, clenching, and tapping habits

Bruxism causes excessive tooth wear characterized by facets on tooth surfaces not ordinarily reached by functional movements, and exaggerated facets in normal functional areas, widening of the occlusal surfaces, and in severe cases reduction in the vertical dimension. Bruxism does not necessarily cause alveolar destruction.[7] The periodontium often responds favorably to the increased function by thickening of the periodontal ligament and increased density of alveolar bone.

However, the repetitive impact created by bruxism and clenching may injure the periodontium by depriving if of function-free periods necessary for normal repair. By traumatizing the periodontium, occlusal habits aggravate existing periodontal disease and lead to tooth mobility.[12, 33, 43] Periodontal injury is most severe around teeth in premature contact. Tapping habits which concentrate on isolated teeth or sections of the arch are more likely to produce injury than are generalized bruxing and clenching.

Occlusal habits may also cause temporo-mandibular joint disorders secondary to hypertonicity of the masticatory muscles, or reduction in vertical dimension from excessive wear uncompensated for by passive eruption.

Tobacco

Ordinarily, smoking does not lead to striking gingival changes. Heat and accumulated products of combustion are local irritants particularly undesirable in periods of post-treatment healing. The following oral changes may occur in smokers:

1. Brownish, tar-like deposits and discoloration of tooth structure.

2. Diffuse grayish discoloration and leukoplakia of the gingiva.

3. "Smoker's palate," characterized by prominent mucous glands with inflammation of the orifices and a diffuse erythema, or wrinkled "cobblestone" surface.

4. Holding a pipe in a fixed location may cause tooth wear, with the formation of an elliptical space between the teeth, drifting and intrusion of teeth, and traumatic changes in the supporting periodontal tissues.

Increased prevalence of chronic gingivitis and acute necrotizing ulcerative gingivitis,[5] as well as increased prevalence and severity of periodontal disease,[4, 24, 80] has been reported in smokers; in addition, plaque accumulation is increased in smokers,[11] with more calculus in pipe smokers than in cigarette smokers.[24, 59, 60] It has been noted that women from the ages of 20 to 39 and men from ages 30 to 59 who smoke cigarettes have about twice the chance of having periodontal disease or becoming edentulous as do nonsmokers.[76]

A specific type of gingivitis termed "gingivitis toxica,"[59] characterized by destruction of the gingiva and underlying bone, has been attributed to the chewing of tobacco.

Keratinized cells in the gingiva are increased in smokers,[15] but no changes other than altered oxygen consumption can be detected in the buccal mucosa. The mucosal response to irritation from tobacco may be modified by experimentally induced systemic disturbance.[42] Daily application of cigarette smoke to the cheek pouch of hamsters for up to 20 months failed to produce any significant change other than occasional slight epithelial hyperplasia.[69] Oral PMN's from smokers show a reduced ability to phagocytize particles.[38]

TOOTHBRUSH TRAUMA

Alterations in the gingiva as well as abrasion of the teeth may result from aggressive brushing in a horizontal or rotary fashion. The deleterious effect of abusive brushing is accentuated when excessively abrasive dentifrices are used.

The gingival changes attributable to toothbrush trauma may be acute or chronic. The acute changes are varied in appearance and duration and include scuffing of the epithelial surface with denudation of the underlying connective tissue to form a painful gingival bruise (Fig. 26–25). Punctate lesions are produced by penetration of the gingiva by perpendicularly aligned bristles. Painful vesicle formation in traumatized areas is also seen. Diffuse erythema and denudation of the attached gingiva throughout the mouth may be a striking sequel of overzealous brushing. The acute gingival changes

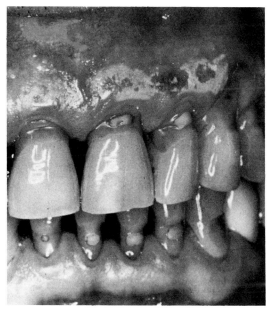

Figure 26–25 Toothbrush Trauma. Surface erosions and hyperkeratosis caused by abusive tooth brushing.

noted above commonly occur when the patient transfers to a new brush. A toothbrush bristle forcibly embedded and retained in the gingiva is a common cause of the acute gingival abscess (Chap. 10).

Chronic toothbrush trauma results in gingival recession with denudation of the root surface. Often the gingival margin is enlarged and appears "piled up," as if it were molded in comformity with the strokes of the toothbrush. Linear grooves may be present that extend from the margin to the attached gingiva. The gingiva in such areas is usually pink and firm.

Improper use of dental floss, toothpicks, or wooden interdental stimulators may result in gingival inflammation. The creation of interproximal spaces by destruction of the gingiva from overzealous use of toothpicks leads to the accumulation of debris and inflammatory changes.

CHEMICAL IRRITATION

Acute gingival inflammation may be caused by chemical irritation, as the result of either sensitivity or nonspecific tissue injury. In allergic inflammatory states, the gingival changes range from simple erythema to painful vesicle formation and ulceration. Severe reactions to ordinarily innocuous mouthwashes or dentifrices or denture materials are often explainable on this basis.

Acute inflammation with ulceration may be produced by the nonspecific injurious effect of chemicals upon the gingival tissues (Chap. 51). The indiscriminate use of strong mouthwashes (Figs. 26–26 and 26–27), the application of aspirin tablets (Fig. 26–28) to alleviate toothache, injudicious use of escharotic drugs, and accidental contact with drugs such as phenol or silver nitrate are representative of the manner in which chemical irritation to the gingiva commonly is produced.

Gingival irritation is also seen in workers in various industries in which chemicals are employed.[71] Gases such as ammonia, chlorine, bromine, acid fumes, and metallic dust are common offenders. The chemical irritation in such occupations is usually of long duration and not necessarily productive of spectacular gingival

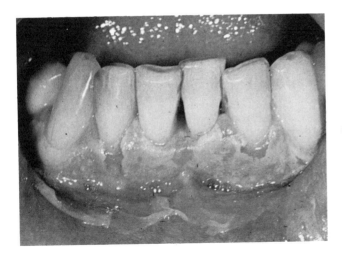

Figure 26–26 Chemical Burn. Necrosis and sloughing produced by undiluted mouthwash.

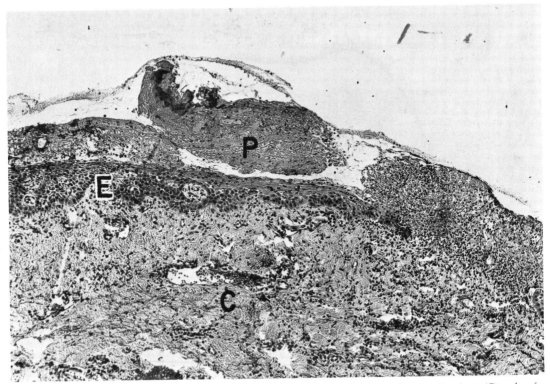

Figure 26–27 Biopsy of Necrotic Area Produced by Chemical Burn. Note inflammed connective tissue (C) and surface pseudomembrane (P). Of particular clinical importance is the newly formed sheet of epithelial cells (E) which undermines the necrotic pseudomembrane and separates it from the underlying connective tissue. This is an important feature of the healing process.

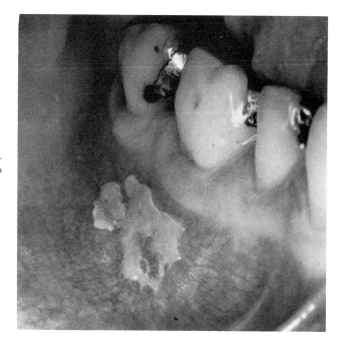

Figure 26–28 Aspirin Burn. Necrosis of mucosa produced by repeated use of aspirin tablets to relieve toothache.

changes. However, in patients with persistent gingival disease that is refractory to treatment, the occupational background should always be explored.

RADIATION

Gingival ulceration, bleeding and suppuration, periodontitis, denudation of roots and bone, and loosening and loss of teeth have been noted following treatment with external and internal radiation in patients with malignancies of the oral cavity and adjacent regions.[6, 21, 78] Periodontal disease is a possible portal of entry for infection and the development of osteoradionecrosis following radiation therapy. Changes that vary in severity from edema and bleeding of the gingiva and widening of the periodontal ligament with disrupted deposition of cementum, to necrosis of the gingiva and periodontal ligament and resorption of alveolar bone, loosening and shedding of the teeth, and the necrosis and sloughing of the oral mucosa, have been reported in experimental animals exposed to single and multiple head or total body roentgen radiation in individual doses of 10 r to 3000 r, to a total dosage of 11,000 r.[23, 27, 28, 46, 47, 72]

REFERENCES

1. Alexander, A. G.: Habitual mouth breathing and its effect on gingival health. Parodontologie, *24*:49, 1970.
2. Anderson, W. S.: The relationship of the tongue-thrust syndrome to maturation and other factors. Am. J. Orthod., *49*:264, 1963.
3. App, G. R.: Effect of silicate, amalgam and cast gold on the gingiva. J. Pros. Dent., *11*:522, 1961.
4. Arno, A., Schei, O., Lovdal, A., and Waerhaug, J.: Alveolar bone loss as a function of tobacco consumption. Acta Odontol. Scand., *17*:3, 1959.
5. Arno, A., Waerhaug, J., Lovdal, A., and Schei, O.: Incidence of gingivitis as related to sex, occupation, tobacco consumption, toothbrushing, and age. Oral Surg., *11*:587, 1958.
6. Aub, J. C., Evans, R. D., Hempelmann, L. H., and Martland, H. S.: The late effects of internally-deposited radioactive material in man. Medicine (Baltimore), *31*:221, 1952.
7. Baer, P. M., Kakehashi, S., Littleton, N. W., White, C. L., and Lieberman, J. E.: Alveolar bone loss and occlusal wear. Periodontics, *1*:91, 1963.
8. Bergman, B., Hugoson, A., and Olsson, C.: Periodontal and prosthetic conditions in patients treated with removable partial dentures and artificial crowns. Acta Odontol. Scand., *29*:621, 1971.
9. Bissada, M. F., Ibrahim, S. I., and Barsoum, W. M.: Gingival response to various types of removable partial dentures. J. Periodontol., *45*:651, 1974.
10. Bjorn, A. L., Bjorn, H., and Grcovic, B.: Marginal

fit of restorations and its relation to periodontal bone level. Odont. Rev., 20:311, 1969.

11. Brandtzaeg, P.: The significance of oral hygiene in the prevention of dental diseases. Odont. T., 72:460, 1964.

12. Bruxism. Report of the 14th Congress of A.R.P.A. Internationale, Venice, Italy. Academy Review, 4:9, 1956.

13. Buckley, L.: The relationship between malocclusion and periodontal disease. J. Periodontol., 43:415, 1972.

14. Burwasser, P., and Hill, T. J.: The effect of hard and soft diets on the gingival tissues of dogs. J. Dent. Res., 18:389, 1939.

15. Calonius, P. E. B.: A cytological study on the variation of keratinization in the normal oral mucosa of young males. J. West. Soc. Periodontol., 10:69, 1962.

16. Carlsson, G. E., Hedegard, B., and Koivumaa, K.: Studies in partial dental prosthesis. IV. Final results of a 4-year longitudinal investigation of dentogingivally supported partial dentures. Acta Odontol. Scand., 23:443, 1965.

17. Carranza, F. A., Sr., and Carraro, J. J.: El empuje lingual como factor traumatizante en periodoncia. Rev. Asoc. Odont. Argent., 47:105, 1959.

18. Chaikin, B. S.: Anterior periodontal destruction due to the loss of one or more unreplaced molars. Dent. Items Int., 61:17, 1939.

19. Dechaume, M.: Importance du sympathique, des troubles de la musculature oro faciale et des ties de succion ou de pulsior, dans les parodontopathies, Rev. Stomatol., 63:701, 1962.

20. Drum, N.: Classification of parafunction. Dtsch. Zahnarztl. Z. 5:411, 1962.

21. Ellinger, F.: Effects of ionizing radiation on the oral cavity. In Ellinger, F. (ed.): Medical Radiation Biology. Springfield, Ill., Charles C Thomas, Publisher, 1957.

22. Eschler, J.: Electrophysiologische and pathologische Untersuchungen des Kausystems. Forum Parodont., 5:1147, 1955.

23. Frandsen, A. M.: Periodontal tissue changes induced in young rats by roentgen irradiation of the molar regions of the head: Acta Odontol. Scand., 20:393, 1962.

24. Frandsen, A. M., and Pindborg, J. J.: Tobacco and gingivitis. III. Difference in the action of cigarette and pipe smoking. J. Dent. Res., 28:404, 1949.

25. Geiger, A., Wasserman, B., and Turgeon, L.: Relationship of occlusion and periodontal disease. VIII. Relationship of crowding and spacing to periodontal destruction and gingival inflammation. J. Periodontol., 45:43, 1974.

26. Gilmore, N., and Sheiham, A.: Overhanging dental restorations and periodontal disease. J. Periodontol., 42:8, 1971.

27. Gowgiel, J. M.: Experimental radio-osteonecrosis of the jaws. J. Dent. Res., 39:176, 1960.

28. Greulich, R. C., and Ershoff, B. M.: Delayed effects of multiple sublethal doses of total body x-irradiation on the periodontium and teeth of mice. J. Dent. Res., 10:1211, 1961.

29. Hirschfeld, I.: Food impaction J. Am. Dent. Assoc., 17:1504, 1930.

30. Hirschfeld, I.: Individual missing tooth. J. Am. Dent. Assoc., 24:67, 1937.

31. Holden, S., Harris, J. E., and Ash, M. M., Jr.: Periodontal disease in Nubian children. I.A.D.R. Abstr., 48th General Meeting, 1970, p. 65.

32. Huttner, G.: Follow-up study of crowns and abutments with regard to the crown edge and the marginal periodontium. Dtsch. Zahnärztl. Z., 26:724, 1971.

33. Ingle, J. L.: Occupational bruxism and its relation to periodontal disease. J. Periodontol., 23:7, 1952.

34. Jacobson, L.: Mouth breathing and gingivitis. J. Periodont. Res., 8:269, 1973.

35. Jacobson, L., and Linder-Aronson, S.: Crowding and gingivitis: A comparison between mouth breathers and non-mouth breathers. Scand. J. Dent. Res., 80:500, 1972.

36. Karlsen, K.: Gingival reactions to dental restorations. Acta Odontol., Scand., 28:895, 1970.

37. Kawakara, H., Yamagani, A., and Nakamura, M., Jr.: Biological testing of dental materials by means of tissue culture. Int. Dent. J., 18:443, 1968.

38. Kenney, E. B., Kraal, J. H., Saxe, S. R., and Jones, J.: The effect of cigarette smoke on human oral polymorphonuclear leukocytes. J. Periodont. Res., 12:227, 1977.

39. King, J. D., and Gimson, A. P.: Experimental investigations of paradontal disease in the ferret and related lesions in man. Brit. Dent. J., 83:126, 1947.

40. Klingsberg, J., Cancellaro, B. A., and Butcher, E. O.: Effects of air drying on rodent oral mucous membrane: A histologic study of simulated mouth breathing. J. Periodontol., 32:38, 1961.

41. Koivamaa, K. K., and Wennstrom, A.: A histological investigation of the changes in gingival margins adjacent to gold crowns. Odont. Tids., 68:373, 1960.

42. Kreshover, S. J.: The effect of tobacco on the epithelial tissues of mice J. Am. Dent. Assoc., 45:528, 1952.

43. Leof, M.: Clamping and grinding habits: Their relation to periodontal disease. J. Am. Dent. Assoc., 31:184, 1944.

44. Lipke, D., and Posselt, U.: Parafunctions of the masticatory system (bruxism): Report of a panel discussion. J. West Soc. Periodontol., 8:133, 1960.

45. Lite, T., et al.: Gingival pathosis in mouth breathers. A clinical and histopathologic study and a method of treatment. Oral Surg., 8:382, 1955.

46. Mayo, J., Carranza, F. A., Jr., Epper, C. E., and Cabrini, R. L.: The effect of total-body irradiation on the oral tissues of the Syrian hamster. Oral Surg., 15:739, 1962.

47. Medak, H., and Burnett, G. W.: The effect of x-ray irradiation on the oral tissues of the macacus Rhesus monkey. Oral Surg., 7:778, 1954.

48. Meyer, J., Shklar, G., and Turner, J.: A compari-

son of the effects of 200 KV radiation and cobalt 60 radiation on the jaws and dental structure of the white rat. Oral Surg., *15*: 1098, 1962.

49. Miller, J., and Hobson, P.: The relationship between malocclusion, oral cleanliness, gingival conditions, and dental caries in school children. Brit. Dent. J.,*111*:43, 1961.

50. Morris, M. L.: Artificial crown contours and gingival health. J. Pros. Dent., *12*:1146, 1962.

51. Mühlemann, H. R., et al.: Okklusion and Artikulation im Atiologiekomplex Parodontaler Erkrankungen. Parodontologie, *11*:20, 1957.

52. Nadler, S. C.: Bruxism, a classification: Critical review. J. Am. Dent. Assoc., *54*:615, 1957.

53. Nadler, S. C.: The importance of bruxism. J. Oral Med., *23*:142, 1968.

54. Norman, R. D., Mehia, R. V., Swartz, M. L., and Phillips, R. W.: Effect of restorative materials on plaque composition. J. Dent. Res., *51*: 1596, 1972.

55. Normann, W., Regolati, B., and Renggli, H. H.: Gingival reaction to well-fitted subgingival proximal gold inlays. J. Clin. Periodontol., *1*:120, 1974.

56. O'Leary, T., Badell, M., and Bloomer, R.: Interproximal contact and marginal ridge relationships in periodontally healthy young males classified as to orthodontic status. J. Periodontol., *46*:6, 1975.

57. O'Leary, T. J., and Sosa, C. E.: Signs of periodontal breakdown in patients with malocclusion. J. Dent. Ed., *10*:172, 1955.

58. Paunio, K.: The role of malocclusion and crowding in the development of periodontal disease. Int. Dent., J., *23*:420, 1973.

59. Pindborg, J. J.: Tobacco and gingivitis. II. Correlation between consumption of tobacco, ulceromembranous gingivitis and calculus. J. Dent. Res., 28:461, 1949.

60. Pindborg, J. J.: Tobacco and gingivitis. I. Statistical examination of the significance of tobacco in the development of ulceromembranous gingivitis and in the formation of calculus. J. Dent. Res., 26:261, 1947.

61. Poulton, D. R., and Aaronson, S. A.: The relationship between occlusion and periodontal status. Am. J. Orthod., *47*:690, 1961.

62. Ramfjord, S. P.: Bruxism, a clinical and electromyographic study. J. Am. Dent. Assoc., *62*:21, 1961.

63. Ray, H. G., and Santos, H. A.: Consideration of tongue-thrusting as a factor in periodontal disease. J. Periodontol., 25:250, 1954.

64. Renggli, H. H.: The influence of subgingival proximal filling borders on the degree of inflammation of the adjacent gingiva. A clinical study. Schweiz. Monatsch. Zahnh., *84*:181, 1974.

65. Renggli, H. H., and Regolati, B.: Gingival inflammation and plaque accumulation by well-adapted supragingival and subgingival proximal restorations. Helv. Odont. Acta, *16*:99, 1972.

66. Robinson, J., Reding, G., Zepelin, H., Smith, V.,

and Zimmerman, S.: Nocturnal teeth-grinding: A reassessment for dentistry. J. Am. Dent. Assoc., 78:1308, 1969.

67. Rosenzweig, K. A., and Langer, A.: Oral disease in Yeshiva students. J. Dent. Res., *40*:993, 1961.

68. Ross, I. F.: The effects of tensional clenching upon the structures of the neck. J. Periodontol., *25*:46, 1954.

69. Salley, J. J., and Kreshover, S. J.: Further studies of the effect of tobacco on oral tissues. J. Dent. Res., *37*:979, 1958.

70. Sanchez-Sotres, L., Van Huysen, G., and Gilmore, H. W.: A histologic study of gingival tissue response to amalgam, silicate and resin restorations. J. Periodontol., *42*:8, 1969.

71. Schour, I., and Sarnat, B. G.: Oral manifestations of occupational origin. J.A.M.A., *120*:1197, 1942.

72. Schüle, H., and Betzold, J.: Experimental investigations on the effect of x-ray irradiation on marginal periodontal tissues. Dtsch. Zahnärztl. Z. *24*:140, 1969.

73. Seeman, S.: Study of the relationship between periodontal disease and the wearing of partial dentures. Austr. Dent. J., 8:206, 1963.

74. Sheppard, I. M.: Tongue dynamics. Dent. Digest, 59:117, 1953.

75. Smoking and Noncancerous Oral Disease. The Health Consequences of Smoking, 1969 Supplement to the 1967 Public Health Service Review. U.S. Department of Health, Education and Welfare, Public Health Service.

76. Solomon, H., Priore, R., and Bross, I.: Cigarette smoking and periodontal disease. J. Am. Dent. Assoc., 77:1081, 1968.

77. Sorrin, S.: Habit: An etiologic factor of periodontal disease. Dent. Digest, *41*:290, 1935.

78. Stafne, E. C., and Bowing, H. H.: The teeth and their supporting structures in patients treated by irradiation. Am. J. Orthod., *33*:567, 1947.

79. Straub, W. J.: Malfunction of the tongue. Part II. The abnormal swallowing habit: Its causes effects, and results in relation to orthodontic treatment and speech therapy. Am. J. Orthod., *47*:596, 1961.

80. Summers, C. J., and Oberman, A.: Association of oral disease with 12 selected variables. I. Periodontal disease. J. Dent. Res., *47*:457, 1968.

81. Sutcliffe, P.: Chronic anterior gingivitis: An epidemiological study in school children. Br. Dent. J., *125*:47, 1968.

82. Takahama, Y.: Bruxism. J. Dent. Res., *40*:227, 1961.

83. Thaller, J. L.: The use of the Cornell index to determine the correlation between bruxism and the anxiety state: A preliminary report. J. Periodontol., *31*:138, 1960.

84. Thaller, J. L., Rosen, G., and Saltzman, S.: Study of the relationship of frustration and anxiety to bruxism. J. Periodontol., 38:193, 1967.

85. Waerhaug, J.: Prevalence of periodontal disease in Ceylon. Association with age, sex, oral hygiene, socioeconomic factors, vitamin defi-

ciencies, malnutrition, betel and tobacco consumption, and ethnic group. Final Report, Acta Odontol. Scand., 25:205, 1967.

86. Waerhaug, J., and Zander, H. A.: Reaction of gingival tissue to self-curing acrylic restorations. J. Am. Dent. Assoc., 54:760, 1957.

87. Wise, M. D., and Dykema, R. W.: The plaque retaining capacity of four dental materials. J. Pros. Dent., 33:178, 1975.

88. Wright, W. H.: Local factors in periodontal disease. Periodontics, 1:163, 1963.

89. Yuodelis, R. A., Weaver, J. D., and Sapkos, S.: Facial and lingual contours of artificial complete crowns and their effect on the periodontium. J. Pros. Dent., 29:61, 1973.

Occlusal Function

Recognition and correction of occlusal relationships that are injurious to the periodontium and may give rise to disorders of the masticatory musculature and temporomandibular joints require an understanding of the principles of occlusion. Fundamentals of occlusal function are presented here; clinical application is described in other chapters.

DEFINITION OF OCCLUSION

The term occlusion *refers to the contact relationships of the teeth resulting from neuromuscular control of the masticatory system (musculature, temporomandibular joints, mandible, and periodontium).*[99] Occlusion is more than just the static relationship of the teeth when the jaws are closed;[14] it consists of all contacts during chewing and swallowing. These are referred to as the *functional contacts* of the dentition. Contacts during gnashing and clenching are called *parafunctional contacts.* **The normality or abnormality of an individual occlusion is determined by the manner in which it functions and by its effect upon the periodontium, musculature, and temporomandibular joints rather than by the alignment of the teeth in each arch and the static relationship of the arches to each other.**

Three functional classes of occlusion are identified:

Physiological Occlusion. *An occlusion that exists in an individual in whom the signs of occlusion-related pathosis are absent is a physiological occlusion.* This implies a range of morphological variability in occlusion of the teeth and, in addition, a sense of psychological and physical comfort. In fact, no occlusion can be considered more ideal than that which exists in a given mouth free of disease and dysfunction.[118] Under conditions of physiological occlusion, there is a controlled adaptive response characterized by minimal muscle hyperactivity and limited stress to the system.

TRAUMATIC OCCLUSION. *A traumatic occlusion is an occlusion judged to be a causal factor in the formation of traumatic lesions or disturbances in the supporting structures of the teeth, muscles, and temporomandibular joints.* **The criterion that determines whether an occlusion is traumatic is whether it produces injury, not how the teeth occlude.** Actually almost any dentition has supracontacts that have traumatic potential under states of altered muscle tonus and stress.

THERAPEUTIC OCCLUSION. *A treatment occlusion employed to counteract problems related to traumatic occlusion is called a therapeutic occlusion.* The term is also used to describe an occlusal scheme employed in restoring or replacing occlusal surfaces so that minimum adaptation is required of the individual and compensatory tissue changes are minimized.

Terminology

Historically, the terminology of occlusion was developed by workers in several biological and dental specialties. This spawned a richly heterogeneous and confusing terminology. The interpretation of the word *centric* seems to a great extent to have contributed to the controversy.[45] Owing to the confusion concerning the terms for the various "centrics," alternative terms are used in this text. The following terms are advocated in an attempt at clarity[58, 122] and in response to research[122] regarding various jaw positions and recording methods.

Intercuspal position, (ICP): (1) The position of the mandible with maximum intercuspation of the teeth; (2) the terminal point of all function contact movement. Synonyms: centric occlusion (CO); habitual occlusion; acquired centric; habitual centric.

Muscular contact position, (MCP): The position of the mandible when it has been lifted from its resting posture to the very first occlusal contact by a minimum of muscular effort. Synonym: neuromuscular centric.

Retruded position, (RP): Any position of the mandible on the terminal hinge path. Synonyms: centric relation (CR); terminal hinge position; ligamentous position.

Retruded contact position (RCP): The end point of terminal hinge closure. Synonym: centric relation contact (CRC).

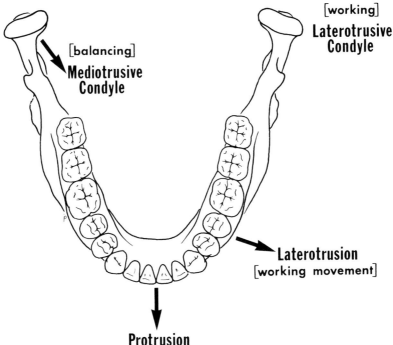

Figure 27–1 Mandibular movement is named after the direction of movement the mandible takes when it moves away from the intercuspal position. Functional parts of the mandible can also be identified by reference to the movement to which they are related.

Excursive movement: * Movement occurring when the mandible moves away from the intercuspal position (Fig. 27–1).

 Protrusion: Movement occurring when the mandible moves anteriorly from intercuspal position.

 Retrusion: Movement occurring when the mandible moves posteriorly from intercuspal position.

 Laterotrusion: Movement occurring when the mandible moves away from the midline. Synonym: working movement.

 Functional segments: (Fig. 27–1).

 Laterotrusive side: The side that moves away from the midline in laterotrusion. Synonyms: working side; functional side.

 Mediotrusive side: The side that moves toward the midline in laterotrusion. Synonyms: balancing side; nonworking side; nonfunctional side; idling side.

Supracontacts and Occlusal Interferences

The term *supracontact* is a general term for any contact that hinders the remaining occlusal surfaces in achieving a many-pointed, stable contact. A supracontact is a morphological relationship and does not necessarily imply a dysfunctional situation. Moreover, a supracontact in relation to one mandibular contact situation is not

---

*The movement of the mandible can be related to the direction in which the mandibular teeth move from ICP during excursion. The Latin word *trudere*, meaning to thrust, is used with appropriate prefixes denoting the direction of movement.

necessarily a supracontact in relation to others.[58] *Occlusal interferences* are supracontacts capable of injuring the supporting periodontal tissues. One type of occlusal interference is that which inhibits or complicates mandibular movement. Interferences that deflect closure in the retruded position are referred to as *retrusive prematurities;* those that interfere with closure in intercuspal position are called *intercuspal prematurities.*

YOUR OWN JAW MOVEMENTS

 Thinking in terms of your own jaw and the movements it can make will help you to understand occlusion. Jaw movement can be classified as **border, intraborder,** and **contact.**

 Border movements are the limits to which the mandible can move in any direction. Posselt, in a classic study,[95] developed a rhomboid figure that represents a sagittal view of the border movement of the mandible. Look at Figures 27–2 and 27–3 and read along as you do the following:

 1. Close your jaw and retrude the mandible as far as you can, keeping your teeth together. If you succeed, you will reach position 1 in Figure 27–2. This is the **retruded contact position (RCP)** of the mandible. For most individuals it would normally be necessary to make a special effort to retrude the jaw to position **1.**

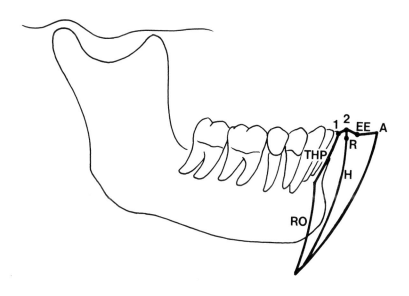

Figure 27–2 Rhomboid Figure of Mandibular Movements in the Sagittal Plane (Posselt). 1, Retruded contact position. 2, Intercuspal position. THP, Terminal hinge path. RO, retruded path beyond terminal hinge opening. The condyles undergo both rotation and translation at this point. A, Border movement with maximum protrusion. H, Habitual (functional) pathway of the mandible. R, The rest (postural) position of the mandible.

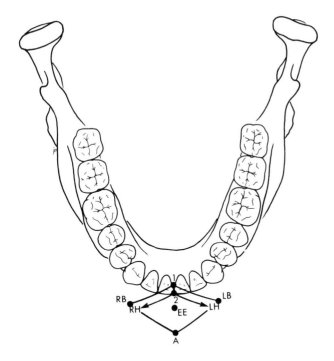

Figure 27–3 Movements of the Mandible at the Incisal Point (Infradentale). 1, Retruded contact position (RCP). 2, Intercuspal position (ICP). EE, Edge-to-edge position. A, Contact at maximal protrusion. RH and LH, Right and left habitual movement position. RB and LB, Right and left border positions. Jaw undergoes maximum lateral movement at RB and LB.

Contact movement is the movement of the mandible with one or more of the opposing occlusal surfaces in contact.

2. Starting from position 1 (RCP), squeeze your teeth slightly forward. This new position which is represented by position **2** in the rhomboid diagram, is called the **intercuspal position (ICP)** or habitual occlusion. The difference between ICP and RCP is about 1 mm. measured at the incisors and 0.5 mm. at the mandibular condyles.[48, 49, 121, 124] Moreover, ICP lies in a symmetrical, forward position relative to RCP in about 85 per cent of young adults (Fig. 27–2).[124] In a small but significant percentage of individuals (10 to 30 per cent), RCP and ICP are coincident or nearly coincident. Although muscular effort is necessary to reach RCP, most individuals with coincident RCP-ICP relationships show no awareness of discomfort when closing to full contacts.

3. Now slide your teeth back to position 1. Hold them there a few seconds and, still trying to retrude your mandible as far as you can, slowly open your mouth. Your mandible is now moving along the line **THP** in Figure 27–2: the **terminal hinge path**. As you open on the THP the con-

dyles remain in position and rotate in a simple hinge movement around the imaginary axis—the **terminal hinge axis**.[64] As you continue to open your jaw, more translation or sliding creeps into the condylar movement, and the mandibular path changes from THP to **RO** in Figure 27–2. Continue to open along line RO to the bottom of the rhomboid. As your mandible moves along line RO, the principal motion of the condyles is a sliding one combined with rotation. The condyles are now at the crest or anterior to the articular eminences.

4. From the bottom of the rhomboid, start to close, protruding your jaw as far as possible. You are now moving along line **A**. Continue to the top of line **A**; your mandibular incisors will now be in front of, and higher than, the incisal edges of the maxillary incisors.

5. Bring your jaw back until your incisors are edge-to-edge and look at Figure 27–2. You are now at **EE** on the protrusive path. Slide back a little more and your teeth will come into the intercuspal position **2**.

Your jaw has traveled the perimeter of the border movements of the mandible.

Intraborder Movement is any mandibular movement within the perimeter of border movement.

6. Now, open your jaw, take a deep breath, exhale, and rest. Then open and close loosely several times. You are now opening and closing on the habitual pathway, line **H** in Figure 27–2. The habitual pathway is the working pathway of the mandible, in which it usually functions. You will notice that it is anterior to the **terminal hinges pathway** (**THP**). This suggests that the habitual pathway is not a border movement of the mandible.

If you wanted to open your jaw along the terminal hinge pathway (line **THP**) the way you did initially, it would be necessary to make a special effort to retrude your mandible and keep it back as you opened. When we want our patients to open and close along the **THP** pathway, we often put pressure on the chin to retrude the jaw passively. Tooth contacts that obstruct the mandible as it tries to reach **RCP** are called "prematurities" or "retrusive interferences." Interfering contacts in the habitual path are called "intercuspal prematurities."

7. Now rest. Wet your lips with your tongue, swallow, and just sit there for a minute. Then bring your posterior teeth gently together until they come into initial contact. This position is termed **muscular contact position** (**MCP**). The chances are that when you swallowed, your MCP was identical to your ICP. One of the characteristics of a physiological occlusion is that the teeth normally contact in ICP when they are closed with a minimum muscular effort from rest position.

"Touch and slide" from MCP to ICP is a sign often found in patients with traumatic or uncomfortable occlusions. While you are resting, your teeth are apart and your mandible is in the **rest position** (**R**). If you look at Figure 27–2 you will notice that this position (**R**) is on the habitual pathway, **H**.

Positions and Movements of the Condyle

Retruded position (**RP**) refers to a position of the mandible and is synonymous with the term *centric relation* (**CR**). The term *intercuspal position* (**ICP**) is synonymous with the term *centric occlusion* (**CO**)[*] and refers to the position of the teeth. When the mandible is in the retruded position (RP) the condyles are in their most retruded, superior position in the mandibular fossae. This retrusive movement is contained by the joint tissues and probably by a stretch of the capsular ligament.[3, 95] There is possibly some muscular involvement.[45] When the teeth are in ICP, the mandible is anterior or anterolateral to RP and the condyles are slightly anterior and inferior to RP. In some individuals RCP and ICP are identical; hence, the position of the condyle does not change. When the mandible is in rest position, the condyles are usually anterior and inferior to their position in ICP.[49, 65, 107]

In opening and closing the jaw, the condyles are capable of rotation or translation or combinations of the two motions. **Rotation** consists of a hinge-like movement of the condyles about an axis without change in their position. **Translation** consists of forward and downward movement of the condyles. On full opening, the condyles glide along the posterior slope of the articular eminence to an average of 1 mm. anterior to the inferior crest of the eminence.[107]

With the jaw opened wide there may be a slight reduction (approximately 0.09 mm.) in the width of the mandible in the molar area.[106] The jaws ordinarily open and close into ICP, rather than into RCP.[116] Opening involves simultaneous rotation and downward and forward translation of the condyle. Closure is usually a simple vertical (elevator) motion.[116]

Movements of the mandible with the teeth in contact, which are termed *excursions*, may be *laterotrusive, protrusive, lateroprotrusive,* or *retrusive* (Fig. 27–1). Laterotrusive (side-to-side) contacts of the mandibular posterior teeth along the buccal cusps of the maxillary teeth (lateral excursions) occur occasionally in chewing and swallowing; they occur often in bruxism. Protrusive excursions are also

---

[*]The term *centric occlusion* was defined in the previous (fourth) edition of this book as the position in which the teeth are intercuspated with the mandible in centric relation. This usage is not followed here.

part of the opening chewing cycle but, similarly, are more extensive in bruxism.

In the lateral movements of the mandible from the closed position, the condyle on the side toward which the mandible is moving either rotates about a vertical axis or combines lateral movement with rotation (Fig. 27–4). The lateral shift of the condyle is called the **Bennett movement** (Fig. 27–4B). The condyle on the mediotru-

sive (balancing) side moves downward, forward, and inward and describes the **Bennett angle** with respect to a saggital line, when viewed in the horizontal plane (Fig. 27–4). As a distinction between the two terms, it should be noted that the Bennett *angle* is always present, but the Bennett *movement* may not be present.

THE FORCES OF OCCLUSION

The forces of occlusion are created by the musculature in chewing, swallowing, and speech, and are transmitted through the teeth to the periodontium. These forces function in synchronized balance. They guide the alignment of the teeth as they erupt and participate in maintaining the position of the teeth in the arches. Tooth position and arch form are not static; they are maintained by the balance among the various forces of occlusion. Disturbance of this balance may lead to altered tooth positions and changes in functional environment that may be injurious to the periodontium.

The following factors are involved in the creation and distribution of the forces of occlusion: (a) muscular activity, (b) inclined planes of the teeth and the anterior component of force, (c) proximal contacts, (d) design and inclination of the teeth, and (e) atmospheric balance.

Muscular activity

The forces of occlusion are created by two groups of muscles: the muscles of mastication and the counteracting oral musculature. The forces created by the muscles of mastication are distributed in several directions by the inclined planes of the teeth. This occurs in chewing, either directly through tooth contact or indirectly through a resistant bolus of food, and in swallowing.[13] The resultant forces tend to displace the maxillary teeth facially and the mandibular teeth lingually, and tend to move all the teeth mesially.

Counteracting forces exerted by the tongue, the lips, and the cheek

These forces balance the tendency toward displacement of the teeth created by

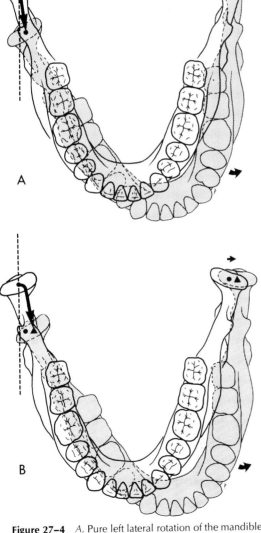

Figure 27–4   *A,* Pure left lateral rotation of the mandible (no Bennett movement). *B,* Lateral movement of the jaw incorporating Bennett movement.

TABLE 27–1 BALANCE BETWEEN ANTAGONISTIC OCCLUSAL FORCES

Lips —————————→	←———Tongue
Cheeks—————————→	←———Tongue
Eruption (growth of teeth)————→	←———Masticatory muscles (masseter, temporalis, internal pterygoid)
Air pressure on skin and nasal cavity———→	←———Tongue in closed mouth, air pressure in open mouth
Masseter—————————→	←———Elasticity of periodontal ligament, particularly of molars, and suprahyoid muscles
Internal pterygoid	
in vertical movement ————→	←———Same as masseter
in lateral movement————→	←———Internal pterygoid of other side
External pterygoid	
in anterior movement————→	←———Posterior third of temporalis, suprahyoid group, digastricus, muscles of the neck
in lateral movement————→	←———External pterygoid of other side

the muscles of mastication. The orbicularis oris counteracts the labially directed force exerted by the mandibular teeth and the tongue against the maxillary anterior teeth. The tongue is a versatile muscle that exerts pressure in various directions, balancing the inward pressure of lips and buccinator muscles and balancing the tendency of inclined planes to force the mandibular premolars and molars lingually. The buccinator balances the tendency of inclined planes to force the maxillary molars buccally.

The balance between the antagonistic forces of occlusion has been summarized by Breitner[11] as shown in Table 27–1.

The inclined planes of the teeth and the anterior component of force

As noted above, the forces exerted by the muscles on closure of the mandible are distributed in several directions by the inclined planes of the teeth. *The resultant of the occlusal forces gives rise to an anterior force, which tends to move the teeth mesially and is termed the anterior component of force* (Fig. 27–5). The forces are anteriorly directed because of the orientation and placement of the occlusal plane below the level of the axis of rotation. The anterior component of force on one side of

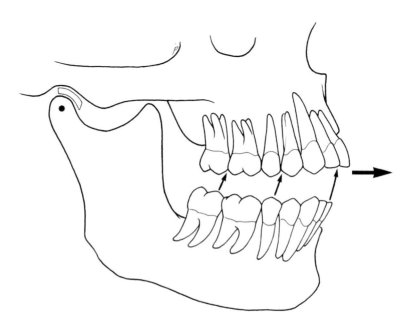

Figure 27–5 Anterior component of force (*large arrow*) is developed as a result of contact along the occlusal plane. The forces are anteriorly directed because of the orientation and placement of the occlusal plane below the level of the axis of rotation.

the arch is transmitted from the molars through the contact points of the teeth to the midline, where it is neutralized by the force from the other side of the arch.

The anterior component of force pushes the teeth mesially in their sockets. When the force is released, the teeth move back to their previous position because of the resilience of the periodontal ligament. With time, the areas of proximal contact are flattened by wear, permitting mesial movement of the teeth, referred to as physiologic mesial migration. The overall effect is a reduction of 0.5 cm. in the length of the dental arch from the third molars to the midline by the age of 40 years.

Proximal contacts

Proximal contact relationships are important in maintaining the stability of the dental arch. The anterior component of force is transmitted through intact proximal contacts. Contacts malpositioned in a cervicoincisal or faciolingual direction deflect the forces of occlusion and may cause displacement of the teeth (Fig. 27–6) and create abnormal forces on the periodontium.

Tooth design and inclination

Certain features of tooth design affect the transmission of occlusal forces.[14] For example, the maxillary central incisor is shaped so that it is inclined mesially to provide maximum efficiency of its cutting edge. In function, the maxillary incisors tend to be driven mesially and buttress each other. The root of the maxillary incisors is shaped so that there is greater area

of attachment of periodontal fibers on the palatal and distal sides, which counteract the tendency toward facial and mesial displacement during function. The molars are inclined mesially so as to transmit a component of the vertical occlusal forces to the premolars and canines.[94]

Atmospheric balance

Breathing is an important factor in maintaining normal atmospheric balance in the nasal and oral cavity. After swallowing with the lips together, a vacuum is created between the tongue and the palate, which is a factor in the development of the palate and the shape of the maxillary dental arch.

THE MUSCULOSKELETAL SYSTEM

The Temporomandibular Joint

The temporomandibular joints differ from other synovial joints in many structural and function aspects (Fig. 27–7). The articulating surfaces are not hyaline as in other weight-bearing joints but consist of a dense, well-organized collagen tissue very sparse in actual cartilage cells. The joint is freely movable and has two compartments separated by an intact articular disc. This functional arrangement allows gliding in the upper compartment. Lower compartment movement between the articulating surface of the condyle and the inferior surface of the disc is a combined movement of both rotation and gliding.[105] The investing capsular tissues are inserted widely over the temporal bone to allow adequate gliding; they attach the disc more securely to the lateral poles of the

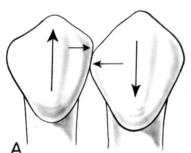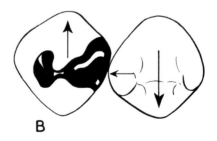

Figure 27–6 *A,* **Improper Proximal Contact Relationship** (*horizontal arrows*). This relationship is a potential source of excessive force in the directions indicated by the vertical arrows. *B,* Improper contact relationship in the faciolingual plane (*horizontal arrows*). This relationship is a potential cause of displacement of the teeth facially and lingually as indicated by the vertical arrows. (After R. A. Jentsch.)

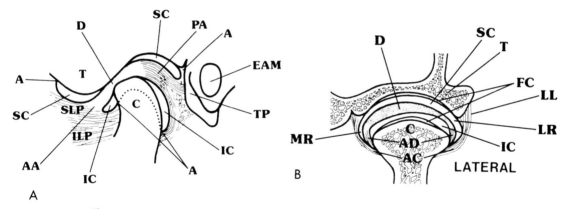

Figure 27-7   Parts of the Temporomandibular Joint. *A,* Lateral view. *B,* Frontal view.

A	attachment of capsule	ILP	inferior head of lateral pterygoid muscle
AA	anterior attachment of disc	LL	lateral capsular wall and lateral ligament
AC	attachments of the capsule	LR	lateral recess
AD	attachments of the articular disc	MR	medial recess
C	condyle	PA	posterior attachment of disc
D	articular disc	SC	superior compartment
EAM	external auditory meatus	SLP	superior head of lateral pterygoid muscle
FC	fibrocartilage	T	temporal bone (articular eminence)
IC	inferior compartment	TP	tympanic plate

condyle for stabilizing a more controlled hinge-gliding function. Under active opening, both a hinge and a glide are observed, whereas in passive opening under manipulation a hinge motion is produced.

Although the joint structures are mainly housed in the mandibular fossa, the functional activity occurs over the biconvex surfaces between the anterosuperior aspect of the mandibular condyle and the posteroinferior aspect of the articular eminence of the temporal bone. The inclination of the posterior surface of the articular eminence is correlated with that of the lingual surface of the maxillary anterior teeth (incisal guidance) but not necessarily with the cuspal inclines of the posterior teeth[57] (Fig. 27-8). The flexible articular disc is the equalizer among these incongruous surfaces and can be divided into two major parts (see Fig. 27-7). The *anterior, dense part* is composed of firmly woven avascular fibrous tissue. The *posterior attachment (bilaminar zone)* is composed of soft, open textured tissue.[24] The extent and nature of innervation suggest that painful stimuli from compression of the posterior attachment or from inflammatory conditions of the joint could give rise to painful joint symptoms.[24] The disc attaches anteriorly to the upper head of the lateral pterygoid muscle. It is returned to its

position by the recoil action of the posterior attachment, which is equipped with true elastic tissue in the superior lamina and regularly folded collagen fibers in the lower lamina. Posteriorly, the posterior attachment fuses with the capsular wall, which in turn attaches to the tympanic plate with its uppermost insertion terminating in the area of the squamotympanic fissure (see Fig. 27-7).

Jaw mobility would be markedly limited without a disc. True fibrous tissue discs occur only where two separate movements occur,[60] hence, the disc facilitates the hinge and glide function. Together with the capsular ligaments, the disc allows for *stabilization* of the mandibular condyle against the articular eminence. This stability is maintained even though the interarticular curvature varies with condyle movement. This stabilizing function could not be served by a stiff, cartilaginous articular disc.

Wherever fibrous discs are found, they do not withstand pressure very well.[60] It has been shown that the condyles and the temporomandibular joints are loaded during function. These loads are normally of short duration and appear adapted to varied light forces rather than unidirectional severe forces.[30, 126] *Under loading condi-*

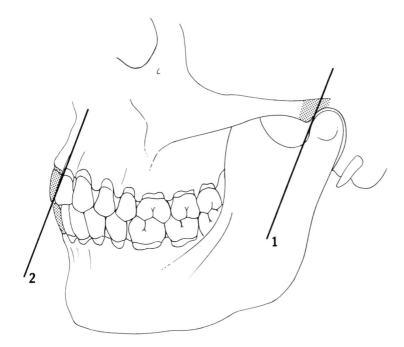

Figure 27–8 Correlation of the Plane of the Articular Eminence (1) with the Lingual Surface of the Maxillary Incisors (2).

tions, the presence of a disc acts as a "buffer" in the transmission of stress to the articular eminence. Further, discs serve a *spreading function* which facilitates lubrication within the joint.[60] Although rupture and degeneration of the disc may create symptoms which make it necessary to remove the disc, this procedure can be done only at compromise to long-term joint function.

The temporomandibular *capsule* covers the joint and unites its parts (see Fig. 27–7). It is composed of (1) an outer dense fibrous layer attached around the periphery of the articular disc and (2) a loose inner vascularized synovial layer. The fibrous capsule of the temporomandibular joint is rather thin. The lateral surface of the fibrous capsule is strengthened by the *lateral (temporomandibular) ligament,* which arises from the articular tubercle and inserts on the lateral pole of the condyle. The lateral ligament is structured into two separate layers, both of which act as a strong "check rein" limiting joint movement.[115] The superficial *oblique band*

prevents downward condyle displacement during protrusion. The deep *horizontal band* prevents posterior displacement further into the mandibular fossa. There is no comparable reinforcement of the medial capsule, probably because the right and left temporomandibular joints function as one articulation. The sphenomandibular and the stylomandibular ligaments are accessory ligaments of the temporomandibular joint and have little influence on the movements of the mandible.[115]

Adaptive remodeling of the temporomandibular joints

Throughout life, mechanical forces produce a slow remodeling of the articular soft and hard tissues of the joint to enable it to adapt to changing occlusal forces.[9, 16, 43, 77, 85, 88]

Remodeling is a rebuilding of adult soft and hard tissue layers. Remodeling occurs in all soft and hard tissues of the joint and is considered to be a subarticular phe-

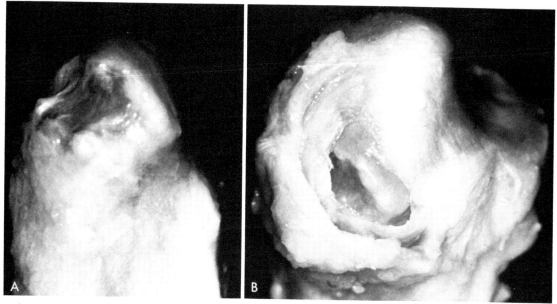

Figure 27–9 *A,* **Right Mandibular Condyle Dissected Free at Autopsy.** Lateral view showing flattening and soft tissue lipping predominantly in the lateral third of the condyle. Even though there are marked changes in the shape of the condyle, the articular surfaces are shiny and intact; hence, this condition is classified as deviation in form (DIF). *B,* **Lateral view of Articular Disc Showing Large Perforation Localized Directly Over the Deviation in Form on the Mandibular Condyle.** By definition, a disc perforation is classified as degenerative joint disease (DJD). (Courtesy of T. Öberg and T. Hansson.)

nomenon not resulting in external changes in form. On the other hand, the changes may be so advanced as to cause an alteration of the joint surfaces, which is termed **deviation in form.**[41]

Deviation in form (DIF) *is deviation from the normally slightly rounded contour of the articular surface, e.g., condyle flattening or enlargement; thickening of the soft tissue layers of the articular components; surface unevenness, or scalloping* (Fig. 27–9A). Continuation of these changes with diminution in the proliferate ability of the articular tissues leads to breakdown of the articulating surfaces of the joints, a process which is termed **degenerative joint disease (DJD)**. Degenerative joint disease is *primarily a non-inflammatory joint disease characterized by wear and tear of the articular soft tissues and by remodeling of the underlying hard tissues. Synonyms: osteoarthritis, arthrosis.*[41]

An increase in the biomechanical loading of a joint stimulates cellular proliferation and cartilage formation from the undifferentiated mesenchyme.[41] This results in thickening of the soft tissue layers, which contributes to the development of deviations in the form of the temporal component and the condyle, with secondary changes of the disc (thinning, ridging). Such deviations in form can cause disturbances of movements and clicking and, with continued unfavorable loading, may gradually lead to degenerative joint disease (arthrosis) with crepitation (grating) as a clinical symptom.[41]

In an analysis of autopsy material (ages 20 to 90), nearly half (47 per cent) of the adult temporomandibular joints revealed some form of DIF or DJD.[42, 43, 88] When DJD lesions occurred in the joint, the subarticular soft tissue of the condyle was significantly thicker laterally than that of normal temporomandibular joints, but the condylar surface usually remained lesion free (Fig. 27–9A). The lateral compression of the disc, which is not regenerative, causes thinning, ridging, and eventual perforation of the disc when the deviation in form is extensive[42, 78] (Fig. 27–9B).

In temporomandibular joints with both

DIF and DJD, disc perforations (Fig. 27–9B) were almost always combined with deviations in form of the condyle and usually accompanied by DJD in the corresponding temporal component. DJD changes are mostly local in nature and usually occur in the lateral one third of the joint.[66, 78, 85, 88]

Experimental studies attempting to create functional remodeling in animals have yielded mixed results. The articulating surfaces of temporomandibular joints in adult monkeys do not appear to be subject to remodeling following change in functional forces.[10] However, morphologic changes were created experimentally in the rat mandibular joint by the removal of quadrants of molar teeth.[28] In another study, experimental distal displacement of the mandible in the rat stimulated growth activity in the embryonic condylar cartilage, but the fossa and disc remained unaltered.[25] In the rabbit, biomechanical factors were shown to play a large role in the occurrence of degenerative joint disease of the knee joint.[131]

Muscles of Mastication*

The lateral (external) pterygoid muscle, especially the inferior belly, is the main trigger muscle in opening the jaw;[53] it is coordinated with the activities of the suprahyoid muscles (the digastric, the mylohyoid, and the geniohyoid), which assist in retracting and depressing the mandible and also in fixing and elevating the hyoid bone. The masseter, medial (internal) pterygoid, and temporal muscles are the principal muscles involved in closing the jaw, and in the regulation of the position of the mandible in space.

Protrusion of the jaw is accomplished by simultaneous bilateral contraction of the lateral pterygoid muscles; the jaw-closing muscle groups may also participate. Retrusion of the jaw is produced by simultaneous contraction of the middle and posterior portions of the temporal muscles, assisted by masseter, posterior digastric, and geniohyoid muscles. Lateral movements are achieved by the contraction of the lateral and medial pterygoid muscle on one side and the contralateral temporal muscle.

THE POSTURAL POSITION OF THE MANDIBLE (PHYSIOLOGIC REST POSITION) AND THE FREE WAY SPACE

When the teeth are not in contact in mastication, swallowing, or speech, the lips are at rest and the jaws are apart. This is termed the *postural position* of the mandible. It is often referred to as the *"physiologic rest position,"*[133] but *"postural position"* is more appropriate.[86] In order to maintain the mandible in this position, it is necessary to support it against the force of gravity; the muscles are in a mild state of contraction, especially the temporalis muscle.[81, 84] The postural position is not constant; it varies with the position of the head and body, and is affected by proprioceptive stimuli from the dentition and emotional factors.[21, 96] Thus, there is no single, constant position of the mandible when the subject is at rest.[73]

The space between the mandibular and maxillary teeth when the mandible is in the postural position is called the free way space. The postural position and free way space are fairly stable and reproducible but are not necessarily constant throughout life. They vary from individual to individual, and even within the same individual with changes in the dentition.[100, 129] A large free way space has been observed in subjects with a deep overbite. Furthermore, a large sagittal difference between postural positions and ICP has been observed in subjects with marked overjet.[130] The average normal space is 1.7 mm.[29, 76] Generally it ranges between 0 and 3 mm.[81] Aging, malocclusion, tooth mobility, periodontal disease, unreplaced posterior teeth, improperly constructed dental restorations, excessive occlusal wear, or unilateral chewing, which change the teeth and their functional relationships, may also change the muscle tonus, which in turn may alter

---

*For a review of the biomechanics of masticatory function, see Sicher and Du Brul.[115]

the postural position and the free way space.[23, 63, 117]

Vertical Dimension of Occlusion

The term vertical dimension of occlusion *designates the distance between the maxilla and mandible when the teeth are in occlusion.* The vertical dimension is maintained by a balance between the rate of occlusal wear and continuous tooth eruption. While the vertical dimension of occlusion should not be changed without a definite biomechanical reason, small changes in the course of dental therapy are usually accommodated by a re-establishment of the free way space. There is no evidence to suggest that the vertical dimension of occlusion should be changed in the presence of a large free way space, since there is considerable variation. One serious problem in increasing the vertical dimension of occlusion could be the intrusion of teeth or a rapid resorption of alveolar bone under dentures. Thus, it may be clinically practical to use the existing structures to establish the vertical dimension of occlusion. In this respect, it may be wise to err on the side of a wider-than-average interocclusal space if no other means are available to assess the proper vertical dimension of occlusion.[101]

NEUROMUSCULAR CONTROL OF MANDIBULAR MOVEMENTS

Knowledge of the neuromuscular control of mandibular movements has developed tremendously through active worldwide research in the area of oral physiology. As a result, dental practitioners have been increasingly interested in the application of these concepts to their daily practice. At this point, however, much information is available but not directly applicable to the complex clinical picture of occlusion in daily practice. The reader is referred to other sources for a detailed presentation of this subject.[54, 55, 68, 73, 114] Clinical observations supported by research investigations have suggested that the following principles be applied when considering occlusal contact relationships.

Most occlusal contact relationships are harmonious in nature (they do not produce inappropriate, guarded, or painful responses in the masticatory muscles). Tooth guidances are likewise passive and unlabored. If a noxious response occurs following occlusal contact, it may be generated from the sensory receptors in the dentition as well as in the joints, the muscles, or the ligaments of the masticatory system.[127] There are many factors which influence reactions to noxious responses (producing a reflex response in the masticatory muscles), among them being the magnitude, direction, and duration of the force, age of dentition, pulpal and periodontal health, muscle and joint health, and central nervous system effects. If a noxious reflex response occurs it will generally be one of the following types: (1) reflexes which reduce closing forces, (2) reflexes initiating mandibular opening, (3) reflexes initiating mandibular closing, (4) reflexes initiating mandibular translation.[62]

Apparently, occlusal interferences are brought into contact and not avoided during function.[112] Normal oral reflex systems prevent damage through increased inhibition of muscle activity. If the interference is of sufficient magnitude to exceed the adaptability of the masticatory system, marked changes in muscular electromyographic activity can be observed.[112] Not enough is known about occlusal interferences to accurately predict which type is most active in masticatory dysfunction. *All occlusal therapy should be directed at preventing and eliminating factors which perpetuate noxious or inappropriate reflex responses.*[127]

ELECTROMYOGRAPHY

The electrical activity of muscles is assessed by electromyography, which is the recording of action potentials from motor units.[82] The significance of the electrical activity in the muscles of mastication springs from its relation to both sensorimotor coordination and motor performance.[82] Electromyography can disclose motor patterns at various levels: coordination of groups of muscles and activity in individual muscles and recently even in individ-

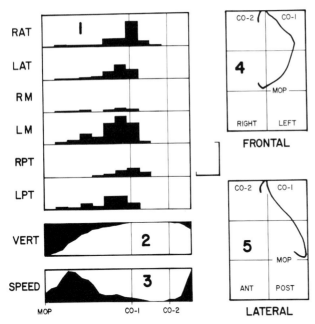

Figure 27–10 Muscle Activity and Jaw Displacement During a Single Chewing Stroke. Data from the closing phase of single, left-sided stroke during a gum-chewing sequence. Electromyographic signals recorded from the right and left anterior temporal (RAT, LAT), posterior temporal (RPT, LPT), and masseter muscles (RM, LM) have been rectified and averaged over continuous 50-msec. periods, and appear as histograms (1). Jaw displacement, measured as movement of an incisor point on the mandible, is shown in three different ways; in time, as the vertical separation of the jaws from the position of maximum intercuspation (2); in time, as the resultant of the speed of jaw movement in three dimensions (3); and as envelopes of jaw displacement seen from frontal (4) and lateral (5) viewpoints. Maximum jaw opening is indicated by MOP, and the points marking the beginning and ending of the intercuspal phase by CO-1 and CO-2. In the frontal and lateral views, this phase is represented by the small flattened area between CO-1 and CO-2. The vertical calibration bar represents 400 μV, 20 mm., and 200 mm./sec. in sections 1, 2, and 3 respectively. The horizontal bar represents 100 msec. Each square in sections 4 and 5 measures 10 mm. by 10 mm. In this instance the planes are referenced to the Frankfort horizontal or at right angles to it.

The speed of jaw movement reaches its maximum early in the closing phase and begins to decline well before the food bolus is crushed by any major muscle contraction. It falls toward zero during the phase when the teeth dwell in maximum intercuspation (2 and 3). Peak muscle activity differs from muscle to muscle both in amplitude (RM, LM) and time (RPT, LPT) and is related to the side chewed upon and the form of the chewing stroke. Activity in all muscles continues well into the intercuspal position (1), and although no vertical movement of the jaw occurs in this area (2), a small anterolateral shift has occurred (3, 4, and 5). Electrical activity in these muscles probably precedes their resultant development of interocclusal force by approximately 7 msec. (Courtesy of A. G. Hannum, 1977.)

ual motor units,[33] which allows a more definitive recording of the factors regulating motor neuron function.[82, 83]

The duration, timing, and amplitude of muscle activity has been documented for the normal functioning occlusion through the use of surface electrodes on the skin.[80] Surface recordings are relatively simple, but the record obtained cannot always be attributed with certainty to one particular muscle.[73] Moreover, the deep muscles (lateral pterygoids) cannot be monitored with this method. As a result, studies on the deep muscles must be conducted with intramuscular needle or fine wire electrodes. Integrated EMG can give a reliable indication of muscle tension provided the electrode is centered over the active muscle fibers in question and provided the muscle contraction is causing no movement but merely a build-up in tension (isometric contraction).[73]

More recently, electromyography has been combined with the measurement of jaw displacement during natural oral function (Fig. 27–10).[40] Moreover, the action of specific muscles has been investigated. Both parts of the lateral pterygoid muscle have been studied on monkeys, using fine wire electrode techniques.[67] This study and others[79, 92] on humans suggest that the lateral pterygoid muscle is functionally separated into two parts, resulting in activity on closing in addition to opening and lateral movements.

Occlusal and psychological factors have been shown to affect muscular activity measured electromyographically. Occlusal interferences were observed to have caused a synchronous and hypertonic muscular activity that returned to normal after the occlusion was corrected.[98] Other studies[27, 56, 112] have demonstrated that occlusal interferences created a disturbance among the jaw muscles, manifesting itself through an altered EMG activity. Psychological stress, both in the experimental and in the natural environment, has been reported to increase the activity of the jaw closing muscles.[109, 137, 138]

THE PHYSIOLOGY OF MASTICATION*

Mastication consists of the coordinated function of various parts of the oral cavity to prepare food for swallowing and digestion. Although the teeth are the most essential unit in mastication, there are other important related factors, such as the lubricating and enzymatic action of the saliva, the lips, the cheeks, the tongue, the hard palate and the gingiva, the muscles of mastication, and the temporomandibular articulation.

Incision

Incision reduces the food to sizes suitable for mastication. It involves coordinated action of the hand, arm, head, neck, and shoulders, as well as the teeth and masticatory musculature.[52] To engage the food the mouth is opened and the mandible is protruded. Shearing strokes of the anterior teeth penetrate the food until it is thinned. The food is not "cut apart" by tooth to tooth contact. The hand and head move in opposite directions to separate the food so that part of it remains in the oral cavity. The tongue and cheek direct the bolus of food to the occlusal table of the posterior teeth for mastication.

Once a bolus has been introduced into the mouth, mastication is automatic and practically involuntary, but can readily be brought under voluntary control. The very act of establishing voluntary control implies a difference between masticatory function under ordinary conditions, and parafunctional jaw movements with the teeth either together or separated.[4]

The Masticatory Cycle

The pathway of the mandible in chewing is referred to as the chewing cycle or the masticatory cycle. The form of the chewing cycle has been observed using

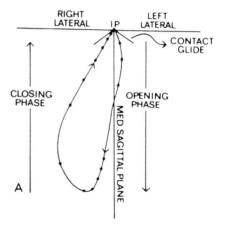

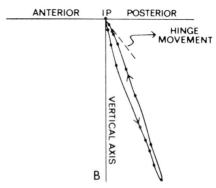

Figure 27–11 Incisal Points During One Chewing Cycle. *A,* Frontal projection. *B,* Sagittal projection. (From Ahlgren, J.,[2] in *Mastication,* D. J. Anderson and B. Mathews (Eds.). J. Wright and Sons, Bristol, 1976.)

photography, graphic methods, radiography, electric and telemetric techniques.[6] The pathway of any point on the mandible in chewing typically has a teardrop shape when viewed in the frontal or sagittal planes[2] (Fig. 27–11). The masticatory cycle consists of three phases: (1) the opening phase, during which the mandible is depressed, (2) the closing phase, during which the mandible is elevated, and (3) the intercuspal phase, during which the mandible is in the intercuspal position (ICP).

The teardrop shape of the chewing cycle is more or less consistent for a given individual but is unique for every person. In

---

*For a comprehensive review of this subject, see Bates[4, 5, 6] and Mathews.[73]

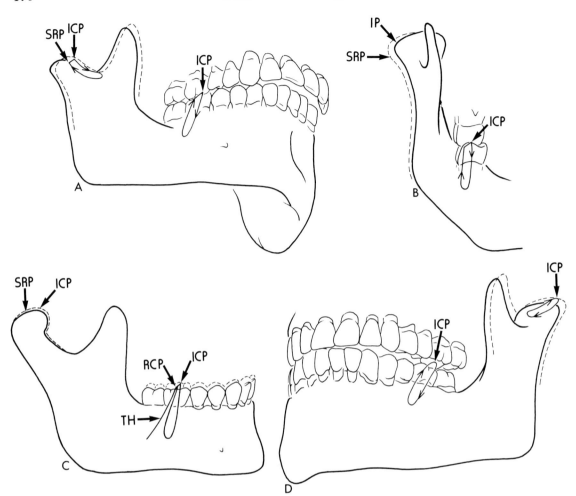

Figure 27–12   Masticatory Cycle. *A,* Seen from the chewing side during one chewing cycle. The chewing side condyle moves upward and rearward and reaches a superior, rearward position (SRP) before the teeth reach the intercuspal phase. The teeth then close along the lateroretrusive cusp inclines on the path to the intercuspal position (ICP). *B,* Frontal view of chewing side, as in A, above. *C,* Sagittal component of the masticatory cycle (chewing side) seen in relation to the terminal hinge path (TH), the retruded contact position (RCP), and the intercuspal position (ICP). Note the retrusive component of the masticatory cycle on the chewing side. *D,* The masticatory cycle seen from the nonchewing side. The nonchewing side condyle (mediotrusive condyle) moves a considerable distance upward and rearward to close directly to the intercuspal position (ICP). Note that closure is along the medioprotrusive maxillary cusp inclines on a path to ICP. The differences between the condyle paths and the paths of the cusps during the chewing cycle for the chewing side and the nonchewing side are significant and have not been taken into account in most chewing studies. (Courtesy of Dr. Harry Lundeen, after Gibbs.[31])

the opening phase, the teeth and the condyles begin movement immediately downward and forward. Early in the closing phase, the entire mandible moves laterally. *The differences between the condyle movement during the chewing cycle on the chewing side and the nonchewing side are significant and have not been taken into account in most chewing studies.* The chewing side condyle moves upward and rearward and reaches a superior, posterior position (SRP, Fig. 27–12A, B, and C) before the teeth reach the intercuspal phase. During the remainder of closing, the chewing side condyle usually demonstrates a slight forward and medial (Bennett) movement. The nonchewing side condyle moves a considerable distance upward and rearward directly to the the intercuspal position[31] (Fig. 27–12D).

On the bolus side, chewing is essentially a two-phased system arising from a lateral-retrusive closing position through the intercuspal position into a medial-protrusive pathway.[6] Subjects chew on the side where there is the most stable intercuspal contact. Where occlusal conditions are similar between sides, chewing takes place on the right and left alternately, and the food is passed from side to side regularly and consistently for the individual.[6]

The chewing pattern of the adult and child differs in the opening movement. In the adult, the opening stroke is medial to the closing stroke. In the child, the opening stroke is typically lateral to the closing stroke.[31]

The chewing pattern is influenced by the consistency, shape, size, and taste of the bolus of food. The occlusion of the tooth is of significant importance for the development of masticatory movements.[2] In general, those individuals with normal occlusion have regular and coordinated chewing movements. Subjects with malocclusion have an irregular chewing pattern.[2] In addition, occlusal alterations or treatments cause changes in the chewing pattern.[6, 30] The occurrence of deep overbite is associated with chopping chewing strokes, whereas in reduced lateral cuspal guidance, the chewing stroke assumes a more horizontal component.[2]

There are about 15 chews in a series from the time of food entry until swallowing. Jaw opening is greatest when food first enters the mouth and decreases in a somewhat linear fashion as chewing continues. The average jaw opening during chewing is between 16 and 20 mm.[2, 75] and the average lateral displacement on chewing is between 3 and 5 mm.[2] The duration of the masticatory cycle varies between 0.6 and 1 second. Different test materials have a significant influence on the duration of the masticatory cycle, with sticky and tough foods increasing it.[2] The duration is decreased and the chewing forces are increased when the subject is stressed or in a hurry to eat.[108]

Deglutition

Swallowing occurs approximately 600 times in a 24-hour period.[61] It occurs most frequently during eating and drinking, at a lesser rate during the usual indoor activities, and least frequently when asleep. The total time of tooth contact in chewing and swallowing in a 24-hour period has been estimated to be 17.5 minutes[34] (Table 27–2).

In swallowing, the palatal muscles seal off the oropharynx from the nasopharynx, the suprahyoid muscles raise and tilt the hyoid bone and larynx, and the tongue forcibly propels the food bolus or liquid posteriorly over the epiglottis into the esophagus. To provide firm anchorage for

TABLE 27–2   TOTAL DURATION OF TOOTH CONTACTS IN A 24-HOUR PERIOD °

Chewing:		
Actual chewing time per meal	450 sec.	
4 meals a day	1800 sec.	
Each second 1 chewing stroke	1800 strokes	
Duration of each stroke	0.3 sec.	
Total chewing forces per day	540 sec. = 9.0 min.	
Swallowing:		
1. Meals		
Duration of 1 deglutition movement	1 sec.	
During chewing 3 × per minute		
⅓ of movements with occlusal force only	30 sec.	0.5 min.
2. Between meals		
Daytime 25 per hour (16 hrs.)	400 sec.	6.6 min.
Sleep 10 per hour (8 hrs.)	80 sec.	1.3 min.
TOTAL	1050 sec. ca. 17.5 min.	

°From Graf, H.[34]

the action of the tongue and to oppose the depressing action of the suprahyoid muscles, the mandible is braced against the maxilla and cranium by the masseter, temporal, and medial pterygoid muscles.[52] *A normal swallow, therefore, generally occurs with the teeth together.*

The act of swallowing may have a profound effect on the development of the orofacial structures, especially in the presence of a deviant swallowing pattern. Prolonged retention of the infantile swallow may contribute to the creation of a malocclusion.[63] It is probable that abnormal swallowing behavior is due to many factors, some being habitual, genetic, mechanical, and neurological.[62]

Masticatory Efficiency

The size of the food platform area, or the total available functional contact surface, is a major factor in determining the chewing efficiency of the dentition.[47, 140] The food platform area is diminished by such factors as missing teeth,[70] cuspal interferences, incomplete eruption, tilting, and other forms of malocclusion, and may be increased by attrition. In mouths with no missing teeth, the first molar provides 36.7 per cent of the total effective chewing area, with the other molar and premolar teeth contributing less.[69]

Loss of the first molar is often compensated for by mesial drifting of the second and third molars, and the dentition performs as if only the third molars were absent. Consideration of the effect of tooth loss on masticatory performance is complicated by the fact that mastication is usually performed on only one side of the dentition at a time.

Pain from caries or periodontal involvement influences the choice of the mastication side, and reduces the masticatory performance as well as the occlusal force that can be exerted on the affected side. Severe bone loss in periodontal disease also appears to reduce the maximum occlusal force.

Tooth Contacts in Chewing and Swallowing

The subject of occlusion presents something of a paradox: there is more informa-tion regarding how to correct and reconstruct the occlusion than there is regarding how the dentition functions. There are many detailed systems for occlusal adjustment and carving tooth cusps in order to attain "proper" occlusion. But there are relatively few facts regarding jaw relationships and tooth contacts during function, which, supposedly, would be the basis for dentistry's corrective and restorative efforts.

It has been difficult to capture and record jaw movements and tooth contacts in the functioning dentition, despite the imaginative techniques used for this purpose (visual studies of attrition facets, photography, graphic methods, radiography, electric and telemetric techniques).[4, 15] A review of these studies has recently been published by Bates et al.[4, 5, 6]

There is some variation in the findings of photographic, graphic, and electronic techniques investigating tooth contact in chewing and swallowing, but the preponderance of evidence indicates that (1) **tooth contacts do occur in chewing and swallowing in the majority of all chewing cycles. The retruded contact position is rarely a terminal occlusal position in chewing or swallowing.**[39] Chewing cycles without tooth contact occur mainly at the beginning of the chewing sequence, i.e., the crushing strokes.[2] When full closure to the intercuspal position is attained, stoppage of movement for about 0.1 to 0.2 second occurs for the subject with good occlusion, but the total contact time, which includes the gliding aspects of the feature, may double this time.[6] Subjects with pathologic occlusions, especially those with mobile teeth, are less likely to reach the intercuspal position and less likely to demonstrate stoppage of jaw movement even when ICP is reached.[30] The chewing force is greatest during the short pause in intercuspal position.[2] (2) **Almost all chewing contacts and most swallowing contacts involve contact in the intercuspal position, and this position is the terminal functional position during the masticatory act.**[2, 39, 87] Chewing contacts in ICP are brief compared with the duration of swallowing contacts.[39] (3) **Gliding contact to and from ICP occurs frequently during mastication, the average glide length being 1 mm. in both the opening and** closing strokes[31, 128] (Fig. 27–12). In some individuals there is no gliding tooth contact at all, but merely a chopping stroke.

The occurrence of lateral tooth contact during the closing phase depends upon the type of food and occlusion. The glide is significantly longer in aborigines chewing tough food. As the attrition proceeds and the cuspal guidance is reduced, the closing stroke assumes a more horizontal direction when moving into ICP.[2]

The angle of approach to and from ICP is steeper than the cuspal inclination; thus the angle within the masticatory cycle always lies within the confines of the cuspal inclines. Teeth are a major guiding factor in the closing phases of the masticatory cycle, but exert little influence in the opening phases.[6]

The Retruded Position and Intercuspal Position in Function

The intercuspal position, formerly considered an acquired or second best occlusion, is really the functional working occlusal position of the human dentition. It is not a detour position into which the jaw is deflected by premature contacts which prevent the teeth from reaching the retruded position (RP). There is conflicting opinion regarding whether the elimination of retrusive prematurities will result in increased use of the retruded contact position.[38, 93] The mandible may follow many paths in opening and closing, but they are normally anterior to RP.[95] The rest (postural) position of the mandible is also anterior to RP.

The retruded position is the posterior border position of the mandible which is reproducible and therefore may be a useful reference position in the analysis and correction of occlusion problems.[20] However, RCP is not the endpoint of most closing jaw movements. After the entire dentition is reconstructed so that RCP is stable and on the same horizontal plane as ICP, a patient may persist in using ICP.[32] Occlusion, like other physiologic body processes, changes with age. The therapist should consider the needs of the individual occlusion at the patient's age, rather than attempt a standard occlusion for all ages. As a further distinction, sliding bruxo-

contacts are developed over lateral and protrusive mandibular positions of greater magnitude than chewing contacts.

OTHER CONCEPTS OF OCCLUSION

Balanced Occlusion

The term *balanced occlusion* refers to simultaneous contact between the right and left posterior segments of the arch in lateral excursions of the mandible, and simultaneous contact between the posterior and anterior segments of the arch in protrusive excursion. At one time considered to be an ideal type of functional relationship, balanced occlusion is rarely encountered in the natural dentition.[12, 50] Balancing tooth contacts introduces a risk of damage to the periodontium, which outweighs the ostensible benefits of attempting to create bilateral balance by occlusal adjustment or prosthetic restorations.[113, 125] In patients with periodontal disease, molars with nonworking side contact (more than 50 per cent of the teeth examined) showed significantly greater mobility, bone loss, and pocket depth than teeth which did not contact on the nonworking side.[139]

Cuspid-protected Occlusion

According to the concept of a cuspid-protected occlusion,[22] the interlocking relation of the maxillary canines between the mandibular canines and first premolars is the most important articulation in the natural dentition. In closure of the jaws in mastication the maxillary canines act as protective stress breakers that bear the brunt of the muscular forces and guide the mandible so that the posterior teeth come into closure with a minimum of horizontal forces (Fig. 27–13A). In lateral and protrusive excursions, the mandibular canines and first premolars engage the lingual surface of the maxillary canines so as to disclude the incisors, premolars, and molars and protect them from undesirable horizontal forces. This concept hypothesizes that the maxillary canines are especially equippped to absorb lateral forces because of the size of the root and radicular bone

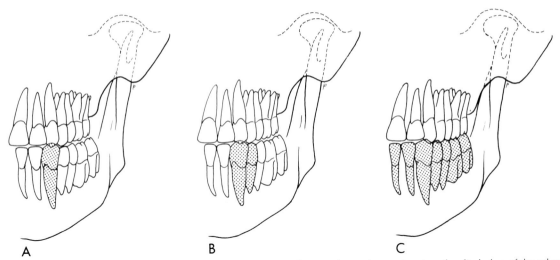

Figure 27–13   Types of Occlusion. A, Cuspid protected occlusion. The canine teeth act as the discluders of the other teeth. B, Canine-premolar disclusion as found in normal young adults.[50] C, Group function occlusion.

and because of an especially sensitive proprioceptive mechanism which reflexly reduces muscle forces when the canines make occlusal contact.

Group Function

Beyron[8] describes "group function," the simultaneous gliding contact of teeth on the laterotrusive side (Fig. 27–13C), as an important feature of optimal occlusion, along with the following: (1) bilateral contact of most teeth in the intercuspal position and in the retruded position. The distance between the two positions should be about 1 mm. or less. (2) Axial loading of the posterior teeth in the retrusive range. (3) Acceptable interocclusal distance.

Hinge Axis Occlusion

This concept is based upon the retruded position and the terminal hinge path as the functional aspects of occlusion. It hypothesizes that the restored occlusion should have the retruded position as the origin of all movements; that excursive movements are functional; and that the factors that govern mandibular movements dictate the occlusal morphology of the teeth.[37]

Functionally Generated Occlusion

According to this concept, the excursive movements of the mandible are the functional pathways of occlusion.[71] The occlusal surfaces of the maxillary posterior teeth are reconstructed in conformity with the individual excursive movements, and in optimal occlusion there is maximum tooth contact on the "working side," with no "balancing side" contact. The occlusion is characterized by a "long centric," in which the mandible can move between the retruded contact position (RCP) and the intercuspal position (ICP) with the dentition in contact.

ORTHOFUNCTION AND DYSFUNCTION

Trauma-producing oral activity has been called **dysfunction** and is a descriptive term for the *forces* causing a wide variety of trauma throughout the stomatognathic system.[110] A more specific term describes dysfunction in the periodontium; namely, **traumatic occlusion.** Dysfunction (traumatic occlusion) is not a pure expression of behavior. It involves both structure (teeth, jaws) and behavior (neuromuscular force). Like two sides of a coin, they can be observed separately, but they are not independent. *Using this concept, trauma generated in the teeth, supporting structures,*

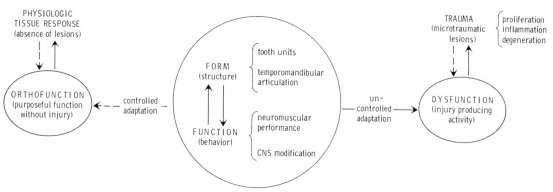

Figure 27–14. The Spectrum of Morpho-functional Harmony and Disharmony. Dysfunction is the immediate cause by which any functional disturbance or microtrauma may arise, including TMJ disorders. The most important determinant of orthofunction is the extent of the individual's adaptive ability, which is determined by host resistance and other nonspecific psychological and physical factors. (From Melcher and Zarb (Ed.): Oral Sciences Reviews, 7, 1976.)

muscles, or temporomandibular joints may be viewed as different manifestations of a basic traumatic phenomenon termed dysfunction.

Orthofunction *is defined as purposeful, noninjurious function.* The patient's adaptive ability appears to be the key determinant in tipping the balance in favor of orthofunction or dysfunction at any point in the patient's life (Fig. 27–14). The effects of dysfunction may be presumed to focus at the site where the greatest forces are exerted and the host resistance is the least.[58] Although not easily observed, the lesions resulting from dysfunction are usually expressed through inflammatory, proliferative, or degenerative tissue responses. In the initial stages, these lesions are largely *reversible* if the stresses that caused them to occur are normalized. Broadly viewed, the adaptive response has far-reaching implications not only as a determinant of injury production and localization, but also in terms of the psychologic host reaction to the symptom itself.[110]

THE SIGNIFICANCE OF OCCLUSAL INTERFERENCES*

There are several possible results of interferences in the retruded or the intercuspal position or both. They may incite muscle activity in an effort to wear away the obstructing tooth surfaces, which become repetitive and develop into bruxism, clamping, or clenching habits.[27, 56, 98] They may cause destruction of the periodontal tissues, loosening of the teeth (trauma from occlusion), and deflection of the pathway of the mandible[132] (Fig. 27–15). They may produce instability of the dentition in closure and disturbed muscle patterns in an effort to overcome instability.[97] This, in turn, may lead to muscle spasm and temporomandibular joint disorders.[102] The fact that most people have occlusal prematurities without necessarily suffering their harmful effects is indicative of the adaptability of the oral tissues.[124]

DENTAL WEAR AND TEAR

Attrition in the English-speaking countries is the term used for wear and tear caused by *teeth against teeth.*[119] Such physical wearing patterns may occur on incisal, occlusal, and approximal tooth surfaces. A certain amount of tooth wear is physiologic, but intensified or even pathologic wear may prevail under abnormal anatomic or unusual functional factors. **Abrasion** *implies teeth against foreign substance* — it is the involvement of an extraneous foreign substance independent of masticatory function per se, as in wear from a hard bristle toothbrush, coarse tooth

---

*For the detection and correction of occlusal interferences, see Chapter 55.

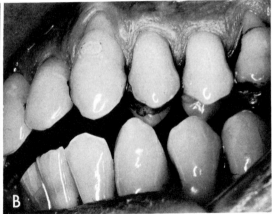

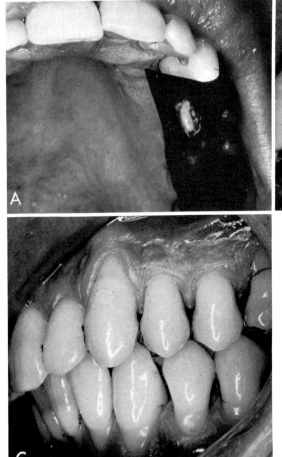

Figure 27–15   Retrusive Prematurity. *A,* Premature contact on the mesiolingual cusp of the maxillary first premolar, encountered when the mandible moves on the terminal hinge path of closure. *B,* Retrusive prematurity prevents closure into a multipointed retruded contact position (RCP). *C,* Upon full closure, the mandible is deflected anteriorly into the intercuspal position (ICP).

powder, the excessive use of tooth picks, or ritual customs.[119]

Excessive wear may result in obliteration of the cusps and the formation of either a flat or cupped-out occlusal surface and reversal of the occlusal plane of the premolars and first and second molars (Fig. 27–16). Occlusal wear increases with age and is characterized by a reduction in cusp height and inclination, and the formation of facets. Tooth surfaces worn by attrition are hard, smooth, and shiny (facets) and if dentin is exposed, a yellowish brown discoloration frequently is present (Fig. 27–17). Facets generally represent occlusal wear from parafunctional tooth contacts such as bruxism, and by premature tooth contacts, but may also be produced through mastication.

Facets vary in size and location, depending upon whether they are produced by physiologic or abnormal wear[3, 7, 135] (Fig.

27–18). They have been reported in 98 per cent of adults and 83 per cent of all teeth examined.[136] Facets are usually not sensitive to thermal and tactile stimulation. Unworn teeth in a mouth with generalized cuspal wear are often sites of premature occlusal contact.

The angle of the facet upon the tooth surface is of potential significance to the periodontium. Horizontal facets tend to direct forces in the vertical axis of the teeth to which the periodontium can adapt most effectively. *Angular facets direct occlusal forces laterally and increase the risk of periodontal injury.*

Erosion, excluding the idiopathic variety, has somewhat unique structural distinctions in being anatomically smooth and clean with more or less clear-cut causative factors, such as those related to the digestive system, medicinal therapy, field of occupa-

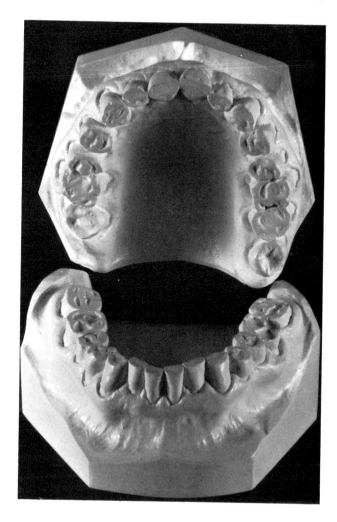

Figure 27–16 Reversed Faciolingual Occlusal Plane (Curve of Pleasure). The normal occlusal plane is sometimes reversed by excessive wear so that in the mandible the occlusal surfaces slope facially instead of lingually, and in the maxilla they are inclined lingually. The third molars are not usually affected.

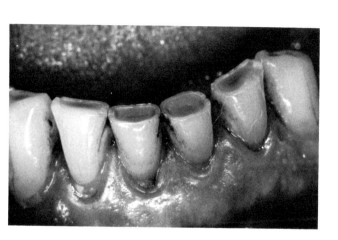

Figure 27–17 Occlusal Wear. Flat shiny discolored surfaces produced by occlusal wear.

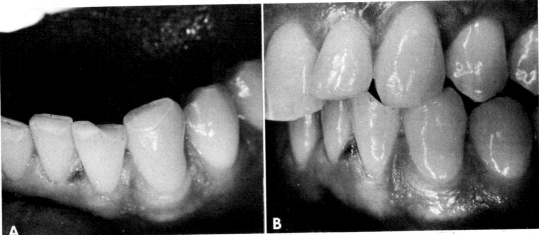

Figure 27-18   Wear Facets. *A,* Flat facets worn on incisal edges of anterior teeth. Note the notch on lateral incisor also produced by wear. *B,* Maxillary canine fits into notch on lateral incisor produced by parafunctional mandibular movements.

tion (acid battery workers), and dietary habits (baking products, citrus fruits, and carbonated drinks). **Idiopathic dental erosion** has long been the subject of much confusion. Some of these cases may be related to **frictional ablation,** a process caused by physical juxtaposition of natural or artificial dental surfaces to hyperfunctional oral soft tissues.[119, 120] Frictional ablation is actually a traumatic activity of the soft tissue against the dentition. It is generated through the vestibular pressures of suction, swallowing, tongue motions, and the intervening forced flow of saliva.[119]

All of the above forms of dental wear exert influences which should be considered in the control and prevention of periodontal disease.

Bruxism

Bruxism is the clenching or grinding of the teeth when the individual is not chewing or swallowing.[99] **Clenching** is the continuous or intermittent closure of the jaws under vertical pressure. *Tapping* and *toothsetting* involve repetitive mandibular movement or placement at isolated contact locations. Bruxism often occurs without any neurologic disorders or defects and could be viewed as a phenomenon present in healthy individuals, provided some other factors eliciting this behavior are present.

Most people are not aware of a bruxism habit until it is brought to their attention. It can be very loud or it can be silent. Individuals who brux generally begin with the teeth in an intercuspal position.[58] They may also lift the teeth apart and press on a more distant contact. If bruxism involves forceful "tooth grinding" with the production of sounds, accelerated wear develops. Wear from bruxism can be observed as facet patterns. The typical pattern is suggestive of side-to-side movements, but small asymmetrical retrusive movements or longer movements protrusively along the lingual surfaces of the maxillary anterior teeth are also common.

There is little known about the prevalence of bruxism in normal populations. It has been reported[112, 124] to be as high as 5 to 20 per cent in some populations with about equal occurrence in men and women. In a clinical population, however, bruxists were more often women.[89] Since nightime bruxism is likely to be under-reported, the prevalence of all bruxism is probably greater.

Etiology

There seems to be a hereditary predisposition to bruxism by certain types of individuals. It has been reported[1] that children of bruxist parents are more apt to be bruxers than children of nonbruxist parents. Olkinuora[89] classifed bruxers into two categories: (1) those whose bruxism was associated with stressful events, and (2) those whose bruxism has no such association. He concluded that hereditary bruxism was much more common in the non–stress-related bruxism group. Evaluations from psychometric and health inventories suggest that "stress" bruxists have more muscular symptoms and seemed more emotionally disturbed.

Sleep studies[91, 104, 111] have shown that bruxism occurs in any stage of sleep, but mostly in stage II. Moreover, bruxism is *not* correlated with rapid eye movement (REM) sleep. Satoh and Harada[111] observed that bruxism tended to occur during the transition from a deeper stage of sleep to a lighter stage of sleep. Thus, bruxism was associated with an arousal phenomenon. These investigators were able to elicit bruxism in sleeping subjects with an auditory stimulus.

There are only a few controlled studies of relationships between bruxism and psychological variables. Bruxism has been considered a multifactorial psychosomatic phenomenon with individuals displaying "aggressive, controlling, precise, energetic personality type on the one hand (non-stress bruxists) and anxious, tense types on the other (stress bruxists)."[90] It is likely that these psychological characteristics fall within the normal limits of personality structure.[103] *There is no evidence to suggest that bruxers have personality derangements or are mentally ill.*

The relationship between emotional states and muscle tension appears better understood. Recent reports have demonstrated that increased masseter muscle tension is directly related to stress situations during the day.[138] One study demonstrated that increased stress levels (as measured by urinary epinephrine content) were strongly correlated to increased levels of masseter muscle activity at night.[18] These studies have consistently shown a strong interrelationship between non-functional masseter muscle activity (bruxism) and stress.

Another interesting aspect of bruxism concerns the perception of stress by bruxism patients. One study[19] suggests that those patients with the greatest amount of bruxism have a diminished ability to recognize when they are under stress. This may occur because chronic bruxism subjects are constantly overacting to stress and cannot therefore determine when it increases. Alternatively, it may be that the bruxist subject simply has never learned to recognize or attend to the physiological changes which occur in the body during stressful situations.

Recent attempts to demonstrate the relationship between stress and bruxism in the natural environment have involved the use of portable electromyographic recording

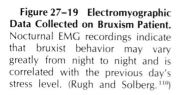

Figure 27–19 Electromyographic Data Collected on Bruxism Patient. Nocturnal EMG recordings indicate that bruxist behavior may vary greatly from night to night and is correlated with the previous day's stress level. (Rugh and Solberg.[110])

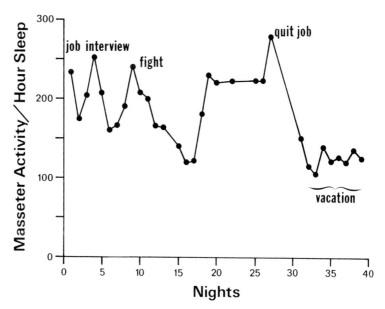

devices. The recordings indicate that brux- ist behavior may vary greatly from night to night, and is correlated with the previous day's stress level (Fig. 27–19).[110] Overall, it may be concluded that both mental strain and predisposing oral factors may act to- gether to produce bruxism.[91]

Not enough is known to say conclusively whether or not occlusal factors are a direct cause of bruxism. It has been suggested that occlusal malrelationships or interferences may precipitate bruxism when combined with nervous tension.[112] In one study,[123] bite splint therapy significantly reduced brux- ism levels while the splints were worn, but returned to previous levels after splint removal. Continuing investigations indicate that the response of bruxism subjects to occlusal therapy is likely to be variable.

Effects of bruxism habits

While bruxism is widespread, it need not be pathologic. Indeed, it can be compatible with states of normal function. In bruxism, the muscles move the mandible over tooth contacts where there is a potential for large forces. Most subjects brux by just playing on the teeth without much forceful contraction. However, under general neuromuscular tension, increased tooth contact pressure will result. This pressure over an extended period may exceed the threshold of the periodontal pressor-receptors and the pa- tient will no longer be aware of increased

muscle activity.[58] The muscles involved will be unable to relax, resulting in fatigue, muscle tenderness, and limited opening (Fig. 27–20).

When muscles contract *isometrically* they are stressed to a greater degree than during *isotonic* contraction. This stress is even worse when the muscle is lengthened while it is contracting tension, as in lateral dis- cluding movements.[58] As a habit, bruxism takes on further significance because as the response strengthens, the likelihood of functional disorders increases. Bruxism can be especially harmful if the threshold of resistance is lowered by persistent neuro- muscular tension or structural weakness from previous pathology.

TEMPOROMANDIBULAR PAIN AND DYSFUNCTION

Temporomandibular joint disorders are characterized by **impaired function** *and* **pain.** At present, there is agreement that the definitional symptoms include one or more of the following: (1) **pain and tenderness** in the region of the muscles of mastication and temporomandibular joints, (2) **sounds** dur- ing condyle movement, (3) **limitation** of mandibular movement.[23, 36, 110, 123, 141] The symptom complex defined above is the musculoskeletal component of a larger group of microtraumatic signs and symp- toms, all of which are manifestations of

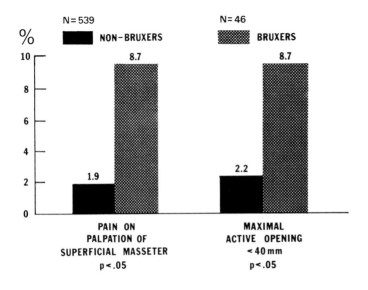

Figure 27–20 **Prevalence of Masseter Muscle Tenderness and Limited Opening in Bruxers and Nonbruxers** (young adult non-patient population). There was a sig- nificant association between bruxism and these symptoms. (Solberg et al.[124])

generalized injury-producing activity called dysfunction (occlusal traumatism).[110]

The term *myofascial pain-dysfunction (MPD) syndrome* has been advocated[59] to identify a subgroup of temporomandibular joint pain and dysfunction. The criteria for inclusion in this subgroup is the triad of symptoms listed above along with the following negative characteristics: (1) absence of clinical or radiographic evidence of organic·changes in the temporomandibular joints, (2) lack of tenderness in the temporomandibular joint when this area is palpated in the external auditory meatus.

The term "syndrome" may be a misnomer, as the symptoms are more apt to be sequential rather than concurrent as in the classic syndromes. The usual sequence of temporomandibular pain and dysfunction is clicking and incoordination followed by acute pain and/or locking at two finger breadths of opening. Limitation and chronic pain are the final complications. Syndromes classically have a specific etiology; most evidence suggests that temporomandibular pain and dysfunction is multicausal.

Temporomandibular disorders may not be a specific entity, even though patients may display similar symptoms.[35, 72, 110] Therefore, the tendency to lump all "TMJ patients" into one group should be avoided. *Careful examination and analysis of patients with temporomandibular pain and dysfunction will reveal that the origin of most complaints can be found in one or more of the following areas:* (1) within the temporomandibular joints, (2) within the masticatory muscles, and (3) from the neck (referred pain). Individual emotional factors can add an additional diagnostic dimension concerning the development and/or persistence of temporomandibular pain and dysfunction.[110]

Clinical Features

The most common causes of *jaw restriction* are intracapsular derangement,[51] capsular contracture and adhesions,[134] muscle spasm, and bony impingement. Therefore, the examiner must attempt to develop this differential diagnosis. Intracapsular restriction usually affects only the sliding function of the condyle. Therefore, most patients with temporomandibular joint problems will be able to hinge their jaws at least two finger breadths (26 mm.). If the active mouth opening is greater than 35 mm., there is increasing likelihood that the problem is mainly muscular in origin, as opposed to intracapsular restriction. Movement preventing full rotation of the condyles (26 mm.) suggests restriction from the temporalis and masseter muscles.

Joint sounds occur as *clicking* (popping, snapping) or *crepitus* (grating). Clicking may be produced by disc displacements influenced by muscular disharmony and a compromised posterior attachment of the disc. The disc may be in a persistent prolapsed relationship at the closed position, which is characteristically identified by reciprocal clicks on opening and closing. Failure of this disc-condyle relationship to self-reduce results in·an abrupt limitation of jaw motion (at about 26 to 30 mm.), termed *locking.* The thickening and flattening process of these changes probably causes a binding effect during condyle translation (through the mechanism of overstretching of the lateral ligament).

Pain from temporomandibular disorders may be limited to the preauricular area or it may radiate to the jaw, teeth, temples, and ear. The symptoms are usually unilateral but the unaffected joint is progressively affected. The pain may be constant or recurrent. It may be precipitated by movement of the mandible or it may occur without provocation. It may be elicited only by digital pressure on a muscle or the capsular structures. Tenderness experienced during joint palpation via the external auditory meatus can be considered capsular pain as opposed to muscular tenderness palpated elsewhere. Painless limitation of joint movement does occur, but infrequently. *Pain referred to the ear and face from the cervical muscles often complicates the clinical picture of temporomandibular pain.*

Prevalence

The vast majority (70 to 90 per cent) of patients with temporomandibular pain and ·dysfunction are women between the ages of 20 and 40.[26] Symptoms of dysfunction are very common in otherwise normal populations. Several studies of normal populations have demonstrated that levels of signs and symptoms approach 25 or 50 per cent.[44] Five per cent of the total patient population of a dental school were treated for temporomandibular joint disorders,[46] suggesting a significant prevalence of this problem among dental patients.

Etiology

Conclusive evidence that there is one major cause for temporomandibular joint disorders is absent even though there are abundant claims to the contrary. The symptoms reported by any one patient develop from a unique set of psychological, structural, and functional factors. Weakness or instability in gnathic structure which make an individual unusually susceptible to temporomandibular joint dysfunction may be inherited, developmental, the result of prior injury, or the result of poor restoration of the occlusion. The possibility that an occlusal interference may activate bruxism cannot be overlooked. It is possible that occlusal interferences as well as traumatic or extensive dental work may focus the subject's attention on the mouth and jaws, making it a vulnerable and potential outlet for emotional tension. *The following factors are thought to be the most significant in the multicausal etiology of temporomandibular pain and dysfunction.*

Macrotrauma

Macrotrauma is a sudden exterior force with subsequent reflex contraction of muscle. External blows to the jaws or whiplash are frequently elicited in the history. Macrotrauma frequently leads to a compromised posterior attachment of the disc and is followed by suboptimal healing of these tissues. Unguarded or excessive forces on the temporomandibular joints during dental procedures are frequently associated with the onset of clinical symptoms. Overstretching or prolonged opening can be macrotraumatic, especially for the individual with incipient dysfunction.

Microtrauma

Microtrauma is a continuing or repetitive mechanical stress. In this process, muscle tonus can be abnormally increased by an interplay of emotional tension, pain, and occlusal interferences.[100] Even the normal forces of function can cause microtrauma in cases of disturbed occlusal support and guidance.

Degenerative joint disease

Deviations in joint contours and lesions of the articular surfaces disturb articular and synovial function and can be associated with production of joint symptoms. The temporomandibular joint is not an uncommon site of focus if the indivdiual is afflicted by rheumatoid arthritis.[17]

Emotional tension

Evidence indicates that emotional factors may play a significant role in the etiology of temporomandibular disorders.[110] Emotional states such as anxiety, frustration, fear, and anger cause increased activity in the masticatory muscles, thereby causing prolonged muscle tension and symptoms characteristic of temporomandibular pain and dysfunction.

OCCLUSAL CONSIDERATIONS IN TREATMENT PLANNING

The main objective in occlusal therapy is to maintain or achieve mandibular stability. The first issue in occlusal treatment planning is whether or not to alter the mandibular position by instituting generalized occlusal changes. If the mandibular position is judged adequate, the goal would be to maintain the existing occlusion, and to remove isolated interferences incident to therapy.

The decision to change the occlusal position should be based upon the positive result of an evaluation of the following two aspects of the patient's oral status.

1. GENERALIZED TRAUMA FROM OCCLUSION. *The presence or absence of signs of trauma from occlusion determine whether your patient's occlusal relationships merit perpetuation in periodontal therapy and ensuing restorative measures. If the trauma is limited to single or few teeth, localized*

TABLE 27-3 OCCLUSAL TREATMENT PLANNING

1. Patient in **ORTHOFUNCTION** (normal function)	Treatments are aimed at preserving the existing occlusion. An effort is made, therefore, to *avoid introducing new occlusal interferences.*
2. Patient in **DYSFUNCTION**	Specific procedures are instituted to remove pathosis related to occlusal interferences. *Partial or total alteration of the occlusion is generally indicated with either reversible or permanent means.* Large scale alterations lead to a therapeutic mandibular position and occlusion.
3. Patient requires **EXTENSIVE OCCLUSAL RECONSTRUCTION** for reasons other than traumatic occlusion.	*Create new intercuspal position to therapeutic occlusal standards,* so that both joints and teeth receive stress with only a slight mesial component.

adjustment of interferences may suffice. No change in the mandibular position would be required. However, if there is generalized trauma from occlusion, faulty maxillo-mandibular relationships are often involved in the production of the trauma. *Normalization of these relationships involves major changes in the mandibular occlusal position in accordance with the standards of therapeutic occlusion* (Table 27-4). Under these conditions, the repetitive and excessive occlusal forces of dysfunction may be minimized.

2. OCCLUSAL RECONSTRUCTION. Coordinated periodontal and restorative therapy sometimes involves massive or total reconstruction of disorganized or unstable occlusion. *Attempts to preserve an acquired, eccentric occlusal position dictated by a few remaining teeth is unwarranted.* Since the reestablishment of a therapeutic occlusal position will involve a significant alteration in the existing intercuspal scheme anyway, a prescribed or "therapeutic" mandibular position is more practical. *That is, the occlusion and mandibular position may be coordinated according to standards of therapeutic occlusion* (Table 27-4). The initial phase of this mandibular reorientation often begins with occlusal adjustment during periodontal therapy.

To summarize, existing occlusal schemes and maxillo-mandibular relationships are altered when it is expected that the resulting changes will (1) normalize the lesions of generalized trauma from occlusion, and (2) facilitate occlusal stabilization (therapeutic occlusion) for future restorative or prosthetic procedures. The change in the

mandibular position need not be permanent; it may be reversible, as in the case of removable bite guards and splints. If a decision is made to maintain the existing intercuspal position, then all occlusal treatments are conservative and are aimed at preserving relationships while removing only traumatic contacts in localized areas. Three categories of patients can be iden-

TABLE 27-4 CHARACTERISTICS OF THERAPEUTIC OCCLUSION (NATURAL DENTITION)

1. **INTERCUSPAL POSITION** (ICP) – Bilateral, simultaneous, well-distributed contacts on the posterior teeth, providing arch stability.
2. **RETRUDED CONTACT POSITION** (RCP) – The RCP-ICP relationship is less than 1 mm along a forward (symmetrical) path measured at incisal levels.
3. **VERTICAL STOPS** – Stable, multiple contacts on the posterior teeth providing individual tooth stability. No buccal-lingual thrust or impact to any tooth in closure to ICP or RCP.
4. **LATERAL EXCURSIONS** – Smooth movement with disclusion controlled by the canine and first premolar on the laterotrusive (working) side. There is little or no contact on the mediotrusive (balancing) side.
5. **PROTRUSIVE EXCURSIONS** – Smooth movement with multiple contacts bilaterally distributed on the anterior teeth.
6. **INTERFERENCES** – Freedom from lateral or protrusive single tooth contacts on the molar teeth; freedom from mediotrusive (balancing) side contacts.
7. **ACCEPTABLE FREE WAY SPACE** – The normal range is 1 to 4 mm. If the free way space measures 8 mm., it then can be reduced. If there are symptoms that can be ascribed to overclosure, then it should be treated.

tified concerning the planning of occlusal positions and maxillo-mandibular relationships. These are noted in Table 27–3.

THERAPEUTIC OCCLUSION

Therapeutic occlusion is a treatment occlusion employed to counteract problems related to traumatic occlusion. It is also an occlusal scheme used in restoring or replacing teeth so that a minimum of adaptation is required of the individual and so that compensatory tissue changes are minimized.

By definition, "therapeutic" implies there are no occlusal interferences and that the new occlusion will be coordinated with the most stable temporomandibular joint position. This insures that jaw closure will be oriented to a functional endpoint where both temporomandibular joints and teeth receive stresses with only a slight mesial component.[101] In constructing a therapeutic occlusion, the dentist will use prevailing principles formulated through his own clinical experience and his evaluation of research reports. In general, the basic characteristics of therapeutic occlusion are generally agreed upon and are summarized in Table 27–3.

Therapeutic occlusal alterations usually include stabilization of the retruded contact position (RCP) and smooth coordination of contacts between RCP and the intercuspal position (ICP). Also smooth, interference-free lateral and protrusive excursions are facilitated from ICP. All disturbing posterior interferences along lateral border paths are usually lessened or removed. These criteria enable the dentist to help individuals with a low tolerance to occlusal interferences or those who have occlusion weakened by bone loss.[100]

Assistance from Mary Kay Penn in the preparation of this chapter is gratefully acknowledged.

REFERENCES

1. Abe, K., and Shimakawa, M.: Genetic and developmental aspects of sleeptalking and teeth-grinding. Acta Paedopsych., 33:336–344, 1966.
2. Ahlgren, J.: Masticatory movements in man. In Anderson, D. J., and Mathews, B. (eds.): *Mastication.* Bristol, Wright and Sons, 1976, p. 119.
3. Arstad, T.: The Capsular Ligaments of the Temporomandibular Joint and Retrusion Facets of the Dentition in Relationship to Mandibular Movements. Oslo, Academisk Forlag, 1954.
4. Bates, J. F., Stafford, G. D., and Harrison, A.: Masticatory function – a review of the literature. I. The form of the masticatory cycle. J. Oral Rehab., 2:281–301, 1975.
5. Bates, J. F., Stafford, G. D., and Harrison, A.: Masticatory function – a review of the literature. II. Speed of movement of the mandible, rate of chewing. J. Oral Rehab., 2:349–361, 1975.
6. Bates, J. F., Stafford, G. D., and Harrison, A.: Masticatory function – a review of the literature. III. Masticatory performance and efficiency. J. Oral Rehab., 3:57–67, 1976.
7. Beyron, H. L.: Occlusal changes in the adult dentition. J.A.D.A., 48:674, 1954.
8. Beyron, H. L.: Optimal occlusion. Dent. Clin. North Am., 13:537, 1969.
9. Blackwood, H. J. J.: Adaptive changes in the mandibular joints with function. Dent. Clin. North Am., 10:559, 1966.
10. Blankenship, J. R., and Ramfjord, S. P.: Lateral displacement of the mandible in rhesus monkeys. J. Oral Rehab., 3:83–99, 1976.
11. Breitner, C.: The tooth-supporting apparatus under occlusal changes. J. Periodontol., 13: 72, 1942.
12. Brenman, H. S., and Amsterdam, M.: Postural effects on occlusion. Dent. Prog., 4:43, 1963.
13. Brill, N., Lammie, G. A., Osborne, J., and Perry, H. T.: Mandibular positions and mandibular movements: A review. Br. Dent. J., 106:391, 1959.
14. Brodie, A. G.: Orthodontics. In Lippincott's Handbook of Dental Practice. Philadelphia, J. B. Lippincott Co., 1948, p. 65.
15. Butler, J. H.: Recent research on physiology of occlusion. Dent. Clin. North Am., 13:555, 1969.
16. Carlsson, G. E., and Oberg, T.: Remodelling of the temporomandibular joints. Oral Sci. Rev., 6:53–86, 1974.
17. Chalmers, I. M., and Blair, G. S.: Rheumatoid arthritis of the temporomandibular joint. Q. J. Med., 42:369–386, 1973.
18. Clark, G. T.: The relationship between stress, nocturnal masseter muscle activity and symptoms of masticatory dysfunction. University of Rochester, Master's thesis, 1977.
19. Clark, G. T., et al.: Stress perception and nocturnal masseter muscle activity. Int. Assoc. Dent. Res. Prog., (Abstr. #436), 1977.
20. Clayton, J. A., Kotowicz, W. E., and Zahler, J. M.: Pantographic tracings of mandibular movements and occlusion. J. Pros. Dent., 25:389–396, 1971.
21. Cohn, L. A.: Factors of dental occlusion pertinent to the restorative and prosthetic problem. J. Pros. Dent., 9:256, 1959.
22. D'Amico, A.: The canine teeth: Normal functional relation of the natural teeth of man. J. South.

Calif. Dent. Assoc., 26:6, 49, 127, 175, 194, 239, 1958.

23. DeBoever, J. A.: Functional disturbances of the temporomandibular joints. Oral Sci. Rev., 2:100–117, 1973.

24. Dixon, A. D.: Structure and functional significance of the intra-articular disc of the human temporomandibular joint. Oral Surg., 15:48, 1962.

25. Folke, L., and Stallard, R.: Condylar adaptation to a change in intermaxillary relationship. J. Peridont. Res., 1:79, 1966.

26. Franks, A. S.: The social character of temporomandibular joint dysfunction. Dent. Practit. Dent. Rec., 15:94, 1964.

27. Funakoshi, M., Fujita, N., and Takehana, S.: Relations between occlusal interference and jaw muscle activities in responses to changes in head position. J. Dent. Res., 55:684–690, 1976.

28. Furstman, L.: The effect of loss of occlusion upon the mandibular joint. Am. J. Orthod., 51:145-161, 1965.

29. Garnick, J., and Ramfjord, S. P.: Rest position. An electromyographic and clinical investigation. J. Pros. Dent., 12:895, 1962.

30. Gibbs, C. H., Messerman, T., Reswick, J. B., and Derda, H. J.: Functional movements of the mandible. J. Pros. Dent., 26:604–620, 1971.

31. Gibbs, C. H.: Summary of jaw movements during chewing. Unpublished research report, 1977.

32. Glickman, I., Haddad, A. W., Martignoni, M., Mehta, N., Roeber, F. W., and Clark, R. E.: Telemetric comparison of centric relation and centric occlusion reconstructions. J. Pros. Dent., 31:527–536, 1974.

33. Goldberg, L. J.: Masseter muscle excitation induced by stimulation of periodontal and gingival receptors in man. Brain Res., 32:369–381, 1971.

34. Graf, H.: Bruxism. Dent. Clin. North Am., 13:659, 1969.

35. Greene, C. S., Lerman, M. D., Sutcher, H. D., and Laskin, D. M.: The TMJ pain-dysfunction syndrome: Heterogeneity of the patient population. J.A.D.A., 79:1168–1172, 1969.

36. Greene, C. S., and Laskin, D. M.: Splint therapy for the myofascial pain-dysfunction (MPD) syndrome; a comparative study. J.A.D.A., 84:624–628, 1972.

37. Guichet, N. F.: Applied gnathology: Why and how. Dent. Clin. North Am., 13:687, 1969.

38. Haddad, A. W., et al.: Effects of occlusal adjustment on tooth contacts during mastication. J. Periodontol., 45:714–724, 1974.

39. Haddad, A. W.: The functioning dentition. In Kawamura; Y. (ed.): Frontiers of Oral Physiology, vol. 2. Basel, S. Karger, 1976.

40. Hannam, A. G.: Unpublished data, 1977.

41. Hansson, T.: Temporomandibular joint changes: Occurrence and development. University of Lund, Sweden, Doctoral dissertation, 1978.

42. Hansson, T., Öberg, T., Carlsson, G. E., and Kopp, S.: Thickness of the soft tissue layers and the articular disk in the temporomandibular joint. Acta Odontol. Scand., 35:77–83, 1977.

43. Hansson, T., and Öberg, T.: Arthrosis and deviation in form in the temporomandibular joint. A microscopic study on a human autopsy material. Acta Odontol. Scand., 35:167–174, 1977.

44. Helkimo, M.: Epidemiological surveys of dysfunction of the masticatory system. In Melcher, A. H., and Zarb, G. A. (eds.): Oral Sciences Reviews: Temporomandibular Joint Function and Dysfunction III. Munksgaard, Copenhagen, 1976.

45. Helkimo, M.: Various centric positions and methods of recording them. In Zarb, G. A., Bergman, B., Clayton, J. A., and MacKay, H. F. (eds.): Prosthodontic Treatment for Partially Edentulous Patients. St. Louis, The C. V. Mosby Co., 1978.

46. Helöe, B., and Helöe, L. A.: Characteristics of a group of patients with temporomandibular joint disorders. Community Dent. Oral Epidemiol., 3:72–79, 1975.

47. Howell, A. H., and Manly, R. S.: An electronic strain gauge for measuring oral forces. J. Dent. Res., 27:705, 1948.

48. Ingervoll, B.: Retruded contact position of the mandible. A comparison between children and adults. Odont. Revy, 15:130, 1964.

49. Ingervoll, B.: Studies of mandibular positions in children. Odont. Revy, 19(Suppl.):15, 1968.

50. Ingervoll, B.: Tooth contacts on the functional and non-functional side in children and young adults. Arch. Oral Biol., 17:191, 1972.

51. Ireland, V. E.: The problem of the clicking jaw. R. Soc. Med., 44:363–372, 1951.

52. Jankelson, B., Hoffman, G. M., and Hendron, J. A.: The physiology of the stomatognathic system. J. Am. Dent. Assoc., 46:375, 1953.

53. Kawamura, Y., Kato, I., and Miyoshi, K.: Functional anatomy of the lateral pterygoid muscle in the cat. J. Dent. Res., 47:1142, 1968.

54. Kawamura, Y.: Physiology of mastication. In Frontiers of Oral Physiology, vol. 1. Basel, S. Karger, 1974.

55. Kawamura, Y.: Physiology of Oral Tissues. In Frontiers of Oral Physiology, vol. 2. Basel, S. Karger, 1976.

56. Kloprogge, M. J., and van Griethuysen, A. M.: Disturbances in contraction and coordination pattern of the masticatory muscles due to dental restoration. J. Oral Rehab., 3:207–216, 1976.

57. Koyoumdjisky, E.: The correlation of the inclined planes of the articular surface of the glenoid fossa with the cuspal and palatal slopes of the teeth. J. Dent. Res., 35:890, 1956.

58. Krogh-Poulsen, W. G., and Olsson, A.: Management of the occlusion of the teeth. In Schwarz, L., and Chayes, C. (eds.). Facial Pain and Mandibular Dysfunction. Philadelphia, W. B. Saunders Co., 1968.

59. Laskin, D. M.: Etiology of the pain-dysfunction syndrome. J. Am. Dent. Assoc., 79:148–153, 1969.

60. Last, R. J.: Personal communication, February, 1977.

61. Lear, C. S. C., Flanagan, J. B., Jr., and Moorees, C. F. A.: The frequency of deglutition in man. Arch. Oral Biol., 10:83, 1965.

62. Lavelle, C. L. B.: Deglutition. *In* Applied Physiology of the Mouth. ·Bristol, John Wright & Sons, Ltd., 1975, pp. 243.

63. Lous, I., Sheik-Ol-Eslam, A., and Møller, E.: Postural activity in subjects with functional disorders of the chewing apparatus. Scand. J. Dent. Res., 78:404–410, 1970.

64. Lucia, V. O.: The fundamentals of oral physiology and their practical application in the securing and reproducing of records to be used in restorative dentistry. J. Pros. Dent., 3:213, 1953.

65. Lundberg, M.: Free movements in the temporomandibular joint. A·cineradiographic study. Acta Radiol., Suppl. 220, 1963.

66. Lysell, L.: Epidemiologic-roentgendiagnostic study on teeth, jaws and temporomandibular joints in 67 year old people in Dalby, Sweden. University of Lund, Doctoral dissertation, 1977.

67. McNamara, J. A.: The independent functions of the two heads of the lateral pterygoid muscle. Am. J. Anat., 138:197–206, 1973.

68. Mahan, P. E.: The Physiology of Occlusion. *In* Clark, J. W. (ed.): Clinical Dentistry, vol. 2. Hagerstown, Md., Harper and Row, Publishers, Inc., 1977, p. 1.

69. Manly, R. S.: Practical Application of Research on Mastication. Monthly Report of Office of Naval Research, Feb. 1, 1950.

70. Manly, R. S., and Shiere, F. R.: The effect of dental deficiency on mastication and food preference. Oral Surg., 3:674, 1950.

71. Mann, A. W., and Pankey, L. D.: Concepts of occlusion – the Pankey-Mann philosophy of occlusal· rehabilitation. Dent. Clin. North Am., 7:621, 1963.

72. Marbach, J. J.: Arthritis of the temporomandibular joints and facial pain. Bull. Rheum. Dis., 27:918–921, 1977.

73. Matthews, B.: Mastication. *In* Lavelle, C. L. B. (ed.): Applied Physiology of the Mouth. Bristol, John Wright & Sons, Ltd., 1975, p. 199.

74. Mayne, J., and Hatch, G.: Arthritis of the temporomandibular joint. J. Am. Dent. Assoc., 79:125, 1969.

75. Mitani, H., and Kawamura, S.: Frontal plane movement of incision inferius during mastication. *In* Functional Movement of the Jaw. Med. J. Osaka Univ., 1971, p. 37.

76. Mitani, H., and Kawazoe, T.: Kinesiological studies on the rest position of the mandible. *In* Functional Movement of the Jaw. Med. J. Osaka Univ., 1971, p. 39.

77. Moffett, B. C., Johnson, L. C., McCabe, J. B., and Askew, H. C.: Articular remodeling in the adult human temporomandibular joint. Am. J. Anat., 115:119, 1964.

78. Mohl, N. D.: Alterations in the temporomandibular joint. Oral Surg., 36:625–631, 1973.

79. Molin, C.: An electromyographic study of the function of the lateral pterygoid muscle. Swed. Dent. J., 66:203–208, 1973.

80. Møller, E.: The chewing apparatus. Acta Physiol. Scand., 69:Suppl. 280, 1966.

81. Møller, E.: Tyggeapparatets naturlige funktioner. *In* Krogh-Poulsen, W., and Carlsen, O. (eds.): Bidfunktion Bettfysiologi. Copenhagen, Munksgaard, 1973.

82. Møller, E.: Quantitative features of masticatory muscle activity. *In* Rowe, N. H. (ed.): Occlusion: Research in Form and Function. Proceed. of Symposium, University of Michigan School of Dentistry, 1975, p. 54.

83. Møller, E.: Human muscle patterns. *In* Sessle, B., and Hannam, A. (eds.): Mastication and Swallowing. Toronto, University of Toronto Press, 1976, p. 128.

84. Møller, E.: Evidence that the rest position is subject to servo-control. *In* Anderson, D. J., and Mathew, B. (eds.): Mastication. Bristol, John Wright and Sons, 1976, pp. 72–80.

85. Mongini, F.: Anatomic and clinical evaluation of the relationship between the temporomandibular joint and occlusion. J. Pros. Dent., 38:539–551, 1977.

86. Moyers, R. E.: Some physiologic considerations of centric and other jaw relations. J. Pros. Dent., 6:183, 1956.

87. Muhlemann, H. R.: Intraoral radiotelemetry. Int. Dent. J., 21:456, 1971.

88. Öberg, T., Carlsson, G. E., and Fajers, C. M.: The temporomandibular joint. A morphological study on a human autopsy material. Acta Odontol. Scand., 29:349–384, 1971.

89. Olkinuora, M.: A psychosomatic study of bruxism with emphasis on mental strain and familiar predisposition factors. Proc. Finn. Dent. Soc., 68:110–123, 1972.

90. Olkinuora, M.: Psychosocial aspects in a series of bruxists compared with a group of non-bruxists. Proc. Finn. Dent. Soc., 68:200–208, 1972.

91. Olkinuora, M.: Bruxism as a psychosomatic phenomenon. Academic dissertation.· Forssan Kirjapaino Oy-Forssa. Helsinki, 1972.

92. Owens, S. E., Lehr, R. P., and Biggs, N. L.: The functional significance of centric relation as demonstrated by electromyography of the lateral pterygoid muscles. J. Prosthet. Dent., 33:5–9, 1975.

93. Pameijer, J. H., Brion, M. A. M., Glickman, I., and Roeber, F. W.: Intraoral occlusal telemetry. V. Effect of occlusal adjustment upon tooth contacts during chewing and swallowing. J. Pros. Dent., 24:492, 1970.

94. Picton, D. C. A.: Tilting movements of teeth during biting. Arch. Oral Biol., 7:151, 1962.

95. Posselt, V.: Studies in the mobility of the human mandible. Acta Odontol. Scand., 10:(Suppl. 10), 1952.

96. Preiskel, H. W.: Some observations on the postural position of the mandible. J. Pros. Dent., 15:625, 1965.

97. Pruzansky, S.: Applicability of electromyographic procedures as a clinical aid in the detection of occlusal disharmony. Dent. Clin. North Am., March, 1960, p. 117.

98. Ramfjord, S. P.: Bruxism, A Clinical and Electromyographic Study. J. Am. Dent. Assoc., 62:21, 1961.

99. Ramfjord, S. P., Kerr, D. A., and Ash, M. M.: World Workshop in Periodontics. Ann Arbor, The University of Michigan Press, 1966.

100. Ramfjord, S. P., and Ash, M. M., Jr.: Occlusion,

2nd ed. Philadelphia, W. B. Saunders Company, 1971.

101. Ramfjord, S. P.: Occlusion. Indent, 1:19–24, 1973.

102. Randow, K., Carlsson, K., Edlund, J., and Oberg, T.: The effect of an occlusal interference on the masticatory system. Odont. Revy, 27:245–256, 1976.

103. Reding, G., Zrpelin, H., and Monroe, L.: Personality study of nocturnal teeth grinders. Percept. Mot. Skills, 26:523–531, 1960.

104. Reding, G., et al.: Sleep pattern of bruxism: A revision. Psychophysiology, 4:396, 1967–68.

105. Rees, L. A.: The structure and function of the mandibular joint. Brit. Dent. J., 96:125–133, 1954.

106. Regli, C. P., and Kelly, E. K.: The phenomenon of decreased mandibular arch width in opening movements. J. Pros. Dent., 17:49, 1967.

107. Ricketts, R. M.: Variations of the temporomandibular joint as revealed by cephalometric laminagraphy. Am. J. Orthod., 36:877–898, 1950.

108. Rugh, J. D.: Variation in human masticatory behavior under temporal constraints. J. Compar. Physiol. Psychol., 80:169–174, 1972.

109. Rugh, J. D., and Solberg, W. K.: Electromyographic studies of bruxist behavior before and after treatment. Cal. Dent. Assoc. J., 3:56–59, 1975.

110. Rugh, J. D., and Solberg, W. K.: Psychological implications in temporomandibular pain and dysfunction. In Melcher, A. H., and Zarb, G. A. (eds.): Oral Sciences Reviews: Temporomandibular Joint Function and Dysfunction III. Munksgaard, Copenhagen No. 7, 1976.

111. Satoh, T., and Harada, Y.: Tooth grinding during sleep as an arousal reaction. Experientia, 27:785–786, 1971.

112. Schärer, P.: Bruxism. Front. Oral Physiol., 1:293–322, 1974.

113. Schuyler, C. H.: Factors contributing to traumatic occlusion. J. Pros. Dent., 11:708, 1961.

114. Sessle, B. J., and Hannam, A. G. (eds.): Mastication and Swallowing. Toronto, University of Toronto Press, 1976.

115. Sicher, H., and DuBrul, E. L. Oral Anatomy, 6th ed. St. Louis, The C. V. Mosby Co., 1975.

116. Silverman, M. M.: Character of mandibular movement during closure. J. Pros. Dent., 15:634, 1965.

117. Sloane, R. B.: Kinesiology and vertical dimension. J. Pros. Dent., 2:12, 1952.

118. Sochat, P., and Schwarz, M. S.: Individualized occlusal adjustment. Part I Rationale. J. South Cal. Dent. Assoc., 40:827, 1972.

119. Sognnaes, R.: Periodontal significance of intraoral frictional ablation. J. West Soc. Periodont. (Periodontal Abst.)25:112–121, 1977.

120. Sognnaes, R.: Frictional ablation—a neglected factor in the mechanisms of hard tissue destruction? In Kuhlencordt, F., and Kruse, H. P. (eds.): Calcium Metabolism, Bone and Metabolic Bone Diseases. Berlin, Springer-Verlag, 1975.

121. Solberg, W. K., Flint, R. T., and Branter, J. P.: Temporomandibular joint pain and dysfunction. A clinical study of emotional and occlusal components. J. Pros. Dent., 28:412–422, 1972.

122. Solberg, W. K.: Terminology in occlusion. In Abou-Rass, M. (ed.): Workshop in Occlusion Education. University of Southern California, 1975.

123. Solberg, W. K., Clark, G. T., and Rugh, J. D.: Nocturnal electromyographic evaluation of bruxism patients undergoing short term splint therapy. J. Oral Rehab., 2:215–223, 1975.

124. Solberg, W. K., Woo, M., and Houston, J. B.: Prevalence of mandibular dysfunction in young adults. (Submitted for publication.)

125. Stallard, H., and Stuart, C. E.: Eliminating tooth guidance in natural dentitions. J. Pros. Dent., 11:47, 1961.

126. Standlee, J. P., Caputo, A. A., and Ralph, J. P.: Stress trajectories within the mandible under occlusal loads. J. Dent. Res., 56:1297, 1977.

127. Storey, A. T.: Physiology of Occlusion. In Rowe, N. H. (ed.): Occlusion: Research in Form and Function. Proceed. of Symposium, University of Michigan School of Dentistry, 1975, p. 38.

128. Suit, S. R., Gibbs, C. H., and Benz, S. T.: Study of gliding tooth contacts during mastication. J. Periodontol., 47:331–334, 1976.

129. Tallgren, A.: Changes in adult face height due to aging, wear and loss of teeth and prosthetic treatment. A roentgen cephalometric study mainly on Finnish women. Acta Odontol. Scand., 15(Suppl.):24, 1957.

130. Tallgren, A.: Muscle activity relative to changes in occlusal jaw relationship: Cephalometric and electromyographic correlation. Occlusion: Research in Form and Function. Proceed. of Symposium, University of Michigan School of Dentistry, 1975, p. 21.

131. Telhaug, H.: Studies in degenerative joint disease. University of Lund, Sweden, Doctoral dissertation. 1973.

132. Thielemann, K.: Biomechanik der Paradentose ins besondere Artikulationsausgleich durch Einschleifen, 2nd ed. Munchen, Barth, 1956.

133. Thompson, J. R.: The rest position of the mandible and its significance to dental science. J. Am. Dent. Assoc., 33:151, 1946.

134. Toller, P. A.: The synovial apparatus and temporomandibular joint function. Br. Dent. J., 111:335–362, 1961.

135. Weinberg, L. A.: Diagnosis of facets in occlusal equilibration. J. Am. Dent. Assoc., 52:26, 1956.

136. Weinberg, L. A.: The prevalence of tooth contact in eccentric movements of the jaw: Its clinical implications. J. Am. Dent. Assoc., 62:402, 1961.

137. Yemm, R.: Some experimental evidence of the aetiology and pathology of masticatory dysfunction. J. Dent. Assoc. S. Afr., 30:213–217, 1975.

138. Yemm, R.: Neurophysiological studies of temporomandibular joint dysfunction. In Melcher, A. H., and Zarb, G. A. (eds.): Oral

Sciences Reviews: Temporomandibular Joint—Function and Dysfunction III. Copenhagen, Munksgaard, No. 7, 1976.

139. Yuodelis, R. A., and Mann, W. V., Jr.: The prevalence and possible role of nonworking contacts in periodontal disease. Periodontics, 3:219, 1965.

140. Yurkstas, A. A.: The masticatory act. J. Pros. Dent., 15:248, 1965.

141. Zarb, G. A., and Thompson, G. W.: The treatment of patients with temporomandibular joint pain dysfunction syndrome. J. Can. Dent. Assoc., 7:410–416, 1975.

Chapter 28

Nutritional Influences in the Etiology of Periodontal Disease

The majority of opinions and research findings on the effects of nutrition on oral and periodontal tissues point to the following:

1. There are nutritional deficiencies that produce changes in the oral cavity; these changes include alterations of lips, oral mucosa, and bone, as well as of the periodontal tissues. These changes are considered as periodontal or oral manifestations of nutritional disease.

2. There are no nutritional deficiencies which by themselves can cause gingivitis or periodontal pockets. There are, however, nutritional deficiencies that can affect the condition of the periodontium and thereby aggravate the injurious effects of local irritants and excessive occlusal forces.

Theoretically it can be assumed that there may be a "border zone" in which local irritants of insufficient severity can cause gingival and periodontal disorders if their effect upon the periodontium were aggravated by nutritional deficiencies. On the basis of this, some clinicians enthusiastically adhere to the theory that would assign a key role in periodontal disease to nutritional deficiencies and imbalances. Although research conducted up to the present does not in general support this view, it has been pointed out[2] that numerous problems in experimental design and data interpretation may render those research findings inadequate.

This chapter will analyze the existing knowledge in the field of nutrition as it relates to periodontal disease, and reference will also be made to other oral changes of nutritional origin.

PHYSICAL CHARACTER OF THE DIET

Numerous experiments in animals have shown that the physical character of the diet may play some role in the accumulation of plaque and the development of gingivitis.[30] Soft diets, nutritionally adequate, may lead to plaque and calculus formation.[6, 14, 15, 17, 26] Hard and fibrous foods provide surface cleansing action and stimulation, which result in less plaque and gingivitis,[9, 31] even if the diet is nutritionally inadequate.[14] On the other hand, studies in humans have been unable to demonstrate reduced plaque formation when hard diets are consumed.[17, 34] The difference may be related to differences in tooth anatomy and to the fact that hard consistency diets are fed to experimental animals as the only diet, while humans also consume soft foods. Human diets also have a high sucrose content which favors the production of a thick plaque.

THE EFFECT OF NUTRITION UPON ORAL MICROORGANISMS

With increased interest in the role of bacterial plaque in periodontal disease, attention has been directed to a relatively unexplored aspect of nutrition—namely, its effect upon the oral microorganisms. Although dietary intake is generally thought of in terms of sustaining the individual, it inadvertently is also the source of bacterial nutrients.

By its effects upon the oral bacteria, the composition of the diet may influence the relative distribution of types of organisms, their metabolic activity, and their pathogenic potential, which in turn affects the occurrence and severity of oral disease. Consideration of the role of nutrition upon the oral flora and of its possible implications in oral disease is in its early stages. Morhart and Fitzgerald[25] present an excellent analysis of the information thus far available on this subject.

It may be that oral changes considered to be the result of nutritional deficiencies upon the oral tissues could be first an effect upon the oral microorganisms, so that their products become increasingly injurious to the oral tissues.

Sources of nutrients for the microorganisms can be endogenous and exogenous. Among the exogenous factors the influence of the sugar content of the diet has been extensively studied; it has been demonstrated that the amount and type of carbohydrates in the diet and the frequency of intake can influence bacterial growth.[7]

VITAMIN A DEFICIENCY

Deficiency of vitamin A results in keratinizing metaplasia of epithelium, increased susceptibility to infection,[12] disturbances in bone growth, shape and texture,[18] abnormalities in the central nervous system,[37] and ocular manifestations—which include night blindness (nyctalopia), xerosis of the conjunctiva, xerosis of the cornea with subsequent corneal turbidity, ulceration, and keratomalacia.[16]

Oral findings in experimental animals

The following changes have been reported in vitamin A deficient rats: widening of the periodontal ligament of the molars and incisors, degeneration of the principal fibers,[4] thickening of the cementum of the molars,[29] apical hypercementosis with imperfect root formation, retarded eruption and malposition of the teeth.[29] Hyperkeratosis of the oral epithelium produced by vitamin A deficiency in experimental animals is comparable to that resulting from prolonged administration of estrogen.[38] Alveolar bone changes in vitamin A deficient animals include increased density with fewer marrow spaces,[19] hypercalcification with retardation in the rate of bone deposition,[29] resorption with fibrosis,[5] atrophy with resorption (most pronounced in the furcation areas),[24] osteophytic formation,[4] osteoporosis and resorption of the crest of the alveolar bone, which may be the result of the deficiency or may occur secondary to gingival changes.[13]

Vitamin A deficiency and periodontal disease

Some studies in experimental animals suggest that vitamin A deficiency may predispose to periodontal disease.[3, 20, 21] Loss of neurotrophic stimulation as a result of peripheral nerve degeneration[13, 23] and atrophy of the salivary glands[3] have been suggested as causative factors.

The gingiva shows epithelial hyperplasia and hyperkeratinization with proliferation of the junctional epithelium.[4, 13, 19] The life cycle of the epithelial cells is shortened as evidenced by early karyolysis.[9] Gingival hyperplasia with inflammatory infiltration and degeneration,[21] pocket formation[3, 4] and the formation of subgingival calculus[13] also occur.

Local irritation is necessary before abnormal epithelial tendencies associated with vitamin A deficiency are manifest in the gingival sulcus.[11] Pocket formation does not occur in vitamin A deficient animals in the absence of local irritation, but when local irritation is present, the pockets are deeper than in nondeficient animals and present associated epithelial hyperkeratosis. Repair of gingival wounds is retarded in vitamin A deficient animals,[10, 22] which are also subject to leukoplakia of the oral mucosa in areas other than the gingiva.[1]

In contrast with the abundance of evidence in experimental animals, there is little information regarding the effects of vitamin A deficiency upon the oral structures in humans. Low daily intake of vitamin A has been associated with periodontal disease.[27] Marshall-Day[8] reported a possible correlation between the incidence of periodontal disease and dermatologic lesions characteristic of vitamin A deficiency, and Russell reported that populations with a high incidence of periodontal disease tend to be deficient in vitamin A.[28] However, several other studies carried out in the Far East, where vitamin A deficiency is common, and in Africa failed to demonstrate any relation between this vitamin and periodontal disease.[33]

Hypervitaminosis A

Large doses of vitamin A in young growing rats produce generalized bone resorptive activity and osteoporosis which result in multiple fractures. Developing dental tissues are not affected, but the alveolar bone shows marked resorption without repair.[36] Hypervitaminosis A may accelerate bone growth.[35] Furthermore, melanin-like pigmentation of the skin, scaling dermatosis, disturbed menstruation, itching, and exophthalmos have been identified with hypervitaminosis A in humans.[32]

REFERENCES

Physical Character of the Diet and Vitamin A

1. Abels, J. C., Rekers, P. E., Hayes, M., and Rhoads, C. P.: Relationship between dietary deficiency and occurrence of papillary atrophy of tongue and oral leukoplakia. Cancer Res., 2:381, 1942.
2. Alfano, M. C.: Controversies, perspectives and clinical implications of nutrition in periodontal disease. Dent. Clin. North Am., 20:519, 1976.
3. Boyle, P. E.: Effect of vitamin A deficiency on the periodontal tissues. Am. J. Orthod., 33:744, 1947.
4. Boyle, P. E., and Bessey, O. A.: The effect of acute vitamin A deficiency on the molar teeth and paradontal tissues, with a comment on deformed incisor-teeth in this deficiency. J. Dent. Res., 20:236, 1941.
5. Burn, C. G., Orten, A. U., and Smith, A. H.: Changes in structure of developing tooth in rats maintained on diets deficient in vitamin A. Yale J. Biol. Med., 13:817, 1941.
6. Burwasser, P., and Hill, T. J.: The effect of hard and soft diets on the gingival tissues of dogs. J. Dent. Res., 18:389, 1939.
7. Carlsson, J., and Egelberg, J.: Effect of diet on early plaque formation in man. Odont. Revy, 16:122, 1965.
8. Day, C. D. M.: Nutritional deficiencies and dental caries in northern India. Br. Dent. J., 76:143, 1944.
9. Egelberg, J.: Local effect of diet on plaque formation and development of gingivitis in dogs. I. Effect of hard and soft diets. Odont. Revy, 16:31, 1965.
10. Frandsen, A. M.: Periodontal tissue changes in vitamin A deficient young rats. Acta Odont. Scand., 21:19, 1963.
11. Glickman, I., and Stoller, M.: The periodontal tissues of the albino rat in vitamin A deficiency. J. Dent. Res., 27:758, 1948.
12. Green, H. N., and Mellanby, E.: Vitamin A as anti-infective agent. Br. Med. J., 2:691, 1928.
13. King, J. D.: Abnormalities in the gingival and subgingival tissues due to diets deficient in vitamin A and carotene. Br. Dent. J., 68:349, 1940.
14. King, J. D., and Glover, N. E.: The relative effects of dietary constituents and other factors upon calculus formation and gingival disease in the ferret. J. Pathol. Bacteriol., 57:353, 1945.
15. Krasse, B., and Brill, N.: Effect of consistency of diet on bacteria in gingival pockets in dogs. Odont. Revy, 11:152, 1960.
16. Kruse, H. D.: Medical evaluation of nutritional

status. IV. The ocular manifestations of avitaminosis A, with especial consideration of the detection of early changes by biomicroscopy. Milbank Mem. Fund. Q., *XIX*:207, 1941.

17. Lindhe, J., and Wicen, P. O.: The effects on the gingivae of chewing fibrous foods. J. Periodont. Res., *4*:193, 1969.

18. Mellanby, E.: A Story of Nutritional Research. Baltimore, Williams & Wilkins Co., 1950.

19. Mellanby, H.: Effect of maternal dietary deficiency of vitamin A on dental tissues in rats. J. Dent. Res., *20*:489, 1941.

20. Mellanby, M.: Dental research, with special reference to parodontal disease produced experimentally in animals. Dent. Record, *59*:227, 1939.

21. Mellanby, M.: Diet and the teeth: An experimental study. Part I. Dental structures in dogs. Med. Res. Council (Brit.) Spec. Rep. Series No. 140, London, 1929.

22. Mellanby, M.: Diet and the teeth: An experimental study. Part II. Diet and dental disease; B. Diet and dental structure in animals other than the dog. Med. Res. Council (Brit.) Spec. Rep. Series No. 153, London, 1930.

23. Mellanby, M., and King, J. D.: Diet and the nerve supply to the dental tissues. Br. Dent. J., *56*:538, 1934.

24. Miglani, D. C.: The effect of vitamin A deficiency on the periodontal structures of rat molars with emphasis on cementum resorption. Oral Surg., *12*:1372, 1959.

25. Morhart, R. E., and Fitzgerald, R. J.: Nutritional determinants of the ecology of the oral flora. Dent. Clin. North Am., *20*:473, 1976.

26. Pelzer, R.: A study of the local oral effect of diet on the periodontal tissues and the gingival capillary structure. J. Am. Dent. Assoc., *27*: 13, 1940.

27. Radusch, D. F.: Nutritional aspect of periodontal disease. Ann. Dent., *7*:169, 1940.

28. Russell, A. L.: International nutrition surveys: A summary of preliminary dental findings. J. Dent. Res., *42*:233, 1963.

29. Schour, I., Hoffman, M. M., and Smith, M. C.: Changes in incisor teeth of albino rats with vitamin A deficiency and effects of replacement therapy. Am. J. Pathol., *17*:529, 1941.

30. Sreebny, L. M.: Effect of the physical consistency of food on the "crevicular complex" and the salivary glands. Intern. Dent. J., *22*:394, 1972.

31. Stralfors, A., Thilander, H., and Bergenholtz, A.: Caries and periodontal disease in hamsters fed cereal foods varying in sugar content and hardness. Arch. Oral Biol., *12*:1681, 1967.

32. Sulzberger, M. B., and Lazar, M. P.: Hypervitaminosis A. J.A.M.A., *146*:788, 1951.

33. Waerhaug, J.: Epidemiology of periodontal disease. Review of Literature. *In* World Workshop in Periodontics, 1966, p. 181.

34. Wilcox, C. E., and Everett, F.: Friction on the teeth and the gingiva during mastication. J. Am. Dent. Assoc., *66*:5, 1963.

35. Wolbach, S. B.: Vitamin A deficiency and excess in relation to skeletal growth. Proc. Inst. Med. Chicago, *16*:118, 1946.

36. Wolbach, S. B., and Bessey, O. A.: Tissue changes in vitamin deficiencies. Physiol. Rev., *22*:233, 1942.

37. Wolbach, S. B., and Bessey, O. A.: Vitamin A deficiency and the nervous system. Arch. Pathol., *32*:689, 1941.

38. Ziskin, D. E., Rosenstein, S. N., and Drucker, L.: Interrelation of large parenteral doses of estrogen and vitamin A and their effect on the oral mucosa. Am. J. Orthod., *29*:163, 1943.

VITAMIN B COMPLEX DEFICIENCY

The vitamin B complex includes the following substances: thiamine (vitamin B_1), riboflavin (vitamin B_2), nicotinic acid (niacin) or nicotinic acid amide (niacinamide), pantothenic acid, pyridoxine (vitamin B_6), biotin, para-aminobenzoic acid, inositol, choline, folic acid (folacin), and vitamin B_{12} (cyanocobalamin).

Oral disease is rarely due to a deficiency in just one component of the B complex group. The deficiency is generally multiple. Oral changes common to deficiencies in the B complex group are gingivitis, glossitis, glossodynia, angular cheilitis, and inflammation of the entire oral mucosa. **The gingivitis in vitamin B deficiencies is nonspecific, caused by local irritation rather than by the deficiency, but it is subject to the modifying effect of the latter.**[1]

Oral Findings Associated with Vitamin B Complex Deficiency

Thiamine (vitamin B_1)

The human manifestations of thiamine deficiency, called beriberi, are characterized by paralysis, cardiovascular symptoms (including edema), and loss of appetite. Frank beriberi is rare in the United States; however, less striking polyneuropathies do result from accompanying conditioning factors that interfere with absorption or utilization of thiamine. Many animals, including man, have microorganisms in their intestinal tracts that have the capacity to synthesize thiamine, thus complicating experimental inducement of deficiency of this vitamin.

The following oral disturbances have been attributed to thiamine deficiency: hypersensitivity of the oral mucosa,[13] minute vesicles (simulating herpes) on the buccal mucosa, under the tongue, or on the palate; and erosion of the oral mucosa.[7] Glossitis could not be produced in humans by deprivation of thiamine.[21] Since thiamine is essential to bacterial and carbohydrate metabolism, it has been postulated that the activity of the oral flora is diminished in thiamine deficiency.[10]

Riboflavin (vitamin B$_2$)

The symptoms of riboflavin deficiency (ariboflavinosis) include glossitis, angular cheilitis, seborrheic dermatitis, and a superficial vascularizing keratitis.[15, 16] The glossitis is characterized by a magenta discoloration and atrophy of the papillae. Disappearance of the papillae of the tongue varies, and depends upon the severity of the deficiency. In mild to moderate cases, the dorsum presents a patchy atrophy of the lingual papillae[1] and engorged fungiform papillae, which project as pebble-like elevations.[8] In severe deficiency, the entire dorsum is flat, having a dry and often fissured surface. The margin of the tongue presents a scalloped appearance, caused by contiguous indentations that conform to the pattern of the interdental spaces of the dentition.

Angular cheilitis is one of the changes most frequently identified with riboflavin deficiency. It begins as an inflammation of the commissure of the lips followed by erosion, ulceration, and fissuring (Fig. 28–1). Riboflavin deficiency is not the only cause of angular cheilitis. Loss of vertical dimension, together with drooling of saliva into the angles of the lips, may produce a condition similar to angular cheilitis. Candidiasis may develop in the commissures of debilitated persons; this lesion has been termed "perlèche."[6]

Changes observed in riboflavin-deficient animals include severe lesions of the gingiva, periodontal tissues, and oral mucosa (including noma),[3, 18] and retarded chondrogenic and osteogenic activity in the condylar growth center of the mandible.[23]

Nicotinic acid (niacin)

Nicotinic acid deficiency, or aniacinosis, results in *pellagra*, which is characterized by dermatitis, gastrointestinal disturb-

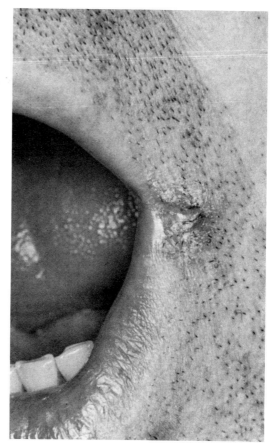

Figure 28–1 Angular Cheilitis in patient with conditioned vitamin B complex deficiency.

ances, neurological and mental disturbances (dermatitis, diarrhea, and dementia), glossitis, gingivitis, and generalized stomatitis.

ORAL CHANGES. Glossitis and stomatitis may be the earliest clinical signs of nicotinic acid deficiency.[14] In the acute form, there are hyperemia of the tongue, enlargement of the papillae, and indentation of the margin, followed by atrophic changes and a resultant glazed surface. The tongue in acute nicotinic acid deficiency is "beefy-red" and painful, with "burning" (glossopyrosis)[11]. In chronic nicotinic acid deficiency the tongue is thinned and fissured, with surface crevices, marginal serrations, and atrophy of the fungiform and filiform papillae.

The gingiva may be involved in aniacinosis[9] with or without tongue changes. The

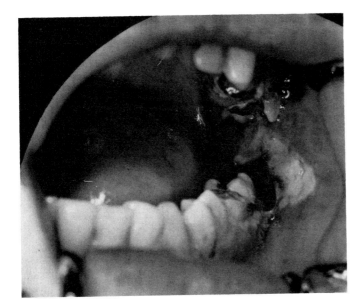

Figure 28–2 Ulceration of Buccal Mucosa in Patient with Nicotinic Acid Deficiency. Note sharp cusp of maxillary molar which initiated the irritation. (Courtesy of Dr. David Weisberger.)

most frequent finding is acute necrotizing ulcerative gingivitis, usually in areas of local irritation (Fig. 28–2).

Oral manifestations of vitamin B complex and nicotinic acid deficiencies in experimental animals include black tongue[1, 4] and gingival inflammation with destruction of the gingiva, periodontal ligament, and alveolar bone.[2] Necrosis of the gingiva and other oral tissues, and leukopenia, are terminal features of nicotinic acid deficiency in experimental animals.

Pantothenic acid

Oral changes caused by pantothenic acid deficiency have been identified in animals but not in humans. These include[20, 23] angular cheilitis, hyperkeratosis with ulceration and necrosis of the gingiva and oral mucosa, proliferation of the basal layer of the oral epithelium, and resorption of the crest of the alveolar bone. Absence of an inflammatory response is a striking finding. Radiographically, narrowing of the periodontal ligament space, alveolar bone loss, and rarefaction of bone may be observed.

The oral mucosa and lips are glistening red, sometimes with ulceration. In the early stages salivary flow is increased and accompanied by drooling, but the dehydration which occurs as the disease progresses leads to reduced salivary flow and dryness.

Pyridoxine (vitamin B₆)

Anemia, cardiovascular disturbances, convulsions, retardation of growth,[22] and patchy atrophy of the dorsum of the tongue (similar to that observed in riboflavin deficiency) have been noted in experimental animals on diets deficient in pyridoxine.[1]

Humans with pyridoxine deficiency present angular cheilitis, and glossitis with swelling, atrophy of the papilla, magenta discoloration and discomfort. When experimentally created in humans, the deficiency results in glossitis resembling that of nicotinic acid, reddening with small ulcerations of the mucosa, and angular cheilitis.[19]

Folic acid (pteroylglutamic acid)

Folic acid deficiency results in macrocytic anemia with megaloblastic erythropoiesis, with oral changes and gastrointestinal lesions, diarrhea, and intestinal malabsorption.[5]

ORAL CHANGES. Folic acid deficient animals present necrosis of the gingiva, periodontal ligament, and alveolar bone without inflammation.[16] The absence of inflammation is the result of deficiency-induced granulocytopenia.

In humans with sprue and other folic acid deficiency states there is generalized stomatitis, which may be accompanied by ulcerated glossitis and cheilitis. Ulcerative stomatitis is an early indication of a toxic effect of folic acid antagonists used in the treatment of leukemia.

In sprue, glossitis may be the presenting complaint; it usually occurs after the onset of steatorrhea. Swelling and redness at the tip and lateral margins are the initial disorders, accompanied in some cases by painful minute ulcers on the dorsum. Disappearance of the filiform and fungiform papillae is followed by the development of a smooth atrophic red tongue. Painful burning symptoms and increased salivation accompany the oral changes.

Vitamin B$_{12}$ (cyanocobalamin)

Vitamin B$_{12}$, the antipernicious anemia factor, is the only vitamin which contains cobalt. It is a patent catalyst and is involved in the synthesis of nucleic acid and folic acid metabolism. Pernicious anemia is the most severe form of vitamin B$_{12}$ deficiency. Other macrocytic anemias are thought to be mild forms of vitamin B$_{12}$ deficiency complicated by deficiency of folic acid. Oral changes in pernicious anemia are described in Chapter 30.

REFERENCES

Vitamin B Complex

1. Afonsky, D.: Oral lesions in niacin, riboflavin, pyridoxine, folic acid and pantothenic acid deficiencies in adult dogs. Oral Surg., 8:207, 315, 867, 1955.
2. Becks, H., Wainwright, W. W., and Morgan, A. F.: Comparative study of oral changes in dogs due to deficiencies of pantothenic acid, nicotinic acid and unknowns of B vitamin complex. Am. J. Orthod. 29:183, 1943.
3. Chapman, O. D., and Harris, A. E.: Oral lesions associated with dietary deficiencies in monkeys. J. Infect. Dis., 69:7, 1941.
4. Denton, J.: A study of tissue changes in experimental black tongue of dogs compared with similar changes in pellagra. Am. J. Pathol., 4:341, 1928.
5. Dreizen, S.: Oral manifestations of human nutritional anemias. Arch. Environ. Health, 5:66, 1962.
6. Goodman, M. H.: Perlèche: A consideration of its etiology and pathology. Bull. Johns Hopkins Hosp., 51:263, 1932.
7. Govier, W. M., and Grieg, M. E.: Prevention of oral lesions in B$_1$ avitaminotic dogs. Science, 98:216, 1943.
8. Jeghers, H.: Riboflavin deficiency. IV. Oral changes. Advances in Internal Medicine I. New York, Interscience Publishers Inc., 1942, p. 257.
9. King, J. D.: Vincent's disease treated with nicotinic acid. Lancet, 2:32, 1940.
10. Kneisner, A. H., Mann, A. W., and Spies, T. D.: Relationship of dental caries to deficiencies of vitamin B group. J. Dent. Res. 21:259, 1942.
11. Kruse, H. D.: Lingual manifestations of aniacinosis with especial consideration of detection of early changes by biomicroscopy. Milbank Mem. Fund Q., 20:262, 1942.
12. Levy, B. M.: The effect of riboflavin deficiency on the growth of the mandibular condyle of mice. Oral Surg., 2:89, 1949.
13. Mann, A. W., Spies, T. D., and Springer, M.: Oral manifestations of vitamin B complex deficiencies. J. Dent. Res., 20:269, 1941.
14. Manson-Bahr, P., and Ransford, O. N.: Stomatitis of vitamin B$_2$ deficiency treated with nicotinic acid. Lancet, 2:426, 1938.
15. Sebrell, W. H., and Butler, R. E.: Riboflavin deficiency in man. Public Health Rep., 53:2282, 1938; 54:2121, 1939.
16. Shaw, J. H.: The relation of nutrition to periodontal disease. J. Dent. Res. (Suppl. 1), 41:264, 1962.
17. Sydenstricker, V. P.: Clinical manifestations of ariboflavinosis. Am. J. Public Health, 31:344, 1941.
18. Topping, N. H., and Fraser, H. F.: Mouth lesions associated with dietary deficiencies in monkeys. Public Health Rep., 54:416, 1939.
19. Vilter, R. W., et al.: The effect of vitamin B$_6$ deficiency induced by desoxypyridoxine in human beings. J. Lab. Clin. Med., 42:335, 1953.
20. Wainwright, W. W., and Nelson, M.: Changes in oral mucosa accompanying acute pantothenic acid deficiency in young rats. Am. J. Orthod., 31:406, 1945.
21. Williams, R. D., Masson, H. L., Wilder, R. M., and Smith, B. F.: Observations on induced thiamine deficiency in man. Arch. Intern. Med., 66:785, 1940; 69:721, 1942.
22. Wolbach, S. B., and Bessey, O. A.: Tissue changes in vitamin deficiencies. Physiol. Rev., 22:233, 1942.
23. Ziskin, D. E., Stein, G., Gross, P., and Runne, E.: Oral, gingival and periodontal pathology induced in rats on a low pantothenic acid diet by toxic doses of zinc carbonate. Am. J. Orthod., (Oral Surg. Sect.), 33:407, 1947.

VITAMIN C (ASCORBIC ACID) DEFICIENCY

Severe vitamin C deficiency in humans results in scurvy, a disease characterized by hemorrhagic diathesis and retardation of wound healing. The hemorrhages commonly occur in areas of trauma or marked function.[18] Clinical features of scurvy include fatigue, breathlessness, lethargy, loss of appetite, sallow complexion, fleeting pains in joints and limbs, skin petechiae (particularly around hair follicles), epistaxis, ecchymosis (mainly in lower extremities), hemorrhage into muscles and deeper tissues (scurvy siderosis), hematuria, edema of the ankles and anemia.[22] Increased susceptibility to infection and impaired wound healing are also features of vitamin C deficiency.[7, 30]

Vitamin C deficiency (scurvy) results in defective formation and maintenance of collagen,[13] mucopolysaccharide ground substance, and intercellular cement substance in mesenchymal tissues.[34] Its effect on bone is marked by retardation or cessation of osteoid formation, impaired osteoblastic function,[25] and osteoporosis.[1, 9, 33] Vitamin C deficiency is also characterized by increased capillary permeability, susceptibility to traumatic hemorrhages, a hyporeactivity of the contractile elements of the peripheral blood vessels, and sluggishness of blood flow.[18] Changes in liver cells and in autonomic ganglion have been reported in chronic marginal vitamin C deficiency.[28]

Periodontal Disease

Gingivitis

Gingivitis with enlarged hemorrhagic bluish red gingiva is described as one of the classic signs of vitamin C deficiency (see Chapter 10), but **gingivitis is not caused by vitamin C deficiency** *per se.* Nor do all vitamin C deficient patients necessarily have gingivitis; it does not occur in the absence of local irritants. **If gingivitis is present in a vitamin C deficient patient it is caused by bacterial plaque.** Vitamin C deficiency may aggravate the gingival response to plaque and worsen the edema, enlargement, and bleeding,[14] and the severity may be reduced by correcting the deficiency; but gingivitis will remain so long as bacterial irritation is present.

The legendary association of severe gingival disease with scurvy led to the presumption that vitamin C deficiency is an etiologic factor in gingivitis which is so common at all ages. Attempts to correlate the ascorbic acid level of the blood with the incidence and severity of gingivitis have produced mixed results. Some claim there is such a relationship,[2, 17, 32] but the majority disagree.[4, 8, 12, 20, 21, 23, 27]

Periodontitis

It has been suggested that in humans alveolar bone loss results from ascorbic acid deficiency[3] and diets without citrus fruit juices,[29] but epidemiologic[24] and chemical[26] studies fail to identify vitamin C deficiency with the prevalence or severity of periodontal disease or tooth mobility.[19] In evaluating clinical studies dealing with ascorbic acid levels, it should be noted that it is the whole blood or leukocyte-platelet method of determination that is the reliable indicator.[5, 8, 23] Blood plasma levels fluctuate with variations in intake; whole blood or leukocyte-platelet levels indicate the nutritional status of the tissues in regard to vitamin C.[5, 22]

Experimental evidence

Changes in the supporting periodontal tissues and gingiva in vitamin C deficiency have been documented extensively in experimental animals.[10, 15, 16, 31, 33] **Acute vitamin-C deficiency results in edema and hemorrhage in the periodontal ligament, osteoporosis of alveolar bone, and tooth mobility; hemorrhage, edema, and degeneration of collagen fibers occur in the gingiva, but acute vitamin C deficiency does not cause or increase the incidence of gingivitis.**

The periodontal fibers that are least affected by vitamin C deficiency are those just below the junctional epithelium and above the alveolar crest, which explains the infrequent apical downgrowth of the epithelium.[31] **Local irritation must be present for gingivitis to occur in experimental animals with acute vitamin C deficiency.[10, 11] The deficiency alters the response to irritation so that the gingiva are enlarged, edematous, and hemorrhagic.** Oral mucosal tissues from scorbutic animals have significantly greater permeability to tritiated endotoxin than tissues from normal animals.[1] This finding appears also in pair-fed animals and is probably therefore multinutrition-dependent.[1] **Vitamin C deficiency also retards gingival healing.**[6, 30]

Vitamin C deficiency does not cause periodontal pockets; local irritating factors are required for pocket formation to occur. However, when pocket formation does occur in vitamin C deficiency, it is of greater depth than that normally produced under comparable local conditions. The occurrence of pocket formation and destruction of underlying tissues in vitamin C deficiency is not attributable to the deficiency alone, but indicates the presence of a complicating local factor.

Acute vitamin C deficiency alters the response of the supporting periodontal tissues to the extent that the destructive effect of gingival inflammation upon the underlying periodontal membrane and alveolar bone is accentuated.[11] The exaggerated destruction results partly from inability to marshal a defensive delimiting reaction to the inflammation and partly from destructive tendencies caused by the deficiency itself. Factors contributing to the destruction of the periodontal tissues in vitamin C deficiency include inability to form a peripheral delimiting connective tissue barrier, reduction in inflammatory cells, diminished vascular response, inhibition of fibroblast formation, and differentiation to osteoblasts, impaired formation of collagen, and mucopolysaccharide ground substance.

REFERENCES

Vitamin C

1. Alfano, M. C., Miller, S. A., and Drummond, J. F.: Effect of ascorbic acid deficiency on the permeability and collagen biosynthesis of oral mucosal epithelium. Ann. N.Y. Acad. Sci., 258:253, 1975.
2. Blockley, C. H., and Baenziger, P. E.: An investigation into the connection between the vitamin C content of the blood and periodontal disturbances. Br. Dent. J., 73:57, 1942.
3. Boyle, P. E.: Dietary deficiencies as a factor in the etiology of diffuse alveolar atrophy. J. Am. Dent. Assoc., 25:1436, 1938.
4. Burrill, D. Y.: Relationship of blood plasma vitamin C levels to gingival and periodontal disease. J. Dent. Res., 21:353, 1942.
5. Butler, A. M., and Cushman, M.: Distribution of ascorbic acid in blood and its nutritional significance. J. Clin. Invest., 19:459, 1940.
6. Cabrini, R. L., and Carranza, F. A., Jr.: Alkaline and acid phosphatase in gingival and tongue wounds in normal and vitamin C deficient animals. J. Periodontol., 34:74, 1963.
7. Cabrini, R. L., and Carranza, F. A., Jr.: Adenosine triphosphatase in normal and scorbutic wounds. Nature, 200:1113, 1963.
8. Crandon, J. H., Lund, C. C., and Dill, D. B.: Experimental human scurvy. N. Engl. J. Med., 223:353, 1940.
9. Follis, R. H.: The Pathology of Nutritional Disease. Springfield, Ill., Charles C Thomas, Publisher, 1948, p. 134.
10. Glickman, I.: Acute vitamin C deficiency and periodontal disease. I. The periodontal tissues of the guinea pig in acute vitamin C deficiency. J. Dent. Res., 27:9, 1948.
11. Glickman, I.: Acute vitamin C deficiency and the periodontal tissues. II. The effect of acute vitamin C deficiency upon the response of the periodontal tissues of the guinea pig to artificially induced inflammation. J. Dent. Res., 27:201, 1948.
12. Glickman, I., and Dines, M. M.: Effect of increased ascorbic acid blood levels on the ascorbic acid level in treated and nontreated gingiva. J. Dent. Res., 42:1152, 1963.
13. Gould, B. S.: Ascorbic acid-independent and ascorbic acid-dependent collagen-forming mechanisms. Ann. N.Y. Acad. Sci., 92:168, 1961.
14. Hodges, R. E., et al.: Experimental scurvy in man. Am. J. Clin. Nutrit., 22:535, 1969.
15. Hojer, J. A.: Studies in scurvy. Acta Paediatr. (Suppl.), 3:119, 1924.
16. Hojer, J. A., and Westin, G.: Jaws and teeth in scorbutic guinea pig. Dent. Cosmos, 67:1, 1925.
17. Keller, S. E., Ringsdorf, W. M., and Cheraskin, E.: Interplay of local and systemic influences in the periodontal diseases. J. Periodontol., 34:259, 1963.
18. Lee, R. E., and Lee, N. Z.: The peripheral vascular system and its reactions in scurvy: An experimental study. Am. J. Physiol., 149:465, 1947.
19. O'Leary, T. J., Rudd, K. D., Crump, P. P., and Kruase, R. E.: The effect of ascorbic acid supplementation on tooth mobility. J. Periodontol., 40:284, 1969.
20. Parfitt, G. J., and Hand, C. D.: Reduced plasma ascorbic acid levels and gingival health. J. Periodontol., 34:347, 1963.
21. Perlitsh, M., Nielsen, A. G., and Stanmeyer, W. R.: Ascorbic acid plasma levels and gingival health in personnel wintering over in Antarctica. J. Dent. Res., 40:789, 1961.
22. Ralli, E. P., and Sherry, S.: Adult scurvy and the metabolism of vitamin C. Medicine, 20:251, 1941.
23. Restarski, J. S., and Pijoan, M.: Gingivitis and vitamin C. J. Am. Dent. Assoc., 31:1323, 1944.
24. Russell, A. L.: International nutrition surveys: A

summary of preliminary dental findings. J. Dent. Res., *42*:233, 1963.

25. Salter, W. T., and Aub, J. C.: Studies of calcium and phosphorus metabolism. IX. Deposition of calcium in bone in healing scorbutus. Arch. Pathol., *11*:380, 1931.

26. Shannon, I., and Gibson, W. A.: Intravenous ascorbic acid loading in subjects classified as to periodontal status. J. Dent. Res., *44*:355, 1965.

27. Spies, T. D.: Nutrition and disease. Postgrad. Med., *17*:2, 1955.

28. Sulkin, N. M., and Sulkin, D. F.: Tissue changes induced by marginal vitamin C deficiency. Ann. N.Y. Acad. Sci., *258*:317, 1975.

29. Thomas, A. E., Busby, M. C., Ringsdorf, W. M., and Cheraskin, E.: Ascorbic acid and alveolar bone loss. Oral Surg., *15*:555, 1962.

30. Turesky, S., and Glickman, I.: Histochemical evaluation of gingival healing in experimental animals on adequate and vitamin C deficient diets. J. Dent. Res., *33*:273, 1954.

31. Waerhaug, J.: Effect of C-avitaminosis on the supporting structures of the teeth. J. Periodontol., *29*:87, 1958.

32. Weisberger, D., Young, A. P., and Morse, F. W.: Study of ascorbic acid blood levels in dental patients. J. Dent. Res., *17*:101, 1938.

33. Wolbach, S. B., and Bessey, O. A.: Tissue changes in vitamin deficiencies. Physiol. Rev., *22*:233, 1942.

34. Wolbach, S. B., and Howe, P. R.: Intercellular substances in experimental scorbutus. Arch. Pathol., *1*:1, 1926.

VITAMIN D (CALCIUM AND PHOSPHORUS) DEFICIENCIES

Vitamin D, a fat-soluble vitamin, is essential for the absorption of calcium from the gastrointestinal tract, and for the maintenance of the calcium-phosphorus balance and the formation of teeth and bones. The metabolism of calcium and phosphorus, and vitamin D, are interrelated. The effects of variations of the calcium, phosphorus and vitamin D intake upon the skeletal and dental structures are influenced by numerous other factors, such as parathyroid function, the presence of carbohydrate, fat, and such inorganic elements as strontium and beryllium, and age. Deficiency in vitamin D and'or imbalance in the calcium-phosphorus intake result in *rickets* in the very young and *osteomalacia* in adults. Their effect upon the periodontal tissues of experimental animals has been described as follows:

Vitamin D deficiency with normal dietary calcium and phosphorus in young dogs is characterized by osteoporosis of alveolar bone;[5] osteoid formed at a normal rate, but remaining uncalcified; failure of osteoid to resorb, leading to its excessive accumulation; reduction in the width of the periodontal space; normal rate of cementum formation but defective calcification and some cementum resorption;[16] and distortion of the growth pattern of alveolar bone. In young rats the periodontium is unaltered in vitamin D deficiency, provided that the diet is adequate in minerals.[13]

In osteomalacic animals there is rapid, generalized, severe osteoclastic resorption of alveolar bone, proliferation of fibroblasts which replace bone and marrow, and new bone formation around remnants of unresorbed bone trabeculae.[7] Radiographically there are generalized partial to complete disappearance of the lamina dura and reduced density of supporting bone, loss of trabeculae, increased radiolucence of trabecular interstices, and increased prominence of remaining trabeculae. Microscopic and radiographic changes in the periodontium are almost identical with those in experimentally induced hyperparathyroidism.

In *vitamin D and calcium deficiency with normal dietary phosphorus* there are generalized bone resorption in the jaws, fibro-osteoid hemorrhage in the marrow spaces, and destruction of the periodontal ligament.[5] The pattern is suggestive of changes in hyperparathyroidism.

Vitamin D and phosphorus deficiency with normal dietary calcium presents rachitic changes characterized by marked osteoid deposition.[11]

In *calcium and phosphorus deficiency with normal vitamin D* there is excessive bone resorption;[1, 5] resorption of alveolar bone and cementum occurs in adult animals on a calcium-deficient diet.[10]

In *phosphorus deficiency with normal dietary vitamin D and calcium,* jaw growth is disturbed, and tooth eruption and condylar growth retarded,[6, 15] accompanied by malocclusion.

Calcium deficiency in young rats produces osteoporosis and reduction in the number and diameter of periodontal fibers and increased cemental resorption.[13]

Hypervitaminosis D

Hypervitaminosis D in humans is characterized by nausea, vomiting, diarrhea, epigastric fullness, polyuria, polydipsia, albuminuria, impaired renal function, hypercalcemia, or hyperphosphatemia. It may terminate fatally. In experimental animals, Follis[9] observed that excessive doses of vitamin D (125,000 units of vitamin D given daily for nine days) resulted in marked osteoblastic activity, and production of large quantities of osteoid about the trabeculae in the shafts of long bones. Baker[2] noted that guinea pigs maintained on hypervitaminotic D diets develop generalized osteoporosis and metastatic calcifications. Weinmann and Sicher[17] suggested that the bone destructive effect of hypervitaminosis D is a phenomenon secondary to renal damage which would create a condition of hyperparathyroidism.

Oral Findings. The periodontal findings in experimental hypervitaminosis D include osteosclerosis characterized by marked endosteal and periosteal bone formation (or deposition of an amorphous highly calcified material), osteoporosis and resorption of alveolar bone,[8] dystrophic calcification in the periodontal ligament and gingiva, severe calculus formation, deposition of a cementum-like substance on the root surfaces (resulting in hypercementosis and the ankylosis of many teeth), and extensive periodontal disease.[3, 4]

Nomura found deposits of dystrophic calcification in the collagen fiber bundles,[12] while Shoshan et al. reported calcification only by combining hypervitaminosis D with osteolathyrism, but not by the vitamin deficiency alone.[14]

REFERENCES

Vitamin D (Calcium and Phosphorus) Deficiencies

1. Arnim, S. S., Clarke, M. F., Anderson, B. G., and Smith, A. H.: Dental changes in rats consuming diet poor in organic salts. Yale J. Biol. Med., 9:117, 1936.
2. Baker, S. L.: The general pathology of bone. In Shanks, S. C., and Kerley, P.: A Textbook of X-ray Diagnosis. 2nd ed. Philadelphia, W. B. Saunders Co., 1950.
3. Becks, H.: Dangerous effects of vitamin D overdosage on dental and paradental structure. J. Am. Dent. Assoc., 29:1947, 1942.
4. Becks, H., Collins, D. A., and Freytog, R. M.: Changes in oral structures of the dogs persisting after chronic overdoses of vitamin D. Am. J. Orthod., 32:463, 1946.
5. Becks, H., and Weber, M.: Influence of diet in bone system with special reference to alveolar process and labyrinthine capsule. J. Am. Dent. Assoc., 18:197, 1931.
6. Burrill, D. Y.: The effect of low phosphorus intake on the growth of the jaws in dogs. J. Am. Dent. Assoc., 30:513, 1943.
7. Dreizen, S., Levy, B. M., Bernick, S., Hampton, J. K., Jr., and Kraintz, L.: Studies on the biology of the periodontium of marmosets. III. Periodontal bone changes in marmosets with osteomalacia and hyperparathyroidism. Israel J. Med. Sci., 3:731, 1967.
8. Fahmy, H., Rodgers, W. E., Mitchell, D. F., and Brewer, H. E.: Effects of hypervitaminosis D on the periodontium of the hamster. J. Dent. Res., 40:870, 1961.
9. Follis, R. H., Jr.: The influence of essential nutrients and hormones on cartilage and bone. Trans. Josiah Macy Jr. Foundation Conference on Metabolic Interrelations, 2:221, 1950.
10. Henrikson, P.: Periodontal disease and calcium deficiency: An experimental study in the dog. Acta Odont. Scand., 26:[Suppl. 50.] 1, 1968.
11. MacCollum, E. V., Simmonds, N., Shipley, P. G., and Park, B. A.: The production of rickets by diets low in phosphorus and fat soluble. A. J. Biol. Chem., 47:507, 1921.
12. Nomura, H.: Histopathological study of experimental hypervitaminosis D_2 on the periodontium of the rat. Shikwa Gaku, 69:1, 1969.
13. Oliver, W. M.: The effect of deficiencies of calcium, vitamin D, or calcium and vitamin D and of variations in the source of dietary protein on the supporting tissues on the rat molar. J. Periodont. Res., 4:56, 1969.
14. Shoshan, S., Pisanti, S., and Sciaky, I.: The effect of hypervitaminosis D on the periodontal membrane collagen in lathyritic rats. J. Periodont. Res., 2:121, 1967.
15. Weinmann, J. P.: Rachitic changes of the mandibular condyle of the rat. J. Dent. Res., 25:509, 1946.
16. Weinmann, J. P., and Schour, I.: Experimental studies in calcification. Am. J. Pathol., 21:821, 1047, 1945.
17. Weinmann, J. P., and Sicher, H.: Bone and bones. St. Louis, The C. V. Mosby Co., 1948, p. 147.

VITAMIN E, VITAMIN K, AND VITAMIN P DEFICIENCIES

Vitamin E

No relationship has been demonstrated between deficiencies in vitamin E and oral disease.[5] Extirpation of the submaxillary and sublingual glands in vitamin E

deficient animals results in gingival bleeding, loosening and exfoliation of the molars, and purulent discharge from the
sockets.[2] In humans, a favorable response
to vitamin E therapy has been reported in
patients having severe periodontal disease,
with a minimum of local irritating factors.[4]

Vitamin K

Vitamin K is necessary for the production of prothrombin in the liver; vitamin K
deficiency results in a hemorrhagic tendency. It may cause excessive gingival
bleeding after toothbrushing, or spontaneously. In humans it is synthesized by
bacteria in the intestinal tract. Antibiotics
and sulfa drugs which inhibit the bacterial
action may interfere with vitamin K synthesis. Bile salts are important in the absorption of vitamin K; obstruction of the
biliary tract may lead to hypoprothrombinemia. Vitamin K is used for the prevention
and control of oral hemorrhage.

Vitamin P (citrin)

Vitamin P is involved in the maintenance of capillary integrity and the prevention of capillary fragility.[1, 6] It has been
used therapeutically for the control of
hemorrhage and in the treatment of blood
dyscrasias.[7] Kreshover and Burket[3] suggested that the capillary fragility frequently encountered in patients with
periodontal disease may be due in part to
vitamin P deficiency. This is based on the
finding of normal blood ascorbic acid levels in patients who manifested a high petechial count in capillary fragility testing.
The use of citrin in the treatment of gingival disease is still in the experimental
stage.

REFERENCES

Vitamin E, Vitamin K, and Vitamin P Deficiencies

1. Bourne, G.: Vitamin P deficiency in guinea pigs.
   Nature, 152:659, 1943.
2. Goldbach, H.: Success of vitamin E therapy in
   periodontal disease. Ztschr. Stomatol., 43:379,
   1946.
3. Kreshover, S., and Burket, L.: Cited in Burket,
   L.: Oral Medicine. Philadelphia, J. B. Lippincott Co., 1946, p. 411.
4. Lieb, H., and Mathis, H.: The treatment of periodontal disease with vitamin E. Ztschr. Stomatol., 47:358, 1950.
5. Nelson, M. A., and Chaudhry, A. P.: Effects of
   tocopherol (vitamin E) deficient diet on some
   oral, para-oral and hematopoietic tissues of the
   rat. J. Dent. Res., 45:1072, 1966.
6. Rusznyák, S., and Szent-Györgyi, A.: Vitamin P:
   flavonals as vitamins. Nature, 138:27, 1936.
7. Scarborough, H.: Vitamin P. Biochem. J., 33:1400,
   1939.

PROTEIN DEFICIENCY

Protein depletion results in hypoprotein-
emia with many pathologic changes including muscular atrophy, weakness,
weight loss, anemia, leukopenia, edema,
impaired lactation, decreased capacity to
form antibodies, decreased resistance to
infection, slow wound healing, lymphoid
depletion, and reduced ability to form certain hormones and enzyme systems.[2] *Kwashiorkor*, a protein deficiency disease of
children with a high mortality rate, is
fairly widespread in malnourished populations.[12]

Oral Manifestations. Protein deprivation
causes the following changes in the periodontium of experimental animals:[4, 6, 9] degeneration of the connective tissue of the gingiva
and periodontal ligament, osteoporosis of alveolar bone,[3] retardation in the deposition of
cementum, delayed wound healing[13] (Fig. 28–
3), and atrophy of the tongue epithelium.[15]
Similar changes occur in the periosteum and
bone in other areas. Osteoporosis results from
reduced deposition of osteoid, reduction in
number of osteoblasts, and retardation in the
morphodifferentiation of connective tissue cells
to form osteoblasts, rather than from increased osteoclasis. These observations are of
interest in that they reveal loss of alveolar
bone that is the result of the inhibition of
normal bone-formative activity rather than
the introduction of destructive factors.

Protein deficiency accentuates the destructive effects of local irritants[14] and occlusal trauma[11] upon the periodontal tissues, but the initiation of gingival
inflammation and its severity depend upon

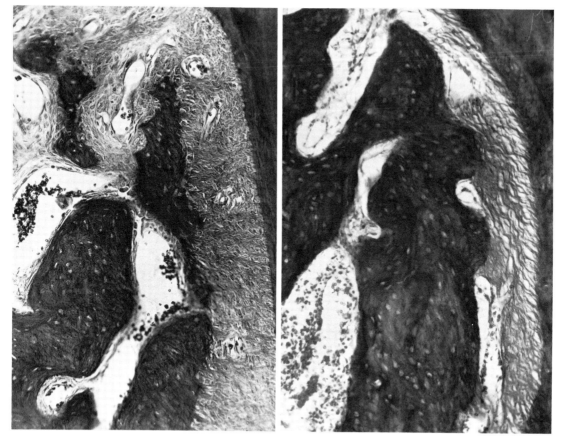

Figure 28–3   The Effect of Protein Deprivation upon the Periodontium of the Albino Rat. *Left,* **Control Animal.** Periodontal ligament and alveolar bone between the molar roots, showing dense collagen fibers. Note continuity of the collagen fibrils of the periodontal ligament with the matrix of the bone and polyhedral cells along the bone margin between the periodontal fibers. *Right,* **Protein Deprivation.** Periodontal ligament and alveolar bone between the molar roots. Note degeneration of the periodontal ligament marked by reduction in number and wavy outline of collagen fibrils. A clear-cut demarcation is seen between the bone matrix and the periodontal ligament (compare with control).

the local irritants. Tryptophan deficiency in rats results in osteoporosis of alveolar bone.[1]

Combined protein-vitamin deficiencies

Protein deficiency commonly produces anemia. However, protein deficiencies are always accompanied by those of hematopoietic vitamins and iron, and vitamin deficiencies include some degree of disturbed protein metabolism, so that anemia is often the result of combined protein-vitamin deficiency.[5] Such deficiency can produce macrocytic anemia with hematologic and oral changes identical with those of pernicious anemia (see Chapter 30). Several types of anemia occur in kwashiorkor, and the oral changes resemble those of pellagra, which is a mixed protein-vitamin deficiency state with severe oral manifestations.

STARVATION

The term "hunger osteopathy" connotes skeletal disturbances that occur in individuals in famine areas. Such disturbances are characterized by a reduction in the amount of normally calcified bone, and have been attributed to deficiencies in calcium, phosphorus, vitamin D, and protein, and to associated hormonal dysfunction. In a study of controlled semi-starvation in

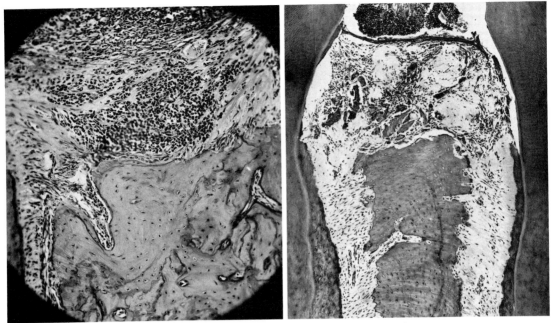

Fig. 28-4   Fig. 28-5

Figure 28-4   Margin of Alveolar Bone beneath area of artificially induced inflammation in albino rat on adequate diet. The bone surface in relation to the leukocytic infiltration presents lacunar resorption and an adjacent layer of osteoid lined with osteoblasts.

Figure 28-5   Interdental Bony Septum subjacent to artificially induced gingival inflammation in albino rat on starvation diet. The bone presents lacunar resorption without any evidence of new bone formation. (Compare with Fig. 28-4.)

young adults,[10] there were no changes in the oral cavity or skeletal system despite a 24 per cent loss of body weight. Another study, however, showed reduction in plaque index and considerable increase in gingival index, as the fasting period lengthened.[12a]

Oral Changes.   In experimental animals acute starvation results in osteoporosis of alveolar bone and other bones, reduction in the height of alveolar bone, and accentuated bone loss associated with gingival inflammation[8] (Figs. 28-4 and 28-5). Furthermore, bone formation associated with extrusion of teeth following the extraction of functional antagonists is impaired by acute starvation.[7]

REFERENCES

Protein Deficiency

1. Bavetta, L. A., and Bernick, S.: Effect of tryptophane deficiency on bones and teeth of rats. III. Effect of age. Oral Surg., 9:308, 1956.
2. Cannon, P. R.: Some Pathologic Consequences of Protein and Amino Acid Deficiencies. Springfield, Ill., Charles C Thomas, Publisher, 1948.
3. Carranza, F. A., Jr., Cabrini, R. L., Lopez Otero, R., and Stahl, S. S.: Histometric analysis of interradicular bone in protein deficient animals. J. Periodont. Res., 4:292, 1969.
4. Chawla, T. N., and Glickman, I.: Protein deprivation and the periodontal structures of the albino rat. Oral Surg., 4:578, 1951.
5. Dreizen, S.: Oral manifestations of human nutritional anemias. Arch. Environ. Health, 5:66, 1962.
6. Frandsen, A. M., et. al.: The effects of various levels of dietary protein on the periodontal tissues of young rats. J. Periodontol., 24:135, 1953.
7. Glickman, I.: The effect of acute starvation upon the apposition of alveolar bone associated with the extraction of functional antagonists. J. Dent. Res., 24:155, 1945.
8. Glickman, I., Morse, A., and Robinson, L.: The systemic influence upon bone in periodontoclasia. J. Am. Dent. Assoc., 31:1435, 1944.
9. Goldman, H. M.: Protein deprivation in rats. J. Dent. Res., 39:690, 1960.
10. Keys, A., et al.: The Biology of Human Starvation. Vol. 1, Chap. 12. Minneapolis, University of Minnesota Press, 1950.
11. Miller, S. C., Stahl, S. S., and Goldsmith, E. D.: The effects of vertical occlusal trauma on the periodontium of protein deprived young adult rats. J. Periodontol., 28:87, 1957.
12. Scrimshaw, N. S., and Béhar, M.: Protein malnu-

trition in young children. Science, *133*:2039, 1961.

12a. Squire, C. F., and Costley, J. M.: Gingival status during prolonged fasting for weight loss. J. Periodontol., *47*:98, 1976.

13. Stahl, S. S.: The effect of a protein-free diet on the healing of gingival wounds in rats. Arch. Oral Biol., 7:551, 1962.

14. Stahl, S. S., Sandler, H. C., and Cahn, L.: The effects of protein deprivation upon the oral tissues of the rat and particularly upon the periodontal structures under irritation. Oral Surg., 8:760, 1955.

15. Stein, G., and Ziskin, D.: The effect of protein free diet on the teeth and the periodontium of the albino rat. J. Dent. Res., 28:529, 1949.

MINERAL DEFICIENCIES AND TOXICITIES

Iron

Pallor of the oral cavity and tongue are the most common and sometimes only oral manifestations of iron deficiency anemia. The tongue may also be swollen with a blotchy or total atrophy of the papillary epithelium.[9, 28] Petechial hemorrhages in the mucosa and angular cheilitis occur in some cases.

Deutsch et al.[10] produced chronic iron deficiency anemias in rats by feeding them liquid and powdered milk diets; the blood studies confirmed the anemic state. Changes observed in the periodontium, however, were related to the physical consistency of the diet and not to the anemia.

Fluoride

Observations in populations using fluoride water supplies do not agree regarding the effects, if any, of ingested fluoride upon the condition of the periodontium (see Chapter 22). Findings in experimental animals vary, with some investigators reporting that fluoride increases periodontal disease,[26, 30] and others that it decreases[8] or protects against it.[27] It has also been shown that fluoride reduces the severity of cortisone-induced alveolar bone resorption,[34] prevents adverse effects of hypervitaminosis D,[14] and inhibits bone resorption in tissue culture.[17] Fluoride in the drinking water in levels used to prevent tooth decay presents no health hazards, although at much higher concentrations fluoride may affect the skeletal system adversely and produce spondylosis deformans characterized by progressive osteo-

sclerosis, ossification of tendon and ligament insertions, and spinal rigidity.[22] In experimental animals fluoride intoxication results in extensive periosteal bone deposition at sites of muscular insertion and generalized osteoporosis of the jaws.[4] Periodontal disease with loss of alveolar bone appeared to be associated with increased fluorine intake in South African natives.[1] Based upon increased bone density associated with high levels of ingested fluoride, as much as 100 mg. per day of sodium fluoride has been tried in the treatment of osteoporosis.[21]

Other intoxications

Reduction in the rate of alveolar bone formation,[11] widening of the periodontal ligament,[11, 23] retarded tooth eruption, and gingival enlargement with connective tissue hyperplasia have also been observed in magnesium-deficient animals.[6] Other changes include altered alveolar bone architecture (with the formation of a mosaic pattern[7]), increased resorption, fibrosis of the marrow, calculus formation, and loosening of the teeth. Molybdenum toxicity in experimental animals causes mandibular exostoses, cemental spurs, hypercementosis, and disorganization of the odontoblastic layer.[29]

Berillium and strontium intoxications result in a hyperproduction of bone, cementum and dentin matrix that do not calcify, leading to a rickets-like lesion.[19]

OSTEOLATHYRISM

Lathyrism is a disease of the nervous system in man and domestic animals caused by the ingestion of certain types of peas, such as *Lathyrus sativus*. It does not produce changes in the jaws or oral tissues. Animals fed diets rich in *Lathyrus odoratus* peas, or administered certain aminonitriles such as aminoacetonitrile, aminopropionitrile, or methyleneaminonitrile develop osteolathyrism, a disease which bears no resemblance to lathyrism in humans.[32] Osteolathyrism is characterized by oral as well as systemic changes.

Exostoses occur on the jaws in areas of muscle attachment, and the condylar cartilage is enlarged. The fibroblasts of the periodontal

ligament exhibit increased cytoplasmic basophilia and palisading, and the collagen fibers
are fine, disoriented, and embedded in amorphous eosinophilic material.[13, 25] Hydroxypro-
line activity and conversion of soluble collagen to the insoluble type are decreased
according to some authors,[33] but in tissue culture studies with a lathyrogenic agent the
synthesis and degradation of collagen are unaffected.[18] The alveolar bone is osteoporotic,
and there are pronounced hypercementosis
and loosening of teeth.[12] Mechanical force is
an important contributing factor in the development of osteolathyritic changes in the
jaws,[24] and systemic conditioning agents modify their severity.[15]

The electron microscope shows mottling of
the bone matrix and disturbed development
of osteoblasts.[3]

CALCIPHYLAXIS

*Calciphylaxis is a condition of induced
systemic hypersensitivity described by
Selye,*[31] in which tissues respond to appropriate challenging agents with precipi-
tous, sometimes evanescent local calcification. Substances which predispose to
calciphylaxis are known as sensitizers;
agents which precipitate the calciphylaxis
phenomenon are known as challengers.
Sensitizers include dihydrotachysterol
(DHT), vitamin D, parathormone, and sodium acetylsulfathiazole among many calcium salts and phosphates.

Challengers may be *direct* or *indirect*.
Direct challengers include mechanical
trauma and various chemical agents (salts
of iron, chromium, aluminum, zinc, manganese, cesium) which cause calcification
at the site of application and may elicit
some form of systemic calciphylaxis when
administered intravenously or intraperiton-
eally. Indirect challengers have little or no
effect at the site of application and produce diverse systemic syndromes of calcification and sclerosis.

Prolonged administration of dihydrotachysterol (DHT) in rats produces a chronic
intoxication syndrome with the following
severe changes in the periodontium: osteosclerosis, pronounced osteoid formation, bulbous distortion in the shape of the
bone, and degeneration of the marrow and
the periodontal ligament. Intraperitoneal

administration of ferric dextran (Fe–Dex)
induced calciphylaxis which reduced the
toxic effects of DHT upon the periodontium.[16]

DISTURBANCES OF THE ACID-BASE BALANCE

The acid-base balance refers to the state
of equilibrium that normally exists between the acid and base components of
the tissues and fluids of the body. Acidosis
is an abnormal state in which there is
accumulation of acids or loss of alkali in
the blood; it may be accompanied by
changes in bone.[2] Acidosis from renal tu-
bular insufficiency without glomerular insufficiency may result in osteomalacia in
adults. Osteoporosis of the jaws has been
described associated with acidosis in experimental animals.[5] Alkalosis is an abnormal state in which there is an accumulation of alkali or loss of acid. Retrograde
changes in alveolar bone have been described in animals maintained on alkaline
diets.[20]

REFERENCES

Mineral Deficiencies and Toxicities

1. Abrahams, L. C.: Masticatory apparatus of the people of Calvinia and Namaqualand in the North-Western Cape of the Union of South Africa. J. Dent. Assoc. South Africa, *1*:5, 1946.
2. Albright, F., and Reifenstein, E. C.: The Parathyroid Glands and Metabolic Bone Disease. Baltimore, Williams & Wilkins Co., 1948, p. 241.
3. Amemiya, A.: Electron microscopic study of periosteal hyperostosis in rats with lathyrism induced by aminoacetonitrile. Bull. Tokyo Med. Dent. Univ., *13*:319, 1966.
4. Bauer, W. H.: Experimental chronic fluorine intoxication: Effects on bones and teeth. Am. J. Orthod., *31*:700, 1945.
5. Bauer, W., and Haslhofer, L.: Veränderung der Kiefer und Zähne durch Zuckerverabreichung. Ztschr. Stomatol., *31*:1359, 1933.
6. Becks, H., and Furuta, W. J.: Effect of magnesium deficient diets on oral and dental tissues. II. Changes in the enamel structure. J. Am. Dent. Assoc., *28*:1083, 1941.
7. Becks, H., and Furuta, W. J.: The effects of magnesium deficient diets on oral and dental tissues. III. Changes in dentine and pulp tissue. Am. J. Orthod., *28*:1, 1942.
8. Costich, E. R., Hein, J. W., Hodge, H. C., and Shourie, K. L.: Reduction of hamster perio-

dontal disease by sodium fluoride and sodium monofluorophosphate in drinking water. J. Am. Dent. Assoc., 55:617, 1957.

9. Darby, W. J.: The oral manifestations of iron deficiency. J.A.M.A., 130:830, 1946.

10. Deutsch, C. M., Dreizen, S., and Stahl, S. S.: The effects of chronic deficiency anemia on the periodontium of the adult rat. J. Periodontol., 40:736, 1969.

11. Gagnon, J. A., Schour, I., and Patras, M. C.: Effect of magnesium deficiency on dentin apposition and eruption in incisor of rat. Proc. Soc. Expr. Biol. Med., 49:662, 1942.

12. Gardner, A. F.: Alterations in mesenchymal and ectodermal tissues during experimental lathyrism. Apposition and calcification of cementum. Paradontology, 20:111, 1966.

13. Gardner, A. F.: Morphologic study of oral connective tissue in lathyrism. J. Dent. Res., 39:24, 1960.

14. Gedalia, I., and Binderman, I.: Effect of fluoride on hypervitaminosis D in rats. J. Dent. Res., 45:825, 1966.

15. Glickman, I., Selye, H., and Smulow, J. B.: Systemic factors which influence the manifestations of osteolathyrism in the periodontium. J. Dent. Res., 42:835, 1963.

16. Glickman, I., Selye, H., and Smulow, J. B.: Reduction by calciphylaxis of the effects of chronic dihydrotachysterol overdose upon the periodontium. J. Dent. Res., 44:374, 1965.

17. Goldhaber, P.: The inhibition of bone resorption in tissue culture by nontoxic concentrations of sodium fluoride. Israel J. Med. Sci., 3:617, 1967.

18. Golub, L., Stern, B., Glimcher, M., and Goldhaber, P.: The effect of a lathyrogenic agent on the synthesis and degradation of mouse bone collagen in tissue culture. Arch. Oral Biol., 13:1395, 1968.

19. Gravina, O., Cabrini, R. L., and Carranza, F. A., Jr.: Effect of a strontium-containing diet on periodontal tissues of rat molars. J. Periodontol., 41:174, 1970.

20. Jones, M. R., and Simonton, F. V.: Mineral metabolism in relation to alveolar atrophy in dogs. J. Am. Dent. Assoc., 15:881, 1928.

21. Jowsey, J., Schenk, R. K., and Reutter, F. W.: Some results of the effect of fluoride on bone tissue in osteoporosis. J. Clin. Endocrinol., Metabol., 28:869, 1968.

22. Kemp, F. H., Murray, M. M., and Wilson, D. C.: Spondylosis deformans in relation to fluorine and general nutrition. Lancet, 243:93, 1942.

23. Klein, H., Orent, E. R., and McCollum, E. V.: Effects of magnesium deficiency on teeth and their supporting structures in rats. Am. J. Physiol., 112:256, 1935.

24. Krikos, G., Beltran, R., and Cohen, A.: Significance of mechanical stress on the development of periodontal lesions in lathyritic rats. J. Dent. Res., 44:600, 1965.

25. Krikos, G. A., Morris, A. L., Hammond, W. S., and McClure, H. H.: Oral changes in experimental lathyrism (odoratism). Oral Surg., 11:309, 1958.

26. Kristoffersen, T., Bang, G., and Meyer, K.: Lack of effect of high doses of fluoride in prevention of alveolar bone loss in rats. J. Periodont. Res., 5:127, 1970.

27. Likins, R. C., Pakis, G., and McClure, F. J.: Effect of fluoride and tetracycline on alveolar bone resorption in the rat. J. Dent. Res., 42:1532, 1963.

28. Monto, R. W., Rizek, R. A., and Fine, G.: Observations on the exfoliative cytology and histology of the oral mucous membranes in iron deficiency. Oral Surg., 14:965, 1961.

29. Ostram, C. A., Van Reen, R., and Miller, C. W.: Changes in the connective tissue of rats fed toxic diets containing molybdenum salts. J. Dent. Res., 40:520, 1961.

30. Ramseyer, W. F., Smith, C. A. H., and McCay, C. M.: Effect of sodium fluoride administration on body changes in old rats. J. Gerontol., 12:14, 1957.

31. Selye, H.: Calciphylaxis. Chicago, University of Chicago Press, 1962.

32. Selye, H.: Lathyrism. Rev. Can. Biol., 16:3, 1957.

33. Smith, D. J.: Biochemical aspects of repair in lathyrism. J. Dent. Res., 45:500, 1966.

34. Zipkin, I., Bernick, S., and Menczel, J.: A morphological study of the effect of fluoride on the periodontium of the hydrocortisone-treated rat. Periodontics, 3:111, 1965.

Chapter 29

Endocrinologic Influences in the Etiology of Periodontal Disease

HORMONAL INFLUENCES ON THE PERIODONTIUM

Hormones are organic substances produced by the endocrine glands. They are secreted directly into the blood stream and exert an important physiologic influence upon the functions of certain cells and systems. The significance of hormonal disturbances in the causation of periodontal disease is presented here.

Hypothyroidism

The effects of hypothyroidism vary with the age at which it occurs. The basal metabolic rate is depressed and growth retarded. Cretinism, juvenile myxedema, and adult myxedema are the three clinical syndromes that result from hypothyroidism.

Cretinism is the manifestation of hypothyroidism that is either congenital or occurs shortly after birth. Delayed physical and mental development is characteristic of the disease. There is understature and disproportion; bone growth is retarded; craniofacial development is abnormal. The cranium is disproportionately large and the face is infantile and coarse; the jaws are small; the rate of tooth eruption is retarded.[13]

Juvenile myxedema occurs between the ages of six and twelve, and may be related to iodine deficiency or other injurious influences on the thyroid gland. Among the first symptoms are physical inactivity, mental dullness, and inability to concentrate.[8] The body tissues have a pseudoedematous appearance. Oral changes may also give an early clue to the disorder. Tooth eruption is retarded, and the formation of the jaws is disturbed. The teeth are poorly formed; delayed formation of the dentin results in incompletely developed roots and patent pulp canals.

Hypothyroidism in the adult results in *myxedema*. The patient is easily fatigued, and usually gains weight in spite of lack of appetite. The characteristic nonpitting edema of subcutaneous tissues is seen. The basal metabolic rate and blood pressure are low, the pulse is slow, and the blood cholesterol is elevated.

Hypothyroidism and the periodontium

Aside from impaired development, no notable changes in the periodontal tissues have been attributed to cretinism. Chronic periodontal disease with severe bone loss has been described in patients with myxedema,[3, 8, 9] with the suggestion that the latter condition contributes to the periodontal destruction. Degenerative changes in the gingiva have been reported in thyroidectomized animals.[1, 20]

In animals with thiouracil-induced hypothyroidism, apposition of alveolar bone is retarded[6] and the size of the haversian systems is reduced,[4] but there is no evidence of periodontal disease.[5] Animals with experimentally induced myxedema present hyperparakeratosis with some keratosis of the gingival epithelium, edema, and disorganization of the collagen bundles in the connective tissue, hydropic degeneration and fragmentation of the fibers of the periodontal ligament, and osteoporosis of the alveolar bone.[11]

Hyperthyroidism

Hyperfunction of the gland is common in young and middle-aged adults. Among the symptoms are cardiovascular effects (increased pulse, hypertension, and cardiac enlargement), nervousness and emotional instability, loss of weight, and exophthalmia. Infants with this disorder show increased growth and development in contrast to the hypothyroid condition, with early eruption of the teeth. The teeth and jaws are well formed and present no unusual irregularities. Alveolar bone appears somewhat rarefied and partially decalcified. In the adult, salivary flow is increased owing to sympathetic hyperstimulation, but there are no notable oral changes.[13]

Hyperthyroidism and the periodontium

Osteoporosis of the alveolar bone, lacunar resorption, increase in the size of the marrow spaces (with fibrosis of the marrow and an increase in the width and vascularity of the periodontal ligament) have been described in experimental animals fed thyroid extract over a period of one to sixteen weeks.[1] Thyroid feeding accentuates the osteoporosis of alveolar bone induced in animals by tryptophane deficiency.[2]

Hypopituitarism

Hypopituitarism, a deficiency in the secretion of the anterior pituitary lobe, is marked by a retardation in the growth of all tissues. The earlier in life the condition occurs, the more severe the clinical changes. Hypopituitarism in children results in dwarfism. The pituitary dwarf is small, underdeveloped, and usually well proportioned, although not always. Disproportion in growth is attributable to other endocrine glands affected by the hyposecretion of adrenotrophic, thyrotrophic, and gonadotrophic hormones of the pituitary. The skeletal and genital systems are affected, but the nervous system is not involved; the patient is alert, and mentally exceeds the developmental age. The latter condition is in contradistinction to cretinism, in which mental as well as physical development is affected.

In dwarfism, the cranium and face develop very slowly, resembling those of a child of a much earlier age. The face is relatively small compared with the cranium, and the sinuses are underdeveloped, especially the frontal. Retardation in development of the teeth and jaws has been noted by many observers. There is delayed resorption of the deciduous teeth and marked retardation in formation and eruption of the permanent teeth. The growth of the maxilla and mandible is arrested, with the mandible showing the greater degree of change. Retardation in the growth of the ramus resulting in failure in increase of the vertical height of the mandible, reduced intermaxillary space, crowding of the teeth, and a tendency toward a distal relationship of the mandible have been attributed to hypopituitarism.

Hypopituitarism and the periodontium

The following is a summary of the microscopic changes observed in the periodontal tissues of experimental animals with artificially induced hypopituitarism:

Resorption of cementum in the molar bifurcation areas, reduced apposition of cementum, resorption of alveolar bone in animals with short postoperative life, with sclerosis and suggestion of mosaic pattern. The vascularity

of the periodontal ligament is reduced and there is degeneration of the ligament with cystic degeneration and calcification of many of the epithelial rests. The junctional epithelium is often atrophic or absent. It has been suggested that the changes observed in these animals may not be specific for hypophysectomy, but may be attributable to an associated reduction in the blood supply, caused either by the hypophysectomy or by resulting changes in other endocrine glands.[12, 14]

Hyperpituitarism

Hyperpituitarism, an increase in the secretion of the anterior lobe of the pituitary, results in giantism or acromegaly, depending upon the age at which it occurs. Hyperpituitarism before the age of six results in *giantism*, characterized by unusual height and disproportion. When hyperpituitarism occurs after the age of six, *juvenile acromegaly* is the result, with abnormal height, huge hands and feet, long face, and prognathic jaw.

In *adults*, hyperpituitarism results in *acromegaly*, which is characterized by a disproportionate overgrowth of the facial bones, with overdeveloped sinuses. The face is large with coarse features. The lips are greatly enlarged and localized areas of hyperpigmentation are often seen along the nasolabial folds. *A marked overgrowth of the alveolar process causes an increase in size of the dental arch and consequently affects the spacing of the teeth. This may affect the periodontium by introducing the irritation of food impaction. Hypercementosis is another feature of the increased rate of growth.*

Hypoparathyroidism

Hypoparathyroidism results from accidental removal of the glands in thyroidectomy or from deficiencies occurring early in life. There is a hypocalcemia and a resultant increased excitability of the nervous system. The condition is known as *parathyroid tetany*.

If the condition occurs in infancy, it causes enamel hypoplasia and disturbances in the calcification of dentin. The developing enamel and dentin show alternate irregular and accentuated zones of undercalcification and overcalcification. Dentin formed and calcified before the onset of the disease is not affected.

Hyperparathyroidism

Parathyroid hypersecretion produces generalized demineralization of the skeleton, the formation of bone cysts and giant cell tumors, increased osteoclasis, occasional osteoid formation, and proliferation of the connective tissue in the marrow spaces and the haversian canals. The serum calcium is increased, serum phosphorus is decreased, and serum phosphatase may be normal or elevated.[19]

Hyperparathyroidism and the periodontium

Different investigators report the percentage of patients with hyperparathyroidism who present oral changes as 25 per cent,[15] 45 per cent,[10] and 50 per cent.[16]

The oral changes include malocclusion and tooth mobility, radiographic evidence of alveolar osteoporosis with closely meshed trabeculae, widening of the periodontal space, absence of the lamina dura and radiolucent cystlike spaces.

Loss of lamina dura and giant cell tumors in the jaws are late signs of hyperparathyroid bone disease, which in itself is uncommon. Complete loss of the lamina dura does not occur often, and there is a danger of attaching too much diagnostic significance to it. Other diseases in which it may occur are *Paget's disease, fibrous dysplasia,* and *osteomalacia.*

In hyperparathyroidism associated with renal insufficiency, Weinmann[18] reported extensive resorption of lamellated bone and its replacement by immature coarse fibrillar spongy bone, and fibrosis of the bone marrow. In experimental animals,[19] small doses of parathormone induce a short period of osteoclasis followed by osteoblastic activity and osteosclerosis of the alveolar bone; massive doses lead to resorption of the bone and its replacement by connective tissue.

A relationship has been suggested between periodontal disease in dogs and hyperparathyroidism secondary to calcium deficiency in the diet.[7] This has not been confirmed by other studies.[17]

REFERENCES

1. Baume, L. J., and Becks, H.: The effect of thyroid hormone in dental and paradental structures. Paradentologie, 6:89, 1952.
2. Bavetta, L. A., Bernick, S., and Ershoff, B.: The influences of dietary thyroid on the bones and periodontium of rats on total and partial tryptophan deficiencies. J. Dent. Res., 36:13, 1957.
3. Becks, H.: Systemic background of paradentosis. J. Am. Dent. Assoc., 28:1447, 1941.
4. English, J. A.: Experimental effects of thiouracil and selenium on the teeth and jaws of dogs. J. Dent. Res., 28:172, 1949.
5. Fisher, R. L., and Mitchell, D. F.: Induced hypothyroidism on the periodontium of the hamster. I.A.D.R. Abstracts of the 40th Meeting, 1962, p. 67.
6. Glickman, I., and Pruzansky, S.: Propyl-thiouracil hypothyroidism in the albino rat. J. Dent. Res., 26:471, 1947.
7. Henrikson, P. A.: Periodontal disease and calcium deficiency in the dog. Acta Odont. Scand., 26:Suppl. 50, 1968.
8. Hutton, J. H.: Relation of endocrine disorders to dental disease. J. Am. Dent. Assoc., 23:226, 1936.
9. Lewis, A. B.: Oral manifestations of endocrine disturbances — myxedema. Dent. Cosmos, 77:47, 1935.
10. Rosenberg, E. H., and Guralnick, W. C.: Hyperparathyroidism. Oral Surg., 15:[Suppl. 2] 84, 1962.
11. Rosenberg, E. H., Goldman, H. M., and Garber, E.: The effects of experimental thyrotoxicosis and myxedema on the periodontium of rabbits. J. Dent. Res., 40:708, 1961.
12. Schour, I.: The effects of hypophysectomy on the periodontal tissues, J. Periodontol., 5:15, 1934.
13. Schour, I., and Massler, M.: Endocrines and dentistry. J. Am. Dent. Assoc., 30:595, 763, 943, 1943.
14. Shapiro, S., and Shklar, G.: The effect of hypophysectomy on the periodontium of the albino rat. J. Periodontol., 33:364, 1962.
15. Silverman, S., Gordan, G., Grant, T., Steinbach, H., Eisenberg, E., and Manson, R.: The dental structures in primary hyperparathyroidism. Oral Surg., 15:426, 1962.
16. Strock, M. S.: The mouth in hyperparathyroidism. N. Engl. J. Med., 224:1019, 1945.
17. Svanberg, G., Lindhe, J., Hugoson, A., and Grondahl, H. G.: Effect of nutritional hyperparathyroidism on experimental periodontitis in the dog. Scand. J. Dent. Res., 81:155, 1973.
18. Weinmann, J. P.: Bone changes in the jaw caused by renal hyperparathyroidism. J. Periodontol., 16:94, 1945.
19. Weinmann, J. P., and Schour, I.: The effect of parathyroid hormone on the alveolar bone and teeth of the normal and rachitic rat. Am. J. Pathol., 21:857, 1945.
20. Ziskin, R. D., and Stein, G.: The gingiva and oral mucous membrane of monkeys in experimental hypothyroidism. J. Dent. Res., 21:296, 1942.

Diabetes

As far back as 1862, Seiffert described an association between diabetes mellitus and pathologic changes in the oral cavity. Despite a voluminous literature on the subject, opinions still differ regarding the exact relationship of diabetes and oral disease. A variety of oral changes have been described in diabetic patients, such as dryness of the mouth; diffuse erythema of the oral mucosa; coated tongue and redness of the tongue, with marginal indentations and a tendency toward periodontal abscess formation; "diabetic periodontoclasia" and "diabetic stomatitis,"[56] enlarged gingiva, "sessile or pedunculated gingival polyps";[26] swollen, tender gingiva papillae that bleed profusely; polypoid gingival proliferations and loosened teeth;[40, 46] and increased incidence of periodontal disease,[49] with both vertical and horizontal bone destruction.[47]

Diabetic patients have a reduced resistance to infections, although it is not clear whether they have a higher actual incidence of infections or, once contracted, the infections become more severe.[45] This susceptibility to infections appears to be a combination of microangiopathy, metabolic acidosis, and ineffective phagocytosis by macrophages.[28]

Periodontal disease in diabetic patients follows no consistent pattern. Unusually severe gingival inflammation, deep periodontal pockets, and periodontal abscesses often occur in patients with poor oral hygiene and calculus accumulation. In juvenile diabetic patients there is often extensive periodontal destruction, which is noteworthy because of their age.

In many diabetic patients with periodontal disease, the gingival changes and bone loss are not unusual, although in others the severity of bone loss is impressive (Fig. 29–1).

The distribution and severity of local irritants and occlusal forces affect the severity of periodontal disease in diabetes. Diabetes does not cause gingivitis or

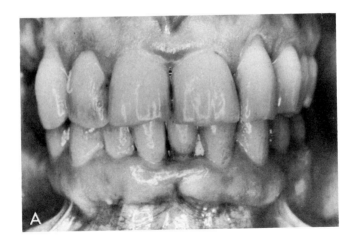

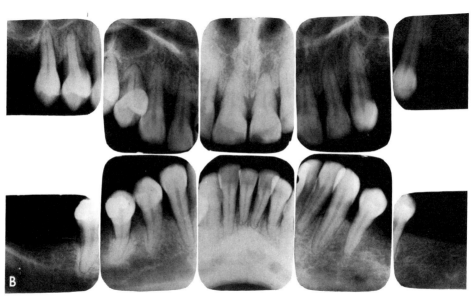

Figure 29–1   Diabetic Patient. *A,* Gingival inflammation and periodontal pockets in 34-year-old diabetic of long duration. *B,* Extensive generalized bone loss in patient shown in *A.* Failure to replace posterior teeth adds to the occlusal burden of the remaining dentition.

periodontal pockets, but there are indications that it alters the response of the periodontal tissues to local irritants and occlusal forces and that it hastens bone loss in periodontal disease and retards postsurgical healing of the periodontal tissues.

STUDIES IN HUMANS

Clinical aspects

Despite the generalized increased susceptibility to infection[44] and severe inflamma-

tion[39] in diabetes, some investigators[2, 8, 34, 41, 43, 53] recognize no relationship between diabetes and oral disease and maintain that when the two conditions exist together, it is a coincidence rather than a specific cause and effect relationship. Others report increased severity of gingivitis[14] and periodontal disease, with increased tooth mobility not related to increased local irritants[3] and an associated increase in tooth loss.[16]

Most of the above-mentioned studies have been highly subjective. In the last few years the utilization of indices to measure local irritants and clinical manifestations of the disease has permitted a more rigorous analysis of the relation between periodontal disease and diabetes. These more recent studies, however, also show no consistency, probably due to the diversity of indices used and differences in patient sampling. The majority of studies, however, show a higher prevalence and severity of periodontal disease in diabetics than in nondiabetic subjects with similar local irritation;[12, 18] other studies found no significant differences.[4] Glavind et al.,[22] after a detailed analysis of 51 diabetics and 51 controls, conclude that up to the age of 30 the rate of destruction is the same for diabetics and nondiabetics; between 30 and 40 years of age diabetics show a slight increase in periodontal breakdown as compared with nondiabetics; and patients suffering overt diabetes for more than 10 years show greater loss of periodontal structures than those with a history of less than 10 years. Also, those diabetics who present retinal changes show greater periodontal destruction. They conclude that the fact that lesions are similar suggests that they are caused by the same bacterial mechanisms; the increased periodontal destruction in patients with long-standing diabetes may reflect some unknown deficiency in the resistance of the diabetic periodontium.[22] In a clinical study of 50 diabetic children and an age-matched control group of 36 children, Bernick et al.[5] found a greater incidence of gingival inflammation in the diabetic group, with both groups having a similar oral hygiene score.

Comparison of the salivary and blood sugar levels with the periodontal condition of diabetics revealed that salivary glucose levels (one hour after breakfast) were higher in diabetics, but not to a degree which was diagnostic.[38] Salivary and blood sugar levels were correlated in nondiabetics, but only in diabetic females.[37] In another study,[17] the glucose content of gingival fluid and blood was found to be higher in diabetics than in nondiabetics with a similar plaque and gingival index; the protein content was found to be similar in both groups. Maider et al.[35] found a significant increase of salivary IgG in diabetic patients.

Microscopic aspects

Microscopic changes described in the gingiva include the following: hyperplasia with hyperkeratosis,[56] or a change from a stippled to smooth surface with diminished keratinization; intranuclear vacuolization in the epithelium; increased intensity of inflammation; fatty infiltration in the inflamed tissue;[21] an increase in calcified foreign bodies;[42] widening of the basement membrane of capillaries and precapillary arterioles[10, 27, 31] but no osteosclerotic changes;[29] PAS fuchsinophilic thickening of small blood vessels;[31] and reduced staining of acid mucopolysaccharides. Oxygen consumption in the gingiva and oxidation of glucose are reduced.[11]

Arteriolar changes consisting of increased fuchsinophilia, thickened walls, narrowed lumen, medial degeneration, and vacuolization have been reported in the gingiva of patients with diabetes and/or hypertensive cardiovascular disease.[52]

Among the microscopic changes described, thickening of the basement membrane of capillaries warrants special attention, because (a) this change in the vessel walls may hamper the transport of nutrients necessary for the maintenance of gingival tissues, and (b) it has been suggested that gingival biopsies may be an important aid for the detection of prediabetic and diabetic states. These procedures have been used in other tissues.[19, 51] The thickness of capillary and arteriolar wall basement membranes has been measured using optical[27, 29, 30] and electron microscopy,[1, 20, 33] but results have been inconsistent.

Listgarten et al.[33] studied with the electron microscope gingival biopsies of 10 diabetic and 10 nondiabetic subjects; each group was composed of 5 normal and 5 inflamed gingivae. A statistically significant increase in thickness of the basement membrane of capillaries was found in diabetics. However, there was considerable overlapping between the two groups, making it very difficult to use it as a diagnostic aid. The thickness of the basement membrane was found to be unrelated to inflammation, age, and duration of diabetes. Frantzis et al.[20] reported greater differences between diabetics and controls and suggested that it may have diagnostic importance.

STUDIES IN ANIMALS

There have been many studies of the periodontium in animals with diabetes induced by (a) injection of the drug alloxan;[23] (b) partial pancreatectomy;[9] or (c) spontaneous development of the disease in hamsters[50] or mice.[15, 48]

The following has been reported: osteoporosis and reduction in the height of alveolar bone (Fig. 29–2) occur in diabetic

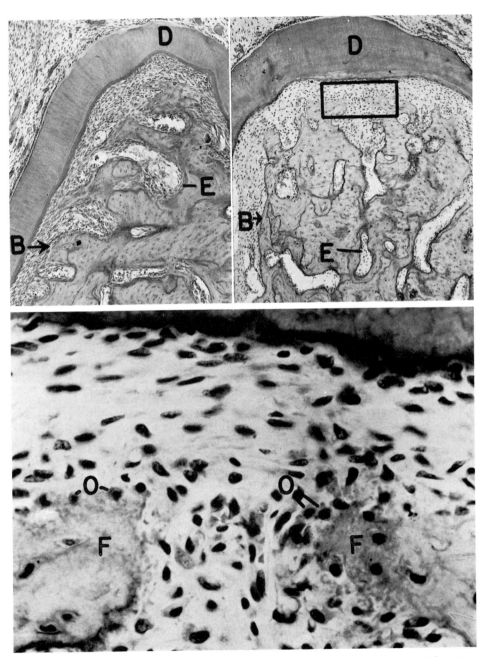

Figure 29–2 Changes in the Periodontium in Experimental Diabetes. *Top Left,* **Control Animal.** Bifurcation area of a mandibular molar (D) showing normal bone deposition adjacent to the periodontal ligament (B). The vessel channels and marrow spaces (E) are lined in part by newly formed bone and in part by resorption lacunae. *Top Right,* **Diabetic Animal.** Bone in bifurcation of a mandibular molar (D). Note absence of normal bone formation adjacent to the periodontal ligament (B) and along the vessel channels and marrow spaces (E). (Compare with control.) *Bottom,* High power study of the area enclosed within the rectangle above, showing fragmentation of the bone matrix (F) and release of the osteocytes (O).

animals, with comparable osteoporosis in other bones. The periodontal ligament and cementum are not affected, but glycogen is depleted in the gingiva. Others report that gingival inflammation and bone destruction associated with local irritants are more severe in diabetic than in nondiabetic animals.[6]

Generalized osteoporosis, resorption of the alveolar crest, and gingival inflammation and periodontal pocket formation associated with calculus have been described in Chinese hamsters with hereditary diabetes under insulin replacement therapy,[50] whereas no periodontal changes were observed in other animals with autosomal recessive diabetes.[48]

Periodontal injury produced by excessive occlusal forces[24] and periodontal atrophy from insufficient forces[32] are worsened in experimental diabetes, and postsurgical gingival healing is retarded.[25]

REFERENCES

1. Anapolle, S. F., Allright, J. T., and Craft, F. D.: The ultrastructure of the gingiva in the diabetic mouse. Microvasc. Res., *14*:132, 1972.
2. Badanes, B. B.: Diabetes acidosis and the significance of acid mouth. Dent. Cosmos, *75*:476, 1933.
3. Belting, C. M., Hinicker, J. J., and Dummett, C. O.: Influence of diabetes mellitus on the severity of periodontal disease. J. Periodontol., *35*:476, 1964.
4. Benveniste, R., Bixler, D., and Cornally, P. M.: Periodontal disease and diabetes. J. Periodontol., *38*:271, 1967.
5. Bernick, S. M., Cohen, D. W., Baker, L., and Laster, L.: Dental disease in children with diabetes mellitus. J. Periodontol., *46*:241, 1975.
6. Bissada, N. F., Schaffer, E. M., and Lazarow, A.: Effect of alloxan diabetes and local irritating factors on the periodontal structures of the rat. Periodontics, *4*:233, 1966.
7. Boenheim, F.: Endocrinen Status bei Paradentose. Zahnarztl. Rundsch., *37*:1002, 1928.
8. Boenheim, F.: The endocrine system in periodontal disease. *In* Miller, S. C.: Textbook of Periodontia. 2nd ed. Philladelphia, The Blakiston Co., 1943, p. 545.
9. Borghelli, R. F., Devoto, F. C. H., Foglia, V., and Erausquin, J.: Periodontal changes and dental caries in experimental prediabetes. Diabetes, *16*:804, 1967.
10. Campbell, M. J. A.: An electron microscope study of the basement membrane of the small vessels from the gingival tissue of the diabetic and non-diabetic patient. J. Dent. Res., *46*:1302, 1967.
11. Campbell, M. J. A.: The oxygen utilization and glucose oxidation rate of gingival tissue from non-diabetic and diabetic patients. Arch. Oral Biol., *15*:305, 1970.
12. Campbell, M. J. A.: Epidemiology of periodontal disease in the diabetic and the non-diabetic. Austr. Dent. J., *17*:274, 1972.
13. Cohen, B., and Fosdick, L. S.: Chemical studies in periodontal disease. VI. The glycogen content of gingival tissues in alloxan diabetes. J. Dent. Res., *29*:48, 1950.
14. Cohen, D. W., Friedman, L. A., Shapiro, J., and Kyle, G. C.: Studies on periodontal patterns in diabetes mellitus. J. Periodont. Res. [Suppl.], *4*:35, 1969.
15. El Geneldy, A. K., Stallard, R. E., Fillios, L. C., and Goldman, H. M.: Periodontal and vascular alterations: Their relationship to the changes in tissue glucose and glycogen in diabetic mouse. J. Periodontol., *45*:394, 1974.
16. Fett, K. D., and Jutzi, E.: Die Bezahnung Bei Diabetiken in Abhangigkeit vom Lebensalter und der Diabetesdaner. Dtsch. Zahnarzt. Z., *20*:121, 1965.
17. Ficara, A. I., Levin, M. P., Grover, M. F., and Kramer, G. D.: A comparison of the glucose and protein content of gingival fluid from diabetics and non-diabetics. J. Periodont. Res., *10*:171, 1975.
18. Finestone, A. J., and Boorujy, S. R.: Diabetes mellitus and periodontal disease. Diabetes, *16*:336, 1967.
19. Friederici, H. H. R., Tucker, W. R., and Schwartz, T. B.: Observations on small blood vessels in normal and diabetic patients. Diabetes, *15*:233, 1966.
20. Frantzis, T. G., Reeve, C. M., and Brown, J. R.: The ultrastructure of capillary basement membranes in the attached gingiva of diabetic and non-diabetic patients with periodontal disease. J. Periodontol., *42*:406, 1971.
21. Gescheff, G.: Einige Lipoiduntersuchungen des Paradentium bei Diabetes. Berlin, Frankf. a. M. Verlangen, 1931, p. 8.
22. Glavind, L., Lund, B., and Löe, H.: The relationship between periodontal state and diabetes duration, insulin dosage and retinal changes. J. Periodontol., *39*:341, 1968.
23. Glickman, J.: The periodontal structures in experimental diabetes. N. Y. J. Dent., *16*:226, 1946.
24. Glickman, I., Smulow, J., and Moreau, J.: Effect of alloxan diabetes upon the periodontal response to excessive occlusal forces. J. Periodontol., *37*:146, 1966.
25. Glickman, I., Smulow, J., and Moreau, J.: Postsurgical periodontal healing in alloxan diabetes. J. Periodontol., *38*:93, 1967.
26. Hirschfeld, I.: Periodontal symptoms associated with diabetes. J. Periodontol., *5*:37, 1934.
27. Hove, K. A., and Stallard, R. E.: Diabetes and the periodontal patient. J. Periodontol., *41*:713, 1970.
28. Khandari, K. C., et al.: Investigations into the causation of increased susceptibility of diabetics to cutaneous infections. Indian J. Med. Res., *57*:1295, 1969.
29. Keene, J. J., Jr.: A histochemical evaluation for

small vessel calcification in human nondiabetic and diabetic gingival biopsy specimens. J. Dent. Res., 48:968, 1969.

30. Keene, J. J., Jr.: Observations of small blood vessels in human nondiabetic and diabetic gingiva. J. Dent. Res., 48:967, 1969.

31. Keene, J. J., Jr.: An alteration in human diabetic arterioles. J. Dent. Res., 51:569, 1972.

32. Kornori, A.: Histological studies of the influence of occlusal function on the periodontal tissues of alloxan diabetic rats. Bull. Tokyo Med. Dent. Univ., 11:207, 1964.

33. Listgarten, M. A., et al.: Vascular basement lamina thickness in the normal and inflamed gingiva of diabetics and non-diabetics. J. Periodontol., 45:676, 1974.

34. MacKenzie, R. S., and Millard, H. O.: Interrelated effects of diabetes, arteriosclerosis and calculus on alveolar bone loss. J. Am. Dent. Assoc., 66:191, 1963.

35. Maider, M. Z., Abelson, D. C., and Mandel, I. D.: Salivary alterations in diabetes mellitus. J. Periodontol., 46:567, 1975.

36. McMullen, J., Gottsegen, R., and Camerini-Davalos, R.: PAS fuchsinophilic thickening of small blood vessels in diabetic gingiva due to accumulation in the periendothelial area. J. Periodontol., 5:61, 1967.

37. Mehrotia, K. K., Chawla, T. N., and Kumar, A.: Correlation of salivary sugar with blood sugar. J. Indian Dent. Assoc., 40:265, 1968.

38. Mehrotia, K. K., Chawla, T. N., and Kumar, A.: Correlation of salivary sugar and blood sugar with periodontal health and oral hygiene status among diabetics and non-diabetics. J. Indian Dent. Assoc., 40:287, 1968.

39. Menkin, V.: Biochemical factors in inflammation and diabetes mellitus. Arch. Pathol., 34:182, 1942.

40. Niles, J. G.: Early recognition of diabetes mellitus through interstitial alveolar resorption. Dent. Cosmos, 74:161, 1932.

41. O'Leary, T. M., Shannon, I., and Prigmore, J. R.: Clinical and systemic findings in periodontal disease. J. Periodontol., 33:243, 1962.

42. Ray, H. G., and Orban, B.: The gingival structures in diabetes mellitus. J. Periodontol., 21:85, 1950.

43. Reeve, C. M., and Winklemann, R. K.: Glycogen storage in gingival epithelium of diabetic and non-diabetic patients. I.A.D.R. Abstracts, 1962, p. 31.

44. Richardson, R.: Influence of diabetes on the development of antibacterial properties in the blood. J. Clin. Invest., 12:1143, 1933.

45. Robbins, S. E.: Pathologic Basis of Disease. Philadelphia, W. B. Saunders Company, 1975.

46. Rudy, A., and Cohen, M. M.: The oral aspects of diabetes mellitus. N. Engl. J. Med., 219:503, 1938.

47. Rutledge, C. E.: Oral and roentgenographic aspects of the teeth and jaws in juvenile diabetics. J. Am. Dent. Assoc., 27:1740, 1940.

48. Shehan, R., and Cohen, M.: The periodontium of diabetic mice. I.A.D.R. Abstracts, No. 251, 1970.

49. Sheppard, I. M.: Alveolar resorption in diabetes mellitus. Dent. Cosmos, 78:1075, 1936.

50. Shklar, G., Cohen, M. M., and Yerganian, G.: Periodontal disease in the Chinese hamster with hereditary diabetes. J. Periodontol., 33: 14, 1962.

51. Siperstein, M. A., Unger, R. H., and Madism, L.: Studies of muscle, capillary basement membrane in normal subjects, diabetics and prediabetic patients. Am. J. Clin. Invest., 47: 1973, 1968.

52. Stahl, S. S., Witkin, G. J., and Scopp, I. W.: Degenerative vascular changes observed in selected gingival specimens. Oral Surg., 15: 1495, 1962.

53. Ulrich, K.: Parodontopathy in diabetes mellitus. Dtsch. Zahnarztl. Z., 4:221, 1962.

54. Williams, J. B.: Diabetic periodontoclasia. J. Am. Dent. Assoc., 15:523, 1928.

55. Williams, R., and Mahan, C. J.: Periodontal disease in diabetic young adults. J.A.M.A., 72: 776, 1960.

56. Ziskin, D. E., Longhlin, W. C., and Seigel, E. H.: Diabetes in relation to certain oral and systemic problems. Part II. Am. J. Orthod., 30: 758, 1944.

The Gonads

Identification of several types of gingival disease with altered secretion of sex hormones has led to increased interest in hormonal effects upon the periodontal tissues and upon periodontal wound healing. There are several types of gingival disease in which modification of the sex hormones is considered to be either the initiating or the complicating factor; these types of gingival alterations are characterized by being associated with physiologic hormonal changes, by a marked hemorrhagic tendency, and by nonspecific inflammatory changes with a predominant vascular component.

EXPERIMENTAL STUDIES

Elevated levels of estrogen and progesterone increase gingival exudation in female animals with and without gingivitis, most likely because of hormone-induced increased permeability of gingival vessels.[33]

Progesterone alone produces dilatation of the gingival microvasculature, which increases susceptibility to injury and exudation, but it does not affect the morphology of the gingival epithelium.[22] Estrogen injections counteract tendencies toward hyperkeratosis of gingival epithelium and fibrosis of vessel walls in castrated female animals.[53] Locally applied progesterone, estrogen, and gonadotropin appear to reduce the acute inflammatory response to chemical irritation.[34]

Ovariectomy results in osteoporosis of alveolar bone, reduced cementum formation, and reduced fiber density and cellularity of the periodontal ligament[17] in young adult mice but not in older animals,[46] and fibrosis of periodontal blood vessels.[52] There is also thinning and reduced cellular activity in the epithelium of the buccal mucosa, but not of the gingiva.[35] Gingival epithelium is atrophic in estrogen-deficient animals.[64]

Repeated injections of estrogen cause increased endosteal bone formation in the jaws[43, 58] and decreased polymerization of mucopolysaccharide protein complexes in the bone ground substance.[1] Estrogen also stimulates bone formation and fibroplasia, which compensate for destructive changes in the periodontium induced by systemic administration of cortisone.[18]

Systemic administration of testosterone retards the downgrowth of sulcus epithelium over the cementum,[51] stimulates osteoblastic activity in alveolar bone, increases the cellularity of the periodontal ligament,[56] and restores osteoblastic activity which is depressed by hypophysectomy.[57] Healing of oral wounds is accelerated by castration in males and is unaffected by ovariectomy.[4]

THE GINGIVA IN PUBERTY

Puberty is frequently accompanied by an exaggerated response of the gingiva to local irritation.[25, 28, 60] Pronounced inflammation, bluish red discoloration, edema, and enlargement result from local irritants that would ordinarily elicit a comparatively mild gingival response (Fig. 29–3). Excessive anterior overbite aggravates these cases because of the complicating effects of food impaction and injury to the gingiva on the labial aspect of the mandibular teeth and palatal aspect in the maxilla.[6]

As adulthood is approached, the severity of the gingival reaction diminishes even when local irritants are still present. Complete return to normal requires their removal. Although the prevalence and severity of gingival disease are increased in puberty, it should be understood that gingivitis is not a universal occurrence during this period; with proper care of the mouth it can be prevented.

GINGIVAL CHANGES ASSOCIATED WITH THE MENSTRUAL CYCLE

As a general rule, the menstrual cycle is not accompanied by notable gingival changes, but occasional problems do occur. During the menstrual period the prevalence of gingivitis increases.[29] The patients may complain of bleeding gums

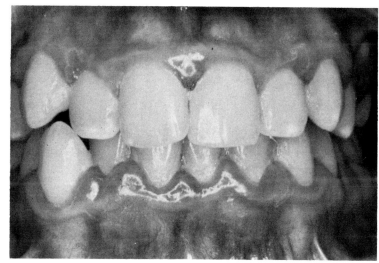

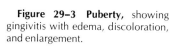
Figure 29–3 Puberty, showing gingivitis with edema, discoloration, and enlargement.

or a bloated, tense feeling in the gums in the days preceding menstrual flow. Horizontal tooth mobility does not change significantly during the menstrual cycle.[15] The salivary bacterial count is increased during menstruation and at ovulation 11 to 14 days earlier.[47] The exudate from inflamed gingiva is increased during menstruation, suggesting that existent gingivitis is aggravated by menstruation, but crevicular fluid of normal gingiva is unaffected.[21]

A variety of oral changes have been reported associated with the menstrual cycle; usually they appear several days before the menstrual period. These include ulcerations of the oral mucosa that seem to have a familial trend,[8, 45] aphthae and vesicular lesions and vicarious bleeding in the oral cavity,[55] "menstruation gingivitis" characterized by periodic recurrent hemorrhage with bright red and rose-colored proliferations of the interdental papillae, and persistent ulceration of the tongue and buccal mucosa that worsens just before the menstrual period. Microscopic examination of the gingiva in a patient with a cyclical recurrent gingivitis revealed desquamation of epithelial cells from the stratum granulosum and the surface.[42]

Periodically recurring ulcers of the mouth and occasionally of the vulva may accompany or precede the menstrual period. The oral lesions heal in three to four days and the vaginal tenderness disappears after menstruation and for the remainder of the cycle.

The lesions do not appear if the patient becomes pregnant, but recur post partum. Improvement has been reported with systemic estrogen[24] or anterior pituitary hormone.[62]

An oral syndrome, termed periodic transitory menogingivitis,[59] has been described, consisting of discomfort, sensitivity, redness, and congestion of the gingiva with bleeding under the normal stress of mastication. The condition was observed just prior to menstruation, in amenorrheas of different types, after hysterectomy, prior to and after ruptured ectopic pregnancy, and during and after menopause. Soreness of the mouth and tongue that appeared a few days prior to menstruation and increased in severity for several days was reported as relieved by systemic estrogen and recurred when the drug was withdrawn.[20] Periodic agranulocytic leukopenia, which may be a factor in the production of oral changes, has also been associated with the menstrual cycle.[23]

Cyclic gingival changes associated with menstruation have been attributed to hormonal imbalances and in some instances are accompanied by a history of ovarian dysfunction.[5] Rhythmic changes in capillary fragility associated with the menstrual cycle and increased tendency to capillary hemorrhage immediately before and during menstruation[3] may affect bleeding of the gingiva.

GINGIVAL DISEASE IN PREGNANCY

Pregnancy itself does not cause gingivitis. Gingivitis in pregnancy is caused by local irritants, just as it is in nonpregnant individuals. Pregnancy accentuates the gingival response to local irritants and produces a clinical picture different from that which occurs in nonpregnant individuals (Figs. 29–4 to 29–6). No notable changes occur in the gingiva in pregnancy in the absence of local irritants. Local irritants cause the gingivitis; pregnancy is a secondary modifying factor.

The severity of gingivitis is increased during pregnancy beginning from the second to third month. Patients with slight chronic gingivitis which attracted no particular attention before pregnancy become aware of the gingiva because previously inflamed areas become excessively enlarged and edematous and more noticeably discolored. Patients with a slight amount of gingival bleeding before pregnancy become concerned about an increased tendency to bleed.

Gingivitis becomes most severe by the eighth month and decreases during the ninth, and plaque accumulation follows a similar pattern.[36] Some report the greatest severity between the second and third trimesters.[7] The correlation between gingivitis and the quantity of plaque is closer after parturition than during pregnancy.[27] This suggests that pregnancy introduces other factors which aggravate the gingival response to local irritants.

The reported incidence of gingivitis in pregnancy—38 per cent,[2] 45.4 per cent,[38]

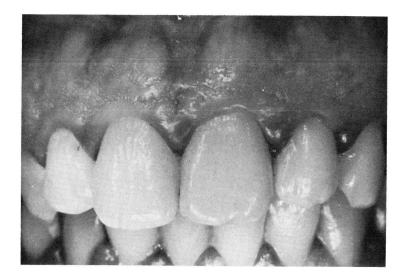

Figure 29–4 Early Changes in the Interdental Papillae in Pregnancy.

52 per cent,[37] 53.8 per cent,[14] 85.9 per cent,[20] 100 per cent,[28, 36]—varies according to the group studied and the method used. The incidence appears to be increased in pregnancy,[54] but this is a difficult determination to make. Pregnancy affects the severity of previously inflamed areas; it does not alter healthy gingiva. Impressions of increased incidence may be created by aggravation of previously inflamed but unnoticed areas.[50, 55] Also increased in pregnancy are tooth mobility,[48] pocket depth, and gingival fluid.[22, 30]

Clinical features

Pronounced vascularity is the most striking clinical feature. The gingiva is inflamed and varies in color from a bright red to a bluish red sometimes described as "old rose."[41, 63, 65] The marginal and interdental gingiva is edematous, pits on pressure, appears smooth and shiny, is soft and pliable, and sometimes presents a raspberry-like appearance. The extreme redness results from marked vascularity, and there is an increased tendency to bleed. The gin-

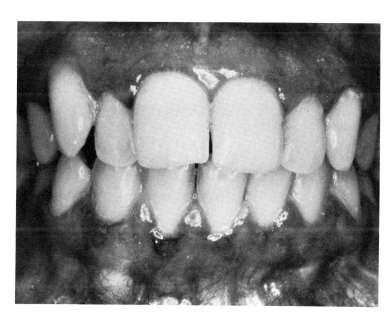

Figure 29–5 Pregnancy, showing edema, discoloration, and bleeding.

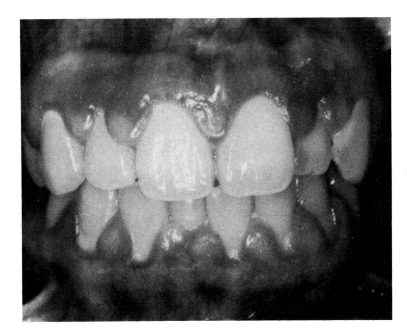

Figure 29–6 Pregnancy, showing edema, discoloration, and enlargement.

gival changes are usually painless unless complicated by acute infection, marginal ulceration, and pseudomembrane formation. In some cases the inflamed gingiva forms discrete "tumor-like" masses, referred to as "pregnancy tumors" (described in Chapter 10).

There is partial reduction in the severity of gingivitis by two months post partum, and after one year the condition of the gingiva is comparable to that of patients who have not been pregnant.[7] However, the gingiva does not return to normal so long as local irritants are present. Also reduced following pregnancy are horizontal tooth mobility, gingival fluid, and pocket depth. In a longitudinal investigation of the periodontal changes during pregnancy and 15 months post partum, no significant loss of attachment was observed.[7]

Histopathology

The microscopic picture[38, 65] of gingival disease in pregnancy is one of nonspecific vascularizing proliferative inflammation. There is marked inflammatory cellular infiltration with edema and degeneration of the gingival epithelium and connective tissue. The epithelium is hyperplastic, with accentuated rete pegs and varying degrees of intracellular and extracellular edema and infiltration by leukocytes. Newly formed, engorged capillaries are present in abundance. Surface ulcerations or pseudomembrane formation is an occasional finding.

Histochemical studies reveal abnormal amounts of water- and alcohol-insoluble glycoprotein residues in the inflamed gingiva.[12] Comparable findings are observed in gingivitis in puberty, in menstruation, and in severe desquamative gingivitis. In an effort to differentiate changes caused by the pregnancy from those caused by local irritation, Turesky et al.[61] studied the attached gingiva that was uninvolved by inflammation, as distinguished from inflamed marginal and interdental areas. They reported that in pregnancy there is diminished surface keratinization, increase in rete peg length, and increase in glycogen in the epithelium. In the connective tissue, the basement layer is thinned and the carbohydrate-protein complexes and glycogen in the ground substance are reduced in density. Electrometric studies indicate a decrease in the density of glycoprotein in the gingiva in the early months of pregnancy, which returns to normal several months after parturition.[16]

The effect of pregnancy upon the gingival response to local irritants is explained on a hormonal basis. There is a marked increase in estrogen and progesterone during pregnancy and a reduction after parturition. The severity of gingivitis varies with the hormonal levels in pregnancy.[22] The aggravation of gingivitis has been attributed principally to the increased progesterone which produced dilatation and tortuosity of the gingival microvasculature, circulatory stasis, and increased susceptibility to mechanical irritation—all of which favor leakage of fluid into perivascular tissues.[40]

The gingiva is a target organ for female sex hormones. Formicola et al.[13] have shown that radioactive estradiol injected into female rats appears not only in the genital tract but also in the gingiva.

It has also been suggested that the accentuation of gingivitis in pregnancy occurs in two peaks: (1) during the first trimester when there is overproduction of gonadotropins and (2) during the third trimester, when estrogen and progesterone levels are highest.[36] Destruction of gingival mast cells by the increased sex hormones and the resultant release of histamine and proteolytic enzymes may also contribute to the exaggerated inflammatory response to local irritants.[32] Other studies have concluded that the hyperactivity of specific steroid enzyme systems and the accumulation of biotransformation products of naturally occurring steroid hormones, progesterone and estrogen, may play a part in the etiology of gingivitis in pregnancy.

HORMONAL CONTRACEPTIVES AND THE GINGIVA

Hormonal contraceptives aggravate the gingival response to local irritants in a manner similar to pregnancy,[10, 31] and when taken for a period of over 1.5 years increase periodontal destruction.[26]

MENOPAUSAL GINGIVOSTOMATITIS (SENILE ATROPHIC GINGIVITIS)

This condition occurs during the menopause or in the postmenopausal period. Mild signs and symptoms sometimes appear associated with the earliest menopausal changes. Menopausal gingivostomatitis is not a common condition. Its designation has led to the erroneous impression that it invariably occurs associated with the menopause, whereas the opposite is true. Oral disturbances are not a common feature of the menopause.

Clinical features

The gingiva and remaining oral mucosa are dry and shiny, vary in color from abnormal paleness to redness, and bleed easily. There is fissuring in the mucobuccal fold in some cases,[49] and comparable changes may occur in the vaginal mucosa. The patient complains of a dry, burning sensation throughout the oral cavity, associated with extreme sensitivity to thermal changes, abnormal taste sensations described as "salty," "peppery," or "sour,"[39] and difficulty with removable partial prostheses.

Histopathology

Microscopically, the gingiva presents atrophy of the germinal and prickle cell layers of the epithelium and, in some instances, areas of ulceration.

When menopausal gingivostomatitis occurs in edentulous patients, they cannot tolerate dentures very well. Normally, when full dentures are inserted there is an initial period of adaptation of the oral mucosa. Thickening of the epithelium is part of the physiologic adaptation that makes toleration of the denture possible. In patients with menopausal gingivostomatitis, the thin, atrophic epithelium offers very little protection. Consequently, the oral mucosa bruises easily in the presence of even slight surface abrasion. Thickening of the epithelium to accommodate the denture does not develop because of the atrophic tendency governing the epithelium. As a result, the patient is continually uncomfortable, even with well-fitting dentures in proper functional relation. The outline of the denture is clearly demarcated by the fiery red and shiny appearance of the underlying sore mucosa.

The signs and symptoms of menopausal gingivostomatitis are in some degree comparable to those of chronic desquamative gingivitis. Signs and symptoms similar to those of menopausal gingivostomatitis occasionally occur following ovariectomy or sterilization by radiation in the treatment of malignant neoplasms.

REFERENCES

1. Bernick, S., and Ershoff, B. H.: Histochemical study of bone in estrogen-treated rats. J. Dent. Res., 42:981, 1963.
2. Biro, S.: Studies regarding the influence of pregnancy upon caries. Vierteljahr. Zahnheilk., 14:371, 1898.
3. Brewer, J. L.: Rhythmic changes in the skin capillaries and their relations to menstruation. Am. J. Obstet. Gynecol., 36:597, 1938.
4. Butcher, E. O., and Klingsberg, J.: Age, gonadectomy and wound healing in the palatal mucosa. J. Dent. Res., 40:694, 1961.
5. Calman, A. S.: Oral complications of pregnancy. Dent. Outlook, 17:2, 1930.
6. Cohen, M.: The gingiva at puberty. J. Dent. Res., 34:679, 1955.
7. Cohen, D. W., Shapiro, J., Friedman, L., Kyle, C. G., and Franlin, S.: A longitudinal investigation of the periodontal changes during pregnancy and fifteen months post-partum. J. Periodontol., 42:653, 1971.
8. Dayton, A. C.: A case of metastasis of menstrual secretion from the uterus to mouth. Am. J. Dent. Sci., 10:42, 1949.
9. Deasy, M. J., Grota, A. J., and Kennedy, J. E.: The effect of estrogen, progesterone and cortisol on gingival inflammation. J. Periodont. Res., 7: 111, 1972.
10. El-Ashiry, G. M., et al.: Comparative study of the influence of pregnancy and oral contraceptives on the gingivae. Oral Surg., 30:472, 1970.
11. El Attar, T. M. A., and Hugoson, A.: Comparative metabolism of female sex steroids in normal and chronically inflamed gingiva of the dog. J. Periodont. Res., 9:284, 1974.
12. Engel, M. B.: Hormonal gingivitis, J. Am. Dent. Assoc., 44:691, 1952.
13. Formicola, A. J., Weatherford, T., and Grupe, H., Jr.: The uptake of H³-estradiol by the oral tissues in rats. J. Periodont. Res., 5:269, 1970.
14. Fraser, G. A.: Pregnancy gingivitis. S. African Dent. J., 10:138, 1944.
15. Friedman, L. A.: Horizontal tooth mobility and the menstrual cycle. J. Periodont. Res., 7:125, 1972.
16. Gans, B. J., Engel, M. B., and Joseph, N. R.: Electrometric studies of human gingiva in pregnancy. J. Dent. Res., 35:566, 1956.
17. Glickman, I., and Quintarelli, G.: Further observations regarding the effect of ovariectomy upon the tissues of the periodontium. J. Periodontol., 31:31, 1960.
18. Glickman, I., and Shklar, G.: The steroid hormones and the tissues of the periodontium. Oral Surg., 8:1179, 1955.
19. Hartzer, R. C., Toto, P. D., and Gargiulo, A. W.: Immune reactions in the gingiva of the pregnant and non-pregnant female. J. Periodontol., 42:239, 1971.
20. Heinemann, M., and Anderson, B. G.: Oral manifestations of certain systemic disorders. Yale J. Biol. Med., 17:583, 1945.
21. Holm-Pederson, P., and Löe, H.: Flow of gingival exudate as related to menstruation and pregnancy. J. Periodont. Res., 2:13, 1967.
22. Hugoson, A.: Gingival inflammation and female sex hormones. J. Periodont. Res., [Suppl.] 5, 1970.
23. Jackson, H., Jr., and Merril, D.: Agranulocytic angina associated with the menstrual cycle. N. Engl. J. Med., 210:175, 1934.
24. Jones, O. V.: Cyclical ulcerative vulvitis and stomatitis. J. Obstet. Gynaecol. Br. Emp., 47:557, 1940.
25. Knapp, E.: An unusual case of periodontitis marginalis progressiva chronica in a thirteen year old girl. Dtsch. Zahnartzl. Wochenschr., 38:1080, 1935.
26. Knight, G. M., and Wade, A. B.: The effects of hormonal contraceptives on the human periodontium. J. Periodont. Res., 9:18, 1974.
27. Kolodzinski, E., Munoa, N., and Malatesta, E.: Clinical study of gingival tissue in pregnant women (Abs.). J. Dent. Res., 53:693, 1974.
28. Kutzleb, H. J.: Changes in the oral mucosa in ovarian disturbances. Dtsch. Zahnartzl., Wochenschr., 42:906, 1939.
29. Larato, D., Stahl, S., Brown, R., Jr., and Witkin, G.: The effect of a prescribed method of toothbrushing on the fluctuation of marginal gingivitis. J. Periodontol., 40:142, 1969.
30. Lindhe, J., and Attstrom, R.: Gingival exudation during the menstrual cycle. J. Periodont. Res., 2:194, 1967.
31. Lindhe, J., and Bjorn, A. L.: Influence of hormonal contraceptives on the gingiva of women. J. Periodont. Res., 2:1, 1967.
32. Lindhe, J., and Branemark, P. I.: Changes in microcirculation after local application of sex hormones. J. Periodont. Res., 2:185, 1967.
33. Lindhe, J., Attstrom, R., and Bjorn, A.: Influence of sex hormones on gingival exudation in gingivitis—free female dogs. J. Periodont. Res., 3:272, 1968.
34. Lindhe, J., and Sonesson, B.: The effect of sex hormones on inflammation II. Progestogen, oestrogen and chorionic gonadotropin. J. Periodont. Res., 2:7, 1967.
35. Litwack, D., Kennedy, J. E., and Zander, H. A.: Response of oral epithelia to ovariectomy and estrogen replacement. I.A.D.R. Abstracts, No. 606, 1970, p. 100.
36. Loe, H.: Periodontal changes in pregnancy. J. Periodontol., 36:209, 1965.
37. Looby, J. P.: Cited by Burket, K. W.: Oral Medicine. Philadelphia. J. B. Lippincott Co., 1946, p. 294.
38. Maier, A. W., and Orban, B.: Gingivitis in pregnancy. Oral Surg., 2:234, 1949.
39. Massler, M., and Henry, J.: Oral manifestations during the female climacteric. The Alpha Omegan, Sept., 1950, p. 105.
40. Mohamed, A. H., Waterhouse, J. P., and Friederici, H. H.: The microvasculature of the rat gingiva as affected by progesterone: An ultrastructural study. J. Periodontol., 45:50, 1974.
41. Monash, S.: Proliferative gingivitis of pregnancy. Surg. Gynecol. Obstet., 42:794, 1926.
42. Muhlemann, H. R.: Gingivitis intermenstrualis. Schweiz. Monatschr. Zahnh., 58:865, 1948.
43. Nutlay, A. G., et al: The effect of estrogen on the gingiva and alveolar bone in rats and mice. J. Dent. Res., 33:115, 1954.
44. Nyman, S.: Studies on the influence of estradiol and progesterone on granulation tissue. J. Periodont. Res., [Suppl. 7] 1971.

45. Pappworth, M. H.: Cyclical mucosal ulceration. Br. Med. J., *1*:271, 1941.
46. Piroshaw, N., and Glickman, I.: The effect of ovariectomy upon the tissues of the periodontium and skeletal bones. Oral Surg., *10*:133, 1957.
47. Prout, R. E. S., and Hopps, R. M.: A relationship between human oral bacteria and the menstrual cycle. J. Periodontol. *41*:98, 1970.
48. Rateitschak, K. H.: Tooth mobility changes in pregnancy. J. Periodont. Res., *2*:199, 1967.
49. Richman, J. J., and Abarbanel, A. R.: Effects of estradiol, testosterone, diethylstilbestrol and several of their derivatives upon the human mucous membrane, J. Am. Dent. Assoc., *30*: 913, 1943.
50. Ringsdorf, W. M., Powell, B. J. Knight, L. A., and Cheraskin, E.: Periodontal status and pregnancy. Am. J. Obstet. Gynecol., *83*:258, 1962.
51. Rushton, M. A.: Epithelial downgrowth: Effect of methyl testosterone. Br. Dent. J., *93*:27, 1952.
52. Schneider, H.: Changes in the periodontium of the rat following ovariectomy. (Ger.) Parodontologie/Acad. Rev., *1*:106, 1967.
53. Schneider, H., and Pose, G.: The effect of estrogen on periodontal conditions in castrated rats. Dtschr. Stomatol. *19*:25, 1969.
54. Schour, F.: Endocrines and teeth. J. Am. Dent. Assoc., *21*:322, 1934.
55. Shelmire, B.: Certain diseases of oral mucous membrane and vermilion border of lips. Intern. J. Ortho., *14*:817, 1928.
56. Shklar, G., Chauncey, H., and Peluso, D.: The effect of testosterone on the periodontium of the male albino rat. I.A.D.R. Abstracts, 1962, p. 68.
57. Shklar, G., Chauncey, H., and Shapiro, S.: The effect of testosterone on the periodontium of normal and hypophysectomy rats. J. Periodontol., *38*:203, 1967.
58. Shklar, G., and Glickman, I.: The effect of estrogenic hormone on the periodontium of white mice. J. Periodontol., *27*:16, 1956.
59. Stoloff, C. I.: Periodic transitory meno-gingivitis incidental in women: A new non-pathological classification of gingival disturbance. J. Dent. Res., *13*:190, 1933.
60. Sutcliffe, P.: A longitudinal study of gingivitis and puberty. J. Periodont. Res., *7*:52, 1972.
61. Turesky, S., Fisher, B., and Glickman, I.: A histochemical study of the attached gingiva in pregnancy. J. Dent. Res., *37*:1115, 1958.
62. Ziserman, A. J.: Ulcerative vulvitis and stomatitis of endocrine origin. J.A.M.A., *104*:826, 1935.
63. Ziskin, D. E., and Blackberg, S. N.: A study of the gingivae during pregnancy. J. Dent. Res., *13*:253, 1933.
64. Ziskin, D. E., and Blackberg, S. N.: The effect of castration and hypophysectomy on the gingiva and oral mucous membranes of Rhesus monkeys. J. Dent. Res., *19*:381, 1940.
65. Ziskin, D. E., Blackberg, S. N., and Stout, A.: The gingivae during pregnancy: An experimental study and a histopathological interpretation. Surg. Gynecol. Obstet., *57*:719, 1933.
66. Ziskin, D. E., and Nesse, G. J.: Pregnancy gingivitis, history, classification, etiology. Am. J. Orthod., *32*:390, 1946.

Corticosteroid Hormones

The systemic administration of cortisone in experimental animals results in osteoporosis of alveolar bone (Fig. 29–7), capillary dilatation and engorgement (with hemorrhage in the periodontal ligament and gingival connective tissue), degeneration and reduction in the number of collagen fibers of the periodontal ligament, and increased destruction of the periodontal tissues associated with inflammation caused by local irritation.[2] Loss of tooth-supporting bone has been noted in adrenalectomized animals.[2] Osteogenesis in alveolar bone which is reduced in adrenalectomized animals was restored by cortisone replacement.[9]

In humans systemic administration of cortisone and ACTH appears to have no effect upon the incidence and severity of gingival and periodontal disease.[4] However, patients with renal transplants and receiving immunosuppressive therapy (prednisone or methyl prednisone and azathioprine or cyclophosphamide) have significantly less gingival inflammation than controls with similar amounts of plaque.[12]

THE GENERAL ADAPTATION SYNDROME AND THE DISEASES OF ADAPTATION

Many forms of stress such as trauma, cold, muscular fatigue, drug intoxication and nervous stimuli affect the body generally, and produce interrelated, nonspecific tissue changes. The composite of the systemic reactions that result from continued exposure to stress is termed the *general adaptation syndrome* (G.A.S.), which is described by Selye as the basis for the pathogenesis of many diseases previously considered to be of unrelated etiology.[6, 7] According to Selye, the general adaptation syndrome is a generalized group of physiologic mechanisms which represent an attempt by the body to resist the damaging effect of stress.

Stress acts through the endocrine glands, particularly the anterior lobe of the pituitary and the adrenal cortex, to produce the morphologic and functional changes that comprise the general adaptation syndrome. Among these changes are enlargement of the adrenal cortex with increased secretion of adrenocorticoid hormones; involution of lymphatic organs; hyalinization and inflam-

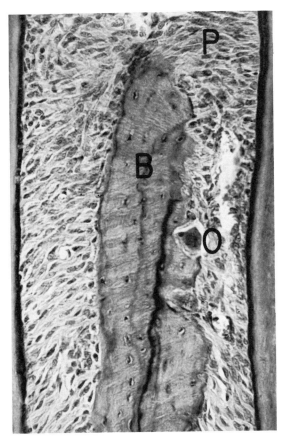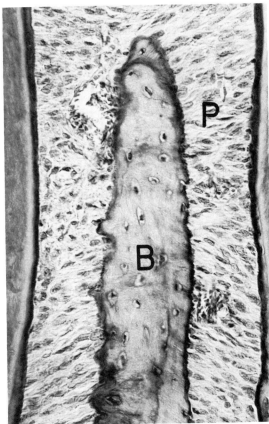

Figure 29–7   The Effects of Systemically Administered Cortisone upon the Periodontium. *Left,* **Control Animal, Interdental Septum.** There is a thin layer of newly formed osteoid bordered by a row of osteoblasts along one surface of the bone (B). The outer surface presents concavities of resorption with an occasional osteoclast (O). The periodontal ligament is shown at P. *Right,* **Cortisone-Injected Animal.** Note absence of normal osteoid and osteoblasts, and irregularly indented deeply staining bone margin (B). The connective tissue cells of the periodontal membrane (P) are reduced in number. The collagen fibers appear fibrin-like and fragmented.

matory changes in blood vessels with hypertension; gastrointestinal ulceration; and malignant nephrosclerosis. The "collagen" diseases of man are benefited by treatment with ACTH and cortisone, and they appear to be part of the general adaptation syndrome. Thus, the adaptive mechanism of the body in response to stress produces recognizable disease entities, referred to as the "diseases of adaptation."

The general adaptation syndrome develops in three stages: (1) the initial response, or "alarm reaction"; (2) the adaptation to stress—the "resistance stage"; and (3) a final stage marked by inability to maintain adaptation to the stress—the "exhaustion stage."

Stress and the periodontal tissues

The following observations have been reported in stressed experimental animals:

In the alarm reaction,[10] no significant changes; in the late stage of the stress syndrome, osteoporosis of alveolar bone,[3] epithelial sloughing, degeneration of the periodontal ligament and reduced osteoblastic activity;[5] in chronic stress, osteoporosis of alveolar bone, apical migration of the epithelial attachment, and the formation of periodontal pockets.[8] Stress results in delayed healing of the connective tissue and bone in artificially induced gingival wounds but does not affect the epithelium.[11]

REFERENCES

1. Applebaum, E., and Seelig, A.: Histologic changes in jaws and teeth of rats following nephritis, adrenalectomy and cortisone treatment. Oral Surg., 8:881, 1955.
2. Glickman, I., Stone, I. C., and Chawla, T. N.: The effect of cortisone acetate upon the periodontium of white mice. J. Periodontol., 24:161, 1953.
3. Gupta, O. P., Blechman, H., and Stahl, S. S.: The effects of stress on the periodontal tissues of young adult male rats and hamsters. J. Periodontol., 31:413, 1960.
4. Krohn, S.: The effect of the administration of steroid hormones on the gingival tissues. J. Periodontol., 29:300, 1958.
5. Ratcliff, P. A.: The relationship of the general adaptation syndrome to the periodontal tissues in the rat. J. Periodontol., 27:40, 1956.
6. Selye, H.: The general adaptation syndrome and the diseases of adaptation. J. Clin. Endocrinol., 6:117, 1946.
7. Selye, H.: The Physiology and Pathology of Exposure to Stress. Acta Endocrinol. (Montreal), 1950.
8. Shklar, G.: Periodontal disease in experimental animals subjected to chronic cold stress. J. Periodontol., 37:377, 1966.
9. Shklar, G.: The effect of adrenalectomy and cortisone replacement on the periodontium of the rat. Periodontics, 3:239, 1965.
10. Shklar, G., and Glickman, I.: The periodontium and the salivary glands in the alarm reaction. J. Dent. Res., 32:773, 1953.
11. Stahl, S. S.: Healing gingival injury in normal and systemically stressed young adult male rats. J. Periodontol., 32:63, 1961.
12. Tollefsen, T., Saltvedt, E., and Koppang, H. S.: The effect of immunosuppressive agents on periodontal disease in man. J. Periodont. Res., 13:240, 1978.

Chapter 30

Hematologic and Other Systemic Disorders in the Etiology of Periodontal Disease

HEMATOLOGIC DISORDERS IN THE ETIOLOGY OF PERIODONTAL DISEASE

Oral changes are often the earliest indication of a hematologic disturbance but cannot be relied upon for the diagnosis of the patient's hematologic disorder. Oral findings suggest the existence of a blood disturbance; specific diagnosis requires complete physical examination and thorough hematologic study. Comparable oral changes occur in more than one form of blood dyscrasia, and secondary inflammatory changes produce a wide range of variation in the oral signs. For these reasons, gingival and periodontal disturbances associated with blood dyscrasias must be thought of in terms of fundamental interrelationships between the oral tissues and the blood and blood-forming organs, rather than as a simple association of dramatic oral changes with hematologic disease.

Abnormal bleeding from the gingiva, or other areas of the oral mucosa, that is difficult to control is an important clinical sign suggesting a hematologic disorder. Hemorrhagic tendencies occur in hematologic disorders whenever the normal hemostatic mechanism is disturbed.[38]

Periodontal Disease in Leukemia

Oral manifestations occur with greatest frequency in acute and subacute monocytic leukemia, less frequently in acute and subacute lymphatic and myelogenous leukemia, and seldom in chronic leukemia. Periodontal changes in leukemia can be (1) *primary changes*, directly attributable to the hematologic disturbance; and (2) *secondary changes*, those superimposed upon the oral tissues by the almost omnipresent local factors, which induce a wide range of inflammatory changes.

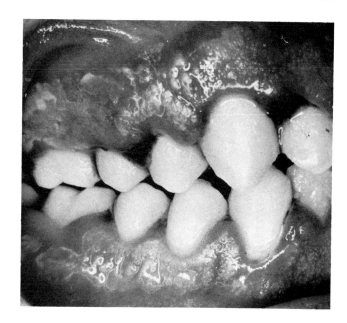

Figure 30–1 Acute Monocytic Leukemia. The gingiva is inflamed, edematous, and discolored.

Acute and subacute leukemia

Clinical changes that may occur in acute and subacute leukemia include a diffuse, cyanotic, bluish red discoloration of the entire gingival mucosa (whose surface becomes shiny), a diffuse edematous enlargement obliterating the details of the normal surface markings (see Chapter 10), a rounding and tenseness of the gingival margin, blunting of the interdental papillae, and varying degrees of gingival inflammation with ulceration, necrosis, and pseudomembrane formation (Figs. 30–1 and 30–2).

Microscopically, the gingiva presents a dense diffuse infiltration of predominantly immature leukocytes in the attached as well as the marginal gingiva (Fig. 30–3). Occasional mitotic figures indicative of ectopic hematopoiesis may be seen. The normal connective tissue components of the gingiva are displaced by the leukemic cells (Figs. 30–3 and 30–4A). The nature of the cells depends on the type of leukemia. The cellular accumulation is denser in the reticular connective tissue layer. In almost all cases, the papillary layer contains comparatively few leukocytes. The blood vessels are distended and contain predominantly leukemic cells. The red blood cells are reduced in number.

The epithelium presents a variety of changes. It may be thinned or hyperplastic.

Degeneration associated with inter- and intracellular edema, and leukocytic infiltration with diminished surface keratinization, are common findings.

The microscopic picture of the marginal gingiva differs from that of the remainder of the gingiva in that it usually presents a notable inflammatory component in addition to the leukemic cells. Scattered foci of plasma cells and lymphocytes with edema and degeneration are common findings. The inner aspect of the marginal gingiva is usually ulcerated, and marginal necrosis with pseudomembrane formation may also be seen.

The periodontal ligament and alveolar bone may also be involved in acute and subacute leukemia (Fig. 30–4B). The periodontal ligament may be infiltrated with mature and immature leukocytes. The marrow of the alveolar bone presents a variety of changes, such as localized areas of necrosis, thrombosis of blood vessels, infiltration with mature and immature leukocytes, occasional red blood cells, and replacement of the fatty marrow by fibrous tissue.[8, 20, 41]

In leukemic mice the presence of infiltrate in marrow spaces and periodontal ligament results in osteoporosis of the alveolar bone with destruction of supporting bone and disappearance of periodontal fibers[7, 9] (Fig. 30–5).

OTHER ORAL MUCOUS MEMBRANE CHANGES. Areas of the oral mucous

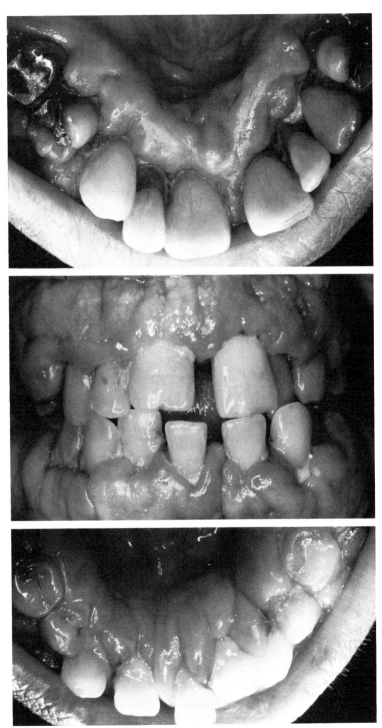

Figure 30–2   Gingival Enlargement in patient with myelocytic leukemia. *Top,* palatal view; *center,* labial view; *below,* lingual view of mandible.

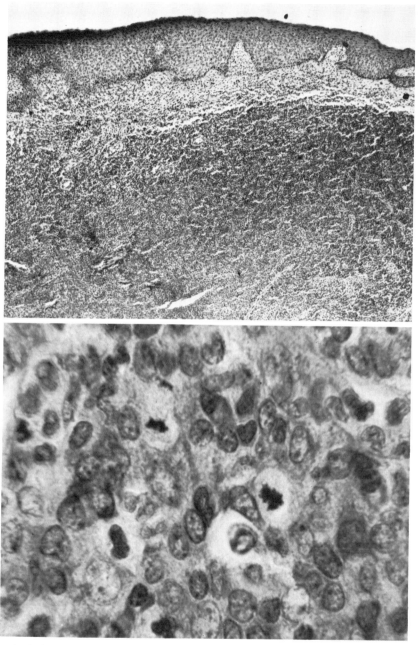

Figure 30–3   Gingival Biopsy of Patient with Acute Monocytic Leukemia. *Above,* Note dense diffuse cellular infiltration in the connective tissue and less cellular zone subjacent to the epithelium. The latter is a common microscopic finding. *Below,* Detailed study showing monocytic cells undergoing mitosis.

membrane other than the gingiva may be involved in acute or subacute leukemia. The site of involvement is generally an area subject to trauma, such as the buccal mucosa in relation to the line of occlusion or the palate. It appears as a *severe ulcer-ation* or *abscess* that is resistant to treatment and spreads rapidly. Because of the difficulty of controlling the extension of infection and the severity of associated toxic complications, fatal termination is occasionally seen in such cases.

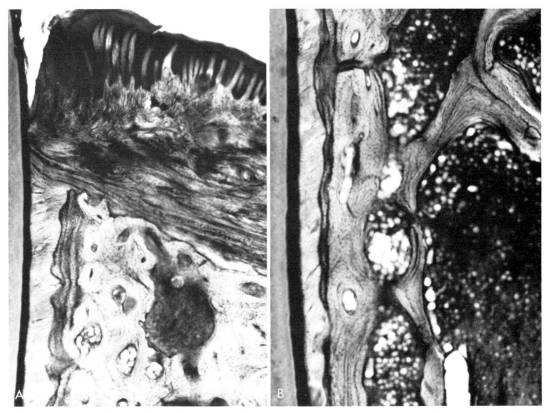

Figure 30–4 *A,* Leukemic infiltrate in gingiva and bone in a human autopsy specimen. *B,* Same case as *A.* Note the dense infiltrate in marrow spaces and lack of extension to the periodontal ligament.

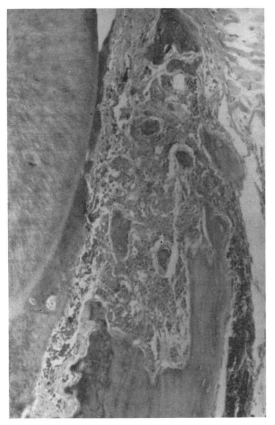

Figure 30–5 Leukemic infiltrate in alveolar bone in AKR mouse. Note the leukemic infiltrate producing destruction of bone and loss of periodontal ligament.

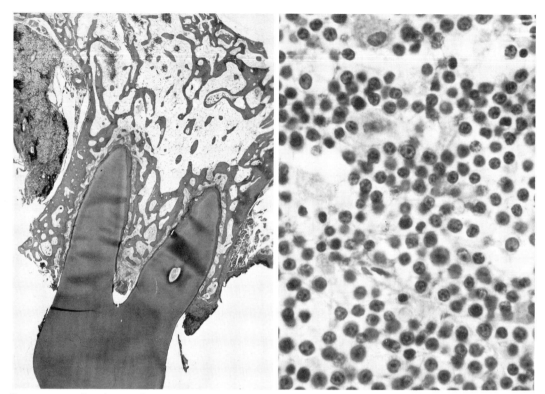

Figure 30–6   Chronic Lymphatic Leukemia. *Left,* Buccopalatal section through the maxilla (molar area) of a patient with chronic lymphatic leukemia, obtained at autopsy. *Right,* Detailed study of lymphocytes in the marrow of the maxilla.

Chronic leukemia

In chronic leukemia there often are no clinical oral changes suggesting a hematologic disturbance. Tumor-like enlargement of the oral mucosa in response to local irritation,[11] generalized alveolar resorption, absence of the lamina dura, diffuse and irregular periodontal spaces, osteoporosis, subperiosteal elevation in the mental region, and analogous changes in other bones may occur in chronic leukemia.[3]

The microscopic changes in chronic leukemia may consist of replacement of the normal fatty marrow of the jaws by islands of mature lymphocytes (Fig. 30–6) or lymphocytic infiltration of the marginal gingiva without dramatic clinical manifestations.

The gingival biopsy and leukemia

The existence of leukemia is sometimes revealed by a gingival biopsy taken to clarify the nature of a troublesome gingival condition. In such cases, the gingival findings must be corroborated by medical examination and hematologic study. The absence of leukemic involvement in a gingival biopsy does not rule out the possibility of leukemia. In chronic leukemia, the gingiva may simply present inflammatory changes with no suggestion of a hematologic disturbance. In patients with recognized leukemia, the gingival biopsy (Fig. 30–3) indicates the extent to which leukemic infiltration is responsible for the altered clinical appearance of the gingiva. Although such findings are of interest, their benefit to the patient is insufficient to warrant routine gingival biopsy in known leukemic patients.

Analysis of the relation of local irritation to gingival and periodontal changes in leukemia

In leukemia, the response to irritation is altered so that the cellular component of the inflammatory exudate differs both quantitatively and qualitatively from that which occurs in nonleukemic individuals. There is pronounced infiltration of immature leukemic cells, and a reduction in the red blood cells (in addition to the usual inflammatory cells). With the cellular infiltration there is degeneration of the gingiva.

The inflamed gingiva differs clinically from that of the nonleukemic individual. It is a peculiar bluish red in color, markedly spongelike and friable, and bleeds persistently upon the slightest provocation, or even spontaneously. This markedly altered and degenerated tissue is extremely susceptible to bacterial infection. Because of the degenerated, anoxemic condition of the gingiva, the bacterial infection is so severe that acute gingival necrosis and pseudomembrane formation are comparatively common findings in acute and subacute leukemia. These oral changes produce associated disturbances that are a source of considerable difficulty to the patient, such as systemic toxic effects, loss of appetite, nausea, blood loss from persistent gingival bleeding, and constant gnawing pain.

There is considerable variation in the gingival and periodontal changes observed in acute and subacute leukemia. The severity of the leukemia affects the extent of cellular infiltration of the gingiva and supporting periodontal structures. The local irritants and the severity of infection account for more striking clinical changes, such as gingival ulceration, necrosis, and pseudomembrane formation, and gingival bleeding. These are the secondary changes superimposed upon the oral tissues altered by the blood disturbance. Differences in the degree of local irritation account for the variation in the oral changes seen in different patients. They also modify the oral picture at different times in the same patient. **By eliminating local irritants it is possible to alleviate severe oral changes in leukemia.**

Oral Changes in Anemia

Anemia refers to any deficiency in the quantity or quality of the blood as manifested by a reduction in the number of red blood cells and in the amount of hemoglobin. Anemia may be the result of blood loss, defective blood formation, or increased blood destruction. *Blood loss* may be acute, as in severe trauma, or chronic, as in gastrointestinal ulcer, or excessive, as in menstrual bleeding. *Defective blood formation* may be due to:

1. Deficiency of protein, iron or hematopoietically active vitamins, folic acid, vitamin B_{12}, pyridoxine, vitamin C, and vitamin K.[15]

2. Depression of bone marrow activity by toxins, chemical substances such as the sulfonamides, physical agents such as roentgen rays, or mechanical interference such as neoplastic disease.

3. Unknown causes, as in "aplastic" anemia.

Increased blood destruction or hemolytic anemia may be due to infections or chemicals or to intrinsic causes.

The anemias are classified according to cellular morphology and hemoglobin content as (1) macrocytic hyperchromic (pernicious anemia), (2) microcytic hypochromic (iron deficiency anemia), and (3) normocytic normochromic anemia (hemolytic anemia; aplastic anemia).

Macrocytic hyperchromic anemia (pernicious or Addison's anemia)

Pernicious anemia is most frequently encountered in individuals past the age of 40. The sexes are equally affected. The disease, which has an insidious onset, is characterized by symptoms referable to the nervous, cardiovascular, and gastrointestinal systems. The usual triad of symptoms includes a numbness and tingling of the extremities, weakness, and a sore tongue. Macrocytic hyperchromic anemia is characterized by a severe decrease in the number of erythrocytes (1,000,000 per cu. mm.) and elevated color index (1.5); a decreased hemoglobin value; a decreased platelet count (40,000); a decrease in the number of white blood cells; anisocytosis, poikilocytosis and polychromatophilia; and the presence of red cells containing nuclei or nuclear fragments.

ORAL CHANGES. Changes occur in the gingiva, the remainder of the oral mucosa, the lips and the tongue, which is involved

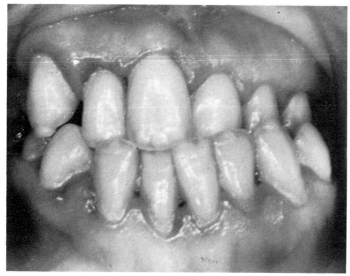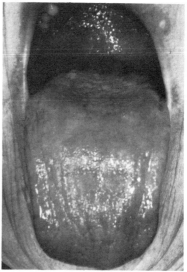

Fig. 30–7   Fig. 30–8

Figure 30–7   Diffuse Pallor of the Gingiva in Patient with Anemia. The discolored inflamed gingival margin stands out in sharp contrast to the adjacent pale attached gingiva.

Figure 30–8   Smooth Tongue in Patient with Pernicious Anemia.

in 75 per cent of the cases.[46] The earliest oral changes may be microscopic and consist of enlargement of epithelial cells with giant nuclei and nuclear pleomorphism.[6] The gingiva and mucosa are pale and yellowish and susceptible to ulceration. The tongue appears red, smooth, and shiny owing to the uniform atrophy of the fungiform and filiform papillae. The tongue is sensitive to hot or spicy foods, and swallowing is painful. The patients complain that the tongue feels raw, and there are sensations of burning and numbness. Atrophy of the tongue may be a manifestation of deficiency of vitamin B complex.[23] *Marked pallor of the gingiva* is a striking finding in pernicious anemia, with a wide variety of inflammatory changes, depending upon the nature of the local irritation[16] (Figs. 30–7 and 30–8).

Pernicious anemia is cyclical, with intermittent symptom-free periods. Remissions may last for a short time or for years, but the glossitis of pernicious anemia persists during all but the most complete remissions. Exacerbation of the glossitis may be a signal of relapse.

Microcytic hypochromic anemia

This form of anemia is caused by a deficiency in iron and other substances concerned with hemoglobin production, occurs in chronic blood loss, and is associated with inadequate iron ingestion or absorption. It is seen more often in females. Weakness, fatigue, and pallor are among the notable clinical features.

Microcytic hypochromic anemia is characterized by a moderate decrease in number of red blood cells (3,000,000), lowered color index (0.5), an increased platelet count (500,000), and a decreased hemoglobin.

ORAL CHANGES. Atrophy of alveolar bone and inflammation of the gingiva occur in animals with experimentally induced anemia.[22] Not all patients with hypochromic anemia present oral changes.[34] When involved, the most conspicuous change is pallor of the gingival mucosa and tongue, followed by erythema of the lateral border of the tongue with papillary atrophy and loss of muscle tone.[14, 19] Areas of gingival inflammation appear purplish red in contrast to the adjacent gingival pallor.

There is an initial erythema of the lateral border of the tongue, followed by pallor and papillary atrophy with loss of normal muscular tone.[14, 19] A correlation has been demonstrated between anemia and moderate to severe periodontal disease.[29] A syndrome consisting of glossitis, ulceration of the oral mucosa and oropharynx, and dysphagia, known as the *Plummer-Vinson syndrome*, may develop in patients with chronic anemia.

Sickle cell anemia

This is a hereditary and familial form of chronic hemolytic anemia and occurs almost exclusively in blacks. It is characterized by pallor, jaundice, weakness, rheumatoid manifestations, leg ulcers, and acute attacks of pain. The blood picture is distinguished by peculiar sickle-shaped and oat-shaped red corpuscles as well as signs of excessive blood destruction and active blood formation. Although not sex-linked, it occurs somewhat more frequently in females. Oral changes include generalized osteoporosis of the jaws, reported in about 80 per cent of the cases, with a peculiar stepladder alignment of the trabeculae of the interdental septa,[39] and pallor and yellowish discoloration of the oral mucosa.[33]

Normochromic normocytic anemia

In this group, the oral changes associated with *Cooley's anemia* are noteworthy. (See Chapter 21.)

Thrombocytopenic Purpura

In thrombocytopenic purpura there is spontaneous bleeding into the skin or from mucous membranes. Petechiae and hemorrhagic vesicles occur in the oral cavity, particularly in the palate and buccal mucosa. The gingiva is swollen, soft, and friable. Bleeding occurs spontaneously or upon the slighest provocation and is difficult to control. Special note should be made of the fact that the gingival changes represent an abnormal response to local irritation; the severity of the gingival condition is dramatically alleviated by removal of the local irritants (Fig. 30–9).

Thrombocytopenic purpura may be idiopathic (e.g., of unknown etiology as in *Werlhof's disease*), or it may occur secondary to some known etiologic factor responsible for a reduction in the amount of functioning marrow and a resultant reduction in the circulating platelets. The latter conditions include aplasia of the marrow; crowding out of the megakaryocytes in the marrow, as in leukemia for example; replacement of the marrow by tumor; destruction of the marrow by x-radiation or radium, or by drugs such as benzene, aminopyrine, and the arsenicals.

Thrombocytopenic purpura is characterized by a low platelet count, a prolonged clot retraction and bleeding time, and by a normal or slightly prolonged clotting time.

Hemophilia

Hemophilia is an inherited sex-linked disease affecting only the male, and transmitted by the female. The afflicted male does not transmit the disease to his male offspring. The defect is passed to the fe-

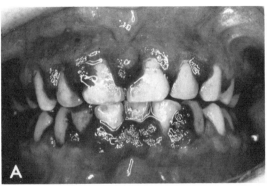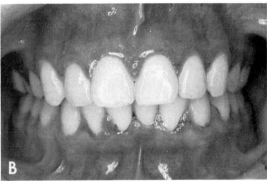

Figure 30–9 Thrombocytopenia Purpura. *A,* Hemorrhagic gingivitis in patient with thrombocytopenia purpura. *B,* Marked reduction in severity of gingival disease after removal of surface debris and careful scaling.

male offspring, who exhibits no symptoms of the disease but who transmits the defect to her son.

Hemophilia is characterized by prolonged hemorrhage from even slight wounds, and by spontaneous bleeding into the skin. Spontaneous bleeding from mucous membranes is not a feature of the disease.

The clotting time is markedly prolonged, but the bleeding time remains normal. The prolonged clotting time is due to a deficiency of serum protein antihemophiliac globulin (AHG; factor VIII), which presumably results from platelet resistance to disintegration. The normal bleeding time may be explained on the following basis:

When a hemophiliac person cuts himself, the capillary, as it would normally, contracts with cessation of bleeding. When the capillary later expands, however, there is no clot present to plug the defect, and bleeding starts again.

Christmas Disease (Pseudohemophilia)

Christmas disease is characterized by abnormal bleeding tendencies that make it clinically indistinguishable from hemophilia. Another resemblance to hemophilia is that it is inherited by the male as a sex-linked recessive trait. It differs from hemophilia in that the hemostatic defect lies in the missing serum fraction, called plasma thromboplastin component (PTC), so named because it affects the production of thromboplastin, without which there is an abnormality in the clotting mechanism.

Mild Christmas disease may escape detection because the bleeding time, coagulation time, and clot retraction time may be within normal limits. In patients with a history of abnormal bleeding, the prothrombin-consumption test or the thromboplastin-generation test may be necessary in order to rule out Christmas disease.[28]

Hereditary Hemorrhagic Telangiectasia

This comparatively rare vascular anomaly, sometimes known as *Rendu-Osler-Weber disease*, is characterized by multiple dilatations of capillaries and venules in the skin and mucous membrane, with a tendency toward hemorrhage. It appears to be transmitted in families as a simple dominant, affecting both sexes.[42]

The most common sites of the lesions, in order of involvement, are nasal mucosa, tongue, palate, lips, mucocutaneous junction, and gingiva.[16] Lesions may occur, however, almost anywhere on the skin and mucous membranes of the body.

The telangiectases may be pinpoint in size or spider-like, with a central nodular pea-sized lesion. Although the condition may be present in childhood, the lesions increase in number as age advances.[43] The blood vessels do not attain their full size until about the age of 35, at which time the telangiectases appear bright-red, violaceous, or purple. Epistaxis is a common symptom, and hemorrhage may occur wherever the lesions exist.

The *Sturge-Weber syndrome* is a congenital condition characterized by capillary angiomas (port-wine stain, nevus flammeus) on the face and on the meninges, with epileptiform symptoms. There are telangiectasis, vascular hyperplasia, and enlargement of the gingiva with associated resorption of alveolar bone.

Infectious Mononucleosis

This is a benign infectious disease of unknown etiology. It usually occurs in children or young adults. The suspicion that it is communicable has not been well substantiated. It is characterized by sudden onset, headache, fever, muscular ache, sore throat, malaise, nausea, vomiting, swelling and tenderness of lymph nodes (particularly in the cervical area), occasional skin rash, and lymphocytosis.

Soreness of the mouth and throat are often the patient's initial complaint. The oral findings include diffuse erythema of the entire mucosa with petechiae in some cases.[13] The marginal and interdental papillae are swollen and markedly reddened, and bleed on slightest provocation or even spontaneously.

After two to four weeks the systemic symptoms usually begin to subside, but the oral changes may persist.

The diagnosis of infectious mononucleosis is based upon the hematologic findings. Leukopenia is seen in the early stages, followed by a marked lymphocytosis. Characteristic of the blood picture are typical "monocytoid" lymphocytes, or Downey cells. The heterophile antibody test (Paul-Bunnell) is used as an aid in diagnosis. This is based on the agglutination of sheep red cells by the patient's serum. Agglutination with serum dilution of 1:64 or above is diagnostic.

Agranulocytosis (Granulocytopenia)

Agranulocytosis is an acute disease characterized by extreme leukopenia and neutropenia, and accompanied by ulceration of the oral mucosa, skin, and gastrointestinal tract.

Drug idiosyncrasy is the most common cause of agranulocytosis, but in some instances its etiology cannot be explained. It has been reported following the administration of drugs such as aminopyrine,[27, 36] barbiturates and their derivatives, benzene ring derivatives,[30] sulfonamides,[32] gold salts, or arsenicals. It generally occurs as an acute disease, but may reappear in cyclical episodes (cyclical neutropenia) that may be correlated with the onset of the menstrual period.[45] It may be periodic with recurring neutropenic cycles.[44]

The onset of the disease is accompanied by fever, malaise, general weakness, and "sore throat." Ulceration in the oral cavity, oropharynx, and throat is characteristic. The mucosa presents isolated necrotic patches that are black and gray and sharply demarcated from the adjacent uninvolved areas.[25, 31] The absence of a notable inflammatory reaction because of lack of granulocytes is a striking feature. The gingival margin may or may not be involved. Gingival hemorrhage, necrosis, increased salivation, and fetid odor are accompanying clinical features.

Bauer[2] described the following microscopic changes in the periodontium: hemorrhage into the periodontal ligament with destruction of the principal fibers; osteoporosis of the cancellous bone with osteoclastic resorption; small fragments of necrotic bone in the hemorrhagic periodontal ligament; hemorrhage in the marrow adjacent to the teeth; areas in which the periodontal ligament is widened and consists of dense fibrous tissue with fibers parallel to the tooth surface, and the formation of new bone trabeculae. In cyclical neutropenia the gingival changes recur with recurrent exacerbation of the disease.[12]

Experimentally, neutropenia has been produced in dogs with heterologous antineutrophil serum. Neutrophilic granulocytes disappeared from the tissues, but ulcerative lesions and bacterial invasion were not observed, probably due to the short duration of the experiment (4 days).[40]

Because infection is a common feature of agranulocytosis, differential diagnosis includes consideration of such conditions as acute necrotizing ulcerative gingivitis, diphtheria, noma, and acute necrotizing inflammation of the tonsils. Definitive diagnosis depends upon the hematologic findings of pronounced leukopenia and almost complete absence of neutrophils.

Polycythemia

Polycythemia refers to an increase in the number of circulating red cells. It is to be distinguished from hemoconcentration ("relative" polycythemia), resulting from the loss of body fluid that accompanies persistent vomiting, diarrhea, or sweating. Polycythemia may be primary or secondary.

Primary polycythemia

Primary polycythemia is also known as polycythemia vera or rubra, or *Vaquez-Osler disease*. It is characterized by increased red cell production in the bone marrow, splenomegaly, and an increase in the red cell count ranging from 7 to 10 million per cubic millimeter. The total red cell volume, as well as the leukocyte and platelet counts, is also increased. The hemoglobin level is between 18 and 24 gm./100 ml., and the range of blood viscosity is 1.075 to 1.085, as compared with the normal range of 1.055 to 1.065.

Secondary polycythemia

Secondary polycythemia may occur as the result of a reduction in oxygen tension of the inspired air, as in elevated altitudes. It may also be due to impaired transport of oxygen, or oxygenation of blood in the lungs, as in congenital or acquired heart disease and pulmonary disease. In secondary polycythemia, there is no increase in total red cell volume per kilogram of body weight, and the red cell count seldom exceeds 7 million per cubic millimeter of blood.

Polycythemia, either primary or secondary, is in most cases characterized by a reddish blue cyanotic discoloration of the skin, with comparable involvement of the oral and pharyngeal mucous membrane.[37, 46] Bright red diffuse discoloration of the gingiva and tongue[10] are sometimes seen with abnormal gingival bleeding.

Arteriosclerosis

In aged individuals arteriosclerotic changes characterized by intimal thickening, narrowing of the lumen, thickening of the media, and hyalinization of the media and adventitia, with or without calcification, are common in vessels throughout the jaws as well as in areas of periodontal inflammation[35, 47] (Fig. 30–10). Periodontal disease and arteriosclerosis both increase with age, and it has been hypothesized that circulatory impairment induced by the vascular changes may increase the susceptibility to periodontal disease.[1]

In experimental animals partial ischemia of more than ten hours' duration, created by arteriolar occlusion, produces changes in the oxidative enzymes and acid phos-

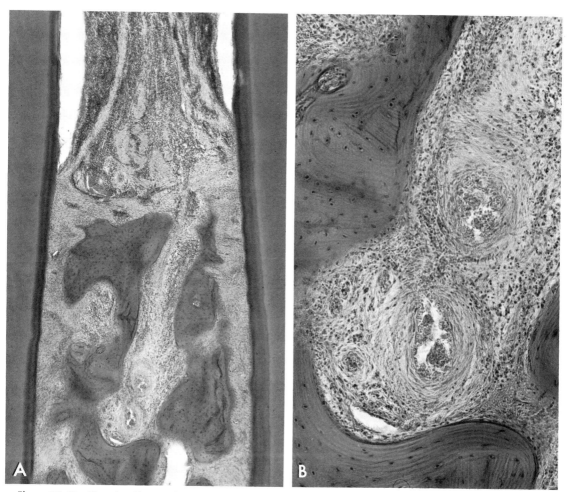

Figure 30–10 **Vascular Changes in Aged Individual with Periodontal Disease.** *A,* **Periodontitis,** showing inflammation extending from the gingiva into the interdental septum. *B,* Detailed view, showing arterioles with thickened walls in the marrow space of the interdental septum.

phatase activity and in the glycogen and lipid content of the gingival epithelium.[24] Focal necrosis followed by ulceration occurs in the epithelium, with the junctional epithelium least affected.[26] DNA duplication is depressed. Changes typical of periodontal disease do not occur. Ischemia is followed by hyperemia, accompanied by metabolic changes and increased DNA synthesis in the epithelium plus epithelial proliferation and thickening—all considered to be part of the gingival response to arteriolar occlusion.

REFERENCES

1. Barrett, R., Cheraskin, E., and Ringsdorf, W., Jr.: Alveolar bone loss and capillaropathy. J. Periodontol., 40:131, 1969.
2. Bauer, W. H.: Agranulocytosis and the supporting dental tissues. J. Dent. Res., 25:501, 1946.
3. Bender, I. B.: Bone changes in leukemia. Am. J. Orthod., 30:556, 1944.
4. Bernick, S.: Age changes in the blood supply to human teeth. J. Dent. Res., 46:544, 1967.
5. Bernick, S., Levy, B. M., and Patek, P. R.: Studies on the biology of the periodontium of marmosets. VI. Arteriosclerotic changes in the blood vessels of the periodontium. J. Periodontol., 40:355, 1969.
6. Boen, S. T.: Changes in the nuclei of squamous epithelial cells in pernicious anemia. Acta Med. Scand., 159:425, 1957.
7. Brown, L. R., et al.: Alveolar bone loss in leukemic and non-leukemic mice. J. Periodontol., 40:725, 1969.
8. Burket, L. W.: A histopathologic explanation for the oral lesions in the acute leukemias. Am. J. Orthod., 30:516, 1944.
9. Carranza, F. A., Jr., Gravina, O., and Cabrini, R. L.: Periodontal and pulpal pathosis in leukemic mice. Oral Surg., 20:374, 1965.
10. Cecil, R. L., and Loeb, R. F.: Textbook of Medicine. 9th ed. Philadelphia, W. B. Saunders Co., 1955.
11. Chaundry, A. P., et al.: Unusual oral manifestations of chronic lymphatic leukemia (report of a case). Oral Surg., 15:446, 1962.
12. Cohen, D. W., and Morris, A. L.: Periodontal manifestations of cyclic neutropenia. J. Periodontol., 32:159, 1961.
13. Cottrell, J. E.: Infectious mononucleosis. J. Periodontol., 9:15, 1938.
14. Darby, W. J.: The oral manifestations of iron deficiency. J.A.M.A., 130:830, 1946.
15. Dreizen, S.: Oral manifestations of human nutritional anemias. Arch. Environ. Health, 5:66, 1962.
16. Durocher, R. T., Morris, A. L., and Burket, L. W.: Oral manifestations of hereditary hemorrhagic telangiectasia. Oral Surg., 14:550, 1961.
17. El Mostehy, M. R., and Stallard, R. E.: The Sturge-Weber syndrome: Its periodontal significance. J. Periodontol., 40:243, 1969.
18. Epstein, I. A.: Clinical indications for the use of blood examinations in the practice of periodontia. J. Periodontol., 6:30, 1935.
19. Frantzell, A., et al.: Examination of the tongue. Acta Med. Scand., 122:207, 1945.
20. Goldman, H. M.: Acute aleukemic leukemia. Am. J. Orthod., 26:89, 1940.
21. Grant, D., and Bernick, S.: Arteriosclerosis in periodontal vessels of aging humans. J. Periodontol., 41:170, 1970.
22. Hall, J. F., and Robinson, H. B. G.: Alveolar atrophy in anemic dogs. J. Dent. Res., 16:345, 1937.
23. Hutter, A. M., Middleton, W. S., and Steenbock, H.: Vitamin B deficiency and the atrophic tongue. J.A.M.A., 101:1305, 1933.
24. Itoiz, M. E., Litwack, D., Kennedy, J. E., and Zander, H. A.: Experimental ischemia in monkeys: III. Histochemical analysis of gingival epithelium. J. Dent. Res. (Part 2), 48:895, 1969.
25. Kastlin, G.: Agranulocytic angina. Am. J. Med. Sci., 173:799, 1927.
26. Kennedy, J. E., and Zander, H. A.: Experimental ischemia in monkeys: I. Effect of ischemia on gingival epithelium. J. Dent. Res. (Part I), 48:696, 1969.
27. Kracke, R. R.: Granulopenia as associated with amidopyrine administration. Report made at Annual Session of A.M.A., June, 1934.
28. Kramer, G., and Griffel, A.: Christmas disease (hemophilia B) in periodontal therapy. Oral Surg., 15:1056, 1962.
29. Lainson, P., Brady, P., and Fraleigh, C.: Anemia, a systemic cause of periodontal disease. J. Periodontol., 39:35, 1968.
30. Madison, F. W., and Squier, T. L.: Primary granulocytopenia after administration of benzene chain derivatives. J.A.M.A., 102:755, 1934.
31. Mark, H. A.: Agranulocytic angina. Its oral manifestations. J. Am. Dent. Assoc., 21:2119, 1934.
32. Meyer, A.: Agranulocytosis. Report of a case caused by sulfadiazine. California and West Med. J., 61:54, 1944.
33. Mittleman, G., Bakke, B. F., and Scopp, I. W.: Alveolar bone changes in sickle cell anemia. J. Periodontol., 32:74, 1961.
34. Monto, R. W., Rizek, R., and Fine, G.: Observations on the exfoliative cytology and histology of the oral mucous membranes in iron deficiency. Oral Surg., 14:965, 1961.
35. Quintarelli, G.: Histopathology of the human mandibular artery and arterioles in periodontal disease. Oral Surg., 10:1047, 1957.
36. Randall, C. L.: Granulocytopenia following barbiturates and amidopyrine. J.A.M.A., 102:1137, 1934.
37. Reznikoff, P., Foot, N., and Bethea, J.: Etiological and pathological findings in polycythemia vera. Am. J. Med. Sci., 189:753, 1935.
38. Robbins, S. L.: Textbook of Pathology. 2nd ed. Philadelphia, W. B. Saunders Co., 1962, p. 156.
39. Robinson, I. B., and Sarnat, B. G.: Roentgen studies of the maxillae and mandible in sickle cell anemia. Radiology, 58:517, 1952.
40. Rylander, H., Attstrom, R., and Lindhe, J.: In-

fluence of experimental neutropenia in dogs with chronic gingivitis. J. Periodont. Res., 10:315, 1975.

41. Schonbauer, F.: Histological findings in the jaw in septicemia and leukemia. Zeit. Stomatol., 27:804, 1929.

42. Schwartz, S., and Armstrong, B.: Familial hereditary hemorrhagic telangiectasia in the Negro. N. Engl. J. Med., 239:434, 1948.

43. Scopp, I. W., and Quart, A.: Hereditary hemorrhagic telangiectasia involving the oral cavity. Oral Surg., 11:1138, 1958.

44. Telsey, B., Beube, F. E., Zegarelli, E. V., and Kutscher, A. H.: Oral manifestations of cyclical neutropenia associated with hypergammaglobulinemia. Oral Surg., 15:540, 1962.

45. Thompson, W. P.: Observations on possible relation between agranulocytosis and menstruation with further studies on a case of cyclic neutropenia. N. Engl. J. Med., 210:176, 1934.

46. Winter, L.: Blood dyscrasias—Their oral manifestations. Am. J. Orthod., 26:67, 1940.

47. Wirthlin, M. R., Jr., and Ratcliff, P. A.: Arteries, atherosclerosis and periodontics. J. Periodontol., 40:341, 1969.

OTHER SYSTEMIC DISORDERS

Metallic Intoxication

Ingestion of metals such as mercury, lead, and bismuth in medicinal compounds and through industrial contact may result in oral manifestations owing to either (1) intoxication or (2) absorption without evidence of toxicity.

Bismuth intoxication

Chronic bismuth intoxication is characterized by gastrointestinal disturbances, nausea, vomiting, and jaundice, as well as an ulcerative gingivostomatitis, generally with pigmentation, accompanied by a metallic taste and burning sensation of the oral mucosa. The tongue may be sore and inflamed. Urticaria, exanthematous eruptions of different types, bullous and purpuric lesions, as well as herpes zoster–like eruptions and pigmentation of the skin and mucous membranes, are among the dermatologic lesions attributed to bismuth intoxication. Acute bismuth intoxication, which is less commonly seen, is accompanied by methemoglobin formation, cyanosis, and dyspnea.

BISMUTH PIGMENTATION IN THE ORAL CAVITY. Bismuth pigmentation usually appears as a narrow blue-black discoloration of the gingival margin in areas of preexistent gingival inflammation (see Chapter 7). Such pigmentation results from the precipitation of particles of bismuth sulfide associated with vascular changes in inflammation. It is not evidence of intoxication, but simply indicates the presence of bismuth in the blood stream. Bismuth pigmentation in the oral cavity also occurs in cases of intoxication. It assumes a linear form if the marginal gingiva is inflamed.

Lead intoxication

The metal is slowly absorbed, and toxic symptoms are not particularly definitive when they do occur. There are pallor of the face and lips and gastrointestinal symptoms consisting of nausea, vomiting, loss of appetite, and abdominal colic. Peripheral neuritis and psychological disorders and encephalitis have been reported. Among the oral signs are salivation, coated tongue, a peculiar sweetish taste, gingival pigmentation and ulceration. The pigmentation of the gingiva is linear (burtonian line), steel-gray, and associated with local irritation. It may occur without toxic symptoms.

Mercury intoxication[1]

Mercury intoxication is characterized by headache, insomnia, cardiovascular symptoms, pronounced salivation (ptyalism), and metallic taste. Gingival pigmentation in linear form results from deposition of mercuric sulfide. The chemical also acts as an irritant which accentuates the pre-existent inflammation and commonly leads to notable ulceration of the gingiva and adjacent mucosa (Fig. 30–11) and destruction of the underlying bone. Mercurial pigmentation of the gingiva also occurs in areas of local irritation in patients without symptoms of intoxication.

Other Chemicals

Other chemicals such as *phosphorous*,[6] *arsenic*,[3] and *chromium*[5] may cause necrosis of alveolar bone with loosening and exfoliation of the teeth. Inflammation and

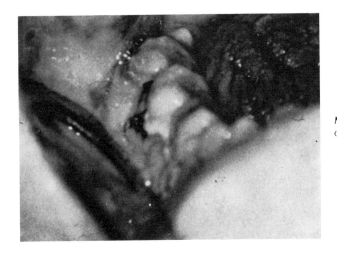

Figure 30–11 Ulceration of the Gingiva in Mercury Intoxication. Note linear pigmentation of the gingival margin adjacent to materia alba.

ulceration of the gingiva are usually associated with destruction of the underlying tissues. *Benzene*[6] intoxication is accompanied by gingival bleeding and ulceration with destruction of the underlying bone.

REFERENCES

Other Systemic Disorders

1. Akers, L. H.: Ulcerative stomatitis following therapeutic use of mercury and bismuth. J. Am. Dent. Assoc., 23:781, 1936.
2. Higgins, W. H.: Systemic poisoning with bismuth. J.A.M.A., 66:648, 1916.
3. Hudson, E. J.: Purpura hemorrhagica caused by gold and arsenical compounds with report of 2 cases. Lancet, 2:74, 1935.
4. Jones, R. R.: Symptoms in early stages of industrial plumbism. J.A.M.A., 104:195, 1935.
5. Liberman, H.: Chrome ulcerations of the nose and throat. N. Eng. J. Med., 225:132, 1941.
6. Schour, I., and Sarnat, B. G.: Oral manifestations of occupational origin. J.A.M.A., 120:1197, 1942.

DEBILITATING DISEASES AND THE PERIODONTIUM

Debilitating diseases such as *syphilis, chronic nephritis,* and *tuberculosis* may predispose to periodontal disease by impairing tissue resistance to local irritants and creating a tendency toward alveolar bone resorption.[23, 26] A type of membranous stomatitis has been described[4] associated with debilitation in uremia; and a sore dry mouth with edema, purulent inflammation, and bleeding of the gingiva has been noted in primary renal disease.[31] The absence of periodontal disease in chronically ill patients has been presented as evidence that in individual cases systemic disease may exert no deleterious effect upon the periodontium.[25]

Difference of opinion exists regarding the relationship of tuberculosis to periodontal disease. Although an increased incidence of gingivitis and chronic destructive periodontal disease as well as alveolar bone changes, characterized by enlargement of the cancellous spaces, has been reported in tuberculous patients,[7, 21] these findings have not been corroborated in other studies.[13, 27] In patients with *leprosy* the chronic destructive periodontal disease has been described as nonspecific in nature and no *M. leprae* have been present in the gingiva.[28]

PSYCHOSOMATIC DISORDERS AND THE PERIODONTIUM

Harmful effects that result from psychic influences in the organic control of tissues are known as psychosomatic disorders.[14] There are two ways in which psychosomatic disorders may be induced in the oral cavity: (1) *through the development of habits which are injurious to the periodontium* and (2) *by the direct effect of the autonomic system upon the physiologic tissue balance.* Giddon[11] has presented an excellent review of experimental evidence which relates psychological factors to oral physiology.

Psychologically, the oral cavity is related directly or symbolically to the major human instincts and passions. In the infant, many oral drives find direct expression, as oral receptive and oral aggressive trends and oral eroticism.[24] In the adult, most of the instinctual drives are normally suppressed by education, and are satisfied in substitutive ways or are taken over by organs more appropriate than the mouth. **However, under conditions of mental and emotional duress, the mouth may subconsciously become an outlet for the gratification of basic drives in the adult.**

Gratification may be derived from neurotic habits, such as grinding or clenching of the teeth,[6, 9] nibbling on foreign objects, such as pencils or pipes, nail biting, or excessive use of tobacco, which are potentially injurious to the periodontium. Correlations have been reported between psychiatric and anxiety states and the occurrence of periodontal disease,[1, 3, 16, 17] and questioned by some.[2] Psychological factors in the etiology of acute necrotizing ulcerative gingivitis are discussed in Chapter 11.

It is necessary to correct local factors which may initiate harmful habits, but investigation of the psychic background is indicated in difficult cases. Saul[24] describes a case of sore throat, bleeding gums, and ulceration of the buccal mucosa traced to mouth breathing and bruxism associated with oral-aggressive dreams. Psychoanalysis resulted in elimination of the underlying difficulty and habit and relief of the oral disease.

Disorders of psychosomatic origin may be produced in the oral cavity by the influence of the autonomic nervous system upon the somatic control of the tissues.[5] Alterations in the vascular supply caused by autonomic stimulation may adversely affect the health of the periodontium by impairing tissue nutrition.[22] Diminution in the secretion of saliva in emotional disorders may lead to xerostomia with painful symptoms. Weiss and English[30] outline the sequence of events whereby psychological disturbances affect tissue alterations as follows:

Psychological disturbance → Functional impairment → Cellular disease → Structural alteration

Autonomic influences upon the muscles of mastication may result in impairment of mandibular movement, which resembles organically induced temporomandibular joint disorders. In such cases, psychiatric management may suffice for the restoration of normal function of the mandible.

HEREDITY IN THE ETIOLOGY OF PERIODONTAL DISEASE

In experimental animals heredity appears to be a factor in calculus formation and periodontal disease.[18] Hypophosphatasia, an inherited disease characterized by rachitic-like skeletal changes, also presents premature loss of deciduous incisors and surrounding alveolar bone by ten months of age, and sometimes without the skeletal changes.[19]

In an investigation of blood types with a view toward the possibility of inheritance of predisposition, it was found that 49 per cent of patients with periodontal disease were of blood type A; the incidence of blood type A in patients without periodontal disease was 40 to 41.1 per cent.[20, 29] Gancotti[10] concluded that inherited tendency was a factor in 62 per cent of the cases of periodontal disease that he studied, whereas other investigators[8] found no indication that heredity affected gingival crevice depth or recession. Gorlin[12] has described numerous genetic disorders which result in oral mucous membrane changes. Heinrich[15] noted that juvenile periodontitis was more common in the pyknic type of individual than in the asthenic type.

REFERENCES

Debilitating Diseases and the Periodontium

1. Baker, E. G., Crook, G. H., and Schwabacher, E. D.: Personality correlates of periodontal disease. J. Dent. Res., 40:396, 1961.
2. Barry, J. R., and Dutkovic, T. R.: Oral pathosis: Exploration of psychological correlates. J. Am. Dent. Assoc., 67:86, 1963.

3. Belting, C. M., and Gupta, O. P.: The influence of psychiatric disturbances on the severity of periodontal disease. J. Periodontol., *32*:219, 1961.

4. Bereston, E. S., and Herb, H.: Membranous stomatitis with debilitation and uremia. Arch. Dermatol. Syph., *44*:562, 1941.

5. Biber, O.: Autonomic symptoms in psychoneurotics. Psychosom. Med., *3*:253, 1941.

6. Burstoen, M. S.: The psychosomatic aspects of dental problems. J. Am. Dent. Assoc., *33*:862, 1946.

7. Cahn, L. R.: Observations in the effect of tuberculosis on the teeth, gums and jaws. Dent. Cosmos, *67*:479, 1925.

8. Ciancio, S., Hazen, S., and Cunat, J.: Periodontal observations in twins. J. Periodont. Res., *4*:42, 1969.

9. Frohman, B. S.: Occlusal neuroses. Psychoanal. Rev., *19*:297, 1932.

10. Gancotti, M.: Hereditary factors in periodontal diseases. Ann. Stomatol. Roma, *5*:117, 1956.

11. Giddon, D. B.: Psychophysiology of the oral cavity. J. Dent. Res., *45*:1627, 1966.

12. Gorlin, R. J.: Genetic disorders affecting mucous membranes. Oral Surg., *28*:512, 1969.

13. Gruber, I. E.: The condition of the teeth and the attachment apparatus in tuberculosis. J. Dent. Res., *28*:483, 1949.

14. Gupta, O. P.: Psychosomatic factors in periodontal disease. Dent. Clin. North Am., 1966, p. 11.

15. Heinrich, E.: Report on sociologic and constitutional typologic examinations on paradentosis of 200 patients. Paradentium, *2*:32, 1933.

16. Manhold, J. H.: Report of a study on the relationship of personality variables to periodontal conditions. J. Periodontol., *24*:248, 1953.

17. Miller, S. C., et al.: The use of the Minnesota Multiplastic Personality Inventory as a diagnostic aid in periodontal disease. A preliminary report. J. Periodontol., *27*:44, 1956.

18. Moskow, B. S. Rennert, M. C., Wasserman, B. H., and Khurana, H.: Interrelationship of dietary factors and heredity in periodontal lesions in the gerbil. Program and Abstracts, 48th General Meeting, I.A.D.R., 1970, p. 134.

19. Poland, C., III, Christian, J. C., and Bixler, D.: Hypophosphatasia: An inherited oral disease. Program and Abstracts, 48th General Meeting, I.A.D.R., 1970, p. 228.

20. Polevitsky, K.: Blood types in pyorrhea alveolaris. J. Dent. Res., *9*:285, 1929.

21. Ramfjord, S.: Tuberculosis and periodontal disease, with special reference to the collagen fibers. J. Dent. Res., *31*:5, 1952.

22. Ryan, E. J.: Psychobiologic Foundation in Dentistry. Springfield, Ill., Charles C Thomas, Publisher, 1946, p. 27.

23. Sandler, H. C., and Stahl, S. S.: The influence of generalized diseases on clinical manifestations of periodontal disease. J. Am. Dent. Assoc., *49*:656, 1954.

24. Saul, L. J.: A note on the psychogenesis of organic symptoms. Psychoanal. Q., *4*:476, 1935.

25. Scopp, I. W.: Healthy periodontium in chronically ill patients. J. Periodontol. *28*:147, 1957.

26. Stahl, S. S., et al.: The influence of systemic diseases on alvolar bone. J. Am. Dent. Assoc., *45*:277, 1952.

27. Tanchester, D., and Sorrin, S.: Dental lesions in relation to pulmonary tuberculosis. J. Dent. Res., *16*:69, 1937.

28. Tochichara, Y.: Pyorrhea alveolaris in leprosy. Nippar No Shikai, *13*:165, 1933.

29. Weber, R., and Pastern, W.: Uber die Frage der konstitutionellen Bereitschaft zur sog. Alveolar Pyorrhea (Alveolarpyorrhoe und Blutgruppen). Dtsch. Monatschr. Zahnheilk., *14*:704, 1927.

30. Weiss, E., and English, O. S.: Psychosomatic Medicine. 2nd ed. Philadelphia, W. B. Saunders Co., 1949.

31. Weller, C. V.: Constitutional factors in periodontitis. J. Am. Dent. Assoc., *15*:1081, 1928.

Chapter 31

The Systemic Condition of Patients with Periodontal Disease

Numerous clinical studies have been conducted to determine whether there are disorders that predispose to periodontal disease and also to determine the effect upon the patient of gingival and periodontal disease. The findings in such studies have been interpreted in the following ways:

1. There may be systemic disorders that predispose to periodontal disease.

2. Periodontal disease may predispose to certain systemic disorders.

3. There may be comparable factors that predispose patients to both periodontal disease and specific systemic disorders.

SYSTEMIC FINDINGS IN PERIODONTAL DISEASE

The following systemic aspects have been investigated in relation to periodontal disease. (Some studies differentiate between systemic findings in patients with periodontitis and those with juvenile periodontitis; others do not make this distinction.)

Metabolism

Patients with periodontitis present no characteristic metabolic pattern.[6-8] In juve-nile periodontitis the metabolism has been reported as both lowered[12] and slightly elevated.[5, 51] Opinions differ as to whether a correlation exists between the periodontal status and glucose tolerance levels.[37, 47]

Endocrine

Dysfunction of the parathyroid and pituitary glands, ovaries and thyroid (particularly hyperthyroidism),[4, 5] and abnormal serum calcium levels have been reported in juvenile periodontitis.[13] Hypothyroidism was observed in 43 out of 80 patients with periodontitis,[3] with and without other endocrine disorders (e.g., diabetes, hypogonadism, and pituitary dysfunction[49]) and reduced urinary estrogen levels[24] have been correlated with increasing severity of periodontal disease.

Blood chemistry

Elevated calcium,[50] lowered calcium with elevated phosphorus,[20] elevated serum glycoprotein,[15] uric acid, glucose, cholesterol, citric acid, and bilirubin have been reported in the blood of patients with juvenile periodontitis.[25, 28, 46, 50] Serum glutamic oxaloacetic transaminase and serum glutamic pyruvic transaminase are not altered.[21]

In periodontitis, elevated blood calcium and lowered phosphorus,[2, 13, 19] elevated serum alkaline phosphatase,[34] and citric acid,[42] and lowered blood catalase[16] levels have been described. Some investigators suggest the possibility of a relationship between dietary inadequacy and deviations in blood chemistry in patients with periodontal disease.[22] Others note no significant changes in periodontal disease.

541

The blood levels of calcium, glucose, cholesterol, ascorbic acid,[23, 45] sodium and potassium,[34] chloride, inorganic phosphate, and urea nitrogen[31] are reported as unaltered. Serum total protein, albumin, globulin, and uric acid show no significant relationship to periodontal status.[38, 39] The level of serum-free 17-hydroxycorticosterone is elevated in periodontal disease, but the significance of this finding has not been established. The glucose content of blood in the gingiva and the finger is the same in patients with periodontal disease,[25] but alkaline phosphatase in gingival blood is greater than in the general circulation.[32] C-reactive protein (CRP) (a nonspecific protein usually associated with diseases causing inflammation and tissue breakdown and not found in healthy individuals) was noted in patients with severe periodontal disease.[40]

A laboratory study of 143 adult patients with advanced periodontal disease included evaluation of calcium, cholesterol, glucose, inorganic phosphorus, total protein, albumin, globulin, urea nitrogen, uric acid, protein-bound iodine, and alkaline phosphatase; oral glucose tolerance tests (fasting, 30 minutes, and 1, 2, and 3 hours); and serum electrophoresis for albumin, alpha-1-globulin, alpha-2-globulin, beta-globulin, gamma globulin, and total protein. There was no indication that the presence of advanced periodontal disease was in any way related to variations in the accepted normal values.[11]

Gastric chemistry

Gastric hyperacidity, hypoacidity, and anacidity[7, 35] occur in patients with periodontal disease. The contention of Broderick,[9] that periodontal disease results from alkalosis and caries is caused by acidosis, has not been confirmed.

Hematologic aspects

Blood studies in patients with periodontal disease reveal the following: normal total and differential leukocyte count and low red blood count,[41] elevated counts, frequent secondary anemia of the hypochromic microcytic type,[18] decrease in hemoglobin values and a low erythrocyte count, as well as a relative lymphocytosis and a decrease in polymorphonuclear leukocytes.[27] Blood type A was noted in 49 per cent of patients with periodontal disease in contrast with 40 to 41.1 per cent of patients without periodontal disease,[33, 48] but no significant relationship between blood grouping and periodontal disease,[1] or between arteriosclerosis and alveolar bone loss[26] has been established.

Comment

The preceding paragraphs reflect the rather unsettled status and sparseness of information regarding the systemic condition of patients with periodontal disease. It is difficult to evaluate many of the investigations because there is no uniformity in the criteria used to judge the periodontal disorders. The inadequacy of available information regarding the possible interrelation of systemic disorders and periodontal disease should not be misinterpreted as indicating an absence of such relationship. One must also guard against attributing too much significance to isolated, unconfirmed findings.

FOCAL INFECTION

According to the concept of focal infection, a primary site of infection in one part of the body may serve as the focus (Latin "hearth") from which infection emanates to other parts of the body. Interest in focal infection has fluctuated considerably from the initial enthusiasm stimulated by the original investigation of Rosenow in 1917. More recently, with the introduction of chemotherapy, attention has again been directed to the subject of focal infection.

In the early days of the focal infection concept, the oral cavity attracted attention because it harbored teeth with chronic apical disease. Physicians confronted with disease elsewhere in the body were drawn to the comparatively easily available "infected teeth." The persistence of disease in other areas of the body even after all the "infected" teeth had been removed, coupled with the revelation that not all pathologic apical lesions were necessarily

TABLE 31-1 THE PERIODONTAL POCKET VS. PERIAPICAL DISEASE

Periodontal Pocket	Periapical Disease
1. Infection is always present.	1. Infection is not necessarily present in long-standing periapical lesions.[10]
2. The bacterial as well as mycotic organisms are of great variety and considerably more numerous as well as of greater pathogenic potentiality.	2. The bacterial organisms are not as varied, numerous nor of equal pathogenic significance.
3. Periodontal pockets are not circumscribed or walled off from the adjacent tissue.	3. Periapical areas are frequently well circumscribed within a fibrotic boundary.
4. Periodontal pockets are subject to constant mechanical stimulation in mastication which could drive bacteria into the blood stream.	4. Periapical areas are located centrally in the bone, in a comparatively undisturbed environment.
5. Periodontal pockets are more prevalent in adults in age groups likely to be subject to ailments requiring medical attention.	5. Less prevalent than periodontal pockets.

infected, exerted a somewhat sobering influence upon the medical and dental professions in regard to the problem of focal infection.

Periodontal disease and focal infection

Interest in the oral cavity as a possible source of focal infection has shifted recently from the periapical areas to the periodontal pocket.[44] Within the limitations which govern the concept of focal infection, **the periodontal pocket represents a greater potential menace than periapical disease for the reasons shown in Table 31-1.**

In patients with periodontal disease and a disturbance elsewhere in the body suspected of being of focal origin, **the responsibility for the decision regarding the fate of the teeth rests with the dentist.** It is reasonable to expect him to understand more about the periodontal tissues than other medical specialists. The physician, on the other hand, is in a position to inform the dentist regarding the likelihood of the patient's medical problem being caused by infection elsewhere in the body. It should be borne in mind that even in a patient with suppurative periodontal disease which the dentist might very well consider a potential focus of infection, there is no assurance that the patient's complaint is related to the oral condition.

BACTEREMIA IN GINGIVAL AND PERIODONTAL DISEASE*

The literature consistently points to disease of the gingiva as a source of bacteremia following mechanical manipulation of the teeth.[30, 36, 43] Murray and Moosnick[29] found positive blood cultures in 55 per cent of the cases in which persons with varying degrees of dental caries and periodontal disease chewed paraffin cubes for 30 minutes. Fish and MacLean[17] reported positive blood cultures after tooth extractions in nine patients with periodontal disease. They assumed that luxation of the teeth in extraction caused alternate compression and stretching of the periodontal ligament and that streptococci were in this way pumped into the lymphatics and blood vessels. Okell and Elliott[30] reported 72 positive blood cultures following extraction in 100 patients with gingival disease. A significantly lower incidence of bacteremia was found in patients with no clinical periodontal disease. In addition, Elliott[14] found that where marked gingival disease was present, rocking of the teeth alone sufficed to produce bacteremia in 86 per cent of the patients. Bacteremia occurred more frequently associated with deep periodontal pockets. *Serratia viridans* was the organism most often seen.

---

*Bacteremia following periodontal treatment is discussed in Chapter 45.

Burket and Burn[10] painted *S. marcescens* into the gingival sulcus prior to extraction and recovered it in postextraction blood cultures in 18 out of 90 cases.

REFERENCES

1. Barros, L., and Witkop, C. S. J.: Oral and genetic study of Chileans 1960 — III Periodontal disease and nutritional factors. Arch. Oral Biol., 8:195, 1963.
2. Becks, H.: Newer aspects in paradentosis. Ann. Intern. Med., 6:65, 1932–3.
3. Becks, H.: Systemic background of paradentosis. J. Am. Dent. Assoc., 28:1447, 1941.
4. Boenheim, F.: Endokriner Status bei Paradentose. Zahnärztl. Rundsch., 37:1326, 1928.
5. Boenheim, F.: Ist das endokrine Druesensystem bei Paradentose gestoert? Paradentium, 3:91, 1930.
6. Boenheim, F.: Pyorrhea alveolaris as systemic disease. Br. Dent. J., 53:12, 1932.
7. Boenheim, F.: Pathogenic importance of the endocrine glands in paradontal disease. J. Dent. Res., 17:19, 1938.
8. Breuer, K.: Metabolic studies in disease of the paradentium. Z. Stomatol., 31:982, 1933.
9. Broderick, F. W.: Pyorrhea Alveolaris. London. John Bale Sons and Danielson, Ltd., 1931.
10. Burket, L. W., and Burn, G. G.: Bacteremia following dental extraction. Demonstration of source of bacteria by means of a nonpathogen. J. Dent. Res., 16:521, 1937.
11. Cattoni, M.. and Shannon, I. L.: Laboratory study of patients with advanced periodontal disease. J. Western Soc. Periodontol., 24:172, 1976–1977.
12. Chiuminatto, L.: Investigation of metabolism in paradentoses. Stomatologie, 27:269, 1929.
13. Citron, J.: Die Paradentose als Symptom von Endokrinen. Z. Clin. Med., 108:331, 1928.
14. Elliott, S. D.: Bacteremia and oral sepsis. Proc. R. Soc. Med., 32:747, 1939.
15. Engle, M. B., Laskin, D. M., and Gans, B. J.: Elevation of a serum glycoprotein in periodontosis. J. Am. Dent. Assoc., 57:830, 1958.
16. Englander, H. R., et al.: The relationship of blood catalase activity and periodontal disease. J. Periodontol., 26:233, 1955.
17. Fish, E. W., and MacLean, L.: Distribution of oral streptococci in the tissues. Br. Dent. J., 61:336, 1936.
18. Goldstein, H.: Systemic and blood picture in several hundred periclasia-free and periclasia-involved individuals. J. Dent. Res., 16:320, 1937.
19. Grove, C. J., and Grove, C. T.: Blood phosphorus insufficiency in pyorrhea. J. Dent. Res., 13:191, 1933.
20. Hawkins, H. F.: Nutritional influences on growth and development. Intern. J. Orthod. 19:307, 1933.
21. Honjo, K., Nakamura, R., Tsunemitsu, A., and Matsummura, T.: Serum transaminases in periodontosis. J. Periodontol., 35:247, 1964.
22. Karshan, M., et al.: Studies in periodontal disease. J. Dent. Res., 31:11, 1952.
23. Karshan, M., and Tenenbaum, B.: Blood studies in periodontoclasia. J. Dent. Res., 25:180, 1946.
24. Karshan, M., Tenenbaum, B., and Friedland, R.: Urinary estrogen in periodontosis. J. Dent. Res., 35:648, 1956.
25. Landgraf, E., et al.: Investigations of uric acid blood level in periodontal disease. Z. Stomatol., 30:91, 1932.
26. Mackenzie, R. S., and Millard, H. D.: Interrelated effects of diabetes, arteriosclerosis, and calculus on alveolar bone loss. J. Am. Dent. Assoc., 66:191, 1963.
27. Martin, D.: The blood associated with pyorrhea alveolaris. Austral. Dent. J., 9:488, 1937.
28. Morelli, G.: The clinical and therapeutic evaluation of the results concerning constitutional factors in cases of paradentoses. Ann. Med., 41:648, 1935.
29. Murray, M., and Moosnick, F.: Incidence of bacteremia in patients with dental disease. J. Lab. Clin. Med., 26:801, 1941.
30. Okell, C. C., and Elliott, S. D.: Bacteremia and oral sepsis. Lancet, 2:869, 1935.
31. O'Leary, T. J., Shannon, I. L., and Prigmore, J. R.: Clinical and systemic findings in periodontal disease. J. Periodontol., 33:243, 1962.
32. Pelzer, R. H.: A method for plasma phosphatase determination for the differentiation of alveolar crest bone types in periodontal disease. J. Dent. Res., 19:73, 1940.
33. Polevitsky, K.: Blood types in pyorrhea alveolaris. J. Dent. Res., 9:285, 1929.
34. Rose, H. P., Kuna, A., and Kraft, E.: Systemic manifestations of periodontal disease. J. Periodontol., 34:253, 1963.
35. Sagal, Z.: Pyorrhea alveolaris and gastric acidity. Dent. Cosmos, 68:1145, 1926.
36. Sand, R.: Periodontal sepsis in relationship to systemic disease. J. Am. Dent. Assoc., 28:710, 1941.
37. Shannon, I. L., and Gibson, W. A.: Oral glucose tolerance responses in healthy young adult males classified as to caries experience and periodontal status. Periodontics, 2:292, 1964.
38. Shannon, I. L., and Gibson, W. A.: Serum total protein, albumin, and globulin in relation to periodontal status and caries experience. Oral Surg., 18:399, 1964.
39. Shannon, I. L., Terry, J. M., and Chauncey, H. H.: Uric acid and total protein in serum and parotid fluid in relation to periodontal status. J. Dent. Res., 45:1539, 1966.
40. Shklair, I., Loving, R., Leberman, O., and Rau, C.: C-Reactive protein and periodontal disease. J. Periodontol., 39:93, 1968.
41. Siegel, E.: Total erythrocyte, lymphocyte and differential white cell counts of blood in chronic periodontal disease. J. Dent. Res., 24:270, 1945.
42. Simon, E., et al.: Citrate content of blood and saliva in relation to periodontal disease in man. Arch. Oral Biol., 13:1243, 1968.
43. Stones, H. H.: Oral and Dental Diseases. Chronic Oral Sepsis and Relation to Systemic Diseases. Baltimore, Williams & Wilkins, 1948, Chap. XXXIII.
44. Stortebecker, T. P.: Dental infectious foci and diseases of the nervous system. Acta Psychiatr. Neurol. Scand., 36(Suppl. 157), 1961.

45. Tenenbaum, B., and Karshan, M.: Blood studies in periodontoclasia. J. Am. Dent. Assoc., *32*: 1372, 1945.

46. Tsunemitsu, A., et al.: Citric acid metabolism in periodontosis. Arch. Oral Biol., *9*:83, 1964.

47. Tuckman, M. A., et al.: The relationship of glucose tolerance to periodontal status. J. Periodontol., *41*:513, 1970.

48. Weber, R., and Pastern, W.: Uber die Frage der Konstitutionellen Bereitschaft zur Sog. Alveolar Pyorrhoe (Alveolarpyorrhoe und Blutgruppen). Deutsch. Monatschr. Zahnheilk., *14*:704, 1927.

49. Weiner, R., Karshan, M., and Tenenbaum, B.: Ovarian function in periodontosis. J. Dent. Res., *35*:875, 1956.

50. Weinmann, J. P.: Study of metabolism in diffuse atrophy. Z. Stomatol., *25*:822, 1927.

51. Weinmann, J. P.: Investigation of metabolism in diffuse atrophy of the alveolar process. Z. Stomatol., *28*:1154, 1930.

THE TREATMENT OF PERIODONTAL DISEASE

Periodontal treatment requires the interrelationship of the care of the periodontium with other phases of dentistry. The concept of **total treatment** includes the following:

1. **The soft tissues** — Elimination of gingival inflammation and the factors that lead to it (plaque accumulation favored by pocket formation, inadequate restorations, areas of food impaction).

2. **The functional aspects** — Establishment of optimal occlusal relationships for the entire dentition.

3. **The systemic aspects** — Systemic adjuncts to local treatment and special precautions in patient management necessitated by systemic conditions.

All these aspects are embodied in a **master plan**, which consists of a rational **sequence of dental procedures** that includes periodontal and other procedures necessary to create a well-functioning dentition in a healthy periodontal environment.

Part I

Diagnosis; Determination of the Prognosis; The Treatment Plan

Diagnosis

Proper diagnosis is essential for intelligent treatment. In addition to recognizing the clinical and radiographic features of different diseases, diagnosis requires an understanding of the underlying disease processes and their etiology. **Our interest is in the patient who has the disease and not simply in the disease itself.** Diagnosis must therefore include a general evaluation of the patient as well as consideration of the oral cavity.

Diagnosis must be systematic, and organized for specific purposes. It is not enough to assemble facts. The findings must be pieced together so that they provide a meaningful explanation of the patient's periodontal problem.

The diagnosis should provide answers to the following questions:

Which factors are responsible for plaque

accumulation leading to gingival inflammation and periodontal pockets? Does the periodontium present evidence of trauma from occlusion? Are there occlusal relationships that account for the traumatic lesions? Are the gingival and periodontal changes explainable by the local factors or do they suggest the possibility of contributing systemic etiology?

The following is a recommended sequence of procedures for the diagnosis of gingival and periodontal disease.

FIRST VISIT

Overall Appraisal of the Patient

From the first meeting, the operator should attempt an overall appraisal of the patient. This includes consideration of the patient's mental and emotional status, temperament, attitude, and physiologic age.

Systemic History

Most of the systemic history is obtained at the first visit and can be enlarged upon by pertinent questions at subsequent visits. The importance of the systemic history should be explained, because patients often omit information that they cannot relate to their dental problem. The systemic history will aid the operator in (1) **the diagnosis of oral manifestations of systemic disease,** (2) **the detection of systemic conditions that may be affecting the periodontal tissue response to local factors,** and (3) **the detection of systemic conditions that require special precautions and modifications in treatment procedures.** The systemic history should include reference to the following:

1. Is the patient under the care of a physician; if so, what is the nature and duration of the illness, and therapy? Special inquiry should be made regarding anticoagulants and corticosteroids—the dosage and duration of therapy.

2. History of rheumatic fever, rheumatic or congenital heart disease, hypertension, angina pectoris, myocardial infarction, nephritis, liver disease, diabetes, fainting spells.

3. Abnormal bleeding tendencies such as nose bleeds, prolonged bleeding from minor cuts, spontaneous ecchymoses, tendency toward excessive bruising, and excessive menstrual bleeding.

4. Infectious disease, recent contact with infectious disease at home or at business, recent chest x-ray.

5. Possibility of occupational disease.

6. History of allergy—hay fever, asthma, sensitivity to foods, sensitivity to drugs such as aspirin, codeine, barbiturates, sulfonamides, antibiotics, procaine, laxatives, or dental materials such as eugenol or acrylic resins.

7. Information regarding the onset of puberty and menopause and menstrual disorders or hysterectomy, pregnancies, miscarriages.

Dental History

Chief complaint

The following are some of the symptoms in patients with gingival and periodontal disease: "bleeding gums," "loose teeth," "spreading of the teeth with the appearance of spaces where none existed before," "foul taste in the mouth," "itchy feeling in the gums, relieved by digging with a toothpick." There may also be pain of varied types and duration, such as "constant dull gnawing pain," "dull pain after eating," "deep radiating pains in the jaws," "acute throbbing pain," "sensitivity to percussion," "sensitivity to heat and cold," "burning sensation in the gums," "extreme sensitivity to inhaled air."

A preliminary oral examination is done to explore the source of the patient's chief complaint and determine whether *immediate emergency care* is required.

The dental history should also include reference to the following:

Visits to the dentist—frequency, date of last visit, nature of the treatment. "Oral prophylaxis" or "cleaning" by a dentist or hygienist—frequency and date of last one.

Toothbrushing—frequency, before or after meals, method, type of toothbrush and dentifrice, intervals at which brushes are replaced. Other methods for mouth care: mouthwashes, finger massage, interdental stimulation, water irrigation, and dental floss.

Orthodontic treatment—duration and approximate time of termination.

Pain "in the teeth" or "in the gums." The manner in which it is provoked, its nature and duration and the manner in which it is relieved.

"Bleeding gums"—when first noted, whether it occurs spontaneously, upon brushing or eating, at night, with regular periodicity. Whether it is associated with the menstrual period or other specific factors. The duration of the bleeding and the manner in which it is stopped.

Bad taste in the mouth, areas of food impaction.

Tooth mobility—do the teeth feel "loose" or insecure? Is there difficulty in chewing?

History of previous "gum" trouble—the nature of the condition, previous treatment, duration, nature, and approximate period of termination.

Habits—"grinding the teeth," "clenching the teeth" during the day or night—do the teeth or muscles feel "sore" in the morning? Other habits such as tobacco smoking or chewing, nail biting, biting on foreign objects.

Intra-oral radiographic survey

The radiographic survey should consist of a minimum of fourteen intra-oral films and posterior bite-wings.

Panoramic radiographs

Panoramic radiographs are a simple and convenient method of obtaining a survey view of the dental arch and surrounding structures (Fig. 32–1). They are helpful for the detection of developmental anomalies, pathologic lesions of the teeth and jaws and fractures, and for dental screening examinations of large groups. They provide an informative over-all radiographic picture of the distribution and severity of bone destruction in periodontal disease, but a complete intra-oral series is required for definitive diagnosis and treatment planning.

Casts

Casts are extremely useful adjuncts in the oral examination. They indicate the position and inclinations of the teeth, proximal contact relationships, and food impaction areas. In addition, they provide a view of lingual cuspal relationships. They are important records of the dentition before it is altered by treatment. They also serve as "visual aids" in discussions with the patient and are useful for pre-

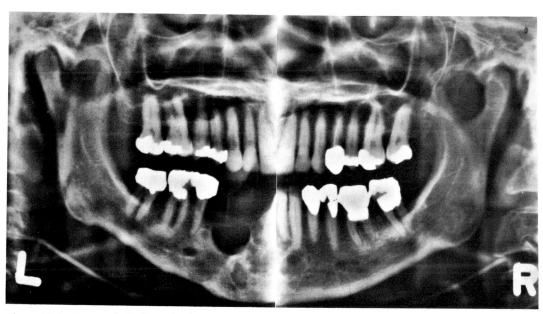

Figure 32–1 Panoramic Radiograph, showing temporomandibular joints, periodontal bone loss, and "cystic" spaces in the jaw.

and post-treatment comparisons as well as reference at check-up visits.

Clinical photographs

Color photographs are not essential but are useful for recording the appearance of the tissue before and after treatment. Photographs cannot always be relied upon for comparing subtle color changes in gingiva; they do depict changes in gingival morphology.

If no emergency care is required, the patient is dismissed and instructed when to report for the second visit. Before this visit, a correlated examination is made of the radiographs and casts to relate the radiographic changes to unfavorable conditions represented on the casts. The casts are checked for evidence of abnormal

wear, plunger cusps, uneven marginal ridges, malposed or extruded teeth, crossbite relationships, or other conditions that could cause occlusal disharmony or food impaction. Such areas are marked on the casts, to be referred to in the detailed examination of the oral cavity to follow. The radiographs and casts are valuable diagnostic aids; however, it is the findings in the oral cavity that constitute the basis for diagnosis.

SECOND VISIT

Oral Examination

Oral hygiene

The "cleanliness" of the oral cavity is appraised in terms of the extent of accumulated food debris, plaque, materia alba,

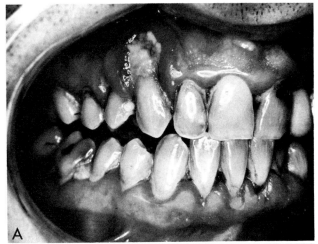
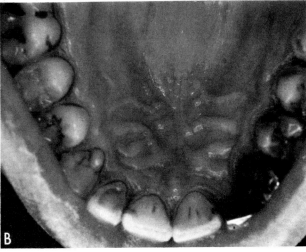

Figure 32–2 Poor Oral Hygiene. *A,* Gingival inflammation associated with plaque, materia alba, and calculus in a patient with hemophilia. *B,* Palatal view of the same patient showing only slight gingivitis because the mechanical action of the tongue and food excursion reduces the accumulation of local irritants.

and tooth surface stains (Fig. 32–2). *Disclosing solution should be used routinely to detect plaque that would otherwise be unnoticed.*

Mouth odors

"Halitosis," also termed "fetor ex ore" or "fetor oris," is foul or offensive odor emanating from the oral cavity.[33] Mouth odors may be of diagnostic significance; their origin may be either (a) local or (b) extra-oral or remote.

LOCAL SOURCES. Retention of odoriferous food particles on and between the teeth,[21] coated tongue, acute necrotizing ulcerative gingivitis, dehydration states, caries, artificial dentures, smoker's breath, healing surgical or extraction wounds. The fetid odor characteristic of acute necrotizing ulcerative gingivitis is easily identified. Chronic periodontal disease with pocket formation may also cause unpleasant mouth odor from accumulated debris and increased rate of putrefaction of the saliva.[5]

EXTRA-ORAL OR REMOTE SOURCES. These may include adjacent structures associated with rhinitis, sinusitis, or tonsilitis; disease of the lungs and bronchi, such as chronic fetid bronchitis, bronchiectasis, lung abscesses, gangrene of the lung, and pulmonary tuberculosis; odors excreted through the lungs from aromatic substances in the blood stream, such as metabolites from ingested foods or excretory products of cell metabolism. Of the latter group, alcoholic breath, acetone odor of diabetes, and uremic breath in kidney dysfunction are examples.

Saliva

Ptyalism or excessive salivary secretion accompanies a variety of conditions such as the use of certain drugs (mercury, pilocarpine, iodides, bromides, phosphorus), acute necrotizing ulcerative gingivitis, various forms of stomatitis, Vincent's angina, irritation from smoking, and psychic stimulation.

Decreased salivary secretion[11, 15] is seen in febrile diseases, chronic diseases such as chronic nephritis, uremia, diabetes mellitus, myxedema, neuropsychiatric disorders, lesions of the salivary glands, Plummer-Vinson and Sjögren syndromes, and pernicious anemia. Xerostomia or "dry mouth" results from decreased salivary secretion and presents various clinical features such as generalized dryness and erythema with fissuring in extreme cases, and varying degrees of discomfort caused by a "burning" sensation.

Lips

Neoplasms, chancre, angular cheilitis, irritation from biting habits, indentations from occlusion, and mucous cysts should be considered in the differential diagnosis of lesions of the lips.

Oral mucosa

A general survey of the color[27] and surface texture of the oral mucosa will indicate pathologic pigmentation, diffuse erythema associated with acute infection, diffuse erythema or bluish red discoloration associated with vitamin B-complex deficiencies, smooth shiny atrophy with fissuring in senile or menopausal gingivostomatitis, patchy gray discoloration and desquamation associated with chronic desquamative gingivitis, and vesicles in pemphigus, erythema multiforme, or benign mucous membrane pemphigoid (Fig. 32–3).

Cheek biting, irritating mouth washes, hot foods, topically applied drugs (Fig. 32–4), and ill-fitting dentures and denture clasps are common causes of painful ulceration. Leukoplakia, lichen planus, Koplik spots, and inflammatory enlargement of the orifice of Stensen's duct are among other mucosal changes.

Floor of the mouth

Ranula, neoplasms, and aphthae are often sources of pain.

Tongue

The tongue should be examined for alterations in the color, size, and nature of the papillae. Leukoplakia, lichen planus, erythema multiforme, pemphigus, pernicious anemia, vitamin B-complex deficiencies, Plummer-Vinson syndrome, syphilis, and tuberculosis are among the systemic conditions in which the tongue may be involved. Other changes include ery-

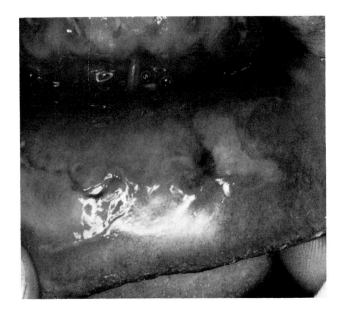

Figure 32-3   Vesicle in Benign Mucous Membrane Pemphigoid.

thema migrans (geographic tongue), moniliasis, congenital fissured tongue, median rhomboid glossitis, and neoplasms. Tongue changes may be painless or accompanied by varying degrees of pain and burning. The operator should check carefully for local sources of irritation before seeking remote explanation of tongue problems. Rough spots on the teeth or margins of restorations, the incisal edges of irregularly aligned teeth, and calculus on the mandibular anterior teeth are common sources of irritation to the tongue.

BURNING TONGUE (OROLINGUAL PARESTHESIA, GLOSSOPYROSIS, GLOSSODYNIA). Burning and tingling tongue symptoms present a diagnostic and therapeutic problem. The tongue may appear normal or atrophic with or without dryness of the mouth (xerostomia) and atrophy and pain of the remainder of the oral mucosa. There are many possible causes of the tongue pain,[25] such as pernicious anemia, vitamin B-complex deficiency, diabetes, hypothyroidism, postmenopausal syndrome, trigeminal neuralgia, mercurialism,

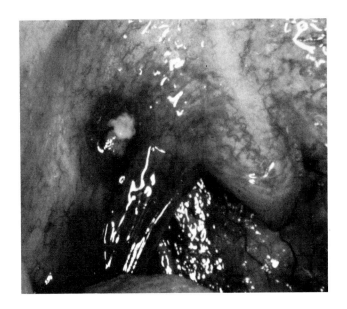

Figure 32-4   Aspirin Burn in the Oropharynx.

use of tobacco and spices, antibiotic therapy, local mechanical irritation, electrogalvanic discharge between dental restorations constructed of different metals, and temporomandibular joint disturbances. Despite the numerous potential etiologic factors, the tongue symptoms are often only explainable on a psychogenic basis.

Palate

Leukoplakia "smoker's palate" with prominent inflamed mucous gland orifices, neoplasms, and exostoses is commonly seen.

Oropharyngeal region

This is the site of pseudomembrane formation in Vincent's angina and diphtheria. Inflamed tonsils often cause radiating pain.

Examination of the Teeth

The teeth are examined for caries, developmental defects, anomalies of tooth form, wasting, hypersensitivity, and proximal contact relationships.

Wasting disease of the teeth

Wasting is defined as any gradual loss of tooth substance characterized by the formation of smooth polished surfaces without consideration of the possible mechanism of this loss. The forms of wasting are erosion, abrasion, and attrition.

Erosion (cuneiform defect) is a sharply defined wedge-shaped depression in the cervical area of the facial tooth surface.[51] The long axis of the eroded area is perpendicular to the vertical axis of the tooth (Fig. 32–5). The surfaces are smooth, hard, and polished. It generally affects a group of teeth. In the early stages, erosion may be confined to the enamel, but it generally extends to involve the underlying dentin as well as the cementum and dentin of the root.

The etiology of erosion is not known. Decalcification by acid beverages[34] or citrus fruits, and the combined effect of acid salivary secretion and friction are suggested causes. Sognnaes[64] refers to these lesions as "dentoalveolar ablation" and attributes them to forceful frictional actions between the oral soft tissues and the adjacent hard tissues. In patients with erosion the salivary pH, buffering capacity, calcium and phosphorus content have been reported as normal, with the mucin level elevated.[31]

Abrasion refers to the loss of tooth substance induced by mechanical wear other than that of mastication. Abrasion results in saucer-shaped or wedge-shaped indentations with a smooth, shiny surface. Abrasion starts on exposed cementum surfaces rather than on the enamel, and extends to involve the dentin of the root. Continued exposure to the abrasive agent, combined with decalcification of the enamel by locally formed acids, may result in a loss of the enamel followed by the dentin of the crown (Fig. 32–6).

Toothbrushing[26] with an abrasive dentifrice and the action of clasps are common causes of abrasion. The former is by far the more prevalent. According to Manly,[29, 30] the degree of tooth wear from

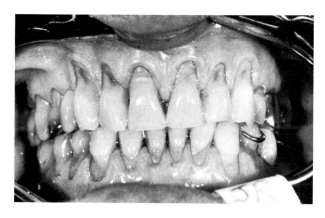

Figure 32–5 Erosion involving the enamel, cementum, and dentin.

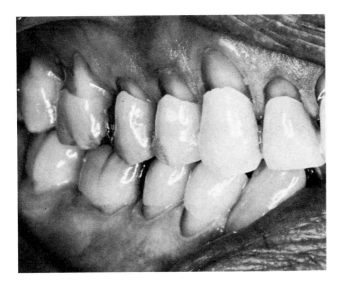

Figure 32–6 Abrasion Attributed to Aggressive Toothbrushing. Involvement of the roots is followed by undermining of the enamel.

toothbrushing depends upon the abrasive effect of the dentifrice and the angle of brushing. Horizontal brushing at right angles to the vertical axis of the teeth results in severest loss of tooth substance. Occasionally abrasion of the incisal edges occurs as a result of habits such as holding a bobby pin or tacks between the teeth.

Attrition. (See Chapter 5.)

Hypersensitivity

Root surfaces exposed by gingival recession may be hypersensitive to thermal changes or tactile stimulation. Patients often direct the operator to the sensitive areas. They may be located by gentle exploration with a probe or cold air.

Proximal contact relations

Because there is a normal tendency toward mesial migration of the teeth, the location of the proximal contact area is important. Abnormal contact relationship may cause a shift in the median line between the central incisors, labial version of the maxillary canine, buccal or lingual displacement of the posterior teeth, and uneven relationship of the marginal ridges.

The location of proximal contact relations is of particular significance in the mandible. Since the mandibular arch is normally contained within the maxillary teeth, displacement of the mandibular teeth due to abnormally located proximal contact leads to a reduction in the circumference of the mandibular arch. This in turn results in increased overbite and loss of vertical dimension, often followed by food impaction, particularly on the lingual surfaces of the maxillary teeth. Proximal contacts are critical factors in the prevention of food impaction. They should be given careful attention when exploring the etiologic factors that contribute to the individual's periodontal problem.

Tooth mobility

All teeth have a slight degree of physiologic mobility. It varies in different teeth (highest in the central and lateral incisors) and at different times of the day.[40] It is highest upon arising in the morning and progressively decreases. The increased mobility in the morning is attributed to slight extrusion of the teeth because of limited occlusal contact during sleep. During the waking hours mobility is reduced by chewing and swallowing forces which intrude the teeth in the sockets.

Tooth mobility beyond the physiologic range (pathologic or abnormal mobility) is increased in periodontal disease as the result of the loss of supporting tissues, in inflammation and trauma from occlusion, and in other conditions. Pathologic mobility is most common in the faciolingual direction; it is less frequent mesiodistally, and vertical mobility occurs only in extreme cases. (For a discussion of tooth mobility see Chapter 20.)

Mobilometers or periodontometers are mechanical or electronic devices for the precise measurement of mobility.[37, 41, 43] They are not widely used despite the fact that standardization of the grading of mobility would be helpful in the diagnosis of periodontal disease and in evaluating the outcome of treatment. As a general rule, mobility is graded clinically with a simple method such as the following:

The tooth is held firmly between the handles of two metal instruments, and an effort is made to move it in all directions; abnormal mobility most often occurs faciolingually. Mobility is graded according to the ease and extent of tooth movement assessed by the individual therapist as follows:

Physiologic mobility.

Pathologic mobility, Grade 1—slightly more than physiologic.

Pathologic mobility, Grade 2—moderately more than physiologic.

Pathologic mobility, Grade 3—severe mobility facio-lingually and/or mesio-distally combined with vertical displacement.

Sensitivity to percussion

Sensitivity to percussion is a feature of acute inflammation of the periodontal ligament. Gently percussing a tooth at different angles to the long axis often aids in localizing the site of the inflammatory involvement. Percussion also serves as a method of "sounding" for detecting teeth with reduced periodontal support.

Pathologic migration of the teeth

Alterations in tooth position should be carefully noted, particularly with a view toward abnormal occlusal forces, tongue

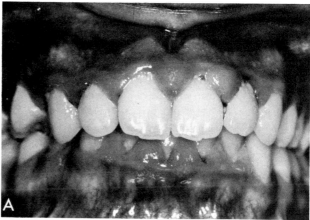
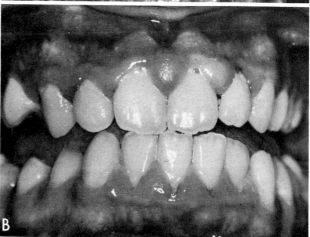

Figure 32–7 Excessive Anterior Overbite. *A,* Excessive anterior overbite with gingival inflammation and enlargement. *B,* Gingival enlargement in anterior region associated with overbite.

thrusting, or other habits that may be contributing factors. Pathologic migration of anterior teeth in young persons is often a sign of juvenile periodontitis.

The dentition with the jaws closed

Examination of the dentition with the jaws closed is not as revealing as examination of the jaws in function, but does indicate conditions of periodontal significance.

Irregularly aligned teeth, extruded teeth, improper proximal contact, and areas of food impaction are all important factors favoring the accumulation of bacterial plaque.

Overbite, *the projection of the maxillary teeth over the mandibular teeth in a vertical direction*, is a normal feature of the dentition. Excessive overbite seen most frequently in the anterior region may cause impingement of the teeth upon the gingiva and food impaction, followed by gingival inflammation, enlargement, and pocket formation (Fig. 32–7). The real significance of excessive overbite on gingival health is, however, controversial.[1]

In open bite relationships, *abnormal vertical spaces exist between the maxillary and mandibular teeth.* The condition occurs most often in the anterior region, although posterior open bite is occasionally seen. Reduced mechanical cleaning by the passage of food may lead to accumulation of debris, calculus formation, and extrusion of teeth.

In crossbite, *the normal relationship of the mandibular teeth to the maxillary teeth is reversed and the maxillary teeth are lingual to the mandibular teeth.* Crossbite may be bilateral, unilateral, or may only affect a pair of antagonists. Trauma from occlusion, food impaction, spreading of the mandibular teeth and associated gingival and periodontal disturbances may be caused by crossbite(Fig. 32–8).

Examination of functional occlusal relationships

Examination of the functional occlusal relationships of the dentition is a critical part of the diagnostic procedure. Dentitions that appear normal when the jaws are closed may present marked functional abnormalities. Systematic procedures for the detection and correction of functional abnormalities are described in Chapter 55.

The temporomandibular joint

The clinical features, etiology, and treatment of temporomandibular joint disorders are presented in Chapters 27 and 55.

Examination of the Periodontium

It is important to look for the earliest signs of gingival and periodontal disease.

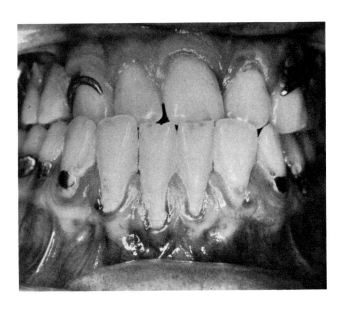

Figure 32–8 Crossbite Relationship with Associated Periodontal Disturbances.

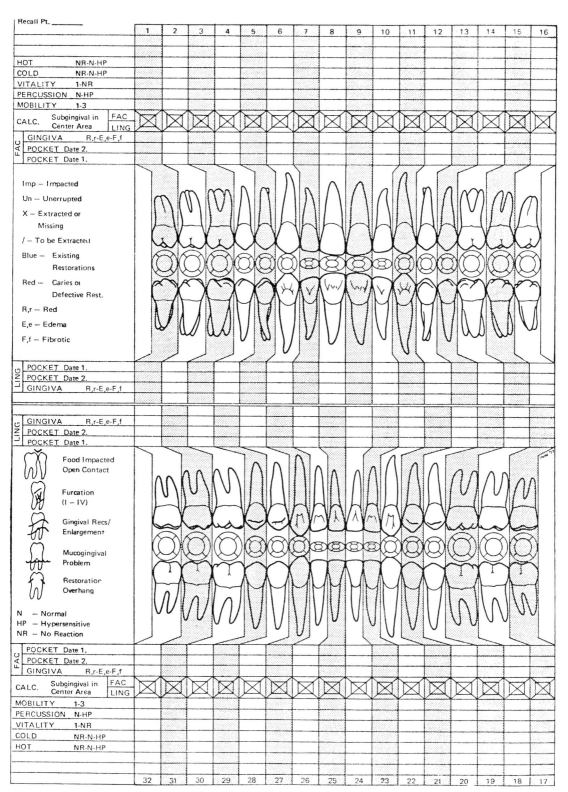

Figure 32–9   U.C.L.A. Periodontal chart.

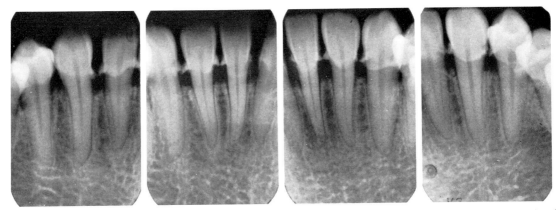

Figure 32–10 Calculus Appears Interproximally as Angular Spurs. The radiopaque image of calculus on the facial and lingual surfaces is superimposed on the teeth.

The examination should be systematic, starting in the molar area in either the maxilla or mandible and proceeding around the arch. This will avoid overemphasis of spectacular findings at the expense of other conditions which, though less striking, may be equally important.

Charts to record the periodontal and associated findings provide a guide for thorough examination and a record of the patient's condition (Fig. 32–9). They are also used for evaluating the response to treatment and for comparison at recall visits. However, excessively complicated mouth charting may lead to a frustrating maze of minutiae rather than clarification of the patient's problem.

Plaque and calculus

There are many methods of assessing plaque and calculus accumulation[13] (Chap. 22). For the detection of **subgingival calculus** each tooth surface is carefully checked to the level of the gingival attachment with a sharp No. 17 probe. Warm air may be used to deflect the gingiva and aid in visualization of the calculus. The amount of **supragingival calculus** may be measured with a calibrated periodontal probe.

The x-ray reveals heavy calculus deposits interproximally (Fig. 32–10) and sometimes on the facial and lingual surfaces, but cannot be relied upon for the thorough detection of calculus.

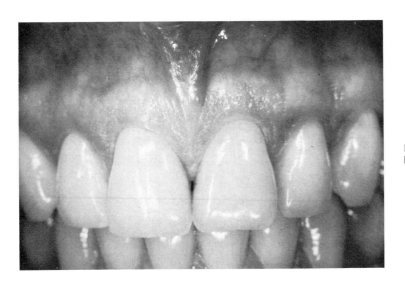

Figure 32–11 Normal Gingiva. Normal surface features are revealed by drying the gingiva.

Gingiva

The gingiva must be dried before accurate observations can be made (Fig. 32–11). Light reflection from moist gingiva obscures detail. In addition to visual examination and exploration with instruments, firm but gentle palpation should be used for detecting pathologic alterations in normal resilience as well as for locating areas of pus formation.

Each of the following features of the gingiva should be considered: **color, size, contour, consistency, surface texture, position** and **ease of bleeding,** and **pain.** (See Chapters 7, 8, 9, and 10.) No deviation from the normal should be overlooked. The distribution of gingival disease and acuteness or chronicity should also be noted.

From a clinical point of view it is very important to recognize that gingival inflammation can produce two basic types of tissue response: (a) **edematous** and (b) **fibrotic.** Edematous tissue response is characterized by a smooth, glossy, soft gingiva. In fibrotic gingiva some of the characteristics of normalcy still persist; the gingiva is more firm, stippled, and opaque, although it is usually thicker and its margin appears rounded.

The position of the gingiva warrants special mention. For accurate appraisal of recession, attention should be given to differentiating between the *apparent position* and the *actual position* of the gingival attachment on each tooth surface (Chap. 9).

Periodontal pockets

Examination for periodontal pockets should include consideration of the following: (1) presence and distribution on each tooth surface, (2) the type of pocket— whether it is suprabony or infrabony, simple, compound, or complex; (3) pocket depth; (4) level of attachment on the root.

The only accurate method of detecting and evaluating periodontal pockets is careful exploration with a pocket probe. Pockets are not detected or measured by radiographic examination. The periodontal pocket is a soft tissue change. Radiographs indicate areas of bone loss where pockets may be suspected. They do not show whether pockets are present in these areas, nor do they reveal pocket depth or the location of the base of the pocket on the tooth surface.

Gutta percha points or calibrated silver points[22] are used with the x-ray to assist in determining the level of the attachment of periodontal pockets and their relationship to the bone (Fig. 32–12). They may be used effectively for individual pockets, but their routine use throughout the mouth would be rather cumbersome. Clinical examination and probing are more direct and efficient.

In the examination for periodontal pockets, check each tooth surface. Probes calibrated in millimeters are available for measuring pocket depth. The probe should be inserted in line with the vertical axis of the tooth until the blunt end con-

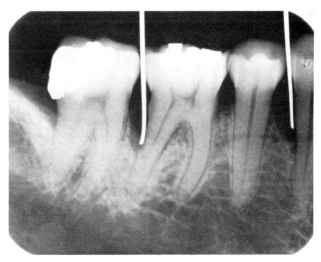

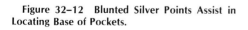

Figure 32–12 Blunted Silver Points Assist in Locating Base of Pockets.

tacts the bottom of the pocket. The probe should not be forced into the underlying tissues*

An attempt should be made to detect the presence of interdental craters. To detect an interdental crater the probe should be placed obliquely from both the facial and the lingual surfaces so as to explore the deepest portion of the pocket located beneath the contact point (Fig. 32–13).

In multirooted teeth the presence of furcation involvements should be carefully explored. Sometimes in these cases probing with especially designed probes (Nabers) or with an explorer or curette may reveal lesions undetected with the probe (Fig. 32–14).

The level of attachment of the base of the pocket on the tooth surface is of greater diagnostic significance than the depth of the pocket. Pocket depth is simply the distance between the base of the

---

*The depth of penetration of the probe into a sulcus and a pocket has recently been studied by several authors.[2,28,34,62] It has been reported[2] that in clinically healthy gingivae a probe inserted with a standardized force of 25 grams penetrates beyond the bottom of the sulcus and into the junctional epithelium to about two thirds of its length, i.e., one third short of its apical end. In cases of periodontitis the probe will go beyond the bottom of the junctional epithelium and into the area of partially destroyed fibers to a depth of about 0.25 millimeter.

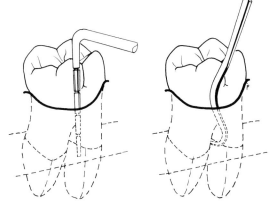

Figure 32–14 Exploring with a periodontal probe *(left)* may not detect furcation involvement; specially designed instruments (Nabers probe) *(right)* can enter the furcation area.

pocket and the gingival margin. It may vary from time to time in untreated periodontal disease. For example, gingival bleeding caused by accidental mechanical irritation results in shrinkage of the pocket wall and some reduction in pocket depth. The level of attachment of the base of the pocket on the tooth surface affords a better indication of the severity of periodontal disease. **Shallow pockets attached at the level of the apical third of the roots connote more severe destruction than deep pockets attached in the coronal third of the roots.**

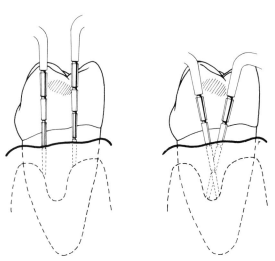

Figure 32–13 Vertical insertion of the probe *(left)* may not detect interdental craters; oblique positioning of the probe *(right)* reaches the depth of the crater.

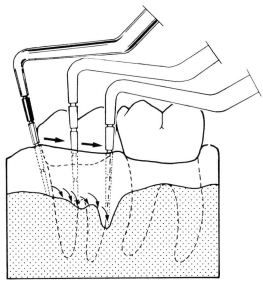

Figure 32–15 "Walking" the probe in order to explore the pocket in all its extent.

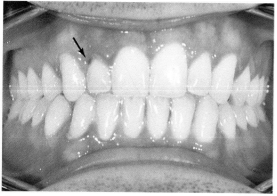

A

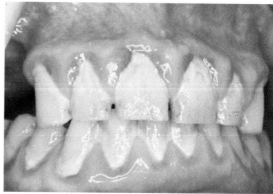

B

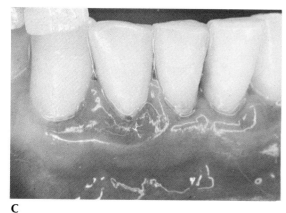

C

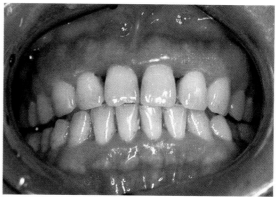

D

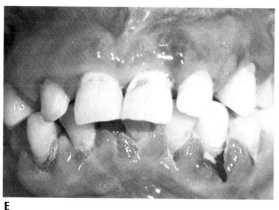

E

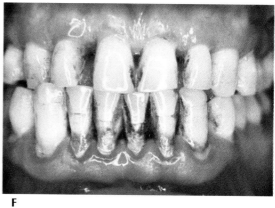

F

Plate IV

A, Incipient marginal gingivitis. Note slight puffiness and bleeding around upper right lateral incisor.

B, Edematous type gingival inflammation. Note loss of stippling, increase in size, abundant plaque and materia alba, and change in color.

C, Close-up view of edematous type of gingival inflammation. Note the red, shiny, smooth gingiva.

D, Fibrotic type of gingival inflammation. Pockets of moderate depth are present, but the gingiva retains its stippling in some areas.

E, Severe generalized gingival inflammation, with migration of teeth and inflammatory gingival enlargement.

F, Fibrotic gingival inflammation. Note the abundant calculus and the gingival recession. The patient has pockets of moderate to severe depth in the mandibular anteriors and shallower pockets in maxillary teeth.

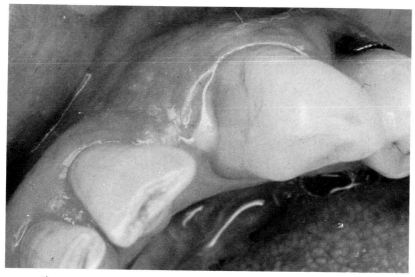

Figure 32–16   Pus Formation on the mesial surface of mandibular canine.

Figure 32–17 Methods to determine the amount of attached gingiva. *A,* Tension test: stretching the lip while the pocket is probed. *B,* Pushing tissue coronally with the probe and comparing with the pocket depth.

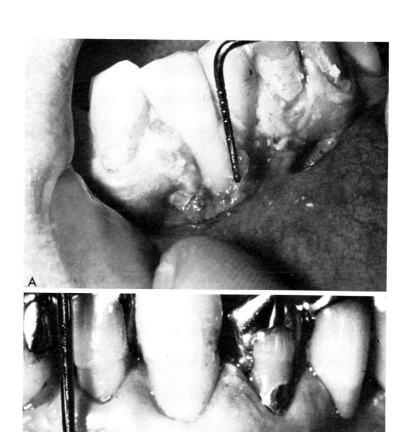

The level of attachment of the base of a periodontal pocket may vary on different surfaces of the same tooth and even on different areas of the same surface. Inserting the probe on all surfaces and in more than one area on individual surfaces reveals the depth and conformation of the pocket (Fig. 32–15).

Suppuration

To determine whether pus is present in a periodontal pocket, the ball of the index finger is applied along the lateral aspect of the marginal gingiva and pressure is applied in a rolling motion toward the crown. Visual examination alone without digital pressure is not enough. Because the purulent exudate is formed on the inner pocket wall, the external appearance of the pocket may give no indication of its presence. Pus formation does not occur in all periodontal pockets but digital pressure often reveals it in pockets where it is not suspected (Fig. 32–16).

Amount of Attached Gingiva

The relation between the bottom of the pocket and the mucogingival line should also be established, in order to determine the amount of attached gingiva that will exist after the pocket is eliminated. The need for mucogingival surgical techniques is therefore determined.

In order to obtain this information the "tension test" is performed. This test consists of stretching the lip or cheek in order to demarcate the mucogingival line while the pocket is probed (Fig. 32–17).

Mucosa in relation to the root apices

Palpating the oral mucosa in the lateral and apical areas of the root is helpful in locating the origin of radiating pain which the patient cannot localize. Infection deep in the periodontal tissues and the early stages of periodontal abscess formation may also be detected by palpation.

Sinus formation

In children a sinus orifice along the lateral aspect of a root is usually the result of periapical infection of a deciduous tooth.

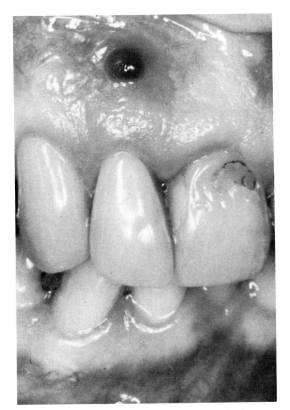

Figure 32–18 **Nodular Mass** at the orifice of a draining sinus.

In the permanent dentition it may be caused by a periodontal abscess as well as apical involvement. The orifice may be patent and draining or it may be closed and appear as a red nodular mass (Fig. 32–18). Exploration of such masses with a probe usually reveals a pinpoint orifice that communicates with an underlying sinus.

Alveolar bone loss

Alveolar bone levels are evaluated by clinical and radiographic examination. Probing is helpful for determining the height and contour of the facial and lingual bone obscured on the radiograph by the dense roots, and for determining the architecture of the interdental bone.

Trauma from occlusion

Trauma from occlusion refers to *tissue injury* produced by occlusal forces—not to the occlusal forces themselves. The criterion that determines whether an occlusal force is injurious is whether it causes damage in the periodontal tissues; therefore the diagnosis of trauma from occlusion is made from the condition of the periodontal tissues. The periodontal findings are then used as a guide for locating the responsible occlusal relationships.

Periodontal findings that suggest the presence of trauma from occlusion are the following: excessive tooth mobility, particularly in teeth with radiographic evidence of widened periodontal space (see Fig. 32–31), vertical or angular bone destruction (see Figs. 32–27 and 32–32), infrabony pockets, and pathologic migration, especially of the anterior teeth.

Additional findings which suggest the presence of abnormal occlusal relationships are neuromuscular disturbances such as impaired function of the masticatory musculature, which in severe cases results in muscle spasm and temporomandibular joint disorders.

Special mention should be made of pathologic migration of the anterior teeth as a sign of trauma from occlusion. Premature tooth contacts in the posterior region

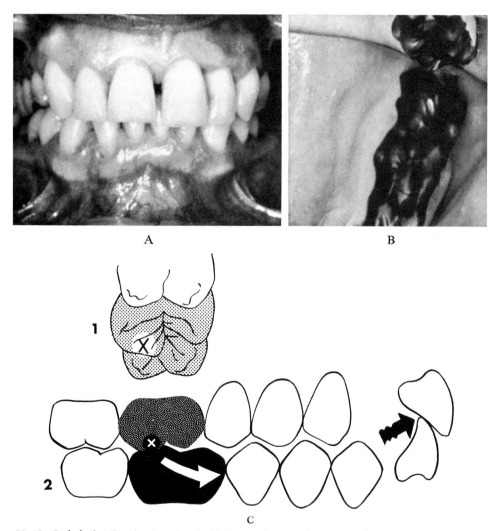

A

B

C

Figure 32–19 Pathologic Migration Associated with Trauma from Occlusion. *A,* Early pathologic migration of maxillary left central incisor. *B,* Mirror view of wax registration, showing prematurity on the mesiolingual incline of the maxillary molar, which deflects the mandible anteriorly and traumatizes the maxillary incisors. *C,* Diagrammatic representation showing (1) Prematurity (X) on the maxillary molar and (2) anterior glide of the mandible *(arrow)* with impact against the maxillary incisors.

Illustration continued on the following page

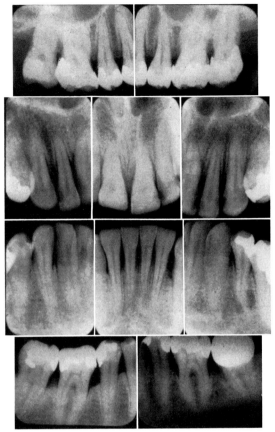

Figure 32–19 *Continued. D,* Radiographs of patient shown in *A.* Note the extensive bone destruction around the maxillary second molars and maxillary and mandibular incisors.

that deflect the mandible anteriorly contribute to destruction of the periodontium of the maxillary anterior teeth and pathologic migration (Figs. 32–19 and 32–20).

THE RADIOGRAPH IN THE DIAGNOSIS OF PERIODONTAL DISEASE

The x-ray is a valuable aid in the diagnosis of periodontal disease, the determination of the prognosis, and the evaluation of the outcome of treatment. **It is an adjunct to the clinical examination, not a substitute for it.** If a choice must be made, a more intelligent diagnosis can be made from the patient without the radiograph, than from radiographs without the patient.

The radiographic image results from the superimposition of tooth, bone, and soft tissues in the pathway between the cone of the machine and the film. The x-ray reveals alterations in calcified tissue; it does not reveal current cellular activity, but shows the effects of past cellular experience upon the bone and roots. Changes in the soft tissues of the periodontium require special techniques which have not as yet attained routine clinical usage.

Normal interdental septa

Because the facial and lingual bony plates are obscured by the relatively dense root structure, radiographic evaluation of bone changes in periodontal disease is based upon the appearance of the interdental septa. The interdental septum normally presents a thin radiopaque border, adjacent to the periodontal ligament and at the crest, referred to as the *lamina dura* (Fig. 32–21). It appears radiographically as a continuous white line, but it is perforated by numerous small foramina containing blood vessels, lymphatics, and nerves which pass between the periodon-

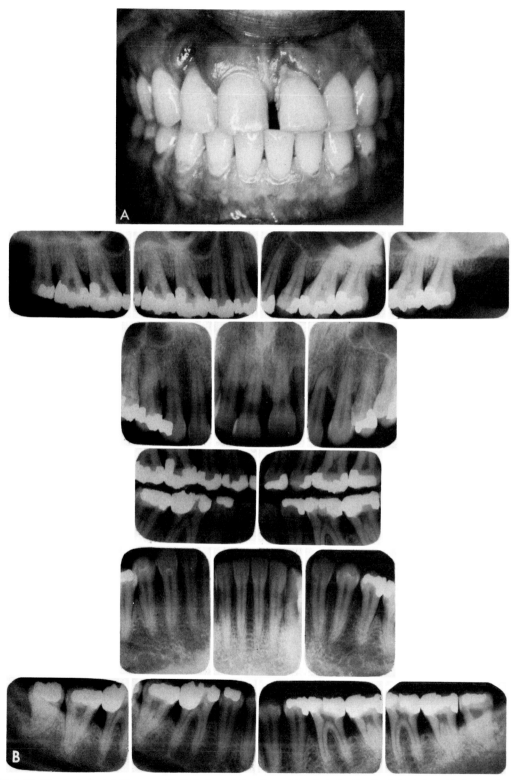

Figure 32–20 Periodontal Disease with Pathologic Migration of the Anterior Teeth. *A,* Periodontal inflammation and tissue loss, and pathologic migration in the anterior maxilla. *B,* Radiograph showing generalized bone loss and the angular pattern of bone destruction in the anterior maxilla.

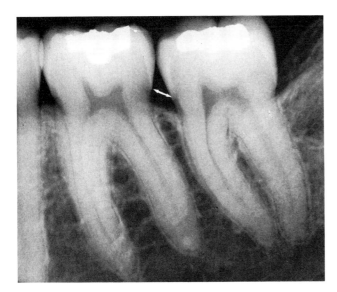

Figure 32–21 Crest of Interdental Septum Normally Parallel to a Line Drawn Between the Cemento-Enamel Junctions of Adjacent Teeth *(arrow).* Note also the radiopaque lamina dura around the roots and interdental septum.

tal ligament and the bone. Since the lamina dura represents the bone surface lining the tooth socket, the shape and position of the root and changes in the angulation of the x-ray beam produce considerable variations in its appearance.[32]

The width and shape of the interdental septum and the angle of the crest normally vary according to the convexity of the proximal tooth surfaces and the level of the cemento-enamel junction of the approximating teeth.[50] The interdental space and the interdental septum between teeth with prominently convex proximal surfaces are wider anteroposteriorly than between teeth with relatively flat proximal surfaces. The faciolingual diameter of the bone is related to the width of the proximal root surface. **The angulation of the crest of the interdental septum is generally parallel to a line between the cemento-enamel junction of the approximating teeth (Fig. 32–21).** When there is a difference in the levels of the cemento-enamel junctions, the crest of the interdental bone is angulated rather than horizontal.

Distortion produced by variation in radiographic technique

Variations in x-ray technique produce artefacts which limit the diagnostic value of the radiograph. The bone level, the pattern of bone destruction, the width of the periodontal ligament space,[69] and the radiodensity, trabecular pattern, and marginal contour of the interdental septum are modified by altering the exposure and development time, the type of film, and the x-ray angulation.[42] Standardized reproducible techniques are required to obtain reliable radiographs for pre- and post-treatment comparisons.[44, 47, 53] A grid calibrated

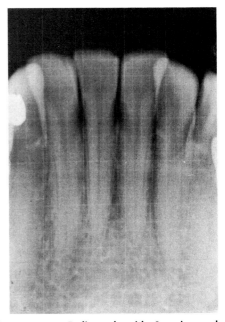

Figure 32–22 Radiograph with Superimposed Grid Calibrated in Millimeters.

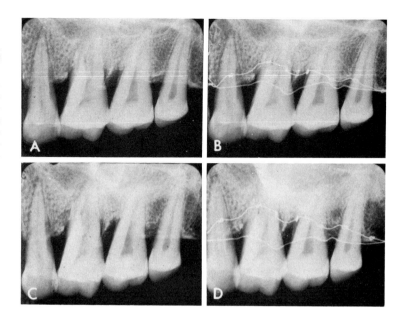

Figure 32–23 Long Cone Paralleling Technique and Bisection of the Angle Technique compared. (Courtesy of Dr. Benjamin Patur, Hartford, Conn.) *A,* Long cone technique. Radiograph of dried specimen. *B,* Long cone technique. Same specimen. The smooth wire is on the margin of the facial plate and the knotted wire is on the lingual plate to show their relative positions. *C,* Bisection of the angle technique. Same specimen. *D,* Bisection of the angle technique. Same specimen. Both bone margins are shifted toward the crown, the facial margin *(smooth wire)* more than the lingual margin *(knotted wire),* creating the illusion that the lingual bone margin has shifted apically.

in millimeters, superimposed upon the finished film, is helpful for comparing bone levels in radiographs taken under similar conditions[10] (Fig. 32–22).

The following are useful facts regarding the effects of angulation:

The long cone paralleling technique projects the most realistic image of the level of the alveolar bone[14] (Fig. 32–23). The bisection of the angle technique increases the projection and makes the bone margin appear closer to the crown; the level of the facial bone margin is distorted more than the lingual (Fig. 32–23). Shifting the cone mesially or distally without changing the horizontal plane projects the x-rays obliquely and changes the shape of the interdental bone, the width of the periodontal ligament space, and the appearance of the lamina dura, and may distort the extent of furcation involvement (Fig. 32–24).

Bone destruction in periodontal disease

Because the radiograph does not reveal minor destructive changes in bone,[3, 4, 48] periodontal disease that produces even slight radiographic changes has progressed beyond its earliest stages. The earliest signs of periodontal disease must therefore be detected clinically. The radiographic image tends to be less severe than the actual bone loss.[67] The difference between

the alveolar crest height and the radiographic appearance ranges from 0 to 1.6 mm.,[49] mostly accounted for by x-ray angulation.

The amount of bone loss

The x-ray is an indirect method for determining the amount of bone loss in periodontal disease. It indicates the amount of remaining bone rather than the amount lost. The amount of bone loss is estimated to be the difference between the physiologic bone level of the patient and the height of remaining bone.

The distribution of bone loss

The distribution of bone loss is an important diagnostic sign. It points to the location of destructive local factors in different areas of the mouth, and in relation to different surfaces of the same tooth.

The pattern of bone destruction

In periodontal disease, the interdental septa undergo changes that affect the **lamina dura, the crestal radiodensity, the size and shape of the medullary spaces, and the height and contour of the bone.** The interdental septa may be reduced in height, with the crest horizontal and per-

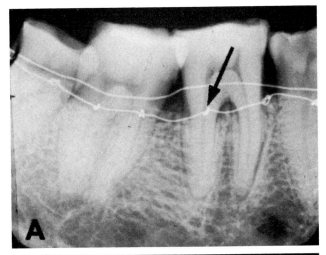

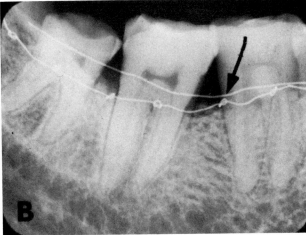

Figure 32-24 Distortion by Oblique Projection. *A,* **Long Cone Technique.** The smooth wire is on the facial bony plate, the knotted wire on the lingual. Note the knot *(arrow)* near the center of the distal root of the first molar, which shows bifurcation involvement. *B,* **Long Cone Technique. Cone Is Placed Distally, Projecting the Rays Mesially and Obliquely.** The oblique projection shifts the image of all structures mesially. *The structures closest to the cone shift the most.* This creates the illusion that the knot *(arrow)* has moved distally. Note that the bifurcation involvement shown in *A* is obliterated in *B.*

pendicular to the long axis of the adjacent teeth (Fig. 32–25), or they may present angular or arcuate defects (Fig. 32–26). The former condition is called **horizontal bone loss,** and the latter, **angular or vertical bone loss.**

Radiographs do not indicate the internal morphology or depth of crater-like interdental defects which appear as angular or vertical defects, nor do they reveal the extent of involvement on the facial and lingual surfaces. There are several reasons for this. Facial and lingual surface bone destruction is obscured by the dense root structure, and bone destruction on the mesial and distal root surfaces may be partially hidden by a dense mylohyoid ridge (Fig. 32–27).

Dense cortical plates on the facial and lingual surfaces of the interdental septa **obscure destruction which occurs in the intervening cancellous bone.** This means that it is possible to have a deep crater in the bone between the facial and lingual plates without radiographic indication of its presence. In order for destruction of the interproximal cancellous bone to be recorded radiographically, the cortical bone must be involved. Reduction of only 0.5 or 1.0 mm. in the thickness of the cortical plate is sufficient to permit radiographic visualization of destruction of the inner cancellous trabeculae.[45]

Passing a probe through the gingiva to the bone helps determine the architecture of osseous defects produced by periodontal disease. It also aids in the location of dehiscences and fenestrations. Gutta percha packed around the teeth increases the usefulness of the radiograph for detecting

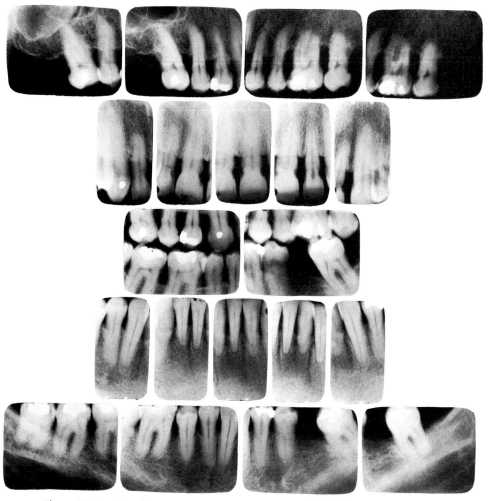

Figure 32–25   Complete Intraoral Series Showing Generalized Horizontal Bone Loss.

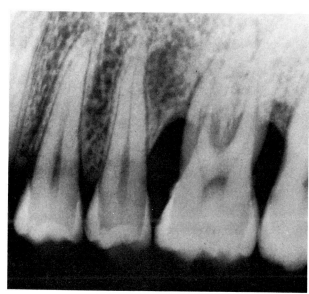

Figure 32–26   Angular Bone Loss on First Molar with Involvement of the Trifurcation.

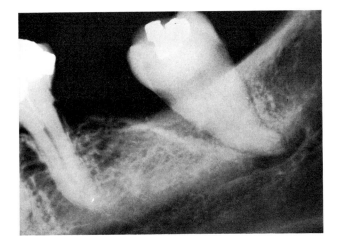

Figure 32-27   Angular Bone Loss on Mandibular Molar Partially Obscured by Dense Mylohyoid Ridge.

the morphology of osseous craters and involvement of the facial and lingual surfaces (Fig. 32–28). However, surgical exposure and visual examination provide the most definitive information regarding the bone architecture produced by periodontal destruction.[46]

Radiographic changes in periodontitis

The following is the sequence of radiographic changes in periodontitis, and the tissue changes which produce them:

Fuzziness and a break in the continuity of the lamina dura at the mesial or distal aspect of the crest of the interdental septum are the earliest radiographic changes in periodontitis (Fig. 32–29).

These result from extension of inflammation from the gingiva into the bone and associated widening of the vessel channels, and a reduction in calcified tissue at the septal margin.

A wedge-shaped radiolucent area is formed at the mesial or distal aspect of the crest of the septal bone (Fig. 32–29B). The apex of the area is pointed in the direction of the root.

This is produced by resorption of the bone of the lateral aspect of the interdental septum with an associated widening of the periodontal space.

The destructive process extends across the crest of the interdental septum and the height is reduced. Finger-like radiolucent projections extend from the crest into the septum (Fig. 32–29C).

The radiolucent projections into the interdental septum are the result of the deeper extension of the inflammation into the bone. Inflammatory cells and fluid, proliferation of connective tissue cells, and increased osteoclasis cause increased bone resorption along the endosteal margins of the medullary spaces. The radiopaque projections, separating the radiolucent spaces, are the composite images of the partially eroded bone trabeculae.

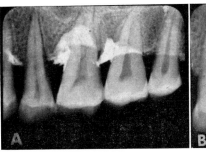
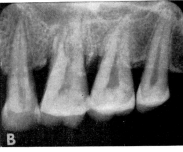

Figure 32-28 Gutta Percha Aids in Detecting Bone Defects. A, Gutta percha packed around teeth shows interproximal and facial and lingual bone loss. B, Same area without gutta percha gives little indication of the extent of bone involvement.

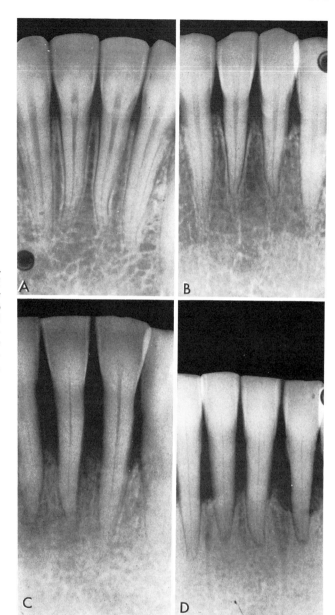

Figure 32–29 Radiographic Changes in Periodontitis. *A,* Normal appearance of interdental septa. *B,* Fuzziness and a break in the continuity of the lamina dura at the crest of the bone distal to the central incisor *(left).* There are wedge shaped radiolucent areas at the crests of the other interdental septa. *C,* Radiolucent projections from the crest into the interdental septum indicate extension of destructive processes. *D,* Severe bone loss.

The height of the interdental septum (Fig. 32–29 *D*) is progressively reduced by extension of inflammation and resorption of bone.

When inflammation is the sole destructive factor in periodontal disease, the crest of the interdental septum is usually horizontal; when the crest appears angular, the possible existence of trauma from occlusion should be explored.

Radiographic changes in juvenile periodontitis

Juvenile periodontitis is characterized by a combination of the following radiographic features:

Loss of alveolar bone is localized in the early stages to a single tooth or group of teeth, and tends to become generalized as the disease progresses. The bone loss occurs initially in the maxillary and man-

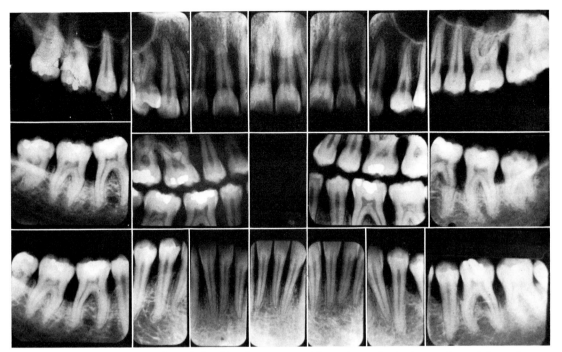

Figure 32–30   Idiopathic Juvenile Periodontitis. The accentuated bone destruction in the anterior and first molar areas is considered characteristic of this disease, formerly called "periodontosis."

dibular incisor and first molar areas, usually bilaterally (Fig. 32–30). The interdental septa present vertical, arclike, or angular destructive patterns. When the bone loss is generalized, it is least pronounced in the mandibular premolar areas.

A generalized alteration in the trabecular pattern of the alveolar bone consists of less clearly defined trabecular markings and increase in the size of the cancellous spaces.

Radiographic changes in trauma from occlusion

Trauma from occlusion can produce radiographically detectable changes in the lamina dura, in the morphology of the alveolar crest, in the width of the periodontal space, and in the density of the surrounding cancellous bone.

Traumatic lesions manifest themselves more clearly in faciolingual aspects, since mesiodistally the tooth has the added stability provided by the contact areas with adjacent teeth. Therefore slight variations in the proximal surfaces may indicate

greater changes in facial and lingual aspects. Radiographic changes listed below are not pathognomonic of trauma from occlusion and have to be interpreted in combination with clinical findings, particularly tooth mobility, presence of wear facets, pocket depth, and analysis of occlusal contacts and habits:

The *injury phase of trauma from occlusion* produces a loss of the lamina dura that may be noted in apices, furcations, and/or marginal areas. This loss of lamina dura will result in widening of the periodontal ligament space (Fig. 32–31). This change, particularly when incipient or very circumscribed, may be easily confused with technical variations owing to angulation of the radiograph or malposition of the tooth; it can be diagnosed with certainty only in radiographs of the highest quality.

The *repair phase of trauma from occlusion* will result in an attempt to strengthen the periodontal structures in order to better support the increased loads. Radiographically this is manifested by widening of the periodontal ligament space, which may be generalized or localized.

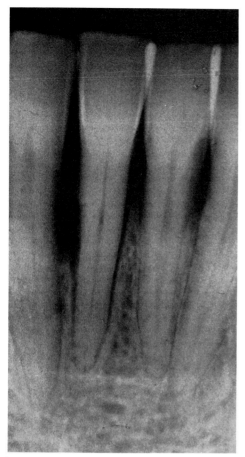

Figure 32–31 **Widened Periodontal Space Caused by Trauma from Occlusion.** Note the increased density of the surrounding bone caused by new bone formation in response to increased occlusal forces.

Although microscopic measurements have determined that there are variations in the width of the periodontal space in the different regions of the root, these are not generally detected in radiographs.

When variations in width between the marginal area and the midroot or between the midroot and the apex are detected, it means that the tooth is being subjected to increased forces.

Successful attempts to reinforce the periodontal structures by widening of the periodontal space will be accompanied by increased width of the lamina dura and sometimes by condensation of the perialveolar cancellous bone.

More advanced traumatic lesions may result in deep angular bone loss (Figs. 32–32 and 32–33) which, when combined with marginal inflammation, may lead to infrabony pocket formation. The very deep combined lesions will extend around the root apex, producing a wide radiolucent periapical image (cavernous lesions).

Root resorption may also occur as a result of excessive forces on the periodontium, particularly derived from orthodontic appliances. Although trauma from occlusion produces many resorption areas, they are usually of a magnitude insufficient to be detected radiographically.

Additional radiographic criteria in the diagnosis of periodontal disease

A radiopaque horizontal line across the roots demarcates the portion of the root where the labial and/or lingual bony plate has been partially or completely destroyed from the remaining bone-supported portion (Fig. 32–33).

Vessel canals in the alveolar bone. Hirschfeld[23] described linear and circular radiolucent areas produced by interdental

Figure 32–32 **Angular Bone Loss Associated with Trauma from Occlusion.** A, Thickening of periodontal space at crest of bone adjacent to central incisors. B, Six years later, angular bone destruction with formation of hemiseptum.

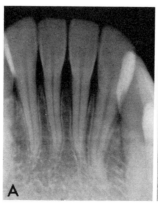
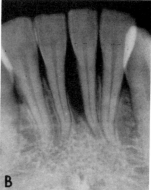

A   B

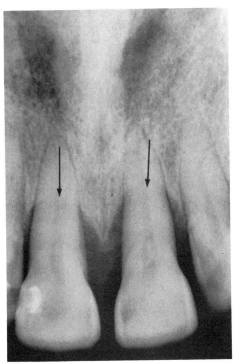

Figure 32-33   Horizontal Line across the roots of the central incisors *(arrows)*. The area of the roots below the horizontal lines are partially or completely denuded of the facial and/or lingual bony plates.

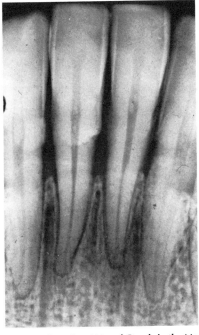

Figure 32-34   Prominent Vessel Canals in the Mandible.

canals and their foramina respectively (Fig. 32-34). These canals indicate the course of the vascular supply of the bone and are normal radiographic findings. The radiographic image of the canals is frequently so prominent, particularly in the anterior region of the mandible, that they might be confused with radiolucence resulting from periodontal disease.

Differentiation between periodontal atrophy and chronic periodontal disease. In older persons it is sometimes necessary to determine whether the bone level is the result of periodontal atrophy or if destructive periodontal disease is a contributory factor. Clinical examination is the basic determinant. However, radiographically detectable alterations in the normal clearcut peripheral outline of the septa are corroborating evidence of periodontal disease.

SKELETAL DISTURBANCES MANIFESTED IN THE JAWS

Skeletal disturbances may produce changes in the jaws[7, 17] that affect the interpretation of radiographs from the periodontal viewpoint. Included among the diseases in which destruction of tooth-supporting bone may occur are the following:

Osteitis fibrosa cystica (von Recklinghausen's disease of bone) causes a diffuse granular mottling, scattered "cystlike" radiolucent areas throughout the jaws, and a generalized disappearance of the lamina dura.[52, 61]

In *Paget's disease*, the radiographic appearance of the jaws varies. The normal trabecular pattern may be replaced by a hazy diffuse meshwork of closely knit, fine trabecular markings, with the lamina dura absent (Fig. 32-35), or there may be scattered radiolucent areas containing irregularly shaped radiopaque zones.[18]

Fibrous dysplasia may appear as a small radiolucent area at a root apex or as an extensive radiolucent area with irregularly arranged trabecular markings.[16] There may be enlargement of the cancellous spaces, with distortion of the normal trabecular pattern and obliteration of the lamina dura (Fig. 32-36).

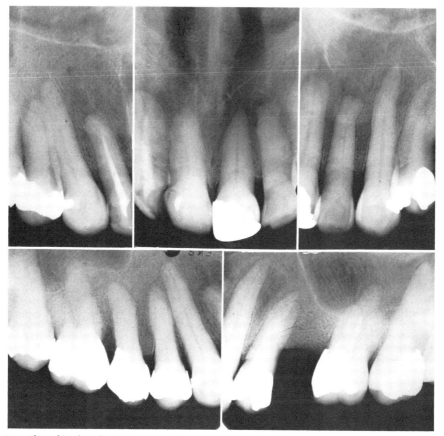

Figure 32–35 Altered Trabecular Pattern and Diminution in the Prominence of the Lamina Dura in Paget's Disease.

In *Hand-Schüller-Christian* disease, the radiographic appearance is that of single or multiple areas of radiolucency. Mobility of the teeth results from loss of bony support. *Letterer-Siwe disease and Gaucher's disease* may present comparable changes (Fig. 32–37).

Eosinophilic granuloma[55, 63] appears as single or multiple radiolucent areas, which may be unrelated to the teeth or entail

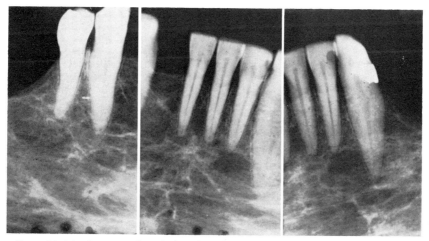

Figure 32–36 Osteoporosis and Altered Trabecular Arrangement in Fibrous Dysplasia.

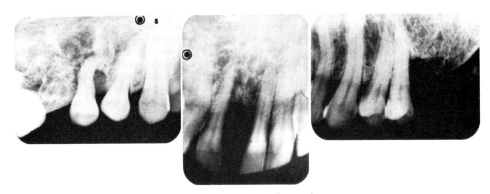

Figure 32–37   Osteoporosis in Gaucher's Disease.

destruction of the tooth-supporting bone (Fig. 32–38).

Numerous radiolucent areas occur when the jaws are involved by *multiple myeloma*.

In *osteopetrosis* (marble-bone disease; Albers-Schönberg's disease),[12] the outlines of the roots may be obscured by diffuse radiopacity of the jaws. In less severe cases, the increased density is confined to the bone in relation to the nutrient canals and the lamina dura.

In *scleroderma* (Chap. 12) the periodontal ligament is uniformly widened at the expense of the surrounding alveolar bone (Fig. 32–39).

LABORATORY AIDS IN DIAGNOSIS

The Biopsy

The biopsy in the diagnosis of neoplasms

The diagnosis of neoplasms should be established by microscopic examination. If it is to serve the purpose for which it is intended, certain principles should govern the biopsy technique.

METHOD OF TAKING A BIOPSY.   *Site of*

Biopsy. 1. Where the lesion is small, it should be totally excised. The excision should be wide enough and deep enough to include a border of healthy tissue along the entire cut surface.

2. Where the size of the lesion is such that complete excision is not possible or feasible, *obtain a specimen representative of the lesion:*

a. *Select that portion of the lesion which demonstrates all of the pathologic changes noted clinically.* If this is not possible with one biopsy, select several areas.

b. *Take thin deep sections rather than broad shallow sections.* A small superficial tab of tissue may show nothing more than degenerative, inflammatory, or necrotic changes.

c. *The section should include tissue at and beyond the lateral margins and base of the lesion.* In this way the transition from healthy to diseased tissue can be followed.

TECHNIQUE FOR OBTAINING TISSUE SPECIMEN.   There are several biopsy techniques.

Incision. Incision can be performed with the scalpel or high frequency cutting current. Removal of the tissue with a sharp blade appears to be the method of choice.

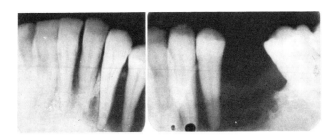

Figure 32–38 Bone Destruction Caused by Eosinophilic Granuloma (Courtesy of Dr. Irving Salman).

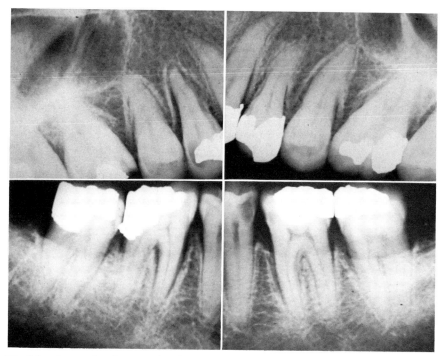

Figure 32–39 Scleroderma, showing typical uniform widening of the periodontal ligament and thickening of the lamina dura. (Courtesy of Drs. David F. Mitchell and Anand P. Chaudhry.)

Electrosurgery may be used to advantage in highly vascular tumors where bleeding may be a difficult complication.

Punch Biopsy. This method is of limited value in the oral cavity. Its greatest applicability is in the removal of small tissue specimens from inaccessible areas, such as the maxillary sinus and lateral or posterior pharyngeal walls.

Curettage. Tissue specimens are curetted from bony cavities and sinus tracts.

HANDLING OF THE TISSUE SPECIMEN.

1. The tissue should not be crushed or mutilated.

2. It should be placed in fixative immediately. Ten per cent formalin is an acceptable fixative. The volume of fixative should be approximately 20 times the volume of the tissue specimen. If the pathologist to whom you submit biopsy specimens prefers another fixative, it would be wise to keep on hand several small bottles containing this fixative.

If the specimen is too thick, only the peripheral portions of the tissue will be completely infiltrated and fixed, while the central area will undergo degenerative changes.

3. The specimen bottle should be properly labeled. Indicate whether the tissue specimen is soft tissue only, or whether it contains bone, and the time at which it was taken.

4. A brief history should accompany the specimen. This should include the name, age, and sex of the patient, a gross description of the lesion, its duration, location, and rate of growth or change in growth rate, and the method used in obtaining the specimen.

The biopsy in the diagnosis of gingival and mucosal disease

The gingival biopsy may be important in the diagnosis of some gingival disturbances. Microscopic study of gingival biopsies is sometimes the only method of detecting local and systemic interrelationships that cannot be discerned by clinical examination. For example, amyloid is present in the gingiva in 78 per cent of patients with amyloidosis,[58] many of whom present no clinical gingival changes.

The amyloid is deposited extracellularly ad-

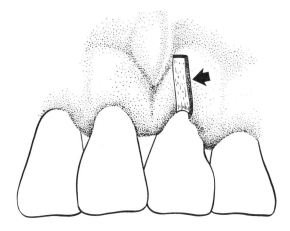

Figure 32–40   Rectangular Gingival Biopsy *(arrow)* Includes Marginal and Attached Gingiva.

jacent to the capillaries in the papillary layer immediately subjacent to the basal layer of the epithelium, and appears as amorphous hyalinized material which stains metachromatically with crystal violet.[35]

The presence of eosinophilic granuloma may be detected by gingival biopsy. In addition to differentiating between different types of gingival enlargement, gingival biopsy is indispensable when the presence of diseases such as desquamative gingivitis, benign mucous membrane pemphigoid, pemphigus, or lichen planus is suspected.

The marginal and attached gingiva should be included in the biopsy (Fig. 32–40). Inflammatory changes in the gingival margin tend to obscure any alterations that may be produced by a systemic disturbance. Inclusion of the attached gingiva, in which the effect of local irritants is less likely to be present, offers an opportunity to investigate tissue changes that may be produced by systemic disturbances.

Exfoliative Cytology

Exfoliative cytology is a diagnostic procedure consisting of the microscopic examination of cells obtained by scraping the surface of the suspected area, or by rinsing the oral cavity. The former is preferred. Its reliability for the diagnosis of cancer is 86 per cent, as compared with the close to 100 per cent reliability of an oral biopsy.[60] Cytology is not a substitute for biopsy but it is valuable if a biopsy cannot be done for some reason, and also in screening large groups of people for the presence of malignancy, provided it is used in conjunction with a careful oral examination. It is also helpful in the diagnosis of bullous and vesicular oral lesions.

To obtain a specimen, the entire surface of the abnormal mucosa is firmly scraped with the edge of a wooden tongue depressor. The material thus removed is spread directly on a glass slide and immediately fixed in 95 per cent alcohol and submitted for microscopic diagnosis.[56]

OTHER AIDS USED IN THE DIAGNOSIS OF ORAL MANIFESTATIONS OF SYSTEMIC DISEASE

When the nature and severity of gingival and periodontal disease cannot be explained by local causes, the possibility of contributing systemic factors must be explored. The dentist must understand the oral manifestations of systemic disease so that he can advise the physician regarding the type of systemic disturbance which may be involved in individual cases.

Numerous laboratory tests aid in the diagnosis of systemic diseases. The manner in which they are performed and the interpretation of findings are found in standard texts on the subject.[68] Those pertinent to the diagnosis of disturbances often manifested in the oral cavity are referred to briefly here.

Nutritional status

Nutrition refers to the complex relationship between the individual's total health status and the intake, digestion, and utilization of nutrients. *Nutritional deficiency connotes an inadequacy in the nutritional status of the tissues.* Malnutrition or poor nutrition may result from excessive food intake and improper nutrient balance as well as from an insufficiency of nutrients.

Nutritional deficiencies may be (1) *primary*, resulting from an overt insufficiency of nutrients; or (2) *secondary (conditioned)*, resulting from bodily conditions which interfere with the ingestion, transport, cellular uptake, or utilization of essential nutrients, in the presence of adequate food intake. Nutritional deficiencies usually develop in stages as follows: (1) *depletion of the tissue nutrient reserve*, (2) *biochemical tissue lesions*, (3) *morphologic and functional abnormalities which are expressed as* (4) *clinical signs and symptoms*, and finally (5) *tissue death.*

Diagnosis of nutritional deficiency

A nutritional diagnosis is based upon four sequential routes of inquiry: (1) medical and social history, and dietary history; (2) clinical examination; (3) laboratory tests; and (4) therapeutic trial.

MEDICAL AND SOCIAL HISTORY. Common complaints of patients with nutritional disorders include general weakness, chronic fatigue, failure of appetite, painful bleeding gums, sore lips, sore tongue and mouth, diarrhea, chronic nervousness, irritability, inability to concentrate, confusion, memory loss, dizziness, lethargy, photophobia, loss of manual dexterity, numbness, pain in the legs, and skin rashes.

Attention should be given to conditions which could lead to secondary nutritional deficiencies such as the following:

Gastrointestinal disturbances which impair the digestion and absorption of nutrients. In diarrhea, hypermotility of the intestine does not permit sufficient time for water-soluble vitamins to be absorbed. Achlorhydria interferes with the absorption of calcium, phosphorus, and iron. In diseases in which fat absorption is impaired, such as sprue, ulcerative colitis, dysentery, and celiac disease, the absorption of the fat soluble vitamins (A, D, E, K) is inhibited. Excessive amounts of oxalic acid (found in spinach) or phytic acid (found in bran) will make minerals unavailable for utilization to the body. The daily use of mineral oil interferes with the absorption of carotene.

Interference with utilization of foods, which occurs as a feature of certain diseases such as diabetes, adrenal dysfunction, cirrhosis of the liver, or thyroid disease.

Increased excretion, such as in polyuria of diabetes or in fever, which affects the nitrogen retention of the tissues as well as the water balance of the body. Lactation tends to reduce the thiamine level.

Factors which increase the nutritional requirements, such as hyperthyroidism, spurt growth periods, pregnancy, lactation, physical exertion, or drug administration.

Factors which interfere with the ingestion of food, such as discomfort from caries and periodontal disease, absence of teeth, loss of appetite caused by infection, food allergy, or nausea of pregnancy.

There is an important relationship between emotional status and appetite. Emotional problems often lead to overeating and obesity. "Breaking the smoking habit" frequently has a similar effect. Loss of appetite may result from bereavement or frustration. In alcoholics, diminished food intake may lead to nutritional deficiency.

DIETARY HISTORY. The dietary history should provide information regarding the patient's usual dietary practices and should include questions regarding the following:

Length of time the present diet has been followed.

History of any special diet, its type and duration. Therapeutic diets such as those prescribed in the treatment of ulcers, biliary disease and colitis, or "reducing diets" may be deficient in one or more essential nutrients.

Use of vitamins or other food supplements.

Regularity of meals.

Food likes, dislikes, and idiosyncrasies.

Living conditions. Young individuals who live away from their families and prepare their own meals, and elderly individuals who live alone and find it difficult to obtain proper foods and prepare well-balanced meals often suffer from malnutrition.

Economic status and education. Inability to afford foods in necessary quantities and variety, and lack of knowledge regarding the requirement of a "good diet" are common causes of nutritional disorder.

After the desired information is obtained, the patient is given a "food diary," in which he is to record his daily food intake for at least five consecutive days which include a weekend.

EVALUATION OF THE DIET.[39] The adequacy of the diet is evaluated by transposing the information in the dietary history into the basic four food groups: (1) *milk*, (2) *meat*, (3) *vegetable and fruit* and (4) *bread and cereal*. The *milk group* (milk, cheese) provides protein, calcium, riboflavin, vitamin A, and other nutrients; the *meat group* (meat, fish, poultry, eggs, dried beans, and peas) provides primarily protein, B complex vitamins, and iron; the *vegetable and fruit group* provides most of the vitamins A and C as well as other minerals and vitamins; and the *bread and cereal group* furnishes B complex vitamins, iron, protein, and carbohydrate. Foods which provide only calories such as sugar and sugar products should be kept to a minimum. The same is true of fats because they are usually contained in the milk and meat groups.

A chart such as that shown in Table 32–1 is helpful for evaluating the diet.[38] It separates the foods into different groups and also records their consistency so that inadequacies in coarse, hard foods which have a helpful cleansing effect upon the teeth and gingiva can be noted and corrected. A person who consumes less food than the amounts recommended in the evaluation chart is not necessarily nutritionally deficient. The recommendations represent amounts considered desirable for maintaining good nutrition in healthy patients, without bodily conditioning factors which interfere with food utilization. They represent goals to be strived for rather than requirements.

CLINICAL EXAMINATION. Certain signs and symptoms have been identified with different nutritional deficiencies.[57] However, many patients with nutritional disease do not exhibit classic signs of deficiency disorders, and different types of deficiency produce comparable clinical findings. Clinical findings are suggestive,

TABLE 32–1   DIETARY EVALUATION CHART

Food Groups	Physical Form	1st Day	2nd Day	3rd Day	4th Day	5th Day	Average per Day	Recommended Intake	Difference
I. Milk	Liquid, soft	/ /		/	/	/ /	2	2 or more servings	OK
	Hard			/	/	/	/			
II. Meat	Soft, chopped	/	/ /	/		/ /	2	2 or more servings	OK
	Solid	/	/	/	/	/			
III. Vegetable and fruit	Juices, soft	/		/ /	/	/ /	2+	4 or more servings	−2
	Raw or slightly cooked	/		/	/	/ /			
IV. Bread and cereal	Soft, cooked	/ / / /	/ / /	/ / /	/ / /	/ / / /	5+	4 or more servings	+1
	Dry, crusty, toasted	/	/ /	/ /	/ /	/ /			

TABLE 32–2 CLINICAL FINDINGS IDENTIFIED WITH NUTRITIONAL DEFICIENCIES*

System	Clinical Findings	Suggested Deficiency
General	Underweight	CHO, fat and protein
	Underheight	Protein, Ca, P, vitamins
	Pallor	Iron, folic acid, B₁₂, intrinsic factor
	Anorexia	Thiamine, niacin
	Weakness and fatigue	Calories, vitamin B complex
Skin	Dermatitis (pellagrous)	Niacin
	Intertrigo	Riboflavin
	Xerosis	Vitamin A
	Hyperkeratosis of hair follicle	Vitamin A
	Acne	Pyridoxine, vitamin A
Eyes	Nyctalopia or night blindness	Vitamin A
	Xerophthalmia	Vitamin A
	Photophobia	Riboflavin, vitamin A
	Bitot's spots	Vitamin A
	Vascular injection of conjunctiva and sclera	Riboflavin
Mouth	Angular cheilosis "Beefy red"	Riboflavin
	Scarlet red glossitis (pellagrous)	Niacin
	Lichen planus	B complex
	Leukoplakia	B complex
	Scorbutic gingivitis	Ascorbic acid
Skeletal	Rachitic deformities	Vitamin D, calcium and phosphorus
Neuromuscular	Muscle cramps	
	(calf tenderness with or without edema)	Thiamine
	Paresthesia	Thiamine

*Comparable clinical findings may result from more than one type of deficiency.

Data from Jolliffe.[24]

but definitive diagnosis of nutritional deficiencies and their nature requires the combined information revealed by the history, clinical and laboratory findings, and therapeutic trial. *Clinical findings* identified with specific nutritional deficiencies are presented in Table 32–2,[24] and the *oral manifestations of nutritional disorders* are described in Chapter 28.

LABORATORY TESTS FOR NUTRITIONAL DEFICIENCY. Blood, serum, and urine tests reflect nutrient intake levels and absorption defects. The following are useful diagnostic aids: In the blood, *macrocytosis* may be the result of *vitamin B₁₂ and folate deficiencies*, whereas a *microcytosis* may indicate lack of *iron* and *vitamin B₆*. *Hypochromia* is associated with *iron deficiency*. The *serum iron-binding capacity*, which normally is 300 to 450 μg per 100 ml., is decreased to less than 18 per cent in *iron deficiency*.

A serum albumin value below 3.5 gm per 100 ml. serum indicates *protein deficiency*. Serum *vitamin A levels* below 10 μg. per 100 ml. suggest deficiency of the vitamin. A serum carotene of 30 μg. per 100 ml. also indicates a vitamin A deficiency. Since *vitamin C* is not stored in the body, *serum ascorbic acid* levels reflect current intake. Serum values below 0.3 mg. per 100 ml. indicate inadequate intake; values below 0.01 mg. per ml. are consistent with a diagnosis of *scurvy*. The normal serum level of *vitamin B₁₂* (cyancobolamine) should range between 7 and 15.9 mμg. per ml. folate activity for *Lactobacillus casei*; below 7 mμg. per ml. is subnormal.

Urinary creatinine is used as a reference unit in tests for several nutrients. Iodine intake is considered inadequate if its level in creatinine is less than 50 mg. per gm. The N-methylnicotinamide content should be above 1.6 mg. per gm. of creatinine. Riboflavin content below 80 μg. per gm. of creatinine in adults and below 300 μg. per gm. of creatinine in children under six, and thiamine values less than 97 to 116 μg. per gm. of creatinine in adults and 120

μg. per gm. of creatinine in children under six are considered indicative of inadequate intake.

The Hemogram

Blood smear

Examination of a stained blood smear reveals information regarding (1) the morphology, staining reaction, and maturity of the red cells, (2) morphology and maturity of the various types of white cells, and (3) presence of parasites in the blood.

Red cell count

In males the average red cell count is 5.4 million per cubic millimeter with a range of 4.6 to 6.2. In females, the count is slightly lower, with an average of 4.8 million per cubic millimeter and a range of 4.2 to 5.4. A lowered red cell count or oligocythemia is present in pernicious anemia (1.5 to 2.5), hemolytic jaundice (1.5 to 3.0), iron deficiency anemia (1.5 to 4.7), acute aplastic anemia (1.0 or less), chronic leukemia (average 4.2) and acute leukemia (1.0). An increased red cell count is seen in polycythemia (7.0 to 12.0).

Hemoglobin content

Total hemoglobin may be measured by the cyanmethemoglobin method. This is a spectrophotometric method and is the preferred technique.[8] Normal values of hemoglobin vary with age and sex. The normal value for adult males is 16 $\pm$ 2.0 gm. per 100 ml., and for adult females is 14 $\pm$ 2.0 gm. per 100 ml. blood.[70]

White cell count

The normal number of leukocytes ranges from 5,000 to 10,000 per cubic millimeter of blood, with an average of 7,500.

The differential white cell count

Leukocytosis is the term applied to an increase in the number of white blood cells. Lymphocytic leukocytosis is an increase in the total white cell count with a predominance in the number of lymphocytes. It usually occurs in chronic inflammatory diseases, such as tuberculosis or syphilis, and in malaria, whooping cough, and Hodgkin's disease. A neutrophilic leukocytosis is observed in a number of pathologic states: (a) diseases caused by a pyogenic or pus-producing organism; (b) tissue necrosis, as, for example, myocardial infarction; (c) acute massive hemorrhage; (d) malignant neoplasms; (e) gout; and (f) nephritis. An eosinophilic leukocytosis (eosinophilia) is seen in (a) parasitic diseases caused by worms (helminthic infestations): (b) allergic diseases, such as asthma, hay fever, and angioneurotic edema; (c) Hodgkin's disease; (d) periarteritis nodosa; and (e) skin diseases, such as pemphigus and psoriasis.

Leukemia represents an unrestrained growth of leukopoietic tissue resulting in the production of excessive numbers of immature white cells. Depending upon the cell type involved, myelogenous, lymphatic, and monocytic leukemia can be distinguished. Leukemia may be either acute, subacute, or chronic. During the course of leukemia, there may be periods when the white cell count is reduced instead of elevated. These periods are referred to as the aleukemic phases of leukemia (aleukemic leukemia), and are thought to be due to the inability of the white cells to leave the markedly hyperplastic marrow or lymphoid tissue. In the bone marrow, the hyperplastic leukopoietic tissue may encroach upon tissue that is forming red cells and blood platelets and cause anemia and thrombocytopenia, with all the complications associated with such deficiencies. Pallor, fatigue and weakness, and

TABLE 32–3   NORMAL VALUES FOR DIFFERENTIAL WHITE CELL COUNT

	Per Cent
Neutrophilic polymorphonuclear leukocytes	60–70
Segmented cells 52–67%; stab cells 3–5%; juveniles 0–1%, myelocytes 0%.	
Eosinophilic polymorphonuclear leukocytes	1–4
Basophilic polymorphonuclear leukocytes	0.25–0.50
Lymphocytes	25–28
Monocytes	2–6

tiny hemorrhages caused by anemia and platelet deficiency are often the presenting symptoms of leukemia.

A reduction in the white cell count below 5000 per cubic millimeter is termed leukopenia. The terms *leukopenia* and *granulopenia* are used interchangeably, because in most cases the granulocytes are the cells that are reduced in number. A leukopenia may be seen in a number of disease processes: bacterial infections, such as typhoid fever; viral diseases, such as measles; protozoal infections; malignant neoplasms; allergic diseases; aleukemic leukemia; and agranulocytosis. *Agranulocytosis* is a severe form of leukopenia in which the granulocytes may be completely absent from the blood, and the white cell count may be reduced to several hundred per cubic millimeter. In the absence of granulocytes, particularly the neutrophils, infections tend to run a rapid and often fatal course.

Erythrocyte sedimentation rate

The sedimentation rate is the rate at which red cells settle in shed blood. Increase in the sedimentation rate occurs in diseases characterized by widespread tissue injury and destruction, as in rheumatic fever, tuberculosis, arthritis, myocardial infarction, and malignant neoplasms. The sedimentation rate is usually normal (Westergren method: 0–15 mm. per hr. in men; 0–20 mm per hr. in women; 0–10 per hr. in children) or only slightly elevated in acute inflammations and infections of a very localized nature.

Laboratory Tests Employed in Exploring the Etiology of Spontaneous or Excessive Bleeding

COAGULATION TIME. The coagulation or clotting time is the time necessary for blood to clot after it has been removed and placed in a test tube or other container. For the determination of the clotting time, blood may be obtained by either skin puncture or venipuncture. The normal clotting time of blood obtained by skin puncture is 2 to 6 minutes. For blood obtained by vein puncture, the normal range is between 5 and 15 minutes. When siliconized tubes are used, the range is 19 to 60 minutes.

BLEEDING TIME. The bleeding time is the time necessary for a small cut to stop bleeding. In the *Duke* method for the determination of the bleeding time, a small cut is made in the ear lobe, and the blood is blotted with filter paper at 30 second intervals until bleeding ceases. The time interval between the first and the last drop is taken as the bleeding time. The normal range is 1 to 6 minutes, with the majority between 1 and 3 minutes. With the *Ivy* method, which entails the use of a cuff, the normal range is 1 to 9 minutes.

CLOT RETRACTION TIME AND CHARACTER OF THE CLOT. The clot retraction time is defined as the time it takes for a blood clot to retract from the wall of a test tube in which the blood is placed. Although the phenomenon of retractility is in some way related to the platelets, it is independent of the coagulation time. Usually the clot begins to retract within a few minutes to one hour after it is formed. Defective clots with prolonged retraction time are indicative of platelet deficiency.

THE PROTHROMBIN TIME. The prothrombin time is the time in seconds required for the formation of fibrin in oxalated plasma that has been recalcified after thromboplastin in excess has been added (Quick's method of determination). The normal prothrombin time is 12 to 14 seconds. The clotting mechanism will usually not be impaired until the prothrombin level has been reduced to approximately 20 per cent of normal.

CAPILLARY FRAGILITY TEST. The test most frequently employed in the determination of increased capillary fragility is the *Rumpel-Leede* test. A blood pressure cuff is placed on the upper arm and a pressure is maintained half way between systolic pressure for eight minutes. The appearance of more than 10 petechiae (tiny hemorrhages) in a circle 5 cm. in diameter below the bend of the elbow is indicative of increased capillary fragility.

The *characteristics of the various hemorrhagic diseases* are presented in Table 32–4.

BONE MARROW STUDIES. Aspiration biopsies are commonly employed in the

TABLE 32-4 CHARACTERISTICS OF THE VARIOUS HEMORRHAGIC DISEASES

Disease	Clotting Time	Clot Retrac- tion Time	Bleeding Time	Platelet Count	Rumpel- Leede Test	Prothrombin Time
1. Idiopathic thrombocytopenic purpura	N	+	+	−	+	N
2. Hemophilia	+	N	N	N	N	N
3. Hereditary hemorrhagic telangiectasia	N	N	N	N	N	N
4. Pseudo-hemophilia	N	N	+	N	N	N
5. Secondary thrombocytopenic purpura	N	+	+	−	+	N
6. Anaphylactic purpura	N	N	±	N	+	N
7. Liver disease	+	N	±	N	N	+

N − normal
+ − prolonged
− − shortened

investigation of blood dyscrasias. Such biopsies are usually taken from the sternum; the other sites are the ileum and spinous processes.

Patients with oral mucous membrane lesions of *suspected allergic origin* may be tested for sensitivity to a wide range of substances. The finding of eosinophilia is suggestive of allergy. A simple patch test for contact sensitivity has been devised for use in the oral cavity.[19] A small rubber suction cup lined with collodion is filled with cotton. The material to be tested is dropped on the cotton, and the cup is fastened to the oral mucosa with dental floss. An average contact time of 20 to 30 minutes is sufficient to elicit a severe localized tissue reaction in cases of sensitivity.

Exploration of Systemic Etiology Factors in Patients with Excessive Bone Loss

In seeking for systemic disturbances in patients with severe and rapid alveolar bone loss, unexplained on the basis of local factors alone, the possibility of metabolic bone disease should be investigated.[59] The following are useful screening procedures:

1. RADIOGRAPHS OF THE SKULL AND SEVERAL LONG BONES.

2. DETERMINATION OF SERUM CALCIUM, SERUM PHOSPHORUS, AND ALKALINE PHOSPHATASE. One must determine the serum calcium (normal values 9 to 11 mg. per 100 ml.), serum phosphorus (normal values 2.5 to 4.0 mg. per 100 ml. in adults; 3.5 to 6.0 mg. per 100 ml. in children) and alkaline phosphatase (normal values 1 to 5 Bodansky units per 100 ml. in adults; 5 to 12 per 100 ml. in children).

3. THYROID FUNCTION. The average basal metabolic rate of men between the ages of 27 and 50 is from 38 to 40 calories per square meter of body surface per hour, which is slightly above the normal for females of a comparable age group. A variation of ± 10 per cent is within normal range. A rise or decrease in the basal metabolic rate of 25 per cent or more is considered indicative of hyperthyroidism or hypothyroidism respectively.

The commonly used thyroid function test is the protein-bound iodine (PBI). This test provides a valid estimate of total hormone bound to protein in peripheral blood in about 90 per cent of cases. The normal range for the PBI is 4.0 to 8.0 μg. per 100 ml. An increased PBI suggests hyperthyroidism; a decreased PBI suggests hypothyroidism.

Another thyroid function test is a radiochemical method that measures displacement of ^{131}I-labeled thyroxine from thyroxine-binding globulin (TBG) by thyroxine released from the patient's serum. This method is relatively unaffected by contamination and may be valuable in the presence of radiographic contrast media. However, phenytoin (Dilantin) may cause interference.

4. LABORATORY STUDIES FOR THE DETECTION OF DIABETES MELLITUS. *Fasting Blood Sugar Level.* The normal level of glucose in venous blood in the fasting state (8 to 14 hours after the last meal) is 60 to 100 mg. per 100 ml. This may normally rise to 160 mg. per 100 ml. after the ingestion of food. In untreated diabetes mellitus, the fasting blood sugar level may be between 200 and 280 mg. per 100 ml.

Postprandial Blood Sugar Level. Because the fasting blood glucose level may be normal in mild diabetics, the postprandial level taken two hours after eating is more reliable. Values between the 120 mg. per 100 (normal) and 140 mg. per 100 ml. are suspicious. Patients with values above 140 mg. per 100 ml. are considered to be diabetic.

Glucose Tolerance Test. The glucose tolerance test provides an indication of the patient's capacity to regulate the blood sugar level following the ingestion of carbohydrate. It is the most reliable laboratory indication of the presence of diabetes. In the Standard Glucose Tolerance Test, the glucose level of the blood rises to a maximum (up to 160 mg. per 100 ml.) within the first hour after the ingestion of a test dose of glucose and returns to normal after two hours. In diabetic patients, the blood glucose rises above 180 mg. per 100 ml. and does not return to normal even after the two-hour interval.

Urinary Glucose. Normally, a very small amount (0.5 to 1.5 gm. daily) of reducing substance is present in the urine, with glucose probably accounting for only a small fraction of this amount. The term glycosuria is applied to the presence of appreciable and abnormal amounts of glucose in urine. Glycosuria is associated with hyperglycemia in diabetes; however, negative urinary findings do not rule out the presence of the disease.

REFERENCES

1. Alexander, A. G., and Tipnis, A. K.: The effect of irregularity of teeth and the degree of overbite and overjet on the gingival health. Br. Dent. J., *128*:539, 1970.
2. Armitage, G. C., Svanberg, G. K., and Loe, H.: Microscopic evaluation of clinical measurements of connective tissue attachment levels. J. Clin. Periodontol., *4*:173, 1977.
3. Bender, I. B., and Seltzer, S.: Roentgenographic and direct observation of experimental lesions in bone. J. Am. Dent. Assoc., *62*:152, 1961.
4. Bender, I. B., and Seltzer, S.: Roentgenographic and direct observations of experimental lesions in bone: II. J. Am. Dent. Assoc., *62*:708, 1961.
5. Berg, M., Burrill, D. Y., and Fosdick, L. S.: Chemical studies in periodontal disease. IV. Putrefactive rate as index of periodontal disease. J. Dent. Res., *26*:67, 1947.
6. Björn, H., and Holmberg, K.: Radiographic determination of periodontal bone destruction in epidemiological research. Odont. Revy, *17*: 232, 1966.
7. Cahn, L.: The jaws in generalized skeletal disease. Ann. R. Coll. Surg. Engl., 8:115, 1951.
8. Cannar, R. K.: Proposal for the distribution of a certified standard for use in hemoglobinometry. Am. J. Clin. Pathol., *25*:376, 1955.
9. Easley, J.: Methods of determining alveolar osseous form. J. Periodontol., *38*:112, 1967.
10. Everett, F. G., and Fixott, H. C.: Use of an incorporated grid in the diagnosis of oral roentgenograms. Oral Surg., 9:1061, 1963.
11. Faber, M.: Causes of xerostomia. Acta Med. Scand., *113*:69, 1943.
12. Fairbank, H. A. T.: Osteopetrosis. J. Bone Joint Surg., *30*:339, 1948.
13. Fischman, S. L., and Picozzi, A.: Review of the literature: The methodology of clinical calculus evaluation. J. Periodontol., *40*:607, 1969.
14. Fitzgerald, G. M.: Dental radiography. IV. The voltage factor (k.p.). J. Am. Dent. Assoc., *41*: 19, 1950.
15. Furstenberg, A. C., and Crosby, E.: Disturbance of the function of the salivary glands. Ann. Otol. Rhinol. Laryngol., *54*:243, 1945.
16. Glickman, I.: Fibrous dysplasia in alveolar bone. Oral Surg., 1:895, 1948.
17. Glickman, I.: The oral cavity. *In* Robbins, S. L.: Textbook of Pathology. Philadelphia, W. B. Saunders Company, 1957, p. 711.
18. Glickman, I., and Glidden, S.: Paget's disease of the maxillae and mandible. Clinical analysis and case reports. J. Am. Dent. Assoc., *29*: 2144, 1942.
19. Goldman, L., and Goldman, B.: Contact testing of the buccal mucous membrane for stomatitis venenata. Arch. Dermatol. Syph., *50*:79, 1944.
20. Grupe, H. E., and Orban, B.: Eosinophilic granuloma diagnosis by gingival biopsy. J. Periodontol., *21*:19, 1950.
21. Haggard, H. W., and Greenberg, L. A.: Breath odors from alliaceous substances. J.A.M.A., *104*:2160, 1935.
22. Hirschfeld, L.: A calibrated silver point for periodontal diagnosis and recording. J. Periodontol., *24*:94, 1953.
23. Hirschfeld, I.: Interdental canals. J. Am. Dent. Assoc., *14*:617, 1927.
24. Jolliffe, N.: Clinical Signs of Malnutrition. Vitamin Methods. New York, Academic Press, Inc., Publishers, 1951, Vol. II.
25. Karshan, M., Kutscher, A. H., Silver, H. G., Stein, G., and Ziskin, D. E.: Studies in the etiolo-

gy of idiopathic orolingual paresthesias. Am. J. Digest Dis., *19*:341, 1952.

26. Kitchen, P. C.: The prevalence of tooth root exposure and the relation of the extent of such exposure to the degree of abrasion in differing age classes. J. Dent. Res., *20*:565, 1941.

27. Kutscher, A. H.: Experiences with a detailed color shade guide for use in the study of the oral mucous membranes in health and disease. Oral Surg., *15*:408, 1962.

28. Listgarten, M. A., Mao, R., and Robinson, P. J.: Periodontal probing: The relationship of the probe tip to periodontal tissues. J. Periodontol., *47*:511, 1976.

29. Manly, R. S.: Abrasion of cementum and dentin by modern dentifrices. J. Dent. Res., *20*:583, 1941.

30. Manly, R. S.: Factors influencing tests on the abrasion of dentin by brushing with dentifrices. J. Dent. Res., *23*:59, 1944.

31. Mannerberg, F.: Saliva factors in cases of erosion. Odont. Revy., *14*:156, 1963.

32. Manson, J. D.: The lamina dura. Oral Surg., *16*: 432, 1963.

33. Massler, M., Emslie, R., and Bolden, T.: Fetor ex ore. Oral Surg., *4*:110, 1951.

34. McCay, C. M., and Wills, L.: Erosion of molar teeth by acid beverages. J. Nutrition, *39*:313, 1949.

35. Meyer, I.: The value of the gingival biopsy in the diagnosis of generalized amyloidosis. J. Oral Surg., *8*:314, 1950.

36. Miller, W. D.: Experiments and observations on the wasting of tooth tissue variously designated as erosion, abrasion, chemical abrasion, denudation, etc. Dent. Cosmos, *49*:1, 1907.

37. Muhlemann, H. R.: Tooth mobility: A review of clinical aspects and research findings. J. Periodontol., *38*:686, 1967.

38. Nizel, A. E.: The role of diet and nutrition in the management of gingival and periodontal disease. *In* Nizel, A. E. (ed.): The Science of Nutrition and Its Application in Clinical Dentistry, Philadelphia, W. B. Saunders Company, 1966.

39. Nizel, A. E.: Nutrition in Preventive Dentistry: Science and Practice. Philadelphia, W. B. Saunders Company, 1972.

40. O'Leary, T. J.: Tooth mobility. Dent. Clin. North Am., *13*:567, 1969.

41. O'Leary, T. J., and Rudd, K. D.: An instrument for measuring horizontal tooth mobility. USAF School of Aerospace Medicine TDR 63–58, August, 1963. Periodontics, *1*:249, 1963.

42. Parfitt, G. J.: An investigation of the normal variations in alveolar bone trabeculations. Oral Surg., *15*:1453, 1962.

43. Parfitt, G. J.: The dynamics of a tooth in function. J. Periodontol., *32*:102, 1961.

44. Patur, B., and Glickman, I.: Roentgenographic evaluation of alveolar bone changes in periodontal disease. Dent. Clin. North Am., March 1960, p. 47.

45. Pauls, V., and Trott, J. R.: A radiological study of experimentally produced lesions in bone. Dent. Pract., *16*:254, 1966.

46. Prichard, J. F.: Role of the roentgenogram in the diagnosis and prognosis of periodontal disease. Oral Med., *14*:182, 1961.

47. Puckett, J.: A device for comparing roentgenograms of the same mouth. J. Periodontol., *39*:38, 1968.

48. Ramadan, A. B. E., and Mitchell, D. F.: A roentgenographic study of experimental bone destruction. Oral Surg., *15*:934, 1962.

49. Regan, J. E., and Mitchell, D. F.: Roentgenographic and dissection measurements of alveolar crest height. J. Am. Dent. Assoc., *66*: 356, 1963.

50. Ritchey, B., and Orban, B.: The crests of the interdental septa. J. Periodontol., *24*:75, 1953.

51. Robinson, H. B. G.: Abrasion, attrition and erosion of teeth. Health Center J., Ohio State Univ., *3*:21, 1949.

52. Rosenberg, E. H., and Guralnick, W. C.: Hyperparathyroidism. Oral Surg., *15*:84 (Suppl. 2), 1962.

53. Rosling, B., Hollender, L., Nyman, S., and Olsson, G.: A radiographic method for assessing changes in alveolar bone height following periodontal therapy. J. Clin. Periodontol., *2*: 211, 1975.

54. Saglie, R., Johanson, J. R., and Flötra, L.: The zone of completely and partially destroyed periodontal fibers in pathological pockets. J. Clin. Periodontol., *2*:198, 1975.

55. Salman, I. and Darlington, C. G.: Eosinophilic granuloma. Am. J. Orthod., *31*:89, 1945.

56. Sandler, H. C., Stahl, S. S., Cahn, L. R., and Freund, H. R.: Exfoliative cytology for the detection of early mouth cancer. Oral Surg., *13*:994, 1960.

57. Sanstead, H. H., Carte, J. P., and Darby, W. J.: How to diagnose nutritional disorders in daily practice. Nutrition Today, *4*:20, 1969.

58. Selikoff, I., and Robitzek, E.: Gingival biopsy for the diagnosis of generalized amyloidosis. Am. J. Pathol., *23*:1099, 1947.

59. Sherwood, L. M., and Parris, E. E.: Physiologic and pharmacologic regulation of bone resorption. N. Engl. J. Med., *282*:909, 1970.

60. Shklar, G., Cataldo, E., and Meyer, I.: Reliability of cytologic smear in diagnosis of oral cancer. A controlled study. Arch. Otolaryngol., *91*: 158, 1970.

61. Silverman, S., Jr., Gordon, G., Grant, T., Steinback, H., Eisenberg, E., and Manson, R.: Dental structures in primary hyperparathyroidism. Oral Surg., *15*:426, 1962.

62. Sivertson, J. F., and Burgett, F. G.: Probing of pockets related to the attachment level. J. Periodontol., *47*:281, 1976.

63. Sleeper, E.: Eosinophilic granuloma of bone. Oral Surg., *4*:896, 1951.

64. Sognnaes, R. F.: Periodontal significance of intraoral frictional ablation. J. Western Soc. Periodontol., *25*:112, 1977.

65. Sponge, J. D.: Halitosis: A review of its causes and treatment. Dent. Practit. Dent. Rec., *14*: 307, 1964.

66. Stallard, H.: Residual food odors of the mouth. J. Am. Dent. Assoc., *14*:1689, 1927.

67. Theilade, J.: An evaluation of the reliability of radiographs in the measurement of bone loss

in periodontal disease. J. Periodontol., *31*: 143, 1960.

68. Todd-Sanford Clinical Diagnosis by Laboratory Methods, Edited by Davidson, I., and Henry, J. B. 14th ed. Philadelphia, W. B. Saunders Company, 1969.

69. Van Der Linden, L. W. J., and Van Aken, J.: The periodontal ligament in the roentgenogram. J. Periodontol., *41*:243, 1970.

70. Wintrobe, M. M.: Clinical Hematology. 5th ed. Philadelphia, Lea & Febiger, 1961, p. 105.

Chapter 33

Determination of the Prognosis

THE PATIENT AND THE PROGNOSIS

The prognosis is the prediction of the duration, course, and termination of a disease and the likelihood of its response to treatment. It must be determined before the treatment is planned. The prognosis of gingival and periodontal disease is critically dependent upon the patient—his attitude, his desire to retain his natural teeth, and his willingness and ability to maintain good oral hygiene. Without these, treatment will not succeed.

THE PROGNOSIS IN PATIENTS WITH GINGIVAL DISEASE

The prognosis of gingival disease depends upon the role of inflammation in the overall disease process. If inflammation is the only pathologic change the prognosis is favorable, provided all local irritants are eliminated, gingival contours conducive to the preservation of health are attained, and the patient cooperates by providing good oral hygiene.

If inflammation is superimposed upon systemically caused tissue changes (such as in gingival enlargement associated with phenytoin therapy, or in patients with nutritional, hematologic, or hormonal disorders), gingival health may be restored temporarily by local therapy alone, but the long-term prognosis depends upon control or correction of the contributing systemic factors.

THE PROGNOSIS IN PATIENTS WITH PERIODONTAL DISEASE

There are two aspects to the determination of the prognosis in patients with periodontal disease: *the overall prognosis* and the *prognosis of individual teeth.*

The Overall Prognosis

The overall prognosis is concerned with the dentition as a whole. It answers the questions, "Should treatment be undertaken?" and "Is it likely to succeed?" The following factors are considered in determining the overall prognosis.

Assessment of the past bone response

The past response of the alveolar bone to local factors is a useful guide for predicting the bone response to treatment and the likelihood of arresting the bone-de-

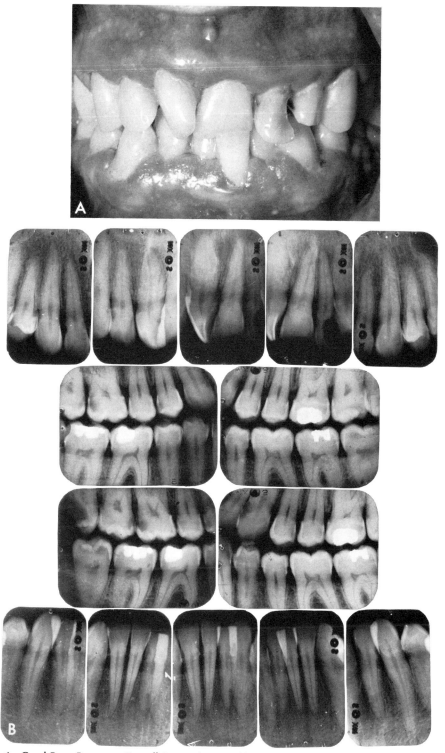

Figure 33–1   Good Bone Response, Overall Prognosis Favorable. *A,* Thirty-two-year-old male with generalized chronic marginal gingivitis and periodontal pocket formation, and excessive anterior overbite. *B,* Excellent bone picture despite unfavorable inflammatory and occlusal factors.

structive process. Assessment of the past bone response entails consideration of severity and distribution of the periodontal bone loss in terms of the following: the patient's age; the distribution, severity, and duration of local irritants such as plaque, calculus, and food impaction; and occlusal abnormalities and habits.

If the amount of bone loss can be accounted for by the local factors, local treatment can be expected to arrest the bone destruction; the overall prognosis for the dentition is good (Fig. 33–1).

If the bone loss is more severe than one would ordinarily expect at the patient's age in the presence of local factors of comparable severity and duration, factors other than those in the oral cavity are contributing to the bone destruction. The overall prognosis is then poor, because of the difficulty generally encountered in determining the responsible systemic factors (Fig.

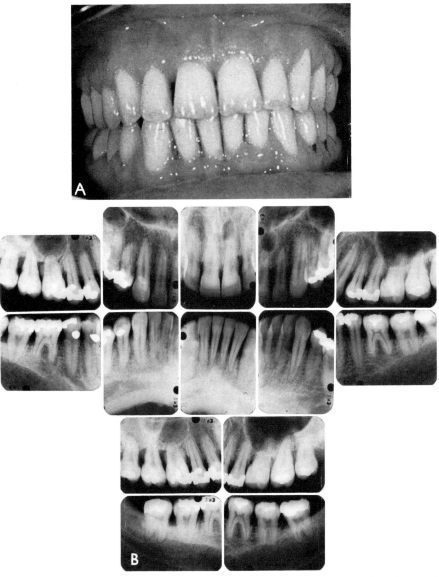

Figure 33–2 Poor Bone Response, Overall Prognosis Poor. *A,* Twenty-seven-year-old male with generalized chronic gingivitis and periodontal pocket formation. *B,* Bone destruction is in excess of that explainable by the local factors. The overall prognosis is poor.

33–2). Local treatment can be relied upon to arrest bone destruction caused by the local factors, but unless the systemic etiologic factors are detected and corrected, bone loss may continue.

The prognosis is not necessarily hopeless without systemic therapy, provided the disease is detected early and sufficient bone remains to support the teeth. In such cases, local treatment often can retain the dentition in useful function for many years by eliminating local destructive factors and limiting the bone destruction to that caused by the systemic conditions.

Application of the "bone factor" concept to periodontal prognosis

The clinical procedure whereby the "bone factor" concept (see p. 252) is applied in the determination of prognosis of periodontal disease is as follows:

1. *Determine the patient's age.*
2. *Evaluate the distribution, severity, and duration of gingival inflammation and occlusal disharmonies, each of which is capable of inducing bone loss.*
3. *Determine the distribution, severity, and rate of bone loss.*

The nature of the individual "bone factor" is determined from the above findings as follows:

A. A diagnosis of *"positive bone factor"* is made when the rate and severity of bone loss can be explained by the existing local factors (Fig. 33–3). It means that the systemic influences upon the alveolar bone are favorable so that new bone is constantly being formed in an effort to compensate for the increased resorption caused by the harmful local factors. Bone loss does occur, but it is maintained at a minimum. *In the presence of a positive bone factor, cessation of bone loss can be expected if the local factors are eliminated.*

B. The diagnosis of *"negative bone factor"* is made when the amount and rate of bone loss are in excess of that which clinical experience would lead one to expect at the patient's age in the presence of local factors of comparable severity and duration (Figs. 33–4 and 33–5). Since local factors are insufficient to account for the bone loss, factors other than those in the oral cavity must share the responsibility for it (Fig. 33–6).

A diagnosis of "negative bone factor" does not mean that the patient has a bone disease or that the periodontal destruction necessarily originated in the alveolar bone. It means that prevailing systemic effects upon one or more of the tissues of the periodontium are such that the amount of bone loss caused by the local factors is accentuated. A diagnosis of "negative bone factor" is also made when alveolar bone loss occurs in the absence of local factors.

In patients with a "negative bone factor" the effectiveness of local treatment in arresting the bone destruction is limited by the extent to which systemic conditions are also responsible for it. However, *local treatment often suffices to retain the teeth in useful function for many years, even if systemic correction is not possible.*

Evaluation of the individual "bone factor" is predicated upon the history and findings at the time of examination. The "bone factor" is an expression of systemic influences and is not necessarily constant; it may be altered by changes in the individual systemic background.

Height of remaining bone

The next question is: "Assuming bone destruction can be arrested, is there enough bone remaining to support the teeth?" The answer is readily apparent in extreme conditions when there is so little bone loss that tooth support is not in jeopardy or when bone loss is severe and generalized and the remaining bone is obviously insufficient for proper tooth support. Most patients, however, do not fit into the extreme categories. The height of remaining bone lies somewhere in between, making the bone level alone inconclusive for determining the overall prognosis.

Patient's age

All other factors being equal, the prognosis is better in the older of two patients with comparable levels of remaining al-

Text continued on page 598

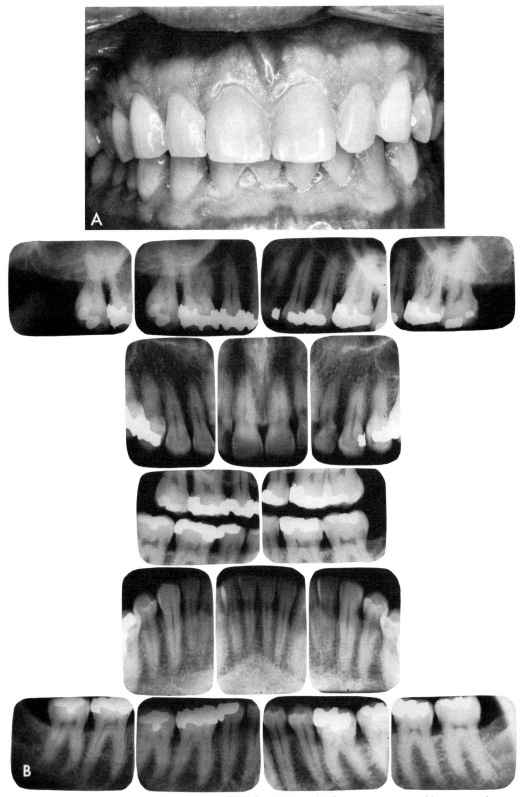

Figure 33–3   Positive Bone Factor in a 42-year-old Male. *A,* Gingival inflammation, poor oral hygiene, and pronounced anterior overbite. *B,* The bone loss is slight considering the age of the patient and the unfavorable local factors. This is a patient with a positive "bone factor."

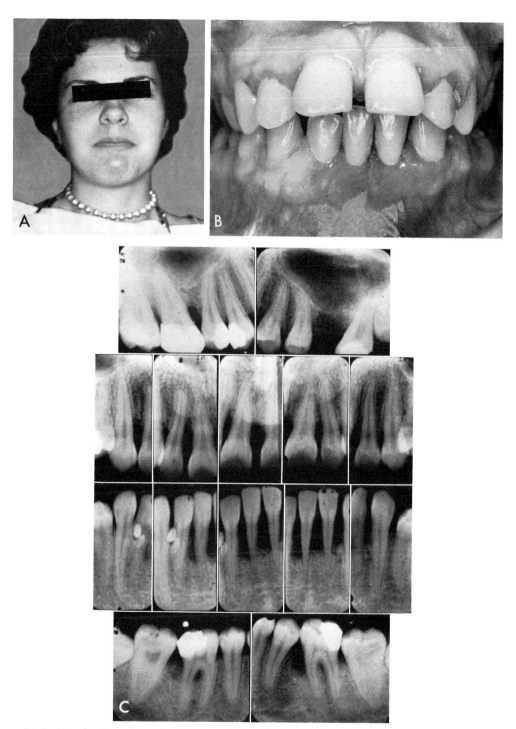

Figure 33–4 Negative Bone Factor in a 17-Year-Old Female Twin. *A,* Clinical appearance of patient. Compare with twin sister (Fig. 33–5*A*). *B,* Gingival inflammation, periodontal pockets, and pathologic migration. *C,* Severe bone destruction exceeds that which ordinarily occurs in 17-year-old patient with comparable local factors. This patient has a "negative bone factor." The distribution of bone loss in the anterior and first molar areas is considered typical of juvenile periodontitis. Note the bifurcation and trifurcation involvement of three remaining first molars.

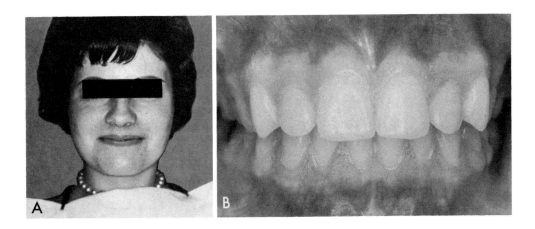

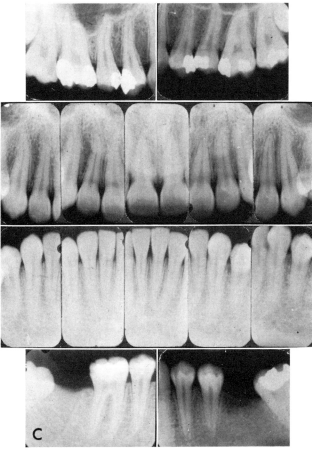

Figure 33–5 Positive Bone Factor. Twin sister of patient shown in 33–4A. A, Clinical appearance. B, Excellent condition of gingiva. C, No bone loss despite missing mandibular first molar (right), tilted second molar, and extruded maxillary first molar. Compare with the first molars in Figure 33–4C.

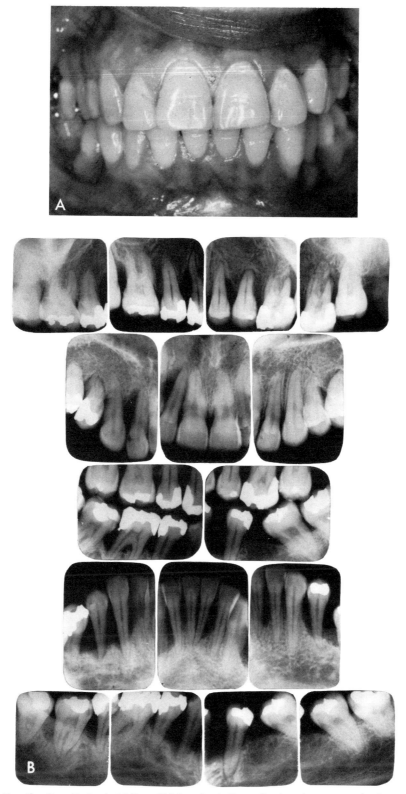

Figure 33–6   Negative Bone Factor in 34-Year-Old Female. *A,* Generalized moderate gingival inflammation with periodontal pocket formation. *B,* Bone loss more severe than ordinarily occurs in patient of this age with comparable local factors.
The bone factor is therefore negative.

veolar bone. The younger patient has suffered a more rapid bone destruction than the older patient owing to the shorter period in which the bone loss has occured. The younger person would ordinarily be expected to have a greater bone-reparative capacity and better post-treatment prognosis. However, the fact that so much bone destruction has occurred in a relatively short period of time reflects unfavorably on the young patient's bone-reparative capacity.

Number of remaining teeth

If the number and distribution of the teeth are inadequate for the support of a satisfactory prosthesis, the overall prognosis is bad. The likelihood of maintaining periodontal health is diminished because of the ability to establish a satisfactory functional environment. An extensive fixed or removable prosthesis constructed on an insufficient number of natural teeth creates periodontal injury which is more likely to hasten the tooth loss than to provide a worthwhile health service.

Patient's systemic background

The patient's systemic background affects the overall prognosis in several ways.[4] In patients with extensive periodontal destruction that cannot be accounted for by local factors alone, it is reasonable to assume contributing systemic etiology. However, the detection of responsible systemic factors is usually difficult, so that the prognosis in such patients is usually poor. However, in patients with known systemic disorders that could affect the periodontium, such as diabetes, nutritional deficiency, hyperthyroidism, and hyperparathyroidism, the prognosis of the periodontal condition benefits from their correction.

The prognosis must be guarded when surgical periodontal treatment is required but cannot be provided because of the patient's health. Incapacitating conditions (such as Parkinson's disease) which prevent the patient from performing oral hygiene procedures also adversely affect the prognosis.

Gingival inflammation

Other factors being equal, the prognosis of periodontal disease is directly related to the severity of inflammation. In two patients with comparable bone destruction, the prognosis is better in the patient with the greater degree of inflammation. A larger component of the bone destruction is attributable to local irritation, and local treatment can be expected to be more effective in arresting the bone destruction.

Periodontal pockets

The location of the base of periodontal pockets is more important than pocket depth in deciding the overall prognosis. Because pocket depth and severity of bone loss are not necessarily related, a patient with deep pockets and little bone loss has a better prognosis than a patient with shallow pockets and severe bone destruction.

Malocclusion

Irregularly aligned teeth, malformation of the jaws, and abnormal occlusal relationships may be important factors in the etiology of periodontal disease inasmuch as they may interfere with plaque control or produce occlusal interferences. In these cases, correction by orthodontic or prosthetic means is essential if periodontal treatment is to succeed. **The overall prognosis is poor in patients with occlusal deformities which cannot be corrected.**

Tooth morphology

The prognosis is poor in patients with short tapered roots and relatively large crowns (Fig. 33–7). Because of the disproportionate crown-root ratio and the reduced root surface available for periodontal support,[1] the periodontium is more susceptible to injury by occlusal forces.

The prognosis of juvenile periodontitis

In patients with periodontal disease diagnosed as juvenile periodontitis, systemic influences are considered to play a significant role in the periodontal destruc-

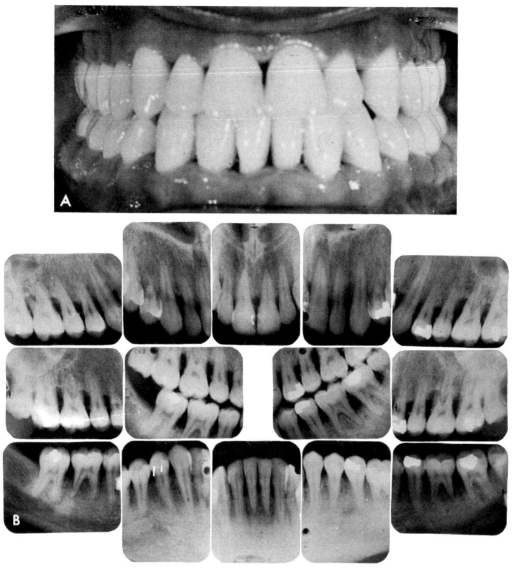

Figure 33–7 Poor Crown-Root Ratio, Overall Prognosis Unfavorable. A, Twenty-four-year-old patient with generalized gingivitis and periodontal pocket formation. B, Severity of bone destruction at this age indicates poor bone response. The contrast between the well-formed crowns and relatively short tapered roots worsens the unfavorable prognosis.

tion. Ideally, treatment should include correction of the responsible systemic conditions, along with local measures, but the former are difficult to determine. However, **except in advanced cases of juvenile periodontitis in which the remaining bone is insufficient to support the teeth, the dentition can be retained in useful function by local treatment alone.**

The Prognosis of Individual Teeth

The prognosis of individual teeth is determined after the overall prognosis and is affected by it. For example, in a patient with a poor overall prognosis one would be disinclined to attempt to retain a tooth which is considered questionable because of local conditions. The following factors are considered in determining the prognosis of individual teeth:

Mobility

The principal causes of tooth mobility are loss of alveolar bone, inflammatory changes in the periodontal ligament, and trauma from occlusion. (Tooth mobility is discussed in detail in Chapter 20.) Tooth mobility caused by inflammation and trauma from occlusion is correctable.[3] Tooth mobility resulting from loss of alveolar bone alone is not likely to be corrected. **The likelihood of restoring tooth stability is inversely proportional to the extent to which it is caused by loss of alveolar bone.**

Periodontal pockets

In suprabony pockets the location of the base of the pocket affects prognosis of individual teeth more than the pocket depth. **Proximity to frenum attachments and to the mucogingival line jeopardizes the prognosis unless corrective procedures are included in the treatment (Chap. 53).**

PROXIMITY OF THE BASE OF THE POCKET TO THE APEX. The prognosis is adversely affected if the base of the pocket is close to the root apex even if there is no evidence of apical disease. **The incidence of degenerative pulp changes is increased in teeth affected by periodontal disease, usually without clinical symptoms or pulp necrosis.** The pulp changes are attributed to irritation from bacterial products

through the dentinal tubules of the exposed root surface wall of periodontal pockets and through lateral pulp canals. If the base of the pocket is close to the apex, injurious bacterial products may reach the pulp through the apical foramina. Root canal therapy is necessary in such cases to obtain optimal results from periodontal treatment.

When the periodontal pocket has extended to involve the apex the prognosis is generally poor. However, striking apical and lateral bone repair is sometimes obtained by combining endodontic and periodontal therapy (Chap. 52).

Teeth adjacent to edentulous areas

Teeth that serve as abutments are subjected to increased functional demands. More rigid standards are required in evaluating the prognosis of teeth adjacent to edentulous areas.

Location of remaining bone in relation to the individual tooth surfaces

When greater bone loss has occurred on one surface of a tooth, the bone height on the less involved surfaces should be taken into consideration in determining the prognosis. Because of greater height of bone in relation to the latter surfaces, the center of rotation of the tooth will be nearer the crown (Fig. 33–8). The leverage upon the periodontium will therefore be

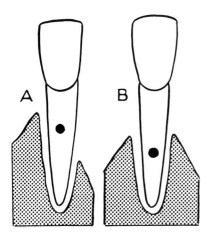

Figure 33–8   The Prognosis for Tooth *A* **Is Better Than That for Tooth** *B,* despite the fact that there is less bone on one of the surfaces. Because the center of rotation of tooth *A* is closer to the crown, the distribution of occlusal forces to the periodontium is more favorable than in *B.*

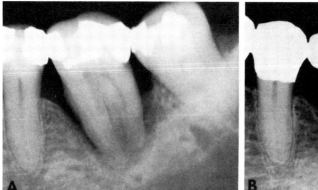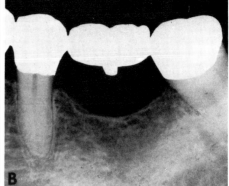

Figure 33–9 Extraction of Severely Involved Tooth to Preserve Bone on Adjacent Teeth. *A,* Extensive bone destruction around mandibular first molar. *B,* Eight and one-half years after extraction of first molar and replacement by prosthesis. Note the excellent bony support.

more favorable than the bone loss on the most severely involved tooth surface suggests.

Relation to adjacent teeth

In dealing with a tooth with questionable prognosis, the chances of successful treatment should be weighed against the benefits that would accrue to the adjacent teeth if the tooth under consideration were extracted. **Heroic attempts to retain a hopelessly involved tooth jeopardizes the adjacent teeth.** Extraction of the questionable tooth is followed by partial restoration of the bone support of the adjacent teeth (Fig. 33–9).

Infrabony pockets

The likelihood of eliminating infrabony pockets depends upon several factors, critical among which are the contour of the osseous defects and the number of the remaining bony walls (see Chapter 51).

Furcation involvement

The presence of bifurcation or trifurcation involvement does not indicate a hopeless prognosis (Chap. 52). However, when a lesion reaches the furcation it adds two important problems: the first is the difficulty of surgical access to the area if bone surgery is to be performed; second is the inaccessibility of the area to plaque removal by the patient. If both these problems can be satisfactorily solved, then prognosis will be similar to or even better than that of single-rooted teeth with a similar degree of bone loss.

Upper first premolars offer the greatest difficulties, and therefore their prognosis is usually unfavorable when the lesion reaches the furcation. Upper molars also offer some degree of difficulty; sometimes their prognosis can be improved by resecting one of the buccal roots (either the mesiobuccal or the distobuccal), thereby improving access to the area. Lower first molars offer good access to the furcation area and therefore their prognosis is usually better.

Caries, nonvital teeth, and tooth resorption

In teeth mutilated by extensive caries the feasibility of adequate restoration and endodontic therapy should be considered before undertaking periodontal treatment. Extensive idiopathic root resorption jeopardizes the stability of teeth and adversely affects the response to periodontal treatment. **The periodontal prognosis of treated nonvital teeth is not different from that of vital teeth.** Reattachment can occur to the cementum of nonvital or vital teeth. However, reattachment to expose root dentin is not likely in nonvital teeth.[2]

REFERENCES

1. Kay, S., Forscher, B. K., and Sackett, L. M.: Tooth root length-volume relationships. An aid to periodontal prognosis. I. Anterior teeth. Oral Surg., 7:735, 1954.
2. Morris, M. L.: Healing of human periodontal tissues following surgical detachment and extirpation of vital pulps. J. Periodontol., 31:23, 1960.
3. Morris, M. L.: The diagnosis, prognosis and treatment of the loose tooth. Oral Surg., 6:1037, 1953.
4. Schulte, W.: Limitations of periodontal therapy due to systemic factors. Dtsch. Zahnärztl. Z., 24:41, 1966.
5. Slatten, R. W.: An evaluation of factors determining prognosis in inflammatory and retrogressive periodontal disease. J. Periodontol., 25:30, 1954.

The Treatment Plan

THE TREATMENT PLAN

After the diagnosis and prognosis have been established, the treatment is planned. *The treatment plan is the blueprint for case management.* It includes all procedures required for the establishment and maintenance of oral health, such as decisions as to teeth to be retained or extracted, decisions on techniques to be used for pocket elimination, the need for mucogingival or reconstructive surgical procedures and occlusal correction, the type of restorations to be employed, which teeth are to be used for abutments, and the indications for splinting.

Unforeseen developments during treatment may necessitate modification of the initial treatment plan. However, it is axiomatic that, except for emergencies, no treatment should be started until the treatment plan has been established.

Periodontal treatment requires long-range planning. Its value to the patient is measured in years of healthful functioning of the entire dentition, not by the number of teeth retained at the time of treatment. It is directed to establishing and maintaining the health of the periodontium throughout the mouth rather than to spectacular efforts to "tighten loose teeth."

The welfare of the dentition should not be jeopardized by a heroic attempt to retain questionable teeth. The periodontal condition of teeth we decide to retain is more important than their number. Teeth that can be retained with a minimum of doubt and a maximum margin of safety provide the basis for the total treatment plan. Teeth on the borderline of hopelessness do not contribute to the overall usefulness of the dentition, even if they can be saved in a somewhat precarious state. Such teeth become sources of recurrent annoyance to the patient and detract from the value of the greater service rendered by the establishment of periodontal health in the remainder of the oral cavity.

THE MASTER PLAN FOR TOTAL TREATMENT

The aim of the treatment plan is *total treatment* — that is, the *coordination of all treatment procedures for the purpose of creating a well-functioning dentition in a healthy periodontal environment.* The "master plan" of periodontal treatment encompasses four different therapeutic objectives for each patient according to his needs.

1. The soft tissue area

This entails elimination of gingival inflammation, periodontal pockets, and the factors which cause them; the establishment of gingival contour and mucogingival relationships conducive to the preservation of periodontal health; restoration of carious areas; correction of the margins of existing restorations; and recontouring proximal, facial, and lingual surfaces and occlusal marginal ridges of existing res-

603

torations to provide proper proximal contact and food excursion pathways.

2. The functional area

An optimal occlusal relationship is one that provides the functional stimulation necessary to preserve periodontal health. To obtain it may require occlusal adjustment; restorative, prosthetic, and orthodontic procedures; splinting; and the correction of bruxism, clamping, and clenching habits.

3. The systemic area

Systemic conditions may necessitate special precautions in the course of periodontal treatment, affect the tissue response to treatment procedures or threaten the preservation of periodontal health after treatment is completed. Such situations should be taken care of in conjunction with the patient's physician. (For a discussion of systemic conditions which require special precautions, see Chapter 48).

4. Case maintenance

This entails all procedures for maintaining periodontal health after it has been attained. It consists of instruction in oral hygiene; recall of the patient at regular intervals according to his needs, to check on the condition of the periodontium, the status of the restorative dentistry, and the need for further occlusal adjustment; and follow-up radiographs.

SEQUENCE OF THERAPEUTIC PROCEDURE

Periodontal therapy is an inseparable part of dental therapy. The sequence of procedures presented here includes periodontal procedures (marked with an asterisk) and other procedures not considered to be within the province of the periodontist.

Preliminary Phase

Treatment of emergencies
    dental or periapical

   *periodontal
   Other
Extraction of hopeless teeth and provisional replacement if needed (may be postponed to a more convenient time).

Phase I Therapy (Etiotropic Phase)

*Plaque control
 Diet control (in rampant caries patients)
*Removal of calculus and root planing
*Correction of restorative and prosthetic irritational factors.
 Excavation of caries and restoration (temporary or final depending on whether a definitive prognosis for the tooth has been arrived at and location of caries)
*Occlusal therapy
*Minor orthodontic movement
*Provisional splinting

Evaluation of response to phase I, rechecking:

*Pocket depth and gingival inflammation
*Plaque and calculus
 Caries

Phase II Therapy (Surgical Phase)

*Periodontal surgery
 Root canal therapy

Phase III Therapy (Restorative Phase)

Final restorations
Fixed and removable prosthodontics

*Evaluation of periodontal response to restorative procedures

Phase IV Therapy (Maintenance Phase)

Periodic recalls, checking
  *Plaque and calculus
  *Gingival condition (pockets, inflammation)
  Caries
  *Occlusion, tooth mobility
  Other pathology

EXPLAINING THE TREATMENT PLAN TO THE PATIENT

The following are suggestions for explaining the treatment plan to the patient:

Be specific. Tell your patient: "You have gingivitis," or "You have periodontitis." Then, explain exactly what these conditions are, how they are treated, and the future for the patient's mouth after treatment. **Avoid vague statements** such as: "You have trouble with your gums," or "Something should be done about your gums." Patients do not understand the significance of such statements and disregard them.

Start your discussion on a positive note. Talk about the teeth which can be retained and the long-term service they can be expected to render. Do not start your discussion with the statement: "The following teeth have to be extracted." This creates a negative impression which adds to the erroneous attitude of hopelessness the patient already may have regarding his mouth.

Make it clear that every effort will be made to retain as many teeth as possible, **but do not dwell on the patient's loose teeth.** Emphasize the fact that the important purpose of the treatment is to prevent the other teeth from becoming as severely diseased as the loose teeth.

Present the entire treatment plan as a unit. Avoid creating the impression that treatment consists of separate procedures, some or all of which may be selected by the patient. **Make it clear that dental restorations and prostheses contribute as much to the health of the gums as does the elimination of inflammation and periodontal pockets.** Do not speak in terms of "having the gums treated" and "then taking care of the necessary restorations later" as if these were unrelated treatments.

Patients frequently seek guidance from the dentist with such questions as: "Are my teeth worth treating?" "Would you have them treated if you were I?" "Why don't I just go along the way I am until the teeth really bother me, and them have them all extracted?"

If the condition is treatable, make it clear that the best results are obtained by prompt treatment. If the condition is not treatable, the teeth should be extracted. Explain that "doing nothing" or holding onto hopelessly diseased teeth as long as possible is inadvisable for the following reasons:

In periodontal disease, proper mastication of food is impaired because of looseness of the teeth and discomfort incurred by chewing. This leads to the "bolting" of food, which complicates the digestive process and may lead to gastrointestinal disturbances.

Exudate from periodontal pockets spoils the taste of food. In addition, the incorporation of purulent material into the food may irritate the mucosa of the stomach and lead to gastritis. Infection in the periodontal area is also a potential source of bacteremia.

Inability to chew properly leads to habits of food selection with preference for soft foods, which are for the most part carbohydrates.

It is not feasible to place restorations or "bridges" on teeth with untreated periodontal disease, because the usefulness of the restoration is limited by the uncertain condition of the supporting structures.

Failure to eliminate periodontal disease not only results in loss of teeth already hopelessly involved, but also shortens the life span of other teeth which, with proper treatment, could serve as the foundation for a healthy, functioning dentition.

It is the dentist's responsibility to advise the patient of the importance of periodontal treatment. However, if treatment is to be successful, the patient must be sufficiently interested in retaining the natural teeth to provide the necessary oral hygiene. Individuals who are not particularly perturbed by the thought of losing their teeth are generally not good patients for periodontal treatment.

Rationale for Periodontal Treatment

There are no forms of gingivitis or periodontal disease in which the removal of local irritants and prevention of their recurrence do not reduce the severity of the disease, lessen the rapidity of the destructive process, and prolong the usefulness of the natural dentition.

The effectiveness of periodontal therapy is made possible by the remarkable healing capacity of the periodontal tissues (Fig. 35–1). Properly performed, periodontal treatment can be relied upon to accomplish the following: eliminate pain, eliminate gingival inflammation[47] and stop gingival bleeding, eliminate periodontal pockets and infection, stop pus formation, arrest the destruction of soft tissue and bone,[48] reduce abnormal tooth mobility,[16] establish optimal occlusal function, in some instances restore tissue destroyed by disease, re-establish physiologic gingival contour necessary for the preservation of periodontal health, prevent the recurrence of disease, and reduce tooth loss[42] (Fig. 35–2).

LOCAL AND SYSTEMIC TREATMENT

Periodontal treatment consists principally of local procedures, because with infrequent exceptions gingival and periodontal diseases are caused by local factors, and local treatment suffices to achieve the desired results. When a systemic cause is suspected, it is generally difficult to determine its nature. Consequently, when systemic therapy is employed, it is usually as an adjunct to local measures and for specific purposes, such as the control of systemic complications from acute infections, chemotherapy to prevent harmful effects of post-treatment bacteremia, supportive nutritional therapy, and the control of systemic diseases which aggravate the patient's periodontal condition or necessitate special precautions during treatment (Chap. 48).

TWO LOCAL DESTRUCTIVE PROCESSES

The local etiologic factors in periodontal disease are numerous and varied, but in the final analysis they are divisible into **two categories: (1) bacterial plaque, which causes gingival inflammation and pocket formation,** and (2) **abnormal occlusal forces which cause trauma from occlusion.**

To be effective, local treatment must eradicate inflammation by totally eliminating plaque and all the conditions that favor plaque accumulation. The thorough elimination of plaque and the prevention of its new formation will, by itself, maintain periodontal health even if traumatic forces are allowed to persist.[31a, 31b] The elimination of trauma from occlusion will serve the purpose of creating occlusal relations

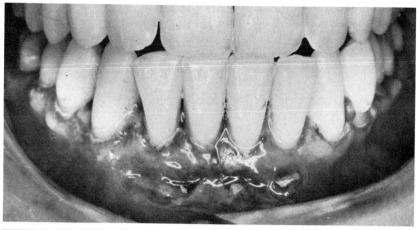

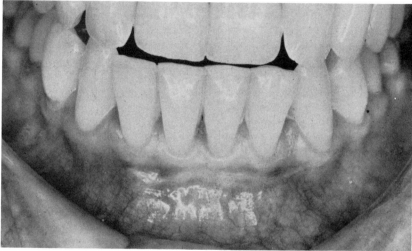

Figure 35–1 Excellent Healing Capacity of the Periodontium. *Above,* One week following periodontal surgery, after removal of periodontal dressing. *Below,* After seven months, showing healed tissues and restoration of physiologic gingival contour.

that are more tolerable to the periodontal tissues and therefore increase the margin of safety of the periodontium to minor build-ups of plaque; it will also reduce tooth mobility. It should be remembered that total plaque elimination as obtained in experimental studies may not be possible in all our human subjects.

FACTORS WHICH AFFECT HEALING *

In the periodontium, as elsewhere in the body, healing is affected by local and systemic factors.

---

*For an excellent discussion of the subject of healing, the reader is referred to the presentation by Robbins.[49]

Local factors

Systemic conditions which impair healing may reduce the effectiveness of local periodontal treatment and should be corrected prior to or along with local procedures. **However, it is the local factors such as contamination by microorganisms, irritation from plaque, food debris, and necrotic tissue remnants, and trauma from occlusion which are the most common deterrents to healing following periodontal treatment.** Healing is also delayed by excessive tissue manipulation during treatment, trauma to the tissues, and repetitive treatment procedures which disrupt the orderly cellular activity in the healing process. Topically applied cortisone and ionizing radiation retard healing.[25]

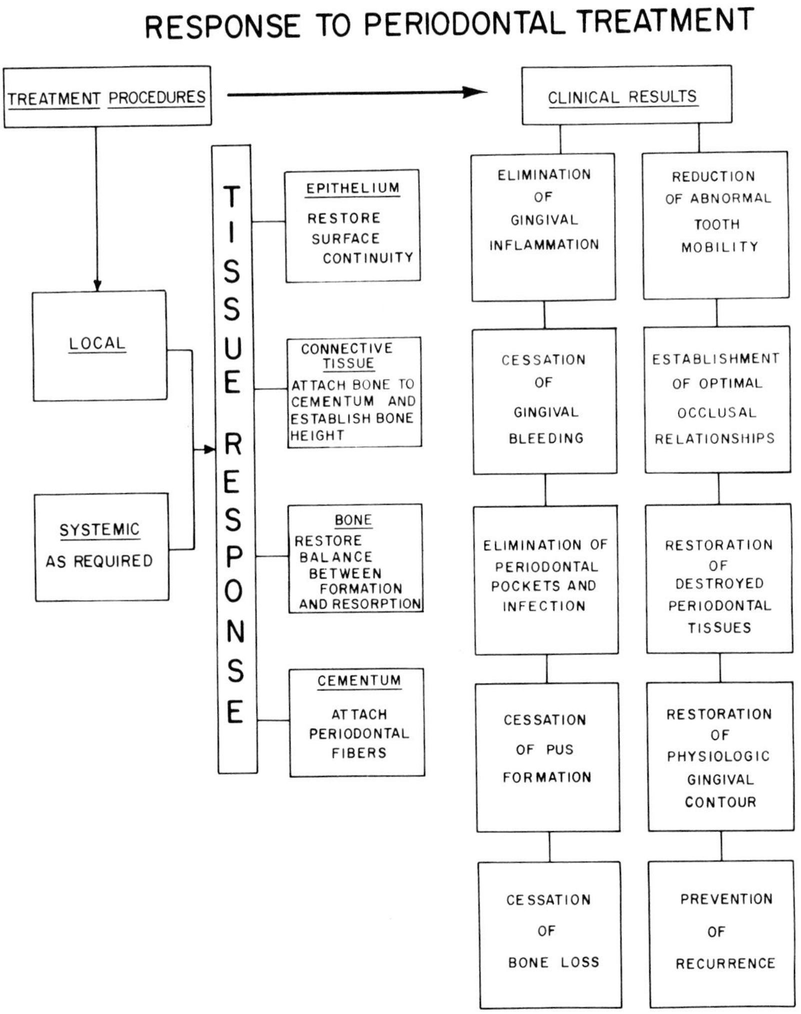

RESPONSE TO PERIODONTAL TREATMENT

Figure 35–2 Tissue Response and Clinical Results Following Periodontal Treatment.

Healing is improved by local increase in temperature, debridement, the removal of degenerated and necrotic tissue, immobilization of the healing area, and pressure on the wound. The cellular activity in healing entails an increase in oxygen consumption, but healing of the gingiva is not accelerated by artificially increasing the oxygen supply beyond the normal requirements.[19]

Systemic factors

The effects of systemic conditions upon healing have been extensively documented in animal experiments, but are less clearly defined in humans. Healing capacity diminishes with age.[9] Atherosclerotic vascular changes which are common in aging and the resultant reduction in blood circulation may be responsible. Healing is delayed in diabetes and in patients with generalized infections and in other debilitating diseases.

The nutrient requirements of the healing tissues in minor wounds such as those created by periodontal surgical procedures are ordinarily satisfied by a well-balanced diet. Healing is retarded by insufficient food intake and by bodily conditions which interfere with the utilization of nutrients. Vitamin C deficiency[1, 10, 15, 63] delays healing by depressing collagen formation and altering the integrity of capillary walls so that they are prone to rupture. Protein deficiency[59] also retards healing by reducing the supply of sulfur-containing amino acids such as cystine and methionine. Healing is also retarded by vitamin A deficiency, by a fat-rich diet, and by overdose of vitamin D. The latter causes necrosis and calcification in the arterioles of the granulation tissue.

Healing is affected by hormones. Systemically administered glucocorticoids such as cortisone hinder repair by depressing the inflammatory reaction or by inhibiting the growth of fibroblasts and the production of collagen and formation of endothelial cells.[49] Systemic stress,[57] thyroidectomy, testosterone, ACTH, and large doses of estrogen suppress the formation of granulation tissue and retard healing.[43] Progesterone increases and accelerates the vascularization of immature granulation tissue[31] and appears to increase susceptibility of gingiva to mechanical injury by producing dilation of marginal vessels.[24] Somatotropic hormone increases fibroplasia during gingival healing.[56]

Systemically administered antibiotics do not improve the epithelization of gingival wounds in experimental animals,[60] nor do systemic antibiotics following gingivectomy in humans ("antibiotic umbrella") appear to prevent the occurrence of marked gingival inflammation.[61] *

HEALING FOLLOWING PERIODONTAL TREATMENT

The basic healing processes are the same following all forms of periodontal therapy. They consist of the removal of degenerated tissue debris and the replacement of tissues destroyed by disease. **Regeneration and reattachment are aspects of periodontal healing which have a special bearing upon the results obtainable by treatment.**

Regeneration

Regeneration is the growth and differentiation of new cells and intercellular substances to form new tissues or parts. It

consists of fibroplasia, endothelial proliferation, the deposition of interstitial ground substance and collagen, epithelial hyperplasia, and the maturation of connective tissue.

Regeneration takes place by growth from the same type of tissue as that which has been destroyed, or from its precursor. In the periodontium, gingival epithelium is replaced by epithelium, and the underlying connective tissue and periodontal ligament are derived from connective tissue. **Bone and cementum are not replaced by existing bone or cementum, but from connective tissue, which is the precursor of both. Undifferentiated connective tissue cells develop into osteoblasts and cementoblasts which form bone and cementum.**

Regeneration of the periodontium is a continuous physiologic process. Under normal conditions new cells and tissues are constantly being formed to replace those which mature and die. This is termed "wear and tear repair."[28] It is manifested by mitotic activity in the epithelium of the gingiva[35] and the connective tissue of the periodontal ligament,[41] by the formation of new bone, and by the continuous deposition of cementum.

Regeneration is also going on during active gingival and periodontal disease. Most gingival and periodontal diseases are chronic inflammatory processes and as such are healing lesions. Regeneration is part of the healing. However, bacteria and bacterial products which perpetuate the disease process, and the inflammatory exudate they elicit are injurious to the regenerating cells and tissues and prevent the healing from proceeding to completion. In supporting periodontal tissues injured by abnormal occlusal forces (trauma from occlusion), the constantly present regenerative process attempts to repair the tissue damage.

By removing bacterial plaque and creating the conditions to prevent its new formation, periodontal treatment removes the obstacles to regeneration, and enables the patient to benefit from the inherent regenerative capacity of the tissues. There is a brief spurt in regenerative activity immediately following periodontal treatment, but there are no local treatment procedures which "promote" or "accelerate" regeneration.

---

* For additional information regarding gingival healing, the reader is referred to a comprehensive review by Stahl.[58]

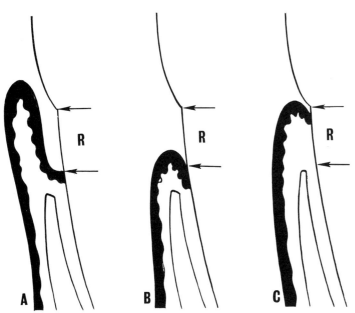

Figure 35–3 Regeneration Following Pocket Elimination — Two Possibilities. *A,* Periodontal pocket before treatment. The root surface *(R)* denuded by periodontal disease is marked by the arrows. *B,* One possibility. Normal sulcus re-established at the level of the base of the pre-existent pocket, the root *(R)* remains denuded. *C,* Another possibility is "reattachment." The periodontium is restored onto the root surface denuded by disease. New fibers and new cementum are formed on formerly denuded root *(R)* with a higher bone level and a healthy gingival sulcus attached closer to the crown.

Regeneration is a microscopic activity which differs in degree from clinically and/or radiographically detectable restoration of destroyed periodontal tissues. In most instances regeneration simply restores the continuity of the diseased marginal gingiva and re-establishes a normal gingival sulcus at the same level on the root as the base of the pre-existent periodontal pocket (Fig. 35–3). It arrests bone destruction without necessarily increasing bone height. Restoration of the destroyed periodontium to a degree which is clinically and/or radiographically detectable (see Fig. 35–6) occurs less frequently, and is dependent upon the occurrence of reattachment.

Reattachment

To obtain clinically significant restoration of destroyed periodontium, reattachment must occur. *Reattachment is the re-embedding of new periodontal ligament fibers into new cementum and the attachment of gingival epithelium to tooth surface previously denuded by disease* (Fig. 35–3). The critical words in this definition are *"tooth surface previously denuded by disease"* (Fig. 35–4). Attachment of gingiva or periodontal ligament to areas of the tooth from which they may be removed in

the course of treatment or during the preparation of teeth for restorations represents *simple healing* of the periodontium, not reattachment. The term *reattachment* has unique usage in the periodontal field and refers specifically to the restoration of the marginal periodontium and not to repair of

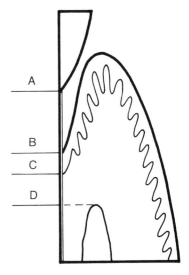

Figure 35–4 *A,* Enamel surface. *B,* Area of cementum denuded by pocket formation. *C,* Area of cementum covered by junctional epithelium. *D,* Area of cementum apical to the junctional epithelium. The term *reattachment* or *new attachment* refers to a new junctional epithelium formed on zone B.

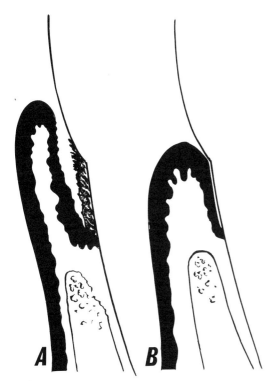

Figure 35–5 "Epithelial Adaptation" Following Periodontal Treatment. *A,* Periodontal pocket. *B,* After treatment; the pocket is closely adapted to, but not attached to, the root.

other areas of the root, such as that following traumatic tears in the cementum, tooth fractures, or the treatment of periapical lesions. Since it is not the existing fibers that reattach but new fibers that are formed and attach to new cementum, there is a tendency to replace the term *reattachment*

with *new attachment.* The two terms are used interchangeably in this text.

Epithelial adaptation is different from reattachment. The former is close apposition of gingival epithelium to the tooth surface without complete obliteration of the pocket.[8, 29] The pocket space does not permit passage of a probe. Although this may be a dangerous situation because bacteria could still penetrate, inducing further loss of attachment and even abscess formation (Fig. 35–5), several recent clinical studies have shown that with an adequate maintenance phase, these deep sulci lined by long thin epithelium may be maintainable. The absence of bleeding or secretion upon probing, the absence of clinically visible inflammation, and the absence of stainable plaque on the root surface when the pocket wall is deflected from the tooth may indicate that the "deep sulcus" persists in an inactive state, causing no further loss of attachment.[11, 46a, 67, 68] A post-therapy depth of 4 or even 5 mm. may therefore appear acceptable in these cases.

Opinions differ regarding the extent and conditions under which reattachment is attainable by periodontal treatment[30] (Fig. 35–6). It occurs more often following the treatment of infrabony pockets[12, 20, 21, 44, 66] than suprabony pockets,[30, 53, 65] except in patients with one-wall infrabony defects (for the treatment of infrabony pockets, see Chapter 51). It has been demonstrated histologically following the treatment of infrabony pockets,[5, 14, 52] but with suprabony pockets both positive[7, 17, 34, 50] and negative

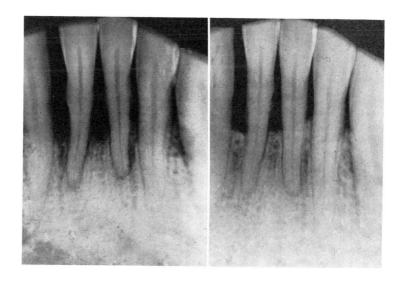

Figure 35–6 Bone Restored Following Periodontal Treatment. *Left,* Before treatment. *Right,* Five years later.

microscopic findings[27, 37] have been reported. Reattachment has been observed
histologically in experimental animals
following healing of artificially created
pockets,[26, 32, 33, 38, 45] and marginal wounds[2,
3, 4, 18, 26, 51] and following the surgical removal of the inflamed gingiva.

FACTORS THAT AFFECT REATTACHMENT

The following factors affect the likelihood of attaining reattachment:

Removal of the junctional epithelium

Removal of the junctional epithelium in
the treatment of deep suprabony and infrabony pockets increases the likelihood of
obtaining reattachment. The post-treatment location of the junctional epithelium
limits the height to which periodontal
fibers become attached to the tooth. The
level of attachment of the periodontal ligament in turn determines the maximum
post-treatment height the bone can attain.
Leaving the junctional epithelium intact

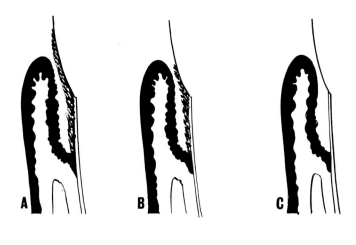

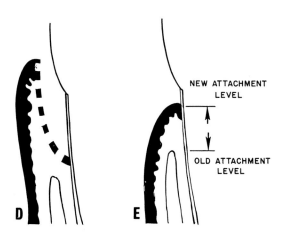

**Figure 35–7 Removal of Epithelial
Attachment Creates Potential for Post-
Treatment Reattachment.** *A,* Periodontal pocket, supragingival calculus removed. *B,* Subgingival calculus removed. *C,* Root smoothed and planed
with hoe scalers. *D,* Pocket wall and
junctional epithelium removed. *E,* Removal of junctional epithelium permits
reattachment of connective tissue fibers
to new cementum on root surface denuded by disease. The gingival sulcus is
attached closer to the crown, and the
bone height is increased.

NEW ATTACHMENT
LEVEL

OLD ATTACHMENT
LEVEL

during periodontal treatment therefore automatically predetermines the post-treatment levels of the periodontal ligament and bone (Fig. 35–7). Removal of the junctional epithelium creates conditions in which connective tissue fibers could reattach to tooth surface coronal to the pretreatment level (Fig. 35–7) and creates the potential for increased bone height, and repair of vertical defects.

In the treatment of periodontal pockets, it cannot be determined by clinical examination whether or not the junctional epithelium has been completely removed. However, histologic studies indicate that it can be completely removed in every case treated by gingivectomy,[46, 64] but opinions differ regarding whether removal can be accomplished consistently by scaling and curettage. Some investigators report complete removal of the junctional epithelium,[40] the sulcal epithelium,[6, 39] and some underlying inflamed connective tissue following gingival curettage, whereas others observe in situ remnants of the junctional epithelium and sulcal epithelium.[50, 62, 65]

Thorough planing of the root surface

Changes in the tooth surface wall of periodontal pockets, such as degeneration of the remnants of Sharpey's fibers, accumulation of bacteria and their products, and disintegration of the cementum and dentin, interfere with reattachment. However, these obstacles can be eliminated by thorough root planing. Periodontally involved root surfaces produce cytotoxic effects on cells in tissue culture; nondiseased root surfaces do not.[23]

The granulation tissue

Granulation tissue adjacent to the pocket wall is removed to provide better visibility and accessibility to the root surface. Its removal does not represent a sacrifice of tissue because it is replaced in the healing process.

The clot

The clot forms the initial protective covering of the treated area. It is replaced by granulation tissue, which may extend up to the clot surface. The vascularity and bulk of the granulation tissue are reduced as it undergoes maturation to connective tissue. The height of the granulation tissue may affect the level at which the epithelium becomes attached to the root, because the proliferating epithelium is guided by the connective tissue surface along which it moves.

Other factors

Trauma from occlusion impairs post-treatment healing of the supporting periodontal tissues and reduces the likelihood of attaining reattachment. Widened periodontal spaces, angular bone defects, and tooth mobility often result when trauma persists during healing.

Reattachment is more likely to occur when the destructive process has been rapid, such as following the treatment of pockets complicated by the formation of acute periodontal abscesses, and acute necrotizing ulcerative gingivitis.

The formation of new cementum and embedding of periodontal ligament fibers can occur on the cementum and dentin of vital teeth; in nonvital teeth it can occur on cementum but is not likely on exposed dentin.[37]

The likelihood of obtaining reattachment is increased by the elimination of infection and the correction of excessive tooth mobility.

REFERENCES

1. Barr, C. E.: Osteogenic activity in acute ascorbic acid deficiency. J. Oral Therap., 4:5, 1967.
2. Beckwith, T. D., Fleming, W. C., and Williams, A.: Repair of the tooth and paradentium in the guinea pig, rabbit and cat. U. of Calif. Publications in Microbiology, V–1, Nov. 1, 1943.
3. Beckwith, T. D., and Williams, A.: Regeneration of the peridental membrane in the cat. Proc. Soc. Exp. Biol. Med., 25:713, 1928.
4. Beckwith, T. D., Williams, A., and Fleming, W. C.: The regeneration of the rodent peridental membrane. Proc. Soc. Exp. Biol. Med., 24:562, 1927.
5. Beube, F. E.: A radiographic histologic study on reattachment. J. Periodontol., 23:158, 1952.
6. Blass, J. L., and Lite, T.: Gingival healing following surgical curettage: A histopathologic study. N.Y. Dent. J., 25:127, 1959.
7. Box, H. K.: Studies in periodontal pathology.

Can. Dent. Res. Found. Bull. 7, May 1924, p. 75.

8. Box, H. K.: Treatment of the periodontal pocket. Toronto, University of Toronto Press, 1928, pp. 94, 105.

9. Butcher, E. O., and Klingsberg, J.: Age, gonadectomy, and wound healing in the palatal mucosa. J. Dent. Res., 40:694, 1961.

10. Cabrini, R. L., and Carranza, F. A., Jr.: Adenosine triphosphatase in normal and scorbutic wounds. Nature, 200:1113, 1963.

11. Caffesse, R. G., Ramfjord, S. P., and Nasjleti, C. E.: Reverse bevel periodontal flaps in monkeys. J. Periodontol., 39:219, 1968.

12. Carranza, F. A., Sr.: A technique for treating infrabony pockets so as to obtain reattachment. Dent. Clin. North Am. March 1960, p. 75.

13. Cheraskin, E., et al.: Resistance and susceptibility to oral disease. II. A study in periodontometry and carbohydrate metabolism. Periodontics, 3:296, 1965.

14. Cross, W. G.: Reattachment following curettage. A histological study. Dent. Pract. 7:38, 1956.

15. Dunphy, J. E.: On the nature and care of wounds. Ann. R. Coll. Surg. Engl., 26:69, 1960.

16. Ferris, R. T.: Quantitative evaluation of tooth mobility following initial periodontal therapy. J. Periodontol., 37:190, 1966.

17. Fleming, W. E.: A Clinical and microscopic study of periodontal tissues treated by instrumentation. Pac. Dent. Gazette, 24:568, 1926.

18. Glickman, I., and Lazansky, J. P.: Repair of the periodontium following gingivectomy in experimental animals. J. Dent. Res. (Abstract), 29:659, 1950.

19. Glickman, I., Turesky, S. S., and Manhold, J.: The oxygen consumption of healing gingiva. J. Dent. Res., 29:429, 1950.

20. Goldman, H. M.: Subgingival curettage—A rationale. J. Periodontol., 19:54, 1948.

21. Gottlieb, B.: The new concept of periodontoclasia. J. Periodontol., 17:7, 1946.

22. Gross, H.: Experiments on the regenerative capacity of the gingiva in dogs. Paradentium, 5:57, 1933.

23. Hatfield, C. G., and Baumhammers, A.: Cytotoxic effects of periodontally involved root surfaces. I.A.D.R. Abstr. 48th General Meeting, 1970, p. 99, No. 203.

24. Hugoson, A.: Gingival inflammation and female sex hormones. J. Periodont. Res., Suppl. No. 5, 1970.

25. Itoiz, M. E., Cabrini, R. L., and Carranza, F. A., Jr.: Histochemical study of healing wounds: Alkaline and acid phosphatase. J. Oral Surg., 27:641, 1969.

26. Jansen, M. T., Coppes, L., and Verdenius, H. H. W.: Healing of periodontal wounds in dogs. J. Periodontol., 26:292, 1955.

27. Kaplan, H., and Mann, J. B.: How is pyorrhea cured? J. Am. Dent. Assoc., 29:1471, 1942.

28. Leblond, C. P., and Walker, B. E.: Renewal of cell populations, Physiol. Rev., 36:255, 1956.

29. Leonard, H. J.: Conservative treatment of periodontoclasia. J. Am. Dent. Assoc., 26:1308, 1939.

30. Leonard, H. J.: In our opinion—Reattachment. J. Periodontol., Supp. to Jan., 1943, p. 5.

31. Lindhe, J., and Brånemark, P. I.: The effect of sex hormones on vascularization of a granulation tissue. J. Periodont. Res., 3:6, 1968.

31a. Lindhe, J., and Ericsson, I.: The influence of trauma from occlusion on reduced but healthy periodontal tissues in dogs. J. Clin. Periodontol., 3:110, 1976.

31b. Lindhe, J., and Nyman, S.: The effect of plaque control and surgical pocket elimination on the establishment and maintenance of periodontal health. A longitudinal study of periodontal therapy in cases of advanced periodontal disease. J. Clin. Periodontol., 2:67, 1975.

32. Linghorne, W. J.: Studies in the reattachment and regeneration of the supporting structures of the teeth. IV. Regeneration in epithelialized pockets following the organization of a blood clot. J. Dent. Res., 36:4, 1957.

33. Linghorne, W. J., and O'Connell, D. C.: Studies in the reattachment and regeneration of the supporting structures of the teeth. III. Regeneration in epithelialized pockets. J. Dent. Res., 34:164, 1955.

34. McCall, J. O.: An improved method of inducing reattachment of the gingival tissues in periodontoclasia. Dent. Items Int., 48:342, 1926.

35. Meyer, J., Marwah, A. S., and Weinmann, J. P.: Mitotic rate of gingival epithelium in two age groups. J. Invest. Derm., 27:237, 1956.

36. Morris, M. L.: Healing of human periodontal tissues following surgical detachment and extirpation of vital pulps. J. Periodontol., 31:23, 1960.

37. Morris, M. L.: Healing of naturally occurring periodontal pockets about vital human teeth. J. Periodontol., 26:285, 1955.

38. Morris, M. L.: The reattachment of the human periodontal tissue following surgical detachment. J. Periodontol., 25:64, 1954.

39. Morris, M. L.: The removal of pocket and attachment epithelium in humans: A histological study. J. Periodontol., 25:57, 1954.

40. Moskow, B. S.: The response of the gingival sulcus to instrumentation. A histologic investigation. II. Gingival curettage. J. Periodontol., 35:112, 1964.

41. Muhlemann, H. R., Zander, H., and Halberg, F.: Mitotic activity in the periodontal tissues of the rat molar. J. Dent. Res., 33:459, 1954.

42. Oliver, R. C.: Tooth mortality following periodontal therapy. (Abstract) J. Periodontol., 41:48, 1970.

43. Perez-Tamayo, Ruy: Mechanisms of Disease and Introduction to Pathology. Philadelphia, W. B. Saunders Company, 1961, p. 105.

44. Prichard, J.: The infrabony technique as a predictable procedure. J. Periodontol., 28:202, 1957.

45. Ramfjord, S. P.: Experimental periodontal reattachment in Rhesus monkeys. J. Periodontol., 22:67, 1951.

46. Ramfjord, S. P., and Costich, E. R.: Healing after simple gingivectomy. J. Periodontol., 34:401, 1963.

46a. Ramfjord, S. P.: Present status of the modified Widman flap procedure. J. Periodontol., 48:558, 1977.

47. Rateitschak, K.: The therapeutic effect of local treatment on periodontal disease assessed

upon evaluation of different diagnostic criteria. 2. Changes in gingival inflammation. J. Periodontol., 35:155, 1964.

48. Rateitschak, K., et al.: The therapeutic effect of local treatment on periodontal disease assessed upon evaluation of different diagnostic criteria. 3. Radiographic changes in appearance of bone. J. Periodontol., 35:263, 1964.

49. Robbins, S. L.: Pathologic basis for disease. Philadelphia, W. B. Saunders Company, 1974, pp. 55–105.

50. Sato, M.: Histopathological study of the healing process after surgical treatment for alveolar pyorrhea. Bull. Tokyo Med. Dent. Univ., 1:71, 1960.

51. Schaffer, E. M., and Korn, N. A.: Comparison of curettage and gingivectomy in dogs. (Abstract) I.A.D.R., 40:69, 1962.

52. Schaffer, E. M., and Zander, H.: Histological evidence of reattachment of periodontal pockets. Paradentologie, 7:101, 1953.

53. Shapiro, M.: Reattachment in periodontal disease. J. Periodontol., 24:26, 1953.

54. Skillen, W. G., and Lundquist, G. R.: An experimental study of peridental membrane reattachment in healthy and pathologic tissues. J. Am. Dent. Assoc., 24:175, 1937.

55. Skillen, W. G., and Lundquist, G. R.: Experimental gingival injuries in dogs. J. Dent. Res., 15:165, 1935.

56. Stahl, S. S.: Effect of oral somatotrophic hormone injections upon gingival wounds in rats. (Abstract) J. Dent. Res., 38:725, 1959.

57. Stahl, S. S.: Healing gingival injury in normal and systemically stressed young adult male rats. J. Periodontol., 32:63, 1961.

58. Stahl, S. S.: Healing of gingival tissues following various therapeutic regimens—a review of histologic studies. J. Oral Therap. Pharm., 2:145, 1965.

59. Stahl, S. S.: The effect of a protein-free diet on the healing of gingival wounds in rats. Arch. Oral Biol., 7:551, 1962.

60. Stahl, S. S.: The influence of antibiotics on the healing of gingival wounds in rats. I. Alveolar bone and soft tissue. J. Periodontol., 33:261, 1962.

61. Stahl, S. S., Soberman, A., and DeCesare, A.: Gingival healing. V. The effects of antibiotics administered during early stages of repair. J. Periodontol., 40:521, 1969.

62. Stone, S., Ramfjord, S., and Waldron, J.: Scaling and gingival curettage. A radioautographic study. J. Periodontol., 37:415, 1966.

63. Turesky, S. S., and Glickman, I.: Histochemical evaluation of gingival healing in experimental animals on adequate and Vitamin C deficient diets. J. Dent. Res., 33:273, 1954.

64. Waerhaug, J.: Depth of incision in gingivectomy. Oral Surg., 8:707, 1955.

65. Waerhaug, J. Microscopic demonstration of tissue reaction incident to removal of subgingival calculus. J. Periodontol., 26:26, 1955.

66. Williams, C. H. M.: Rationalization of periodontal Pocket Therapy. J. Periodontol., 14:67, 1943.

67. Yukna, R. A.: A clinical and histologic study of healing following the excisional new attachment procedure in Rhesus monkeys. J. Periodontol., 47:701, 1976.

68. Yukna, R. A., Bowers, G. M., Lawrence, J. J., and Fedi, P. F.: A clinical study of healing in humans following the excisional new attachment procedure. J. Periodontol., 47:696, 1976.

Part II

Instrumentation

The Periodontal Instrumentarium

Periodontal instruments are designed for specific purposes, such as removal of calculus, planing of root surfaces, curettage of the gingiva, or removal of diseased tissue. Upon first examination, the number of instruments available for similar purposes appears confusing. With experience, however, one selects a relatively small set that fulfills all requirements.

CLASSIFICATION OF PERIODONTAL INSTRUMENTS

Periodontal instruments are classified according to the purposes they serve, as follows.

Periodontal probes are used to locate, measure, and mark pockets and determine their course on individual tooth surfaces.

Explorers are used to locate deposits and caries.

Scaling and curettage instruments serve the following purposes: removal of calcified deposits from the crown and root of a tooth[8]; removal of necrotic, altered cementum from the subgingival root surface;[13] and débridement of the soft tissue lining the pocket. Scaling and curettage instruments are classified as follows.

Sickle scalers are heavy instruments used to remove supragingival calculus.

Curettes are fine instruments used for subgingival scaling, root planing, and removal of the soft tissue lining the pocket.

Hoe, chisel, and file scalers are used to remove tenacious subgingival calculus and necrotic cementum. Their use is limited as compared with curettes.

Ultrasonic instruments are used for scaling and cleansing tooth surfaces and curetting the soft tissue wall of the periodontal pocket.[10]

Cleansing and polishing instruments. Rubber cups, brushes, portepolishers, and dental tape are used to cleanse and polish tooth surfaces.

The wearing and cutting qualities of some types of steel used in periodontal instruments have been tested,[17,18] but specifications vary among manufacturers. Each group of instruments has characteristic features; individual therapists often develop variations with which they operate most effectively. Small instruments are recommended to fit into pockets without injuring the soft tissues.[21,25,26]

The parts of each instrument, referred to as the *blade, shank,* and *handle,* are shown in Figure 36–1.

PERIODONTAL PROBES

Periodontal probes are used to measure the depth of pockets and to determine

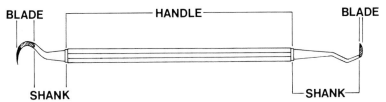

Figure 36–1   Parts of a Typical Periodontal Instrument.

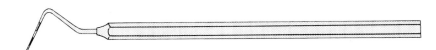

Figure 36–2   The periodontal probe is composed of the handle, the shank, and the calibrated working end.

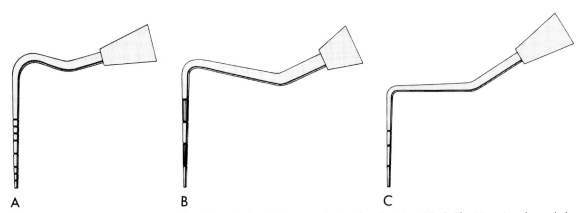

A   B   C

Figure 36–3   Types of Periodontal Probes. *A*, The Glickman periodontal probe No. 26G. *B*, The Marquis color-coded probe. Calibrations are in 3-mm. sections. *C*, The University of Michigan "O" probe.

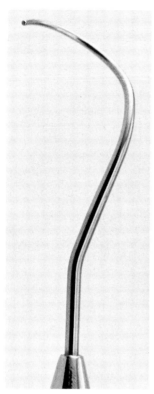

Figure 36–4   The Nabers Curved Probe for Detection of Furcation Areas.

their configuration. The typical feature is a tapered rod-like portion calibrated in millimeter markings, with a blunt, rounded tip (Fig. 36–2). There are several other designs with varying millimeter calibrations (Fig. 36–3). Ideally, these probes are thin, and the shank is angled to allow easy insertion into the pocket. Furcation areas can best be evaluated by the curved Nabers probe (Fig. 36–4).

In measuring a pocket, the probe is inserted with a firm, gentle pressure to the bottom of the pocket (Fig. 36–5). The shank should be aligned with the long axis of the tooth. Several measurements are made to determine the course of the pocket along the surface of the tooth.

EXPLORERS

Explorers are used to locate subgingival deposits and carious areas. They are also used to check the smoothness of the root surfaces after root planing. Explorers are designed with different shapes and angles for a variety of uses. Some of the most commonly used explorers are shown in

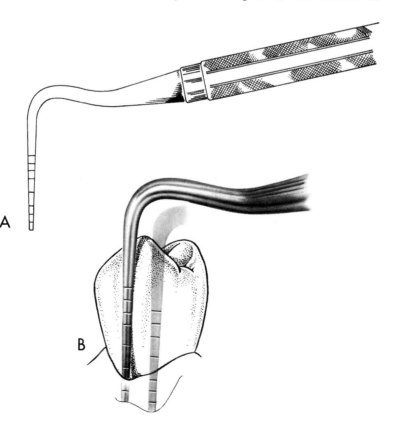

Figure 36–5 The Glickman Periodontal Probe. *A,* Calibrated blade offset from the shank. *B,* Pocket probed across the facial surface.

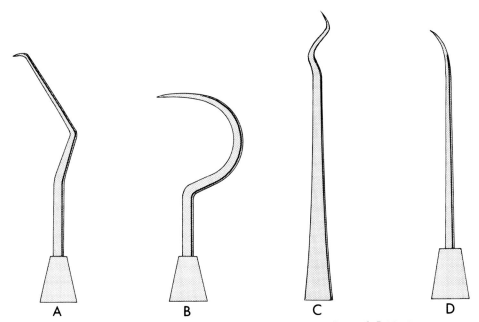

Figure 36–6   Four Typical Explorers. *A,* No. 17. *B,* No. 23. *C,* Pigtail. *D,* No. 3.

Figure 36–6. Their uses and limitations are shown in Figure 36–7. The periodontal probe can also be very useful in the detection of subgingival deposits (Fig. 36–7).

SCALING AND CURETTAGE INSTRUMENTS

Scaling and curettage instruments are illustrated in Figure 36–8.

Sickle Scalers (Superficial Scalers)

The sickle scaler is used to remove supragingival deposits (Fig. 36–9). Because of the design of this instrument, it would be difficult to insert the blade under the gingiva without damaging the surrounding gingival tissues (Fig. 36–10). The sickle scaler is triangular, with a pointed tip, and it has cutting edges on both sides of the blade (Fig. 36–11). It is used with a pull

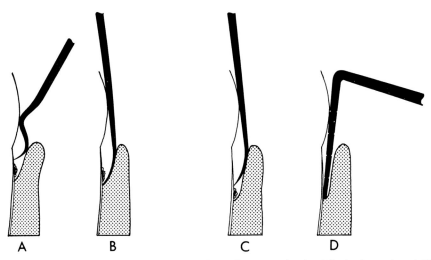

Figure 36–7   Insertion of Several Types of Explorers and a Probe in a Pocket for Calculus Detection. *A,* The limitations of the pigtail explorer in a deep pocket. *B,* Insertion and *C,* limitation of the No. 3 explorer. *D,* Insertion of the probe.

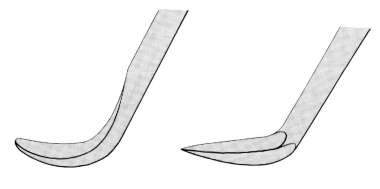

Figure 36–8 The Five Basic Scaling Instruments: curette, sickle, file, chisel, and hoe.

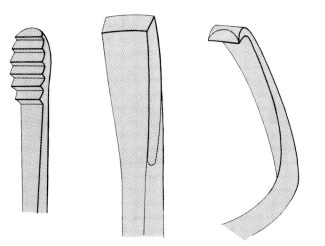

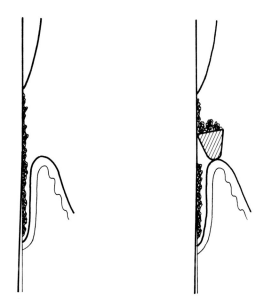

Figure 36–9 Use of Sickle Scaler for Removal of Supragingival Calculus.

stroke. Both the sickle scaler and the curette consist of a handle, shank, and blade (see Fig. 36–1). The shank may have several sections, depending on the number of turns incorporated into the design. The portion of the shank closest to the blade is called the lower or working shank.

Sickle scalers have varying sizes and shapes. Glickman has designed a series of three double-ended scalers, Nos. 1G–2G,

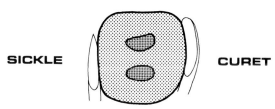

SICKLE   **CURET**

Figure 36–10 Subgingival adaptation around the root is better with the curette than with the sickle.

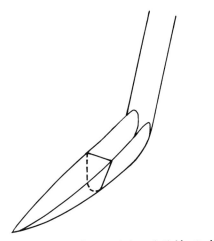

Figure 36–11   Basic Characteristics of Sickle Scaler: triangular shape, double cutting edge, and pointed tip.

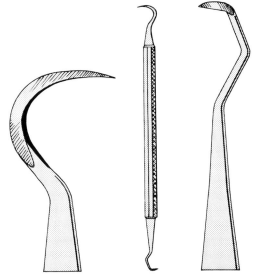

Figure 36–13   Sickle Scaler U15/30. Blade on *left* is a U15; blade on *right* is a jaquette 30. Both instruments are widely used for supragingival scaling.

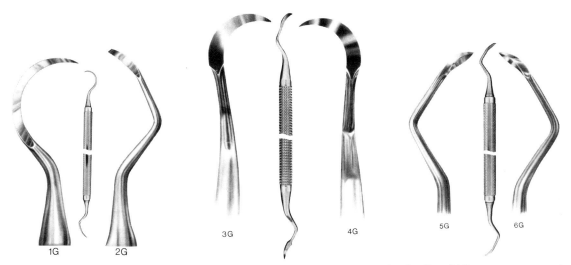

1G   2G   3G   4G   5G   6G

Figure 36–12   Sickle Scalers of the Glickman Series: 1G, 2G, 3G, 4G, 5G, and 6G.

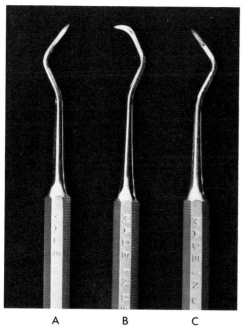

Figure 36–14 Jaquette Scalers. A, No. 2. B, No. 1. C, No. 3.

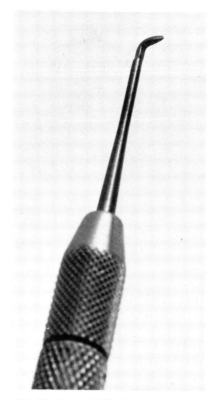

Figure 36–15 Morse Sickle Scaler. Blades are replaceable.

3G–4G, and 5G–6G (Fig. 36–12). The U15/30 (Fig. 36–13) and the Jaquette Nos. 1, 2, and 3 (Fig. 36–14) are other popular sickle scalers.

The Morse sickle (Fig. 36–15) is very useful in the mandibular anterior area when there is very little interproximal space. The blade is replaceable and can be obtained in various sizes (0, 00, and so forth). The miniature blades enable the instrument to engage tight interproximal areas and, to some extent, subgingival areas.[22a]

It is important to note that sickle scalers with the same basic design can be obtained with different blade sizes and shank types to adapt to specific uses. The No. 1G–2G, No. 3G–4G, and Ball sickles are very large. The Jaquette Nos. 1, 2, 3 and the No. 5G–6G sickles are medium-bladed. The Morse sickles with their small blades (0, 00) are miniature instruments. The selection of these instruments should be based on the area to be scaled.

Curettes

The curette is the instrument of choice for removing deep subgingival calculus,

root planing the altered cementum, and removing the soft tissue lining the periodontal pocket (Fig. 36–16). It is finer than the sickle scalers and does not have any sharp points or corners other than the cut-

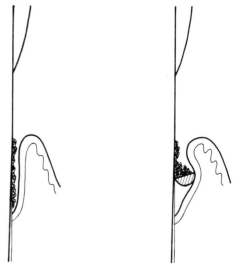

Figure 36–16 The curette is the instrument of choice for subgingival scaling and root planing.

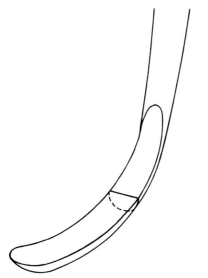

Figure 36-17　Basic Characteristics of a Curette: spoon-shaped blade and rounded tip.

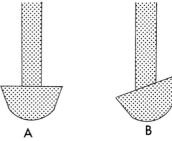

Figure 36-18　Principal Types of Curettes As Seen from the Toe of the Instrument. *A,* Universal curette. *B,* Gracey curette. Note the offset blade angulation of the Gracey curette.

ting edges of the blade (Fig. 36-17). Therefore, curettes provide better access to deep pockets with a minimum of soft tissue trauma (see Figure 36-10). The design of the curette is such that in cross section, the blade appears semi-circular with a convex base. The two lateral borders of the convex base form a cutting edge with the face of the semi-circular blade. The tip of the blade is rounded, unlike the sickle scaler, which is pointed. The blade may have either one or two cutting edges, and the instrument may be single- or double-ended, depending on the preference of the operator.

As seen in Figure 36-10, the curved design of the curette allows the blade to hug the root surface, unlike the straight blade and pointed end of a sickle scaler.

The curettes are of two basic types, universal and specific. *Universal curettes* are designed so that they may be inserted in most areas of the dentition by altering and adapting the finger rest, the fulcrum, and the hand position of the operator. The blade size and the angle and length of the shank may vary, but all universal curettes are at a 90° angle (perpendicular) with the lower shank when seen in cross section from the tip (Fig. 36-18A). The Glickman No. 7G-8G (Fig. 36-19), the Barnhart Nos. 1-2 and 5-6, and the Columbia Nos. 13-14, 2R-2L,

and 4R-4L (Fig. 36-20) are examples of universal curettes.

Gracey curettes are representative of the *specific curettes;* they are a set of several instruments designed and angled to adapt to specific anatomical areas of the dentition (Fig. 36-21). *These curettes are probably the best for subgingival scaling and root planing.* Double-ended Gracey curettes are paired in the following manner:

Gracey No. 1-2 ⎫
Gracey No. 3-4 ⎭ Anterior teeth
Gracey No. 5-6 ⎱ Anterior teeth and bicuspids
Gracey No. 7-8 ⎫
Gracey No. 9-10 ⎭ Posterior teeth: buccal and lingual
Gracey No. 11-12 ⎱ Posterior teeth: mesial (Fig. 36-22)
Gracey No. 13-14 ⎱ Posterior teeth: distal (Fig. 36-23)

Single-ended Gracey curettes can also be obtained, in which case a set would be composed of fourteen instruments. Although these curettes are designed to be used in specific areas as shown in the foregoing list, an experienced operator can adapt each instrument for use in several different areas by altering the position of his hand and the position of the patient.

The Gracey curette also differs from the universal curettes in that the blade is not at a 90° angle to the lower shank. The term *offset blade* is used for Gracey curette, since they are angled approximately 60 to 70° from the lower shank (Fig. 36-18B). This unique angulation allows the blade to be inserted in the precise posi-

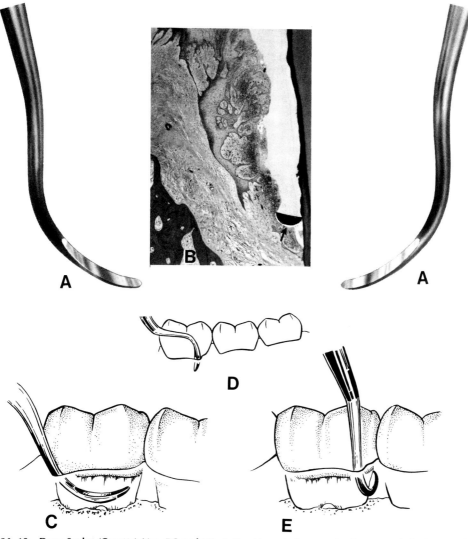

Figure 36–19　Deep Scaler (Curette) Nos. 7G and 8G. *A,* Double-ended curette for the removal of subgingival calculus. *B,* Cross-section of the scaler blade against cemental wall of a deep periodontal pocket. *C,* Curette in position at the base of a periodontal pocket on the facial surface of a mandibular molar. *D,* Curette inserted in pocket with tip directed apically. *E,* Curette in position at base of pocket on distal surface of mandibular molar.

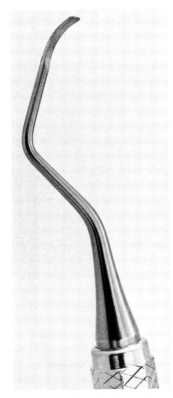

Figure 36–20   Columbia 4R and 4L.

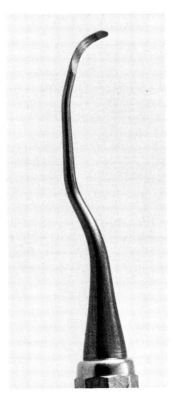

Figure 36–22   Gracey 11/12 Curette. Note the double turn of the shank.

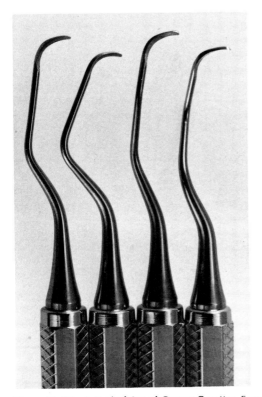

Figure 36–21   A Typical Set of Gracey Curettes. From left, No. 5/6, No. 7/8, No. 11/12, and No. 13/14.

tion for subgingival scaling and root planing, provided that the lower shank is parallel with the long axis of the tooth being scaled. Another difference in the blade is seen from the top. Specific curettes have a curved blade, whereas the blade of the universal curette is straight (see Fig. 36–24). Thus, a pull stroke can be utilized. Some of the major differences between Gracey (specific) curettes and universal curettes can be seen in Table 36–1.

Hoe Scalers

Hoe scalers are used for planing and smoothing root surfaces, which entails removal of calculus remnants and softened cementum. The No. 11G–12G and No. 13G–14G hoes are double-ended instruments designed to provide access to all root surfaces (Fig. 36–25A). The blade is bent at a 99° angle; the cutting edge is formed by the junction of the flattened terminal surface with the inner aspect of the blade. The cutting edge is beveled at 45°. The blade is slightly bowed so that it

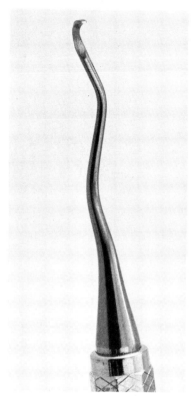

Figure 36–23 **Gracey 13/14 Curette.** Note the acute turn of the blade.

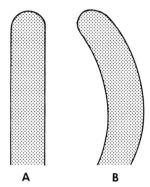

Figure 36–24 *A,* **Universal Curette As Seen from the Blade.** Note that blade is straight. *B,* **Gracey Curette As Seen from the Blade.** The blade is curved; only the convex cutting edge is used.

can maintain contact at two points on a convex surface. The back of the blade is rounded, and the blade has been reduced to minimum thickness to permit access to the roots of deep pockets without interference from the adjacent tissues.

Hoe scalers are used as follows:

1. The blade is inserted to the base of the periodontal pocket so that it makes two-point contact with the tooth (Fig. 36–25*B* and *C*). This stabilizes the instrument and prevents nicking of the root.

2. The instrument is activated with a firm motion toward the crown, with every effort being made to preserve the two-point contact with the tooth.

McCall's Hoe Scalers Nos. 3, 4, 5, 6, 7, and 8 are a set of six hoe scalers designed to provide access to all tooth surfaces (Fig. 36–26). Each instrument has a different angle between shank and handle.

Files

Files were popular at one time, but they are no longer used very much for scaling

TABLE 36–1 COMPARISON OF SPECIFIC (GRACEY) AND UNIVERSAL CURETTES*

	Gracey Curette	Universal Curette
Area of Use	*Area-specific.* Set of many designed for specific areas and surfaces.	*Universal.* One curette designed for all areas and surfaces.
Cutting Edge		
Use	*One cutting edge used.* Work with outer edge only.	*Both cutting edges used.* Work with either outer or inner edge.
Curvature	*Curved in two planes.* Blade curves up and to the side.	*Curved in one plane.* Blade curves up, not to side.
Blade Angle	*Offset blade.* Face of blade beveled at 60° to shank.	*Not offset.* Face of blade beveled at 90° to shank.

*Modified from Pattison, G., and Pattison, A.: *Periodontal Instrumentation.* Reston, Virginia: Reston Publishing Company, 1978.

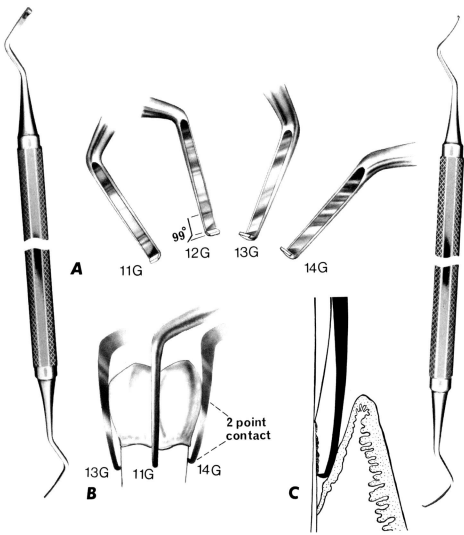

Figure 36–25   Hoe Scalers No. 11G–12G and No. 13G–14G. *A,* Double-ended hoe scalers with beveled cutting edge. *B,* Hoe scalers designed for different tooth surfaces, showing "two point" contact. *C,* Hoe scaler in a periodontal pocket. The back of the blade is rounded for easier access. The instrument contacts the tooth at two points for stability.

and root planing, because they gouge and roughen root surfaces.[15] They are sometimes used for removing overhanging margins of dental restorations.

Chisel Scalers

The chisel scaler, designed for proximal surfaces of teeth too closely spaced to permit the use of other scalers, is usually used in the anterior part of the mouth. The No. 15G–16G is a double-ended instrument with a curved and a straight shank (Fig. 36–27); the blades are slightly curved with a straight cutting edge beveled at 45°.

The scaler is inserted from the facial surface. The slight curve of the blade makes it possible to stabilize it against the proximal surface, whereas the cutting edge engages the calculus without nicking the tooth. The instrument is activated with a push motion while the side of the blade is held firmly against the root.

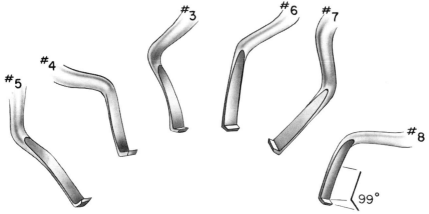

Figure 36–26   McCall's Hoe Scalers.

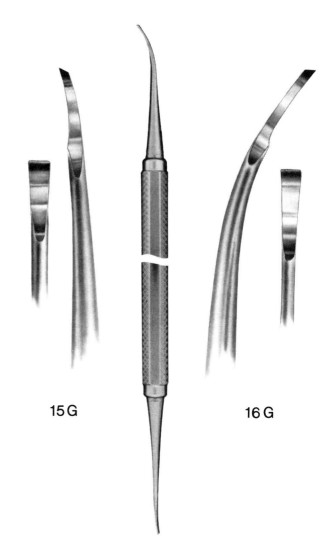

Figure 36–27   Chisel Scaler No. 15G and 16G with Curved and Straight Shanks.

15 G

16 G

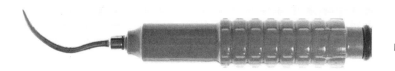

Figure 36–28   Ultrasonic Tip.

Ultrasonic Instruments

Ultrasonic instruments may be used for scaling, curettage, and stain removal.[31] Their action is derived from physical vibrations of particles of matter, similar to sound waves, at frequencies ranging from 20,000 to many million cycles per second, above the range of human hearing. ("Cycles per second" are also referred to as Hertz or H_z.) In periodontal instrumentation, tipped instruments producing up to 29,000 vibrations per second are used.

Ultrasonic tips of different shapes are available for scaling, curettage, root planing, and gingival surgery (Fig. 36–28). All tips are designed to operate in a wet field and have attached water outlets (Fig. 36–29). The spray is directed at the end of the tip to dissipate the heat generated by the ultrasonic vibrations.

The instrument is used with a light touch and a limited number of strokes per unit of area. Improper use may produce gouging and roughening of root surfaces. The tips work best against hard tooth surfaces but can also be used against gingival tissue. The gingiva can be made more rigid by injecting anesthetic solution directly into it.[5] When placed against a tooth or soft tissue surface, the instrument mechanically debrides surface accumulations or necrotic tissue. The liquid sprayed on the vibrating tip reinforces the mechanical cleansing effect of the vibrations. The instrument should be kept away from bone to avoid the possibility of necrosis and sequestration. Ultrasonic instruments should not be used on young growing tissues; thus, their use in the treatment of children is not recommended.[10]

When applied to the gingiva of experimental animals, ultrasonic vibrations disrupt tissue continuity, lift off epithelium, dismember collagen bundles, and alter the morphology of fibroblast nuclei.[12] However, the simple application of ultrasonic vibration to the gingiva produces no clini-

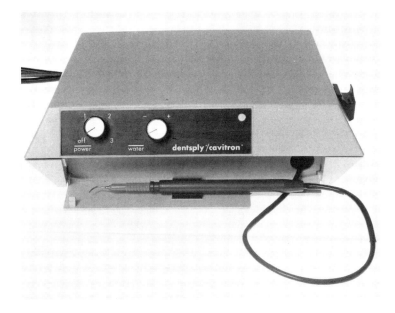

Figure 36–29   Ultrasonic Unit.

cally discernible morphologic changes, and use following gingivectomy does not appear to retard gingival healing.[11]

Ultrasound is effective for removing calculus[5, 14, 19, 24] and debriding the epithelial lining of periodontal pockets.[12] It produces a narrow band of necrotic tissue (microcauterization), which strips off from the inner aspect of the pocket. The Morse-type scaler and the rod-shaped instrument are used for this purpose. Some investigators find ultrasonic instruments as effective as manual instruments for curettage[20] with less inflammation but more pronounced disruption of the uppermost periodontal fibers.[27] When debriding the gingival wall of periodontal pockets, these instruments tend to remove less of the underlying connective tissue than manual instruments, but they do not smooth the root as well.[23] They tend to produce a stippled root with greater removal of tooth substance.[3] The volume and depth of tooth structure loss may be reduced by using a medium setting on the instrument and applying only slight tactile force.[6]

There are reports that ultrasonic instruments roughen dentin surfaces[4] and cause more gouging and nicking of the roots than manual instruments,[1, 14] and that they are not as effective as manual instruments for root planing.[24] The roughness scores of teeth planed with ultrasound have been reported as twice those of teeth planed with hand curettes.[15]

Opinions differ regarding the effectiveness of ultrasound for removing stains as compared with conventional methods of oral prophylaxis.[5, 14, 20] There is no significant difference between manual and ultrasonic instruments in the incidence of bacteremia following subgingival procedures.[2]

The EVA System

Probably the most efficient and least traumatic instruments for correcting overhanging or overcontoured proximal alloy and resin restorations are motor-driven diamond files (Fig. 36–30).* These files, which come in symmetrical pairs, are made of aluminum in the shape of a wedge protruding from a shaft; one side of the wedge is diamond-coated, the other side is smooth. The files can be mounted

---

*EVA prophylaxis instrument, designed by Dr. Per Axelsson, Karlstadt, Sweden.

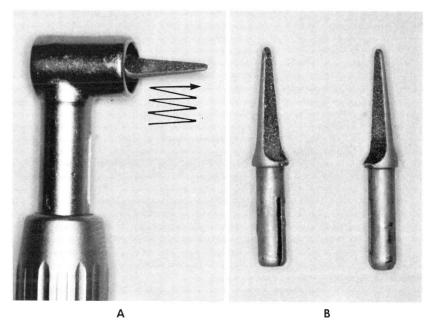

A **B**

Figure 36–30 *A,* **EVA Handpiece.** Zig-zag arrows indicate direction of motion. *B,* **EVA Tips.**

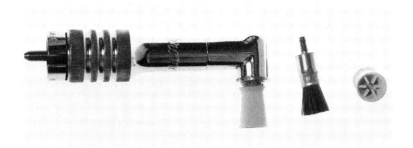

Figure 36–31   Prophylaxis Handpiece with Rubber Cup and Brush.

on a special dental handpiece attachment that generates reciprocating strokes of variable frequency. When the unit is activated interproximally, with the diamond-coated side of the file touching the restoration and the smooth side adjacent to the papilla, the oscillating file swiftly planes the contour of the restoration and reduces it to the desired shape.

CLEANSING AND POLISHING INSTRUMENTS

The rubber cup, portepolisher, bristle brush, and dental tape are employed in the dental office for cleansing and polishing the tooth surfaces.

Rubber cups consist of a rubber shell with or without web-shaped configurations in the hollow interior (Fig. 36–31). They are used in the handpiece with a special prophylaxis angle. There are many types of cleansing and polishing pastes, which should be kept moist to minimize frictional heat as the cup revolves. Aggressive use of the rubber cups may remove the layer of cementum, which is very thin in the cervical area.

The portepolisher is a hand instrument constructed to hold a wooden point with which polishing paste is applied to the tooth with a firm burnishing action. The Ivory straight portepolisher with the wood point set at an angle of 45° with the handle fulfills most needs (Fig. 36–32). A contra-angle portepolisher, angulated at 60° for use in the posterior part of the mouth, is also available.

Bristle brushes are available in wheel and cup shapes (Fig. 36–31). The brush is used in the handpiece with a polishing paste. Because the bristles are very stiff, use of the brush should be confined to the crown to avoid injuring the cementum.

Dental tape with polishing paste is used for polishing proximal surfaces inaccessible to the other polishing instruments. The tape is passed interproximally while being kept at a right angle to the long axis of the tooth and is activated in a firm labiolingual motion. Particular care is taken to avoid injury to the gingiva. The area should be cleansed with warm water to remove all remnants of paste.

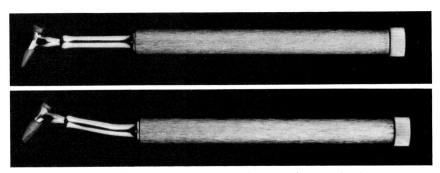

Figure 36–32   **Portepolishers.** *Above,* Straight type. *Below,* Angulated type.

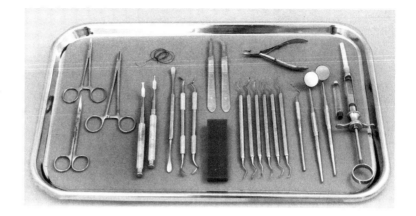

Figure 36–33 A Typical Surgical Instrument Tray.

SURGICAL INSTRUMENTS

Periodontal surgery is accomplished with numerous instruments. Figure 36–33 shows a typical surgical tray. Periodontal surgical instruments are classified as follows:

1. Excisional and incisional instruments
2. Surgical curettes and sickles
3. Periosteal elevators
4. Surgical chisels
5. Surgical files
6. Scissors
7. Hemostats and tissue forceps

Excisional and Incisional Instruments

Periodontal Knives (Gingivectomy Knives). The No. 20G–21G and No. 15K–16K are representative examples of knives commonly used for gingivectomy. They can be obtained as either double- or single-ended instruments. The entire periphery of these kidney-shaped knives is a cutting edge (Fig. 36–34).

Interdental Knives. The No. 22G–23G (Fig. 36–35), the Orban No. 1–2, and the Merrifield Nos. 1, 2, 3, and 4 are examples of knives that are used for the interdental areas. These spear-shaped knives have cutting edges on both sides of the blade and are designed with either double- or single-ended blades.

Surgical Blades. Scalpel blades of different shapes and sizes are used in periodontal surgery. These blades are used in flap, mucogingival, and graft operations. The most commonly used blades are Nos. 11, 12, and 15 (Fig. 36–36). The blades are usually used once and are considered disposable.

Electrosurgery (Surgical Diathermy)°

The term *electrosurgery* is currently used to identify surgical techniques performed on soft tissue by using controlled high-frequency electrical (radio) currents in the range of 1,500,000 to 7,500,000

°The reader is referred to Oringer[22] for a more extensive discussion on electrosurgery.

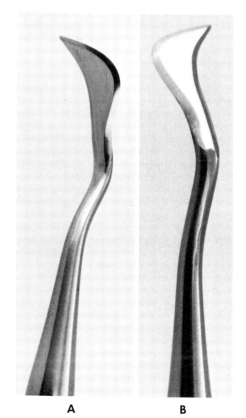

A   **B**

Figure 36–34   Kirkland Gingivectomy Knife. *A,* 15K. *B,* 16K.

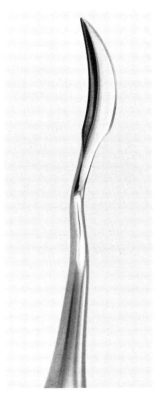

Figure 36–35   The 22G–23G Interdent Knife.

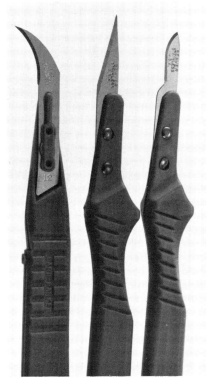

Figure 36–36   Surgical Blades. From left to right, Nos. 12, 11, and 15.

cycles per second. Modern electronic research has produced a new generation of electrosurgical equipment capable of precise, safe management of soft tissue (Fig. 36–37).

Since their initial use in 1900 for coagulation and in 1908 for tissue cutting, progress in the use of high-frequency currents has been very slow. Early electrosurgical units primarily developed for the medical and veterinary professions were over-powered and did not possess the refinement of current or currents required for the multitude of soft tissue procedures performed within the oral cavity. Significant improvement in the equipment designed for dental use did not occur until the 1960's. In late 1973, filtered, fully rectified currents

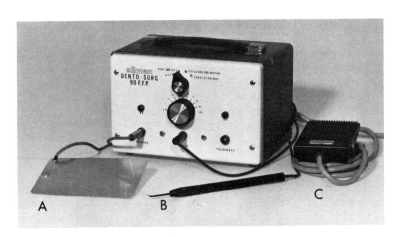

Figure 36–37 Electrosurgical Unit. *A,* Passive or conductive plate. *B,* Active electrode handle and tip electrode. *C,* Foot switch.

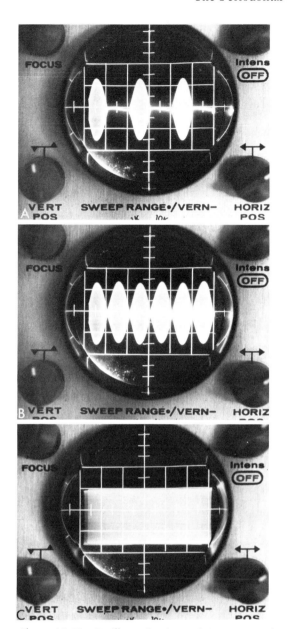

Figure 36–38 Oscilloscopic Views of Currents Used in Electrosurgery. A, Partially rectified current wave train. B, Fully rectified current. C, Filtered, fully rectified current wave train.

became available. The three types of current (partially rectified, fully rectified, and filtered fully rectified) offer a wide range of control over tissue management and hemorrhage (Fig. 36–38).

There are three classes of active electrodes (Fig. 36–39): (1) single-wire electrodes for incising or excising, (2) loop electrodes for planing tissue, and (3)

heavy, bulkier electrodes for coagulation procedures.

Basically, there are four types of electrosurgical techniques:

Electrosection, also referred to as electrotomy or acusection, requires an undamped (fully rectified) or continuous (filtered fully rectified) wave train. Three classes of procedures are included in electrosection: incisions, excisions, and planing. Incisions and excisions are performed with single-wire active electrodes that can be bent or adapted to perform any type of cutting procedure. Planing of tissue can be accomplished by correct selection of the appropriate loop electrode.

Electrocoagulation uses a damped or interrupted wave train such as the partially rectified current or modified fully rectified current. A very wide range of coagulation or hemorrhage control can be obtained by utilizing the electrocoagulation current with different techniques. It must be clearly understood that electrocoagulation can *prevent* bleeding or hemorrhage at the initial entry into soft tissue. It cannot *stop* bleeding once blood is present. All forms of hemorrhage must be stopped first by some form of direct pressure: air, compress, or hemostat. Once bleeding has momentarily stopped, final sealing of the capillaries or large vessels can be accomplished by short application of the electrocoagulation current. The active electrodes used for coagulation are much bulkier than the fine tungsten wire used for electrosection. There are three types of coagulation electrodes. Ball electrodes are used for general hemostasis, bar electrodes for controlling petechial or slight hemorrhage in restricted areas. The bar electrode can also be used to desensitize hypersensitive dentin. Cone electrodes can be used for sulcular bleeding.

Electrosection and electrocoagulation are bi-terminal techniques that require the use of a large conductive plate electrode, which is referred to as the passive electrode. (Sometimes it is called the indifferent plate or dispersive plate or electrode.) The closer the passive plate is to the operative site, the more effective any given current value will be. The passive plate is needed for predictable and refined cutting. Best results are obtained when the

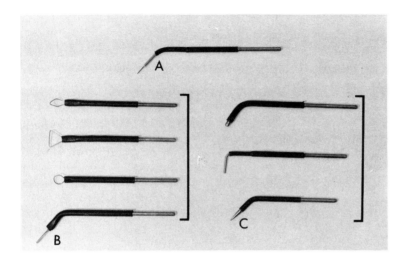

Figure 36–39 Active Electrodes. A, Single-wire cutting tip. B, Loop electrodes for planing. C, Coagulation electrodes.

passive plate has direct contact with skin, but it may be placed in a close but less obvious location for psychological reasons.

Electrosection and electrocoagulation are the procedures most commonly used in all areas of dentistry. The two mono-terminal techniques, electrofulguration and electrodessication, are seldom used. In mono-terminal procedures, only the active electrode is used; the passive plate is not used.

Electrofulguration uses a high-voltage, low-current, damped wave train or, less often, an interrupted wave train. No passive plate is used. This technique somewhat resembles the hyprecator techniques of the 1950's. The active electrode is held just slightly out of tissue contact and moved over the tissue, spraying sparks to produce an eschar. It has limited application in dentistry.

Electrodesiccation, which employs a dehydrating current, is the least used, as well as the most dangerous technique. The active electrode is inserted into the tissue, and the tissue surrounding the electrode is mass coagulated in situ. This procedure is useful in dermatology and cancer surgery and for cavernous hemangiomas.

It is well to remember that the electrosurgical unit is a radio transmitter. Just as a radio station must be fine tuned for good reception, successful electrosurgical procedures also require fine tuning. Each kind of body tissue has a different impedance or resistance value. Electrosurgical units, even from the same manufacturer, differ in wave form and output characteristics. Impedance and electrolyte content vary in different areas of the body and in different patients. Operatory environments differ in grounding potential. Also, current output varies with local demand for electrical energy. All these factors govern the final result of electrosurgery.

The local heat generated in the tissues immediately lateral to the operative site is called *lateral heat.* It is directly under the control of the operator. Lateral heat is directly related to five controlling factors: the duration of current exposure to any one point, the dosage of current, the size and shape of the electrode, the type of current, and the tissue impedance. An excess of any one of these factors must be offset with a reduction of one or more of the other factors to prevent accumulation of destructive heat within the tissues.

The most important basic rule of electrosurgery is *always keep the tip moving.* Prolonged or repeated application of current to tissue induces heat accumulation and undesired tissue destruction, whereas interrupted application at intervals adequate for tissue cooling (5 to 10 seconds) reduces or eliminates heat build-up. Electrosurgery is *not* intended to destroy tissue; it is a controllable means of sculpturing or modifying oral soft tissue with the least discomfort and hemorrhage for the patient.

The advantages of electrosurgery are:
1. The active electrodes are flexible fine wires that:
   a. Can be bent or shaped to fit any requirement
   b. Never need sharpening
   c. Are self-sterilizing
   d. Require no pressure; in fact, pressure is contraindicated.
2. It permits any degree of hemorrhage control desired.
3. It prevents seeding of bacteria into the incision site.
4. It permits tissue planing—a procedure unique to electrosurgery.
5. It provides a better view of the operative site because bleeding is controlled and no pressure is needed for cutting.
6. It eliminates scar formation.

The disadvantages of electrosurgery are:
1. It is contraindicated for patients who have noncompatible or poorly shielded cardiac pacemakers.

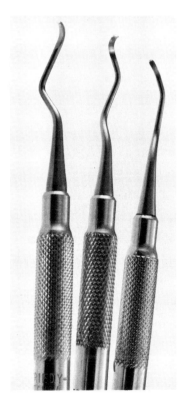

Figure 36–40 Kramer Heavy Surgical Curettes Nos. 1, 2, and 3.

2. It produces an odor and sometimes a taste that must be controlled.

The indications for electrosurgery in periodontal therapy and a description of wound healing after electrosurgery are presented in Chapter 49.

Surgical Curettes and Sickles

Larger and heavier curettes and sickles are often needed during surgery for the removal of granulation tissue, fibrous interdental tissues, and tenacious subgingival deposits. The Kramer Nos. 1, 2, and 3 (Fig. 36–40) and the Kirkland surgical instruments are curettes, whereas the Glickman Nos. 3G and 4G (Fig. 36–41) and the Ball scaler No. B2–B3 are popular heavy sickles. The wider, heavier blades of these instruments make them suitable for surgical procedures.

Periosteal Elevators

These instruments are necessary to reflect and move the flap after the incision has been made for flap surgery. The No. 24G (Fig. 36–42) and the Goldman-Fox No. 14 are two very well-designed periosteal elevators.

Surgical Chisels and Hoes

Chisels and hoes are used during periodontal surgery for removing and reshaping bone. The No. 19G (Fig. 36–43) is an example of a hoe, which has a curved shanked blade as compared with the straight-shanked Wiedelstadt and Todd-Gilmore chisels (Fig. 36–44A). The surgical hoe No. 19G has a flattened, fishtail-shaped blade with a pronounced convexity in its terminal portion. The cutting edge is beveled with rounded edges and projects beyond the long axis of the handle to preserve the effectiveness of the instrument when the blade is reduced by sharpening. The surgical hoe is generally used for detaching pocket walls after the gingivectomy incision, but it is also useful for smoothing root and bone surfaces made accessible by any surgical procedure. The Ochsenbein No. 1–2 (Fig. 36–44B) is a

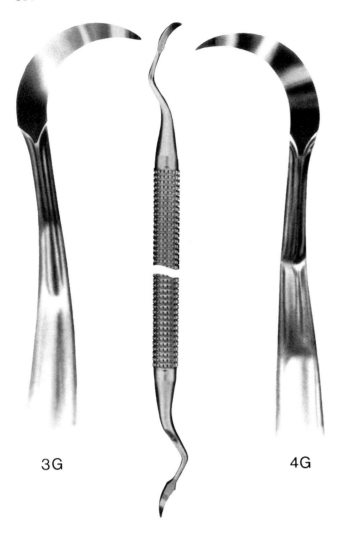

3G   4G

Figure 36–41   Glickman Heavy Sickle No. 3G and 4G.

very useful chisel with a semi-circular indentation on both sides of the shank to allow the instrument to engage around the tooth into the interdental area. Surgical hoes are usually used with a pull stroke, whereas chisels are engaged with a push stroke.

Surgical Files

Periodontal surgical files are used primarily to smooth rough bony ledges and to remove small areas of bone. The Schluger and Sugarman files are similar in design (Fig. 36–45) and can be used with a push and pull stroke, primarily in the interdental areas.

Scissors

Scissors are used in periodontal surgery for such purposes as removing tabs of tissue during gingivectomy, trimming the margins of flaps, enlarging incisions in periodontal abscesses, and removing muscle attachments in mucogingival surgery. There are many types; the choice is a matter of individual preference. Illustrated

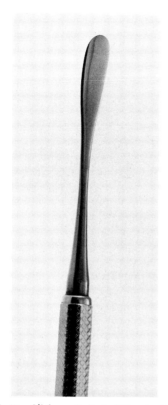

Figure 36–42   Glickman Periosteal Elevator No. 24G.

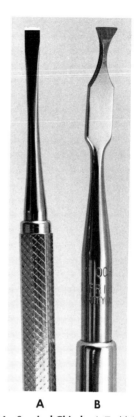

A   B

Figure 36–44   Surgical Chisels. *A,* Todd Gilmore chisel. *B,* Ochsenbein chisel.

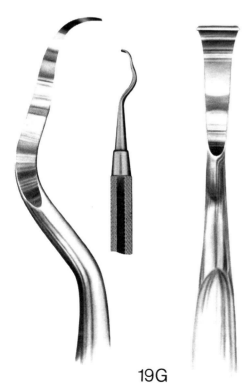

19G

Figure 36–43   Surgical Hoe No. 19G.

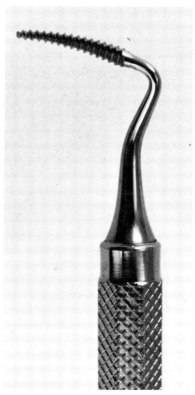

Figure 36–45   Schluger No. 9/10 Surgical File.

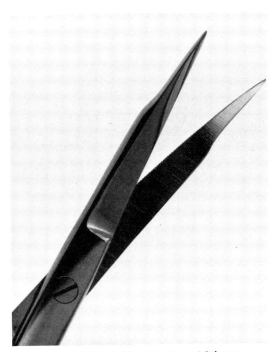

Figure 36–46   Goldman-Fox No. 16 Scissors.

in Fig. 36–46 is the Goldman-Fox No. 16 with a curved beveled blade with serrations.

REFERENCES

1. Allen, E. F., and Rhoads, R. H.: Effects of high speed periodontal instruments on tooth surface. J. Periodontol., 34:352, 1963.
2. Bandt, C. L., et al.: Bacteremias from ultrasonic and hand instrumentation. J. Periodontol., 35:214, 1964.
3. Belting, C. M.: Effects of high speed periodontal instruments on the root surface during subgingival calculus removal. J. Am. Dent. Assoc., 69:578, 1964.
4. Björn, H., and Lindhe, J.: The influence of periodontal instruments on the tooth surface. Odont. Rev., 13:355, 1962.
5. Burman, L. R., Alderman, N. E., and Ewen, S. J.: Clinical application of ultrasonic vibrations for supragingival calculus and stain removal. J. Dent. Med., 13:156, 1958.
6. Clark, S. M.: The effect of ultrasonic instrumentation on root surfaces. J. Periodontol., 39:135, 1968.
7. Clark, S. M.: The ultrasonic dental unit: a guide for the clinical application of ultrasonics in dentistry and in dental hygiene. J. Periodontol., 40:621, 1969.
8. Everett, F. G., Foss, C. L., and Orban, B.: Study of instruments for scaling. Periodontol., 16:61, 1962.
9. Ewen, S. J.: The ultrasonic wound – some microscopic observation. J. Periodontol., 32:315, 1961.
10. Ewen, S. J., and Glickstein, C.: Ultrasonic therapy in periodontics. Springfield, Ill., Charles C Thomas, 1968.
11. Frisch, J., et al.: Effect of ultrasonic instrumentation on human gingival connective tissue. Periodontics, 5:123, 1967.
12. Goldman, H. M.: Histologic assay of healing following ultrasonic curettage versus hand instrument curettage. Oral Surg., 14:925, 1961.
13. Green, E., and Ramfjord, S. J.: Tooth roughness after subgingival root planing. J. Periodontol., 37:44, 1966.
14. Johnson, W. N., and Wilson, J. R.: The application of the ultrasonic dental units to scaling procedures. J. Periodontol., 28:264, 1957.
15. Kerry, G. J.: Roughness of root surfaces after use of ultrasonic instruments and hand curettes. J. Periodontol., 38:340, 1967.
16. Klug, R. G.: Gingival tissue regeneration following electrical retraction. J. Prosthet. Dent., 16:955, 1966.
17. Lindhe, J.: Evaluation of periodontal scalers. II. Wear following standardized or diagonal cutting tests. Odont. Rev., 17:121, 1966.
18. Lindhe, J., and Jacobson, L.: Evaluation of periodontal scalers. I. Wear following clinical use. Odont. Rev., 17:1, 1966.
19. McCall, C. M., and Szmyd, L.: Clinical evaluation of ultrasonic scaling. J. Am. Dent. Assoc., 61:559, 1960.
20. Nadler, H.: Removal of crevicular epithelium by ultrasonic curettes. J. Periodontol., 33:220, 1962.
21. Orban, B., and Manella, V. B.: A macroscopic and microscopic study of instruments designed for root planing. J. Periodontol., 27:120, 1956.
22. Oringer, M. J.: Electrosurgery in Dentistry. Philadelphia, W. B. Saunders Co., 2nd ed., 1975.
22a. Romanelli, J. H.: Raspaje subgingival; su técnica. Rev. Odont. (B.A.), 36:501, 1948; 37:113, 277, 1949.
23. Sanderson, A. D.: Gingival curettage by hand and ultrasonic instruments – a histologic comparison. J. Periodontol., 37:279, 1966.
24. Stende, G. W., and Schaffer, E. M.: A comparison of ultrasonic and hand scaling. J. Periodontol., 32:312, 1961.
25. Waerhaug, J., et al.: The dimension of instruments for removal of subgingival calculus. J. Periodontol., 25:281, 1954.
26. Wentz, F. M.: Therapeutic root planing. J. Periodontol., 28:59, 1957.
27. Zach, L., and Cohen, G.: The histology of the response to ultrasonic curettage. J. Dent. Res., 40:751, 1961.
28. Zinner, D. D.: Recent ultrasonic dental studies, including periodontia, without the use of an abrasive. J. Dent. Res., 34:748, 1955 (abstract).

Chapter 37

Principles of Periodontal Instrumentation

GENERAL PRINCIPLES OF INSTRUMENTATION

Effective instrumentation is governed by a number of general principles which are common to all periodontal instruments. Proper positioning of the patient and the operator, illumination and retraction for optimum visibility, and sharp instruments are fundamental prerequisites. A constant awareness of tooth and root morphology and of the condition of the periodontal tissues is also essential. Knowledge of instrument design enables the clinician efficiently to select the proper instrument for the procedure and the area in which it will be performed. In addition to all these principles, the basic concepts of grasp, finger rest, adaptation, angulation, and

stroke must be understood before clinical instrumentation skills can be mastered.

Accessibility (Positioning of Patient and Operator)

Accessibility facilitates thoroughness of instrumentation. The position of the patient and operator should provide maximum accessibility to the area of operation. Inadequate accessibility impedes thorough instrumentation, prematurely tires the operator, and diminishes his effectiveness.

The clinician should be seated in a comfortable operating stool that has been positioned so that the clinician's feet are flat on the floor and the thighs parallel to the floor. The clinician should be able to observe the field of operation while keeping his back straight and head erect.[18]

The patient should be in a supine position and placed so that the mouth is close to the resting elbow of the clinician. For instrumentation on the maxillary arch, the patient should be asked to raise his chin slightly to provide optimum visibility and accessibility. For instrumentation on the mandibular arch, it may be necessary to raise the back of the chair slightly and request that the patient lower his chin until the mandible is parallel to the floor. This will especially facilitate work on the lingual surfaces of the mandibular anterior teeth.

Visibility, Illumination, and Retraction

Whenever possible, direct vision with direct illumination from the dental light

---

Material in this chapter was drawn freely from Pattison, G., and Pattison A., *Periodontal Instrumentation*, Reston, Va., Reston Publishing Co., 1978.

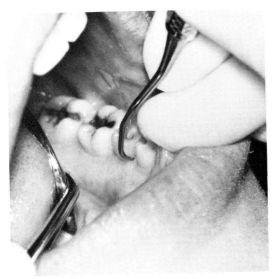

Figure 37-1   Direct Vision and Direct Illumination in the Mandibular Left Premolar Area.

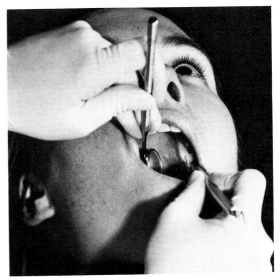

Figure 37-3   Indirect Illumination Using the Mirror to Reflect Light onto the Maxillary Left Posterior Lingual Region.

is most desirable (Fig. 37-1). If this is not attainable, indirect vision may be obtained by using the mouth mirror (Fig. 37-2), and indirect illumination may be obtained by using the mirror to reflect light to where it is needed (Fig. 37-3). Indirect vision and indirect illumination are often used simultaneously (Fig. 37-4).

Retraction provides visibility, accessibility, and illumination. The fingers, the mir-

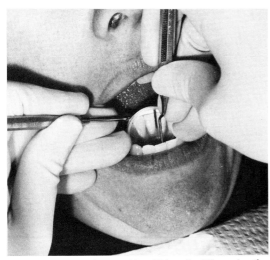

Figure 37-2   Indirect Vision Using the Mirror for the Lingual Surfaces of the Mandibular Anterior Teeth.

ror, or both are used for retraction, depending on the location of the area of operation. The mirror may be used for retraction of the cheeks or the tongue. The index finger is used for retraction of the lips or cheeks. The following illustrated methods are effective for retraction:

1. Use of the mirror to deflect the cheek while the fingers of the nonoperating hand retract the lips and protect the angle of the mouth from irritation by the mirror handle (Fig. 37-5).
2. Use of the mirror only to retract the lips and cheek (Fig. 37-6).
3. Use of the fingers of the nonoperating hand to retract the lips (Fig. 37-7).
4. Use of the mirror to retract the tongue (Fig. 37-8).
5. Combinations of the above.

When retracting, care should be taken to avoid irritation to the angles of the mouth. If the lips and skin are dry, softening the lips with petroleum jelly before beginning instrumentation is a helpful precaution against cracking and bleeding. Careful retraction is especially important for patients with a history of recurrent herpes labialis because these patients may easily develop herpetic lesions following instrumentation.

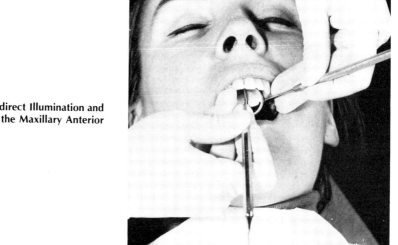

Figure 37–4 Combination of Indirect Illumination and Vision for the Lingual Surfaces of the Maxillary Anterior Teeth.

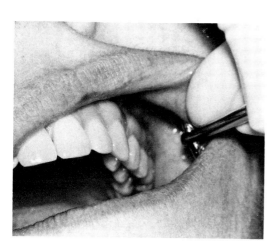

Figure 37–5 Retracting the cheek with the mirror and fingers of the nonoperating hand.

Figure 37–6 Retracting the Cheek with the Mirror.

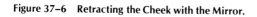

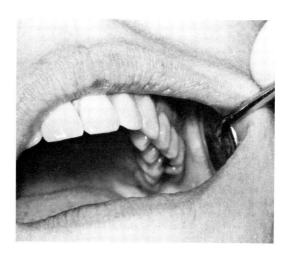

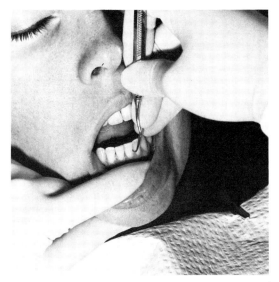

Figure 37–7   Retracting the Lip with the Index Finger of the Nonoperating Hand.

Condition of Instruments (Sharpness)

Prior to any instrumentation, all instruments should be inspected to make sure that they are clean, sterile, and in good condition. The working ends of pointed or bladed instruments must be sharp to be effective. Sharp instruments enhance tactile sensitivity and allow the clinician to work more precisely and efficiently. Dull instruments may lead to incomplete calculus removal and unnecessary trauma be-

cause of the excess force usually applied to compensate for their ineffectiveness. (See Chapter 39, "Sharpening of Periodontal Instruments.")

Maintaining a Clean Field

Despite good visibility, illumination, and retraction, instrumentation can be hampered if the operative field is obscured by saliva, blood, and debris. Pooling of saliva interferes with visibility during instrumentation and impedes control because a firm finger rest cannot be established on wet, slippery tooth surfaces. Adequate suction with a saliva ejector or, if working with an assistant, an aspirator, is essential.

Gingival bleeding is an unavoidable consequence of subgingival instrumentation. In areas of inflammation this is not necessarily an indication of trauma from incorrect technique; rather, it is an indication of ulceration of the pocket epithelium. Blood and debris can be removed from the operative field with suction and by wiping or blotting with gauze squares. The operative field should also be flushed occasionally with water.

Compressed air and gauze squares can be used to facilitate visual inspection of tooth surfaces just below the gingival margin during instrumentation. A jet of air directed into the pocket will deflect a retractable gingival margin. Retractable tissue can also be deflected away from the tooth by gently packing the edge of the gauze square into the pocket with the back of a curette. Immediately after the gauze is removed, the subgingival area should be clean, dry, and clearly visible for a brief interval.

Instrument Stabilization

Stability of the instrument and the hand is the primary requisite for controlled instrumentation. Stability and control are essential for effective instrumentation and avoidance of injury to the patient or the clinician. The two factors of major importance in providing stability are the instrument grasp and the finger rest.

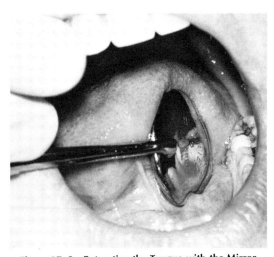

Figure 37–8   Retracting the Tongue with the Mirror.

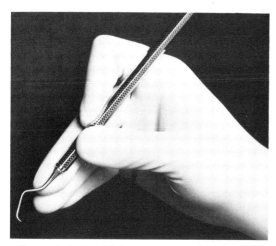

Figure 37–9 Modified Pen Grasp. Pad of the middle finger rests on the shank.

Instrument grasp

A proper grasp is essential for the precise control of movements made during periodontal instrumentation. The most effective and stable grasp for all periodontal instruments is the *modified pen grasp* (Fig. 37–9). Although other grasps are possible, this modification of the *standard pen grasp* (Fig. 37–10) insures the greatest control in performing intraoral procedures. The thumb, index finger, and middle finger are used to hold the instrument as a pen is held, but the middle finger is positioned so that the pad rather than the side of the finger is resting on the instrument shank. The index finger is bent at the second joint from the fingertip and is positioned well above the middle finger on the same side of the handle. The pad of the thumb is placed *midway* between the middle and index fingers on the opposite side of the handle. This creates a triangle of forces or *tripod effect* that enhances control because it counteracts the tendency for the instrument to turn uncontrollably between the fingers when scaling force is applied to the tooth. This stable modified pen grasp also enhances control because it enables the clinician to roll the instrument in precise degrees against the index and middle fingers with the thumb in order to adapt the blade to the slightest changes in tooth contour. The modified pen grasp also enhances tactile sensitivity because slight irregularities on the tooth surface are best perceived when the tactile sensitive pad of the middle finger is placed on the shank of the instrument.

The *palm and thumb grasp* (Fig. 37–11) is useful for stabilizing instruments during sharpening or for manipulating air and water syringes, but it is not recommended for periodontal instrumentation. Maneuverability and tactile sensitivity are so inhibited by this grasp that it is unsuitable for the precise and controlled movements necessary during periodontal procedures.

Figure 37–10 Standard Pen Grasp. Side of the middle finger rests on the shank.

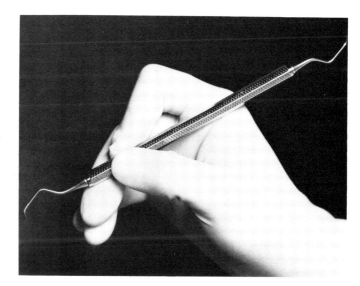

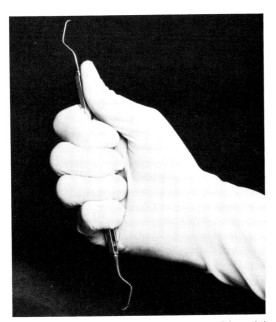

Figure 37-11   Palm and Thumb Grasp. Used for stabilizing instruments during sharpening.

Finger rest

The finger rest serves to stabilize the hand and the instrument by providing a firm fulcrum as movements are made to activate the instrument. A good finger rest prevents injury and laceration of the gingiva and surrounding tissues by poorly controlled instruments. The fourth or ring finger is preferred by most clinicians for the finger rest. Although it is possible to use the third or middle finger for the finger rest, this is not recommended because it restricts the arc of movement during the activation of strokes and severely curtails the use of the middle finger for both control and tactile sensitivity. Maximum control is achieved when the middle finger is kept between the instrument shank and the fourth finger. This "built-up fulcrum" is an integral part of the wrist-forearm action that activates the powerful working stroke for calculus removal. Whenever possible, these two fingers should be kept together during scaling and root planing, to work as a one-unit fulcrum. The separation of the middle and fourth finger during scaling strokes results in a loss of power and control because the separation of the fingers forces the clini-

cian to rely solely on finger-flexing for activation of the instrument.

Finger rests may be generally classified as *intraoral* finger rests or *extraoral* fulcrums. Intraoral finger rests on tooth surfaces are ideally established close to the working area. Variations of intraoral finger rests and extraoral fulcrums are utilized whenever good angulation and a sufficient arc of movement cannot be achieved by a finger rest close to the working area. The following examples illustrate the different variations of the intraoral finger rest:

1. *Conventional.* The finger rest is established on tooth surfaces immediately adjacent to the working area (Fig. 37-12).
2. *Cross-arch.* The finger rest is established on tooth surfaces on the other side of the same arch (Fig. 37-13).
3. *Opposite arch.* The finger rest is established on tooth surfaces on the opposite arch, e.g., mandibular arch finger rest for instrumentation on the maxillary arch (Fig. 37-14).
4. *Finger-on-finger.* The finger rest is established on the index finger or thumb of the nonoperating hand (Fig. 37-15).

Extraoral fulcrums are essential for ef-

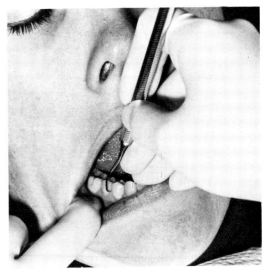

Figure 37-12 Intraoral Conventional Finger Rest. Fourth finger rests on the occlusal surfaces of adjacent teeth.

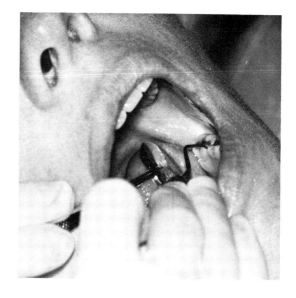

Figure 37–13   Intraoral Cross-Arch Finger Rest. Fourth finger rests on the incisal surfaces of teeth on the opposite side of the same arch.

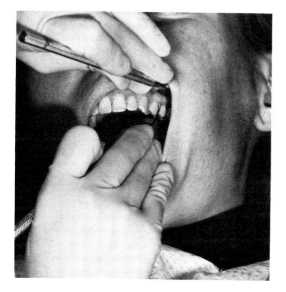

Figure 37–14   Intraoral Opposite Arch Finger Rest. Fourth finger rests on mandibular teeth while maxillary posterior teeth are instrumented.

Figure 37–15   Intraoral Finger-on-Finger Rest. Fourth finger rest on the index finger of nonoperating hand.

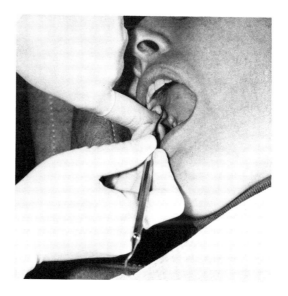

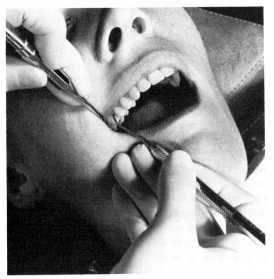

Figure 37–16 Extraoral Palm-up Fulcrum. Backs of fingers rest on right lateral aspect of mandible while maxillary right posterior teeth are instrumented.

patient's face to provide the greatest degree of stability. The two most commonly used extraoral fulcrums are shown.

1. *Palm-up.* The fulcrum is established by resting the backs of the middle and fourth fingers on the skin overlying the lateral aspect of the mandible on the right side of the face (Fig. 37–16).

2. *Palm-down.* The fulcrum is established by resting the front surfaces of the middle and fourth fingers on the skin overlying the lateral aspect of the mandible on the left side of the face (Fig. 37–17).

Both intraoral finger rests and extraoral fulcrums may be reinforced by applying the index finger or thumb of the nonoperating hand to the handle or shank for added control and pressure against the tooth. The reinforcing finger is usually employed for opposite arch or extraoral fulcrums where precise control and pressure are compromised by the longer distance between the fulcrum and the working end of the instrument. Figure 37–18 shows the index finger reinforced, and Figure 37–19 shows the thumb reinforced.

fective instrumentation of some aspects of the maxillary posterior teeth (see Chapter 38). When properly established, they allow optimal access and angulation while providing adequate stabilization. Extraoral fulcrums are not finger rests in the literal sense because the tips or pads of the fingers are not used for extraoral fulcrums as they are for intraoral finger rests. Instead, as much of the front or back surface of the fingers as possible is placed on the

Instrument Activation

Adaptation

Adaptation refers to the manner in which the working end of a periodontal

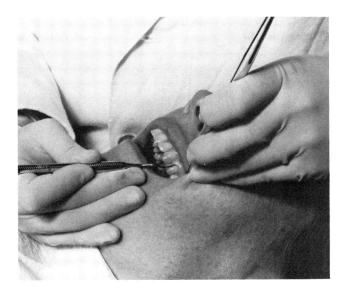

Figure 37–17 Extraoral Palm-down Fulcrum. Front surfaces of fingers rest on left lateral aspect of mandible while maxillary left posterior teeth are instrumented.

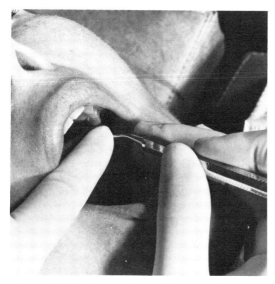

Figure 37–18 Index Finger Reinforced Rest. Index finger placed on shank for pressure and control in maxillary left posterior lingual region.

and to insure maximum effectiveness of instrumentation.

Correct adaptation of the probe is quite simple. The tip and side of the probe should be flush against the tooth surface as vertical strokes are activated within the crevice. Bladed instruments such as curettes and sharp-pointed instruments such as explorers are more difficult to adapt. The ends of these instruments are sharp and can lacerate tissue, so adaptation in subgingival areas becomes especially important. The lower third of the working end, which is the last few millimeters adjacent to the toe or tip, must constantly be kept in contact with the tooth while moving over varying tooth contours (Fig. 37–20). Precise adaptation is maintained by carefully rolling the handle of the instrument against the index and middle fingers with the thumb. This rotates the instrument in slight degrees so that the toe or tip leads into concavities and around convexities. On convex surfaces such as line angles, it is not possible to adapt more than a millimeter or two of the working end against the tooth. On broad flat surfaces, however, more of the working end may be adapted.

instrument is placed against the surface of a tooth. The objective of adaptation is to make the working end of the instrument conform to the contour of the tooth surface. Precise adaptation must be maintained with all instruments to avoid trauma to the soft tissues and root surfaces

If only the middle third of the working

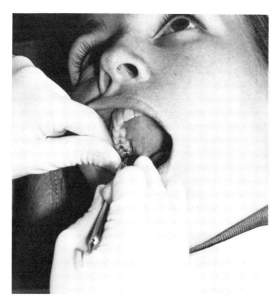

Figure 37–19 Thumb Reinforced Rest. Thumb placed on handle for control in maxillary right posterior lingual region.

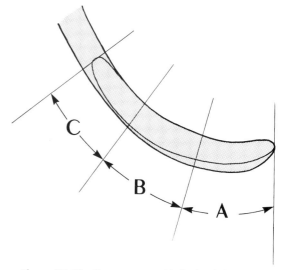

Figure 37–20 Gracey curette blade divided into three segments: the lower one third of the blade consisting of the terminal few millimeters adjacent to the toe; the middle one third; and the upper one third which is adjacent to the shank.

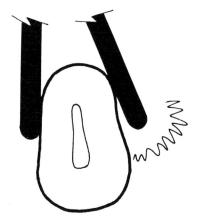

Figure 37–21   Blade Adaptation. The curette on the left is properly adapted to the root surface. The curette on the right is incorrectly adapted so that the toe juts out, lacerating the soft tissues.

end is adapted on a convex surface, so that it contacts the tooth at a tangent, the toe or sharp tip will jut out into soft tissue, causing trauma and discomfort (Fig. 37–21). If the instrument is adapted so that *only* the toe or tip is in contact, the soft tissue can be distended or compressed by the back of the working end, also causing trauma and discomfort. A curette that is improperly adapted in this manner can be particularly damaging because the toe can gouge or groove the root surface.

Angulation

Angulation refers to the angle between the face of a bladed instrument and the tooth surface. It may also be called the "tooth-blade relationship."

Correct angulation is essential for effective calculus removal. For subgingival insertion of a bladed instrument such as a curette, angulation should be as close to 0° as possible (Fig. 37–22). The end of the instrument can be inserted to the base of the pocket more easily with the face of the blade flush against the tooth. During scaling and root planing, optimal angulation is between 45° and 90° (Fig. 37–22). The exact blade angulation depends on the amount and nature of the calculus, the procedure being performed, and the condition of the tissue. Blade angulation is diminished or closed by tilting the lower shank of the instrument toward the tooth. It is increased or opened by tilting the lower shank away from the tooth.

During scaling strokes on heavy tenacious calculus, angulation should be just less than 90° so that the cutting edge "bites" into the calculus. With angulation of less than 45°, the cutting edge will not "bite" into or engage the calculus properly (Fig. 37–22). Instead, it will slide over the calculus, smoothing or "burnishing" it. If angulation is more than 90° the lateral surface of

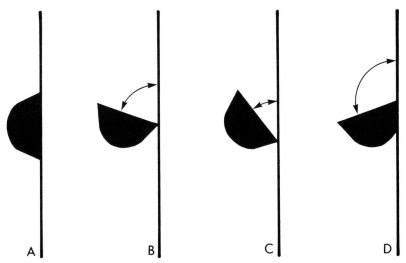

Figure 37–22   Blade Angulation. *A,* 0°—correct angulation for blade insertion. *B,* 45°–90°—correct angulation for scaling and root planing. *C,* Less than 45°—incorrect angulation for scaling and root planing. *D,* More than 90°—incorrect angulation for scaling and root planing, correct angulation for gingival curettage.

the blade, rather than the cutting edge, is against the tooth and the calculus is not removed or becomes burnished (Fig. 37–22). After the calculus has been removed, angulation of just less than 90° may be maintained or the angle may be slightly closed as the root surface is smoothed with light root planing strokes.

When gingival curettage is indicated, angulation greater than 90° is deliberately established so that the opposite cutting edge will engage and remove the pocket lining.

Lateral pressure

Lateral pressure refers to the pressure created when force is applied against the surface of a tooth with the cutting edge of a bladed instrument. The exact amount of pressure applied must be varied according to the nature of the calculus and according to whether the stroke is intended for initial scaling to remove calculus or for root planing to smooth the root surface.

Lateral pressure may be described as being firm, moderate, or light. When removing calculus, firm or moderate lateral pressure is used initially and is progressively diminished until light lateral pressure is applied for the final root planing strokes. When insufficient lateral pressure is applied for

the removal of heavy calculus, rough ledges or lumps may be shaved to thin, smooth sheets of burnished calculus that are very difficult to detect and remove. This burnishing effect often occurs in areas of developmental depressions and along the cemento-enamel junction.

Although firm lateral pressure is necessary for thorough removal of calculus, the indiscriminate, unwarranted, or uncontrolled application of heavy forces during instrumentation should be avoided. Repeated application of excessively heavy strokes will nick or gouge the root surface.

The careful application of varied and controlled amounts of lateral pressure during instrumentation is an integral part of effective scaling and root planing technique and is absolutely critical to the success of both of these procedures.

Strokes

Three basic types of strokes are used during instrumentation: the exploratory stroke, the scaling stroke, and the root planing stroke. Any of these basic strokes may be activated by a pull or a push motion in a vertical, oblique, or horizontal direction (Fig. 37–23). Vertical and oblique strokes are used most frequently. Horizontal

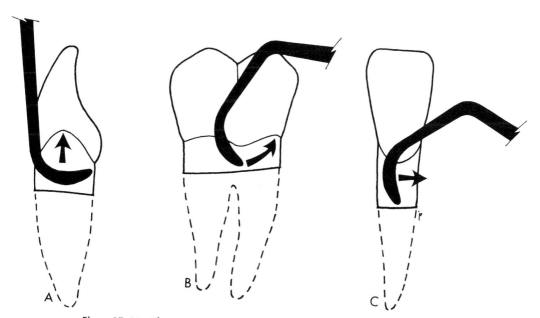

Figure 37–23 **Three Basic Stroke Directions.** *A,* Vertical. *B,* Oblique. *C,* Horizontal.

strokes are used selectively on line angles or deep pockets that cannot be negotiated with vertical or oblique strokes. The direction, length, pressure, and number of strokes necessary for either scaling or root planing are determined by four major factors: gingival position and tone, pocket depth and shape, tooth contour, and the amount and nature of the calculus or roughness.

The exploratory stroke is a light, "feeling" stroke that is used with probes and explorers to evaluate the dimensions of the pocket and to detect calculus and irregularities of the tooth surface. With bladed instruments such as the curette, the exploratory stroke is alternated with scaling and root planing strokes for these same purposes of evaluation and detection. The instrument is grasped lightly and adapted with light pressure against the tooth to achieve maximum tactile sensitivity.

The scaling stroke is a short, powerful, pull stroke that is used with bladed instruments for the removal of both supragingival and subgingival calculus. The muscles of the fingers and hand are tensed to establish a secure grasp, and lateral pressure is firmly applied against the tooth surface. The cutting edge engages the apical border of the calculus and dislodges it with a firm movement in a coronal direction. The scaling motion should be initiated in the forearm and transmitted from the wrist to the hand with slight flexing of the fingers. Rotation of the wrist is synchronized with movement of the forearm. The scaling stroke is not initiated in the wrist or fingers, nor is it carried out independently without the use of the forearm.

It is possible to initiate the scaling motion by rotating the wrist and forearm or by flexing the fingers. The use of wrist and forearm action versus the finger motion has long been debated among clinicians. Perhaps the strong feelings on both sides should be the most valid indication that there is a time and place for both. Neither method can be advocated exclusively because a careful analysis of effective scaling and root planing technique reveals that, indeed, both types of stroke activation are necessary for complete instrumentation. The wrist and forearm motion, pivoting in an arc on the finger rest, produces a more powerful stroke and is therefore preferred for scaling. Finger flexing is indicated for precise control over stroke length in areas such as line angles and when horizontal strokes are used on the lingual or facial aspects of narrow-rooted teeth.

The push scaling motion has been advocated by some clinicians. In the push stroke, the instrument engages the lateral or coronal border of the calculus and the fingers provide a thrust motion that dislodges the deposit. Because the push stroke may force calculus into the supporting tissues, its use, especially in an apical direction, is not recommended.

The root planing stroke is a moderate to light pull stroke that is used for final smoothing and planing of the root surface. Although hoes, files, and ultrasonic instruments have been used for root planing, curettes are widely acknowledged as the most effective and versatile instruments for this procedure.[3, 5, 6, 8, 10, 12, 16, 19] The design of the curette, which allows it to be more easily adapted to subgingival tooth contours makes curettes particularly suitable for root planing of periodontal patients who have deep pockets and furcation involvements. With a moderately firm grasp, the curette is kept adapted to the tooth with even lateral pressure. A continuous series of long, overlapping, shaving strokes is activated. As the surface becomes smoother and resistance diminishes, lateral pressure is progressively reduced.

PRINCIPLES OF SCALING AND ROOT PLANING

Definitions and Rationale for Scaling and Root Planing

Scaling is the process by which plaque and calculus are removed from both supragingival and subgingival tooth surfaces. There is no deliberate attempt to remove tooth substance along with the calculus. *Root planing* is the process by which residual embedded calculus and portions of cementum are removed from the roots to produce a smooth, hard, clean surface.

The primary objective of scaling and root planing is to restore gingival health by completely removing from the tooth surface factors that provoke gingival inflammation: plaque, calculus, and altered cementum. Scaling and root planing are not separate procedures. All the principles of scaling apply equally to root planing. The difference between scaling and root planing is only a matter of degree. The nature of the tooth surface determines the degree to which the surface must be scaled or planed.

On enamel surfaces, plaque and calculus provoke gingival inflammation. Unless grooved or pitted, enamel surfaces are relatively smooth and uniform. When plaque and calculus form on enamel, the deposits are usually superficially attached to the surface and not locked into irregularities. Scaling alone is sufficient to completely remove plaque and calculus from enamel, leaving a smooth, clean surface.

Root surfaces exposed to plaque and calculus pose a different problem. Studies by Zander[20] and Moskow[9] have shown that deposits of calculus on root surfaces are frequently embedded in cemental irregularities; scaling alone is therefore insufficient to remove them. A portion of the cementum itself must be removed to eliminate these deposits. Furthermore, when cementum is exposed to plaque and the pocket environment, its surface is permeated by toxic substances, notably endotoxins.[1, 2, 7] Recent evidence suggests that this altered cementum is a source of gingival irritation and must be removed by root planing to produce a hard, clean, unaltered surface that is free of toxic substances.[1] The removal of the altered cementum may expose dentin. Although this is not the aim of treatment, it may be unavoidable.[12, 16]

Scaling and root planing should not be thought of or practiced as separate procedures. It is apparent that scaling *without* root planing will often be inadequate to remove from root surfaces all the factors responsible for gingival inflammation.

As the rationale for scaling and root planing is thoroughly understood, it becomes apparent that mastery of these skills is essential to the ultimate success of any course of periodontal therapy. Of all clinical dental procedures, subgingival scaling and root planing in deep pockets are the most difficult and exacting skills to master. It has been argued that such proficiency in

instrumentation cannot be attained; therefore, periodontal surgery is necessary to gain access to root surfaces. Others have argued that although proficiency is possible, it need not be developed because access to the roots can be gained more easily with surgery. However, without mastering subgingival scaling and root planing skills, the clinician will be severely hampered and unable to treat adequately those patients for whom surgery is contraindicated.

Detection Skills

Good visual and tactile detection skills are required for accurate initial assessment of the extent and nature of deposits and root irregularities before scaling and root planing. Valid self-evaluation upon completion of instrumentation depends on these detection skills.

Visual examination of supragingival calculus or of subgingival calculus just below the gingival margin is not difficult with good lighting and a clean field. Light deposits of supragingival calculus are often difficult to see when wet with saliva. Compressed air may be used to dry supragingival calculus until it is chalky white and easily visible. It may also be directed into the pocket in a steady stream to deflect the marginal gingiva away from the tooth so that subgingival deposits near the surface can be seen.

Tactile exploration of the tooth surfaces in subgingival areas of pocket depth, furcations, and developmental depressions is much more difficult than visual examination of supragingival areas and requires the skilled use of a fine-pointed explorer or probe. The explorer or probe is held with a light but stable modified pen grasp. This provides maximum tactile sensitivity for detection of subgingival calculus and other irregularities. The pads of the thumb and fingers, especially the middle finger, should perceive the slight vibrations conducted through the instrument shank and handle as irregularities of the tooth surface are encountered.

After a stable finger rest is established, the tip of the instrument is carefully inserted subgingivally to the base of the pocket. Light exploratory strokes are activated vertically up and down on the root surface. When calculus is encountered, the tip of the instrument should be advanced apically over the deposit until the termination of the calculus on the root is felt. The distance between the apical edge of the calculus and the bottom of the pocket usually ranges from 0.2 to 1.0 millimeters. The tip is adapted closely to the tooth to insure the greatest degree of tactile sensitivity and to avoid tissue trauma. When exploring a proximal surface, strokes must be extended at least halfway across that surface past the contact area to insure complete detection of interproximal deposits. When an explorer is used at line angles, convexities, and concavities, the handle of the instrument must be rolled slightly between the thumb and fingers to keep the tip constantly adapted to the changes in tooth contour.

Although exploring technique and good tactile sensitivity are very important, interpreting varying degrees of roughness and making clinical judgments based on these interpretations also requires much expertise. The beginning student usually has difficulty detecting fine calculus and altered cementum. One must begin by recognizing ledges, lumps, or spurs of calculus, then smaller spicules, then slight roughness, and finally, a slight graininess that feels like a sticky coating or film covering the tooth surface. Overhanging or deficient margins of dental restorations, caries, decalcification, and root roughness caused by previous instrumentation are all commonly found during exploration. These and other irregularities must be recognized and differentiated from subgingival calculus. Because this requires a great deal of experience and a high degree of tactile sensitivity, many clinicians agree that the development of detection skills is equally as important as the mastery of scaling and root planing technique.

Supragingival Scaling Technique

Supragingival calculus is generally less tenacious and less calcified than subgingival calculus. Since instrumentation is performed coronal to the gingival margin, scaling strokes are not confined by surrounding tissues. This makes adaptation and angulation easier. It also allows direct visibility as well as a freedom of movement that is not possible during subgingival scaling.

Sickles, curettes, and ultrasonic instruments are most commonly used for the removal of supragingival calculus. Hoes and chisels are less frequently used. To perform supragingival scaling, the sickle or curette is held with a modified pen grasp, and a firm finger rest is established on the teeth adjacent to the working area. The blade is adapted with an angulation of slightly less than 90° to the surface being scaled. The cutting edge should engage the apical margin of the supragingival calculus while short, powerful, overlapping scaling strokes are activated coronally in a vertical or oblique direction. The sharp pointed tip of the sickle can easily lacerate marginal tissue or gouge exposed root surfaces, so careful adaptation is especially important when this instrument is being used. The tooth surface is instrumented until it is visually and tactilely free of all supragingival deposits. If the tissue is retractable enough to allow easy insertion of the bulky blade, the sickle may be used slightly below the free gingival margin. If the sickle is used in this manner, final scaling and root planing with the curette should always follow.

Ultrasonic instrumentation for removal of supragingival calculus is described on page 662.

Subgingival Scaling and Root Planing Technique

Subgingival scaling and root planing are far more complex and difficult to perform than supragingival scaling. Subgingival calculus is usually harder than supragingival calculus, and it is often locked into root irregularities, making it more tenacious and therefore more difficult to remove.[9, 13, 20]

The overlying tissue creates significant problems in subgingival instrumentation. Vision is obscured by the bleeding that inevitably occurs during instrumentation as well as by the tissue itself. The clinician must rely heavily on tactile sensitivity to detect calculus and irregularities, to guide the instrument blade during scaling and root planing, and to evaluate the results of instrumentation.

In addition, the direction and length of the strokes are limited by the adjacent pocket wall. The confines of the soft tissue make careful adaptation to tooth contours imperative in order to avoid trauma. Such precise adaptation cannot be accomplished without a thorough knowledge of tooth morphology. The clinician must form a mental image of the tooth surface to anticipate variations in contour, continually confirming or modifying the image in response to tactile sensations and visual cues like the position of the instrument handle and shank. The clinician must then instantaneously adjust the adaptation and angulation of the working end to the tooth. It is this complex and precise coordination of visual, mental, and manual skills that makes subgingival instrumentation one of the most difficult of all dental skills.

The curette is preferred by most clinicians for subgingival scaling and root planing because of the advantages afforded by its design. The curved blade, rounded toe, and curved back allow the curette to be inserted to the base of the pocket and to be adapted to variations in tooth contour with a minimum of tissue displacement and trauma.

Hoes, files, and ultrasonic instruments are also used for subgingival scaling of heavy calculus but are not recommended for root planing. Although some delicate files may be inserted to the base of the pocket to crush or initially fracture tenacious deposits, heavier files, hoes, and ultrasonic instruments are bulky and cannot be easily inserted into deep pockets or where tissue is firm and fibrotic. Hoes and files are not able to produce as smooth a surface as curettes.[3, 12] Ultrasonics are effective for removal of readily accessible calculus, but curettes have been shown to be clearly superior for the removal of subgingival cementum.[16] Hoes, files, and ultrasonic instruments are all more hazardous than is the curette in terms of trauma to the root surface and surrounding tissues.[3, 10, 12]

Subgingival scaling and root planing are accomplished with either universal or area-specific (Gracey) curettes by the following basic procedure. The curette is held with a modified pen grasp, and a stable finger rest is established. The correct cutting edge is lightly adapted to the tooth, with the lower shank kept parallel with the tooth surface. The lower shank is moved toward the tooth so that the face of the blade is nearly flush with the tooth surface. The blade is then inserted under the gingiva and advanced to the base of the pocket by a light exploratory stroke. When the cutting edge reaches the base of the pocket, a working angulation between 45 and 90° is established, and pressure is applied laterally against the tooth surface. Calculus is removed by a series of controlled, overlapping, short, powerful strokes primarily utilizing wrist-arm motion (Fig. 37–24). As calculus is removed, resistance

Figure 37–24 Subgingival Scaling Procedure.
A, Curette inserted with face of blade flush against tooth. *B,* Working angulation (45°−90°) is established at base of pocket. *C,* Lateral pressure is applied and scaling stroke is activated in coronal direction.

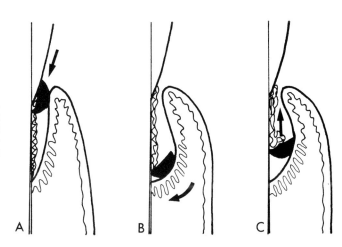

to the passage of the cutting edge diminishes until only slight roughness remains. Longer, lighter root planing strokes are then activated with less lateral pressure until the root surface is completely smooth and hard. The instrument handle must be rolled carefully between the thumb and fingers to keep the blade adapted closely to the tooth surface as line angles, developmental depressions, and other changes in tooth contour are followed.

Scaling and root planing strokes should be confined to the portion of the tooth where calculus or altered cementum is found. This zone is known as the "instrumentation zone." Sweeping the instrument over the crown where it is not needed wastes operating time, dulls the instrument, and causes loss of control.

The amount of lateral pressure applied to the tooth surface depends on the nature of the calculus and whether the strokes are for initial calculus removal or for final root planing. If heavy lateral pressure is continued after the bulk of calculus has been removed, and if the blade is repeatedly readapted with short, "choppy" strokes, the result will be a root surface roughened by numerous nicks and gouges, resembling the rippled surface of a washboard.[11] If heavy lateral pressure is continued with long, even strokes, the result will be excessive removal of root structure, producing a smooth but "ditched" or "riffled" root surface. To avoid these hazards of overinstrumentation, a deliberate transition from short, powerful scaling strokes to longer, lighter root planing strokes must be made as soon as calculus and initial roughness have been eliminated.

When scaling strokes are used to remove calculus, force can be maximized by concentrating the lateral pressure onto the lower third of the blade (Fig. 37–20). This small section, the terminal few millimeters of the blade, is positioned slightly apical to the lateral edge of the deposit, and a short vertical or oblique stroke is used to split the calculus from the tooth surface. Without withdrawing the instrument from the pocket, the lower third of the blade is advanced laterally and repositioned to engage the next portion of the remaining deposit. Another vertical or oblique stroke is made, slightly overlapping the previous stroke. This process is repeated in a series

of powerful scaling strokes until the entire deposit has been removed. The overlapping of these pathways or "channels" of instrumentation[11] insures that the entire instrumentation zone is covered.

Engaging a large tenacious ledge or piece of calculus with the entire length of the cutting edge is not recommended, because the force is distributed through a longer section of the cutting edge rather than being concentrated. Far more lateral pressure is required to dislodge the entire deposit in one stroke. Although some clinicians may possess the strength to remove calculus completely in this manner, the heavier forces that are required diminish tactile sensitivity and contribute to a loss of control that results in tissue trauma. A single heavy stroke usually is not sufficient to remove calculus entirely. Instead, the blade skips over or skims the surface of the deposit. Subsequent strokes made with the entire cutting edge tend to shave the deposit down layer by layer, and when a series of these repeated whittling strokes is applied, the calculus may be reduced to a thin, smooth, "burnished" sheet that is very difficult to distinguish from the surrounding root surface.

A common error in instrumenting proximal surfaces is failing to reach the mid-proximal region apical to the contact because this area is relatively inaccessible and requires more instrumentation skill than do buccal or lingual surfaces. It is extremely important to extend strokes at least halfway across the proximal surface so that no calculus or roughness remains in the interproximal area. With properly designed curettes, this can be accomplished by keeping the lower shank of the curette parallel to the long axis of the tooth (Fig. 37–25). With the lower shank parallel to the long axis, the blade of the curette will reach the base of the pocket and the toe will extend beyond the midline as strokes are advanced across the proximal surface. This extension of strokes beyond the midline insures thorough exploration and instrumentation of these surfaces. If the lower shank is angled or tilted away from the tooth, the toe will move toward the contact area. Because this prevents the blade from reaching the base of the pocket, calculus apical to the contact will not be detected or removed. Strokes will be hampered because

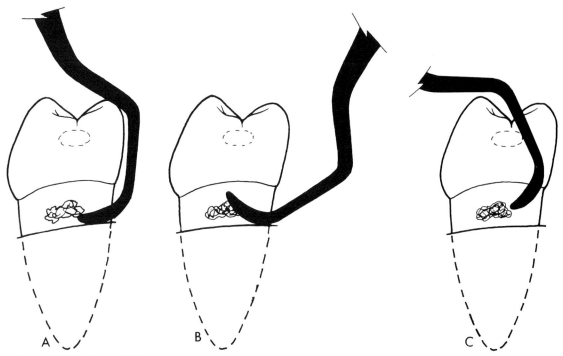

Figure 37–25   Shank Position for Scaling Proximal Surfaces. *A,* Correct shank position, parallel to long axis of the tooth. *B,* Incorrect shank position, tilted away from tooth. *C,* Incorrect shank position tilted too far toward the tooth.

the toe tends to become lodged in the contact (Fig. 37–25). If the instrument is angled or tilted too far toward the tooth, the lower shank will hit the tooth or the contact area, preventing extension of strokes to the mid-proximal region (Fig. 37–25).

The relationship between the location of the finger rest and the working area is important for two reasons. First, the finger rest or fulcrum must be positioned to allow the lower shank of the instrument to be parallel or nearly parallel to the tooth surface being treated. This parallelism is a fundamental requirement for optimal working angulation.

Second, the finger rest must be positioned to enable the operator to use wrist-arm motion to activate strokes. On some aspects of the maxillary posterior teeth, these requirements can only be met with the use of extraoral or opposite arch fulcrums. When intraoral finger rests are used in other regions of the mouth, the finger rest must be close enough to the working area to fulfill these two requirements. A finger rest that is established too far away

from the working area forces the clinician to separate the middle finger from the fourth finger in an effort to obtain parallelism and proper angulation. Effective wrist-arm motion is only possible when these two fingers are kept together in a "built-up" fulcrum. Separation of the fingers commits the clinician to the exclusive use of finger flexing for the activation of strokes.

As instrumentation proceeds from one tooth to the next, the location of the finger rest must be frequently adjusted or repositioned to allow parallelism and wrist-arm motion.

Instruments for Scaling and Root Planing

Universal curettes

The working ends of the universal curette are designed in pairs so that all surfaces of the teeth can be treated with one double-ended instrument or a matched pair of single-ended instruments.

In any given quadrant, when approaching from the facial aspect, one end of the universal curette will adapt to the mesial surfaces and the other end will adapt to the distal surfaces. When approaching from the lingual aspect in the same quadrant, the double-ended universal curette must be turned end-for-end because the blades are mirror images. This means that the end that adapts to the mesial surfaces on the facial aspect also adapts to the distal surfaces on the lingual aspect and vice versa. Both ends of the universal curette are used to instrument the anterior teeth. On posterior teeth, however, owing to limited access to distal surfaces, a single working end can be used to treat both mesial and distal surfaces by using both of its cutting edges. To do this, the instrument is first adapted to the mesial surface with the handle nearly parallel to the mesial surface. Because the face of the universal curette blade is honed at 90° to the lower shank, if the lower shank is positioned so that it is absolutely parallel to the surface being instrumented, the tooth-blade angulation is 90°. In order to close this angle and thus obtain proper working angulation, the lower shank must be tilted slightly toward the tooth. The distal surface of the same posterior tooth can be instrumented with the opposite cutting edge of the same blade. This cutting edge can be adapted at proper working angulation by positioning the handle so that it is *perpendicular* to the distal surface (Fig. 37–26).

When adapting the universal curette blade, as much of the cutting edge as possible should be in contact with the tooth surface, except on narrow convex surfaces such as line angles. Although the entire cutting edge should contact the tooth, pressure should be concentrated to the lower third of the blade during scaling strokes. During root planing strokes, however, lateral pressure should be evenly distributed along the cutting edge.

The primary advantage of these curettes is that they are designed to be used universally on all tooth surfaces, in all regions of the mouth. However, universal curettes have limited adaptability for treatment of periodontal patients with deep pockets in which apical migration of the attachment has exposed furcations, root convexities, and developmental depressions. For this

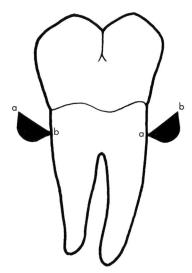

Figure 37–26   Adaptation of the Universal Curette on a Posterior Tooth. Cross-sectional representations of the same universal curette blade as its cutting edges are adapted to the mesial and distal surfaces of a posterior tooth.

reason, the Gracey curettes, which are area-specific and specially designed for subgingival scaling and root planing of periodontal patients, are preferred by many clinicians.

Gracey curettes

Gracey curettes are a set of area-specific instruments that were designed by Dr. Clayton H. Gracey of Michigan in the mid-1930's.

Four design features make the Gracey curettes unique: (1) they are area-specific; (2) only one cutting edge on each blade is used; (3) the blade is curved in two planes; and (4) the blade is "offset." (These features have been summarized in Chapter 36 in a table shown on page 627.) Each of these features directly influences the manner in which the Graceys are used and should be discussed individually.

Area specificity. There are seven pairs of curettes in the set. The Gracey 1–2 and 3–4 are used on anterior teeth. The Gracey 5–6 may be used on both anterior and premolar teeth. The facial and lingual surfaces of posterior teeth are instrumented with the Gracey 7–8 and 9–10. The Gracey 11–12 is designed for mesial surfaces of posterior teeth, and the Gracey 13–14 adapts to the distal surfaces of posterior teeth. Although these guidelines for areas of use were originally established by Dr. Gracey, it is possible to use a Gracey curette in an area of the mouth other than the one for which it was specifically designed if the general principles are understood and applied. Gracey curettes need not be reserved exclusively for periodontally involved patients. In fact, many clinicians prefer Gracey curettes for general scaling because of their excellent adaptability.

Single Cutting Edge Used. Like a universal curette, the Gracey curette has a blade with two cutting edges. Unlike the universal curette, however, the Gracey instrument is designed so that only one cutting edge is used. In order to determine which of the two is the correct cutting edge to adapt to the tooth, the blade should be held face up and parallel to the floor. When viewed from this angle, the blade can be seen to curve to the side. One cutting edge forms a larger outer curve and the other forms a shorter, smaller inner curve. The larger outer curve, which has also been described as the inferior cutting edge or as the cutting edge further away from the handle, is the correct cutting edge (Fig. 37–27).

Blade Curves in Two Planes. Like the toe of the universal curette, the toe of the Gracey curette curves upward. However, the toe of the Gracey curette also curves to the side as previously mentioned. This

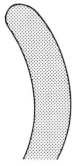

Figure 37–27 Determining the Correct Cutting Edge of a Gracey Curette. When viewed from directly above the face of the blade, the correct cutting edge is the one forming the larger, outer curve on the right.

unique curvature enhances the blade's adaptation to convexities and concavities as the working end is advanced around the tooth. Only the lower third or half of the Gracey blade is in contact with the tooth during instrumentation. The cutting edge of a universal curette blade, on the other hand, is straight and does not curve to the side. This makes it less adaptable to root concavities.

Offset Blade. Gracey curette blades are honed at an "offset" angle. This means that the face of the blade is not perpendicular to the lower shank as it is on a universal curette. Rather, Gracey curettes are designed so that the tooth-blade working angulation is 60 to 70° when the *lower shank* is held *parallel* to the tooth surface. Gracey curettes were originally designed to be used with push strokes and were beveled to provide tooth-blade angulation of 40° when the lower shank is parallel to the tooth surface. For many years, Graceys were only available in this form. Gracey curettes are now available not only in the original push design but also in a modified version to be used with pull strokes. It is important to understand this when purchasing Gracey curettes to avoid instruments that are not properly designed for pull strokes. When Graceys that are designed to be used with push strokes are used with pull strokes instead, they are very likely to burnish calculus rather than completely remove it. The design of the Gracey curette was modified to create an instrument that can be used with pull strokes in response to requests from clinicians who liked the shank design and adaptability of the original Gracey instruments but were opposed to the use of push strokes for scaling and root planing. The push stroke is not recommended, especially for the novice clinician, because it is very likely to cause undue trauma to the junctional epithelium and to embed fragments of dislodged calculus in the soft tissues.

The general principles of use of the Gracey curettes are essentially the same as those for the universal curette. (Those italicized apply only to Gracey curettes.)

1. *Determine the correct cutting edge.* The correct cutting edge should be determined by visually inspecting the blade and confirmed by lightly adapting this cutting

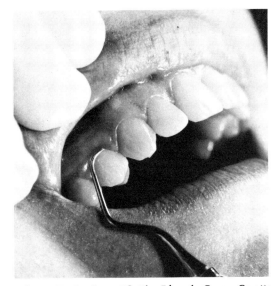

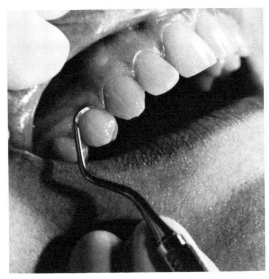

Figure 37–28 Correct Cutting Edge of a Gracey Curette Adapted to the Tooth.

Figure 37–29 Wrong Cutting Edge of a Gracey Curette Adapted to the Tooth.

edge to the tooth with the lower shank parallel to the surface of the tooth. With the toe pointed in the direction to be scaled, e.g., mesially with a 7–8, only the back of the blade can be seen if the correct cutting edge has been selected (Fig. 37–28). If the wrong cutting edge has been adopted, the flat, shiny face of the blade will be seen instead (Fig. 37–29).

2. *Make sure the lower shank is parallel with the surface to be instrumented.* The lower shank of a Gracey is that portion of the shank between the blade and the first bend in the shank. Parallelism of the handle

or upper shank is not an acceptable guide with Graceys because the angulations of the shanks vary. On anterior teeth, the lower shank of the Gracey 1–2, 3–4, or 5–6 should be parallel to the mesial, distal, facial, or lingual surfaces of the teeth (Fig. 37–30). On posterior teeth, the lower shank of the 7–8 or 9–10 should be parallel to the facial or lingual surfaces of the teeth (Fig. 37–31), the lower shank of the 11–12 should be parallel to the mesial surfaces of the teeth (Fig. 37–32), and the lower shank of the 13–14 should be parallel to the distal surfaces of the teeth (Fig. 37–33).

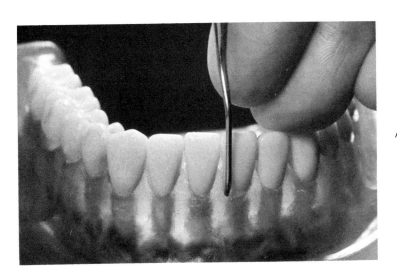

Figure 37–30 Gracey 5/6 Curette Adapted to an Anterior Tooth.

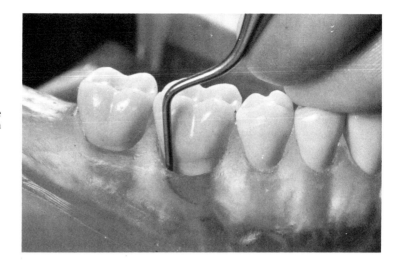

Figure 37–31 Gracey 7/8 Curette Adapted to the Facial Surface of a Posterior Tooth.

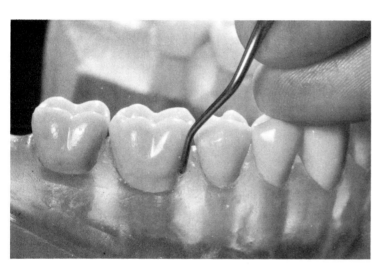

Figure 37–32 Gracey 11/12 Curette Adapted to the Mesial Surface of a Posterior Tooth.

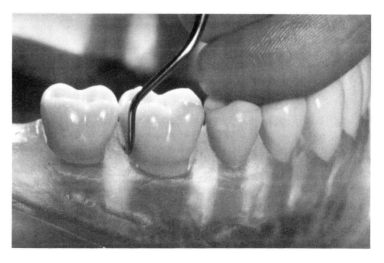

Figure 37–33 Gracey 13/14 Curette Adapted to the Distal Surface of a Posterior Tooth.

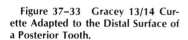

3. When using intraoral finger rests, keep the fourth and middle fingers together in a "built-up" fulcrum for maximum control and wrist-arm action.

4. Use extraoral fulcrums or mandibular finger rests when working on the maxillary posterior teeth for optimal angulation.

5. *Concentrate on using the lower third of the cutting edge for calculus removal,* especially on line angles or when attempting to remove a calculus ledge by breaking it away in sections beginning at the lateral edge.

6. Allow the wrist and forearm to carry the burden of the stroke rather than flexing the fingers.

7. Roll the handle slightly between the thumb and fingers to keep the blade adapted as the working end is advanced around line angles and into concavities.

8. Modulate lateral pressure from firm to moderate to light depending on the nature of the calculus, and reduce pressure as the transition is made from scaling to root planing strokes.

Ultrasonic scaling instruments

When properly utilized, the ultrasonic scaling device is a useful adjunct to conventional hand instrumentation. Owing to several limitations, however, it should never be considered or utilized as a substitute for hand instruments in scaling and root planing.

The vibrational energy produced by the ultrasonic instrument makes it useful for removing heavy, tenacious deposits of calculus and stain. Such deposits can be removed more quickly and with less effort than they can be manually. When ultrasonic instruments are properly manipulated, there is less tissue trauma and therefore less postoperative discomfort. This makes ultrasonic instrumentation useful for initial débridement in patients suffering from acute, painful conditions such as necrotizing ulcerative gingivitis.

Despite their effectiveness for gross supragingival scaling, ultrasonic instruments are significantly limited for subgingival scaling and root planing procedures. The working ends of the instruments are bulky and blunt. This makes subgingival insertion to the base of the pocket possible only when the tissue is extremely inflamed and retractable. It also greatly diminishes tactile sensitivity compared with hand instruments. The working end of the instrument must come into contact with the calculus deposit in order to fracture and remove it. Small pieces of calculus, particularly subgingival calculus, may easily be missed.

It has been shown that ultrasonic instruments will remove root substance.[1] Although cementum removal with ultrasonics is possible in easily accessible areas, the curette has been established as a far more effective instrument for overall root planing.[5, 6, 8, 16]

Visibility is hampered by the constant water spray that is necessary for the operation of the instrument. During ultrasonic instrumentation the tooth surface should be frequently examined with an explorer to evaluate the completeness of calculus removal; and the use of ultrasonics should always be followed by hand instrumentation for removal of residual deposits. These factors limit the use of ultrasonic instruments to the gross removal of heavy calculus, stain, and debris. Once this has been accomplished, curettes should be used to remove residual deposits and to root plane.

With these points in mind, the ultrasonic device is used in the following manner.

1. The instrument should be properly tuned to produce a light mist of water at the working tip. Adequate aspiration will be necessary to remove this water as it accumulates in the mouth. The power setting should be no higher than necessary to remove calculus. The clinician and the assistant should wear masks to minimize inhalation of the contaminated aerosol that is produced during instrumentation.

2. The instrument is grasped with a modified pen grasp, and a finger rest or fulcrum should be established as for conventional hand instrumentation.

The handle of the instrument is kept in the long axis of the tooth and the working end is adapted to conform to the contour of the tooth surface.

3. The instrument is switched on by stepping on the foot pedal. Short, light, vertical strokes are activated and the working end is passed over the deposit. Heavy lateral pressure is unnecessary because it

is the vibrational energy of the instrument that dislodges the calculus. However, the working end must touch the deposit for this to occur.

4. The working end should be kept in constant motion and the tip should never be held perpendicular to the surface of the tooth, as this would etch or groove the surface.

5. The foot pedal should be released periodically to allow for aspiration of water, and the tooth surface should be examined frequently with an explorer.

6. Scaling and root planing is completed with curettes or other hand instruments.

Evaluation of Scaling and Root Planing

The adequacy of scaling and root planing is evaluated when the procedure is performed and later, after a period of soft tissue healing.

Immediately following instrumentation, the tooth surfaces should be carefully inspected visually with optimum lighting and the aid of the mouth mirror and compressed air. They should also be examined with a fine explorer or probe. Subgingival surfaces should be hard and smooth. Although complete removal of calculus is definitely necessary for the health of the adjacent soft tissue,[17] there is little documented evidence that root smoothness is necessary.[5] Nevertheless, relative smoothness is still the best immediate clinical indication that calculus and altered cementum have been completely removed.[5]

Even though smoothness is the criterion by which scaling and root planing are immediately evaluated, the ultimate evaluation is based on tissue response.[17] Clinical evaluation of the soft tissue response to scaling and root planing, including probing, should not be conducted earlier than two weeks postoperatively. Stahl and associates[14, 15] have shown that re-epithelialization of the wounds created during instrumentation takes from one to two weeks. Until then, gingival bleeding on probing can be expected even when calculus has been completely removed, because the soft tissue wound is not epithelialized. Any gingival bleeding on probing that is noted after this interval is

more likely to be due to persistent inflammation produced by residual deposits that were not removed during the initial procedure or to inadequate plaque control.

There may be times when the clinician finds that some slight root roughness remains after scaling and root planing. If sound principles of instrumentation have been followed, the roughness may not be calculus. Since calculus removal, *not* root smoothness per se, has been shown to be necessary for tissue health, it might be more prudent in such a case to stop short of perfect smoothness and reevaluate the patient's tissue response after two weeks. This avoids overinstrumentation and removal of excessive root structure in a pursuit of smoothness for smoothness' sake. If the tissue is healthy after a two week interval, no further root planing is necessary. If the tissue is inflamed, the clinician must determine to what extent this is due to plaque accumulation or the presence of residual calculus and to what degree further root planing is necessary.

REFERENCES

1. Aleo, J., DeRenzis, F., Farber, P.: In vitro attachment of human gingival fibroblasts to root surfaces. J. Periodontol., 46:639, 1975.
2. Aleo, J., DeRenzis, F., Farber, P., and Varboncoeur, A.: The presence and biological activity of cementum bound endotoxin. J. Periodontol., 45:672, 1974.
3. Barnes, J. E., and Schaffer, E. M.: Subgingival root planing: a comparison using files, hoes, and curets. J. Periodontol., 31:300, 1960.
4. Clark, S., Group, H., and Mabler, D.: The effect of ultrasonic instrumentation on root surfaces. J. Periodontol., 39:125, 1968.
5. Garrett, J. S.: Root planing: a perspective. J. Periodontol., 48:553, 1977.
6. Green, E., and Ramfjord, S. R.: Tooth roughness after subgingival root planing. J. Periodontol., 37:396, 1966.
7. Hatfield, C. G., and Baumhammers, A.: Cytotoxic effects of periodontally involved surfaces of human teeth. Arch. Oral Biol., 16:465, 1971.
8. Kerry, G. J.: Roughness of root surfaces after use of ultrasonic instruments and hand curets. J. Periodontol., 38:340, 1967.
9. Moskow, B. S.: Calculus attachment in cemental separations. J. Periodontol., 40:125, 1969.
10. Orban, B., and Manella, V.: Macroscopic and microscopic study of instruments designed for root planing. J. Periodontol., 27:120, 1956.
11. Parr, R., Green, E., Madsen, L., and Miller, S.: *Subgingival Scaling and Root Planing.* Berkeley, California, Praxis Publishing Co., 1976.

12. Schaffer, E. M.: Histologic results of root curettage on human teeth. J. Periodontol., *27*:269, 1956.

13. Selvig, K.: Attachment of plaque and calculus to tooth surfaces. J. Periodontol. Res., *5*:8, 1970.

14. Stahl, S. S., Weiner, J. M., Benjamin, S., and Yamada, L.: Soft tissue healing following curettage and root planing, J. Periodontol., *42*:678, 1971.

15. Stahl, S. S., Slavkin, H. C., Yamada, L., and Levine, S.: Speculations about gingival repair. J. Periodontol., *43*:395, 1972.

16. Van Volkinburg, J., Green, E., and Armitage, G.: The nature of root surfaces after curette, cavi-tron, and alpha-sonic instrumentation. J. Periodontol. Res., *11*:374, 1976.

17. Waerhaug, J.: Healing of the dento-epithelial junction following subgingival plaque control. J. Periodontol., *49*:1, 1978.

18. Wilkins, E. M.: *Clinical Practice of the Dental Hygienist,* 4th ed., Philadelphia, Lea & Febiger, 1976, pp. 49–50.

19. Wilkinson, R. F., and Maybury, J.: Scanning electron microscopy of the root surface following instrumentation. J. Periodontol., *44*:559, 1973.

20. Zander, H. A.: The attachment of calculus to root surfaces. J. Periodontol., *24*:16, 1953.

Chapter 38

Instrumentation in Different Areas of the Mouth

Various approaches to instrumentation in different areas of the mouth are illustrated here in atlas form. The examples shown provide maximum efficiency for the clinician and comfort for the patient. For most areas, more than one approach is presented. Other approaches are possible and are acceptable if they provide equal efficiency and comfort.

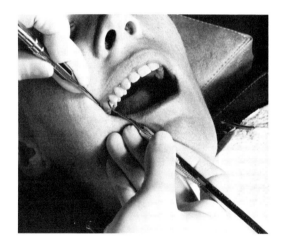

Figure 38–1 Maxillary Right Posterior Sextant; Facial Aspect.
Operator Position: Side position.
Illumination: Direct.
Visibility: Direct. Indirect for distal surfaces of molars.
Retraction: Mirror or index finger of nonoperating hand.
Finger Rest: Extra-oral, palm-up. Backs of the middle and fourth fingers on the lateral aspect of the mandible on the right side of the face.

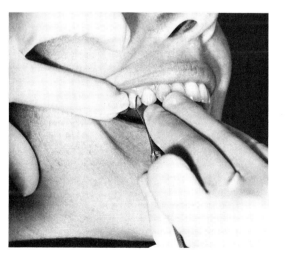

Figure 38–2 Maxillary Right Posterior Sextant; Facial Aspect.
Operator Position: Side or front position.
Illumination: Direct.
Visibility: Direct. Indirect for distal surfaces of molars.
Retraction: Mirror or index finger of nonoperating hand.
Finger Rest: Intra-oral, palm-down. Fourth finger on incisal or facial surfaces of maxillary anterior teeth or on occlusal or facial surfaces of maxillary bicuspid teeth.

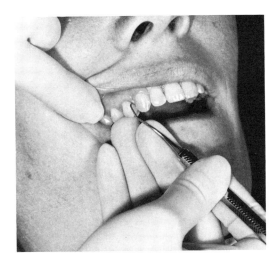

Figure 38–3 Maxillary Right Posterior Sextant, Premolar Region Only; Facial Aspect.

Operator Position: Side or back position.
Illumination: Direct.
Visibility: Direct.
Retraction: Mirror or index finger of nonoperating hand.
Finger Rest: Intra-oral, palm-up. Fourth finger on the occlusal surfaces of the adjacent maxillary posterior teeth.

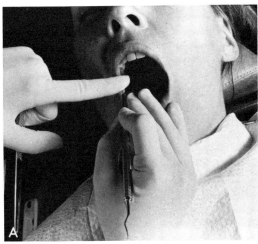

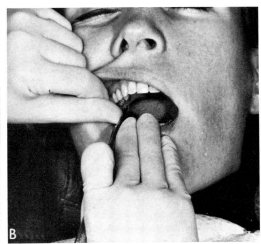

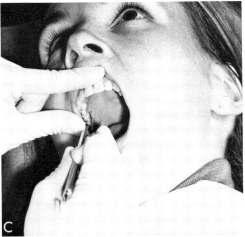

Figure 38–4 Maxillary Right Posterior Sextant; Lingual Aspect.

Operator Position: Front position.
Illumination: Direct.
Visibility: Direct.
Retraction: Index finger of nonoperating hand or no retraction.
Finger Rest: Intra-oral, palm-down, opposite arch, reinforced. Fourth finger on incisal edges of mandibular anterior teeth, reinforced with the thumb or index finger of the nonoperating hand.

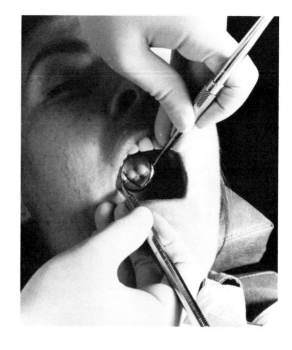

Figure 38–5 Maxillary Right Posterior Sextant; Lingual Aspect.
Operator Position: Side or front position.
Illumination: Direct and indirect.
Visibility: Direct or indirect.
Retraction: None.
Finger Rest: Extra-oral, palm-up. Backs of middle and fourth fingers on the lateral aspect of the mandible on the right side of the face.

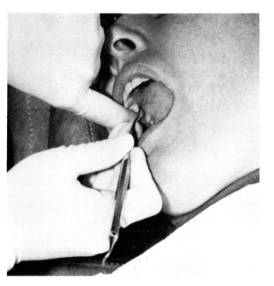

Figure 38–6 Maxillary Right Posterior Sextant; Lingual Aspect.
Operator Position: Front position.
Illumination: Direct.
Visibility: Direct.
Retraction: None.
Finger Rest: Intra-oral, palm-up, finger-on-finger. Index finger of nonoperating hand on occlusal surfaces of maxillary right posterior teeth. Fourth finger of operating hand on index finger of nonoperating hand.

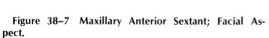

Figure 38–7 Maxillary Anterior Sextant; Facial Aspect.
Operator Position: Back position.
Illumination: Direct.
Visibility: Direct.
Retraction: Index finger of nonoperating hand.
Finger Rest: Intra-oral, palm-up. Fourth finger on incisal edges or occlusal surfaces of adjacent maxillary teeth.

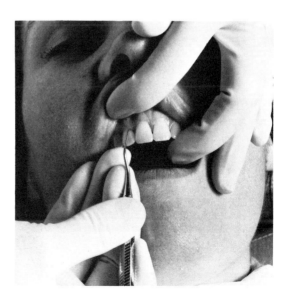

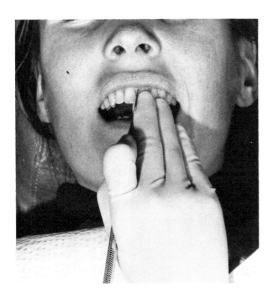

Figure 38–8 Maxillary Anterior Sextant; Facial Aspect.

Operator Position: Front position.
Illumination: Direct.
Visibility: Direct.
Retraction: Index finger of nonoperating hand.
Finger Rest: Intra-oral, palm-down. Fourth finger on incisal edges or occlusal or facial surfaces of adjacent maxillary teeth.

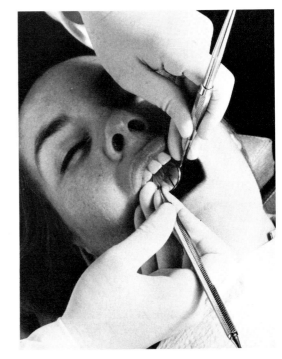

Figure 38–9 Maxillary Anterior Sextant; Lingual Aspect.

Operator Position: Back position.
Illumination: Indirect.
Visibility: Indirect.
Retraction: None.
Finger Rest: Intra-oral, palm-up. Fourth finger on incisal edges or occlusal surfaces of adjacent maxillary teeth.

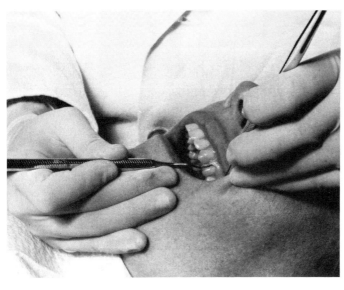

Figure 38–10 Maxillary Left Posterior Sextant; Facial Aspect.

Operator Position: Side or back position.
Illumination: Direct or indirect.
Visibility: Direct or indirect
Retraction: Mirror.
Finger Rest: Extra-oral, palm-down. Front surfaces of middle and fourth fingers on lateral aspect of mandible on left side of the face.

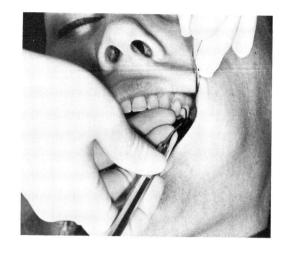

Figure 38–11 Maxillary Left Posterior Sextant; Facial Aspect.

Operator Position: Back or side position.
Illumination: Direct or indirect.
Visibility: Direct or indirect.
Retraction: Mirror.
Finger Rest: Intra-oral, palm-up. Fourth finger on incisal edges or occlusal surfaces of adjacent maxillary teeth.

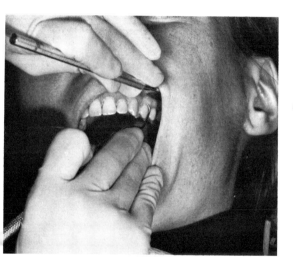

Figure 38–12 Maxillary Left Posterior Sextant; Facial Aspect.

Operator Position: Front position.
Illumination: Direct or indirect.
Visibility: Direct or indirect.
Retraction: Mirror.
Finger Rest: Intra-oral, palm-down, opposite arch. Fourth finger on incisal edges or occlusal or facial surfaces of mandibular left teeth.

Figure 38–13 Maxillary Left Posterior Sextant; Lingual Aspect.

Operator Position: Front position.
Illumination: Direct.
Visibility: Direct.
Retraction: None.
Finger Rest: Intra-oral, palm-down, opposite arch, reinforced. Fourth finger on incisal edges of mandibular anterior teeth or facial surfaces of mandibular premolars, reinforced with the index finger of the nonoperating hand.

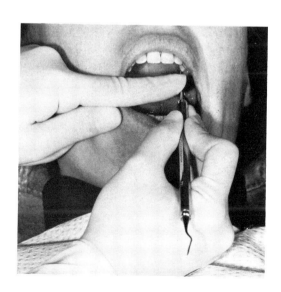
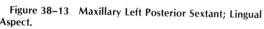

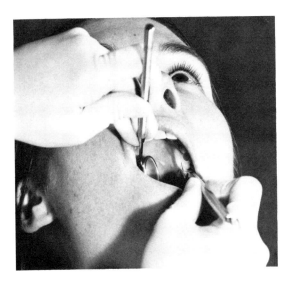

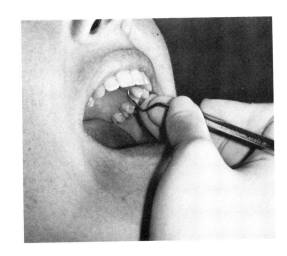

Figure 38–14   Maxillary Left Posterior Sextant; Lingual Aspect.
Operator Position: Front position.
Illumination: Direct and indirect.
Visibility: Direct and indirect.
Retraction: None.
Finger Rest: Intra-oral, palm-down, opposite arch. Fourth finger on incisal edges of mandibular anterior teeth or facial surfaces of mandibular premolars. Nonoperating hand holds mirror in position for indirect illumination.

Figure 38–15   Maxillary Left Posterior Sextant; Lingual Aspect.
Operator Position: Side or front position.
Illumination: Direct.
Visibility: Direct.
Retraction: None.
Finger Rest: Intra-oral, palm-up. Fourth finger on occlusal surfaces of adjacent maxillary teeth.

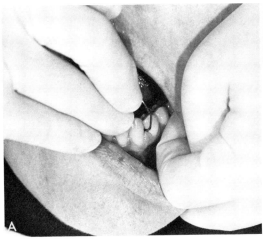

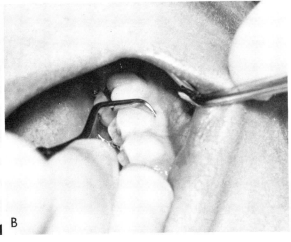

A   B

Figure 38–16   Mandibular Left Posterior Sextant; Facial Aspect.
Operator Position: Side or back position.
Illumination: Direct.
Visibility: Direct or indirect.
Retraction: Mirror or index finger of nonoperating hand.
Finger Rest: Intra-oral, palm-down. Fourth finger on incisal edges or occlusal or facial surfaces of adjacent mandibular teeth.

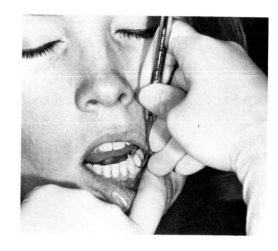

Figure 38–17   Mandibular Left Posterior Sextant, Premolar Region Only; Facial Aspect.
Operator Position: Front position.
Illumination: Direct.
Visibility: Direct.
Retraction: Index finger of nonoperating hand.
Finger Rest: Intra-oral, palm-down, finger-on-finger. Index finger of nonoperating hand is placed in mandibular left vestibule. Fourth finger of operating hand rests on index finger of nonoperating hand.

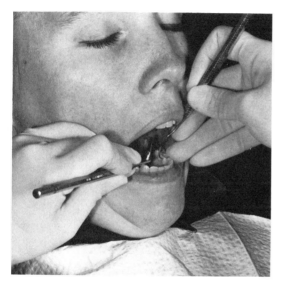

Figure 38–18   Mandibular Left Posterior Sextant; Lingual Aspect.
Operator Position: Front or side position.
Illumination: Direct and indirect.
Visibility: Direct.
Retraction: Mirror retracts tongue.
Finger Rest: Intra-oral, palm-down. Fourth finger on incisal edges or occlusal surfaces of adjacent mandibular teeth.

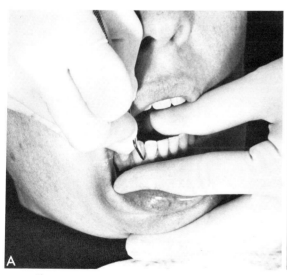
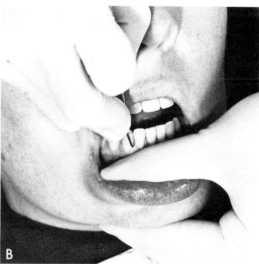

Figure 38–19   Mandibular Anterior Sextant; Facial Aspect.
Operator Position: Back position.
Illumination: Direct.
Visibility: Direct.
Retraction: Index finger or thumb of nonoperating hand.
Finger Rest: Intra-oral, palm-down. Fourth finger on incisal edges or occlusal surfaces of adjacent mandibular teeth.

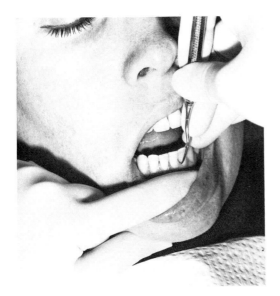

Figure 38–20 Mandibular Anterior Sextant; Facial Aspect.
Operator Position: Front position.
Illumination: Direct.
Visibility: Direct.
Retraction: Index finger of nonoperating hand.
Finger Rest: Intra-oral, palm-down. Fourth finger on incisal edges or occlusal surfaces of adjacent mandibular teeth.

Figure 38–21 Mandibular Anterior Sextant; Lingual Aspect.
Operator Position: Back position.
Illumination: Direct and indirect.
Visibility: Direct and indirect.
Retraction: Mirror retracts tongue.
Finger Rest: Intra-oral, palm-down. Fourth finger on incisal edges or occlusal surfaces of adjacent mandibular teeth.

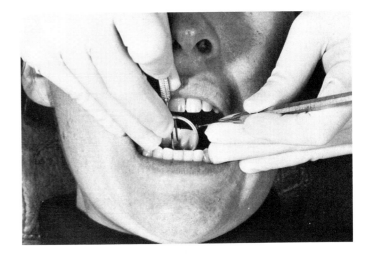

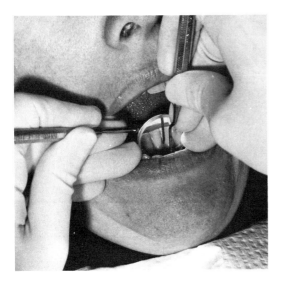

Figure 38–22 Mandibular Anterior Sextant; Lingual Aspect.
Operator Position: Front position.
Illumination: Direct and indirect.
Visibility: Driect or indirect.
Retraction: Mirror retracts tongue.
Finger Rest: Intra-oral, palm-down. Fourth finger on incisal edges or occlusal surfaces of adjacent mandibular teeth.

Figure 38–23 Mandibular Right Posterior Sextant; Facial Aspect.

Operator Position: Side or front position.

Illumination: Direct.

Visibility: Direct.

Retraction: Mirror or index finger of nonoperating hand.

Finger Rest: Intra-oral, palm-down. Fourth finger on incisal edges or occlusal surfaces of adjacent mandibular teeth.

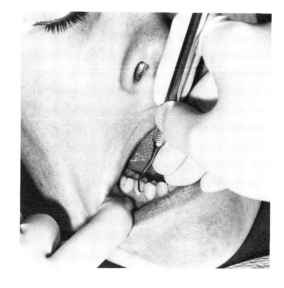

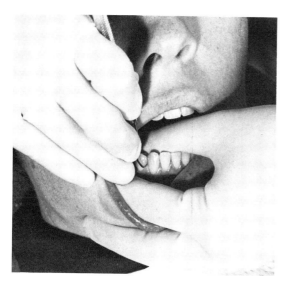

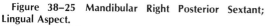

Figure 38–24 Mandibular Right Posterior Sextant, Premolar Region Only; Facial Aspect.

Operator Position: Back position.

Illumination: Direct.

Visibility: Direct.

Retraction: Index finger of nonoperating hand.

Finger Rest: Intra-oral, palm-down, finger-on-finger. Index finger of nonoperating hand is placed in mandibular right vestibule. Fourth finger of operating hand rests on index finger of nonoperating hand.

Figure 38–25 Mandibular Right Posterior Sextant; Lingual Aspect.

Operator Position: Front position.

Illumination: Direct and indirect.

Visibility: Direct and indirect.

Retraction: Mirror retracts tongue.

Finger Rest: Intra-oral, palm-down. Fourth finger on incisal edges or occlusal surfaces of adjacent mandibular teeth.

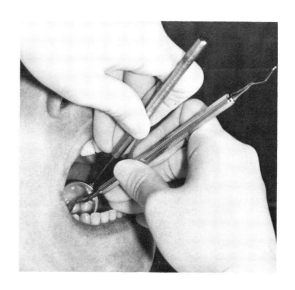

Chapter **39** _____

Sharpening of Periodontal Instruments

It is impossible to carry out periodontal procedures efficiently with dull instruments. A sharp instrument cuts more precisely and quickly than a dull instrument. To do its job at all, a dull instrument must be held more firmly and pressed harder than a sharp instrument. This reduces tactile sensitivity and increases the possibility that the instrument will inadvertently slip. Therefore, to avoid wasting time and operating haphazardly, one must be thoroughly familiar with the principles of sharpening and able to apply them to produce a keen cutting edge on the instruments one is using. Developing this skill requires patience and practice, but one cannot attain clinical excellence without it.

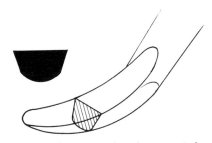

Figure 39–1 The cutting edge of a curette is formed by the angular junction of the face and lateral surfaces of the instrument. When the instrument is sharp, the cutting edge is a fine line.

674

SHARPNESS AND HOW TO EVALUATE IT

The cutting edge of an instrument is formed by the angular junction of two surfaces of its blade. The cutting edges of a curette, for example, are formed where the face of the blade meets the lateral surfaces (Fig. 39–1).

When the instrument is sharp, this junction is a fine line running the length of the cutting edge. As the instrument is used, metal is worn away at the cutting edge, and the junction of the face and lateral surface becomes rounded or dulled (Fig. 39–2).[1, 3] Instead of an acute *angle*, the cutting edge is now a rounded *surface*. This is why a dull instrument cuts less efficiently and requires more pressure to do its job.[2]

Sharpness can be evaluated by sight and touch in one of the following ways.

1. When a dull instrument is held under a light, the rounded surface of its cutting edge reflects light back to the observer. It appears as a white line running the length of the cutting edge (Fig. 39–3). The acutely angled cutting edge of a sharp instrument, on the other hand, has no surface area to reflect light. When a sharp instrument is held under a light, no white line can be observed (see Fig. 39–1).

2. Tactile evaluation of sharpness is performed by drawing the instrument lightly across the thumbnail. A dull instrument will slide smoothly without "biting" into the

Figure 39–2 The cutting edge of a dull curette is rounded.

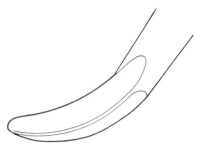

Figure 39–3 Light reflected from the rounded cutting edge of a dull instrument appears as a white line.

surface and raising a light shaving as a sharp instrument would.[5]

3. Tactile evaluation of sharpness can also be accomplished by gently drawing the pad of the thumb across the cutting edge.[2] A sharp instrument will produce a "grabbing" sensation on the skin. Naturally, care should be taken not to lacerate the thumb when using this method with extremely sharp periodontal knives.

SHARPENING STONES

Sharpening stones may be quarried from natural mineral deposits or may be pro-

duced artificially. In either case, the surface of the stone is made up of abrasive crystals that are harder than the metal of the instrument to be sharpened. Coarse stones have larger particles and cut more rapidly. They are used on instruments that are very dull. Finer stones with smaller crystals cut more slowly and are reserved for final sharpening to produce a finer edge and for sharpening instruments that are only slightly dull. India and Arkansas oilstones are examples of natural, abrasive stones. Carborundum and ruby stones are man-made and are produced by impregnating nonmetallic substances with abrasive particles (Fig. 39–4).

Sharpening stones can also be categorized by their method of use.

Mounted rotary stones. These stones are mounted on a metal mandrel and are used in a motor-driven handpiece. They may be cylindrical, conical or disc-shaped. These stones are generally not recommended for routine use because they are difficult to control precisely and can ruin the shape of the instrument, they tend to wear the instrument down quickly, and they can generate quite a bit of frictional heat which may affect the temper of the instrument.

Unmounted stones. These come in a

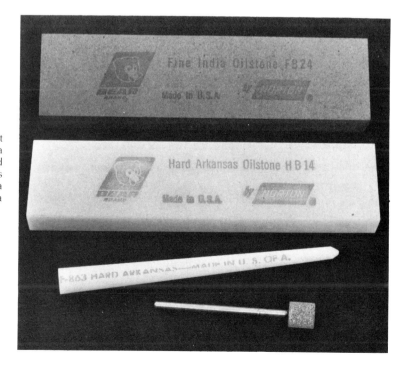

Figure 39–4 Sharpening Stones. At the top of the photograph is a flat India stone. Next is a flat Arkansas stone, and below that is a cone-shaped Arkansas stone. At the bottom of the photo is a mandrel-mounted ruby stone used in a handpiece.

variety of sizes and shapes. Some are rectangular with flat or grooved surfaces, whereas others are cylindrical or cone-shaped. Unmounted stones may be used in two ways: the instrument may be stabilized and held stationary while the stone is drawn across it, or the stone may be stabilized and held stationary while the instrument is drawn across it.

THE OBJECTIVE OF SHARPENING

The objective of sharpening is to restore the fine, thin linear cutting edge of the instrument. This is done by grinding the surfaces of the blade until their junction is once again sharply angular rather than rounded. For any given instrument, several sharpening techniques may produce this result. A technique is acceptable if it produces a sharp cutting edge without unduly wearing the instrument or altering its original design. To maintain the original design, the operator must understand the location and course of the cutting edges and the angles between the surfaces that form them. It is important to restore the cutting edge without distorting the original angles of the instrument. When these angles have been altered, the instrument does not function as it was designed to function. This limits its effectiveness.

PRINCIPLES OF SHARPENING

1. Choose a stone suitable for the instrument to be sharpened, one that is of appropriate shape and abrasiveness.
2. Use a sterilized sharpening stone if the instrument to be sharpened is being used on a patient or is about to be used on a patient.
3. Establish the proper angle between the sharpening stone and the surface of the instrument on the basis of an understanding of its design.
4. Maintain a stable, firm grasp of both the instrument and the sharpening stone. This ensures that the proper angulation is maintained throughout the controlled sharpening stroke. In this manner, the entire surface of the instrument can be reduced evenly, and the cutting edge will not be improperly beveled.

5. Avoid excessive pressure. Heavy pressure will cause the stone to grind the surface of the instrument more quickly and may shorten the instrument's life unnecessarily.
6. Avoid the formation of a "wire edge" with minute filamentous projections of metal extending as a roughened ledge from the sharpened cutting edge.[1, 2, 4, 5] When the instrument is used on root surface, these projections will produce a grooved rather than a smooth surface. A wire edge occurs when the direction of the sharpening stroke is away from, rather than into or toward, the cutting edge.[1, 4] When back-and-forth or up-and-down sharpening strokes are used, formation of a wire edge can be avoided by finishing with a down-stroke toward the cutting edge.[3]
7. Lubricate the stone during sharpening. This minimizes clogging of the abrasive surface of the sharpening stone with metal particles removed from the instrument.[2, 4, 5] It also reduces heat produced by friction. Use oil for natural stones and water for synthetic stones.
8. Sharpen at the first sign of dullness. A grossly dull instrument is very inefficient and requires more pressure when used, which hinders control. Furthermore, sharpening such an instrument requires the removal of a great deal of metal to produce a sharp cutting edge. This shortens the effective life of the instrument.

SHARPENING INDIVIDUAL INSTRUMENTS

Universal Curettes

Several techniques will produce a properly sharpened curette. Whichever tech-

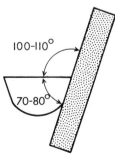

Figure 39–5 When the sharpening stone forms a 100 to 110° angle with the face of the blade, the 70 to 80° angle between the face and lateral surface is automatically preserved.

Figure 39–6 At the *left* is a properly sharpened curette that maintains a 70 to 80° angle between its face and lateral surface. The curette in the *center* has been sharpened so that one of its cutting edges is less than 70°. This fine edge is quite sharp but dulls easily. One of the cutting edges of the curette on the *right* has been sharpened to 90°. Heavy lateral pressure must be applied to the tooth to remove deposits with such an instrument.

nique is employed, one must keep in mind that the angle between the face of the blade and the lateral surface of any curette is 70 to 80° (Fig. 39–5). This is the most effective design for calculus removal and root planing. Changing this angle distorts the design of the instrument and makes it less effective. A cutting edge of less than 70° is quite sharp but also very thin (Fig. 39–6). It wears down quickly and becomes dull. A cutting edge of 90° or more requires heavy lateral pressure to remove deposits. Calculus removal with such an instrument is often incomplete and root planing cannot be done effectively (Fig. 39–6). The following technique is recommended because it enables one to visualize the critical 70–80° angle easily, thereby consistently restoring an effective cutting edge.

Sharpening the Lateral Surface. When a flat hand-held stone is correctly applied to the lateral surface of a curette to maintain the 70 to 80° angle, the angle between the face of the blade and the surface of the stone will be 100 to 110° (See Figure 39–5).

This can best be visualized by holding the curette so that the face of the blade is parallel to the floor. Use a palm grasp and brace the upper arm against the body for support.

1. Apply the sharpening stone to the lateral surface of the curette so that the angle between the face of the blade and the stone is 100 to 110° (Figs. 39–5 and 39–7). If the curette is dull, there will be a gap between the face of the blade and the surface of the stone (Fig. 39–8).

2. Beginning at the shank end of the cutting edge and working toward the toe, activate the stone with short up-and-down strokes. Use consistent, light pressure and keep the stone continuously in contact with the blade. Make sure that the 100 to 110° angle is constantly maintained (Fig. 39–9). As metal is ground away from the lateral surface during sharpening, the gap between the cutting edge and the surface of the sharpening stone will gradually diminish until the stone reaches the cutting edge. If sharpening is then continued, a

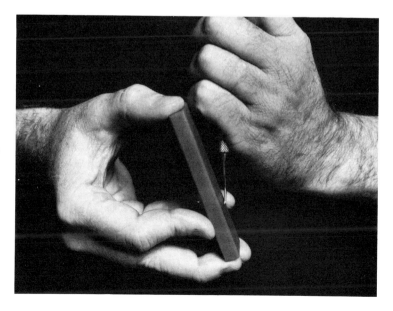

Figure 39–7 Using a palm grasp, the universal curette is held so that the face of the blade is parallel with the floor. The stone makes a 100 to 110° angle with the face of the blade.

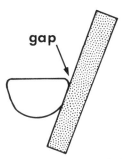

Figure 39–8 Note the gap between the face of the blade and the stone caused by the rounded cutting edge of a dull curette.

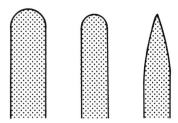

Figure 39–10 At the left is a new, unsharpened curette viewed from directly above the face of the blade. The curette in the center has been correctly sharpened to maintain the rounded toe. The curette at the right has been incorrectly sharpened, producing a pointed toe.

sludge of metal shavings and oil may develop on the face of the blade. These signs indicate that sharpening is nearly complete.

3. Check for sharpness as previously described, and continue sharpening as necessary. To prevent the toe of the curette from becoming pointed, sharpen the entire blade from shank end to toe. When approaching the toe, be sure to sharpen around it to preserve its rounded form (Fig. 39–10).

4. As the stone is moved along the cutting edge, finish each section with a downstroke into or toward the cutting edge. This will minimize the formation of a wire edge. Check the cutting edge under a light.

5. Sharpening the curette in this manner tends to flatten the lateral surface. This can be corrected by lightly grinding the lateral surface and back of the instrument, away from the cutting edge, each time the instrument is sharpened.

6. When one edge has been properly sharpened, the opposite cutting edge can be sharpened in the same manner.

Some clinicians can produce the same result with curved up-strokes or down-strokes. Usually these are performed as a rapid series of separate strokes in which the stone is removed from the instrument at the end of each stroke and reapplied to

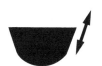

Figure 39–9 Maintaining the 100 to 110° angle, activate short up-and-down strokes.

begin a new stroke. Some clinicians will combine these up and down strokes into a continuous series in which the stone never leaves the instrument (Fig. 39–11).

Performing these sharpening operations properly requires a great deal of experience, because the angles cannot be directly seen during the sharpening movement. This, coupled with the fact that the angulation of the stone to the instrument is constantly changing during the sharpening stroke, leads to a tendency to produce a cutting edge that is 90° or more—a very inefficient curette design. Therefore, these sharpening methods are not recommended for novices or anyone who cannot use them to produce a properly sharpened curette.

Sharpening the Face of the Blade. This may be done moving a hand-held cylindrical or cone-shaped stone back and forth across the face of the blade. A cylindrical or cone-shaped stone mounted in a handpiece may also be used by applying it to the face of the blade with the stone rotating toward the toe. These methods are not recommended for routine use because: 1. The angulation between the instrument and the stone is difficult to maintain, and therefore the blade may be improperly beveled (Fig. 39–12).[1] 2. Sharpening the face of the blade narrows the working end from face to back. This weakens the blade and makes it likely to bend or break while in use (Fig. 39–12).[1, 3, 4, 5] 3. Sharpening the face of the blade with a hand-held stone using a back and forth motion will produce a wire edge that interferes with the sharpness of the blade.[1]

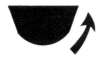

Figure 39–11 It is difficult to maintain proper angulation when a rapid series of curved up or down strokes is used to sharpen. The result is often an instrument with a distorted cutting edge as shown at the right.

Gracey Curette

Like a universal curette, a Gracey curette has an angle of 70 to 80° between the face and lateral surface of its blade. Therefore, the technique described for sharpening a universal curette can be used to sharpen a Gracey. However, there are several unique design features that distinguish a Gracey from a universal curette, and these must be understood to avoid distorting the design of the instrument while sharpening.

Gracey curettes have what is known as an offset blade, i.e., the face of the blade is not perpendicular to the shank of the instrument, as it is on a universal curette, but is offset at a 70° angle (Fig. 39–13). A Gracey curette is further distinguished by the curvature of its cutting edges. When viewed from directly above the face of the blade, the cutting edges of a universal curette extend in straight lines from shank to toe. Both cutting edges can be used for scaling and root planing. The cutting edges of a Gracey curette, on the other hand, gently curve from shank to toe. Only the larger, outer cutting edge is used for scaling and root planing (Fig. 39–14).

With these points in mind, a Gracey curette is sharpened in the following manner.

1. Hold the curette so that the face of the blade is parallel to the floor. Because the blade is offset, the shank of the instru-ment will not be perpendicular to the floor as it is with universal curettes (Fig. 39–15).

2. Identify the edge to be sharpened. Remember that only one cutting edge is used, so only that edge needs to be sharpened. Apply the stone to the lateral surface so that the angle between the face of the blade and the stone is 100 to 110°.

3. Activate short up-and-down strokes, working from the shank end of the blade to the curved toe. Finish with downstrokes.

4. Remember that the cutting edge is curved. Preserve the curve while sharpening from shank to toe by turning the stone. If the stone is kept in one place for too many strokes, the blade will be flattened (Fig. 39–16).

5. Evaluate sharpness as previously described. Continue sharpening as necessary.

Sickle Scalers

There are two types of sickle scalers, the straight sickle and the curved sickle. The face of the blade on a straight sickle is flat from shank to tip, whereas on the curved sickle the face of the blade forms a gentle curve (Fig. 39–17). Both the straight and

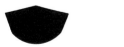

Figure 39–12 Angulation is difficult to control when sharpening the face of the blade and often results in un-wanted beveling as shown at the *left*. Sharpening the face also weakens the blade by narrowing it from face to back as shown at the *right.*

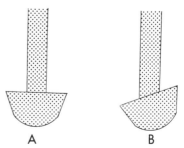

A   B

Figure 39–13 The face of a universal curette is 90° to its shank. The face of a Gracey curette is offset, forming a 70° angle with its shank.

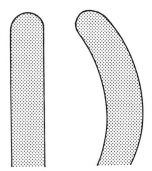

Figure 39–14 The cutting edges of a universal curette extend straight from shank to toe. The cutting edge of a Gracey curette gently curves from shank to toe. Only the larger, outer cutting edge at the right is used for scaling and needs to be sharpened.

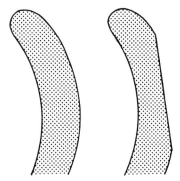

Figure 39–16 The Gracey curette on the left has been properly sharpened to maintain a symmetrical curve to its outer cutting edge. On the right the sharpening stone was activated too long in one place, thereby flattening the blade.

curved sickle have similar cross-sectional designs, however. As in the curette, the angle between the face of the blade and the lateral surface of a sickle is 70 to 80° (Fig. 39–18). When a sharpening stone is correctly applied to the lateral surface to preserve this angle, the angle between the face of the blade and the surface of the stone is 100 to 110°. With this in mind, the sickle scaler can be sharpened in a manner very much like that described for the curette.

1. Grasp the sickle with a palm grasp so that the face of the blade is parallel with the floor.

2. Apply the sharpening stone to the lateral surface of the sickle so that the angle between the face of the blade and the surface of the stone is 100 to 110°.

3. Sharpen with short up-and-down strokes. Use consistent light pressure and keep the stone continuously in contact with the blade. On most sickles, the stone will contact the entire cutting edge from shank to toe. To sharpen a sickle whose blade is longer, begin sharpening at the shank end of the blade and work toward the toe. Sickles have a sharp, pointed toe. Do not make it rounded.

4. Look for a sludge of oil and metal shavings forming on the face of the blade. This indicates that sharpening is nearly complete. Finish with a down-stroke to avoid producing a wire edge.

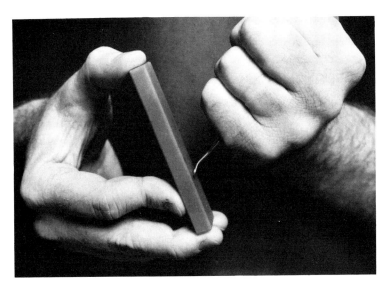

Figure 39–15 Note that when held in proper sharpening position, the shank of a Gracey curette is not perpendicular to the floor, owing to its offset blade angle. The stone meets the blade at an angle of 100 to 110°. Compare this photo to the sharpening position of a universal curette in Figure 39–7.

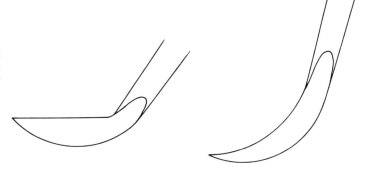

Figure 39–17 The face of the blade on a straight sickle is flat from shank to tip, whereas on the curved sickle the blade face forms a gentle arc.

5. Check for sharpness as previously described. Continue sharpening as necessary.

6. When one edge has been properly sharpened, sharpen the opposite edge in the same manner.

7. A large flat stone may also be used to sharpen sickles (Fig. 39–19). The stone is stabilized on a table or cabinet, with the left hand. The sickle is held in the right hand with a modified pen grasp and applied to the stone so that the angle between the face of the blade and the stone is 100 to 110°. The fourth finger is placed on the right-hand edge of the stone to stabilize and guide the sharpening movement. The right hand then pushes and pulls the sickle across the surface of the stone. To avoid a wire edge, finish with a pull stroke. Be sure that proper angulation is always maintained.

A mounted stone can also be used to sharpen the lateral surface of a sickle.

However, as with curettes, mounted stones are not recommended for routine use. Sickles can also be sharpened by grinding the face of the blade. Again, as with curettes, this is not recommended, because proper angulation is difficult to maintain, leading to unwanted beveling of the face of the blade, and because sharpening the face narrows the instrument face to back, thereby weakening the blade.

Hoe Scalers

Hoe scalers have a single straight cutting edge. The face of the hoe forms a 100° angle with the shank of the instrument. The cutting edge is formed by the juncture of the beveled lateral surface and the face of the blade, which meet at a 45° angle. The cutting edge is perpendicular to the shank of the instrument (Fig. 39–20).

To sharpen the hoe, stabilize a flat sharpening stone on a flat surface. Grasp the instrument with a modified pen grasp. Establish a finger rest with a pad of the third and fourth fingers against the straight edge of the sharpening stone (Fig. 39–21). Apply the flat beveled surface of the hoe to the surface of the stone. If the entire lateral surface is contacting the stone, the 45° angle between the lateral surface and the face of the blade will be maintained, and the instrument design will not be altered (Fig. 39–20).

Using moderate, steady pressure with the hand and arm held rigid and the finger rest on the edge of the stone as a guide, pull the instrument toward you. Release pressure slightly and push the instrument

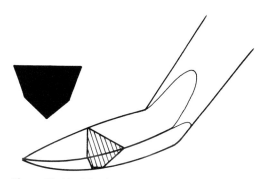

Figure 39–18 Like the curette, the sickle has an angle of 70 to 80° between the face of the blade and the lateral surface.

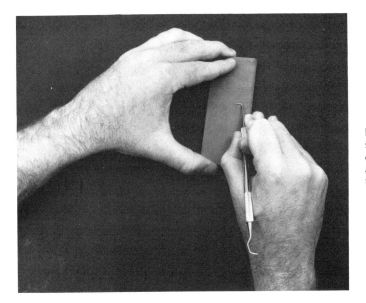

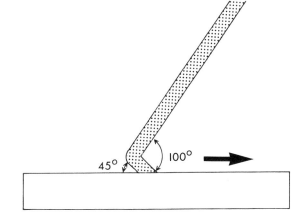

Figure 39-19 A large flat stone may also be used to sharpen the sickle. The stone is stabilized on a flat surface. The fourth finger of the right hand guides the sharpening stroke as the instrument is pulled toward the operator across the face of the stone.

Figure 39-20 The angle between the face of the blade of a hoe and its shank is 100°. The 45° angle of the cutting edge will be maintained if the entire lateral surface is kept in contact with the stone as the instrument is pulled toward the operator.

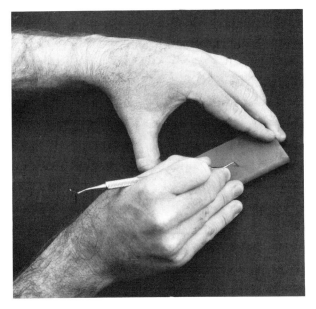

Figure 39-21 When sharpening a hoe, a large flat stone is stabilized on a flat surface. The instrument is applied to the stone at proper angulation. The fourth finger on the side of the stone guides the sharpening motion as the instrument is pulled toward the operator.

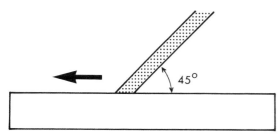

Figure 39–22 When the entire bevel on a chisel contacts the sharpening stone the angle between the instrument and the stone is 45°. The cutting edge will be properly sharpened if this angle is maintained as the instrument is pushed across the stone.

back to its starting point. Repeat the sharpening stroke until a sharp edge has been obtained. Remember to end with a pull stroke to prevent formation of a wire edge. Check for sharpness as previously described. Examine the instrument carefully to be sure its design has not been inadvertently altered.

Chisels

Chisels have a single straight cutting edge that is perpendicular to the shank. The face of the blade is continuous with the shank of the instrument, which may be directly in line with the handle or slightly curved. The end of the blade is beveled at 45° to form the cutting edge.

To sharpen a chisel, stabilize a flat sharpening stone on a flat surface. Grasp the instrument with a modified pen grasp. Establish a finger rest with the pad of the third and fourth fingers against the straight edge of the sharpening stone. Apply the flat beveled surface of the chisel to the surface of the stone. If the entire surface of the bevel is contacting the stone, the 45° angle between the beveled surface and the face of the blade will be maintained and the design of the instrument will not be altered (Figs. 39–22 and 39–23).

Using moderate, steady pressure, with the hand and arm acting as a unit and the finger resting on the edge of the stone as a guide, push the instrument across the surface of the sharpening stone. Release pressure slightly and draw the instrument back to its starting point. Repeat the sharpening stroke until a sharp edge has been obtained. Remember to finish with a push stroke to prevent formation of a wire edge. Check for sharpness as previously described. Examine the instrument carefully to be sure that its design has not been inadvertently altered.

Periodontal Knives

There are two general types of periodontal knives. The first are the disposable scalpel blades that come prepackaged. They are presharpened and sterilized by

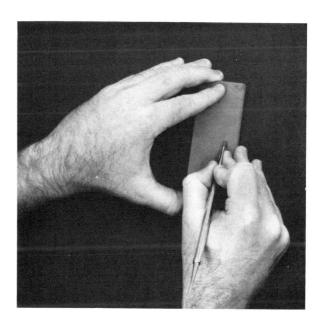

Figure 39–23 The chisel is also sharpened on a stationary flat sharpening stone.

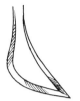

Figure 39–24 Flat-bladed gingivectomy knives like this Kirkland knife have a cutting edge that extends around the entire blade. The entire cutting edge must be sharpened.

the manufacturer. These are not resharpened when they become dull but are discarded and replaced with a new blade.

A second group of periodontal knives are reusable and must be sharpened when they become dull. The most commonly used knives in this group are the flat-bladed gingivectomy knives (of which the Glickman No. 20G and 21G, the Goldman-Fox No. 7, the Orban No. 1–2, and the Kirkland 15K and 16K are examples) and the narrow, pointed interproximal knives (of which the Goldman-Fox No. 11 and the Buck No. 5–6 are examples).

FLAT-BLADED GINGIVECTOMY KNIVES. These knives have broad, flat blades that are nearly perpendicular to the lower shank of the instrument. The curved cutting edge extends around the entire outer edge of the blade and is formed by bevels on both the front and back surfaces of the blade (Fig. 39–24).

When sharpening these instruments, only the bevel on the back surface of the instrument need be ground. This can be done by drawing the blade across a stationary flat sharpening stone or by holding the instrument stationary and drawing the stone across its blade.

Stationary Stone Technique. Stabilize a flat sharpening stone on a flat surface. Grasp the handle of the instrument with a modified pen grasp. Apply the bevel on the back surface of the blade to the flat

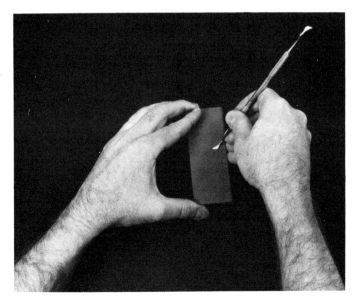

Figure 39–25 The gingivectomy knife may be sharpened on a stationary flat stone. The instrument is held with a modified pen grasp. The fourth finger guides the sharpening stroke as the instrument is drawn toward the operator. The instrument is rolled between the fingers so that all sections of the blade are sharpened.

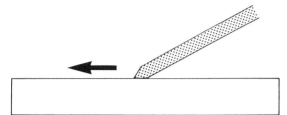

Figure 39–26 This cross section of a gingivectomy knife shows the two short bevels that form the cutting edge. The bevel on the back of the blade is applied to the surface of the stone and the instrument is drawn toward the cutting edge.

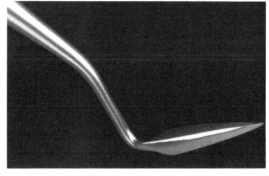

Figure 39–27 The two cutting edges of an interproximal knife are formed by bevels on the front and back surfaces of the blade.

surface of the sharpening stone. With moderate pressure, pull the instrument toward you (Figs. 39–25 and 39–26). Release pressure slightly and return to the starting point. Begin at one end of the cutting edge and continue around the blade by rolling the handle of the instrument slightly between the thumb and first and second fingers. Finish each section of the blade with a pull stroke to prevent formation of a wire edge. Check for sharpness as described previously.

Stationary Instrument Technique. Grasp the instrument with the palm. Apply the flat surface of a hand-held sharpening stone to the bevel on the back surface of the blade. Begin at one end of the cutting edge and, with moderate pressure, draw the stone back and forth across the instrument. To prevent the formation of a wire edge, finish each section with a

stroke into or toward the cutting edge. Proceed around the entire length of the cutting edge by gradually rotating the instrument and stone in relation to one another.

Interproximal Knives

The blades of interproximal knives have two long, straight cutting edges that come together at the sharply pointed tip of the instrument. The cutting edges are formed by bevels on the front and back surfaces of the blade. The entire blade is roughly perpendicular to the lower shank of the instrument (Fig. 39–27). As with the flat-bladed gingivectomy knives, only the bevels on the back surface of the interproximal knives need be sharpened. Again, this can be ac-

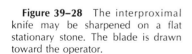

Figure 39–28 The interproximal knife may be sharpened on a flat stationary stone. The blade is drawn toward the operator.

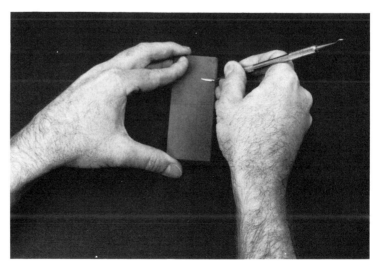

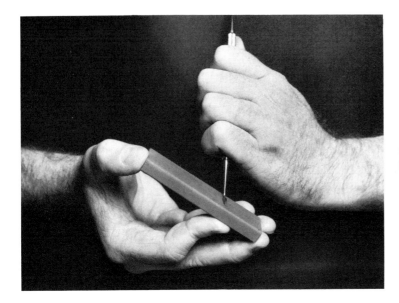

Figure 39-29 The interproximal knife may also be sharpened with a hand-held stone. The instrument is held with a palm grasp and the stone is applied to the entire cutting edge.

complished by drawing the instrument across a stationary stone or by holding the instrument stationary and moving the stone across it.

Stationary Stone Technique. Grasp the instrument and stone as described for the flat bladed gingivectomy knife. Apply the beveled cutting edge to the stone. Be sure the entire cutting edge is contacting the surface of the stone (Fig. 39-28). With moderate pressure, pull the instrument toward you. Release pressure slightly and return to the starting point. Continue until a sharp edge has been obtained. Evaluate sharpness as previously described. Be sure to finish with a pull stroke to prevent formation of a wire edge. When one cutting edge has been properly sharpened, sharpen the opposite edge.

Stationary Instrument Technique. Grasp the handle of the instrument with the palm. Apply a flat hand-held stone to the beveled cutting edge (Fig. 39-29).

Sharpen the instrument using moderate pressure and up-and-down strokes. Be sure the entire cutting edge is contacting the surface of the stone. Finish with a down-stroke to prevent a wire edge. Check for sharpness as before and proceed to the opposite cutting edge.

REFERENCES

1. Antonini, C. J., Brady, J. M., Levin, M. P., and Garcia, W. L.: Scanning electron microscope study of scalers, J. Periodontol., 48:45, 1977.
2. Green, E., and Seyer, P. C.: *Sharpening Curets and Sickle Scalers*, 2nd ed. Berkeley, California: Praxis Publishing Co., 1972.
3. Lindhe, J., and Jacobson, L.: Evaluation of periodontal scalers: I. Wear following clinical use. Odontol. Rev., 17:1, 1966.
4. Parquette, O. E., and Levin, M. P.: The sharpening of scaling instruments: I. An examination of principles. J. Periodontol., 48:163, 1977.
5. Wilkins, E. M.: *Clinical Practice of the Dental Hygienist*, 4th ed. Philadelphia: Lea & Febiger, 1976.

Part III

Treatment of Emergencies

Treatment of the Periodontal Abscess

The most effective way to treat periodontal abscesses is with surgical procedures which provide the necessary visibility and access to the responsible local irritants. There are two types of periodontal abscesses: (1) abscesses deep in the supporting tissues, which are usually treated with the simple (unrepositioned) flap operation; and (2) abscesses contained in the walls of periodontal pockets, which are usually treated by scaling and curettage or by gingivectomy.

The abscess may be either acute or chronic. If it is acute, preliminary measures are instituted, following which the condition is treated as a chronic lesion.

The Acute Periodontal Abscess

Day one

After the diagnosis is established, the patient's temperature is taken and the general systemic reaction is evaluated. The abscess is isolated with gauze sponges and dried and swabbed with an antiseptic solution, followed by a topical anesthetic. After waiting two or three minutes for the anesthetic to become effective, the abscess is palpated gently to locate the most fluctuant area.

With the Bard-Parker No. 12 blade, a vertical incision is made through the most fluctuant part of the lesion, extending from the mucogingival fold to the gingival margin (Fig. 40–1). If the swelling is on the lingual surface, the incision is started just apical to the swelling and extended through the gingival margin. The blade should penetrate to firm tissue to be sure to reach deep purulent areas. After the initial extravasation of blood and pus, irrigate with warm water and gently spread the incision to facilitate draining.

If the tooth is extruded, it should be ground slightly to avoid contact with its antagonists. Stabilize the tooth with the index finger to reduce vibration and discomfort. It is often preferable to relieve the teeth in the opposing jaw to avoid discomfort.

After drainage stops, the area is dried and painted with an antiseptic. Patients without systemic complications are instructed to rinse hourly with a solution of a teaspoonful of salt in a glass of warm water, and to return the next day. Penicillin or other antibiotics are prescribed for patients with elevated temperatures, in addition to the rinses (See Chap. 45). The patient is also instructed to avoid exertion and is put on a copious fluid diet. If necessary, bed rest is recommended. Analgesics are prescribed for pain.

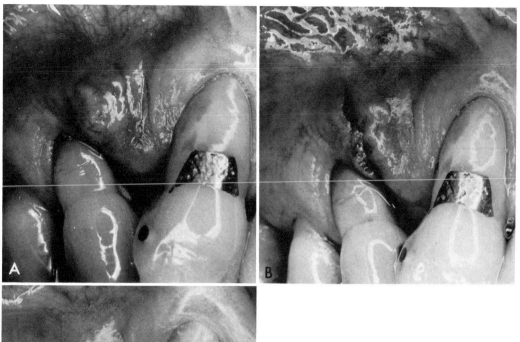

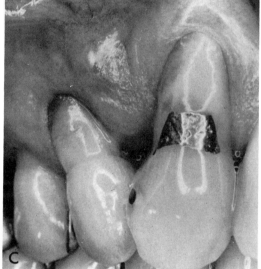

Figure 40–1 Incision of Acute Periodontal Abscess. A, Fluctuant acute periodontal abscess. B. Abscess incised. C, After acute signs subside.

Day two

The next day, the swelling is generally markedly reduced or absent, and the symptoms have subsided. If acute symptoms persist, the patient is instructed to continue the regimen prescribed the previous day, and return in 24 hours. The symptoms invariably disappear by then and the lesion is ready for usual treatment for a chronic periodontal abscess (Fig. 40–2).

Chronic Periodontal Abscess

Treatment by flap operation*

The area is isolated with gauze, dried, painted with antiseptic facially and lingually, and injected to ensure adequate anesthesia.

---

*General principles of periodontal surgery are presented in Chapter 48, and general considerations on the flap technique in Chapter 50.

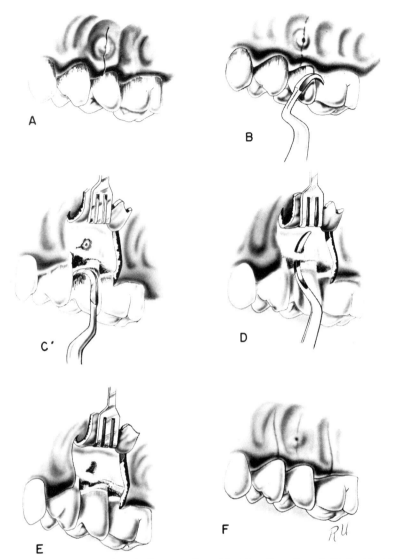

Figure 40–2 Incision of Acute Periodontal Abscess Followed by Flap Operation. A, Vertical incision of acute periodontal abscess deep in the supporting periodontal tissues. B, Superficial calculus removed. C, Flap is elevated, revealing sinus in the bone. Calculus revealed by elevating the flap is removed. D, Continuity between the alveolar crest, the abscess on the root, and the external surface of the facial plate. E, Root surface scaled and smoothed. F, Flap replaced.

Determining the operation approach

The first requirement is to determine the relative facial or lingual location of the purulent focus of the abscess. Lingual abscesses may produce swelling on the facial surface and vice versa. To locate the abscess area, probe around the gingival margin following tortuous pockets to their termination. If a sinus is present, the abscess may be probed through it.

Because it offers better accessibility and visibility, the facial approach is preferred and is the one that is used unless the abscess is close to the lingual surface.

The incisions

After the approach is decided upon, the superficial calculus is removed and two vertical incisions are made from the gingival margin to the mucobuccal fold, outlining the field of operation (Fig. 40–3A). If the lingual approach is used, the incisions are made from the gingival margin to

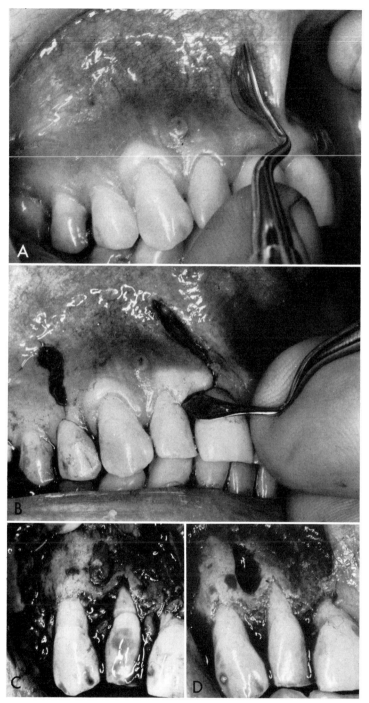

Figure 40–3   Simple Full Thickness Flap Operation for Periodontal Abscess. *A,* Chronic periodontal abscess with sinus between the maxillary canine and lateral. No. 20G periodontal knife in position for vertical incision. *B,* Operative field is outlined with two vertical incisions. Horizontal incision being made across the interdental papilla with a periodontal knife preparatory to elevating a full thickness flap. Note how the knife is stabilized by the finger rest. *C,* Full thickness flap is elevated, showing granulation tissue at the gingival margin and sinus opening filled with spongy purulent tissue. *D,* Sinus curetted. Note the narrow marginal bridge of bone which is usually infected and removed to facilitate healing.

the level of the root apices. The operative field should be large enough to allow unhampered visibility and accessibility. A flap that is too narrow or too short jeopardizes the outcome of treatment.

Elevating the flap

After the vertical incisions are made, a mesiodistal incision is made across the interdental papilla with a periodontal knife to facilitate detachment of the flap (Fig. 40–3B). A full thickness flap is raised with a periodontal knife or periosteal elevator and held in position with a retractor. A flap on either the facial or lingual surface usually suffices. In the case of an abscess which was initially acute, the edges of the incision made the previous day are usually united so that the flap may be raised in one piece. An aspirator is essential to maintain a clean field and provide the necessary visibility.

Elevation of the flap reveals some or all of the following conditions (Fig. 40–3C):

1. Granulation tissue at the gingival margin.

2. Calculus on the root surface.

3. Bony surfaces with multiple pinpoint bleeding areas.

4. A sinus opening on the external bone, which can be probed inwardly to the tooth.

5. Purulent spongy tissue in the orifice of the sinus.

Removal of the granulation tissue and calculus and root planing

After the field is carefully surveyed, the granulation tissue is removed with cu-

rettes to provide a clear view of the root. All deposits are scaled from the teeth, and the root surfaces are planed with hoe scalers and smoothed with curettes. If a sinus is present, it is explored and curetted (Fig. 40–3D).

The location of the sinus determines the manner in which the bone is managed. The bone is not disturbed except in cases in which only a thin rim of bone separates the sinus from the crest of the alveolar bone (Fig. 40–4). Thin marginal bridges of bone are removed, because they are usually pathologically involved and act as foreign bodies which impair healing.

Replacing the flap

The area is cleansed with warm water preparatory to replacing the flap. The margin of the flap usually contains a periodontal pocket lined by epithelium which prevents the flap from reattaching to the tooth. To remove the pocket epithelium the margin of the flap is everted and an internal bevel is cut along the margin with a scissors (Fig. 40–5).

The facial and lingual surfaces are covered with a piece of gauze shaped into a "U," which is held in position until bleeding stops. The gauze is removed and the flap is sutured and covered with a periodontal pack.

The patient is instructed not to rinse until the next day, when a pleasant-tasting mouthwash diluted one to three in warm water is used every two hours. The area should be cleansed gently with a soft toothbrush and water irrigation under medium pressure. The patient is to return in one week, at which time the pack and sutures are removed and the patient is

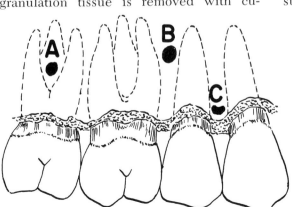

Figure 40–4 Various Levels at Which the Sinus from a Periodontal Abscess May Be Located. In the case of C, the narrow marginal bridge of bone is removed during treatment.

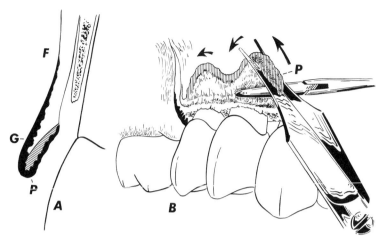

Figure 40–5   Simple Flap for the Treatment of Periodontal Abscess. *A,* Flap (F) elevated from the bone. The marginal gingiva is shown at G. P is the inner surface of the periodontal pocket *(shaded area). B,* Flap everted with hemostat. Inner pocket wall (P) *(shaded area)* removed with scissors.

instructed in plaque control. Repacking is usually not necessary.

The normal appearance of the gingiva is attained within six to eight weeks; repair of the bone requires approximately nine months. The prospects for bone repair and fill are better for osseous defects produced by rapidly destructive periodontal disease[1] (Fig. 40–6).

Treatment by Gingivectomy*

After the acute symptoms have subsided, the treatment is the same as that employed if the patient presented initially with a chronic abscess.

---

*The gingivectomy technique is described in detail in Chapter 49.

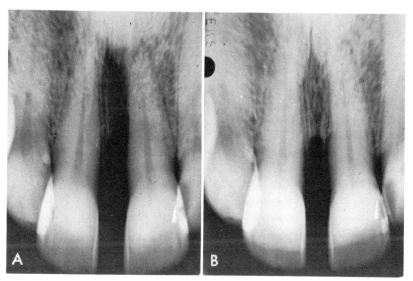

Figure 40–6   Repair of Osseous Defect Following Treatment of Periodontal Abscess. *A,* Bone destruction and osseous defect produced by periodontal abscess. *B,* Bone repair one year after treatment by flap operation without osseous surgery.

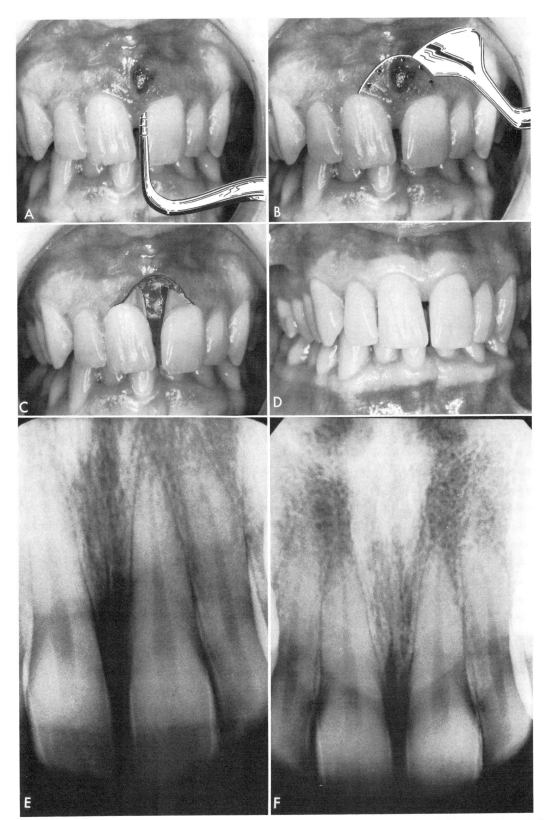

Figure 40–7 Chronic Periodontal Abscess Treated by Gingivectomy. *A,* Chronic periodontal abscess in the wall of a deep pocket is explored with Glickman periodontal probe No. 26G. *B,* Semilunar incision approximately 2 mm. apical to bleeding points made by pocket marker (composite illustration). *C,* Removal of pocket wall reveals abscess tract along incisor root (composite illustration). *D,* Appearance of healed gingiva after one year. *E,* Radiograph before treatment. *F,* Bone repair one year after treatment.

The area is isolated, dried, and painted with an antiseptic solution and injected to ensure adequate anesthesia. The abscess is probed to determine the extent of involvement, and the pocket is marked with a pocket marker (Fig. 40–7A).

The incision

The supragingival calculus is removed and a semilunar incision is made approximately 2 mm. peripheral to the pinpoint markings with the periodontal knives No. 20G and No. 21G (Fig. 40–7B). The incised gingiva is removed with a surgical hoe No. 19G, exposing the following: granulation tissue, calculus, and a tract of bone destruction along the root (Fig. 40–7C).

The granulation tissue and calculus are removed and the roots are smoothed. The bone is not disturbed.

The area is cleansed with warm water and covered with a gauze pad until bleeding stops, after which a periodontal pack is applied. Both the lingual and facial surfaces should be packed to provide better retention of the pack. The patient is dismissed with a list of instructions usually provided after surgery and instructed to return in one week, when the pack is removed. It is not necessary to replace the pack for another week, unless the area is particularly sensitive. The patient is instructed in plaque control (see Chap. 43). Gingival health is restored within six to eight weeks (Fig. 40–7D); bone repair may be observed radiographically after about nine months (Fig. 40–7E and F).

REFERENCE

1. Nabers, J. M., Meador, H. L., and Nabers, C. L.: Chronology, an important factor in the repair of osseous defects. Periodontics, 2:304, 1964.

The Treatment of Acute
Gingival Disease

The treatment of acute gingival disease entails the alleviation of the acute symptoms and the elimination of all other periodontal disease, chronic as well as acute, throughout the oral cavity. **Treatment is not complete so long as periodontal pathology or factors capable of causing it are still present.**

Acute necrotizing ulcerative gingivitis

occurs in a mouth essentially free of any other gingival involvement, or superimposed upon underlying chronic gingival disease. **The simplest part of clinical treatment is the alleviation of the acute symptoms; correction of underlying chronic gingival disease requires more comprehensive procedures.**

The treatment of acute necrotizing ulcerative gingivitis consists of the following phases:

1. LOCAL. Alleviation of the acute inflammation plus treatment of chronic disease either underlying the acute involvement or elsewhere in the oral cavity.

2. SYSTEMIC. *A. Supportive Treatment.* Alleviation of generalized toxic symptoms such as fever and malaise.

B. Etiotropic Treatment. The correction of systemic conditions which contribute to the initiation or progress of the gingival changes.

Treatment should follow an orderly sequence, as described in the following paragraphs.

COMPREHENSIVE TREATMENT OF ACUTE NECROTIZING ULCERATIVE GINGIVITIS

At the **first visit** the dentist should obtain a general impression of the patient's background, including information regarding recent illness, living conditions, dietary background, type of employment, hours of rest, and mental stress. Observe the general appearance, the apparent nutritional status, responsiveness or lassitude, and **take the patient's temperature.** Palpate the submaxillary and submental areas for enlarged lymph glands.

Examine the oral cavity for the "characteristic lesion" of acute necrotizing ulcerative gingivitis (Chap. 11), its distribution, and possible involvement of the oropharyngeal region. Evaluate the oral hygiene; check for the presence of pericoronal flaps, periodontal pockets, and local irritants. A bacterial smear may be made from the material in the involved areas, but this is merely corroboratory and is not to be relied upon for diagnosis.

Examine the occlusion and check for bruxism, clamping, or clenching.

Question the patient regarding the history of the acute disease, its onset and duration. Is it recurrent? Are the recurrences associated with specific factors such as menstruation or foods, exhaustion or mental stress? Has there been any previous treatment? When, and for how long? Inquire as to the type of treatment and the patient's impression regarding its effect.

After the diagnosis is established, the patient is treated as either "nonambulatory" or "ambulatory," based upon the following criteria:

NONAMBULATORY PATIENTS. These are patients with symptoms of generalized toxicity, such as high fever, malaise, and lassitude; bed rest is often necessary, and extensive office treatment should not be undertaken until the systemic symptoms subside.

AMBULATORY PATIENTS. In these patients, there may be localized adenopathy and a slightly elevated temperature, but no serious systemic complications.

Preliminary Treatment for Nonambulatory Patients

Day one

1. Local treatment is limited to gently removing the necrotic pseudomembrane with a pellet of cotton saturated with hydrogen peroxide.

2. The patient is advised to rest in bed and rinse the mouth every two hours with a glass of an equal mixture of warm water and 3 per cent hydrogen peroxide. For systemic antibiotic action, penicillin is administered either intramuscularly in a dose of 300,000 units or as 250 mg. tablets every four hours.

For penicillin-sensitive patients, other antibiotics such as erythromycin (250 mg. every four hours) are prescribed. Keep a carbon copy of the prescription in the patient's file for future reference. The patient is to report to the dentist after 24 hours.

Always stipulate the period for which the instructions are intended, and check the condition of the patient the next day. It is poor practice to place the patient on a home regimen for a protracted period of time. There may be a severe reaction to the antibiotic, and the peroxide mouthwash may produce diffuse erythema and ulceration of the oral mucosa and swelling of the tongue.

Day two

If the patient's condition has improved, proceed to the treatment described below under Treatment for Ambulatory Patients. If there is no improvement at the end of 24 hours, a bedside visit should be made. **The instrumentarium required for this visit includes a mirror, explorer, cotton pliers, flashlight, thermometer, a container of cotton pellets, and a glass-stoppered bottle of peroxide.** At the bedside, the oral condition, the possibility of oropharyngeal involvement, and the patient's temperature are checked. The involved gingiva is again gently swabbed with peroxide, and the instructions for the previous day are repeated. The patient is to communicate with the dentist after 24 hours.

Day three

In most instances, the patient is improved by this time and is started on the treatment for ambulatory patients described below.

Treatment for Ambulatory Patients

The following is the procedure for ambulatory patients and for initially nonambulatory patients after satisfactory response to preliminary treatment:

Day one

Instrumentarium: two dappen dishes, one containing topical anesthetic, the other 3 per cent hydrogen peroxide; cotton pellets and cotton rolls, mirror, explorer, cotton pliers, and superficial scalers.

Treatment is confined to the acutely involved areas, which are isolated with cotton rolls and dried. Topical anesthetic is applied, and after two or three minutes the areas are gently swabbed with a cotton pellet to remove the pseudomembrane and nonattached surface debris. Each cotton pellet is used in a small area and is then discarded; sweeping motions over large areas with a single pellet are not used. After cleansing with warm water, the superficial calculus is removed. Ultrasonic scalers are very useful for this purpose.

Deep scaling and curettage are contraindicated at this time because of the possibility of extending the infection into deeper tissues, and also of causing a bacteremia. Unless an emergency exists, surgical procedures such as extractions or periodontal surgery are postponed until the patient has been symptom-free for a period of four weeks in order to minimize the likelihood of exacerbation of the acute symptoms.

The patient should be advised of the extent of the total treatment the condition requires and that treatment is not complete when the pain stops. He should be informed of the presence of chronic gingival and periodontal disease which must also be eliminated in order to prevent recurrence of acute symptoms. The patient is to return in 24 hours.

INSTRUCTIONS TO THE PATIENT. The patient is dismissed with the following instructions: **Avoid tobacco, alcohol, and condiments.** Heat and the products of tobacco irritate the inflamed tissue and retard healing. If the patient is a heavy smoker, it is preferable to recommend less smoking, rather than complete abstinence. A heavy smoker who might disregard a drastic order to discontinue smoking entirely may be more cooperative if he is permitted to indulge in tobacco occasionally. The occasional use of tobacco is obviously better than total disregard of unacceptable instructions.

Rinse with a glassful of an equal mixture of 3 per cent hydrogen peroxide and warm water every two hours.

Pursue usual activities, but avoid excessive physical exertion or prolonged exposure to sun as required in golf, tennis, swimming, or sunbathing.

Confine toothbrushing to the removal of surface debris with a bland dentifrice; overzealous brushing will be painful. Dental floss, interdental cleaners, and water irrigation under medium pressure are recommended.

The patient need not be placed in isolation but **use of a separate set of dishes is recommended and intimate contacts are discouraged.** The contagiousness of acute necrotizing ulcerative gingivitis has not been demonstrated; but until such time as it

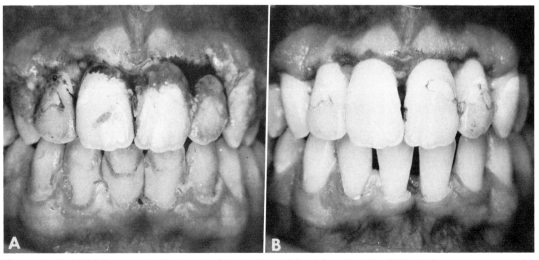

Figure 41–1 Initial Response to Treatment of Acute Necrotizing Ulcerative Gingivitis. *A,* Severe acute necrotizing ulcerative gingivitis. *B,* Third day. There is still some erythema but the condition is markedly improved.

is conclusively ruled out, methods of transmitting organisms should be avoided as a precautionary measure.

Day two

The patient's condition is usually improved; the pain is diminished or no longer present. The gingival margins of the involved areas are erythematous, but without a superficial pseudomembrane.

Deep scalers and curettes are added to the instrumentarium, and the procedures performed on Day One are repeated. Shrinkage of the gingiva may expose previously covered calculus, which is removed along with gentle curettage of the gingiva. Instructions to the patient are the same as the previous day. If there have been undesir-

able effects of the peroxide, warm water alone is used for rinsing.

Day three

The patient is essentially symptom-free. There is still some erythema in the involved areas, and the gingiva may be slightly painful to tactile stimulation (Fig. 41–1). Scaling and curettage are repeated. The patient is instructed in plaque control procedures (described in Chap. 43) which are essential for the success of the treatment and maintenance of periodontal health. The peroxide rinses are discontinued.

Day four

Tooth surfaces in the involved areas are scaled and smoothed, and plaque control by

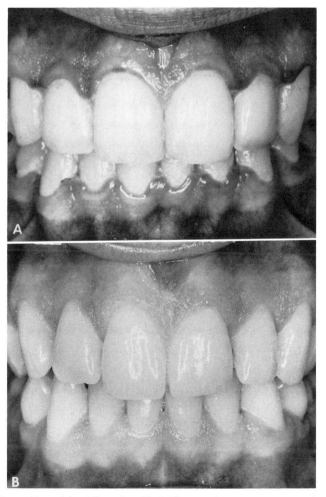

Figure 41–2 Treated Acute Necrotizing Ulcerative Gingivitis. A, Before treatment. Note the characteristic interdental lesions. B, After treatment, showing restoration of gingival health contour.

the patient is checked and corrected if necessary.

Day five

Unfortunately, treatment is often stopped at this time because the acute condition has subsided, but this is when comprehensive treatment of the patient's chronic periodontal problem should start. Appointments are scheduled for the treatment of chronic gingivitis, periodontal pockets and pericoronal flaps, and the elimination of all forms of local irritation, plus occlusal adjustment if necessary.

Patients without gingival disease other than the treated acute involvement are dismissed for one week. If the condition is satisfactory at that time, the patient is dismissed for one month when the schedule for subsequent recall visits is determined according to the patient's needs.

Gingival Changes with Healing

The characteristic lesion of acute necrotizing ulcerative gingivitis undergoes the following changes in the course of healing in response to treatment:

Removal of the surface pseudomembrane exposes the underlying red hemorrhagic crater-like depression in the gingiva.

In the next stage the bulk and redness of the crater margins are reduced, but the surface remains shiny.

This is followed by the early signs of the restoration of normal gingival contour and color.

In the final stage the normal gingival

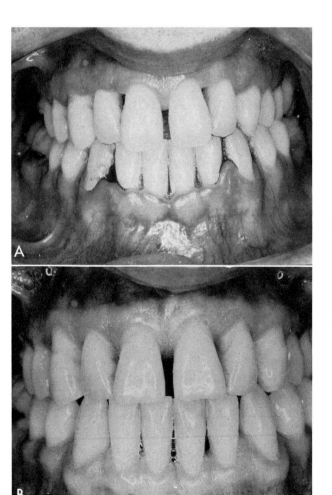

Figure 41–3 Physiologic Contour and Reattachment of Gingiva Following Treatment of Acute Necrotizing Ulcerative Gingivitis. *A,* Acute necrotizing ulcerative gingivitis showing the characteristic punched-out eroded gingival margin with surface pseudomembrane. *B,* After treatment. Note the restoration of physiologic gingival contour and reattachment of the gingiva to the surfaces of the mandibular teeth, which had been exposed by the disease.

color, consistency, surface texture, and contour are restored. Portions of the root exposed by the acute disease are covered by healthy gingiva (Figs. 41–2 and 41–3).

CONTOURING THE GINGIVA AS AN ADJUNCTIVE TREATMENT PROCEDURE

Even in the cases of severe gingival necrosis, healing ordinarily leads to restoration of the normal gingival contour (Fig. 41–4). However, if the teeth are irregularly aligned, healing sometimes results in the formation of a shelf-like gingival margin which favors the retention of food and recurrence of gingival inflammation. This can be corrected by reshaping the gingiva with a periodontal knife or electrosurgery (Figs. 41–5 to 41–7). Effective plaque control by the patient is particularly important to establish and maintain normal gingival contour in areas of tooth irregularity.

SURGICAL PROCEDURES AND ACUTE NECROTIZING ULCERATIVE GINGIVITIS

Tooth extraction or extensive gingival surgery should be postponed until four weeks after the acute signs and symptoms of necrotizing ulcerative gingivitis have subsided. If emergency surgical interference is required in the presence of acute symptoms, prophylactic chemotherapy with penicillin or other antibiotics is indicated to prevent worsening or spread of the acute disease. Penicillin is administered systemically either by intramuscular injection of phenoxymethyl penicillin, 300,000 units once daily for three days beginning the evening before the surgical procedure, or by oral administration of 250 mg. tablets, one every four hours beginning the evening before the operation and continuing for 48 hours after it.

THE MENSTRUAL PERIOD AND THE TREATMENT OF ACUTE NECROTIZING ULCERATIVE GINGIVITIS

When the menstrual period occurs in the course of treatment, there is a tendency for exacerbation of the acute signs and symptoms, giving the appearance of a "relapse." Patients should be informed of this possibility and spared unnecessary anxiety regarding their oral condition.

A

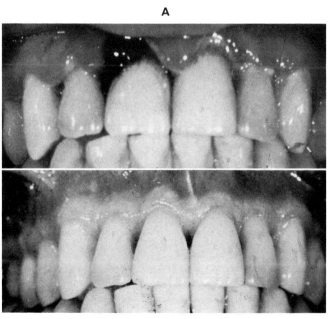

Figure 41–4 Gingival Healing Following Treatment. *A*, Before treatment. Severe acute necrotizing ulcerative gingivitis with crater formation. *B*, After treatment. Note the restored gingival contour.

B

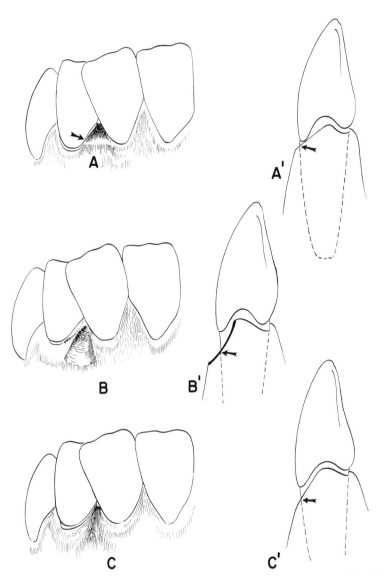

Figure 41–5 Contouring the Gingiva as an Adjunct in Treating Some Cases of Acute Necrotizing Ulcerative Gingivitis.
A, "Gingival shelf" *(arrow)* which remains in an area of tooth irregularity, after the acute symptoms are alleviated. *A',* Faciolingual view showing outline of the gingival shelf. *B,* The gingiva is contoured to eliminate the shelf. *B',* Corrected contour of the gingiva. *C,* Physiologic gingival contour after healing. *C',* Faciolingual view of healed gingiva.

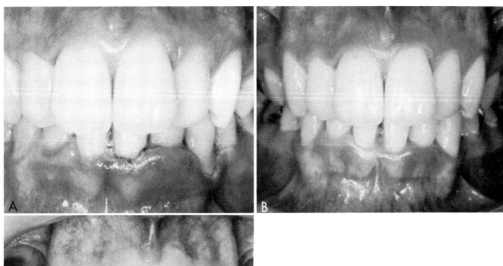

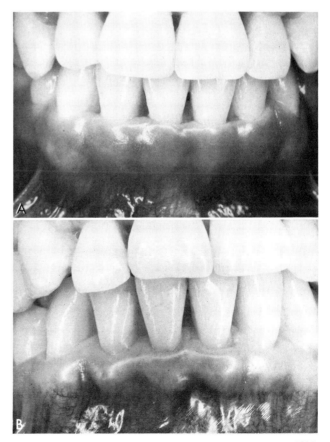

Figure 41–6 Reshaping the Gingiva in the Treatment of Acute Necrotizing Ulcerative Gingivitis. A, Before treatment, showing bulbous gingiva and interdental necrosis in the mandibular anterior area. B, After treatment, gingival contours still undesirable. C, Final result; physiologic contours obtained by reshaping the gingiva.

Figure 41–7 Craters Corrected by Reshaping the Gingiva. A, Gingival craters which remain after the treatment of acute necrotizing ulcerative gingivitis. B, Healed gingiva after recontouring with a periodontal knife.

TABLE 41–1 TOPICALLY APPLIED DRUGS USED IN TREATMENT OF ACUTE NECROTIZING ULCERATIVE GINGIVITIS

Oxygen-Liberating Agents	*Escharotics (Caustics)*
Zinc peroxide	Copper sulfate and zinc chloride
Hydrogen peroxide	Chromic acid 8%
Sodium perborate	Negatan
Potassium chlorate	Zinc chloride 8%
Potassium permanganate	Phenol 95%
Sodium peroxyborate[26]	Trichloroacetic acid 50%
	Iodine 16.5% and silver nitrate 35%
Mercurial Derivaties	*Aniline Dyes*
Tinct. Metaphen 1:200 (untinted)	Viogen (Berwick's solution)
Mercuric cyanide 1%	Acriviolet 1%
Merthiolate 1:1,000	Gentian violet 1%
Mercuric chloride 1:2,000	Acriflavine 1%
	Methylene blue 1%
Spirocheticides	*Other Agents*
Sodium carbonate 10% aqueous	Ascoxal[5]
Arsphenamine 10% aqueous	Copper sulfate, phenol, glycerin and water
Mapharsen	Metronidazole[7, 27]
Neoarsphenamine	Penicillin[8]
Fuadin	Sulfonamide in paraffin—especially sulfadiazine
	Surgical pack (zinc oxide–resin, eugenol)
	Vancomycin[6, 19]

ROLE OF DRUGS IN THE TREATMENT OF ACUTE NECROTIZING ULCERATIVE GINGIVITIS

A large variety of drugs have been used topically in the treatment of acute necrotizing ulcerative gingivitis, some of which are listed in Table 41–1. **Topical drug therapy is only an adjunctive measure in the treatment of acute necrotizing ulcerative gingivitis;**[3] **no drug, when used alone, can be considered complete therapy.**

Escharotic drugs such as phenol, silver nitrate, and chromic acid should not be used. They are necrotizing agents that alleviate the painful symptoms by destroying the nerve endings in the gingiva. They also destroy the young cells necessary for repair and delay healing. Their repeated use results in loss of gingival tissue, which is not restored when the disease subsides.[15]

SYSTEMIC ANTIBIOTICS IN THE TREATMENT OF ACUTE NECROTIZING ULCERATIVE GINGIVITIS

Antibiotics are administered systemically in patients with toxic systemic complications or local adenopathy but are not recommended for topical use because of the risk of sensitization. Phenoxymethyl penicillin is the drug of choice. It may be administered as follows: (1) in tablet or capsule form, 250 mg every four hours (V-Cillin K, Pen-Vee, and other effective preparations); (2) intramuscular injection, 300,000 units, repeated at 24-hour intervals until the systemic symptoms subside. In penicillin-sensitive patients, other antibiotics such as erythromycin or lincomycin, 250 mg. four times daily, may be used.

Antibiotics are continued until the systemic complications or local lymphadenopathy subside. Systemic penicillin also effects some reduction in the oral bacterial flora and temporary alleviation of the oral symptoms,[25, 27] but it is only an adjunct to the complete local treatment the disease requires. Patients treated by systemic antibiotics alone should be cautioned that the acute painful symptoms may recur after the drug is discontinued.

SUPPORTIVE SYSTEMIC TREATMENT

In addition to systemic antibiotics, supportive treatment consists of copious fluid consumption and analgesics for relief of pain. Bed rest is necessary for patients with toxic systemic complications such as high fever, malaise, anorexia, and general debility.

Nutritional supplements

The role of nutritional therapy in the treatment of gingival and periodontal disease in general is considered in Chapter 45. The rationale for nutritional supplements in the treatment of acute necrotizing ulcerative gingivitis is based upon the following: (1) Experimental evidence that lesions resembling acute necrotizing ulcerative gingivitis have been produced in animals in certain nutritional deficiencies (Chap. 11); (2) the possibility that difficulty in chewing raw fruits and vegetables in a painful condition such as acute necrotizing ulcerative gingivitis could lead to the selection of a diet inadequate in vitamins B and C. Because these are water-soluble vitamins which are not stored in the body and require continual replenishment, daily supplements may be needed to prevent a nutritional deficiency; (3) there are isolated clinical studies[17, 18] reporting fewer recurrences when local treatment of acute necrotizing ulcerative gingivitis is supplemented with vitamin B or vitamin C.

When the intake of water-soluble vitamins B and C has been severely curtailed because of pain in acute necrotizing ulcerative gingivitis, nutritional supplements may be indicated along with local treatment in order to ward off deficiencies in the aforementioned vitamins. Under such circumstances the patient may be started on a standard multivitamin preparation combined with a therapeutic dose of vitamins B and C.

The patient should be placed on a natural diet with the required detergent action and nutritional content as soon as the oral condition permits. Nutritional supplements may be discontinued after two months.

Local procedures are the keystone of the treatment of acute necrotizing ulcerative gingivitis. Inflammation is a local conditioning factor which impairs the nutrition of the gingiva regardless of the systemic nutritional status. Local irritants should be eliminated in order to foster normal metabolic and reparative processes in the gingiva. Persistent or recurrent acute necrotizing ulcerative gingivitis is more likely to be caused by failure to remove local irritants and inadequate plaque control than by nutritional deficiency.

ETIOTROPIC SYSTEMIC TREATMENT

Etiotropic treatment consists of measures for the correction of systemic conditions which contribute to the initiation or progress of acute necrotizing ulcerative gingivitis. Since the role of systemic etiologic factors has not been established, the indications for and value of systemic therapy are not clearly defined.

SEQUELAE THAT MAY FOLLOW TREATMENT OF ACUTE NECROTIZING ULCERATIVE GINGIVITIS

Persistent or "nonresponsive" cases

If the dentist finds himself changing from drug to drug in an effort to relieve a "stubborn" case of acute necrotizing ulcerative gingivitis, something is wrong with the over-all treatment regimen which is not likely to be corrected by changing drugs. **When confronted with such a problem: (1) All local drug therapy should be discontinued so that the condition may be studied in an uncomplicated state.** (2) Careful differential diagnosis is undertaken to rule out diseases which resemble acute necrotizing ulcerative gingivitis. (See Chapter 11.) (3) A search is made for contributing local and systemic etiologic factors that may have been overlooked. (4) Special attention is given to instructing the patient in plaque control before undertaking comprehensive local treatment.

Recurrent acute necrotizing ulcerative gingivitis

The following factors should be explored in patients with recurrent acute necrotizing ulcerative gingivitis:

INADEQUATE LOCAL THERAPY. Too frequently, treatment is discontinued when the symptoms have subsided, without eliminating the chronic gingival disease and periodontal pockets which remain after the superficial acute condition is relieved. Persistent chronic inflammation causes degenerative changes which predispose the gingiva to recurrence of acute involvement.

PERICORONAL FLAP. **Recurrent acute involvement in the mandibular anterior area is often associated with persistent pericoronal inflammation arising from difficult eruption of third molars.**[12] The anterior involvement is less likely to recur after the third molar situation is corrected.

ANTERIOR OVERBITE. Marked overbite is often a contributing factor in the recurrence of disease in the anterior region. Where the incisal edges of the maxillary teeth impinge upon the labial gingival margin, or the mandibular teeth strike the palatal gingiva, the resultant tissue injury predisposes to recurrent acute disease. Less severe overbite produces food impaction and gingival trauma. Correction of the overbite is necessary for the complete treatment of acute necrotizing ulcerative gingivitis.

Inadequate plaque control and heavy use of tobacco are also common causes of recurrent disease.

TREATMENT OF ACUTE PERICORONITIS

The treatment of pericoronitis depends upon the severity of the inflammation, the

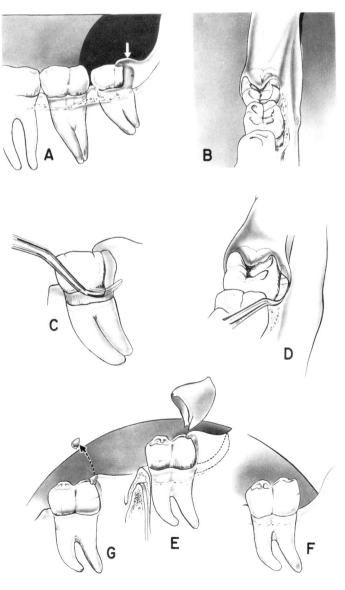

Figure 41–8 Treatment of Acute Pericoronitis. *A,* Inflamed pericoronal flap in relation to the mandibular third molar. *B,* Anterior view of third molar and flap. *C,* Lateral view with Younger-Good scaler in position to gently remove debris under flap. *D,* Anterior view of scaler in position. *E,* Removal of section of the gingiva distal to the third molar, after the acute symptoms subside. The line of incision is indicated by the dotted line. *F,* Appearance of the healed area. *G,* Incorrect removal of the tip of the flap, permitting deep pocket to remain distal to the molar.

systemic complications, and the advisability of retaining the involved tooth. All pericoronal flaps should be viewed with suspicion. **Persistent symptom-free pericoronal flaps should be removed as a preventive measure against subsequent acute involvement.**

The following is the procedure for the treatment of acute pericoronitis:

Visit 1

1. Determination of the extent and severity of involvement of adjacent structures and toxic systemic complications (Fig. 41–8).

2. The area is gently flushed with warm water to remove superficial debris and surface exudate, and a topical anesthetic is applied.

3. The area is swabbed with antiseptic, and the flap is gently elevated from the tooth with a scaler. The underlying debris is removed, and the area is flushed with warm water (Fig. 41–8). Extensive curettage or surgical procedures are contraindicated at the initial visit. Instructions to the patient include hourly rinses with a solution of a teaspoonful of salt in a glass of warm water, rest, copious fluid intake, and systemic antibiotics for fever. The patient is to return in 24 hours.

4. If the gingival flap is swollen and fluctuant, an anteroposterior incision is made with a No. 15 Bard-Parker blade to establish drainage, followed by insertion of a 1/4" gauze wick.

Visit 2

After 24 hours, the condition is usually markedly improved. If a drain had been inserted, it is removed. The flap is gently separated from the tooth and the area flushed with warm water. The patient is to continue with the instructions of the previous day and return in 24 hours.

Visit 3

At this visit, a determination is made as to whether the tooth is to be retained or extracted. This decision is governed by the likelihood of further eruption into a good functional position. Bone loss on the distal surface of the second molars is a hazard following the extraction of partially or completely impacted third molars[2] which is significantly greater if the third molars are extracted after the roots are formed or in patients beyond their early twenties. **To reduce the risk of bone loss around second molars, partially or completely impacted third molars should be extracted as early as possible in their development.**

If it is decided to retain the tooth, the necessary surgical procedures are performed at this visit, provided there are no acute symptoms. Periodontal knives or electrosurgery is used for this purpose. Under anesthesia, an incision is begun just anterior to the border of the ramus and brought downward and forward to the distal surface of the crown, as close as possible to the level of the cemento-enamel junction. This will detach a wedge-shaped section of tissue that includes the gingival flap (Fig. 41–8).

It is necessary to remove the tissue distal to the tooth as well as the flap on the occlusal surface. Incising only the occlusal portion of the flap leaves a deep distal pocket which invites recurrence of acute pericoronal involvement.

After the tissue is removed, a periodontal pack is applied. The pack may be retained by bringing it forward along the facial and lingual surfaces into the interproximal space between the second and third molars. The pack is removed after one week.

Pericoronitis and Acute Necrotizing Ulcerative Gingivitis

Pericoronal flaps which are chronically inflamed may become the sites of acute necrotizing ulcerative gingivitis. The disease is treated in the same manner as elsewhere in the mouth and, after acute symptoms have subsided, the flap is removed. Pericoronal flaps are often referred to as "primary incubation zones" in acute necrotizing ulcerative gingivitis; their elimination is one of many measures required to minimize the likelihood of recurrent disease.

TREATMENT OF ACUTE HERPETIC GINGIVOSTOMATITIS

Various medications have been used in the treatment of this condition, including local applications of 8 per cent zinc chloride, camphorated phenol, spirits of camphor, Talbot's iodine, phenol, sulfonamide solutions, moccasin snake venom,[10] systemically administered yeast,[13] riboflavin, vitamin B complex,[4] thiamine, and radiation therapy. Aureomycin has been used successfully as a mouthwash,[1] applied topically in a 3 per cent ointment,[9] or administered systemically in the form of 250 mg. capsules for a total dosage of 3 grams.[16] Vaccination with smallpox vaccine or a vaccine prepared from the contents of the vesicles has been described both as a thera-

peutic measure and as a measure for the prevention of recurrence,[11, 21] but the results are doubtful.

Treatment consists of palliative measures to make the patient comfortable until the disease runs its course (seven to ten days).

Plaque, food debris, and superficial calculus are removed to reduce gingival inflammation which complicates the acute herpetic involvement. Extensive periodontal therapy should be postponed until the acute symptoms subside in order to avoid the possibility of exacerbation (Fig. 41–9). Painful, swollen herpetic infection of a dentist's finger after preparing a crown in a patient with herpetic lesions on the lower lip has been reported.[23]

Relief of pain to enable the patient to

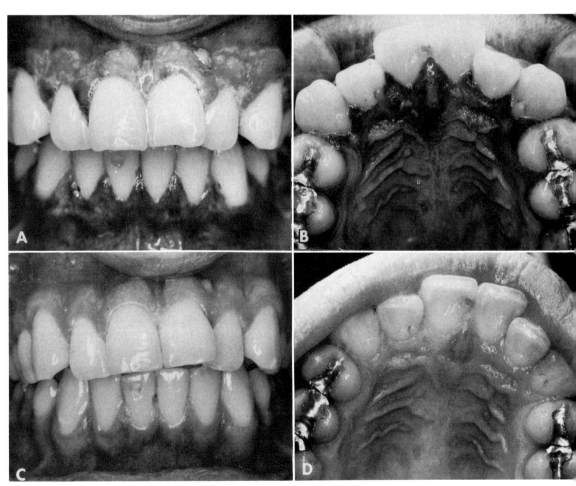

Figure 41–9   Treatment of Acute Herpetic Gingivostomatitis. *A,* Before treatment, diffuse erythema and surface vesicles. *B,* Before treatment, lingual view showing gingival edema and ruptured vesicle on palate. *C,* One month after treatment showing restoration of normal gingival contour and stippling. *D,* One month after treatment, lingual view.

eat comfortably is obtained with Dyclone (dyclonic hydrochloride), a topical anesthetic mouthwash[28] which is available in 0.5 per cent solution which may be diluted 1 to 1 with water. It is held in the mouth for one or two minutes and swished around, to produce an anesthetic effect that lasts for 40 minutes. It is helpful when used before meals, but may be used more often without toxic effects.

Supportive treatment

Supportive measures include copious fluid intake and systemic antibiotic therapy (Aureomycin, 250 mg. four times daily) for the management of toxic systemic complications. For the relief of pain, systemically administered aspirin is usually sufficient. A dosage of 10 grains every three hours may be prescribed for adults, with smaller doses used for children.

REFERENCES

1. Arnold, H. L., Domzalski, C. A., and Austin, E. R.: Aureomycin mouthwash for herpetic stomatitis. Proc. Staff Meet. Honolulu, 15:85, 1949.
2. Ash, M. M., Jr., Costich, E. R., and Hayward, J. R.: A study of periodontal hazards of third molars. J. Periodontol., 33:209, 1962.
3. Burket, L. W.: Oral Medicine. 3rd ed. Philadelphia, J. B. Lippincott Co., 1946, p. 53.
4. Burket, L. W., and Hickman, G. C.: Oral herpes (simplex) manifestations: Treatment with vitamin B complex. J. Am. Dent. Assoc., 29:411, 1942.
5. Clausen, F. P.: Local treatment of acute necrotizing ulcerative gingivitis with ascoxal: Clinical experiences from treatment of military personnel. Tandlaegebladet, 70:1009, 1966.
6. Collins, J., and Hood, H. M.: Topical antibiotic treatment of acute necrotizing ulcerative gingivitis. J. Oral Med., 22:59, 1967.
7. Duckworth, R., Waterhouse, J. P., Britton, D. E. R., Nuki, K., Sheiham, A., Winter, R., and Blake, G. C.: Acute ulcerative gingivitis: A double-blind controlled clinical trial of Metronidazole. Br. Dent. J., 120:599, 1966.
8. Emslie, R.: Treatment of acute ulcerative gingivitis. A clinical trial using chewing gum containing metronidazole or penicillin. Br. Dent. J., 122:307, 1967.
9. Everett, F. G.: Aureomycin in the therapy of herpes simplex labialis and recurrent oral aphthae. J. Am. Dent. Assoc., 40:555, 1950.
10. Fisher, A. A.: Treatment of herpes simplex with moccasin snake venom. Arch. Derm. Syph., 43:444, 1941.
11. Frank, S. B.: Formalized herpes virus therapy and the neutralizing substance in herpes simplex. J. Invest. Dermatol., 1:267, 1940.
12. Frankl, Z.: Dentitio difficilis and parodontosis. Paradentologie, 1:107, 1947.
13. Gerstenberger, H. J.: The etiology and treatment of herpetic (aphthous and aphthoulcerative) stomatitis and herpes labialis. Am. J. Dis. Child., 26:309, 1923.
14. Glickman, I.: The use of penicillin lozenges in the treatment of Vincent's infection and other acute gingival inflammations. J. Am. Dent. Assoc., 34:406, 1947.
15. Glickman, I., and Johannessen, L. B.: The effect of a six per cent solution of chromic acid on the gingiva of the albino rat—A correlated gross, biomicroscopic, and histologic study. J. Am. Dent. Assoc., 41:674, 1950.
16. Jacobs, H. G., and Jacobs, M. H.: Aureomycin: Its use in infections of the oral cavity. Oral Surg., 2:1015, 1949.
17. King, J. D.: Nutritional and other factors in "trench mouth" with special reference to the nicotinic acid component of the vitamin B_2 complex. Br. Dent. J., 74:113, 1943.
18. Linghorne, W. J., McIntosh, W. G., Tice, J. W., Tisdall, F. F., McCreary, J. F., Drake, T. G. H., Greaves, A. V., and Johnstone, W. M.: The relation of ascorbic acid intake to gingivitis. J. Can. Dent. Assoc., 12:49, 1946.
19. Mitchell, D. F., and Baker, B. R.: Topical antibiotic control of necrotizing gingivitis. J. Periodontol., 39:81, 1968.
20. Roth, H.: Vitamins as an adjunct in the treatment of periodontal disease. J. Am. Dent. Assoc., 32:60, 1945.
21. Savitt, L. E., and Ayres, S., Jr.: Persistent multiple herpes-like eruption. Response to repeated intradermal injections of smallpox vaccine. Arch. Derm. Syph., 59:653, 1949.
22. Shinn, D. L. S., Squires, S., and McFadzean, A.: The treatment of Vincent's disease with metronidazole. Dent. Practit., 15:275, 1965.
23. Snyder, M. L., Church, D. H., and Rickles, N. H.: Primary herpes infection of right second finger. Oral Surg., 27:598, 1969.
24. Stephen, K. W., McLatchie, M. F., Mason, D. K., Noble, H. W., and Stevenson, D. M.: Treatment of acute ulcerative gingivitis (Vincent's type). Br. Dent. J., 121:313, 1966.
25. Wade, A. B., Blake, G. C., Manson, J. D., Berdon, J. K., Mathieson, F., and Bate, D. M.: Treatment of the acute phase of ulcerative gingivitis (Vincent's type). Br. Dent. J., 115:372, 1963.
26. Wade, A. B., and Mirza, K. B.: The relative effectiveness of sodium peroxyborate and hydrogen peroxide in treating acute ulcerative gingivitis. Dent. Practit., 14:185, 1964.
27. Wade, A. B., Blake, G., and Mirza, K.: Effectiveness of metronidazole in treating the acute phase of ulcerative gingivitis. Dent. Practit. Dent. Rec. 16:440, 1966.
28. Weisberger, D.: Treatment of some diseases of the soft tissues of the mouth. Dent. Clin. North Am., March 1960, p. 215.

Part IV

Phase I Therapy

Preparation of the Tooth Surface

RATIONALE

Initial therapy or *phase I therapy* is the first therapeutic step in the chronological sequence of procedures that constitute periodontal treatment. The objective of initial therapy is the reduction or elimination of gingival inflammation (Color Plate 6); it is achieved by complete removal of calculus, correction of defective restorations, obturation of carious lesions, and institution of a comprehensive plaque control regimen.[4, 10, 23, 24, 26, 41]

There has been considerable controversy regarding the necessity of an "initial preparation of the mouth" in cases requiring surgical therapy.[16] Preparatory therapy, especially prior to gingivectomy, does not seem to improve postoperative healing or gingival architecture[2, 15, 40] and subjects the patients twice, for each treated area, to the risk of systemic complications caused by postoperative bacteremia.[18, 22] Current data from clinical research, however, indicate that in the last analysis, long-term success of periodontal treatment is principally dependant on maintaining the results achieved with phase I therapy and depends much less on what specific surgical procedure is employed.[25, 30, 31, 36] In addition, phase I therapy provides an opportunity for the periodontist to evaluate tissue response as well as the patient's attitude toward periodontal care, both of which are crucial to the prognosis of a periodontal condition.

The purpose of eliminating overt gingival inflammation with phase I therapy is (1) to restore gingival health, (2) to inhibit the transition of gingivitis to periodontitis, (3) to inhibit the progression of periodontitis, (4) to eliminate periodontal pockets produced by edematous enlargement of inflamed gingiva, or (5) to achieve surgical manageability of the gingiva, i.e., firm consistency of the tissue and reduced bleeding.

Based on the concept that microbial dental deposits (plaque) produce the primary pathogens of gingival inflammation, the specific aim of phase I therapy is to facilitate the daily removal of such accretions from the teeth by eliminating rough and irregular contours from the tooth surfaces and then establishing a suitable plaque control regimen (see Chapter 43). The institution of effective plaque control being the ultimate objective of every therapeutic periodontal procedure, phase I therapy is primarily concerned with the fact that the presence of smooth and regular tooth surfaces is a major prerequisite for achieving this goal. Adequate plaque removal by the patient can be expected only if the tooth surfaces are unobstructed by rough deposits or irregular contours but readily accessible for oral hygiene aids.

The following sequence of procedures is recommended (Color Plate 5).

711

Color Plate V   Top. Effect of Phase I Therapy on the Gingiva. Edematous gingiva *(A)* before, and *(B)* after treatment. Fibrotic gingiva *(C)* before and *(D)* after treatment.

Color Plate V   Bottom. Phase I Therapy. Sequence of Procedures. *A,* Supragingival treatment: *(1)* limited plaque control instructions; *(2)* supragingival calculus removal; *(3)* recontouring of existing restorations; *(4)* obturation of carious lesions. *B,* Subgingival extension of treatment: *(5)* comprehensive plaque control instructions; *(6)* subgingival calculus removal, elimination of necrotic cementum, and root planing. *C,* Tissue re-evaluation for surgical treatment, following completion of surface recontouring and institution of plaque control. *Green,* Plaque zones to be cleaned by the patient. *Blue,* Plaque zones to be corrected by the therapist prior to plaque control instructions. *Red,* Gingival inflammation.

Color Plate V   Top

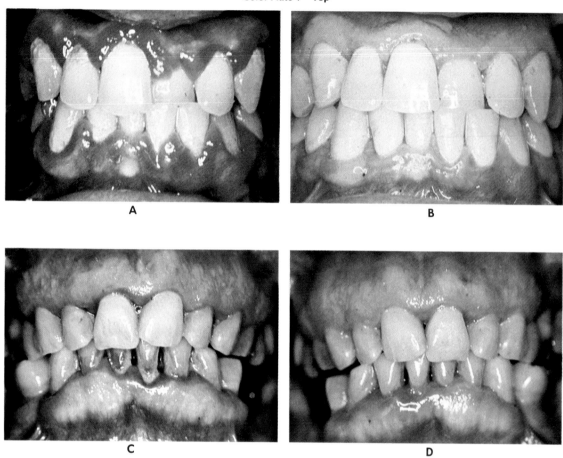

A

B

C

D

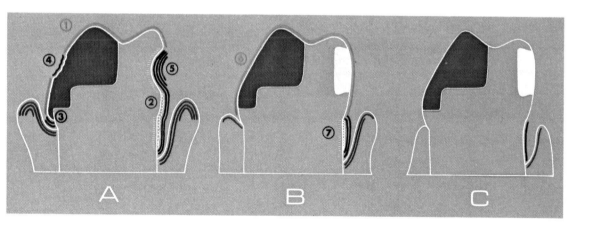

Color Plate V   Bottom

Legend on opposite page

After careful analysis of the case, the number of appointments needed to complete this phase of treatment is estimated. Patients with only slight amounts of calculus and relatively healthy tissues can be completed in one appointment. Most other cases will require several appointments. The dentist should estimate the number of appointments on the basis of number of teeth in the mouth, amount and location of calculus, depth of pockets, presence of furcation involvements, etc.

Step 1. LIMITED PLAQUE CONTROL INSTRUCTIONS (See Chapter 43.)

Introducing an oral hygiene program to the patient is of high priority in every periodontal treatment plan. Plaque control instructions should begin at the first therapeutic appointment. The patient is taught how to clean all smooth and regular surfaces of the teeth. When therapy is begun, a number of tooth surfaces frequently are altered by calculus, defective restorations, carious lesions, or necrotic cementum (Color Plate V Bottom, A), preventing sufficient access for oral hygiene aids. The patient should not be expected to control plaque in such areas.

The toothbrush is often the only hygiene aid indicated at this stage of therapy. Dental floss should be used on *smooth* proximal tooth surfaces only, since flossing around sharp edges and coarse surfaces of calculus or overhanging restorations causes the floss to shred and break, leads to ineffective plaque removal as well as persistence of inflammatory bleeding (see Figure 42–3D), and is often a frustrating experience for the patient.

Step 2: SUPRAGINGIVAL REMOVAL OF CALCULUS

Dental calculus is a mineralized aggregate of non-vital microorganisms embedded in an intermicrobial matrix.[23] Although not injurious to the periodontium by itself,[3, 46] it provides a highly retentive surface for the oral microflora and thus promotes the accumulation of injurious dental plaque.[26] Since adequate removal of plaque from calculus surfaces is not feasible with current oral hygiene techniques,

calculus must be eliminated entirely in order to facilitate effective plaque control.

In the presence of inflamed, friable gingiva adjacent to deep periodontal pockets, calculus is first dislodged from all *supra*gingival tooth surfaces. This leads to a substantial improvement of the marginal gingiva. Removal of *sub*gingival calculus from these areas, prior to the resolution of pronounced marginal gingivitis, is not recommended since it may produce undue laceration of the diseased gingiva and provoke an acute inflammatory tissue reaction.

Calculus is dislodged by scaling the tooth surfaces with instruments especially designed for that purpose (see Chapter 36). For supragingival calculus removal, ultrasonic scalers, hand scalers, and curettes are the instruments of choice.[37] Special prophylaxis burs in the shape of a hexagonal cone, attached to a dental handpiece, are also effective,[11] but may cause undesirable gouging of the tooth surface.

Scaling consists of a "pull" motion, except on the proximal surfaces of closely spaced anterior teeth, where thin chisel scalers are used with a "push" motion. In the "pull" motion, the instrument engages the apical border of the calculus and dislodges it with a firm movement through the entire instrumentation zone in the direction of the crown (Fig. 42–1).

The scaling motion is initiated in the forearm and transmitted from the wrist to the hand with slight flexing of the fingers. Rotation of the wrist is synchronized with movement of the forearm. The scaling motion is not initiated in the wrist or fingers, nor is it carried out independently without the use of the forearm.

In the "push" scaling motion, the fingers activate the instrument. This method is used with the chisel scaler on the proximal surfaces of crowded anterior teeth. The instrument engages the lateral border of the calculus and the fingers provide a thrust motion, which dislodges the calculus.

The removal of calculus is not a whittling operation. Calculus is dislodged in its entirety, starting below its border; it is not "pared down" until the tooth surface is reached. After calculus is removed from one section of the tooth, the instrument is moved laterally to engage the adjacent deposits.

Scaling is confined to a small area of the

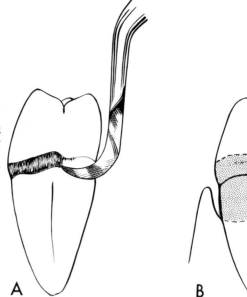

Figure 42–1 Instrumentation Zones for Calculus Removal and Root Planing. *A,* Supragingival calculus removal by engaging lower border of concrement with cutting edge of scaler. *B,* Apical extension of instrumentation zone (shaded area) for subgingival calculus removal and root planing.

tooth on both sides of the cemento-enamel junction where the calculus and other deposits are located. Sweeping the instrument over the crown where it is not needed lengthens operating time, dulls the instrument, and is contrary to the careful attention to detail required for effective instrumentation.

Complete interproximal access for scaling instruments is often difficult, especially between incisor teeth with narrow embrasures. In those areas, sharp-pointed sickle scalers rather than round-ended curettes should be used to reach close to the contact zones. Crowding of anterior teeth frequently results in very long, tight contact zones and extremely narrow embrasures. This prevents adequate access even for sharp-pointed sickle scalers. Abrasive finishing strips inserted between the teeth can be used for effective removal of calculus and stain from such areas (Fig. 42–2).

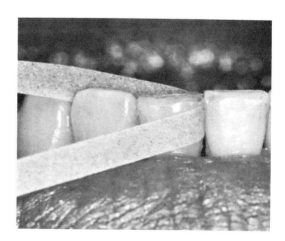

Figure 42–2 Finishing Strips. Effective for removing stain and calculus from proximal tooth surfaces adjacent to tight contact areas and narrow embrasures.

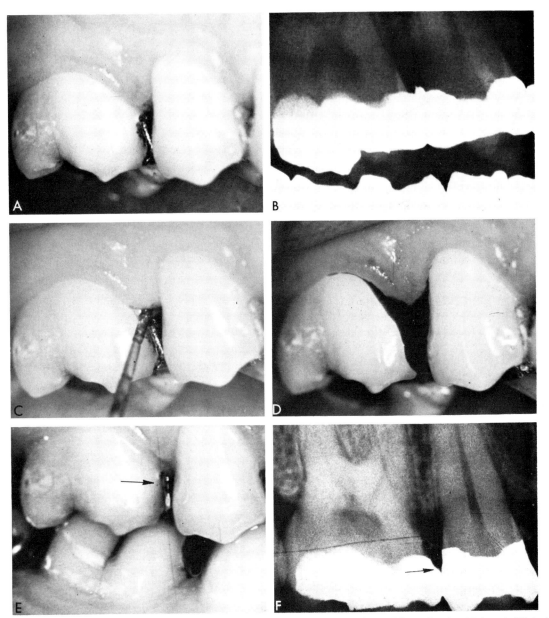

Figure 42–3 Effect on the Gingiva of an Overhanging Amalgam Restoration Mesial on the First Molar. *A,* Clinical aspect. *B,* Radiographic aspect. *C,* Interproximal probing provokes (*D*) profuse bleeding from the col area, a sign of gingival inflammation. *E,* Clinical and (*F*) radiographic aspects of recontoured restoration.

Scaling invariably leaves the treated tooth, especially cementum and dentin, with a rough and scratched surface favoring quick re-establishment of plaque and calculus. Following calculus removal, the tooth surface must therefore be planed with suitable scalers or curettes[9, 12, 13, 17, 20, 28, 35, 43, 47] and polished with abrasive paste on a rotary rubber cup or brush. Smooth, polished tooth surfaces are highly conducive to effective plaque control and resist calculus formation considerably better than rough surfaces.[44]

Step 3. RECONTOURING OF DEFECTIVE RESTORATIONS

With few exceptions,[34] rough, overcontoured, overhanging, or subgingivally located restorations and orthodontic appliances are associated with pronounced accumulation of plaque[6, 8, 45, 46] and periodontal inflammation[1, 5, 19, 21, 27, 29, 32, 33, 48] (Fig. 42–3), as well as loss of alveolar bone and periodontal attachment.[7, 14, 39, 42] Like calculus, such restorations or appliances interfere with efficient plaque control and must therefore be corrected or removed to allow for reduction or elimination of gingival inflammation. Correction of existing restorations is as important as the removal of calculus and should therefore be completed at the same time. *Adequate plaque control by the patient on teeth with restorations is feasible only if the restorations are well contoured and their surface is smooth* (see Figure 42–5C and D).

Defective restorations, especially overhanging margins, are detected clinically by running a fine explorer along their periphery, moving the explorer tip continuously back and forth across the margins of the restoration (Fig. 42–4). In the presence of an overhanging margin, a clicking sound is produced when the explorer is run from the restoration to the tooth, and a definitive catch is felt when moving the explorer from the tooth to the restoration. Bite wing radiography may be a helpful diagnostic adjunct to determine the approximate mesio-distal and occluso-apical dimension of a proximal overhang (see Fig. 42–3B).

Special attention is given to restorations on root surfaces of molars and premolars. Frequently, the contours of such restorations do not reproduce the concave interradicular depressions usually found on these teeth. Instead, the restorations exhibit overhanging margins or over-contoured surfaces (Fig. 42–5A), making it difficult for the patient to reach the subjacent tooth surface with an oral hygiene instrument (Fig. 42–5B).

Overhanging margins are eliminated either by replacing the entire restoration or by correcting the contour of the existing restoration. The latter, although often only a temporary means, is preferred, whenever feasible, because it involves considerably less time and effort than replacing an entire restoration. Thus, it does not unneces-

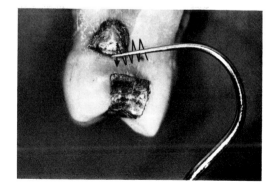

Figure 42–4 Identification of Defective Restorations. Rough surfaces and overhanging margins can be detected with the tip of a fine explorer.

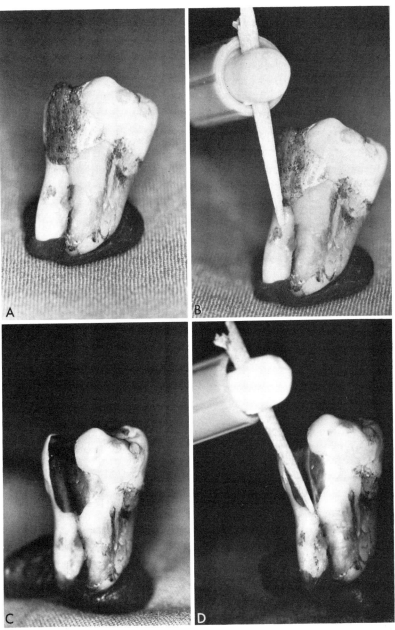

Figure 42–5 Effect of restoration contours on plaque control. *A,* Overcontoured amalgam restoration, causing (*B*) poor accessibility for oral hygiene aid in furcation area. *C,* Recontoured restoration, providing (*D*) adequate access for oral hygiene aid.

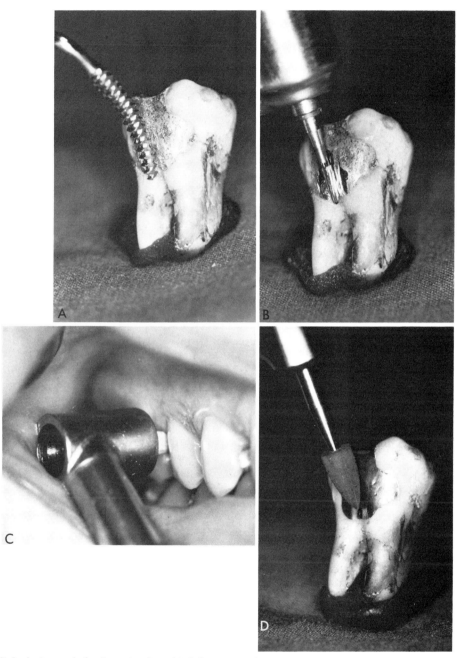

Figure 42–6 Instruments for Recontouring of Existing Restorations. *A,* Periodontal file. *B,* Finishing bur. *C,* Diamond file mounted on a handpiece. *D,* Rubber cone for final polishing.

sarily prolong this phase of periodontal therapy.

Overhanging portions of *alloy* and *resin* restorations are removed with scalers or periodontal files (Fig. 42-6A), finishing burs (Fig. 42-6B), or diamond files mounted on a special handpiece attachment that generates reciprocating strokes of high frequency (Fig. 42-6C; see also Chapter 36, Figure 36-1).

Scalers and periodontal files are efficient for gross removal of overhangs from accessible areas such as lingual and facial tooth surfaces or large interproximal embrasures. They leave a relatively rough surface on the restoration that needs to be smoothed with abrasive discs or finishing strips.

Finishing burs and handpiece-mounted files are more versatile owing to their small size, which makes them accessible to narrow spaces. Their high working speed allows them to remove large overhangs efficiently, leaving a relatively smooth restoration surface. When a bur is used, the instrument is pressed gently against the restoration and moved across the overhanging ledge to the tooth surface. The procedure is repeated until the overhang is eliminated. The bur should not be guided from the tooth toward the restoration, as this is likely to undermine the restoration and traumatize subjacent tooth structures. Final polishing of the recontoured restoration is accomplished with abrasive discs, finishing strips, or rubber cones (Fig. 42-6D). When a handpiece-mounted diamond file is used, it is centered with a continuous circular burnishing motion over the ledge of the restoration until all excess material has been shaved down. For polishing, the procedure is repeated after replacing the file in the handpiece with a plastic tip of similar shape, coated with polishing paste.

Overhanging *gold* restorations are corrected like alloy and resin restorations, but with thin, tapered *diamond* burs instead of finishing burs.

Step 4: OBTURATION OF CARIOUS LESIONS

Caries in the vicinity of the gingiva interferes with gingival health, even in the absence of adjacent calculus or defective restorations, because it acts as a large and usually inaccessible reservoir of microorganisms. Obturation of carious lesions is therefore an integral part of phase I therapy. Complete removal of such lesions and permanent closure of the cavities is desirable whenever possible. Temporary restorations are also acceptable. However, their purpose in phase I of periodontal therapy is primarily to eliminate microbial reservoirs that are injurious to the gingiva, and not to restore form and function of the affected teeth. They should therefore be placed only in cases where (1) permanent restorative care is not immediately available to the patient, or (2) the prognosis of a decayed tooth depends upon the result of periodontal therapy.

In preparing a tooth for temporary restoration, the main emphasis is placed on achieving a tight seal between tooth and restoration along the cavo-surface line of the lesion. All carious material is eliminated from the tooth surface in immediate proximity to the cavity. A shallow carious lesion is removed entirely. In extensive lesions, sometimes, the deepest portions of carious dentin are not removed completely in order to avoid potential complications such as pulp exposure or fracture of undermined enamel that would necessitate endodontic or restorative emergency care. The cavity is lined with a calcium hydroxide base and sealed with temporary restoration material. Fracture of a temporary restoration is best prevented by undercontouring rather than overcontouring its surface, especially if reproducing the original tooth contour left large portions of the restoration unsupported by the tooth while under the forces of mastication. Final cavity preparation and replacement of the temporary filling with a permanent restoration should be performed as soon as periodontal therapy of the affected tooth is completed.

Step 5: COMPREHENSIVE PLAQUE CONTROL INSTRUCTION (See Chapter 43.)

Following removal of supragingival calculus, recontouring of defective restorations, and sealing of carious lesions, a dentition is restored to the point where a comprehensive plaque control regimen can be instituted. The patient is now expected to remove plaque from the entire clinical crown of all of his teeth except from root surfaces adjacent to deep periodontal pockets (Color Plate V Bottom, *B*).

Step 6: SUBGINGIVAL ROOT TREATMENT

When the patient is able to control supragingival plaque and marginal gingivitis, subgingival root treatment consisting of calculus removal, elimination of necrotic cementum, and root planing is initiated. This constitutes the final step in achieving smooth and regular contours on all oral tooth surfaces (Color Plate V Bottom, *C*).

Subgingival calculus is removed with curettes (see Chapter 3). Since these concrements are much harder and more tenacious than supragingival calculus,[38] subgingival scaling requires considerable force and good control of the working instrument (see Chapters 37 and 38). Accidental injury to the soft periodontal tissues adjacent to the root surface being treated is not uncommon. Therefore, inflammation of the marginal gingiva should be under control before subgingival root therapy is initiated; this reduces the friability of the tissue and the risk of severe

tissue laceration from subgingival instrumentation.

The extent of subgingival calculus should be appraised before an effort is made to remove it. This entails sliding a fine instrument (probe or explorer) gently along the calculus in the direction of the apex until the termination of the calculus on the root is felt. The distance between the apical edge of the calculus and the bottom of the pocket usually ranges from 0.2 to 1.0 mm. The operator should try to see the entire calculus mass by blowing warm air between the tooth and the gingival margin or deflecting the gingiva with a probe or small pellet of cotton. Although subgingival calculus is generally brown or dark gray and can be readily distinguished from the color of the tooth, it is often difficult to see calculus in deep pockets because of the bulk of the soft tissue wall.

The complete removal of subgingival calculus requires the development of a delicate sense of touch. With the toe of the curette sliding along the tooth surface, the instrument is gently inserted in the pocket and moved apically, beyond the deepest portion of the calculus (Fig. 42–7A). The curette should never be pushed hard in an apical direction, since this often forces calculus and other debris into the tissue and may elicit an acute inflammatory response. Calculus is dislodged from the tooth and the pocket by firmly press-

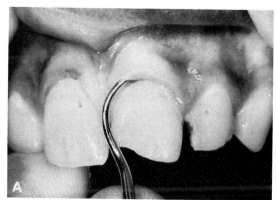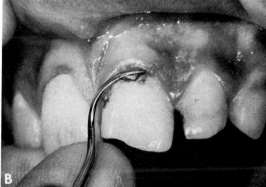

Figure 42–7   Removal of Subgingival Calculus. *A,* Curette inserted below gingival margin. *B,* Flint-like subgingival calculus removed.

ing the tip of the curette sideways against the root surface and removing the instrument from the pocket with a long, swift stroke (Fig. 42–7B). Short, abrupt "sweeps" at the tooth should be avoided because they result in "nicking" of the root surface, which requires extensive planing, leads to undue loss of tooth structure, and causes postoperative sensitivity.

In the course of the scaling procedure, the smoothness of the root must be checked and rechecked with a fine probe or explorer (Figure 42–4). It should be borne in mind that there is often a slight vertical groove on proximal root surfaces of posterior teeth.Calculus lodged in these grooves often gives the root a regular contour, thus conveying the erroneous impression that the root surface is clean.

It is not enough to eliminate the calculus from the root surface. After subgingival calculus has been completely removed, there may be areas in which the root feels softened or rough (where the cementum has undergone necrotic changes, or heavy instrumentation has produced grooves and scratches in the surface). *The root must be planed until it is smooth. Smoothness of the root surface is essential for optimal plaque control and is one of the most reliable clinical signs to diagnose absence of calculus or necrotic cementum.*

Root planing requires the same instruments and procedures that are used for subgingival calculus removal. Initially, pull strokes with firm pressure against the tooth are indicated for efficient removal of necrotic cementum or roughened dentin. As the surface becomes smoother, the pressure is gradually reduced while length and frequency of the strokes are increased; in addition, vertical strokes are combined with oblique and horizontal strokes. This produces the required smoothness of the root.

Within three to four weeks following removal of calculus, elimination of necrotic cementum, recontouring or planing of irregular tooth surfaces, and institution of plaque control, substantial reduction or elimination of gingival inflammation usually occurs. This healing process is frequently accompanied by transient root hypersensitivity, as well as a marked recession of the gingival margin (Color Plate V Top, A to D) that may have an unaesthetic effect. The patient must be informed in advance of these therapeutic sequelae to prevent his potential distrust and loss of motivation regarding periodontal therapy.

Step 7: TISSUE RE-EVALUATION

The periodontal tissues are now re-examined for further therapy. Occlusal and functional dental relationships are analyzed and corrected where indicated (see Chapter 56). Pockets are re-probed to decide if surgical treatment is indicated. However, further improvement of a periodontal condition by means of surgery can be expected only if phase I therapy has been successfully completed. Therefore, surgical reduction or elimination of periodontal pockets should be attempted only if a patient is exercising effective plaque control and if the periodontal tissues are free of overt inflammation.

REFERENCES

1. Alexander, A. G.: Periodontal aspects of conservative dentistry. Br. J. Dent., *124*:111, 1968.
2. Ambrose, J. A., and Detamore, R. J.: Correlation of histologic and clinical findings in periodontal treatment. Effect of scaling on reduction of gingival inflammation prior to surgery. J. Periodontol., *31*:238, 1960.
3. Allen, D. L., and Kerr, D. A.: Tissue response in the guinea pig to sterile and non-sterile calculus. J. Periodontol., *36*:121, 1965.
4. Axelsson, P., and Lindhe, J.: The effect of a preventive programme on dental plaque, gingivitis and caries in school children. Results after one and two years. J. Clin. Periodontol., *1*:126, 1974.
5. Bergman, B., Hugoson, A., and Olsson, C-O.: Periodontal and prosthetic conditions in patients treated with removable partial dentures and artificial crowns. A longitudinal study. Acta. Odont. Scand., *29*:621, 1971.
6. Björby, A., and Löe, H.: The relative significance of different local factors in the initiation and development of periodontal inflammation. J. Periodontol. Res., *2*:76, 1967.
7. Björn, A. L., Björn, H., and Grkovic, B.: Marginal fit of restorations and its relation to periodontal bone level. I. Metal fillings. Odontol. Rev., *20*:311, 1969.
8. Brebou, M., and Mühlemann, H. R.: The role of surface roughness of plastic foils in the collec-

tion of early calculus deposits. Helv. Odontol. Acta, 10:137, 1966.

9. Burke, S. W., and Green, E.: Effectiveness of periodontal files. J. Periodontol., 41:39, 1970.

10. Chawla, T. N., Nanda, R. S., and Kapoor, K. K.: Dental prophylaxis procedures in control of periodontal disease in Lucknow (rural) India. J. Periodontol., 46:498, 1975.

11. Ellman, I. A.: Safe high-speed periodontal instrument. Dent. Survey, 36:759, 1960.

12. Ewen, S. J.: A photomicrographic study of root scaling. Periodontics, 4:273, 1966.

13. Ewen, S. J., and Gwinnett, A. J.: A scanning electron microscopic study of teeth following periodontal instrumentation. J. Periodontol., 48:92, 1977.

14. Gilmore, N., and Sheiham, A.: Overhanging dental restorations and periodontal disease. J. Periodontal., 42:8, 1971.

15. Glickman, I.: The effect of prescaling upon healing following periodontal surgery. A clinical and histologic study. J. Dent. Med., 16:19, 1961.

16. Gottsegen, R.: Should the teeth be scaled prior to surgery? J. Periodontol., 32:301, 1961.

17. Green, E., and Ramfjord, S. P.: Tooth roughness after subgingival root planing. J. Periodontol., 37:396, 1966.

18. Gutverg, M., and Haberman, S.: Studies on bacteremia following oral surgery: some prophylactic approaches to bacteremia and the results of tissue examination of excised gingiva. J. Periodontol., 33:105, 1962.

19. Karlsen, K.: Gingival reactions to dental restorations. Acta Odontol. Scand., 28:895, 1970.

20. Kerry, G. J.: Roughness of root surfaces after use of ultrasonic instruments and hand curettes. J. Periodontol., 38:340, 1967.

21. Koivumaa, K. K., and Wennstrom, A.: A histological investigation of the changes in gingival margins adjacent to gold crowns. Odontol. T., 68:373, 1960.

22. Korn, N. A., and Schaffer, E. M.: A comparison of the postoperative bacteremias induced following different periodontal procedures. J. Periodontol., 33:226, 1962.

23. Lightner, L. M., O'Leary, T. J., Drake, R. B., Crump, P., and Allen, M. F.: Preventive periodontics treatment procedures: results over 46 months. J. Periodontol., 42:555, 1971.

24. Lindhe, J., and Koch, G.: The effect of supervised oral hygiene on the gingiva of children. Progression and inhibition of gingivitis. J. Periodontol. Res., 1:260, 1966.

25. Lindhe, J., and Nyman, S.: The effect of plaque control and surgical pocket elimination on the establishment and maintenance of periodontal health. A longitudinal study of periodontal therapy in cases of advanced disease. J. Clin. Periodontol., 2:67, 1975.

26. Löe, H., Theilade, E., and Jensen, S. B.: Experimental gingivitis in man. J. Periodontol., 36:177, 1965.

27. Marcum, J. S.: The effect of crown margin depth upon gingival tissue. J. Prosth. Dent., 17:479, 1967.

28. Pameijer, C. H., Stallard, R. E., and Hiep, N.: Surface characteristics of teeth following periodontal instrumentation: a scanning electron microscope study. J. Periodontol., 43:628, 1972.

29. Perel, M. L.: Axial crown contours. J. Prosth. Dent., 25:642, 1971.

30. Ramfjord, S. P., Knowles, J. W., Nissle, R. R., Burgett, F. G., and Shick, R. A.: Results following three modalities of periodontal therapy. J. Periodontol., 46:522, 1975.

31. Ramfjord, S. P.: Present status of the modified Widman flap procedure. J. Periodontol., 48:558, 1977.

32. Renggli, H. H.: Reaktion der Gingiva auf überhängende Füllungsränder. Dtsch. zahnärztl. Z., 27:322, 1972.

33. Renggli, H. H.: Auswirkungen subgingivaler approximaler Füllungsränder auf den Etzündungsgrad der benachbarten Gingiva. Thesis, Dental Institute, Zürich, Switzerland, 1974.

34. Richter, W. A., and Ueno, H.: Relationship of crown margin placement to gingival inflammation. J. Prosth. Dent., 30:156, 1973.

35. Rosenberg, R. M., and Ash, M. M., Jr.: The effect of root roughness on plaque accumulation and gingival inflammation. J. Periodontol., 45:146, 1974.

36. Rosling, B., Nyman, S., Lindhe, J., and Jern, B.: The healing potential of the periodontal tissues following different techniques of periodontal surgery in plaque-free dentitions. A 2-year clinical study. J. Clin. Periodontol., 3:233, 1976.

37. Schaffer, E. M.: Periodontal instrumentation: scaling and root planing. Int. Dent. J., 17:297, 1967.

38. Schroeder, H. E.: Formation and Inhibition of Dental Calculus. Hans Huber Publishers: Berne, Stuttgart, Vienna, p. 15, 1969.

39. Silness, J.: Periodontal conditions in patients treated with dental bridges. III. The relationship between the location of the crown margin and the periodontal condition. J. Periodontol. Res., 5:225, 1970.

40. Stahl, S. S., Witkin, G. J., Cantor, M., and Brown, R.: Gingival healing. II. Clinical and histologic repair sequences following gingivectomy. J. Periodontol., 39:109, 1968.

41. Suomi, J. D., Greene, J. C., Vermillion, J. R., Doyle, J., Chany, J. J., and Leatherwood, E. C.: The effect of controlled oral hygiene procedures on the progression of periodontal disease in adults: results after third and final year. J. Periodontol., 42:152, 1971.

42. Valderhaug, J., and Birkeland, J. M.: Periodontal conditions in patients 5 years following insertion of fixed prostheses. I. Pocket depths and loss of attachment. J. Oral Rehab., 3:237, 1976.

43. Van Volkinburg, J. W., Green, E., and Armitage, G. C.: The nature of root surfaces after curette, cavitron and alpha sonic instrumentation. J. Periodontol. Res., 11:374, 1976.

44. Villa, P.: Degree of calculus inhibition by habitual

tooth brushing. Helv. Odontol. Acta, *12*:31, 1968.
45. Waerhaug, J.: Tissue reactions around artificial crowns. J. Periodontol., *24*:172, 1953.
46. Waerhaug, J.: Effect of rough surfaces upon gingival tissue. J. Dent. Res., *35*:323, 1956.

47. Wilkinson, R. F., and Maybury, J. E.: Scanning electron microscopy of the root surface following instrumentation. J. Periodontol., *44*:559, 1973.
48. Wright, W. H.: Local factor in periodontal disease. Periodontics, *1*:163, 1963.

Plaque Control

hibitors incorporated in mouthwashes or dentifrices.

Plaque control is one of the keystones of the practice of dentistry. Without it oral health can neither be attained nor preserved, although there is probably a minimal plaque level that the gingiva can tolerate, beyond which plaque accumulation need not be reduced to prevent gingival and periodontal disease. Every patient in every dental practice should be on a plaque control program. For the patient with a healthy periodontium, plaque control means the preservation of health. For the patient with periodontal disease it means optimal healing following treatment. For the patient with treated periodontal disease, plaque control means the prevention of recurrence of disease.

Plaque control is the removal of microbial plaque[38, 44, 95, 146, 185] and the prevention of its accumulation on the teeth and adjacent gingival surfaces. Plaque control also retards the formation of calculus.[153, 190] Removal of microbial plaque leads to the resolution of gingival inflammation in its early stages.[32] Cessation of tooth cleaning leads to its recurrence.[93, 108] Thus, plaque control is an effective way of treating and preventing gingivitis and is therefore a critical part of all the procedures involved in the prevention of periodontal disease.[27, 31, 76, 102, 170]

To date, the most dependable mode of controlling plaque is by mechanical cleansing with a toothbrush and other cleansing aids. Considerable progress has also been made with chemical plaque in-

MANUAL TOOTHBRUSHES AND BRISTLES

Toothbrushes vary in size and design as well as in length, hardness, and arrangement of the bristles (Fig. 43–1).[19, 49] The American Dental Association has described the range of dimensions of acceptable brushes: brushing surface from 1 to 1¼ inches (25.4 to 31.8 mm.) long and 5/16 to 3/8 inch (7.9 to 9.5 mm.) wide, 2 to 4 rows, 5 to 12 tufts per row.[2] A toothbrush should be able to reach and clean efficiently most areas of the mouth. The choice is a matter of individual preference rather than a demonstrated superiority of any one type. Ease of manipulation by the patient is an important factor in brush selection. The effectiveness of or potential injury from different types of brushes depends to a great degree on how the brushes are used.[29]

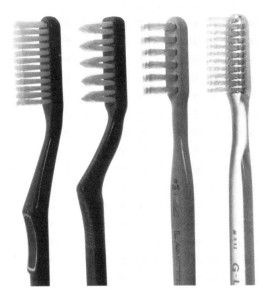

Figure 43–1   Types of manual brushes. The two brushes on the left have contra-angle shanks.

There are two kinds of bristle material used in toothbrushes, *natural* (hog bristle) and *nylon.* The cleaning effect of either type seems to be equally satisfactory.[19, 79] However, while natural bristles vary considerably in size in the same brush and tend to soften in a wet environment, nylon bristles retain their firmness longer, are more uniform in size and shape, and are easier to keep clean. Also, patients accustomed to the softness of an old natural bristle brush often traumatize the gingiva when using new nylon bristles with comparable vigor. Careful instruction is therefore necessary when changing from natural to nylon bristles.

The bristles are grouped in tufts arranged usually in three to four rows (Fig. 43–1). Four-row brushes (multi-tufted) contain more bristles and therefore tolerate more working pressure without flexing. Rounded bristle-ends are assumed to be safer than flat-cut bristles with sharp ends. But this has been questioned,[73] since cut bristle tips also round over after being used for one to two weeks. The question of the most desirable bristle hardness is not settled. Bristle hardness is proportional to the square of the diameter and inversely proportional to the square of bristle length.[69] Diameters of commonly used bristles range from 0.007 inch (0.2

mm.), soft to 0.012 inch (0.3 mm.), medium, and 0.014 inch (0.4 mm.), hard.[73] Soft bristle brushes of the type described by Bass[16] have been gaining wide acceptance. Bass recommended a straight handle, nylon bristles 0.007 inch, (0.2 mm.) in diameter, 13/32 inch (10.3 mm.) long, with rounded ends arranged in three rows of tufts, six evenly spaced tufts per row, with 80 to 86 bristles per tuft (Fig. 43–1). For children, the brush is smaller, with thinner (0.005 inch or 0.1 mm.) and shorter (11/32 inch or 8.7 mm.) bristles.

Opinions regarding the merits of hard and soft bristles are based upon studies carried out under different conditions and are often inconclusive and not in agreement with each other.[74] Medium bristles seem to cleanse better than soft bristles.[40] Soft bristles are more flexible, cleanse beneath the gingival margin (sulcus cleansing),[17] and reach more of the proximal tooth surface, but may not completely remove heavy plaque deposits.[56] Soft bristles seem to cleanse better than hard bristles because of the "matting effect" produced by the combination of soft bristles and dentifrice.[23] This increases tooth/dentifrice contact and adds to the cleansing action, but could also increase tooth abrasion.[69] However, the manner in which a brush is used and the abrasiveness of a dentifrice[1, 149] affect the cleansing action and abrasion to a greater degree than the bristle hardness itself.[125]

Patients should be advised that, in order to maintain the cleaning efficiency of a toothbrush, it must be replaced as soon as the bristles begin to fray. With conscientious, regular use of a brush, this should occur within three months. If a brush is "worn out" after one week, tooth cleaning is usually performed too vigorously; if the bristles are still straight after six months, the brushing is either done too gently or the brush has not been used every day. Unfortunately, there is a tendency to use a brush "as long as it lasts" which often is long after the bristles have lost their cleaning effectiveness or have become injurious to the gingiva.

Selecting the handle shape of a toothbrush is a matter of individual preference. A handle should be long enough to fit the palm of the hand. Straight handles are most common. Handles with contra-angle shanks (Fig. 43–1) may provide the grasping hand with a better feeling of touch, since the working surface of the brush, i.e., the bristle ends, is placed along the direct imaginary extension of the long axis of the handle. Also, the stretching of the lip when brushing facial molar surfaces is less with contra-angle handles than with straight handles.

For the routine patient, a short-headed brush with straight-cut, round-ended, soft-to-medium nylon bristles arranged in three or four tuft rows is recommended.

POWERED TOOTHBRUSHES

There are many types of electric toothbrushes, some with a reciprocal arcuate or back-and-forth motion, some with a combination of both, some with a circular motion, and some with an elliptical motion (Figs. 43–2 and 43–3). Regardless of the type, best results are obtained if the patient is instructed in its proper use.[10, 124] Patients who can develop the ability to use a toothbrush properly usually do equally well with both a manual and electric toothbrush. Less

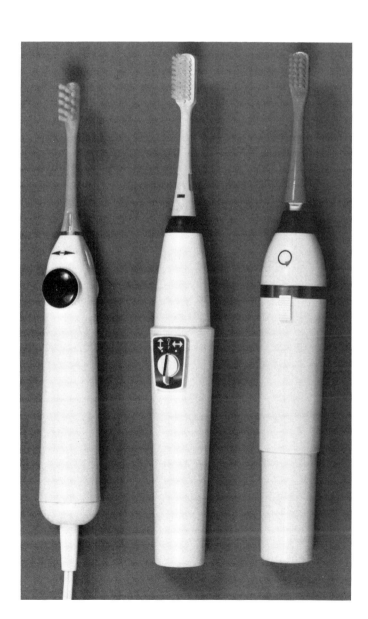

Figure 43–2 Types of powered brushes.

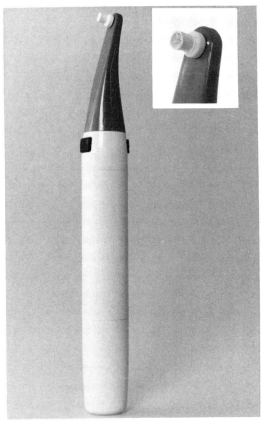

Figure 43–3   Powered tooth cleaner with rotary rubber cup.

diligent brushers do better with an electric toothbrush, which compensates somewhat for their inadequacy. Electric brushes are recommended (1) for individuals lacking manual dexterity, (2) for small children or handicapped or hospitalized patients who need to have their teeth cleaned by someone else, and (3) for patients with orthodontic appliances.

A number of researchers report that electrically powered toothbrushes are su-

perior to manual toothbrushes in terms of removing plaque, reducing plaque and calculus accumulation, and improving gingival health.[95, 102, 123, 146, 153] Others claim that manual and powered brushes are equally effective.[11, 62, 129, 186] Electric brushes seem to produce less abrasion of tooth substance and restorative materials than manual brushing,[126, 128] unless the manual brush is used in a vertical rather than a horizontal direction.[69]

DENTIFRICES

Dentifrices are aids for cleaning and polishing tooth surfaces. They are used mostly in the form of a paste. Tooth powders and liquids are also available. The cleansing effect of a dentifrice is related to its content of (1) abrasives such as calcium carbonate, calcium phosphate, calcium sulfate, sodium bicarbonate, sodium chloride, aluminum oxide, and silicate, and (2) detergents such as sodium lauryl sulfate and sodium lauroyl sarcosinate. In addition, a paste contains humectants (glycerin, sorbitol), water, thickening agents (carboxymethyl cellulose, alginate, amylose), flavoring, and coloring agents.

There is considerable interest in improving dentifrices by using them as vehicles for chemotherapeutic agents to inhibit plaque, calculus, caries, or root hypersensitivity. Except for the pronounced caries-prophylactic effect of fluorides incorporated in dentifrices.[126a] substances such as chlorhexidine,[46] penicillin, dibasic ammonium phosphate, vaccines, vitamins, chlorophyll, formaldehyde, and strontium chloride have proven to be of little therapeutic value.

If a dentifrice is to be an effective ad-

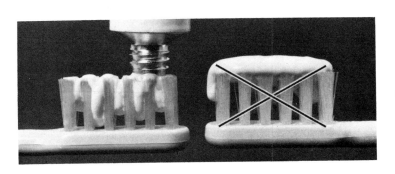

Figure 43–4   Correct and incorrect (×) application of dentifrice.

junct to oral hygiene, it must come in intimate contact with the teeth. This is achieved best by depositing the paste *between* the bristles of the toothbrush rather than on top of the bristles (Fig. 43–4), from which large portions of the dentifrice often are displaced before reaching the tooth surfaces.

Dentifrices should be sufficiently abrasive for satisfactory cleansing and polishing but should provide a margin of safety to protect the aggressive toothbrusher from wearing away tooth substance and soft restorative materials.[149, 156] The abrasive quality of dentifrices affects enamel, but it is more of a concern in patients with exposed cementum and dentin because it can lead to surface abrasion and root hypersensitivity.[178] However, the fact that abrasions are more prevalent on maxillary than on mandibular teeth and are found more frequently on the left than on the right half of the dental arch[48, 86, 94] indicates that abrasion may be caused by a *number of factors.* Dentifrices that provide the cleansing effectiveness required for plaque control, with a minimum of abrasion, should be selected for periodontal patients. Inasmuch as the formulations of dentifrices are occasionally changed, the most current information should be obtained from the Council on Dental Therapeutics of the American Dental Association.[2]

TOOTHBRUSHING METHODS

There are many methods of toothbrushing.[18, 21, 37, 54, 72, 75, 169, 177] **Except for overtly**

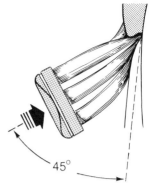

Figure 43–6 Bass Method. Intrasulcus position of brush, at 45 degree angle to long axis of tooth.

traumatic methods, thoroughness rather than technique is the important factor in determining the effectiveness of toothbrushing. Three methods of toothbrushing are presented here, each of which, if properly performed, can accomplish the desired results.

The Bass Method (Sulcus Cleansing)[18]

Maxillary teeth: Facial and facio-proximal surfaces

Place the head of a soft-to-medium brush parallel to the occlusal plane with the "tip" of the brush distal to the last molar (Fig. 43–5). Place the bristles at the gingival margin, establish an apical angle of 45 degrees to the long axis of the teeth, **exert gentle vibratory pressure in the long axis of the bristles,** and force the bristle ends into the facial gingival sulci (Fig. 43–6) as well as into the interproximal embrasures (Fig. 43–7). This should pro-

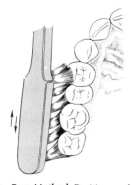

Figure 43–5 Bass Method. Position on facial and facio-proximal surfaces of maxillary molars.

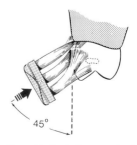

Figure 43–7 Bass Method. Interproximal position of brush at 45 degree angle to long axis of tooth.

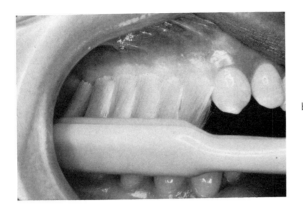

Figure 43–8 Bass Method. Correct application of brush should produce perceptible blanching of the gingiva.

duce perceptible blanching of the gingiva (Fig. 43–8). Activate the brush with a short back-and-forth motion *without dislodging the tips of the bristles.* Complete 20 such strokes in the same position. This cleans the teeth facially within the apical third of their clinical crowns as well as within their adjacent gingival sulci and along their proximal surfaces as far as the bristles reach. Lift the brush, move it anteriorly, and repeat the process in the premolar and canine area (Fig. 43–9); place the brush so that its "heel" is still distal to the canine prominence. This cleans the premolars and the distal half of the canine.

Then lift the brush and move it so that its "tip" is mesial to the canine prominence (Figs. 43–10 and 43–11). This cleans the mesial half of the canine and the incisors.

Continue on the opposite side of the arch, section by section covering three teeth at a time, until the whole maxillary dentition is completed.

COMMON ERRORS. The following errors in the use of the brush often result in unsatisfactory cleansing or soft tissue injury:

1. When the arm holding the brush becomes tired, there is a tendency to relax and let the brush slide down, creating an

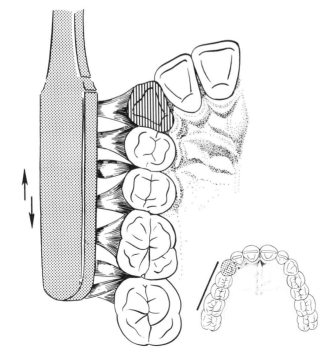

Figure 43–9 Bass Method. Position on facial and facio-proximal surfaces of maxillary premolars and distal half of canine.

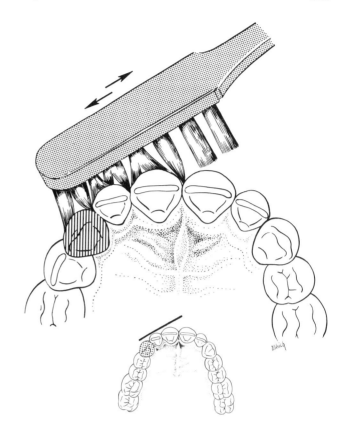

Figure 43–10 Bass Method. Position on facial and facio-proximal surfaces of maxillary incisors and mesial half of canine.

angle between the occlusal plane and the long axis of the brush (Fig. 43–12). This prevents the main bulk of the bristles from adequate penetration interproximally and into the gingival sulci. The error is corrected by raising the elbow as far as necessary.

2. The bristles are placed on the attached gingiva rather than into the gingival sulci (Fig. 43–13). When the brush is activated, the gingival margin and the tooth surfaces are neglected while the attached gingiva and the alveolar mucosa are traumatized (Fig. 43–14). The error is corrected by practicing correct positioning of the brush under visual guidance, using the brush dry without dentifrice.

3. The bristles are pressed sideways

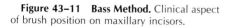

Figure 43–11 Bass Method. Clinical aspect of brush position on maxillary incisors.

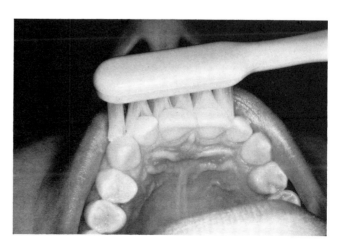

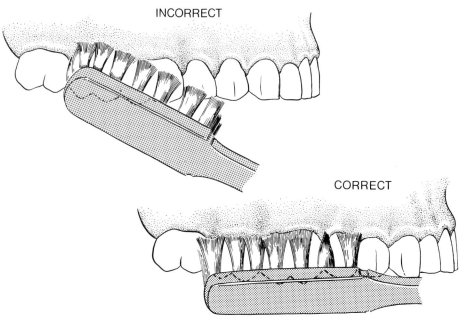

Figure 43–12   Bass Method. Incorrect brush position (top) due to low position of elbow. Error corrected (bottom) by raising elbow.

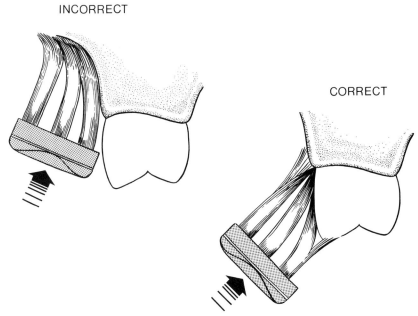

Figure 43–13   Bass Method. Incorrect brush position (left) due to poor instruction. Position corrected (right) by practicing under visual guidance with a dry brush.

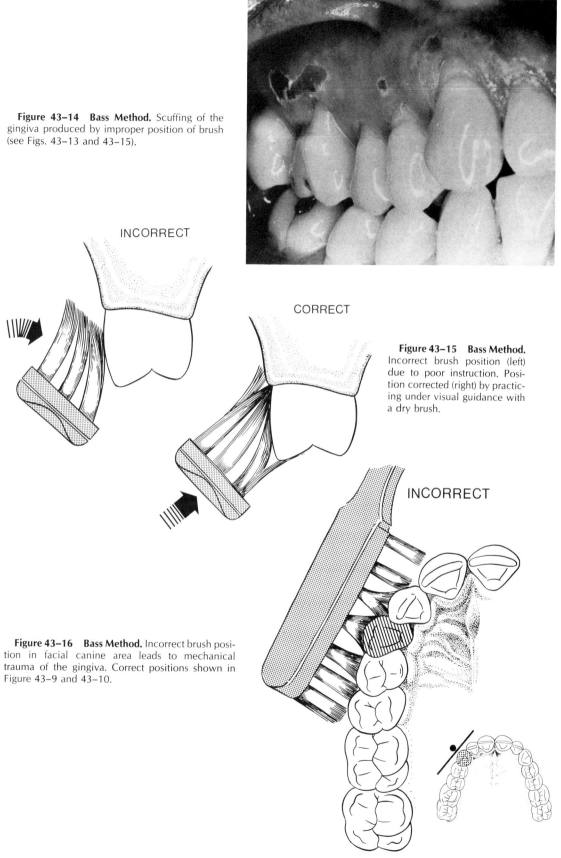

Figure 43–14 Bass Method. Scuffing of the gingiva produced by improper position of brush (see Figs. 43–13 and 43–15).

INCORRECT

CORRECT

Figure 43–15 Bass Method. Incorrect brush position (left) due to poor instruction. Position corrected (right) by practicing under visual guidance with a dry brush.

INCORRECT

Figure 43–16 Bass Method. Incorrect brush position in facial canine area leads to mechanical trauma of the gingiva. Correct positions shown in Figure 43–9 and 43–10.

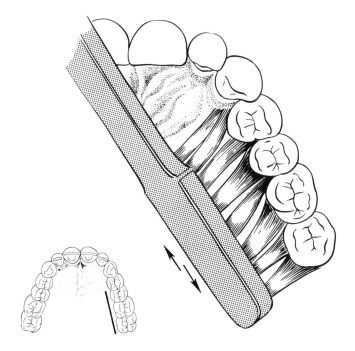

Figure 43–17 Bass Method. Palatal position on molars and premolars.

against the teeth rather than straight into the gingival sulci (Fig. 43–15). Activating the brush cleanses facial tooth surfaces but neglects the highly plaque-retaining areas interproximally and along the gingival margin. The error is corrected by practicing with the dry brush.

4. The brush is placed against the canine prominence (Fig. 43–16). This traumatizes the gingiva when attempting to force the bristles into the interproximal embrasures of adjacent teeth and could lead to gingival recession at the canine

prominence. The correct positions are shown in Figures 43–9 and 43–10.

Maxillary teeth: Palatal and palato-proximal surfaces

Engage the brush at a 45 degree apical angle in the molar and premolar areas, covering three teeth at a time (Figs. 43–17 and 43–18). Clean each segment with 20 short back-and-forth strokes. To reach the palatal surface of the anterior teeth, insert the brush vertically (Figs. 43–19 and 43–

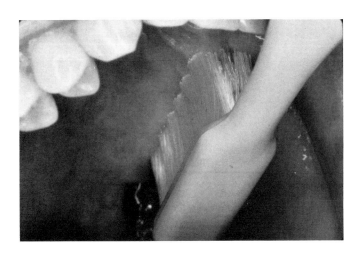

Figure 43–18 Bass Method. Clinical aspect of palatal position on molars and premolars.

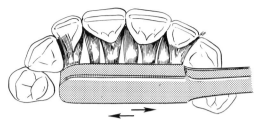

Figure 43–21   Bass Method. Variation of palatal brush position on incisors if space permits.

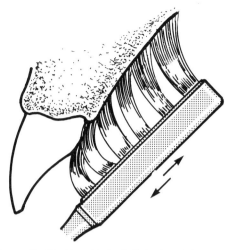

Figure 43–19   Bass Method. Palatal position on incisors. Hard palate is used as guide plane for the brush.

20). Press the "heel" of the brush into the gingival sulci and interproximally at a 45 degree angle to the long axis of the teeth, using the anterior portion of the hard palate as a guide plane. Activate the brush with 20 short up-and-down strokes. If the shape of the arch permits, the brush may be inserted horizontally between the canines with the bristles angulated into the gingival sulci of the anterior teeth (Fig. 43–21).

Mandibular teeth: Facio-proximal, lingual, and linguo-proximal surfaces

The mandibular teeth are cleaned in the same way as the maxillary teeth, section by section, 20 strokes in each position. In the anterior lingual region the brush is inserted vertically, using the lingual surface of the mandible as a guide plane, and with the bristles angulated into the gingival sulci (Fig. 43–22). If space permits, the brush may also be inserted horizontally between the canines (Fig. 43–23).

COMMON ERROR.   The brush is placed on the incisal edge with the bristles on the lingual surface but not reaching into the sulci (Fig. 43–24). When the brush is moved back and forth, only the incisal edges and a portion of the lingual surfaces are cleaned. This error is due to insufficient opening of the mouth and too relaxed position of the arm. To achieve the proper position, the mouth is opened wide and the elbow is raised high enough so that the hand holding the brush touches the tip of the nose.

Occlusal surfaces

Press the bristles firmly on the occlusal surfaces with the ends as deeply as possible into the pits and fissures (Fig. 43–25).

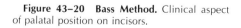

Figure 43–20   Bass Method. Clinical aspect of palatal position on incisors.

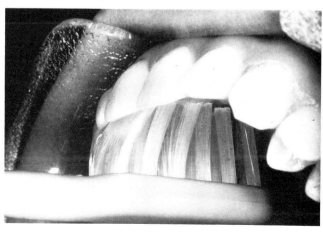

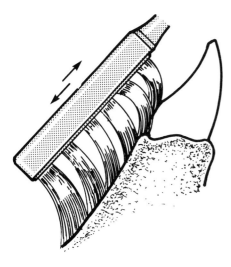

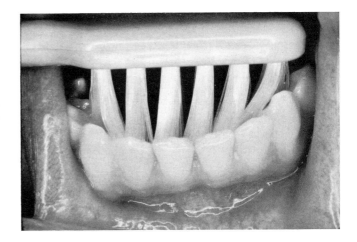

Figure 43–22 Bass Method. Lingual position on mandibular incisors. Lingual surface of mandible is used as guide plane for the brush.

Figure 43–23 Bass Method. Variation of brush position to clean lingual surfaces of mandibular incisors.

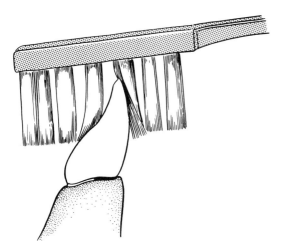

Figure 43–24 Bass Method. Incorrect application of brush due to insufficient opening of mouth and low elbow position. Error is corrected by opening wide and raising elbow.

INCORRECT

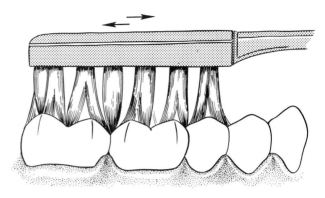

Figure 43–25 Brush position on occlusal surfaces used with the Bass, Stillman, or Charters method.

Activate the brush with 20 short back-and-forth strokes, advancing section by section until all posterior teeth in all four quadrants are cleaned.

COMMON ERROR. The brush is "scrubbed" across the teeth in long horizontal strokes instead of short back-and-forth movements.

To reach the distal surface of the most distal molars, open the mouth wide and thrust the tip of the brush against that surface, 20 times for each molar (Fig. 43–26).

The Bass technique requires approxi-mately 40 different toothbrush positions to cover a full dentition. The mouth of each patient should, therefore, be divided into sections and a systematic cleaning sequence individually prescribed giving areas with high plaque-retention priority over those with less deposits (Fig. 43–27).

The Bass method has the following distinctive advantages over other techniques.

1. The short back-and-forth motion is **easy**

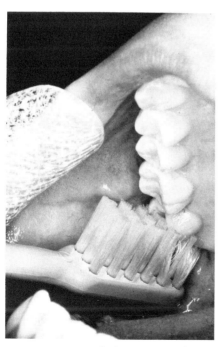

Figure 43–26 Bass Method. Position on distal surface of the most distal molars.

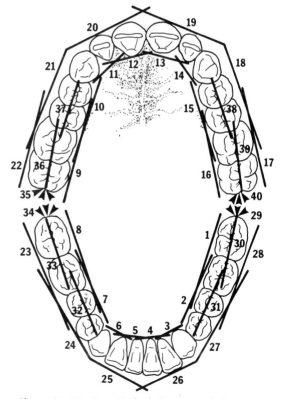

Figure 43–27 Bass Method. Recommended sequence of brush positions.

to learn because it requires the same simple elbow movement familiar to most patients who are accustomed to the still popular long-stroke scrubbing technique. Except for the 45 degree sulcus position of the bristles and a considerably shorter stroke, there is no difference between the two methods.

2. It concentrates on the **cervical and interproximal portions of the teeth** where microbial plaque is most detrimental to the gingiva.

This technique can be **recommended for the routine patient** with or without periodontal involvement.

The Modified Stillman Method[75, 177]

A medium-to-hard two- or three-row brush is placed with the bristle ends resting partly on the cervical portion of the teeth and partly on the adjacent gingiva, pointing in an apical direction at an oblique angle to the long axis of the teeth (Fig. 43–28). Pressure is applied laterally against the gingival margin so as to produce a perceptible blanching. The brush is activated with 20 short back-and-forth strokes and is simultaneously moved in a coronal direction along the attached gingiva, the gingival margin, and the tooth surface.

This process is repeated on all tooth surfaces, proceeding systematically around the mouth. To reach the lingual surfaces of maxillary and mandibular incisors, the handle of the brush is held in a vertical position, engaging the "heel" of the brush.

The occlusal surfaces of molars and premolars are cleaned with the bristles perpendicular to the occlusal plane and penetrating deeply into the sulci and interproximal embrasures (see Fig. 43–25). With this technique, the sides rather than the ends of the bristles are used and penetration of the bristles into the gingival sulci is avoided. The Stillman method is therefore **recommended for cleaning in areas with progressing gingival recession** and root exposure in order to prevent abrasive tissue destruction.

The Charters Method[37]

A medium-to-hard two- or three-row brush is placed on the tooth with the bristles pointed toward the crown at a 45 degree angle to the long axis of the teeth (Fig. 43–29). To cleanse the occlusal surfaces, the bristle tips are placed into the pits and fissures and the brush activated with **short** back-and-forth strokes (see Fig. 43–25). The procedure is repeated until all chewing surfaces are cleansed, segment by segment.

The Charters method is **especially suit-**

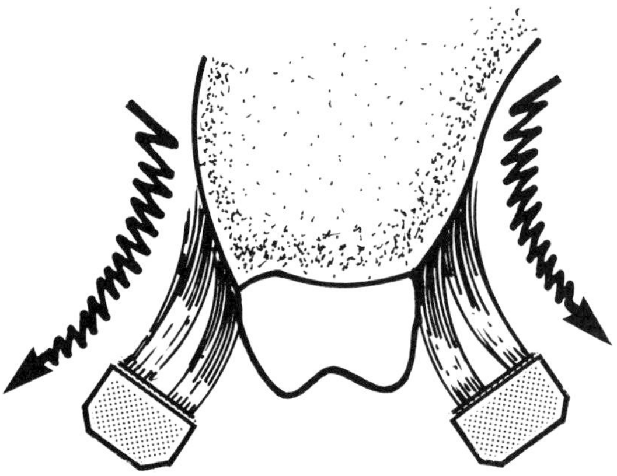

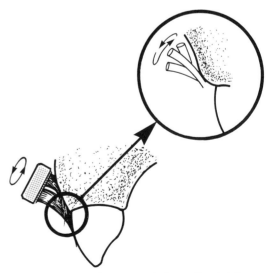

Figure 43–28 Stillman Technique, modified. The sides of the bristles are pressed against teeth and gingiva while moving the brush with short back-and-forth strokes in a coronal direction.

Figure 43–29 Charters Technique. The bristles are pressed sideward against teeth and gingiva. The brush is activated with short circular or back-and-forth strokes.

able for gingival massage. When used in conjunction with a soft-to-medium brush, this technique is also recommended for temporary cleaning in areas of healing gingival wounds, e.g., following gingivectomy or flap surgery.

Methods of Cleaning with Powered Brushes

The various mechanical motions built into electric brushes do not require special techniques of application provided the vibratory excursions of the bristle ends are small enough.

The three methods described for manual brushing are also suitable for powered tooth cleaning (Fig. 43–30).

INTERDENTAL CLEANSING AIDS

Removal of interproximal plaque is probably far more important than cleaning facial and lingual tooth surfaces because the prevalence of inflammation is highest there.[30, 85, 127, 163, 164, 173]

It has been shown that a toothbrush, regardless of the method used, does not completely remove interdental plaque accumulation, neither in persons with healthy periodontal conditions nor in periodontally treated patients with open embrasures.[24, 59, 65, 162] For optimal plaque control, toothbrushing should therefore be supplemented with a more effective way of interdental cleaning. The specific aids required for this procedure depend upon various criteria such as the size of the interdental spaces, the presence of open furcations, the individual rate of plaque formation, smoking habits, tooth alignment, and presence of orthodontic appliances or fixed prostheses.

Among the numerous aids available, dental floss and interdental cleansers such as wooden or plastic tips and interdental brushes are the most commonly used.

Dental Floss

Dental flossing is the most widely recommended method of cleansing proximal tooth surfaces.[57, 133] Many prefer unwaxed, high-tenacity nylon,[17] because it is often considerably finer than waxed floss and therefore passes more easily between teeth with tight contact areas. In addition, unwaxed floss produces a distinct squeaking sound when moved over a tooth surface that is devoid of soft deposits. This acoustic phenomenon can serve as a practical indicator of a clean tooth surface. It is

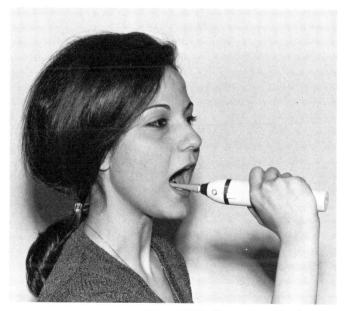
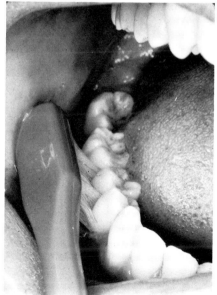

Figure 43–30 Powered toothbrushing using the Bass method.

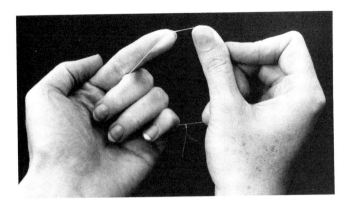

Figure 43–31   Dental flossing using the loop technique.

particularly helpful for interproximal areas where the effect of cleaning cannot be readily demonstrated with the use of a conventional disclosing agent. A difference in effectiveness between waxed and unwaxed floss, however, is not demonstrable.[71, 80, 81]

There are several ways of using dental floss. The following is recommended:

Cut a piece of floss about one foot long and tie the ends together to form a loop. Stretch the floss tightly between thumb and forefinger (Fig. 43–31) and pass it gently through each contact area with a firm sideward sawing motion. Do not forcibly snap the floss past the contact area, because this will injure the interdental gingiva. Wrap the floss around the proximal surface of one tooth, at the base of the gingival sulcus. Move the floss **firmly** along the tooth **up** to the contact area and **gently down** into the sulcus again, repeating this up-and-down stroke five or six times (Fig. 43–32). Displace the floss across the interdental gingiva and repeat the procedure on the proximal surface of the adjacent tooth. Continue through the whole dentition, including the distal surface of the last tooth in each quadrant. When the working portion of the floss becomes soiled or begins to shred, move index finger and thumb along the loop to a fresh portion of floss.

The manipulation of dental floss can be simplified by using a floss holder (Fig. 43–33). Such a device, although considerably more time-consuming to use than the loop, is especially recommended for patients lacking manual dexterity and for nursing personnel assisting handicapped and hospitalized patients in cleaning their teeth. A floss holder should feature (1)

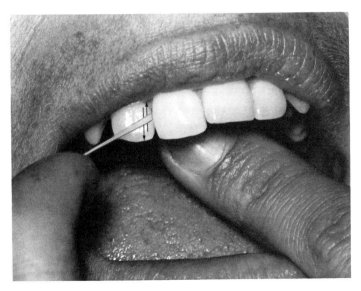

Figure 43–32   Dental Flossing. The floss is wrapped around each proximal surface and activated with repeated up-and-down strokes.

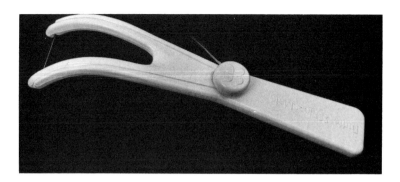

Figure 43–33 Floss Holder. It simplifies the manipulation of dental floss.

one or two forks that are rigid enough to keep the floss taut even when it is moved past tight contact areas, and (2) an effective and simple mounting mechanism that holds the floss firmly in place yet allows quick rethreading of the floss whenever its working portion becomes soiled or begins to shred.

The purpose of flossing is to remove plaque, not to dislodge fibrous threads of food wedged in between two teeth or impacted into the gingiva. Chronic food impaction should be treated by correcting proximal tooth contacts and "plunger" cusps. Removing impacted food with dental floss simply provides temporary relief but permits the condition to become worse.

Interdental Cleansers

For cleaning in narrow gingival embrasures that are occupied by intact papillae and bordered by tight contact zones, dental floss is probably the most effective dental hygiene aid, although a superiority over the toothbrush has been questioned.[162] Proper application of the floss requires good manual dexterity, intensive instruction, and repeated monitoring. Furthermore, concave root surfaces cannot be reached with dental floss (Fig. 43–34A). Therefore, special cleaning devices that are easy to handle and that adapt themselves to irregular tooth surfaces better than does dental floss (Fig. 43–34B) are recommended for proximal cleaning of teeth with large or open

Figure 43–34 Cleaning of concave or irregular proximal tooth surfaces. Dental floss (A) is less effective than an interdental brush (B).

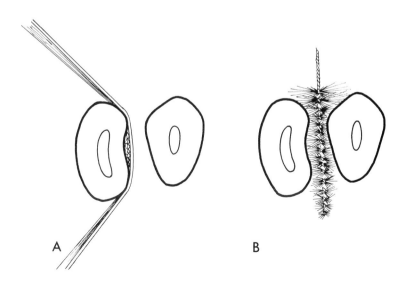

A   B

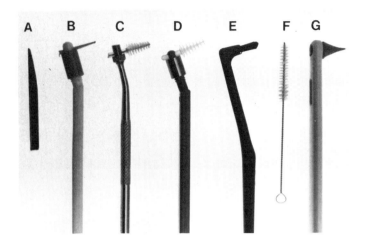

Figure 43–35   Interdental Cleansers. *Wooden tips:* A, Stimu-U-Dent; B, Perio-Aid. *Interdental brushes:* C, cone-shaped bristle-brush; D, cone-shaped plastic brush; E, uni-tufted brush; F, miniature bottle brush. *Rubber tip:* G, for gingival massage.

interdental spaces such as those found in periodontally treated dentitions.

A wide variety of interdental cleansers is available for efficient removal of soft debris from proximal tooth surfaces that are not accessible to a fullsize toothbrush (Fig. 43–35).[26, 162]

Wooden tips

Wooden tips are used either with (e.g., Perio-Aid) or without (e.g., Stim-U-Dent) the aid of a special holder.

A *Stim-U-Dent* (Fig. 43–35A) consists of a soft wooden tip that is triangular in cross-section. Held between middle finger, index finger, and thumb, it is introduced in the interdental spaces in such a way that the base surface of the triangle rests tangentially on the interproximal gingiva and the sides are in contact with the proximal tooth surfaces (Fig. 43–36). The Stim-U-Dent is then repeatedly forced in and out of the embrasure, removing soft deposits from the teeth and mechanically stimulating the papillary gingiva.

The *Perio-Aid* (Fig. 43–35B) consists of a round, tapered end of a toothpick that is inserted in a handle for convenient application. Deposits are removed by using either the side (Fig. 43–37A) or the end of the tip (Fig. 43–37B). This device is particularly efficient for cleaning along the gingival margin,[162] and within gingival sulci or periodontal pockets. The small dimensions of the tip allow for exceptionally good visibility of the tooth surface being

cleaned, which contributes substantially to the effectiveness of the Perio-Aid.

Interdental Brushes

These are cone-shaped brushes made of bristles or plastic discs mounted on a handle (Fig. 43–35C and D), uni-tufted brushes (Fig. 43–35E), or miniature bottle brushes (Fig. 43–35F). Interdental brushes are

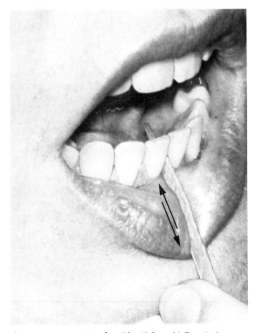

Figure 43–36   Wooden Tip (Stimu-U-Dent). Interproximal cleaning and massage with the tip inserted tangentially to the facial surface of the gingival papilla.

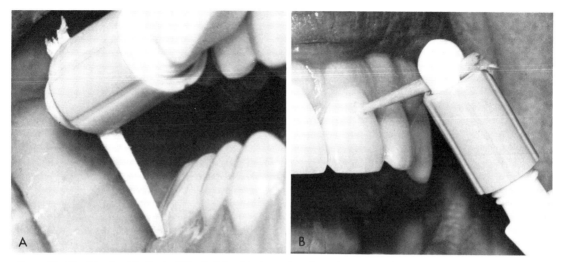

Figure 43–37   Wooden Tip (Perio-Aid). *A,* Side of tip is used to clean along gingival margins and subgingivally. *B,* Frayed end of tip cleans large surface areas.

particularly suitable for cleaning large, irregular, or concave tooth surfaces adjacent to wide interdental spaces. They are inserted interproximally and activated with short back-and-forth strokes in a linguo-facial direction. For best cleansing efficiency, the diameter of the brush should be slightly larger than the gingival embrasures so that the bristles or plastic discs can exert pressure on the tooth surfaces.

Selection of Interdental Cleansing Aids

With the purpose of selecting the most adequate interdental cleansing device,

three types of interproximal embrasures can be distinguished.

Type I embrasures are totally occupied by the interdental papillae. *Type II* embrasures are characterized by a slight to moderate recession of the interdental papillae. *Type III* embrasures are created by extensive recession or complete loss of the interdental papillae.

In type I embrasures, dental floss should be used[65] (Fig. 43–38A). It is the only device that can be passed through such narrow spaces without forcing the papillae apically, which could induce undesired gingival recession.

In type II embrasures, small interdental

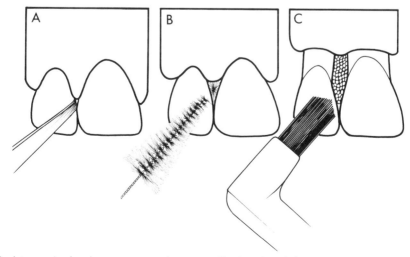

Figure 43–38   Interproximal embrasure types and corresponding interdental cleansers. *A,* Type I—no gingival recession: dental floss. *B,* Type II—moderate papillary recession: interdental brush. *C,* Type III—complete loss of papillae: uni-tufted brush.

brushes (Prox-a-brush) should be used (Fig. 43–38B). Dental floss is less effective in these cases because interproximal gingival recession usually leads to the exposure of concave root depressions (Fig. 43–34). Wooden tips can also be used.

In type III embrasures, larger brushes such as a uni-tufted brush are recommended (Fig. 43–38C).

In general, the largest applicable device should always be selected.

GINGIVAL MASSAGE

Massaging the gingiva with a toothbrush or interdental cleansers produces epithelial thickening, increased keratinization, and increased mitotic activity in the epithelium and connective tissue.[28, 33, 35, 36, 64, 148, 174, 175] It is claimed that massage improves blood circulation, the supply of nutrients and oxygen to the gingiva, tissue metabolism, and the removal of waste products.[143, 177] Whether epithelial thickening, increased keratinization, and improved blood circulation provide substantial protection against microorganisms and other local irritants and are therefore beneficial or necessary for gingival health is questionable.[63, 120] Since keratinization occurs in the oral gingiva and not in the sulcular gingiva, which is more vulnerable to microbial attack, it appears that improved gingival health provided by toothbrushing and other oral hygiene procedures results predominantly from the removal of microbial pathogens and not from gingival massage. In addition, studies with chemotherapeutic mouth rinses have demonstrated that gingival health can be maintained in the absence of mechanical oral hygiene procedures.[111]

Gingival massage is recommended as an aid to stimulate and accelerate the re-establishment of firm and keratinized gingiva following surgical interventions such as gingivectomies or flap procedures. It is administered with a toothbrush by placing the side of the bristles against the gingival surface (see Figs. 43–28 and 43–29), with stimulators such as Stim-U-Dents (see Fig. 43–35A), or with rubber tips which are inserted in the handle of a toothbrush (see Fig. 43–35G) or are mounted on a separate holder. A stimulator is inserted interdentally with the end of the tip slanted toward the occlusal surface so that its side rests tangentially against the interdental gingiva (see Fig. 43–36). In this position, the tip is likely to create or preserve the normal slope of the interdental papillae. The brush or tip is activated with a rotary motion that is repeated 20 times, pressing the instrument into the interproximal space. Each interdental area is treated from both the facial and lingual sides. This technique is also applicable to supragingival furcation areas. It is a common error to insert the Stim-U-Dent or rubber tip perpendicular to the long axis of the teeth. This creates flattened, cupped-out interdental gingival contours, which are less desirable esthetically and are more conducive to interproximal food trapping than is a sloped gingival surface produced by proper angulation of the instrument.

ORAL IRRIGATION DEVICES

Oral irrigators work on the principle of a high-pressure steady or pulsating stream of water that is directed through a nozzle to the tooth surfaces. The pressure is generated by a built-in pump or by attaching the device to the water faucet (Fig. 43–39). Oral irrigators clean non-adherent bacteria and debris from the oral cavity more effectively than toothbrushes and mouth rinses.[145, 187] They are particularly helpful for removing non-structured debris from inaccessible areas around orthodontic appliances and fixed prostheses. Also, gingival keratinization increases with the use of oral irrigators.[88] When used as adjuncts to toothbrushing, these devices can have a beneficial effect on periodontal health by retarding the accumulation of plaque and calculus.[25, 45, 77, 104, 150] and reducing gingival inflammation and pocket depth.[20, 34, 41, 90, 150] **However, water irrigation removes only negligible amounts of stainable plaque from tooth surfaces.**[51]

In the near future, oral irrigators may prove to be of considerable value as vehicles for administering chemotherapeutic agents that inhibit microbial growth, especially in inaccessible regions such as inter-

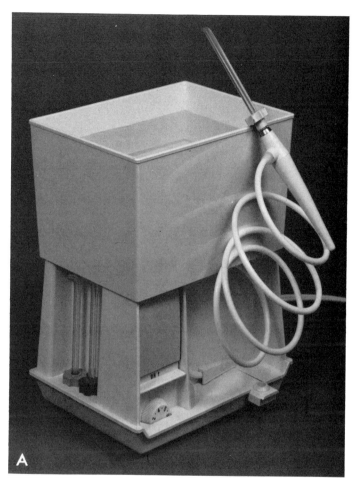

Figure 43–39   Oral Irrigation Devices.
A, Type with built-in pump. *B,* Type which attaches to water faucet.

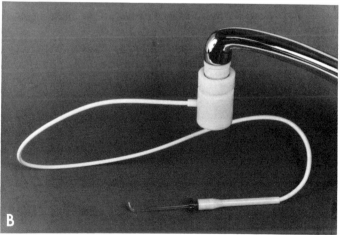

dental areas or periodontal pockets.[3] Water irrigation may cause minimal damage to soft oral tissues[140] but does not induce bacteremia when used according to the manufacturer's instructions in patients with healthy gingiva or gingivitis.[90, 105, 183] Transient bacteremia following its use in periodontitis has been reported.[50] However, bacteremia as well as gingival trauma has also been found following toothbrushing.[141, 167]

CHEMICAL PLAQUE AND CALCULUS INHIBITORS

To date, mechanical tooth cleaning with manual or powered toothbrushes, interdental cleansing aids, and rotary brushes or rubber cups is still the most effective method available for controlling plaque, calculus, and ultimately periodontal disease. But since this is a tedious procedure that cannot be relaxed without risking the establishment of new accumulations and the onset of periodontal inflammation, there is an increasing search for chemical aids which could prevent or significantly influence plaque and inflammation, thus lessening our dependence upon mechanical cleansing.[5, 43, 122, 144, 165, 166, 179]

Many agents have been tested systemically or topically for their capability of inhibiting the quantitative or qualitative development of microbial deposits, calculus, or periodontal inflammation.[118] Promising results have been reported with fluorides,[115, 117] chlorhexidine,[61, 111] alexidine,[107, 171, 172] antibiotics[109] such as erythromycin,[103] kanamycin,[114, 116] niddamycin (cc 10232),[191] penicillin,[194] spiramycin[70] and vancomycin,[132] metronidazole and nitrimidazine,[119] urea,[22, 134a, 147] bradosol,[84] victamin C,[84, 188, 189] chlorides,[84, 160] ascoxal,[134] sodium rincinoleate,[165] enzymes such as dextranase,[83, 106] mucinase,[6, 97, 176] and hyaluronidase,[192] and acetate compounds of zinc, manganese, and copper.[7] The most commonly used mode of applying these agents has been topical in the form of mouthwashes, dentifrices, gels, lozenges, and chewing gum.

The agent that has attracted the most attention to date is **chlorhexidine,** a diguanidohexane with pronounced antiseptic properties. Since the discovery that **two daily rinses with 10 ml. of a 0.2 per cent aqueous solution of chlorhexidine gluconate** almost completely inhibit the development of dental plaque, calculus, and gingivitis[111] in the human model for experimental gingivitis,[108] a number of short-term clinical investigations have confirmed this observation.[61, 110, 137-139, 182] In most of the studies, a mouth rinse has been employed as the preferred mode of application.[51, 58, 111, 165, 166] Chlorhexidine incorporated into dentifrices, gels, and lozenges has proved so far to be considerably less, if at all, effective.[46, 53, 61, 68, 78, 155] This may be due to lower concentrations of chlorhexidine in, or partial inactivation of the agent by, these carriers.[60, 155]

Aside from some local, reversible side effects such as brown staining of teeth, tongue, and silicate and resin restorations,[47, 53, 113] transient impairment of taste perception,[112, 165, 166] and discrete desquamation of the oral mucosa,[52] chlorhexidine appears to be one of the safest antiseptics known.[121, 135, 182] It has not so far shown any evidence of systemic toxic activity in humans,[159] nor produced any appreciable resistance of oral microorganisms.[131, 157, 158]

Similarly promising results have been reported with alexidine, another bis-guanide that is closely related to chlorhexidine,[14, 107, 171, 172] and with fluorides.[115, 117]

As evidence of a specific microbial etiology of inflammatory periodontal diseases is increasing (see Chap. 24), it seems likely that some antimicrobial agents that have so far proved to be effective against acute gingivitis may also be applicable to prevent or reduce the severity of long-standing chronic gingivitis and periodontitis.

DISCLOSING AGENTS

These are **solutions** and **wafers** capable of staining bacterial deposits on the surfaces of teeth, tongue, and gingivae. They are excellent oral hygiene aids because they provide the patient with a self-educational and self-motivational tool to improve his efficiency of plaque control (Fig. 43–40).[9]

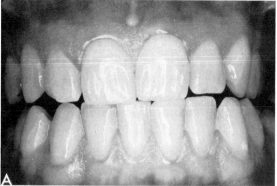
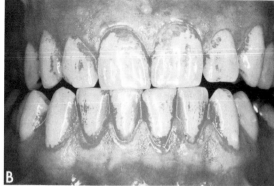
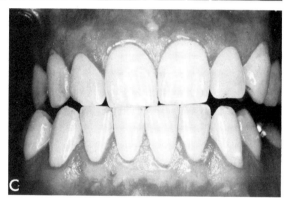

Figure 43–40 Effect of a Disclosing Agent. *A,* Unstained. *B,* Stained with a 6 per cent solution of basic fuchsin; plaque shows as dark particulate patches. *C,* Restained with basic fuchsin after thorough tooth cleaning.

Solutions

1. Basic fuchsin   6 gm.
   Ethyl alcohol, 95%   100 ml.
   Add two drops to water in a
     dappen dish

2. Potassium iodide   1.6 gm.
   Iodine crystals   1.6 gm.
   Water   13.4 ml.
   Glycerin   to make   30.0 ml.

Solutions are applied to the teeth as concentrates on cotton swabs or as dilutes in mouthwashes. They usually produce heavy staining of bacterial plaque, gingivae, tongue, lips, fingers, and sink. Therefore, they are useful in the dental office only where an impressive demonstration of bacterial deposits is desirable and excessive staining can be controlled or readily removed with prophylaxis instruments. Except for a sodium fluorescein dye, which produces a yellow glowing of dental plaque only when exposed to a light source of a certain wavelength,[39, 55, 91] solutions are not recommended for home use due to this inconvenient intensive staining effect, which may act as a deterrent rather than as a motivator.

Wafers

F.D.C. red #3 (erythrosine)	15 mg.
Sodium chloride	0.747%
Sodium sucaryl	0.747%
Calcium stearate	0.995%
Soluble saccharin	0.186%
White oil	0.124%
Flavoring (F.D.A. approved)	2.239%
Sorbitol to make	7.0 gr.

Wafers are crushed between the teeth and swished around the mouth for about 30 seconds without swallowing. Because of the convenient form of application, wafers are recommended specifically for home use.

It is obvious that the mere addition of disclosing agents to oral health instructions is not sufficient motivation for a patient to clean his teeth more effectively.

Visual feedback can, however, be an important aspect of health education if used in conjunction with other methods.

FREQUENCY OF TOOTH CLEANING

Recent studies have shown that maintenance of gingival health is compatible with conscientious plaque removal once every 24 to 48 hours.[82, 92, 110] Hence, the validity of the classic recommendation to brush the teeth after every meal and at bedtime is questionable. Numerous studies have reported on improved periodontal health associated with increasing frequency of brushing up to twice per day.[4, 67, 89, 130, 168, 180, 184] Higher cleaning frequencies, i.e., three or more per day, did not produce significantly better periodontal conditions. For practical purposes, **two brushings per day**, one of them performed with detailed thoroughness, are recommended.

Although of doubtful practicality to date, it is noteworthy that **periodontal health can be maintained** and **treated periodontal disease is arrested** over periods of several years when personal oral hygiene is supplemented **by professional tooth cleaning**, i.e., complete removal of stainable deposits, **once every two to four weeks.**[11, 12, 98, 99, 136, 151, 152]

In conclusion, emphasis must be placed on efficiency rather than frequency of tooth cleaning.

STEP-BY-STEP PROCEDURE FOR PLAQUE CONTROL INSTRUCTION

In periodontal therapy, plaque control serves three important purposes: (1) to minimize gingival inflammation prior to periodontal surgery, (2) to facilitate optimal healing following periodontal surgery, and (3) to prevent the recurrence or progression of periodontal disease in the treated mouth. In view of many socio-economic barriers still associated with the application of other successful modes of administering plaque control, such as professional tooth cleaning once every two to four weeks,[11, 12, 98, 99, 136, 151, 152] the daily mechanical removal of plaque by the pa-

tient appears so far to be the only practical means for improving oral hygiene on a long-term basis. The following step-by-step procedure to teach a patient this self-therapeutic approach to oral health is suggested.

Step I. Motivation

Motivation for effective plaque control is one of the most critical and most difficult elements of long-term success of periodontal therapy because, in most cases, it requires from a patient the following efforts: (1) receptiveness, i.e., understanding the concept of the pathogenesis, the treatment, and the prevention of periodontal disease; (2) change of habits, i.e., adopting a self-administered *daily* plaque control regimen, and (3) *behavioral changes*, i.e., adjusting the hierarchy of one's beliefs, practices, and values so as to accommodate the required new oral hygiene habits.

A patient must understand what periodontal disease is, what its effects are, that he is susceptible to it, and what he can do to achieve and maintain oral health.[42] He must be willing and able to develop and use the manual skills that are necessary to establish a plaque-control regimen. He must then want to keep his mouth clean for his own benefit (and not only to please his dentist). If these efforts are not made by the patient, long-term failure of any individual plaque-control program is inevitable and leads to frustration of the dentist and the patient. It should be recognized that effective long-range motivation within the realm of a dental office is often extremely difficult, if not impossible, to achieve. Therefore, the dentist should be prepared to alter his original treatment plan if a patient is not able to cooperate satisfactorily.

Step II. Education

Most patients think of toothbrushing only in terms of removing food debris and preventing tooth decay.[101] Its importance in the prevention and treatment of periodontal disease is rarely recognized and must therefore be explained. **Toothbrush-**

ing is the most important patient-administered preventive and therapeutic procedure. In no other field of medicine can the patient so effectively assist in controlling a disease as can be done in relation to periodontitis by conscientious plaque control. If a person maintained good oral hygiene from 5 to 50 years of age, he very likely could avoid the destructive effects of periodontal disease during this major period of his life.[67, 100]

Patients must be informed that periodic scaling and cleansing of the teeth in the dental office are helpful protective measures against periodontal disease, but only if combined with continuous, daily oral hygiene procedures at home. Therefore, time spent in the dental office teaching the patient how to cleanse his teeth is as valuable a service as cleaning his teeth for him. It must be explained that dental visits two or three times a year are not nearly as effective as is the daily oral home care. Only a combination of regular office visits with conscientious home care significantly reduces gingivitis and loss of supporting periodontal tissues.[100, 136, 181]

A periodontal patient should be shown that periodontal disease has manifested itself in his own mouth. Stained dental plaque, bleeding of inflamed gingiva, and a periodontal probe inserted into a pocket are impressive and convincing documentation of the presence of pathogens and actual disease.[13] It is of even higher educational value to a patient to have his oral cleanliness and periodontal condition recorded periodically.[15]

He can utilize this as feedback information about his level of performance. The following indices are recommended:

Plaque control record[142]

Disclosing solution is applied to all supragingival tooth surfaces. After the patient has rinsed, each tooth surface (except occlusal surfaces) is examined for presence or absence of stained deposits at the dentogingival junction. If present, they are recorded by coloring the appropriate box in a diagram (Fig. 43–41). After all teeth have been scored, an index is calculated by dividing the number of surfaces with plaque by the total number of teeth scored.

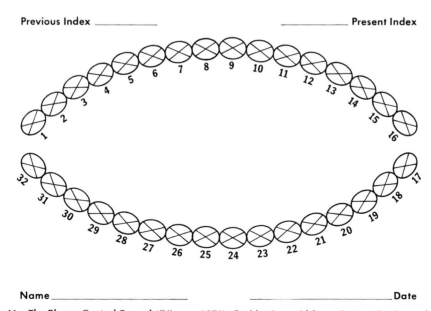

Figure 43–41   **The Plaque Control Record** (O'Leary, 1972). Oral hygiene aid for patient motivation and instruction.

Papillary bleeding index,[154] Modified

A periodontal pocket probe is inserted facially into the distal col area of each tooth (except third molars). Keeping the tip in light touch with the bottom of the sulcus, the probe is gently moved along the distofacial surface of one tooth and withdrawn at the distofacial line angle. The tip is re-inserted in the col and the procedure is repeated along the mesiofa-

cial surface of the adjacent tooth. In this way, the facial papilla distal to each tooth is probed. When probing is completed in one arch, the margin of each probed papilla is scored as follows:

  x = absence of corresponding tooth
  0 = no bleeding
  1 = minute blood spot
  2 = large blood spot (or line)
  3 = hemorrhagic oozing

The scores are entered in an index chart (Fig. 43–42). The procedure is repeated in

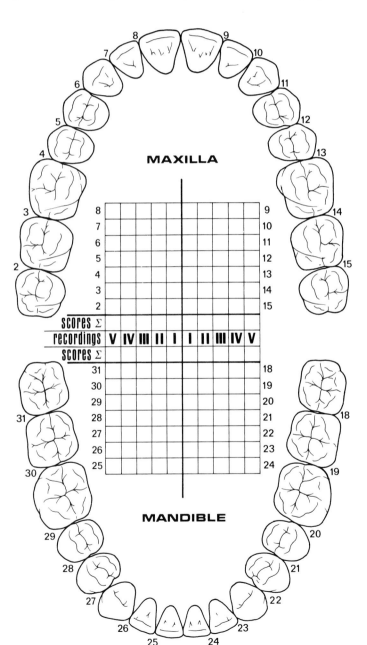

Figure 43–42 Papillary Bleeding Index (Saxer and Mühlemann, 1975), modified. Oral hygiene aid to patient motivation and instruction.

the opposite arch and the score total tabulated for each quadrant. Five consecutive recordings spaced over the entire periodontal treatment period can be made on one chart. By teaching a patient how to probe with a thin toothpick, a weekly scoring of anterior papillae can even be incorporated in his oral hygiene regimen as a self-educational tool.

The papillary bleeding index is designed to demonstrate a clinical **effect**, i.e., bleeding gingiva, rather than the cause of periodontal inflammation. Since bleeding is commonly associated with trauma or disease, papillary bleeding may well have a strong educational and motivational impact on a patient.

Step III. Instruction

With instruction and supervision, patients can reduce the incidence of plaque and gingivitis far more effectively than with self-acquired oral hygiene habits.[66, 87, 161, 181, 193] However, instruction in how to clean teeth must be more than a cursory chairside demonstration in the use of a toothbrush and oral hygiene aids. It is a painstaking procedure that requires patient participation, careful supervision with immediate correction of developing mistakes, and re-instruction during return visits until the patient demonstrates that he has developed the necessary proficiency.[8, 13, 96]

At the **first instruction visit**, the patient is presented a new toothbrush, an interdental cleanser, and a disclosing agent. First, the patient's plaque is located. Unstained, small amounts of bacterial deposits are difficult to see (Fig. 43–40A); heavier accumulations of plaque and unstructured debris (materia alba) may be visible as gray, yellow, or white material on the teeth, along the gingival margin, and in faciolingual embrasures. Loose food debris and materia alba are washed off with a strong water spray. Then a disclosing agent (solution or wafer)[9] is applied to stain all otherwise invisible plaque. After a brief water rinse to remove stained saliva which would obscure the picture, the stained plaque and pellicle can now be clearly demonstrated to the patient (Fig. 43–40B). Illuminated mouth mirrors especially designed for this purpose will give an impressive close-up view (Fig. 43–43). Polished dental restorations do not take up the stain, but the oral mucosa and the lips may retain it up to several hours. Covering the lips lightly with Vaseline before using the stain is helpful.

Toothbrushing is now demonstrated on a cast, stressing the exact placement and activation of the bristles. This is followed by a demonstration in the patient's mouth while he observes with a hand mirror. The patient then takes over and repeats on his own teeth what he has been shown, with the instructor assisting and correcting him. This exercise should not be carried out in the dental chair but rather in front of a

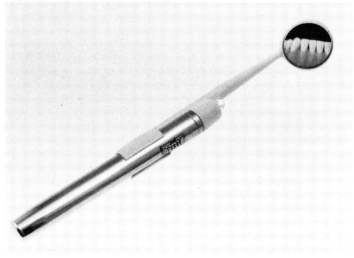

Figure 43–43 Illuminated Mouth Mirror. Oral hygiene aid for the patient to locate stained plaque.

well-illuminated wall mirror and a sink with running water. This enables the patient to have good visibility, to use both of his hands if necessary, and to rinse out freely. The procedure is repeated with dental floss and interdental cleansing aids according to the patient's needs. After one cleaning exercise is completed, the teeth are re-stained to evaluate the efficiency of plaque removal. Even after vigorous cleaning some stain usually remains on proximal surfaces. The instruction procedures are repeated until the patient is able to remove all stainable soft material from his teeth (Fig. 43–40C). Teaching machines with film strips or transparencies can be used as an adjunct to person-to-person instruction—but not as a substitute for it.

When the first visit is terminated, the patient is given the hygiene aids that were demonstrated to him, including a supply of disclosing wafers for self-evaluation of his cleaning performance at home. He is instructed to clean his teeth at least once a day with thorough attention to all details. Such a cleansing exercise in a full dentition takes 5 to 10 minutes. The patient is advised to choose for his oral hygiene a convenient time and place in his daily schedule, for instance while taking a shower. Generally, bed time is considered not to be the best choice, since one's mental and physical state before retiring at night is often not conducive to a vigorous cleaning exercise.

Subsequent instruction visits are used to re-enforce or modify previous instructions. The state of gingival health and oral cleanliness is recorded using first the papillary bleeding index (Fig. 43–42) and then the plaque control record (Fig. 43–41).

Following the recording of both indices, the patient is asked to remove the stained deposits, with special emphasis on areas that stained the heaviest. This exercise should be supervised. If corrections are indicated, they must be instituted immediately, making sure the patient understands how and why they are made. During the first few weeks, a patient often has considerable technical or motivational difficulties with a new oral hygiene regimen. He should be encouraged to comment on his own experience so that potential deficiencies or aversions can be identified and

corrected. Painful toothbrush lacerations of the gingiva (see Fig. 43–14) commonly occur with the use of a new toothbrush. They should not be overlooked. The patient is informed that the condition is transient and can be cured within a few days by temporarily cleaning with the sides rather than the ends of the bristles (see Fig. 43–29). If such a condition is overlooked, a patient could lose his confidence in the new regimen and go back to his previous cleaning habits, often without telling the dentist about it.

A patient is not dismissed until he has demonstrated some improvement over his performance at the outset of the visit. However, instruction visits should not be longer than 10 minutes each. Long visits tend to tire the patient and may lead to embarrassment, frustration, and loss of motivation.

Subsequent instruction visits are scheduled, lengthening the intervals between them, until the patient attains the proficiency required to keep his mouth healthy. Patience and repetition are the secrets of instruction in oral hygiene.

REFERENCES

1. Abrasivity of Current Dentifrices: Report of the Council of Dental Therapeutics. J. Am. Dent. Assoc., *81*:117, 1970.
2. Accepted Dental Therapeutics, 3rd ed. Chicago, American Dental Association, 1969/70, p. 225.
3. Agerbaek, N., Melsen, B., and Rölla, G.: Application of clorhexidine by oral irrigation systems. Scand. J. Dent. Res., *83*:284, 1975.
4. Ainamo, J.: The effect of habitual tooth cleaning on the occurrence of periodontal disease and dental caries. Suom. Hammaslääk, *67*:63, 1971.
5. Alderman, E. J., Jr., and Scallon, V. L.: An in vivo study of the effect of the prolonged use of a specific mouthwash on the oral flora. Chron. Omaha Dent. Soc., *28*:284, 1965.
6. Aleece, A. A., and Forscher, B. K.: Calculus reduction with a mucinase dentifrice. J. Periodontol., *25*:122, 1954.
7. Amdur, B., Brudevold, F., and Messer, A. C.: Observations on the calcification of salivary sediment. I.A.D.R. Abstr., 1962, p. 18.
8. Anderson, J. L.: Integration of plaque control into the practice of dentistry. Dent. Clin. North Am., *16*:621, 1972.
9. Arnim, S. S.: The use of disclosing agents for

measuring tooth cleanliness. J. Periodontol., *34*:227, 1963.

10. Ash, M. M.: A review of the problems and results of studies on manual and power toothbrushes. J. Periodontol., *35*:202, 1964.

11. Axelsson, P., and Lindhe, J.: The effect of the preventive programme on dental plaque, gingivitis and caries in schoolchildren: Results after one and two years. J. Clin. Periodont., *1*:126, 1974.

12. Axelsson, P., Lindhe, J., and Waseley, J.: The effect of various plaque control measures on gingivitis and caries in schoolchildren. Community Dent. Oral Epidemiol., *4*:323, 1976.

13. Barkley, R. F.: Successful Preventive Practices. Macomb, Ill., Preventive Dentistry Press. 1972, pp. 75ff, 209ff.

14. Barnes, G. P., et al.: Dental plaque reduction with an antimicrobial mouth rinse. Part I. Oral Surg., *34*:553, 1972.

15. Barrikman, R., and Penhall, O.: Graphing indexes reduces plaque. J. Am. Dent. Assoc., *87*:1904, 1973.

16. Bass, C. C.: The optimum characteristics of toothbrushes for personal oral hygiene. D. Items Int., *70*:696, 1948.

17. Bass, C. C.: Optimum characteristics of dental floss for personal oral hygiene. D. Items Int., *70*:921, 1948.

18. Bass, C. C.: An effective method of personal oral hygiene, Part II. J. Louisiana St. Med. Soc., *106*:100, 1954.

19. Bay, I., Kardel, K., and Skougaard, M. R.: Quantitative evaluation of the plaque-removing ability of different types of toothbrushes. J. Periodontol., *38*:526, 1967.

20. Beget, B. C., and Bram, M.: Oral Irrigation and Inflammation. Forty-fifth General Meeting, International Association for Dental Research, Washington, D.C., March, 1967, p. 36.

21. Bell, D. G.: Teaching home care to the patient. J. Periodontol., *19*:140, 1948.

22. Belting, C. M., and Gordon, D. L.: In vitro effect of a urea containing dentifrice on dental calculus formation, II. J. Periodontol., *37*:26, 1966.

23. Bergenholtz, A., Hugoson, A., and Sohlberg, F.: An evaluation of the plaque-removing ability of some aids to oral hygiene. Svensk. Tandlák. T., *60*:447, 1967.

24. Bergenholtz, A., Hugoson, A., Lundgren, D., and Ostgren, A.: The plaque-removing ability of various toothbrushes used with the roll technique. Svensk. Tandlák. T., *62*:15, 1969.

25. Bergenholtz, A.: Mechanical cleaning. *In* Frandsen, A. (ed.): Oral Hygiene. Copenhagen, Munskgaard, 1971, pp. 27–60.

26. Bergenholtz, A., Bjorne, A., and Vikström, B.: The plaque-removing ability of some common interdental aids. J. Clin. Periodontol., *1*:160, 1974.

27. Berman, C. L., Hosiosky, E. N., Kutscher, A. H., and Kelly, A.: Observations of the effect of an electric toothbrush; preliminary report. J. Periodontol., *33*:195, 1962.

28. Bertolini, A.: Experimental research on the effects of mechanical gingival massage. Parodontol., *9*:144, 1955.

29. Bjórn, H., and Lindhe, J.: On the mechanics of toothbrushing. Odont. Revy, *17*:9, 1966.

30. Black, A. D.: Something of the etiology and early pathology of the diseases of the periodontal membrane with suggestions as to tooth treatment. Cosmos, *55*:1219, 1913.

31. Brandtzaeg, P.: The significance of oral hygiene in the prevention of dental diseases. Odont. T., *72*:460, 1964.

32. Brandtzaeg, P., and Jamison, H. C.: The effect of controlled cleansing of the teeth on periodontal health and oral hygiene in Norwegian army recruits. J. Periodontol., *35*:308, 1964.

33. Cantor, M. T., and Stahl, S. S.: The effects of various interdental stimulators upon the keratinization of the interdental col. Periodontics, *3*:243, 1965.

34. Cantor, M. T., and Stahl, S. S.: Interdental col tissue responses to the use of a water pressure cleansing device. J. Periodontol., *40*:292, 1969.

35. Carter, S. B.: The masticatory mucosa and its response to brushing; Findings in the Merion rat, meriones libycus, at different ages. Br. Dent. J., *101*:76, 1956.

36. Castenfelt, T.: Toothbrushing and massage in periodontal disease. An experimental clinical histologic study. Stockholm, Nordisk Rotegravyr, 1952, p. 109.

37. Charters, W. J.: Eliminating mouth infections with the toothbrush and other stimulating instruments. Dent. Digest, *38*:130, 1932.

38. Chilton, N. W., Didio, A., and Rothner, J. T.: Comparison of the clinical effectiveness of an electric and a standard toothbrush in normal individuals. J. Am. Dent. Assoc., *64*:777, 1962.

39. Cohen, D. W., et al.: A comparison of bacterial plaque disclosants in periodontal disease. J. Periodontol., *43*:333, 1972.

40. Conroy, C. W.: Comparison of automatic and hand toothbrushes: Cleaning effectiveness. J. Am. Dent. Assoc., *70*:921, 1965.

41. Crumley, P. J., and Sumner, C. F.: Effectiveness of a water pressure cleansing device. Periodontics, *3*:193, 1965.

42. Derbyshire, J. C.: Methods of achieving effective hygiene of the mouth. Dent. Clin. North Am., *8*:231, 1964.

43. Dudding, N. J., et al.: Patient reactions to brushing teeth with water, dentifrice, or salt and soda. J. Periodontol., *31*:386, 1960.

44. Elliot, J. R.: A comparison of the effectiveness of a standard and an electric toothbrush. J. Periodontol., *34*:375, 1963.

45. Elliot, J. R., Bowers, G. M., Clemmer, B. A., and Rovelstad, G. H.: A comparison of selected oral hygiene devices in dental plaque removal. J. Periodontol., *43*:217, 1972.

46. Eriksen, H. M., Gjermo, P., and Johansen, J. R.: Results from two years' use of chlorhexidine(CH)–containing dentifrices. Helv. Odontol. Acta, *17*:52, 1973.

47. Eriksen, H. M., and Gjermo, P.: Incidence of stained tooth surfaces in students using chlorhexidine-containing dentifrices. Scand. J. Dent. Res., 81:533, 1973.

48. Ervin, J. C., and Bucher, E. T.: Prevalence of tooth root exposure and abrasion among dental patients. Dent. Items of Interest, 66:760, 1944.

49. Fanning, E. A., and Henning, F. R.: Toothbrush design and its relation to oral health. Australian Dent. J., 12:464, 1967.

50. Felix, J. A., Rosen, S., and App, G. R.: Detection of bacteremia after the use of an oral irrigation device in subjects with periodontitis. J. Periodontol., 42:785, 1971.

51. Fine, D. H., and Baumhammers, A.: Effect of water pressure irrigation on stainable material on the teeth. J. Periodontol., 41:468, 1970.

52. Flötra, L., et al.: A four-month study on the effect of chlorhexidine mouth washes on 50 soldiers. Scand. J. Dent. Res., 80:10, 1972.

53. Flötra, L.: Different modes of chlorhexidine application and related local side effects. J. Periodont. Res. 8 (Suppl. 12):41, 1973.

54. Fones, A. C.: Mouth Hygiene, 4th ed. Philadelphia, Lea and Febiger, 1934, p. 300.

55. Friedman, L., et al.: Bacterial plaque disclosure survey. J. Periodontol., 45:435, 1974.

56. Gilson, C. M., Charbeneau, G. T., and Hill, H. C.: A comparison of physical properties of several soft toothbrushes. J. Mich. Dent. Assoc., 51:347, 1969.

57. Gjermo, P., and Flötra, L.: The plaque-removing effect of dental floss and toothpicks: A group comparison study. J. Periodont. Res., 4:170, 1969.

58. Gjermo, P., Baastad, K. L., and Rölla, G.: The plaque-inhibiting capacity of 11 antibacterial compounds. J. Periodont. Res., 5:102, 1970.

59. Gjermo, P., and Flötra, L.: The effect of different methods of interdental cleaning. J.Periodont. Res., 5:230, 1970.

60. Gjermo, P., and Rölla, G.: The plaque-inhibiting effect of chlorhexidine-containing dentifrices. Scand. J. Dent. Res., 79:126, 1971.

61. Gjermo, P.: Chlorhexidine in dental practice. J. Clin. Periodontol., 1:143, 1974.

62. Glass, R. L.: A clinical study of hand and electric toothbrushing. J. Periodontol., 36:322, 1965.

63. Glickman, I., Petralis, R., and Marks, R.: The effect of powered toothbrushing plus interdental stimulation upon the severity of gingivitis. J. Periodontol., 35:519, 1964.

64. Glickman, I., Petralis, R., and Marks, R.: The effect of powered toothbrusing and interdental stimulation upon microscopic inflammation and surface keratinization of the interdental gingiva. J. Periodontol., 36:108, 1965.

65. Goldman, H. M.: The effect of single and multiple toothbrushing in the cleansing of the normal and periodontally involved dentition. Oral Surg., 9:203, 1956.

66. Gravelle, H. R., Shackelford, N. F., and Lovett, J. T.: The oral hygiene of high school students as affected by three different educational programs. J. Pub. Health Dent., 27:91, 1967.

67. Gray, P. G., et al.: Adult dental health in England and Wales in 1968. London, H.M.S.O., 1970.

68. Hansen, F., Gjermo, P., and Eriksen, H. M.: The effect of a chlorhexidine-containing gel on oral cleanliness and gingival health in young adults. J. Clin. Periodontol., 2:153, 1975.

69. Harrington, J. H., and Terry, I. A.: Automatic and hand toothbrushing abrasion studies. J. Am. Dent. Assoc., 68:343, 1964.

70. Harvey, R. F.: Clinical impressions of a new antibiotic in periodontics: Spiramycine. J. Can. Dent. Assoc., 27:576, 1961.

71. Hill, H. C., Levi, P. A., and Glickman, I.: The effects of waxed and unwaxed dental floss on interdental plaque accumulation and interdental gingival health. J. Periodontol., 44:411, 1973.

72. Hine, M. K.: The use of the toothbrush in the treatment of periodontitis. J. Am. Dent. Assoc., 41:158, 1950.

73. Hine, M. K.: Toothbrush. Int. Dent. J., 6:15, 1956.

74. Hiniker, J. J., and Forscher, B. K.: The effect of toothbrush type on gingival health. J. Periodontol., 25:40, 1954.

75. Hirschfeld, I.: The toothbrush, its use and abuse. D. Items of Interest, 3:833, 1931.

76. Hoover, D. R., and Lefkowitz, W.: Reduction of gingivitis by toothbrushing. J. Periodontol., 36:193, 1965.

77. Hoover, D. R., Robinson, H. B. G., and Billingsley, A.: The comparative effectiveness of the Water-Pik in a non-instructed population. J. Periodontol., 39:43, 1968.

78. Johansen, J. R., Gjermo, P., and Eriksen, H. M.: A longitudinal study on the effect of chlorhexidine containing dentifrices. J. Periodont. Res., (Suppl.) 10:36, 1972.

79. Kardel, K. M., Olesen, K. P., and Bay, I.: Tanborstens evne til at fjerne plaque. II. B tydningen af borstehovedets storrelse og fiberbundtplaceringin. Tandlaege, 75:189, 1971.

80. Keller, S. E., and Manson-Hing, L. R.: Clearance studies of proximal tooth surfaces. Part II. In vivo removal of interproximal plaque. Ala. J. Med. Sci., 6:266, 1969.

81. Keller, S. E., and Manson-Hing, L. R.: Clearance studies of proximal tooth surfaces. Part III and IV. In vivo removal of interproximal plaque. Ala. J. Med. Sci., 6:399, 1969.

82. Kelner, R. M., Wahl, B. R., Deasy, M. J., and Formicola, A. J.: Gingival inflammation as related to frequency of plaque removal. J. Periodontol., 45:303, 1974.

83. Keyes, P. H., et al.: Dispersion of dextranous bacterial plaques on human teeth with dextranase. J. Am. Dent. Assoc., 82:136, 1971.

84. Keyes, P. H., and McCabe, R. M.: The potential of various compounds to suppress microorganisms in plaques produced in vitro by streptococcus or an Actinomycete. J. Am. Dent. Assoc. 86:396, 1973.

85. King, J. D.: Gingival disease in Dundee. Dent. Record, 65:9, 32, 55, 1945.

86. Kitchin, P.: The prevalence of tooth root exposure

and the relation of the extent of such exposure to the degree of abrasion in different age classes. J. Dent. Res., 20:565, 1941.

87. Koch, G., and Lindhe, J.: The effect of supervised oral hygiene on the gingiva of children. The effect of toothbrushing. Odont. Revy., 16:327, 1965.

88. Krajewski, J., Giblin, J., and Gargiulo, A. W.: Evaluation of the water pressure cleansing device as an adjunct to periodontal treatment. Periodontics, 2:76, 1964.

89. Kristofferson, T.: Periodontal conditions in Norwegian soliders. An epidemiological and experimental study. Scand. J. Dent. Res., 78:34, 1970.

90. Lainson, P. A., Berquist, J. J., and Fraleigh, C. M.: A longitudinal study of pulsating water pressure cleansing devices. J. Periodontol., 43:444, 1972.

91. Lang, N. P., Ostergaard, E. Q., and Löe, H.: A fluorescent plaque disclosing agent. J. Periodont. Res., 7:59, 1972.

92. Lang, N. P., Cumming, B. R., and Löe, H.: Toothbrushing frequency as it relates to plaque development and gingival health. J. Periodontol., 44:396, 1973.

93. Larato, D., Stahl, S., Brown, R., Jr., and Witkin, G.: The effect of a prescribed method of toothbrushing on the fluctuation of marginal gingivitis. J. Periodontol., 40:142, 1960.

94. Larsson, B. T.: Tandsubstansforlusten och Tandborstning i ett Folkstandvards klientel. Severiges Tandlak. Tidn., 61:58, 1969.

95. Lefkowitz, W., and Robinson, H. B. G.: Effectiveness of automatic and hand brushes in removing dental plaque and debris. J. Am. Dent. Assoc., 65:351, 1962.

96. Less, W.: Mechanics of teaching plaque control. Dent. Clin. North Am., 16:647, 1972.

97. Leung, S. W., and Draus, F. J.: Effect of certain enzymes on calculus deposition (Abstr.). J. Dent. Res., 38:709, 1959.

98. Lindhe, J., and Axelsson, P.: The effect of controlled oral hygiene and topical fluoride application on caries and gingivitis in Swedish schoolchildren. Community Dent. Oral Epidemiol., 1:96, 1973.

99. Lindhe, J., Axelsson, P., and Tollskog, G.: Effect of proper oral hygiene on gingivitis and dental caries in Swedish schoolchildren. Community Dent. Oral Epidemiol., 3:150, 1975.

100. Lindhe, J., and Nyman, S.: The effect of plaque control and surgical pocket elimination on the establishment and maintenance of periodontal health. A longitudinal study of periodontal therapy in cases of advanced disease. J. Clin. Periodontol., 2:67, 1975.

101. Linn, E. L.: Oral hygiene and periodontal disease: Implications for dental health programs. J. Am. Dent. Assoc., 71:39, 1965.

102. Lobene, R. R.: The effect of an automatic toothbrush on gingival health. J. Periodontol., 35:137, 1964.

103. Lobene, R. R., Brion, M., and Socransky, S. S.: Effect of erythromycin on dental plaque and plaque forming microorganisms of man. J. Periodontol., 40:287, 1969.

104. Lobene, R. R.: The effect of a pulsed water pressure cleaning device on oral health. J. Periodontol., 40:667, 1969.

105. Lobene, R. R., and Soparkar, P. M.: Effect of a pulsed water pressure cleansing device on oral health. I.A.D.R., Abstr. No. 344:126, 1969.

106. Lobene, R. R.: A clinical study of the effect of dextranase on human dental plaque. J. Am. Dent. Assoc., 82:132, 1971.

107. Lobene, R. R., and Soparkar, P. M.: The effect of an alexidine mouthwash on human plaque and gingivitis. J. Am. Dent. Assoc., 87:848, 1973.

108. Löe, H., Theilade, E., and Jensen, S. B.: Experimental gingivitis in man. J. Periodontol., 36:177, 1965.

109. Löe, H., et al.: Experimental gingivitis in man: III. The influences of antibiotics on gingival plaque development. J. Periodont. Res., 2:282, 1967.

110. Löe, H.: A review of the prevention and control of plaque. In McHugh, W. D. (ed.): Dental plaque; a symposium held in the University of Dundee. Edinburgh, E & S Livingstone, 1969, p. 259.

111. Löe, H., and Schiött, C. R.: The effect of mouthrinses and topical application of chlorhexidine on the development of dental plaque and gingivitis in man. J. Periodont. Res., 5:79, 1970.

112. Löe, H.: Does chlorhexidine have a place in the prophylaxis of dental disease? J. Periodont. Res., 8 (Suppl. 12):93, 1973.

113. Löe, H., Schiött, C. R., Glavind, L., and Karring, T.: Two years oral use of chlorhexidine in man. I. General design and clinical effects. J. Periodont. Res., 11:135, 1976.

114. Loesche, W. J., et al.: Effect of topical kanamycin sulfate in plaque accumulation. J. Am. Dent. Assoc., 83:1063, 1971.

115. Loesche, W. J., Murray, R. J., and Mellberg, J. R.: The effect of topical fluoride on percentage of Streptococcus mutans and Streptococcus sanguis in interproximal plaque samples. Caries Res., 7:283, 1973.

116. Loesche, W. J., and Nafe, D.: Reduction of supragingival plaque accumulations in institutionalized Down's syndrome patients by periodic treatment with topical kanamycin. Arch. Oral Biol., 18:1131, 1973.

117. Loesche, W. J., et al.: Effect of topical acidulated phosphate fluoride on percentage of Streptococcus mutans and Streptococcus sanguis in plaque. II. Pooled occlusal and pooled approximal samples. Caries Res., 9:139, 1975.

118. Loesche, W. J.: Chemotherapy of dental plaque infections. Oral Sci. Rev., 9:65, 1976.

119. Lozdan, J., et al.: The use of nitrimidazine in the treatment of acute ulcerative gingivitis. A double-blind controlled trial. Br. Dent. J., 130:294, 1971.

120. Lyons, H.: Fiction and facts in periodontology: An appraisal. J. Am. Dent. Assoc., 39:513, 1949.

121. MacKenzie, I. C., Nuki, K., Löe, H., and Schiött, C. R.: Two years oral use of chlorhexidine in

man. V. Effects on stratum corneum of oral mucosa. J. Periodont. Res., 11:165, 1976.

122. Manhold, J. H., Jr., Parker, L. A., and Manhold, B. S.: Efficacy of a commercial mouthwash: In vivo study. N. Y. J. Dent., 32:165, 1962.

123. Manhold, J. H.: Gingival tissue health with hand and power brushing: A retrospective with corroborative studies. J. Periodontol., 38:23, 1967.

124. Manhold, B. S., Manhold, J. H., and Weisinger, E.: A study of total oral debris clearance. J. New Jersey State Dent. Soc., 38:64, 1967.

125. Manly, R. S., and Brudevold, F.: Relative abrasiveness of natural and synthetic toothbrush bristles on cementum and dentin. J. Am. Dent. Assoc., 55:779, 1957.

126. Manly, R. S., Wiren J., Manly, P. J., and Keene, R. C.: A method for measurement of abrasion of dentin by toothbrush and dentifrice, J. Dent. Res., 44:533, 1965.

126a. Marthaler, T. M.: Caries inhibition after seven years of unsupervised use of an amine fluoride dentifrice. Brit. Dent. J., 124:510, 1968.

127. Massler, M., Ludwick, W., and Schour, I.: Dental caries and gingivitis in males 17-20 years old (at the Great Lakes Naval Training Center). J. Dent. Res., 31:195, 1952.

128. McConnel, D., and Conroy, C. W.: Comparisons of abrasion produced by a simulated manual versus a mechanical toothbrush. J. Dent. Res., 46:1022, 1967.

129. McKendrick, A. J. W., Barbenel, L. M. H., and McHugh, W. D.: A two year comparison of hand and electric toothbrushes. J. Periodont. Res., 3:224, 1968.

130. McKendrick, A. J. W., Barbenel, L. M. H., and McHugh, W. D.: The influence of time of examination, eating, smoking, and frequency of brushing on the oral debris index. J. Periodont. Res., 5:205, 1970.

131. Mikkelsen, L., Jensen, S. B., Schiött, C. R., and Löe, H.: Studies on human plaque—Streptococci after two years of oral chlorhexidine hygiene. I.A.D.R., Scand. Div., Abstr. No. 23:992, 1973.

132. Mitchell, D. F., and Holmes, L. A.: Topical antibiotic control of dentogingival plaque. J. Periodontol., 36:202, 1965.

133. Mohammed, C.: Dental plaque removed by floss. J. New Jersey Dent. Soc., 36:419, 1965.

134. Müller, E., et al.: The effect of two oral antiseptics on early calculus formation. Helv. Odont. Acta, 6:42, 1962.

134a. Newman, M. G., Chaconas, S., and Newman, S. L.: Effect of oxygenating agents on the periodontium of orthodontic patients. J. Orthodont., 73:108, 1978.

135. Nuki, K., Schlenker, R., Löe, H., and Schiött, C. R.: Two years oral use of chlorhexidine in man. VI. Effect on oxidative enzymes in oral epithelia. J. Periodont. Res., 11:172, 1976.

136. Nyman, S., Rosling, B., and Lindhe, J.: Effect of professional tooth cleaning on healing after periodontal surgery. J. Clin. Periodontol., 2:80, 1975.

137. Ochsenbein, H.: Chlorhexidin in der Zahnheil-

kunde—eine Literaturübersicht. Schweiz. Mschr. Zahnheilk., 83:113, 1973.

138. Ochsenbein, H.: Chlorhexidin in der Zahnheilkunde—Fortsetzung einer Literaturübersicht. Schweiz. Mschr. Zahnheilk., 83:819, 1973.

139. Ochsenbein, H.: Chlorhexidin in der Zahnheilkunde—Aktueller Stand der Forschung. Schweiz. Mschr. Zahnheilk., 84:459, 1974.

140. O'Leary, T. S., Shafer, W. G., Swenson, H. M., Nesler, D. C., and Van Dorn, P. R.: Possible penetration of crevicular tissue from oral hygiene procedures. I. Use of oral irrigation devices. J. Periodontol., 41:158, 1970.

141. O'Leary, T. J., Shafer, W. G., Swenson, H. M., and Nesler, D. C.: Possible penetration of crevicular tissue from oral hygiene procedures. II. Use of the toothbrush. J. Periodontol., 41:163, 1970.

142. O'Leary, T. J., Drake, R. B., and Naylor, J. E.: The plaque control record. J. Periodontol., 43:38, 1972.

143. O'Rourke, J. T.: The relation of the physical character of the diet to the health of the periodontal tissues. Am. J. Orthod., 33:687, 1947.

144. Ostrolenk, M., and Weiss, W.: Effect of mouthwashes on the oral flora. Dent. Abstr., 5:51, 1960.

145. Phillips, J. E.: Effect of Water Irrigation on Oral Flora and Gingival Health. Masters Thesis, Graduate School, Marquette University, Milwaukee, Wisconsin, June, 1967.

146. Quigley, G. A., and Hein, J. W.: Comparative cleansing efficacy of manual and power brushing. J. Am. Dent. Assoc., 65:26, 1962.

147. Reddy, J., and Salkin, L. M.: The effect of a urea peroxide rinse on dental plaque and gingivitis. J. Periodontol., 47:607, 1976.

148. Robinson, H. B. G., and Kitchin, P. C.: The effect of massage with the toothbrush on keratinization of the gingiva. Oral Surg., 1:1042, 1948.

149. Robinson, H. B. G.: Individualizing dentifrices: The dentist's responsibility. J. Am. Dent. Assoc., 79:633, 1969.

150. Robinson, H. B. G., and Hoover, P. R.: The comparative effectiveness of a pulsating oral irrigator as an adjunct in maintaining oral health. J. Periodontol., 42:37, 1971.

151. Rosling, B., Nyman, S., and Lindhe, J.: The effect of systematic plaque control on bone regeneration in infrabony pockets. J. Clin. Periodontol., 3:38, 1976.

152. Rosling, B., Nyman, S., Lindhe, J., and Jern, B.: The healing potential of periodontal tissues following different techniques of periodontal surgery in plaque-free dentitions. A 2-year clinical study. J. Clin. Periodontol., 3:233, 1976.

153. Sanders, W. E., and Robinson, H. B. G.: The effect of toothbrushing on deposition of calculus. J. Periodontol., 33:386, 1962.

154. Saxer, U. P., and Mühlemann, H. R.: Motivation und Aufklärung. Schweiz. Mschr. Zahnheilk., 85:905, 1975.

155. Saxer, U. P., and Schmid, M. O.: The plaque

inhibiting effect of chlorhexidine lozenges. J. West. Soc. Periodontol., 24:56, 1976.

156. Saxton, C. A.: The effects of dentifrices on the appearance of the tooth surface observed with the scanning electon microscope. J. Periodont. Res., 11:74, 1976.

157. Schiött, C. R., Briner, W. W., and Löe, H.: Two years oral use of chlorhexidine in man. II. The effect on the salivary bacterial flora. J. Periodont. Res., 11:145, 1976.

158. Schiött, C. R., Briner, W. W., Kirkland, J. J., and Löe, H.: Two years oral use of chlorhexidine in man. III. Changes in sensitivity of the salivary flora. J. Periodont. Res., 11:153, 1976.

159. Schiött, C. R., Löe, H., and Briner, W. W.: Two years oral use of chlorhexidine in man. IV. Effect on various medical parameters. J. Periodont. Res., 11:158, 1976.

160. Schmid, M. O., Schait, A., and Mühlemann, H. R.: Effect of a zinc chloride mouthrinse on calculus deposits formed on foils. Helv. Odont. Acta, 17:22, 1974.

161. Schmid, M. O., and Cuvilovic, Z.: Die Wirkung von Instruktion und Motivation auf die Mundhygiene. Schweiz. Mschr. Zahnheilk., 85:457, 1975.

162. Schmid, M. O., Balmelli, O., and Saxer, U. P.: The plaque-removing effect of a toothbrush, dental floss and a toothpick. J. Clin. Periodontol., 3:157, 1976.

163. Schour, I., and Massler, M.: Gingival disease in Postwar Italy (1945). I. Prevalence of gingivitis in various age groups. J. Am. Dent. Assoc., 35:475, 1947.

164. Schour, I., and Massler, M.: Prevalence of gingivitis in young adults. J. Dent. Res. (Abstr.), 27:733, 1948.

165. Schroeder, H. E., Marthaler, T. M., and Mühlemann, H. R.: Effect of some potential inhibitors on early calculus formation. Helv. Odont. Acta, 6:6, 1962.

166. Schroeder, H. E.: Formation and Inhibition of Dental Calculus. Berne, Hans Huber Publishers, 1969.

167. Sconyers, J. R., Crawford, J. J., and Moriarty, J. D.: Study of bacteremia following toothbrushing using sensitive culture methods. I.A.D.R., Abstr. No. 757, 1971.

168. Sheiham, A.: Dental cleanliness and chronic periodontal disease: Studies in British populations. Br. Dent. J., 129:413, 1970.

169. Smith, T. S.: Anatomic and physiologic conditions governing the use of the toothbrush. J. Am. Dent. Assoc., 27:874, 1940.

170. Smith, W. A., and Ash, M. M.: Effectiveness of an electric toothbrush. I.A.D.R., Abstr. No. 207, 1963.

171. Spolsky, V. W., et al.: The effect of an antimicrobial mouthwash on dental plaque and gingivitis in young adults. J. Periodontol., 46:685, 1975.

172. Spolsky, V. W., and Forsyth, A. B.: Effects of alexidine-2HCl mouthwash on plaque and gingivitis after six months. J. Dent. Res., 56:805, 1977.

173. Stahl, S. S., and Goldman, H. M.: The incidence of gingivitis among a sample of Massachusetts school children. Oral Surg., 6:707, 1953.

174. Stahl, S. S., Wachtel, N., DeCastro, C., and Pelletier, G.: The effect of toothbrushing on the keratinization of the gingiva. J. Periodontol., 24:20, 1953.

175. Stanmeyer, W. R.: A measure of tissue response to frequency of toothbrushing. J. Periodontol., 28:17, 1957.

176. Stewart, G. G.: Mucinase — A possible means of reducing calculus formation. J. Periodontol., 23:85, 1952.

177. Stillman, P. R.: A philosophy of the treatment of periodontal disease. Dent. Digest, 38:314, 1932.

178. Stookey, G. K., and Muhler, J. C.: Laboratory studies concerning the enamel and dentin abrasion properties of common dentifrice polishing agents. J. Dent. Res., 47:524, 1968.

179. Strålfors, A., Thilander, H., and Bergenholtz, A.: Simultaneous inhibition of caries and periodontal disease in hamsters by disinfection, toothbrushing or phosphate addition. Arch. Oral Biol., 12:1367, 1967.

180. Suomi, J. D.: Periodontal disease and oral hygiene in an institutionalized population: Report of an epidemiology study. J. Periodontol., 40:5, 1969.

181. Suomi, J. D., et al.: The effect of controlled oral hygiene procedures on the progression of periodontal disease in adults: Results after two years. J. Periodontol., 40:416, 1969.

182. Symposium on chlorhexidine in the prophylaxis of dental diseases. J. Periodont. Res., Suppl. No. 12, 1973.

183. Tamimi, H. A., Thomassen, P. R., and Moser, E. H., Jr.: Bacteremia study using a water irrigation device. J. Periodontol., 40:424, 1969.

184. Todd, J. E., and Whitworth, A.: Adult dental health in Scotland, 1972. London, H.M.S.O., 1974.

185. Toto, P. D., and Farchione, A.: Clinical evaluation of an electrically powered toothbrush in home periodontal therapy. J. Periodontol., 32:249, 1961.

186. Toto, P. D., Goljan, K. R., Evans, J. A., and Sawinski, V. J.: A study on the uninstructed use of an electric brush. J. Am. Dent. Assoc., 72:904, 1966.

187. Toto, P. D., Evans, C. L., and Sawinski, V. J.: Effects of water jet rinse and toothbrushing on oral hygiene. J. Periodontol., 40:296, 1969.

188. Turesky, S., Gilmore, N. D., and Glickman, I.: Calculus inhibition by topical application of the chloromethyl analogue of victamin C. J. Periodontol., 38:142, 1967.

189. Turesky, S., Gilmore, N. D., and Glickman, I.: Reduced plaque formation by the chloromethyl analogue of victamin C. J. Periodontol., 41:41, 1970.

190. Villa, P.: Degree of calculus inhibition by habitual toothbrushing. Helv. Odontol. Acta, 12:31, 1968.

191. Volpe, A. R., et al.: Antimicrobial control of bacterial plaque and calculus and the effects of these agents on oral flora. J. Dent. Res., 48:832, 1969.

192. Wasserman, B. H., Mandel, I. D., and Levy, B. M.: In vitro calcification of dental calculus. J. Periodontol., 29:144, 1958.

193. Williford, J. W., Johns, C., Muhler, J. C., and Stookey, G. K.: Report of a study demonstrating improved oral health through education. J. Dent. Child., 34:183, 1967.

194. Zander, H. A.: The effect of penicillin dentifrice on caries incidence in schoolchildren. J. Am. Dent. Assoc., 40:569, 1950.

Chapter 44

Treatment of Uncomplicated Chronic Gingivitis

Treatment

Causes of Failure

Uncomplicated chronic gingivitis is the most common disease of the gingiva. It affects the interdental and marginal gingiva. **It should be detected in its earliest stages and treated as soon as it is detected** (Figs. 44–1 and 44–2). Usually painless, it is the most common cause of gingival bleeding. Failure to treat it invites destruction of the underlying periodontal tissues and premature tooth loss.

Separation of the treatment of chronic gingivitis from the scaling and root planing technique described in Chapter 42 (Preparation of the Tooth Surface) is somewhat artificial. However, chronic gingivitis is the initial stage in periodontitis and should be treated before pockets develop.

Chronic gingivitis is always caused by local irritation. Systemic conditions may aggravate the inflammation caused by local irritants and should be appropriately dealt with (Chap. 45), but **no systemic conditions of themselves cause chronic gingivitis.**

TREATMENT

Treatment should be preceded by careful examination to detect all sources of local irritation, such as dental plaque, calculus, food impaction, overhanging or improperly contoured restorations, or irritating removable prostheses. The teeth should be stained with disclosing solution to detect plaque, and carefully probed with the No. 17 or No. 21 explorers to locate small particles of calculus.

Step 1. Treatment of uncomplicated gingivitis is started by explaining the importance of plaque control and teaching the patient how to achieve it. **This gives the patient a realistic perspective regarding the treatment of gingivitis: that it includes something he must do for himself, as well**

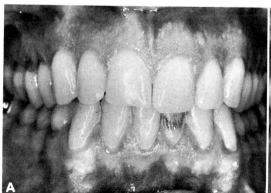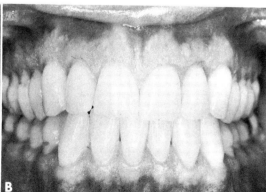

Figure 44–1   Slight Chronic Marginal Gingivitis. *A,* Before treatment. *B,* After treatment.

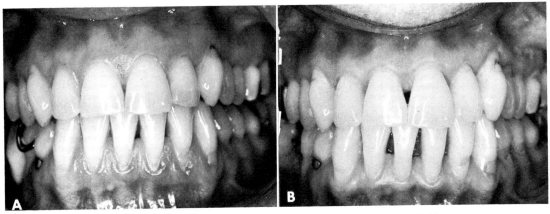

Figure 44–2   Chronic Marginal Gingivitis and Recession. A, Before treatment. B, After treatment.

as something the dentist does for him. It also provides an opportunity to demonstrate that plaque control really benefits his gums. After the patient is instructed in plaque control, he is given an appointment for the next visit.

Step 2.   The condition of the gums is reviewed with the patient, and improvement is pointed out to him. The teeth are stained with disclosing solution and plaque control is reviewed, with the patient demonstrating the various procedures he used.

The teeth are scaled to remove all deposits, and all tooth surfaces are polished with a paste of fine pumice or Improved Zircate.

Polishing is an important preventive measure against the recurrence of gingivitis. Plaque, the most important cause of gingivitis and the initial stage in the formation of calculus, tends to form more readily on rough surfaces.

Other sources of local irritation referred to earlier should be eliminated.

Step 3.   The gingivae are examined and plaque control is reviewed. Special attention is given to areas of persistent inflammation, which usually entails rescaling and emphasis on patient technique for cleansing the area.

These procedures are repeated at subsequent visits until the gingivae are healthy. The patient is then placed on "recall," **with a careful explanation of the reasons for peri-** odic visits and the importance of the care he gives his mouth in the intervening periods.

CAUSES OF FAILURE

Treatment of chronic gingivitis should present no problems. However, if disease persists, the following are the most likely causes:

1. Failure to remove minute particles of calculus, often just beneath the cemento-enamel junction.

2. Failure to polish the tooth surfaces after deposits are removed.

3. Failure to eliminate sources of irritation other than deposits on the teeth. Food impaction is one of the frequently overlooked factors.

4. Inadequate plaque control because of one or more of the following: (a) insufficient patient instruction, (b) premature dismissal of the patient before he demonstrates competence in plaque control, or (c) lack of patient cooperation.

5. A tendency to seek remote systemic etiology for persistent gingivitis caused by overlooked local irritants.

6. Dependence upon vitamins, mouthwashes, and topical application of drugs, particularly hormones, antibiotics, and oxidizing agents. **Except for topical anesthetics, drugs serve no significant purpose in the treatment of chronic gingivitis.**

Systemic Aspects of
Periodontal Therapy

The treatment of gingival and periodontal disease consists for the most part of local procedures. This is understandable because the local factors so important in the etiology are accessible for correction, whereas, in many cases in which systemic causative factors are suspected, it is frequently difficult to establish their nature.

The following are conditions requiring systemic therapy as part of their overall management: (1) oral manifestations of certain dermatologic diseases (Chap. 12); (2) gingival disturbances attributed to hormonal imbalance (Chap. 29); (3) systemic toxicity in patients with acute gingival disease (Chap. 41); (4) systemic conditions requiring special precautions; (Chap. 48) (5) nutritional deficiencies, and (6) infections. Of these, the last two are presented in this chapter.

ANTIMICROBIAL THERAPY*

The prolonged morbidity and occasional mortality from infections related to oral and

---

*The information, recommendations, and procedures presented in this section have been adapted in whole or part from references 1, 3, 9, 13, and 25. The reader is urged to refer to these sources for more in-depth considerations.

periodontal surgical interventions and sepsis require preventive and therapeutic measures based upon biologic knowledge of the infective agents and their effects upon the host.

Infection usually develops as a diffuse inflammatory process without suppuration (cellulitis), which is characterized by edema, erythema, pain, and interference with function. The tissues undergo cellular infiltration by red blood cells, leukocytes, histiocytes, and macrophages. Suppuration often follows, being the result of liquefaction of tissues and the formation of pus. Abscesses which may form in the infected area are usually walled off by a pyogenic membrane which produces induration about the abscess. Cellulitis in varying degrees usually extends beyond the wall of the abscess. Regional infections may develop from the direct extension of microorganisms along areolar, fascial, muscular, or other anatomic planes. Bacterial proteolytic enzymes, including proteinases, aid in the process of tissue liquefaction.[1]

Clinical Considerations

The following aspects of the biology of infection are of clinical importance:

1. The nature, source, and invasive qualities of microorganisms.

2. The inflammatory and immunologic responses of the body, as well as the dose of microorganisms, play a major role in determining whether an infection will become established. Devitalized tissue and foreign bodies are the keys to invasion in many instances.

3. Severity of infection is directly related to the balance between the injury inflicted and the physiologic responses which limit the septic process until it can be brought under control and eliminated.

Infection in clinical practice is due to the

entrance, growth, metabolic activities, and resultant pathophysiologic effects of microorganisms in the tissues of a patient. Although most periodontal lesions are in essence infections, we shall refer here only to the infections that may result as a complication of surgical procedures. Other acute periodontal infections such as the periodontal abscesses and the acute gingival infections are dealt with in Chapters 40 and 41.

Surgical wounds are considered uninfected if they heal *per priman* without discharge.[1] They are definitely infected if there is a purulent discharge, even if organisms are not cultured from the purulent material. Wounds that are inflamed without discharge and wounds that drain culture-positive serous fluid are considered possibly infected.

Suture abscesses are excluded from definite or possible infections if (1) inflammation and discharge are minimal and confined to points of suture penetration, or (2) the incision heals *per priman* without drainage. Clinical judgment is most important in the diagnosis of infections.

The precise and complete identification of microorganisms present in a surgical infection is important and advisable. Emphasis has frequently been placed on infections produced by the hemolytic *Staphylococcus*, and by the streptococci.[1] It is extremely important to point out, however, that a **considerable number of surgically associated infections of the oral cavity are mixed bacterial infections produced by a variety of bacteria, both aerobic and anaerobic, gram-positive and gram-negative** (see Chap. 24).

The incidence of various fungal and viral infections has also been increasing with the expanding clinical use of steroids, immunosuppressive agents, and multiple antibiotic agents.

Aerobic and anaerobic infections of oral and dental tissues may extend locally or spread widely to produce serious infection in other parts of the body.[13] There are numerous examples of serious infection arising from the oral cavity. Table 45–1 is a partial listing.

Many factors may predispose patients undergoing periodontal surgery to severe infections. These factors include trauma, injection of local anesthetic, severe periodontal infection, systemic or primary metabolic disease, radiation, vitamin deficiency, and malignancy.

Systemic infections are related to the dissemination of microorganisms into the circulation, resulting in either bacteremia or septicemia. In bacteremia, bacteria enter once or intermittently. The old concept suggested that the actual growth or reproduction of microorganisms within the circulating bloodstream was a septicemia in contrast to the bacteremia where microorganisms could not reproduce within the circulating bloodstream. The newer concept, however, indicates that the difference is in the rate at which organisms enter into the bloodstream. When the distribution is more or less constant, it is a *septicemia*; when it is intermittent or occurs once, it is considered to be a *bacteremia*.[1]

Therapeutic Considerations

Antimicrobial therapy is of great importance in the proper management of infection, but it is only one aspect of the multifaceted approach necessary for successful management.[1] The principles of treatment are directed toward altering the environment for pathogenic bacteria and reducing the invasion of these bacteria into healthy areas.

To control the local environment, useful measures include removal of dead tissue, drainage of collections of pus, elimination of obstructions, decompression of tissues where indicated, release of trapped gas, improvement of circulation to the part, and improved oxygenation of tissues.

Adherence to important surgical principles such as achievement of good hemostasis, avoidance of dead space, gentle handling of tissues during surgery, and avoidance of contamination of clean body cavities is very important.

When localization of infection has occurred, surgical decompression is necessary. *In the presence of suppuration, antimicrobial agents do not replace the scalpel.*[1] When the infection is localized by the body's inflammatory defenses as an abscess, the surgical method is required. Antibiotics are administered only to prevent invasive or systemic infection. If the infection is localized by anatomic boundaries, antibiotics may be effective if used early while an intact blood supply exists, but progression of the infection, causing limitation of blood supply, necessitates surgical intervention. The diminished blood flow prevents access of the drug to the area of bacterial activity.

Many patients receive antibiotics unnecessarily or receive antibiotics to which the infecting organisms are resistant. It is important that clinicians monitor and in some instances restrict antibiotic uses, withholding selected antibiotics for specifically defined infections and limiting broad-spectrum antibiotic therapy to patients with specific indications.[1]

Equally important is the regulation of the

TABLE 45–1 POTENTIAL SERIOUS INFECTIONS ARISING FROM BACTERIA IN THE ORAL CAVITY*

Infection	Oral Bacteria	Oral Cavity Source	References
Meningitis Metastatic lung abscess	Fusiforms, spirochetes	Maxillary periostitis	31
Orbital & brain abscess	*B. corrodens, F. fusiform, S. faecalis*	ANUG & extractions	10, 29
Fever, meningeal signs Epidural abscess in lumbar area Eventual paraplegia	*Actinomyces* and *B. melaninogenicus*	Tooth extraction	16
Orbital cellulitis	Anaerobic streptococci	Submandibular cellulitis following extraction	21
Cellulitis of face	*Bacteroides necrophorus B. melaninogenicus, Staphylococcus albus,* fusiforms, streptoccoci	Extractions	23, 31
Endocarditis	Buday bacillus, *B. fragilis,* streptococci, *B. melaninogenicus,* anaerobic streptoccoci	Periapical abscess, extraction and periodontitis	12, 32, 24
Ludwig's angina	*Fusobacterium*	Extractions, dental manipulation, dental disease	10
Pulmonary infection: pneumonia, empyema necrotizing pneumonia	*S. fragilis, Peptococcus, Propionibacterium, Fusobacterium, B. oralis,* microaerophillic streptococci, *Bifidobacterium, B. melaninogenicus*	Dental disease, dental manipulation, juvenile periodontitis	17
Fatal bacteremia	*Fusobacterium*	Severe periodontitis	18
Bacteremia	Streptococcus, other		8, 20 7, 22, 26
Maxillary sinusitis	*Bacillus* sp.	Dental cyst	5

* Information derived and modified from Finegold.[13]

TABLE 45–2 FACTORS RELATING TO THE
EFFICACY OF ANTIBIOTICS IN
PERIODONTAL SURGERY*

1. Degree of susceptibility of the invading microorganism.
2. Concentration of drug obtained at the site of the
   infection (dosage, or biologic and pharmacologic
   properties of the particular drug preparation being
   used).
3. Location of the infection.
4. Pathophysiologic state of the patient.
5. Natural history of the infection.
6. Nature and severity of the infection.
7. Application of other supportive therapeutic measures, e.g., prompt incision and drainage of abscesses.

*From Barry, L.: The Antimicrobic Susceptibility
Test: Principles and Practices. Philadelphia, Lea &
Febiger, 1977.

duration of antibiotic therapy, which is
determined by the patient's response and
the character of the infection, including the
site and nature of the infecting organisms.
For most acute surgical infections, it is
unusual to require antibiotic therapy for
more than 10 days, but more chronic infections, such as osteomyelitis, subacute bacterial endocarditis, tuberculosis, and perhaps aggressive forms of periodontal disease, may require prolonged antimicrobial
therapy. Antibiotics are of great value, but
they are only a part of the surgeon's armamentarium. They must not be omitted when
indicated nor relied upon to the exclusion
of other methods.[1]

The use of antibiotics in surgery may be
divided into two categories: (1) to prevent
potential infection, and (2) to treat established infection. In both cases the efficacy
of a particular antimicrobial agent depends
upon a number of factors, some of which
are listed in Table 45–2. Each factor must
be carefully considered if successful control of infection is to occur.

Since antimicrobial drugs act by killing
or inhibiting the growth of bacteria, therapy
is successful only if the organisms causing
the infection are susceptible to the drug.
This is best achieved when there is a single
kind of organism that is very sensitive to
the antimicrobial agent. When multiple
organisms are involved, the effectiveness of
antibiotics is diminished. Of primary importance in the selection of antibiotics is the
monitoring of occurrence and sensitivity of
the organisms causing infections.[3]

Once selected, the agent should be given
in sufficient quantity and by a route that
affords establishment and maintenance of
an effective concentration in the contaminated tissue. *There are no "prophylactic"
doses, as opposed to "therapeutic" doses.*
(Doses for adults are given in Tables 45–4
and 45–5.)

Treatment of Acute Infections

General guidelines for the clinical diagnosis of infection include both local and
systemic signs and symptoms (Table 45–3).
Presence of these factors will guide the
clinician in the immediate treatment of the
patient.

Patients of concern are those considered treatable in a private office who do not require hospitalization. Antibiotic therapy is usually prescribed for such patients who have: (1) some
systemic as well as local signs of infection, and
(2) local signs of infection but also present a high
risk (e.g., patients with a heart murmur, diabetes
or history of rheumatic fever, endocarditis or
cardiac prosthesis, etc.).[9]

Antibiotic therapy should not be initiated
before a diagnosis of infection has been
established. Immediate microscopic examination of an exudate is very helpful in the
final diagnosis and in deciding which of
several organisms cultured predominate in
the infection. Candidiasis can often be diagnosed by microscopic means alone. However, most severe deep oral tissue infections require that antibiotics be prescribed
empirically. *Culture and antibiotic susceptibility testing is obtained to confirm whatever antibiotic was chosen.*[9]

If the patient presents with acute infec-

TABLE 45–3 CLINICAL DIAGNOSIS OF
INFECTION*

Local Signs and Symptoms of Infection
1. Swelling   5. Loss of function
2. Pain   6. Pus formation
3. Erythema   7. Loss of structure
4. Heat
Systemic Signs and Symptoms of Infection
1. Regional lymphadenopathy 5. Chills
2. Elevated temperature   6. Elevated blood leukocyte
3. Increased respiration rate   count
4. Increased pulse rate   7. Increase in young PMN
                                 cells (shift to left)
                             8. General malaise

*From Crawford, J. J.: General Guidelines for Initiating
Antibiotic Treatment of Acute Oral Infections. University of
North Carolina Dental School, 1974.

TABLE 45–4

Antibiotics	Form	Usual Dosage °
1. Penicillin V-potassium	Tbs.	250–500 mg. 4 times daily
Penicillin G-potassium	I.M. for rapid initial blood level	600,000 μ initial dose followed by oral admin.
2. Erythromycin	Caps or Tbs.	250–500 mg. 4–6 times daily
3. Keflex (cephalexin-H_2)	Caps.	250 ml 4 times daily
4. Ampicillin	Caps., liquid	250 mg 4–6 times daily
5. Tetracycline†	Caps.	250 mg 4 times daily
6. Cleocin (clindamycin)†	Caps.	125 mg 1–2 caps, 3 times
Antifungal (against *Candida albicans*)		
1. Nystatin (Mycostatin)	Solution	500,000 μ 3 times daily. Hold solution in mouth 2 min. and swallow.
	Troches	100,000 μ troches dissolved in mouth 4 times daily

° Doses indicated are for a 150 lb adult. Higher doses are prescribed for more severe infections, or as initial doses to establish a high initial drug level. Lower doses for an "average adult" are not recommended. Adult doses are usually used for children over 5 years of age, but consult the child's pediatrician.

† These agents have potential side effects which must be considered prior to administration or prescription.

Modified from Crawford, J. J.: General Guidelines for Initiating Antibiotic Treatment of Acute Oral Infections. University of North Carolina Dental School, 1974.

tion, including surgically related problems, usually an initial dose of 600,000 to 1,200,000 units of penicillin (e.g., procain penicillin) is given intramuscularly. Or 500 mg. or more of penicillin V-potassium, erythromycin, or tetracycline is given orally. This may be followed by 500 mg. every six hours for 5 to 10 days. For more severe or extreme infections the continuing dose may be increased, and the patient is usually hospitalized.[9]

Surgical drainage of well-localized lesions with distinct fluctuant mass (a "pointed lesion") is essential. Penetration of walled-off abscessed tissues by antibiotics is extremely difficult.[9]

Patients with less severe forms of infection may be treated with the antibiotics listed in Table 45–4. The *general principles* of the treatment of infections as briefly discussed in this chapter must be carefully and conscientiously followed. The drugs and dosage regimens suggested here are only general guidelines which undoubtedly will change with the advent of new agents, the emergence of resistant bacteria, and new knowledge. *Culture and antibiotic susceptibility testing should be performed to con-* *firm the choice of antibiotic and guide treatment, especially in severe cases.*

The empirical selection of antimicrobial agent and dosage regimen is based on knowledge of potential pathogens and clinical experience. The drugs listed in Table 45–4 are those chosen on the basis that the infecting agents are probably a mixed bacterial population (aerobic, anaerobic, grampositive, and gram-negative). Circumstances may alter the selection and use of a particular drug.

The method of administration and the route whereby the agent travels to make contact with bacteria are of great importance. The unique opportunity afforded by open wounds and abscesses and accessible normal body cavities and structures offers the surgeon optional modalities for drug administration. As a result, topical application of antimicrobial drugs has been popular not only for treatment of established infection but also for prophylaxis in surgical wounds, as well as in the wounds of trauma. Agents such as chlorhexidine, alexidine, and hydrogen peroxide have been used successfully following periodontal surgical procedures to prevent postoperative infection and im-

TABLE 45–5   PROPHYLAXIS FOR DENTAL PROCEDURES*

	Most congenital heart disease,[c] rheumatic or other acquired valvular heart disease; idiopathic hypertrophic subaortic stenosis; mitral valve[d] prolapse syndrome with mitral insufficiency.	Prosthetic heart valves[e]
All dental procedures that are likely to result in gingival bleeding.[a, b]	Regimen A or B	Regimen B

Regimen A – Penicillin
1. Parenteral-oral combined:
   Adults: Aqueous crystaline penicillin G (1,000,000 units intramuscularly) mixed with procaine penicillin G (600,000 units intramuscularly). Give 30 minutes to one hour prior to procedure; then give penicillin V (formerly called phenoxymethyl penicillin) 500 mg orally every 6 hours for 8 doses.
2. Oral:
   Adults: Penicillin V (2.0 gm. orally) 30 minutes to one hour prior to the procedure and then 500 mg. orally every 6 hours for 8 doses.
   Children: Penicillin V (2.0 gm. orally) 30 minutes to one hour prior to procedure and then 500 mg. orally every 6 hours for 8 doses. For children less than 60 lbs., use 1.0 gm. orally 30 minutes to one hour prior to the procedure and then 250 mg. orally every 6 hours for 8 doses.

   For patient allergic to penicillin:
   Either use vancomycin (see Regimen B) or use:
   Adults: Erythromycin (1.0 gm. orally 1½ to 2 hours prior to the procedure and then 500 mg. orally every 6 hours for 8 doses.
   Children: Erythromycin (20 mg./kg. orally 1½ to 2 hours prior to the procedure and then 10 mg./kg. every 6 hours for 8 doses.

Regimen B – Penicillin plus Streptomycin
   Adults: Aqueous crystalline penicillin G (1,000,000 units intramuscularly) mixed with procaine penicillin G (600,000 units intramuscularly plus streptomycin (1 gm. intramuscularly). Give 30 minutes to one hour prior to the procedure; then penicillin V 500 mg. orally *every* 6 hours for 8 doses.
   Children: Aqueous crystalline penicillin G (30,000 units/kg. intramuscularly) mixed with procaine penicillin G (600,000 units intramuscularly plus streptomycin (20 mg./kg. intramuscularly). Timing of doses for children is the same as for adults. For children less than 60 lbs. the recommended oral dose of penicillin V is 250 mg. every 6 hours for 8 doses.

TABLE 45–5   PROPHYLAXIS FOR DENTAL PROCEDURES (*Continued*)

For patients allergic to penicillin:
Adults: Vancomycin (1 gm. intravenously over 30 minutes to one hour). Start initial vancomycin infusion ½ to one hour prior to procedure; then erythromycin 500 mg. orally every 6 hours for 8 doses.
Children: Vancomycin (20 mg./kg. intravenously over 30 minutes to one hour). Timing of doses for children is the same as for adults. Erythromycin dose is 10 mg./kg. every 6 hours for 8 doses.

Footnotes to Regimens

In unusual circumstances or in the case of delayed healing, it may be prudent to provide additional doses of antibiotics even though available data suggest that bacteremia rarely persists longer than 15 minutes after the procedure. The physician or dentist may also choose to use the parenteral route of administration for all of the doses in selected situations.

Doses for children should not exceed recommendations for adults for a single dose or for a 24-hour period.

For vancomycin the total dose for children should not exceed 44 mg./kg./24 hours.

For those patients receiving continuous oral penicillin for secondary prevention of rheumatic fever, alpha-hemolytic streptococci which are relatively resistant to penicillin are occasionally found in the oral cavity. While it is likely that the doses of penicillin recommended in regimen A are sufficient to control these organisms, the physician or dentist may choose one of the suggestions in Regimen B or may choose oral erythromycin.

° Modified from J. Am. Dent. Assoc., 95:600, 1977.

a Does not include shedding of deciduous teeth.

b Does not include simple adjustment of orthodontic appliances.

c Ventricular septal defect, tetralogy of Fallot, aortic stenosis, pulmonic stenosis, complex cyanotic heart disease, patent ductus arteriosus, or systemic to pulmonary artery shunts. Does not include uncomplicated secundum atrial septal defect.

d Although cases of infective endocarditis in patients with mitral valve prolapse syndrome have been documented, the incidence appears to be relatively low and the necessity for prophylaxis in all of these patients has not yet been established.

e Some patients with a prosthetic heart valve in whom a high level of oral health is being maintained may be offered oral antibiotic prophylaxis for routine dental procedures except the following: parenteral antibiotics are recommended for patients with prosthetic valves who require extensive dental procedures, especially extractions, or oral or gingival surgical procedures.

prove the environment for the healing tissues.

In addition to general principles of control and treatment of infections, the dental structures form many unique microenvironments which are important for the control of colonizing bacteria. The choice of drug, and route of administration depend upon these complex factors. For a complete discussion, see Loesche.[19]

PERIODONTAL TREATMENT. The use of antibiotics to control and potentially stop progressive forms of periodontal disease has aroused interest since the beginning of the antibiotic era. Several clinicians have suggested the use of antibiotics in order to improve the chances of obtaining reattachment and bone fill of vertical bony lesions.[6, 15]

Recently, interest has focused on the use of systemic tetracycline in advanced cases of periodontal disease.[28] Much of the impetus came from observations on the excretion of tetracycline through the gingival sulcus in dogs[2] and its prolonged use in low doses in patients with dermatologic disorders[11] and particularly from unpublished information on pilot studies conducted by Socransky and Newman.[27] No definitive publications have appeared on this subject to date (1977). At the present time, there is insufficient evidence to support the "long-term, low-dose" approach advocated by some clinicians.

Prophylactic Use of Antibiotics

"Prophylaxis" implies that microorganisms are prevented from contamination prior to colonization or, if colonization has occurred, before infection begins. Its major goal is to prevent the development of clinical infection rather than to treat infection that is already established.

Dental surgical procedures are usually associated with transitory bacteremia (see Chap. 48). Bacteria in the bloodstream may lodge on damaged or abnormal valves, such as those found in rheumatic or congenital heart defects, causing bacterial endocarditis.

Since this infection will not occur without a preceding bacteremia, antibiotics are prophylactically recommended.

Periodically the American Heart Association revises its recommendations for the prevention of *bacterial endocarditis*.* The 1977 revision and guidelines are presented in part below.

When selecting antibiotics for prophylaxis of bacterial endocarditis, one should consider the variety of bacteria that are likely to enter the bloodstream. Certain species of microorganisms cause the majority of cases of infective endocarditis, and their antimicrobial sensitivity patterns have been defined.

Since alpha-hemolytic streptococci are the organisms most commonly implicated in bacterial endocarditis following dental procedures, antibiotic prophylaxis should be specifically directed toward them.

In general, parenteral administration of antibiotics is preferred, since it provides more predictable blood levels. Close cooperation with the patient's physician is needed for optimal prophylaxis.[25]

Antibiotic prophylaxis is recommended with *all* dental procedures (including routine professional cleaning) that are likely to cause gingival bleeding. Chemoprophylaxis for dental procedures in children should be managed in a similar manner to the way in which it is handled in adults.[25]

Even in the absence of dental procedures, the presence of periodontal disease can induce, with toothbrushing and even with mastication, transient bacteremia that may seed bacteria in the heart valves. Patients at risk to develop bacterial endocarditis should therefore maintain good oral health. Even edentulous patients may be at risk due to ulcers from ill-fitting dentures.[25]

Patients who will undergo open heart surgery, particularly those who will be given prosthetic heart valves or other intracardiac materials, are at risk to develop endocarditis. The required periodontal treatment should be performed in these patients several weeks in advance.[25]

Table 45–5 contains regimens for chemoprophylaxis for dental procedures sug-

---

*The remaining portion of this section has been drawn freely from the summary of the committee report of the American Heart Association as published by the Journal of the American Dental Association, 95:600, 1977. The reader is urged to consult this publication, as well as the complete report published in Circulation, 65:139A, 1977. The clinician is also urged to keep up to date on the periodic changes which occur in the guidelines.

gested by the American Heart Association. The order of listing does not imply superiority of one regimen over another, although parenteral administration is favored when practical.[25]

The following warning, also taken from the ADA publication,[25] appears to be of utmost importance:

It is not possible to make recommendations for all possible clinical situations. Practitioners should exercise their clinical judgment in determining the duration and choice of antibiotic(s) when special circumstances apply. Furthermore, since endocarditis may occur despite antibiotic prophylaxis, physicians and dentists should maintain a high index of suspicion in the interpretation of any unusual clinical events following the above procedures. Early diagnosis is important to reduce complications, sequelae, and mortality.[25]

REFERENCES

1. Altemeir, W. A.: Manual on Control of Infection in Surgical Practice. American College of Surgeons. Philadelphia, J. B. Lippincott, 1977.
2. Bader, H. J., and Goldhaber, P.: The passage of intravenously administered tetracycline in the gingival sulcus of dogs. J. Oral Ther. Pharmacol., 2:324, 1966.
3. Barry, L.: The Antimicrobic Susceptibility Test: Principles and Practices. Philadelphia, Lea & Febiger, 1977.
4. Bartlett, J. B., and Finegold, S. M.: Anaerobic pleuropulmonary infections. Medicine (Baltimore), 51:413, 1972.
5. Boez, L., Kehlstadt, A., and Schreiber, J.: Les bacteriemies anaerobies a bacillus ramosus (Sept Observations). Ann. Med. (Paris), 23:340, 1928.
6. Carranza, F. A., Sr.: A technique for reattachment. J. Periodontol., 25:272, 1954.
7. Chow, A. W., and Guze, L. B.: Bacteriodaceae bacteremia: Clinical experience with 1212 patients. Medicine (Baltimore), 53:93, 1974.
8. Connor, H. D., Haberman, S., Collins, C. K., and Winford, T. E.: Bacteremias following periodontal scaling in patients with healthy appearing gingiva. J. Periodontol., 38:466, 1967.
9. Crawford, J. J.: General Guidelines for Initiating Antibiotic Treatment of Acute Oral Infections. University of North Carolina Dental School, 1974.
10. Crystal, D. K., Day, S. W., Wagner, C. L., and Krantz, J. M.: Emergency treatment in Ludwig's angina. Surg. Gynecol. Obstet., 129:755, 1969.
11. Delaney, T. J., Heppard B. J., and MacDonald, D. M.: Effects of long term treatment with tetracycline. Acta Derruatovener, 54:487, 1974.
12. Felner, J. M., and Dowell, V. R., Jr.: "Bacteriodes" bacteremia. Am. J. Med. 50:787, 1971.
13. Finegold, S. M.: Anaerobic Bacteria in Human Disease. New York, Academic Press, Inc., 1977.
14. Francis, L. E., and de Vries, J. A.: Therapeutics and the management of common infections. Dent. Clin. North Am., 1968, p. 243.
15. Harvey, R. F.: Clinical impressions of a new antibiotic in periodontics: Spiramycine. J. Can. Dent. Assoc., 27:576, 1961.
16. Ikemoto, H., Hazato, N., and Matsumura, F.: Actinomycosis of the central nervous system. Naika, 21:754, 1968.
17. Khairat, O.: The non-aerobes of post-extraction bacteremia. J. Dent. Res., 45:1191, 1966.
18. Larson, W. P., and Barron, M.: Report of a case in which the fusiform bacillus was isolated from the blood stream. J. Infect. Dis., 13:429, 1913.
19. Loesche, W.: Chemotherapy of dental plaque infections. Oral Sci., Rev., 9:65, 1976.
20. Marseille, A.: Bacteriaemie NA Kiesextractie, Geneeskd. Tijdschr. Med. Indie, 77:2491, 1937.
21. Mason, D. A.: Steroid therapy and dental infection. Case report. Dr. Dent. J., 128:271, 1970.
22. McEntegart, M. G., and Porterfield, J. A.: Bacteremia following dental extractions. Lancet, 2:596, 1949.
23. Meleney, F. L.: Treatise on Surgical Infections. London, Oxford University Press, 1948.
24. Nobles, E. R., Jr.: Bacteroides infections. Ann. Surg., 177:601, 1973.
25. Prevention of Bacterial Endocarditis: A Committee Report of the American Heart Association. J. Am. Dent. Assoc., 95:600, 1977.
26. Rogosa, M., Hampp, E. G., Nevin, T. A., Wagner, H. N., Driscoll, E. J., and Baer, P. N.: Bloodsampling and cultural studies in the detection of postoperative bacteremias. J. Am. Dent. Assoc., 60:181, 1960.
27. Socransky, S. S., and Newman, M. G.: Unpublished data.
28. Tetracycline Use in Periodontal Therapy. Bull. Northeast Soc. Periodontol., 6:4, 1976.
29. Thompson, L. E.: A fatal case of brain abscess from Vincent's angina following extraction of a tooth under procaine hydrochloride. J.A.M.A. 93:1063, 1929.
30. Veszpremi, D.: Kultur- und Tierversuche mit dem Bacillus fusibormis und dem Spirillum. Zentralbl. Bakteriol., Parasitenkd., Infektionskr. Hyg., Abt. 1: Orig., 38:136, 1905.
31. Vic-Dupont, M., Laufer, J., and Cartier, F.: Onze maladies d'Osler d'origine dentaire. Bull. Mem. Soc. Med. Hop. Paris, 114:869, 1963.
32. Weiss, C.: The pathogenicity of bacteroides melaninogenicus and its importance in surgical infections. Surgery, 13:683, 1943.

NUTRITIONAL THERAPY IN THE TREATMENT OF GINGIVAL AND PERIODONTAL DISEASE

Nutritional therapy may be required as an adjunct in the treatment of the following: chronic gingivitis, chronic periodontal disease, acute necrotizing ulcerative gingivitis, and other acute conditions of the oral mucous membrane. When indicated, nutritional therapy serves two basic functions in regard to the periodontium: (1) it satisfies the chemical requirements of the tissues by supplying the necessary nutriments, and (2) it provides mechanical stimulation to the tissues in the course of mastication.

Nutritional therapy in chronic periodontal disease

Nutritional therapy[11,24] **in the treatment of gingival and periodontal problems should be based upon a demonstrated need,** which is determined as follows:

If when examining a patient it is the operator's impression that the response of the periodontium to existing local factors varies from what he would ordinarily expect, then he may suspect the existence of contributing systemic factors, one of which may be nutritional.

This suspicion must be corroborated by evaluation of the patient's nutritional status (Chap. 32). This entails the medical and dietary history and a physical examination for signs of nutritional disturbances in areas other than the oral cavity. In some instances biochemical tests are indicated.

When existence of a nutritional disturbance has been established, nutritional therapy should be provided as follows:

1. Modify the patient's diet so as to include the necessary nutriments and also satisfy caloric requirements. Standard texts are useful aids in diet analysis and construction.[19] It is preferable to use a protective natural diet rather than to continue a poor diet and attempt to supplement it.

2. Consideration should be given to the physical character of foodstuffs; the mechanical stimulation from hard and detergent foods such as raw fruits and vegetables, as well as chewy foods, such as meat, aids in the maintenance of periodontal health.

Nutritional supplements may improve the effectiveness of local periodontal treatment, provided the patient has a nutritional deficiency. The evidence that **nutritional supplements** (protein,[5,17,26] fats,[25] multivitamins, trace minerals,[27,28] and water-soluble bioflavonoids[4]) prevent gingival or periodontal disease in man or improve the response to local treatment is not conclusive.[10] Some clinical studies[8] indicate that scaling and polishing reduce the severity of gingivitis by 30 per cent, whereas 45 per cent reduction is obtained by the systemic administration of **synthetic vitamin C alone,** and 67 per cent reduction follows the combination of scaling and polishing with systemic **synthetic vitamin C.** Others[21] note that **increasing the plasma ascorbic acid levels** by dietary supplements in patients with gingival disease and below average plasma ascorbic levels does not improve the condition of the gingiva, and find no significant relationship between either whole blood or urine **ascorbic acid** levels and the periodontal status.[29] It has also been reported that elevating the **ascorbic acid** level of the blood by dietary supplements does not decrease **tooth mobility** or affect the ascorbic acid level of inflamed gingiva or influence the outcome of local treatment.[12,20]

It has been suggested that gingivitis is more severe and the response to oral prophylaxis is poor in individuals with inadequate **carbohydrate metabolism** as reflected in **nonfasting blood glucose levels,**[6] whereas other investigators find no significant relationship between the periodontal status and either **fasting or postprandial serum glucose levels.**[29]

Some investigators have suggested beneficial effects from **fluoride in the treatment of osteoporosis and other human metabolic bone disease,**[2,7] and fluoride concentrations from 4 to 5.8 p.p.m. in water have been shown to reduce the prevalence and severity of osteoporosis.[1] Others[15] have found that the addition of **fluoride** to the diet has no effect on osteoporosis induced in dogs by feeding low calcium–high phosphorus diets. Periodontal disease has been reported to be less severe in individuals using drinking water with 1.2 p.p.m. **fluoride,** compared with those using water containing 0.1 p.p.m.[9] X-ray diffraction studies of human bone indicate that a rise in fluoride content is accompanied by an increase in apatite crystal size, which produces a more stable bone apatite.[23] In tissue cultures, low concentrations of **fluoride** inhibit bone resorption without any apparent effect on bone formation, but high concentrations of fluoride inhibit both bone formation and resorption.[13] Systemic **fluoride** has been recommended for the treatment of alveolar atrophy,[18] but there are conflicting reports regarding the effectiveness of high doses of fluoride in preventing alveolar bone loss in rats.[16, 31]

Oral mucosal lesions caused by nutritional deficiency respond to nutritional therapy alone (Fig. 45–1). However, in nutritionally deficient patients with periodontal disease nutritional therapy is only an adjunct to local treatment. **The eradication of gingivitis and periodontal pockets requires removal of all forms of local irritation and the maintenance of effective oral hygiene.**[21, 22]

Removal of local irritants is essential for other reasons. **The chronic inflammation and circulatory congestion they produce interfere with the transport of nutrients.** This may create a local conditioned nutritional deficiency in the periodontium of individuals with a satisfactory nutritional status — and prevent the periodontium from benefiting from nutritional therapy where nutritional deficiencies exist. In addition, the degeneration that often accompanies inflammation or is caused by injurious occlusal forces impairs the capacity of the periodontal tissues to utilize nutrients.

Patients on special diets for medical reasons

Patients on low-residue, nondetergent diets often develop gingivitis because the foods lack cleansing action and the tendency for plaque and food debris to accumulate on the teeth is increased. Because fibrous foods are contraindicated, special effort is made to compensate for the soft diet by emphasizing the patient's oral hygiene procedures. Patients on salt-free diets should not be given saline mouthwashes, nor should they be treated with saline preparations without consulting the patient's physician. Diabetes, gallbladder disease, and hypertension are examples of conditions in which particular care should be taken to avoid the prescription of contraindicated foodstuffs.

Supportive nutritional therapy in acute necrotizing ulcerative gingivitis and other acute conditions of the oral mucous membrane

Nutritional considerations in the treatment of acute necrotizing ulcerative gingivitis in nutritionally deficient patients were presented in Chapter 41. Severe

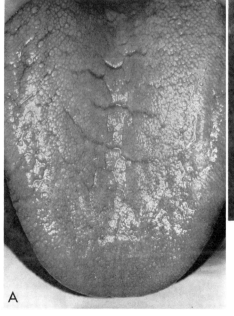
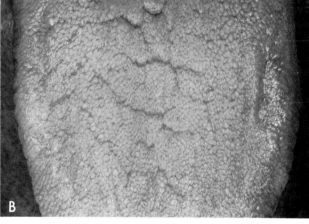

Figure 45–1 Tongue Changes Following Nutritional Therapy. *A,* Atrophy of the papillae in patient with vitamin B-complex deficiency. *B,* Regeneration of papillae after nutritional therapy.

cases of acute necrotizing ulcerative gingivitis or other painful conditions, such as acute herpetic gingivostomatitis, aphthous stomatitis, desquamative gingivitis, erythema multiforme, bullous lichen planus, or pemphigus, are often accompanied by poor appetite, inability to chew or swallow food, and excessive loss of fluids, nitrogen, and water-soluble vitamins (vitamin B complex and vitamin C). In such patients nutritional therapy may be indicated as a supportive measure to restore a chemically adequate nutrition in order to obtain maximum benefits from local treatment.

SYSTEMIC THERAPY FOR CHRONIC PERIODONTAL DISEASE

There are two aspects of systemic therapy to supplement local procedures in the treatment of chronic periodontal disease. The first deals with **patients with a known systemic disease, such as hyperthyroidism, osteoporosis, or diabetes, in which the effectiveness of local treatment in attaining cessation of bone destruction depends upon treatment of the systemic disturbance.** The desired results are obtained by a close working relationship with the patient's physician.

The second aspect of systemic therapy for chronic periodontal disease is still in its experimental stage. It consists of the systemic use of drugs or tissue extracts (Herosteon L3532, Vaduril, Alveoactive, Ebosone, Siccacel, and Insadol[3, 14]) for the purpose of stimulating cellular activity in the periodontium in an effort to improve the response to local treatment.

REFERENCES

1. Bernstein, D. S., et al.: Prevalence of osteoporosis in high- and low-fluoride areas in North Dakota. J.A.M.A., 198:499, 1966.
2. Bernstein, D. S., et al.: The use of sodium fluoride in metabolic bone disease. In Proceedings of the American Society for Clinical Investigation. J. Clin. Invest., 42:916, 1963.
3. Bertolini, A. G.: Behandlung parodontaler Kollagenopathien mit lebenden Liophilzellen Siccacel. Parodontol., 16:66, 1962.
4. Carvel, R. I., and Halperin, V.: Therapeutic effect of water-soluble bioflavonoids in gingival inflammatory conditions. Oral Surg., 14:847, 1961.
5. Cheraskin, E., and Ringsdorf, W. M., Jr.: Periodontal pathosis in man. X. Effect of combined versus animal protein supplementation upon sulcus depth. J. Oral Ther., 1:497, 1965.
6. Cheraskin, E., and Ringsdorf, W. M., Jr.: Resistance and susceptibility to oral disease. I. A study in gingivitis and carbohydrate metabolism. J. Dent. Res., 44:374, 1965.
7. Cohen, P., and Gardner, F. H.: Induction of subacute skeletal fluorosis in a case of multiple myeloma. N. Engl. J. Med., 271:1129, 1964.
8. El-Ashiry, G. M., Ringsdorf, W. M., Jr., and Cheraskin, E.: Local and systemic influences in periodontal disease: II. Effect of prophylaxis and natural versus synthetic vitamin C upon gingivitis. J. Periodontol., 35:250, 1964.
9. Englander, H. R., Kesel, R. G., and Gupta, O. P.: The Aurora-Rockford, Illinois, study. II. Effect of natural fluoride on the periodontal health of adults. Am. J. Public Health, 53:1233, 1963.
10. Glickman, I.: Nutrition in the prevention and treatment of gingival and periodontal disease. J. Dent. Med., 19:179, 1964.
11. Glickman, I.: The role of nutritional therapy in the management of periodontal disease. J. Am. Dent. Assoc., 52:275, 1956.
12. Glickman, I., and Dines, M. M.: Effect of increased ascorbic acid blood levels on the ascorbic acid level in treated and non-treated gingiva. J. Dent. Res., 42:1152, 1963.
13. Goldhaber, P.: The inhibition of bone resorption in tissue culture by nontoxic concentrations of sodium fluoride. Israel J. Med. Sci., 3:617, 1967.
14. Held, A. J.: Endogenous therapy in parodontolysis. Paradentologie, 3:7, 1949.
15. Henrikson, P., et al.: Fluoride and nutritional osteoporosis: Physicochemical data on bones from an experimental study in dogs. J. Nutr., 100:631, 1970.
16. Kristoffersen, T., Bang, G., and Meyer, K.: Lack of effect of high doses of fluoride in prevention of alveolar bone loss in rats. J. Periodont. Res., 5:127, 1970.
17. Lederman, N. J., and Hazen, S. P.: Relationship between supplementary dietary protein and periodontal health. I.A.D.R. Abst., 1965, p. 53, No. 66.
18. Lukomsky, E. H.: Fluorine therapy for exposed dentin and alveolar atrophy. J. Dent. Res., 20:649, 1941.
19. Nizel, A. E.: The Science of Nutrition and Its Application in Clinical Dentistry, 2nd ed. Philadelphia, W. B. Saunders Company, 1966, p. 185.
20. O'Leary, T. J., Rudd, K. D., Crump, P. P., and Krause, R. E.: The effect of ascorbic acid supplementation on tooth mobility. J. Periodontol., 40:284, 1969.
21. Parfitt, G. J., and Hand, C. D.: Reduced plasma ascorbic acid levels and gingival health. J. Periodontol., 34:347, 1963.
22. Pierce, H. B., Newhall, C. A., Merrow, S. B., Lamden, M. P., Schweiker, C., and Laughlin, A.: Ascorbic acid supplementation: I. Re-

sponse of gum tissue. Am. J. Clin. Nutr., 8:353, 1960.

23. Posner, A. S., et al.: X-Ray diffraction analysis of the effect of fluoride on human bone apatite. Arch. Oral Biol., 8:549, 1963.

24. Radusch, D. F.: The periodontal benefits of well-planned diets. J. Am. Dent. Assoc., 47:14, 1953.

25. Rao, S. S., Shourie, K. L., and Shankwalker, G. B.: Effect of dietary fat variations on the periodontium. An experimental study on rats. Periodontics, 3:66, 1965.

26. Ringsdorf, W. M., Jr., and Cheraskin, E.: Periodontal pathosis in man: IV. Effect of protein versus placebo supplementation upon gingivitis. J. Dent. Med., 18:92, 1963.

27. Ringsdorf, W. M., Jr., and Cheraskin, E.: Periodontal pathosis in man. VI. Effect of multivitamin-trace minerals versus placebo supple-mentation on gingivitis. J. West. Soc. Periodont., 11:85, 1963.

28. Ringsdorf, W. M., Jr., and Cheraskin, E.: Periodontal pathosis in man. VII. Effect of multivitamin-trace mineral versus placebo supplementation on sulcus depth. J. Am. Dent. Assoc., 68:1, 1964.

29. Shannon, I. L., and Gibson, W. A.: Intravenous ascorbic loading in subjects classified as to periodontal status. J. Dent. Res., 44:355, 1965.

30. Shannon, I. L., and Gibson, W. A.: Relationship of oral health to fasting and postprandial serum glucose levels. J. Dent. Med., 20:3, 1965.

31. Zipkin, I., Larson, R. H., and Bernick, S.: Blocking of the nutritionally induced periodontal disease syndrome with fluoride. I.A.D.R. Abst., 1970, p. 134.

Surgical Phase

Pocket Elimination

Pocket elimination consists of reducing the depth of periodontal pockets to that of a physiologic sulcus. It is important in the overall management of periodontal disease, but it is not the total treatment. Additional measures indicated by the requirements of the individual case must also be employed.

Elimination of the periodontal pocket is a critical factor in restoring periodontal health and arresting destruction of the supporting periodontal tissues. The purpose of reducing the depth of the pocket to that of the normal gingival sulcus is to facilitate access by the patient to keep the area free of plaque. The presence of a pocket creates areas which are impossible for the patient to keep clean and therefore a vicious cycle is established.

Periodontal pocket deepening ⟶ Plaque accumulation

Total pocket elimination has traditionally been considered one of the main goals of periodontal therapy. Another viewpoint has emerged in recent years, supported by clinical longitudinal studies. It has been shown that after therapy, pockets of 4 and even 5 mm. can be maintained in a healthy state and without radiographic evidences of advancing bone loss. This was accomplished by scaling and root planing and oral hygiene reinforcement performed at regular intervals of not more than three months after pocket therapy. In these cases the residual defect can be penetrated with a thin periodontal probe but with no pain, exudate, or bleeding; no plaque appears to form on the subgingival tooth surfaces.

Pocket depth is an extremely useful and widely used clinical parameter but has to be evaluated together with level of attachment and presence of bleeding, exudation, and pain. The most important parameter to evaluate whether a pocket (or deep sulcus) is progressive or not is the *level of attachment* measured in millimeters from the cemento-enamel junction; in the last analysis it is the displacement of the level of attachment that places the tooth in jeopardy, not the increase in pocket depth that may be due to coronal displacement of the gingival margin. Therefore a periodontal pocket that can be maintained free of plaque and that does not result in progressive loss of attachment can be considered a satisfactory result of treatment.

Ramfjord et al.[1, 2] and Rosling et al.[3] have shown that regardless of the technique used for pocket elimination, a certain pocket depth will recur. This depth appears to depend on the original pocket depth and not too much on the technique of treatment. In the last analysis, therefore, *maintenance of this depth without any further loss of attachment becomes the real goal.*

This does not minimize the need for pocket therapy and the indications for pocket elimination, but rather emphasizes the importance of the maintenance phase and the close monitoring of both level of attachment and pocket depth, together with the other clinical parameters (bleeding, secretion, tooth mobility). *The transformation of the initial, deep, active lesion into a shallower, inactive, maintainable one requires some form of definitive pocket therapy and a constant supervision thereafter.*

METHODS OF POCKET ELIMINATION

An understanding of the underlying pathologic processes is helpful in the treatment of periodontal disease. However, pocket elimination per se is a technical procedure that must be mastered along with the many other techniques of general dentistry. The methods of pocket elimination are classified under three main headings:

(1) *Reattachment techniques*: these methods offer the ideal result, since they eliminate pocket depth by reunion of the gingiva to the tooth at a position coronal to the bottom of the pre-existing pocket; it is usually associated with filling-in of bone and regeneration of periodontal ligament and cementum.

(2) *Removal of the lateral wall of the pocket*: these are the most commonly performed methods. The lateral wall of the pocket can be removed by (a) *retraction or shrinkage*: this is the result when scaling and root planing resolves the inflammatory process and the gingiva therefore shrinks, reducing the pocket depth; (b) *surgical removal*: this is performed by the gingivectomy technique; and (c) *apical displacement* with an apically positioned flap.

(3) *Removal of the tooth side of the pocket*, which is accomplished by tooth extraction or by partial tooth extraction (hemisection or root resection).

The techniques, what they accomplish, and the factors governing their selection are presented in the next chapters.

Criteria for Method Selection

Scientific criteria to establish the indications for each technique are difficult to determine. Longitudinal studies following a significant number of cases over a significant number of years, standardizing multiple factors and different parameters, would be needed. Clinical experience, however, has suggested the following criteria to select in individual cases the method to be used to eliminate the pocket:

1. *Gingival Pockets.* Two factors are taken into consideration: (a) the character of the pocket wall and (b) the pocket accessibility.

The pocket wall can be either edematous or fibrotic. Edematous tissue will shrink after elimination of local factors, thereby reducing or totally eliminating pocket depth. Pockets having a fibrotic wall will not appreciably reduce their depth after scaling and root planing; after considerably longer periods of time of adequate plaque control their depth may become somewhat reduced; however, chances of recurrence are greater.

Pocket elimination has to be based on total elimination of the responsible local factors. Accessibility then becomes an important consideration. The following table will clarify the rationale for selection of pocket eradication method in gingival pockets.

Accessibility	Pocket Wall — Edematous	Fibrotic
Good	Curettage	Gingivectomy
Poor	Gingivectomy	Gingivectomy

2. *Suprabony Pockets.* Two problems have to be considered: (1) the presence or absence of an adequate band of attached gingiva, and (2) the presence of bone deformities requiring some type of surgical correction. The following table will summarize the rationale for selection of treatment technique in suprabony pockets.

Adequate Attached Gingiva		Inadequate Attached Gingiva	
No Bone Deformities	*Bone Deformities*	*No Bone Deformities*	*Bone Deformities*
Closed or open curettage or gingivectomy	Muco-periosteal flap with osseous contouring	Mucosal apically positioned flap or gingival extension with free soft tissue autograft	Muco-periosteal apically positioned flap with osseous contouring

3. *Infrabony Pockets.* Treatment of infrabony pockets may be directed to obtaining bone regeneration and reattachment, or to contouring the remaining bone to an acceptable morphology. The decision depends mainly on the exact shape of the

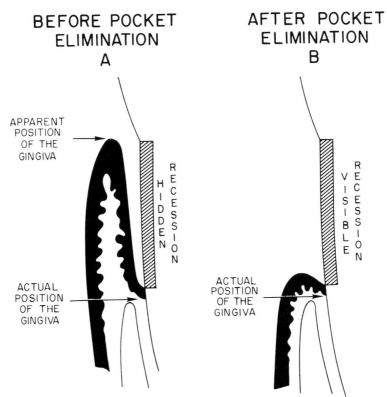

Figure 46–1   Amount of Recession is Determined by the Actual Position of the Gingiva, Not by the Apparent Position.
A, Before periodontal pocket is eliminated. Recession (**Hidden Recession**) is present, but it is covered by the disease pocket wall. *B,* After the periodontal pocket is eliminated, the recession which was present but hidden before treatment becomes visible (**Visible Recession**).

bony defect (number of walls, width, and general configuration of the defect). The only way to determine the shape of bone is visual inspection. Therefore, the technique indicated for the treatment of infrabony pockets will be the mucoperiosteal flap, with osseous surgery aimed at bone regeneration or bone removal according to the morphology of the defect. This technique may also be combined with mucogingival procedures when an inadequate amount of attached gingiva is present. Other indications for the solution of mucogingival problems will be given in Chapter 53.

RECESSION AND POCKET ELIMINATION

The fact that more of the root surface is often visible after periodontal pockets are eliminated has led to the erroneous impression that periodontal treatment causes recession. This impression is based upon a misconception of what recession is. **The amount of recession depends upon the location of the junctional epithelium on the tooth surface, not the position of the crest of the gingiva.** *The former is the actual position of the gingiva; the latter is the apparent position* (Fig. 46–1).

Judging pre- and post-treatment recession by the location of the crest of the gingival margin is misleading. Recession is present before the periodontal pocket is treated, but the denuded root is hidden by the diseased pocket wall (Fig. 46–1). After the pocket is eliminated, the previously denuded root surface becomes exposed to view. **What happens is that hidden recession becomes visible recession** (Fig. 46–1).

Most often the amount of recession before and after the treatment of periodontal pockets is essentially the same. In some instances there may be more recession after treatment, and if reattachment occurs there is less. **However, in all instances the amount of recession is determined by the location of the junctional epithelium.**

RECURRENCE OF POCKET DEPTH

After treatment to eliminate periodontal pockets, some of the depth tends to return with time, regardless of the treatment technique.[1, 2] This occurs in patients with apparently good oral hygiene who are recalled at three-month intervals for maintenance prophylaxis and reinstruction in home care. The clinical significance of this has not yet been fully understood. As mentioned previously, a "deepened" sulcus could be considered an acceptable result of therapy as long as its depth remains stable, there are no signs of bleeding, secretion, or pain upon probing, and periodic radiographs show no further bone loss.

REFERENCES

1. Ramfjord, S. P.: Present status of the modified Widman flap procedure. J. Periodontol., 48:558, 1977.
2. Ramfjord, S. P., Knowles, J. W., Nissle, R. R., Burgett, F. G., and Shick, R. A.: Results of following three modalities of periodontal therapy. J. Periodontol., 46:522, 1975.
3. Rosling, B., Nyman, S., Lindhe, J., and Jern, B.: The healing potential of the periodontal tissues following different techniques of periodontal surgery in plaque-free dentitions. A 2-year clinical study. J. Clin. Periodontol., 3:233, 1976.

Gingival Curettage

The scaling and curettage technique is the basic, most commonly employed procedure for the elimination of periodontal pockets and the treatment of gingival disease. It consists of *scaling* to remove calculus, plaque, and other deposits, *planing* the root to smooth it and remove necrotic tooth substance, and *curetting* the inner surface of the gingival wall of periodontal pockets to separate away diseased soft tissue.

The term curettage is sometimes used to designate smoothing of root surfaces; however, we use it only in connection with treatment of soft tissues. Smoothing of root surfaces is referred to as root planing.

Curettage hastens healing by reducing the task of the body enzymes and phagocytes, which ordinarily remove tissue debris during healing. Also, by removing the epithelial lining of the periodontal pocket, curettage removes a barrier to reattachment of the periodontal ligament to the root surface. Some degree of irritation and trauma to the gingiva is unavoidable with scaling and curettage, even if it is performed with extreme care. The injurious effects are of microscopic proportion and generally do not significantly affect the healing. Over-zealous scaling and curettage causes postoperative pain and retards healing.

Scaling and root planing are done routinely for every patient as preparation for pocket elimination techniques. They constitute the so-called Phase I therapy (see Chap. 42). Curettage is considered one of the surgical techniques; however, when curettage is done it is usually performed in one operation with the treatment of the hard tissue side of the pocket by scaling and root planing. In these cases, therefore, Phase I and Phase II therapy (surgical phase) are combined in one operation.

INDICATIONS

Scaling and curettage is the technique of choice for the following:

1. Elimination of suprabony pockets in which the depth is such that the calculus on the root can be completely visualized by deflecting the pocket wall with a blast of warm air or a probe. For scaling and curettage to succeed, the pocket wall must be edematous so that it can shrink to normal

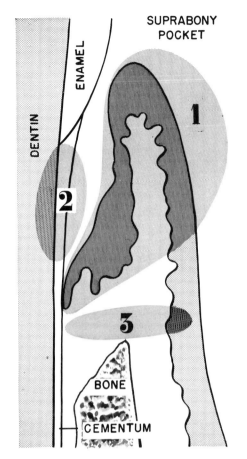
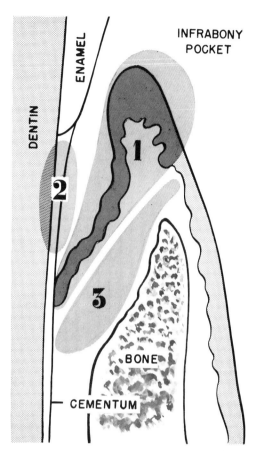

Figure 47–1   Critical Zones in Pocket Eradication. *Left.* Suprabony pocket; *Right,* infrabony pocket. Zone 1: Soft tissue wall and junctional epithelium. Zone 2: Tooth surface. Zone 3: Connective tissue between the pocket wall and bone.

sulcus depth. If the pocket wall is firm and fibrous, surgical treatment is required to eliminate the pocket because the fibrous pocket wall will not shrink sufficiently following scaling and curettage.

2. Most types of gingivitis, except gingival enlargement.

Scaling and curettage is also one of several techniques for the treatment of infrabony pockets.

POCKET ELIMINATION BY SCALING AND CURETTAGE

In pocket elimination, just as in the preparation of a carious tooth for a restoration, it is necessary to have a plan of procedure before the operation is begun. As a guide to treatment, periodontal pockets may be subdivided into three critical zones (Fig. 47–1).

Critical Zones in Pocket Elimination

Zone 1. The soft tissue wall and junctional epithelium

The soft tissue wall of the pocket is inflamed and presents varying degrees of degeneration and ulceration with engorged blood vessels close to the surface, often separated from the contents of the pocket by only a thin layer of tissue debris. In this zone determine the following:

Whether the pocket wall extends in a straight line from the gingival margin or follows a tortuous course around the tooth.

The number of tooth surfaces involved by the pocket.

The location of the bottom of the pocket on the tooth surface, and the pocket depth.

The relationship of the pocket wall to the alveolar bone (Fig. 47–1). Is the entire pocket coronal to the crest of the bone (suprabony pocket), or is there bone lateral to the pocket wall (infrabony pocket)?

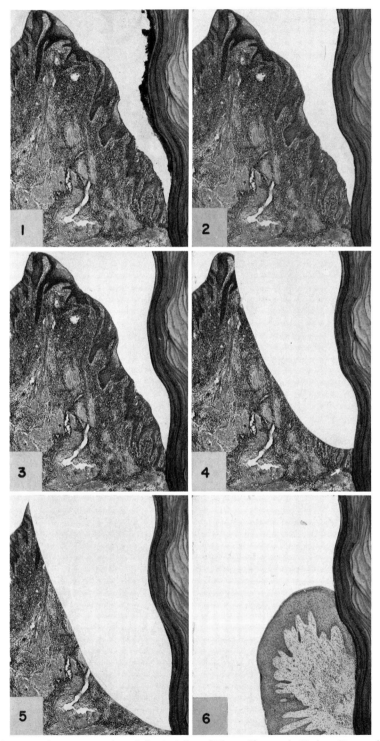

Figure 47–2   Diagrammatic Representation of the Anticipated Tissue Changes in Various Stages of Pocket Eradication Using Scaling and Curettage. *1,* The periodontal pocket with calculus on the root surface. *2,* Calculus removed. Note contour of the cementum. *3,* Root surface smoothed. *4,* Pocket wall curetted. Junctional epithelium *(arrow)* not disturbed. *5,* Alternate procedure to that shown in *4.* Pocket wall curetted. Junctional epithelium also removed. *6,* Pocket eradicated.

Zone 2. The tooth surface

Adherent to the tooth are calculus and other tooth surface deposits of varying amounts and texture. The superficial calculus is generally claylike in consistency, obvious, and easily detached by well-directed instrumentation. However, deep in the pocket the calculus is hard, flint-like, and tenaciously adherent to the surface. In the coronal portion of the root the cementum is extremely thin, and a ledge is often formed at the cemento-enamel junction, which must be taken into consideration when the tooth is scaled. The cementum surface may be softened by caries. It may be deformed by adherent cementicles.

The pocket itself contains bacteria, bacterial products, the products of food decomposition, and calculus, all bathed in a slimy mucous medium. Pus may or may not be present.

In this zone determine the following:

1. The extent and location of deposits.
2. The condition of the tooth surface; the presence of softened, eroded areas.
3. The accessibility of the root surface to the necessary instrumentation.

Zone 3. The connective tissue between the pocket wall and the bone

In this zone, determine whether the connective tissue is soft and friable, or firm and bound to the bone. This is a significant consideration in the treatment of infrabony pockets.

Scaling and Curettage Technique

The following is a step-by-step procedure for eliminating pockets by scaling and curettage, with an explanation of what each step accomplishes.

Pocket elimination should be systematic, beginning in one section and proceeding in orderly sequence until the entire mouth is treated. Treatment is usually started in the right maxillary molar area, unless it is urgently needed in another section. The number of teeth included at each visit varies with the skill of the operator, the type of patient, and the severity of periodontal involvement (see Chapters 37 and 42).

Step 1. Isolate and anesthetize the area

The field is isolated with cotton rolls or gauze pads and swabbed with a mild antiseptic such as Merthiolate or Metaphen. Throughout the scaling and curettage procedure the area is cleansed intermittently with pellets of cotton saturated with an equal mixture of warm water and 3 per cent peroxide. Strong antiseptics or escharotic drugs are not used because they may induce tissue injury and retard healing.

Topical or infiltration and block anesthesia are used according to the needs. Topical anesthetics are usually adequate for the elimination of shallow pockets, but for deep pockets more profound anesthesia by injection is advised. It is better to have slightly more anesthesia than not enough.

A fetish is sometimes made of not using any form of anesthetic for scaling and curettage. The removal of supragingival calculus does not require anesthesia, and experienced clinicians can perform subgingival scaling and curettage with a minimum of discomfort. The presence of anesthesia may foster abuse of the tissues. Judicious use of topical and injected anesthetics, however, is appreciated by the patient and precludes the likelihood of sacrificing thoroughness in an effort to avoid pain when anesthesia is not used.

Step 2. Remove the supragingival calculus

Remove the visible calculus and debris with superficial scalers. This will result in shrinkage of the gingiva because of bleeding elicited by even slight instrumentation.

Step 3. Remove the subgingival calculus

A curette is inserted to the bottom of the pocket just beneath the lower border of the calculus and the calculus dislodged. The chisel type of scaler is used for proximal surfaces too close together to be reached with other types of scalers (Fig. 47–2, *1* and 2).

Step 4. Plane the tooth surface

Curettes are then used to ensure removal of the deep deposits, removal of necrotic cementum, and smoothing the root surface[8] (Fig. 47–2, *3*).

The bacterial flora of the periodontal pocket is reduced after subgingival calculus is removed.[21, 22] The removal of necrotic cementum and dentin, in addition to removing local irritants, prepares the root so that new connective tissue may be deposited on its freshened surface. In the course of healing, new cementum is more likely to be deposited on a clean dentin surface than on necrotic cementum.

Step 5. Curette the soft tissue wall

Curettage is employed to remove the diseased inner lining of the pocket wall, including the junctional epithelium (Fig. 47–2, *4* and 5). If the junctional epithelium is permitted to remain, epithelium from the crest of the gingiva will proliferate along the curetted pocket wall to join it and prevent any possibility of reattachment of the connective tissue to the root surface.[11] Curettes are used for this purpose with cutting edges on two sides of the blade so that the root is smoothed in the same operation.

Removal of the inner pocket lining and the junctional epithelium is a two-stage procedure. The curette is inserted to engage the inner lining of the pocket wall and carried along the soft tissue to the crest of the gingiva. The pocket wall is supported by gentle finger pressure on the external surface. The curette is then placed under the cut edge of the junctional epithelium so as to undermine it. The junctional epithelium is separated away with a scooping motion of the curette to the tooth surface. Curettage removes degenerated tissue, proliferating epithelial buds, and granulation tissue, which will go to form the inner aspect of the pocket wall, and creates a cut, bleeding connective tissue surface. The bleeding causes shrinkage in the height of

the gingiva and reduction in pocket depth and facilitates healing by removing tissue debris.

Opinions differ regarding whether scaling and curettage consistently remove the pocket lining and junctional epithelium. Some report that scaling and root planing tear the lining epithelium, without removing it or the junctional epithelium,[13] but that both epithelial structures,[2, 3, 11] sometimes including underlying inflamed connective tissue,[14] are removed by curettage. Others report that the removal of lining and junctional epithelium is not complete.[19, 23, 25]

Step 6. Polish the tooth surface

Using a rubber polishing cup with Improved Zircate or a paste of fine pumice in water, the root surface and adjacent coronal surface are polished. The flexibility of the rubber cup permits access to the subgingival area without traumatizing the tissues. Brushes are not used for polishing the root surfaces at this stage because of the difficulty of avoiding soft tissue injury. After the root surfaces are polished, the field is cleansed with warm water and slight pressure is applied to adapt the gingiva to the tooth. The use of tissue varnish to cover the area is optional.

The patient is dismissed and advised to pursue his usual eating habits, but to be mindful that there may be some discomfort for a few days. He is to pay particular attention to keeping his teeth clean, gently at first, but gradually increasing the vigor of brushing, interdental cleansing, and flossing, followed by water irrigation.

HEALING FOLLOWING SCALING AND CURETTAGE

Immediately after scaling and curettage, a blood clot fills the gingival sulcus. This is followed by a rapid proliferation of granulation tissue with a decrease in the number of small blood vessels as the tissue matures. Restoration and epithelization of the sulcus generally require from two to seven days,[10, 14, 15, 23] and restoration of the junctional epithelium occurs in animals as early as five days. Immature collagen fibers appear within 21 days after treatment. Healthy gingival fibers inadvertently severed from the tooth by scaling, root planing, and curettage,[16] and tears in the sulcular epithelium[13, 17] and junctional epithelium are repaired in the healing process.

Electromicroscopic studies reveal the following regarding roots which have been thoroughly scaled and planed.[20]

Immediately after treatment the surfaces are smooth; there may be some cracked and fragmented areas. In some sections the cementum is completely removed.

Pellicle and bacterial plaque are deposited on the surface within a few hours, followed by calcification of the root. Caries sometimes develops within seven days.

Within three to four weeks after exposure to the oral cavity a hypermineralized surface zone and a subsurface cuticle develop. These are produced by an interchange of minerals and organic components at the saliva-root interface. Remineralization occurs more frequently following scaling and root planing in periodontally diseased teeth than in periodontally healthy teeth.

Appearance of the gingiva after one week

The gingiva is reduced in height because of shrinkage and shift in the position of the gingival margin. The gingiva is also slightly redder than normal because of increased vascularity associated with healing.

Appearance of the gingiva after two weeks

At this time, with proper oral hygiene by the patient, the normal color, consistency, surface texture, and contour of the gingiva are attained and the gingival margin is well adapted to the tooth (Fig. 47–2, 6).

Sequelae of pocket elimination with the scaling and curettage technique

Healing is usually uneventful, but several types of complications may develop.

1. SENSITIVITY TO PERCUSSION. Inflammation of the periodontal ligament may develop within a day or two after treatment. The tooth is slightly extruded and sensitive to percussion and the patient complains of a throbbing pain. There may be localized lymphadenopathy. In such cases, antibiotics are administered systemically (Chap. 45) as a prophylactic measure. The involved tooth or its antagonist is ground slightly to relieve the occlusion. Using a topical anesthetic, the gingival margin is gently probed to stimulate bleeding and examined for any fragments of calculus that may be lodged in the tissues. The patient is instructed to avoid exertion and to rinse every hour with warm solution of a teaspoonful of salt in a glass of water. When the patient is seen after 24 hours, the condition is generally alleviated. The antibiotic therapy is continued for another 24 hours and rinsing reduced to three times a day.

2. BLEEDING. Bleeding may occur after two or three days. This results from inflammation around surface vessels, with rupture of the vessel walls. The area is generally partially covered with a small berry-like clot when the patient appears. To correct this condition, the clot is removed with a pellet of cotton saturated with peroxide, 3 per cent, and the bleeding point located. The surface is gently curetted and irritants are removed. Pressure is applied with either a gauze pad or a cotton pellet wedged interproximally for 20 minutes.

3. SENSITIVITY TO THERMAL CHANGES AND TACTILE STIMULATION. The patient may complain about sensitivity to cold and tactile stimulation. This is caused either by removal of cementum and exposure of the extremely sensitive granular layer of Tomes at the periphery of the root dentin,[5] or by exposure of root surface previously insulated from thermal changes by heavy calculus deposits.

Root sensitivity is treated with sodium fluoride desensitizing paste or other desensitizing agents. Burnishing the clean root surface with a slightly warmed ball burnisher is frequently helpful in eliminating localized areas of sensitivity. Except in extreme cases, desensitization should not be undertaken the first week after treatment. It is advisable to postpone its use until shrinkage of the gingiva is complete and a well-developed epithelial covering is present. If the desensitizing agent is used the first week after treatment, gingival bleeding elicited in an effort to reach the denuded root surfaces diminishes the effectiveness of the desensitizing agent. There is also a tendency for post-treatment sensitivity to diminish spontaneously after two or three weeks have elapsed.

OTHER TECHNIQUES

The following techniques have been described to facilitate calculus removal and shrinkage of the pocket wall. They are not in general use at present and are described here with the purpose of offering a historic perspective to the methods suggested in this chapter.

Packing Technique (Box)

Box[6, 7] advocated a variation of the scaling and curettage technique for pocket eradication which included the use of periodontal packs. The packs consist of boracic acid, oil of peppermint, oxygen, and other medicinals incorporated in a paraffin base, which is formed into sticks. The paraffin is heated and forced into the pocket areas by digital pressure or with a syringe designed for this purpose, where it remains for 24 to 48 hours. When it is removed, calculus exposed by separation of the gingiva is removed by scaling.

A second application is made at this time or later, and repeated until gingival disease is eliminated. Individual packs may be changed daily or every other day, but may be left on longer. The period of treatment may be two or three weeks, at the end of which time excellent results are obtained. The effectiveness of the aforementioned procedure is enhanced if it is preceded by flushing the pockets with a special glycerin mixture (Mentho-Borate).

Advantages claimed for this technique include the following: It favors repair by covering the inflamed gingiva with a bland coating and separating it from the tooth. The pack also acts as a protective seal which prevents reinfection during healing. Mechanical pressure results in atrophy of the gingival margin and dilatation of the pocket which facilitates scaling with a minimum of trauma to the gingiva.

"Conservative Surgical" Technique (Barkann)

Barkann[1] describes a modification of the scaling and curettage technique for pocket elimination which includes excision of the inner pocket wall and a phenol-camphor coagulating mixture. The following is the procedure:

Use a topical anesthetic and, after swabbing the pocket with an antiseptic, pack it with a cotton strand impregnated with a mixture of 25 per cent phenol and 75 per cent camphor. The strand remains in the pocket for an instant, and on its removal curetting is begun. The process of packing the strands and curetting is repeated, enlarging the pocket opening. As much coagulated tissue and pocket contents as possible are removed.

With a curved knife designed for this purpose, the papilla is excised with a semilunar incision and an internal bevel. With the sharp blade, the tissue walls within the pocket are scraped to create fresh bleeding surfaces. Special care must be exercised to retain the facial and lingual walls of the pocket, which form a trough for the retention of the blood clot through which regeneration of connective tissue proceeds.

After all extraneous matter has been removed, and the inner wall is bleeding freely, the pocket is packed with 1/4 inch gauze dressing, about 1 1/2 to 2 inches long, which has been moistened with sterile water and into which the phenol-camphor coagulating mixture has been incorporated. It is rarely necessary to pack a broad, hollow marginal pocket.

The following day the gauze is removed and the area is irrigated with normal saline solution and swabbed with an antiseptic. If very deep, the pocket is packed for another day with gauze saturated with an antiseptic such as Metaphen or Merthiolate. Plaque control is started as soon as the condition permits.

REFERENCES

1. Barkann, L.: A conservative surgical technic for the eradication of a pyorrhea pocket. J. Am. Dent. Assoc., 26:61, 1939.
2. Beube, F. E.: Treatment methods for marginal gingivitis and periodontitis. Texas Dent. J., 71:427, 1953.
3. Blass, J. L., and Lite, T.: Gingival healing following surgical curettage: A histopathologic study. N.Y. Dent. J., 25:127, 1959.

4. Bodecker, C. F.: The difficulty of completely removing subgingival calculus. J. Am. Dent. Assoc., 30:703, 1943.

5. Bodecker, C. F.: The most sensitive areas of the teeth and their operative treatment. Trans. Seventh International Dental Congress I, 751, 1926.

6. Box, H. K.: Twelve Periodontal Studies. Toronto, University of Toronto Press, 1946, p. 138.

7. Cripps, S.: The elimination of the periodontal pocket by pressure packing. Br. Dent. J., 90:235, 1951.

8. Green, E., and Ramfjord, S. P.: Tooth roughness after subgingival root planing. J. Periodontol., 37:396, 1966.

9. Hirschfeld, L.: Subgingival curettage in periodontal treatment. J. Am. Dent. Assoc., 44:301, 1952.

10. Kon, S., et al.: Visualization of microvascularization of the healing periodontal wound. II. Curettage. J. Periodontol., 40:96, 1969.

11. Morris, M. L.: The removal of the pocket and attachment epithelium in humans: A histological study. J. Periodontol., 25:7, 1954.

12. Moskow, B. S.: Calcifications in gingival biopsies. Dent. Progress, 1:30, 1960.

13. Moskow, B. S.: The response of the gingival sulcus to instrumentation: A histologic investigation. I. The scaling procedure. J. Periodontol., 33:282, 1962.

14. Moskow, B. S.: The response of the gingival sulcus to instrumentation: A histologic investigation. II. Gingival curettage. J. Periodontol., 35:112, 1964.

15. O'Bannon, J. Y.: The gingival tissues before and after scaling the teeth. J. Periodontol., 35:69, 1964.

16. Ramfjord, S., and Costich, E. R.: Healing after simple gingivectomy. J. Peridontol., 34:401, 1963.

17. Ramfjord, S., and Kiester, G.: The gingival sulcus and the periodontal pocket immediately following scaling of the teeth. J. Periodontol., 25:167, 1954.

18. Riffle, A. B.: The cementum during curettage. J. Periodontol., 23:170, 1952.

19. Sato, M.: Histopathological study of the healing process after surgical treatment for alveolar pyorrhea. Bull. Tokyo Dent. College, 1:71, 1960.

20. Selvig, K. A.: Biological changes at the tooth-saliva interface in periodontal disease. J. Dent. Res., 48:846, 1969.

21. Simonton, F. V.: The most significant findings of the California stomatological research group in the study of pyorrhea. J. Dent. Res., 8:235, 1928.

22. Steen, E.: The occurrence of bacteria in gingival pockets. Norske Tannlaegefore. Tid., 65:230, 1955.

23. Stone, S., Ramfjord, S. P., and Waldron, J.: Scaling and gingival curettage. A radioautographic study. J. Periodontol., 37:415, 1966.

24. Thebaud, J.: Some microscopic aspects of the curetted surface of the cementum after the subgingival curettage. J. Can. Dent. Assoc., 17:127, 1951.

25. Waerhaug, J.: Microscopic demonstration of tissue reaction incident to removal of subgingival calculus. J. Periodontol., 26:26, 1955.

General Principles of
Periodontal Surgery

This chapter will present some general considerations, important to all periodontal surgical techniques. The following chapters will deal with the different surgical techniques that may be used.

GENERAL CONTRAINDICATIONS AND CONDITIONS REQUIRING SPECIAL PRECAUTIONS

Periodontal surgery will be contraindicated by some systemic diseases as well as in patients with acute oral infections. In other conditions special precautions may be taken in order to reduce the risks introduced by surgery.

Hemorrhagic disorders

HEMOPHILIA. Scaling and curettage and periodontal surgery can be performed on patients with hemophilia provided sufficient precautions are taken;[33] it is preferable to avoid surgery. The precautions include hospitalization before treatment, transfusions with fresh whole blood, fresh human plasma or intravenous Factor VIII (2.5 ml. per kg. per hour) for 10 hours to achieve a 30 per cent blood level of Factor VIII. Factor VIII may be given postoperatively (1 ml. per kg. per hour) until bleeding has stopped.

After scaling and curettage or surgery, dried thrombin and oxidized cellulose are packed around the area previous to insertion of the periodontal pack. Other local measures for the control of the bleeding include electrocautery and Monsel's solution.

Christmas Disease (Hemophilia B). **Periodontal therapy should present no problems, since the clotting defect responds to administration of blood or plasma.**[36] Surgery should be confined to small areas. Before the periodontal pack is inserted, bleeding points should be controlled by cotton pellets saturated with Monsel's solution applied under pressure or electrocautery.

PROTHROMBIN DEFICIENCY. **Bleeding tendencies caused by prothrombin deficiency**[39] **can be remedied by the systemic administration of vitamin K, except in patients with advanced liver disease.** Vitamin K, 50 mg., or menadione sodium bisulfite, a synthetic vitamin K analogue, 72 mg., is administered intravenously immediately preceding treatment, and may be repeated daily if necessary. In patients with advanced liver disease, daily intravenous doses of vitamin K, 150 mg., may be tried, but administration of fresh whole blood or plasma may also be required.

It should be emphasized that difficulties in patients with bleeding tendencies can be reduced by operating with extreme care with a minimum of tissue laceration.

The topical use of clorhexidine or other similar substances not yet accepted by the F. D. A. would be extremely useful for the periodontal treatment of patients with hemorrhagic diseases.

Diabetes

Special precautions are indicated in the periodontal care of diabetic patients.[22] **Treatment should not be undertaken until the diabetes is under control.** Dental visits should not interfere with the patient's eating schedule so as to minimize the likelihood of diabetic acidosis, coma, or insulin reaction. Elderly chronic diabetics are prone to arteriosclerosis, hypertension, and coronary artery disease. In such patients the need for periodontal surgery should be weighed against the risk involved. It is preferable to perform the surgery in a hospital where cardiovascular complications can be handled properly.

In diabetics, resistance to infection is reduced. The causes are not understood, but the decreased resistance has been attributed to impaired antibody formation, reduced phagocytic activity, and a lowered state of cellular nutrition.[35] Therefore, antibiotics should be prescribed before and after extensive scaling and curettage or surgical procedures (see Chap. 45).

Controlled diabetics should respond well to periodontal therapy. All local etiologic factors must be eliminated, and the patient must provide fastidious oral hygiene. In young adult diabetics elimination of gingival and periodontal disease may reduce the insulin required to control the diabetes.[62]

Cardiac disorders

Patients with a history of **coronary insufficiency** or **hypertensive heart disease,** which may be accompanied by symptoms of **angina pectoris,** are ordinarily under medical care and required to avoid exertion and excitement, or excessive activity. **The patient's physician should be consulted before undertaking periodontal treatment.** The patient should be sedated at home before leaving for the office or sedated at the office 30 minutes before beginning treatment. If barbiturates are used, someone should accompany the patient; if this is not feasible, the patient should be hospitalized. Treatment done at each visit should be limited. Local anesthetics should be used without vasoconstrictor drugs,[2] or with a minimal adequate amount (epinephrine, 1:100,000).[15]

In patients with a history of **congenital cardiac defects, plastic valve replacements, or rheumatic heart disease, premedication with antibiotics or chemotherapeutic agents is indicated before scaling and curettage or surgical periodontal procedures**[18] (see Chap. 45).

Patients on anticoagulant therapy

Anticoagulants are used as continuous therapy in patients with coronary artery disease for the purpose of preventing intravascular clotting. Drugs used for this purpose are heparin, bishydroxycoumarin (Dicumarol), warfarin sodium (Coumadin), phenindione derivatives (Hedulin and

Danilone), cyclocumarol (Cumopyran), and ethyl biscoumacetate (Tromexan ethyl acetate).[32, 55]

Heparin inactivates thrombin and has an almost immediate anticoagulant effect; the other drugs depress prothrombin synthesis in the liver, and require a longer period to develop their anticoagulant effect.[8] Dosage is generally adjusted so that the patient's normal prothrombin time (Quick test) is increased one and a half to two and a half times. Vitamin K, or a synthetic analogue, is used to reduce the prothrombin time if it becomes excessive.

An increasing number of patients are being placed on anticoagulant therapy, and appropriate inquiry should be included in every case history. **The patients are on a scheduled recall program for check of prothrombin time and physical examination by their physician, who should be consulted before periodontal treatment is begun.** The danger of clotting if the anticoagulant is stopped is greater than the problem of bleeding under drug therapy, provided proper precautions are taken.[60] **The range within which moderate scaling procedures can be safely performed is one and one half to two times the average normal prothrombin time (12 to 14 seconds).**[18] Aspirin should not be prescribed for these patients, because when combined with anticoagulants it may lead to excessive bleeding.

Scaling and curettage can usually be performed without difficulty, but patients should not be dismissed until bleeding has stopped. A gauze sponge is applied under moderate pressure to hasten the clotting. Periodontal surgery may be performed in such patients, but factors other than the risk of hemorrhage should be considered. Because of the cardiac condition for which the anticoagulants are being used, elective surgery may be contraindicated. In older patients scaling and curettage is often an advisable compromise.

It is preferable to perform periodontal surgery in a hospital, where emergency care is available, but it may also be performed in small segments in the dental office. Resection of the gingiva with electrosurgery reduces the bleeding. Local anesthesia with epinephrine or other vasoconstrictors 1:100,000 is preferred to general anesthesia. Before the periodontal pack is applied, bleeding is stopped by packing cotton pellets interproximally and applying pressure facially and lingually with a gauze sponge. The periodontal pack is inserted over the cotton pellets.

Patients on corticosteroid therapy

Corticosteroid hormones are used widely for the long-term treatment of a variety of conditions such as rheumatoid arthritis, lupus erythematosus, periarteritis nodosa, dermatomyositis, scleroderma, bronchial asthma, allergic vasomotor rhinitis, pulmonary fibrosis, sarcoidosis, ulcerative colitis, regional ileitis, pemphigus, psoriasis, atopic dermatitis, acute gouty arthritis, and certain renal diseases and hematologic disorders.

The prolonged administration of potent corticosteroids may lead to inactivity and atrophy of the adrenals, resulting in hypoadrenalism. Sustained hormonal therapy with cortisone or ACTH results in a variety of side effects, many of which resemble naturally occurring Cushing's syndrome,[66] are characterized by fever, hypertension, and anoxia, and may be fatal. In addition, these patients cannot tolerate the stress of an operative procedure[46] and are less capable of coping with infection. Topically applied corticoids in the form of ointments or eyedrops may not have this depressant effect upon the adrenals.[61]

Patients on prolonged corticosteroid therapy should be given an additional 100 mg. of cortisone acetate or 20 mg. of Prednisone administered orally two hours before periodontal surgery to prevent acute adrenal crisis. As a precautionary measure Solu-Cortef should be available for intravenous administration. Prophylactic antibiotic therapy (250 mg. of penicillin orally three times a day, or other antibiotics) should begin 24 hours before each periodontal treatment and continue for 48 hours postoperatively.

ADDISON'S DISEASE. Patients with Addison's disease ordinarily receive a daily oral dose of 25 to 37.5 mg. of cortisone, which is equivalent to 5 to 7.5 mg. of prednisolone. For periodontal surgery, these patients should receive 100 to 200 mg. of cortisone intramuscularly, 18 to 24 hours before operation. The regular oral dose is omitted. On the day of surgery, the patients receive 100 mg. of cortisone intramuscularly. The next day they return to their regular daily oral dose.

Hyperthyroidism

In hyperthyroidism the patient's condition should be under control before extensive periodontal treatment is undertaken. Periodontal surgery may be performed in an uncontrolled or unsuspected hyperthyroid without complication but thyrotoxic episodes characterized by angina, tachycardia, or other cardiac arrhythmias may occur.

Acute and subacute leukemia

Patients with acute and subacute leukemia often present periodontal problems which, in addition to being painful, jeopardize the systemic management of the patient. Gingival enlargement that interferes with mastication, persistent gingival bleeding, and acute gingival and periodontal infection that causes severe systemic complications are examples of conditions requiring immediate periodontal care.

Periodontal treatment in acute and subacute leukemia introduces risks of troublesome hemorrhage and severe infection and should be approached with proper precautions.[50] The hematologic findings should be checked with particular reference to bleeding and clotting time, platelet count, and prothrombin time.

One of the most common problems in these patients is gingival enlargement (Chap. 30), which produces deepened gingival crevices in which plaque, food debris, and bacteria accumulate. The resulting gingival inflammation is usually aggravated by the fact that the patients have stopped toothbrushing, either because they were frightened by gingival bleeding or preoccupied with concern regarding their "blood condition," or because of physical weakness.

In most cases, the first thing to do is to remove the accumulated plaque and debris, and carefully cleanse around the necks of the teeth with a pellet of cotton saturated with 3 per cent hydrogen peroxide. Place the patient on a plaque control regimen, preparing the patient to expect some gingival bleeding during the cleansing procedures. After 24 to 48 hours the gingival condition is usually improved. Superficial scaling is carried out to further reduce the inflammation and the enlargement.

In patients with persistent gingival bleeding the source is usually deep in a periodontal pocket. Surface hemostatics alone are not effective in controlling such bleeding. The following procedure is recommended: Carefully cleanse the area with a pellet of cotton saturated with 3 per cent hydrogen peroxide to remove partially clotted debris. Locate the bleeding point in the periodontal pocket. Carefully explore along the tooth surface adjacent to the bleeding point to locate calculus and other deposits and remove them, making every effort to avoid injury to the gingiva. Clean the area again with hydrogen peroxide. Place a cotton pellet saturated with thrombin or dipped in ferric subsulfate (Monsel's salt) against the bleeding point. Cover the area with a gauze sponge and maintain it in position under pressure for at least 20 minutes. Remove the gauze; if there are still signs of oozing, a periodontal pack should be applied for at least 24 hours.

Acute necrotizing ulcerative gingivitis often complicates the oral picture in acute and subacute leukemia. The regular treatment (Chap. 41) is followed; its primary purpose is to make the patient comfortable and eliminate a source of systemic toxicity. Systemic antibiotics are essential to prevent complications.

Acute gingival or periodontal abscesses are common sources of pain in these patients, with regional adenopathy and systemic complications. The latter are controlled by systemic antibiotics. Under topical anesthesia—using a Bard-Parker No. 11 or No. 12 blade—the abscess is incised to provide drainage, and cleaned with cotton pellets saturated with 3 per cent peroxide. Bleeding is stopped with a gauze sponge held under pressure for 20 minutes. The acute symptoms generally subside after 24 hours.

In chronic leukemia gingival and periodontal disorders may be treated by scaling and curettage without complications, but an effort should be made to avoid periodontal surgery. Adherent superficial deposits not dislodged with cotton pellets are removed with the scalers, making every effort to avoid injuring the gingiva, and the patient is instructed in plaque control.

Apprehensive and neurotic patients

Apprehensive and neurotic patients require special management. The former are premedicated with Nembutal or Seconal, 100 mg. 30 minutes before operating, or are treated with tranquilizing drugs. Neurotic patients with deep-seated anxieties are more complicated problems. The success of treatment may be jeopardized by a peculiar reaction of such patients to some aspect of the case management.

BARBITURATES

The barbiturates are effective sedatives and hypnotics for preoperative sedation of apprehensive patients; they are not used for relief of pain. These drugs should not be administered in the office unless someone is available to accompany the patient home.

Pentobarbital (Nembutal) is a short-acting barbiturate; a 100 mg. capsule approximately 30 minutes before operative procedures is usually effective. Seconal (100 mg. capsule) is another barbiturate that may be used in this way.

Promethazine hydrochloride (Phenergan hydrochloride) is an effective sedative and antihistaminic. The preoperative dosage for adult patients is 25 to 50 mg. It should not be given to ambulatory patients who are going to drive after they leave the office.

Phenobarbital is a long-acting sedative and hypnotic. Large doses may cause severe circulatory depression. Patients with toxic goiter react with severe rashes. The average dosage is 50 mg.

TRANQUILIZERS

These drugs are useful for the relief of anxiety, tension, and fear. Among the commonly used tranquilizers are chlordiazepoxide (Librium), adult dosage 5 to 10 mg., three or four times daily; meprobamate (Miltown), a tranquilizer with muscle relaxant action, adult dosage 200 to 400 mg., three times a day; diazepam (Valium), adult dosage 2 to 10 mg., two to four times daily;

and hydroxyzine hydrochloride (Vistaril), 25 to 100 mg., three or four times daily. Patients using tranquilizers sometimes complain of having a dry mouth.

SEQUENCE OF SURGICAL INTERVENTIONS

A mouth with generalized pocket formation is treated in quadrants or sextants at weekly or biweekly intervals. All periodontal conditions in the quadrant or sextant are treated, often combining different surgical procedures.

ANESTHESIA

Periodontal surgery should be painless. The patient should be assured of this at the outset and should be thoroughly anesthetized, using local block and infiltration injections. Injection directly into the interdental papillae may be helpful.

Anesthetic Agents

These are used by injection or topically to prevent pain during surgical procedures or subgingival scaling and curettage. Those commonly administered by injection are procaine hydrochloride, lidocaine hydrochloride, butethamine hydrochloride (Monocaine),[26] and mepivacaine hydrochloride (Carbocaine).

There are many topical anesthetics, in liquid, gel, and aerosol forms (Topanol, Butyn, Cetacaine, Xylocaine); butacaine sulfite, benzyl alcohol, and benzocaine are the usual components. Applied liberally to the field of operation these are helpful in scaling and curettage, and in incising acute periodontal abscesses or pericoronitis. Care must be exercised in the use of spray anesthetics to prevent inhalation, which may cause a toxic reaction.

Dyclone (0.5 per cent dyclonine hydrochloride) is used as a topical anesthetic mouthwash. A small amount swished thoroughly around the mouth five minutes before eating provides sufficient anesthesia to enable patients with painful mucous membrane lesions to eat comfortably. It lasts for about 40 minutes and may be repeated to provide continuous relief from pain.

HEMOSTASIS

An aspirator is indispensable for performing periodontal surgery. It provides the clear view of each root surface, which is necessary for thorough removal of deposits and planing. Further, it permits accurate appraisal of the extent and pattern of soft tissue and bone involvement and prevents seepage of blood into the floor of the mouth and oropharynx.

Periodontal surgery produces profuse bleeding in its initial incisional steps. However, after the existing granulation tissue has been removed, the bleeding disappears or is considerably reduced. Packing gauze squares and the use of an aspirator are necessary to keep a dry field.

Hemostatics and vasoconstrictors

Hemostatics are drugs that stop bleeding from lacerated capillaries and arterioles by producing a rapid coagulation of the blood about the vessels. They are ineffective in cases of severe hemorrhage, where sutures or compression must be employed.

Ferric subsulfate powder is useful to arrest gingival bleeding. A cotton pellet dipped in the powder is applied to the bleeding area and kept there for about 20 minutes.

Thrombin is a drug capable of hastening the process of blood clotting. It is intended for topical application only and is applied as a liquid or a powder.

Oxidized cellulose (Novacell, Oxycel) and absorbable gelatin sponge (Gelfoam) are useful hemostatics in deep wounds, rather than for gingival surface bleeding. Epinephrine is sometimes used to control bleeding during scaling and curettage (1:25,000) and in gingival retraction (1:10,000). Because it increases the blood pressure and heart rate it must be used guardedly; allergic manifestations have also been reported.

PERIODONTAL PACKS (PERIODONTAL DRESSINGS)

These are used for postoperative care following surgical periodontal procedures. Two principal types are in use (with and without eugenol), and plastics are being investigated.

Eugenol packs

Most periodontal packs consist of zinc oxide and eugenol, with varied ingredients. The Kirkland-Kaiser periodontal pack is in this group. The pack is prepared from a powder and liquid.

The powder consists of zinc oxide, powdered rosin, and tannic acid flakes. It is prepared as follows: Mix the zinc oxide and powdered rosin in equal proportion by weight. To four parts of this mixture add one part by weight of tannic acid flakes. Mix thoroughly. The liquid is a mixture of one part peanut oil and two parts eugenol. It is prepared as follows: Pour the eugenol into a test tube, add a lump of rosin about the size of the last joint of the thumb and warm over a burner flame until the rosin is liquefied. After this is cooled, add the peanut oil.

The pack is ready for use immediately after it is mixed. Wrapped in wax paper it retains its working qualities for an entire day. It may also be frozen and stored for longer periods and removed from the freezer prior to use.

Another pack in this group is the following:

Powder	
Zinc oxide	63 gm.
Rosin	30 gm.
Asbestos fiber	5 gm.
Zinc acetate	2 gm.
Liquid	
Eugenol	80 ml.
Olive oil	20 ml.

Non-eugenol packs

A typical non-eugenol, fat-containing pack consists of:

Powder
Zinc oxide
Rosin powder

Zinc bacitracin
Ointment
Zinc oxide
Hydrogenated fat

Coe-Pack is a non-eugenol pack with demonstrated antimicrobial action (in vitro)[49] which is well accepted by patients. It is supplied in two tubes and must be used when it is mixed.

Cyanoacrylate pack

N-butyl cyanoacrylate is a periodontal dressing which is applied in drops or as a spray and solidifies in five to ten seconds.[5, 10] Polymerization from liquid to solid state is catalyzed by moisture, heat, and pressure. It adheres to smooth and irregular surfaces for periods of from two to seven days. N-butyl cyanoacrylate has been studied extensively in clinical trials, but has not as yet been released for general periodontal use.

Each of the above packs has its proponents, but the choice is often a matter of individual preference. Some claim that non-eugenol packs produce less inflammation when used on exposed bone,[4, 6] but others find no such differences.[21, 44] No differences have been observed in the tissue reaction around eugenol and non-eugenol implants.[24] Degenerative changes occur in healing epithelium beneath eugenol and non-eugenol packs,[48] and they produce no difference in postoperative sequelae following scaling and curettage or gingivectomy.[45] Comparable healing has been reported following gingivectomy with or without a pack.[57] Comparison of the effects of eugenol, non-eugenol, and N-butyl cyanoacrylate on denuded bone, partial thickness flaps, and mucoperiosteal flaps reveals no microscopic differences in healing, but the cyanoacrylate-packed areas appear better clinically.[44] Cyanoacrylate is normally phagocytized by leukocytes, but some report that it may delay healing by producing foreign body granulomas.[65]

Antibiotics in packs

Improved healing and patient comfort,[3] with less odor and taste,[5] have been obtained by including zinc bacitracin (3000 units per gram) in the pack. Other antibiotics such as Terramycin[20] (125 mg. powdered drug in six drops of liquid), neomycin, and nitrofurazone have also been tried, but all produce hypersensitivity reactions.[40]

An "intraoral adhesive bandage" (consisting of pectin, gelatin, sodium carboxymethyl cellulose, and polyisobutylene, coated on the outside with a polyethylene film) has been tried to secure periodontal grafts without suturing.

Our preference at present is the Kirkland-Kaiser type pack. It is easy to manipulate and apply, affords adequate working time before it sets, is firm enough to withstand mastication, is well tolerated by the tissues, and is easily removed.

When a non-eugenol pack is needed because the patient is allergic to eugenol, Coe-Pack can be used. It is also recommended to cover free mucosal autografts and displaced flaps because it can be applied in a softer state. Hard packs may displace the flap.

Preparation of Kirkland-Kaiser pack

The pack consists of a powder and liquid which are mixed on a wax paper pad with a wooden throat stick. The powder is gradually incorporated into the liquid until a thick paste is formed. More powder is kneaded into the paste with the fingers until it becomes a thick, not tacky, putty. **Proper consistency is important. The initial tendency is to make a mix which is too soft and, therefore, difficult to apply.** Tincture of green soap or orange solvent effectively removes the pack from the fingers.

How to apply the periodontal pack

The pack is rolled into two strips approximately the length of the treated area. The end of one strip is bent into a hook shape and fitted around the distal surface of the last tooth, approaching it from the facial surface (Fig. 48–1). The remainder of the strip is brought forward along the facial surface to the midline, gently pressing it into place along the incised gingival margin and interproximally. The second strip of pack is applied from the lingual surface. It is

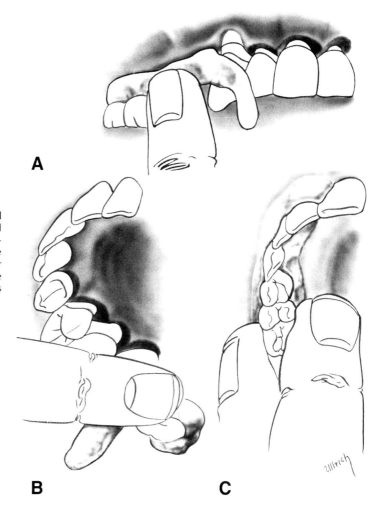

A

Figure 48–1   Inserting the Periodontal Pack. *A,* Strip of pack is hooked around last molar and pressed into place anteriorly. *B,* Lingual pack joined to the facial strip at the distal of the last molar and fitted into place anteriorly. *C,* Gentle pressure on facial and lingual surfaces joins pack interproximally.

B   **C**

joined to the pack at the distal surface of the last tooth, then brought forward along the cut gingival margin to the midline. The strips are joined interproximally by applying gentle pressure on the facial and lingual surfaces of the pack (Fig. 48–1).

For isolated teeth separated by edentulous spaces, the pack should be made continuous from tooth to tooth, covering the edentulous area. Joining the teeth with a loop of dental floss aids retention of the pack over the edentulous area (Fig. 48–2). When the edentulous space is long, isolated teeth may be packed separately to reduce the likelihood of displacement. To do this, a strip of one-fourth inch gauze is loosely fitted around the tooth. The gauze loop is removed, embedded with pack, replaced on the tooth and tightened (Fig. 48–3). The

ends of the gauze are cut and pack is added.

The pack should completely cover the gingiva (Fig. 48–4), but overextension onto uninvolved mucosa should be avoided. **Excess pack irritates the mucobuccal fold and floor of the mouth, and interferes with the tongue.** Overextension also jeopardizes the remainder of the pack because it tends to break off, taking pack from the operated area with it. **Pack that interferes with the occlusion should be trimmed away before the patient is dismissed** (Fig. 48–5). Failure to do this causes discomfort and jeopardizes retention of the pack.

The operator should wait 15 minutes after the pack is applied before trimming it. This permits the lips, cheeks, and tongue to mold the pack while it is soft. Excess will be

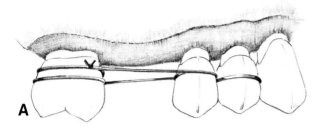

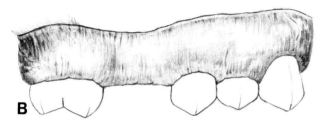

Figure 48-2   Dental Floss Loop Aids Retention of Pack Over Edentulous Area. *A,* Dental floss across edentulous space. *B,* Pack in place.

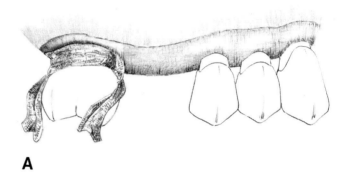

Figure 48-3   Pack Retained With Gauze Strip Around Isolated Tooth. *A,* Strip of ¼" gauze loosely fitted to molar. *B,* Gauze embedded with pack is replaced on tooth, tightened and trimmed with scissors. *C,* Pack completed.

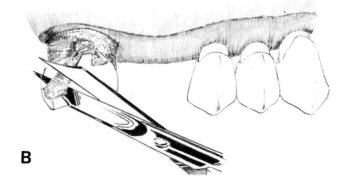

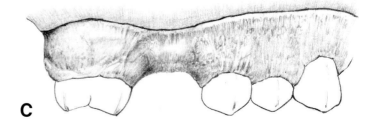

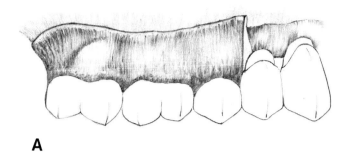

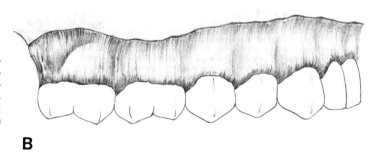

Figure 48–4   **Pack in Place.** *A,* Cutaway view of pack extending just beyond the cut surface, without overextension onto uninvolved mucosa. *B,* Pack in place. *C,* Lingual pack in place; overextension onto palate will detach the pack and should be avoided.

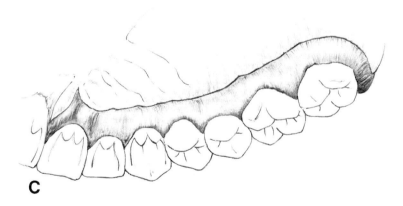

forced into areas where it is not needed and from which it can be easily removed.

The patient should not be dismissed until oozing of blood from beneath the pack has stopped.

As a general rule, the pack is kept on for one week after surgery. The one-week period is based upon the timetable of healing and clinical experience. It is not a rigid requirement; it may be extended, or the area may be repacked for an additional week.

If hemorrhage occurs through the pack at any time in the course of the week, the operator should remove the pack, locate the bleeding point, and treat as indicated on page 797.

Fragments of the surface of the pack may come off during the week, but this presents no problem. If a portion of the pack is lost from the operated area and the patient is uncomfortable, it is usually best to repack the area. Remove the remaining pack, wash the area with warm water, and apply a topical anesthetic before replacing the pack, which is then to be retained for a week.

Patients may develop pain from an overextended margin which irritates the

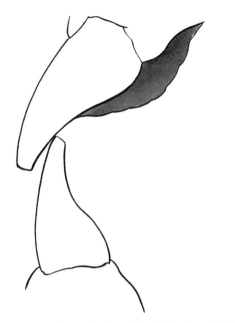

Figure 48–5   The Pack Should Not Interfere with the Occlusion.

vestibule, floor of the mouth, or tongue. The excess pack should be trimmed away, making sure that the new margin is not rough, before the patient is dismissed.

Patients report that the mouth feels unclean when the pack is on. Rinsing with a pleasant-tasting mouthwash diluted 1:3 with warm water, beginning on the second postoperative day, is helpful.

Functions of the periodontal pack

There are no packs with any demonstrated curative properties. The value of the pack is indirect. It assists healing by protecting the tissue rather than by providing "healing factors." The pack serves the following functions:

1. Controls postoperative bleeding.
2. Minimizes the likelihood of postoperative infection and hemorrhage.
3. Provides some splinting of mobile teeth.
4. Facilitates healing by preventing surface trauma during mastication and irritation from plaque and food debris.

INSTRUCTIONS FOR THE PATIENT AFTER SURGERY

After the pack is placed, the following printed instructions are given to the patient to be read before leaving the chair:

INSTRUCTIONS FOR

Mrs. Jane Smith

The operation which has been performed on your gums will help you keep your teeth. The following information has been prepared to answer questions you may have about how to take care of your mouth. Please read the instructions carefully—our patients have found them very helpful.

When the anesthesia wears off, you may have slight discomfort—not pain. Two 5-grain aspirin tablets will usually keep you comfortable. You may repeat every three hours if necessary.

We have placed a periodontal pack over your gums to protect them from irritation. The pack prevents pain, aids healing, and enables you to carry on most of your usual activities in comfort. The pack will harden in a few hours, after which it can withstand most of the forces of chewing without breaking off. It may take a little while to become accustomed to it.

For your benefit the pack should remain in place as long as possible. **Do not remove it.** If particles of the pack chip off during the week do not be concerned as long as you do not have pain. If a piece of the pack breaks off and you are in pain, or if a rough edge irritates your tongue or cheek, please call the office. The problem can be easily remedied by replacing the pack. The pack will be removed at your next appointment.

For the first three hours after the operation avoid hot foods in order to permit the pack to harden. After this eat anything you can manage without chipping off the pack. Eggs, Jell-O, cereals, soups, milk, fish, hamburger or any semi-solid or finely minced foods are suggested. Avoid citrus fruits or fruit juices, highly spiced foods, and alcoholic beverages. They will cause pain. Food supplements and/or vitamins are generally not necessary. We will prescribe them if needed.

Do not smoke—the heat and smoke will irritate your gums and delay healing. If at all possible, use this opportunity to give up smoking. Smokers have more gum disease than nonsmokers.

Rinsing is not part of the treatment, but it will help make your mouth feel refreshed. **Do not rinse today.** Beginning tomorrow, you may rinse as often as you wish with one of the popular, pleasant-flavored mouthwashes. Do not use it in concentrated form, dilute it — ⅓ mouthwash to ⅔ warm water.

Clean the parts of your mouth which have been treated on previous weeks using the methods in which you were instructed. The gums most likely will bleed more than they did before the operation. This is perfectly normal in the early stage of healing and will gradually subside. Do not stop cleaning because of it.

Follow your regular daily activities, but avoid excessive exertion of any type. Golf, tennis, skiing, bowling, swimming, or sunbathing should be postponed for two days after the operation.

You may experience a slight feeling of weakness or chills during the first 24 hours. This should not be cause for alarm but should be reported at the next visit.

Swelling is not unusual, particularly in areas which required extensive surgical procedures. The swelling generally subsides in three or four days. If the swelling is painful or appears to become worse, please call the office.

There may be occasional blood stains in the saliva for the first four or five hours after the operation. This is not unusual and will correct itself. If there is considerable bleeding beyond this, take a piece of gauze, form it into the shape of a "U," hold it in the thumb and index finger, apply it to both sides of the pack and hold it under pressure for 20 minutes. Do not remove it during this period to examine it. If the bleeding does not stop at the end of 20 minutes, please contact the office. **Do not try to stop the bleeding by rinsing.**

If any other problems arise, please call the office.

THE PATIENT DURING THE FIRST POSTOPERATIVE WEEK

Properly performed, periodontal surgery presents no serious postoperative problems.

Unfavorable sequelae are the exception rather than the rule; the following may arise in the first postoperative week:

1. PERSISTENT BLEEDING AFTER GINGIVECTOMY. The pack should be removed, the bleeding points located, and the bleeding stopped with either pressure, electrosurgery, or electrocautery. After the bleeding is stopped the pack is replaced.

2. SENSITIVITY TO PERCUSSION. Sensitivity to percussion may be caused by extension of inflammation into the periodontal ligament. The patient should be questioned regarding the progress of the symptoms. Progressively diminishing severity is a favorable sign. The pack should be removed and the gingiva checked for localized areas of infection or irritation which should be cleaned or incised to provide drainage. Particles of calculus that may have been overlooked should be removed. Relieving the occlusion is usually helpful.

Sensitivity to percussion may also be caused by excess pack which interferes with the occlusion. Removal of the excess usually corrects the condition.

3. SWELLING. Sometimes within the first two postoperative days patients report with a soft painless swelling of the cheek in the area of operation. There may be lymph node enlargement and the temperature may be slightly elevated. The area of operation itself is usually symptom-free. This type of involvement results from a localized inflammatory reaction to the operative procedure. It generally subsides by the fourth postoperative day, without necessitating removal of the pack. Penicillin, 250 mg. every four hours for 48 hours, is helpful as a prophylactic measure following the next operation.

4. FEELING OF WEAKNESS. Occasionally patients report having experienced a "washed-out" weakened feeling for about 24 hours after the operation. This represents a systemic reaction to a transient bacteremia induced by the operative procedure. It is prevented by premedication with penicillin, 250 mg. every four hours, beginning 24 hours before the next operation and for a 24-hour postoperative period. Prophylactic chemotherapy is ordinarily not used except for patients with a history of rheumatic fever, cardiovascular disease, diabetes, or prolonged corticosteroid therapy (see Chap. 45).

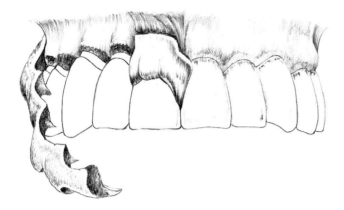

Figure 48–6 Removal of the Periodontal Pack.

Removal of the Periodontal Pack and Return Visit Care

When the patient returns after one week, the pack is taken off by inserting a surgical hoe along the margin and exerting gentle lateral pressure (Fig. 48–6). Pieces of pack retained interproximally and particles which adhere to the tooth surfaces are removed with scalers. Particles may be enmeshed in the cut surface and should be carefully picked off with fine cotton pliers. The entire area is syringed with warm water to remove superficial debris.

What to Look for at the Time of Pack Removal

The following are the usual findings when the pack is removed (see Fig. 49–20):

If a gingivectomy has been performed, the cut surface will be covered with a friable meshwork of new epithelium which should not be disturbed. After a flap operation, the areas corresponding to the incisions will be epithelized but may bleed readily upon touching; they should not be disturbed. Pockets should not be probed. The facial and lingual mucosa may be covered with a gray-yellow or white granular layer of food debris that has seeped under the pack. It is easily removed with a moist cotton pellet.

The root surfaces may be sensitive to a probe or thermal changes, and the teeth may be stained. There may be prominent beadlike remnants of calculus and granulation tissue.

Persistent granulation tissue

Red, beadlike protuberances of granulation tissue persist if calculus has not been completely removed. The granulation tissue is removed with a curette which exposes the calculus so that it can be removed and the root can be planed. Removal of the granulation tissue without removing the calculus will be followed by recurrence.

Calculus

Fragments of calculus delay healing. Each root surface should be rechecked visually to be certain no calculus is present. Sometimes the color of the calculus is similar to that of the root. The grooves on proximal root surfaces and the furcations are areas in which calculus is likely to be overlooked.

After the pack is removed, it is usually not necessary to replace it. However, it is advisable to repack for an additional week for patients with (1) a low pain threshold who are particularly uncomfortable when the pack is removed, (2) unusually extensive periodontal involvement, or (3) slow healing. Clinical judgment will help decide whether to repack the area or leave the initial pack on longer than one week.

Tooth mobility

Tooth mobility is increased immediately after surgery,[14] but by the fourth week it diminishes beyond the pretreatment level.[34]

Final check on smoothness of the root surfaces

One week after the pack is removed from the final quadrant, all root surfaces are checked to see that they are smooth and firm. A rubber cup with fine pumice or Improved Zircate, and polishing strips are used for the final smoothing of the root at this time.

CARE OF THE MOUTH WHILE PERIODONTAL SURGERY IS IN PROGRESS

Care of the mouth by the patient between the treatment of the first and final areas, as well as after surgery is completed, is extremely important. It begins after the pack is removed from the first operation. The patient has been through a presurgical period of instructed plaque control and should be reinstructed at this time.

Vigorous brushing during the first week after the pack is removed is not feasible. However, the patient is informed that plaque and food accumulation will retard healing and he is advised **to try to keep the area as clean as possible** by the gentle use of interdental cleansers and dental floss and light water irrigation. Brushing is introduced when healing of the tissues permits; vigor of the overall hygiene regimen is increased as healing progresses. Patients should be told that there will most likely be more gingival bleeding than before the operation; that it is perfectly normal and will subside as healing progresses; and that it should not deter them from following their oral hygiene regimen.

Clorhexidine mouthwashes or topical application with Q-tips is indicated for the first few postoperative weeks in those countries where its use is permitted.

Treatment of Sensitive Roots*

When the pack is removed, there is a feeling of "emptiness" around the teeth because the patient has become accustomed to the pack. The roots may be sensitive to

thermal changes and to touch. It is preferable to allow about two weeks to see if the sensitivity subsides. After this, sensitivity may be relieved by having the patient use the following solution:

Sodium fluoride 2% aqueous solution. . . . 8 oz. Color and flavor
Directions: Dip the toothbrush in a small amount of solution contained in a glass. Use the solution instead of a dentrifice. DO NOT SWALLOW.

The patient is usually comfortable by the time the solution is completely used. Areas of persistent sensitivity are treated with sodium fluoride paste or another desensitizing agent. Elimination of sensitivity caused by root caries requires excavation and restoration.

There are many office methods for desensitizing cervical areas of teeth. Our choice is sodium fluoride paste. It is prepared by mixing 10 gm. each of sodium fluoride and kaolin with sufficient glycerin to form a paste which is stored in a closed container, and is used as follows:

The tooth surface is dried and the paste burnished with a metal instrument and left in position for two minutes. The patient may report an initial sensation of cold. The paste is removed with warm water, and the mouth is thoroughly rinsed. Burnishing is important; comparable results are not obtained when the paste is applied with a rubber cup. It may be repeated after two weeks if necessary. Sodium fluoride paste is effective and does not injure the gingiva or discolor the teeth; it should not be used on freshly cut tooth surfaces.

Other desensitizing agents for office use are zinc chloride, 8 per cent solution; liquid phenol; formaldehyde; ammoniacal silver nitrate; a mixture of sodium carbonate monohydrate, 2.5 gm., with potassium carbonate, 12.5 mg.; and sodium silicofluoride.[28, 37] Except for the last two, these chemicals are not to be used on freshly cut dentin to avoid injury to viable tissue.

Reduction in sensitivity has also been reported with a stannous fluoride–containing gel used as a dentifrice[41] and with a sodium monofluorophosphate dentifrice.[29] Some patients report relief with dentifrices containing formalin (Thermodent)[19] and strontium chloride (Sensodyne).[12, 54] Corticosteroid hormones have also been tried for desensitizing exposed root surfaces.[43]

---

*The reader is referred to the excellent review by Peden[47] on dental hypersensitivity.

COMPLETE-MOUTH PERIODONTAL SURGERY

Ordinarily, periodontal surgery is an office procedure performed in quadrants or sextants at weekly or biweekly intervals. Under certain circumstances, however, it is in the best interest of the patient to treat the mouth in one operation with the patient hospitalized.

Indications

PATIENT PROTECTION. There are patients with systemic conditions that are not severe enough to contraindicate elective surgery but that may require special precautionary measures, best provided in a hospital. This group includes patients with cardiovascular disease, diabetes, hyperthyroidism, those undergoing prolonged steroid therapy, and those with a history of rheumatic fever or abnormal bleeding tendencies.

The purpose of hospitalization is to protect patients by anticipating their special needs — not to perform periodontal surgery when it is contraindicated by the patients' general condition. There are patients for whom elective surgery is contraindicated regardless of whether it is performed in the dental office or the hospital. When consultation with the patients' physician leads to this decision, palliative periodontal therapy, in the form of scaling and curettage if permissible, is the necessary compromise.

THE APPREHENSIVE PATIENT. Gentleness, understanding, and preoperative sedation usually suffice to calm the fears of most patients. For some patients, however, the prospect of a series of surgical procedures is sufficient stress to trigger disturbances that jeopardize the well-being of the patient and hamper treatment. Explaining that the treatment at the hospital will be performed painlessly, and that it will be preceded by a depth of sedation that is not practical for ambulatory patients visiting a dental office, are important steps toward allaying their fears. The thought of completing the necessary surgical procedures in one session rather than in repeated visits is an added comfort to the patient, because it eliminates the prospect of repeated anxiety in anticipation of each treatment.

With complete-mouth surgery, there is less stress for the patient. It is performed after a night's rest in the hospital and under ample sedation rather than after coming from the street into the dental office (sometimes after rushing to be on time for the appointment). The patient is returned to his room after surgery for a check of his physical condition and for a restful postoperative sleep, instead of leaving the dental office and making the trip home.

PATIENT CONVENIENCE. For patients whose occupation entails considerable contact with the public, surgery performed at weekly intervals sometimes presents a special problem. It means that for a period of several weeks, some area of the mouth will be covered by the periodontal pack. With the complete-mouth technique, the pack is ordinarily retained for only one week. Patients find this a very acceptable alternative to several weeks of involvement with the pack. For a variety of other reasons, patients may desire to attend to their surgical needs in one session under optimal conditions.

Hospital admission and presurgical medical examination

If, after consideration of all factors, complete-mouth operation is selected as the procedure of choice, a hospital appointment is made. The days immediately preceding and during the menstrual period are avoided because there may be excessive postoperative bleeding at that time.

The length of the hospital stay is 48 hours. The patient enters early in the afternoon preceding the morning of the operation, to allow time for a physical examination, hemogram and other laboratory procedures, and medical consultations.

Preparations are made for special precautionary measures that may be required before, during, or after surgery. For example, diabetics who consider themselves to be "under control" sometimes require a short period of dietary supervision and regulation of insulin before surgery. The medical examination occasionally reveals disease of which the patient is not aware as well as conditions which the patient felt were not relevant to his dental problem and were thus omitted from the case history taken in the dentist's office.

Premedication and anesthesia

PREMEDICATION. Many combinations of drugs may be used for sedation. The following has been found to be effective.

The night before surgery, before retiring: Seconal 100 mg.; one hour before surgery: Nembutal, intramuscular; one half hour before anesthesia: scopolamine, 0.4 mg., and morphine sulfate, 10 mg. Patients with a history of rheumatic fever, cardiovascular disease, diabetes, or prolonged corticosteroid therapy are premedicated with antibiotics.

ANESTHESIA. Local or general anesthesia may be used. Local anesthesia is our method of choice, except for especially apprehensive patients. It permits unhampered movement of the head which is necessary for optimal visibility and accessibility to the various root surfaces.

The following injections are used for the mandible: bilateral mandibular and long buccal injections; for the maxilla: bilateral anterior palatine nerve injections at the posterior palatine foramen and the nasopalatine nerve injection in the incisive foramen, plus buccal infiltration in the molar, premolar, and anterior regions. Injection directly into the interdental papillae is not ordinarily required; it may be used in areas in which sensitivity persists.

The operation

Surgery is performed on the operating table with the patient's back elevated at an angle of approximately 30 degrees and the head at the level of the operator's elbows. The assistant responsible for the aspirator stands on the side of the table opposite the operator.

Postoperative instructions at the hospital

The patient is returned to his room; the following postoperative instructions are entered in the record:

Cold semi-solid foods only
Demerol, 50 mg. every four hours if necessary
Discharge tomorrow (date) morning
Periodontal pack is to remain in place, to be removed at the doctor's office

The patient is discharged from the hospital the morning following the operation, with an appointment for a week later at the dentist's office.

Instructions for the patient following complete-mouth surgery

The patient is given a printed booklet containing the following instructions:

INSTRUCTIONS FOR

Mr. Alan Jones

The operation which has been performed on your gums will help you keep your teeth. The following information has been prepared to answer questions you may have about how to take care of your mouth. Please read the instructions carefully — our patients have found them very helpful.

We have placed a periodontal pack over your gums to protect them from irritation. The pack prevents pain, aids healing, and enables you to carry on most of your usual activities in comfort.

For your benefit the pack should remain in place as long as possible. **Do not remove it.** If particles of the pack chip off during the week, do not be concerned as long as you do not have pain. If a piece of the pack breaks off and you are in pain, or if a rough edge irritates your tongue or cheek, please call the office. The problem can be easily remedied.

Eat anything you can manage without chipping off the pack. Eggs, Jell-O, cereals, soups, milk, fish, and hamburger or any semi-solid or finely minced foods are suggested. **Avoid citrus fruits or fruit juices, highly spiced foods, and alcoholic beverages. They will cause pain.** You may supplement your diet with a multivitamin preparation for the next two weeks.

Do not smoke — the heat and smoke will irritate your gums and delay healing. If at all possible, use this opportunity to give up smoking. Smokers have more gum disease than nonsmokers.

Rinsing is not part of the treatment, but it will help make your mouth feel refreshed. At home you may rinse gently as often as you wish with one of the popular mouthwashes. Do not use it in concentrated form;

dilute it—$1/3$ mouthwash to $2/3$ warm water.

Cleanse the surface of the pack with a soft toothbrush moistened with water, without a dentifrice. A water irrigation device used at low pressure with room temperature water is also helpful.

Please remain at home the day you return from the hospital. After this you may follow your regular daily activities, avoiding excessive exertion of any type. Golf, tennis, skiing, bowling, swimming, or sunbathing should be postponed for four days after the operation.

For the first two days you will be unaccustomed to having the pack in your mouth and it may be uncomfortable. Should you have pain take two aspirin tablets, 5 grains every three hours. If the pain is not relieved, please call the office.

Swelling is not unusual, particularly in areas which required extensive surgical procedures. The swelling generally subsides in three or four days. If the swelling is painful or appears to become worse, please call the office.

There may be occasional blood stains in the saliva for the first four to five hours after the operation. This is not unusual and will correct itself. If there is considerable bleeding beyond this, take a piece of gauze, form it into the shape of a "U," hold it in the thumb and index finger, apply it to both sides of the pack and hold it under pressure for 20 minutes. Do not remove it during this period to examine it. If the bleeding does not stop at the end of 20 minutes, please contact the office. **Do not try to stop the bleeding by rinsing.**

If other problems arise, please call the office.

First postoperative office visit

The patient is seen at the office one week after the operation. The pack is usually removed and the patient is instructed in plaque control. If it appears advisable, one or more areas may be repacked for another week.

BACTEREMIA FOLLOWING PERIODONTAL TREATMENT

Bacteremia may occur in as many as 88 per cent of patients following periodontal treatment,[53] but lower incidences have been reported (16 to 46 per cent following prophylaxis;[58] 8 per cent[52] and 83.8 per cent[31] following scaling; 26.3 per cent following scaling and curettage;[63] and 24.56,[58] 38.18,[25] and 83.3[31] per cent following gingivectomy). The size of the blood sample, the time at which it is taken, the ratio of sample to medium, and the nature of the culture media may account for the differences in the findings in the various studies.[53] Bacteremia has also been noted in patients with periodontal disease previous to treatment.[31]

Post-treatment bacteremias are transient, with most of the bacteria eliminated within 10 minutes by the natural defense mechanisms. The bacteremia is likely to persist as long as surgical manipulation of the tissues is in progress. In some cases, bacteria are recovered from the blood stream more than two hours after gingivectomy.[58] The incidence of bacteremia is related to the duration of the treatment, and may[16, 64] or may not[25, 59] be related to the severity of the disease or the mobility of the teeth.

Seventy different strains of organisms have been recovered at different times following scaling and curettage and gingivectomy,[53] including strains of *Streptococcus*, diphtheroid, *Vibrio*, *Spirillum*, *Tetracoccus*, *Bacteroides*, *Veillonella*, *Fusobacterium*, *Actinomyces*, *Micrococcus*, *Leptotrichia* and two nontypable anaerobes. Streptococci and diphtheroids were found most frequently.[25, 58]

The greatest interest is in S. *viridans*, the most common organism. Transient bacteremia is usually unattended by clinical sequelae, but in patients with a history of rheumatic fever or congenital heart valve injury, it constitutes a real menace. The circulating bacteria may lodge and vegetate on the injured valve and establish bacterial endocarditis. S. *viridans* is almost always the responsible organism. Two cases of subacute bacterial endocarditis associated with *Lactobacillus acidophilus* have been reported,[11] and one with S. *mitis*.[17] Pretreatment with chemotherapy is the most effective way of reducing the incidence of bacteremia.

The effectiveness of chemotherapeutic agents results from retardation of the rate of multiplication of microorganisms (inhibitory), cessation of multiplication (bacteriostatic or fungistatic), and/or destruction of viable organisms (bactericidal or fungicidal). Antibiotics and sulfonamides are the commonly used chemotherapeutic agents.[1, 7, 9, 13, 23, 51] (see Chap. 45).

REFERENCES

1. Alder-Hradecky, C., and Kelentey, B.: Salivary excretion and inactivation of some penicillins. Nature, 198:792, 1963.
2. American Dental Association and American Heart Association: Management of dental problems in patients with cardiovascular disease. J.A.M.A., 187:848, 1964, Summary.
3. Baer, P. N., Goldman, H. M., and Scigliano, J.: Studies on a bacitracin periodontal dressing. Oral Surg., 11:712, 1958.
4. Baer, P. N., Sumner, C. F., III, and Scigliano, J.: Studies on a hydrogenated fat-zinc bacitracin periodontal dressing. Oral Surg., 13:494, 1960.
5. Baer, P. N., Sumner, C. F., III, and Miller, G.: Periodontal dressings. Dent. Clin. North Am., 13:181, 1969.
6. Baer, P. N., and Wertheimer, F. W.: A histologic study of the effects of several periodontal dressings on periosteal-covered and denuded bone. J. Dent. Res., 40:858, 1961.
7. Bartels, H. A., Cohen, G., and Scopp, I. W.: Alterations in the oral microbial flora accompanying local and systemic drug therapy. J. Periodontol., 40:421, 1969.
8. Behrman, S. J., and Wright, I. S.: Dental surgery during continuous anticoagulant therapy. J. Am. Dent. Assoc., 62:172, 1961.
9. Bender, I. B., Pressman, R. S., and Tashman, S. G.: Studies on excretion of antibiotics in human saliva. I. Penicillin and streptomycin. J. Am. Dent. Assoc., 46:164, 1953.
10. Bhaskar, S. N., Frisch, J., Margetis, P. M., and Leonard, F.: Oral surgery–oral pathology conference number 18, Walter Reed Army Medical Center. Oral Surg., 22:526, 1966.
11. Biocca, E., and Seppilli, A.: Human infections caused by lactobacilli. J. Infect. Dis., 18:112, 1947.
12. Blitzer, B.: A consideration of the possible causes of dental hypersensitivity: Treatment by a strontium-ion dentifrice. Periodontics, 5:318, 1967.
13. Borzelleca, J. F., and Cherrick, H. M.: The excretion of drugs in saliva. Antibiotics. J. Oral Therap. Pharm., 2:180, 1965.
14. Burch, J., et al.: Tooth mobility following gingivectomy. A study of gingival support of the teeth. Periodontics, 6:90, 1960.
15. Chamberlain, F. L.: Management of medical-dental problems in patients with cardiovascular diseases. Mod. Concepts Cardiovasc. Dis., 30:697, 1961.
16. Conner, H., Haberman, S., Collings, C., and Winford, T.: Bacteremias following periodontal scaling in patients with healthy appearing gingiva. J. Periodontol., 38:466, 1967.
17. Eisenbud, L.: Subacute bacterial endocarditis precipitated by non-surgical dental procedures. Oral Surg., 15:624, 1962.
18. Fay, J. T.: Dental procedures for the patient with cardiovascular disease. J. Am. Dent. Assoc., 78:105, 1969.
19. Forrest, J. O.: A clinical assessment of three desensitizing toothpastes containing formalin. Br. Dent. J., 114:103, 1963.
20. Fraleigh, C. M.: An evaluation of topical terramycin in postgingivectomy pack. J. Periodontol., 27:201, 1956.
21. Frisch, J. E., and Bhaskar, S. N.: Tissue response to eugenol-containing periodontal dressings. J. Periodontol., 38:402, 1967.
22. Gottsegen, R.: Dental and oral considerations in diabetes. In Ellenberg, M., and Rifkin, H. (eds.): Clinical Diabetes Mellitus. New York, McGraw-Hill, 1962.
23. Gross, A., and Uotinen, K. G.: Elimination of antibiotics in submaxillary and parotid saliva of unanaesthetized dogs. Pharm. Therap. Dent., 1:46, 1970.
24. Guglani, L. M., and Allen, E. F.: Connective tissue reaction to implants of periodontal packs. J. Periodontol., 36:279, 1965.
25. Gutverg, M., and Haberman, S.: Studies on bacteremia following oral surgery: Some prophylactic approaches to bacteremia and the results of tissue examination of excised gingiva. J. Periodontol., 33:105, 1962.
26. Hiatt, W.: Local anesthesia: History; potential toxicity: Clinical investigation of mepivacaine. Dent. Clin. North Am., July, 1961, p. 243.
27. Hirschfeld, I.: Vincent's infection of mouth: Clinical incidents in its diagnosis and treatment. J. Am. Dent. Assoc., 21:768, 1934.
28. Hunter, G. C., Jr., Barringer, M., and Spooner, G.: Analysis of desensitization of dentin by sodium silico-fluoride and Gottlieb's solution by use of radioactive silver nitrate. J. Periodontol., 32:333, 1961.
29. Kanouse, M. C., and Ash, M. M., Jr.: The effectiveness of a sodium monofluorophosphate dentifrice on dental hypersensitivity. J. Periodontol., 40:38, 1969.
30. Kaplan, S. I., and Hurwitz, G.: Reactions to penicillin. Oral Surg., 2:21, 1949.
31. Kom, N. A., and Schaffer, E. M.: A comparison of the post-operative bacteremias induced following different periodontal procedures. J. Periodontol., 33:226, 1962.
32. Kwapis, B. W.: Anticoagulant therapy and dental practice. J. Am. Dent. Assoc., 66:172, 1963.
33. Leonard, M. E.: Hemophilia. In Conn, H. F. (ed.): Current Therapy. Philadelphia, W. B. Saunders Co., 1957, p. 183.
34. Majewski, I., and Sponholz, H.: Ergebnisse nach parodontal therapeutischen Massnahmen unter besonderer Berucksich tigung der Zahnbeweglichkeitssung mit dem Makroperiodontometer nach Muhlemann. Zahnarztl. Rundschaw, 75:57, 1966.
35. Marble, A., White, H. J., and Fernald, A. T.: The nature of the lowered resistance to infection in diabetes mellitus. J. Clin. Invest., 17:423, 1938.
36. McIntyre, H., Nour-Eldin, F., Israels, M. C. G., and Wilkinson, J. F.: Dental extractions in

patients with haemophilia and Christmas disease. Lancet, 2:642, 1959.

37. Massler, M.: Desensitization of cervical cementum and dentin by sodium silicofluoride. J. Dent. Res., *34*:761, 1955.

38. McCall, J. O.: The measure of success in periodontic practice. J. Am. Dent. Assoc., *15*:279, 1928.

39. Meyers, M. C.: Hemorrhagic disorders. *In* Conn, H. F. (ed.): Current Therapy. Philadelphia, W. B. Saunders Co., 1957, p. 184.

40. Meyler, L.: Side effects of drugs, Vol. 5. Amsterdam, Excerpta Medica Foundation, 1966.

41. Miller, J. T., Shannon, I. L., Kilgore, W. G., and Bookman, J. E.: Use of a water-free stannous fluoride–containing gel in the control of dental hypersensitivity. J. Periodontol., *40*:490, 1969.

42. Mopsik, E. R.: Infections and antibiotics. Dent. Clin. North Am., *15*:327, 1971.

43. Mosteller, J. H.: Use of prednisolone in the elimination of postoperative thermal sensitivity. J. Pros. Dent., *12*:1176, 1962.

44. Ochstein, A. J., Hansen, N. M., and Swenson, H. M.: A comparative study of cyanoacrylate and other periodontal dressing on gingival surgical wound healing. J. Periodontol., *40*:515, 1969.

45. Oliver, W. M., and Heaney, T. G.: Sequelae following the use of eugenol or non-eugenol dressings after gingivectomy and subgingival curettage. Dent. Pract. (Bristol), *21*:49, 1970.

46. Parnell, A. G.: Adrenal crisis and the dental surgeon. Br. Dent. J., *116*:294, 1964.

47. Peden, J. W.: Dental hypersensitivity. J. Western Soc. Periodontol., *25*:75, 1977.

48. Persson, G., and Thilander, H.: Experimental studies of surgical packs. 1. *In vivo* experiments on antimicrobial effect. Odont. T., 76:147, 1968.

49. Persson, G., and Thilander, H.: Experimental studies of surgical packs. 2. Tissue reaction to various packs. Odont. T., 76:157, 1968.

50. Prichard, J. F.: Periodontal case management in hemorrhagic disease. J. Periodontol., 26:247, 1955.

51. Rammelkamp, C. H., and Keefer, C. S.: The absorption, excretion, and distribution of penicillin. J. Clin. Invest., 22:425, 1943.

52. Robinson, L., et al.: Bacteremias of dental origin. Oral Surg., 3:519, 923, 1950.

53. Rogosa, M., Hampp, E. G., Nevin, T. A., Wagner, H. N., Jr., Driscoll, E. J., and Baer, P. N.: Blood sampling and cultural studies in the detection of post-operative bacteremias. J. Am. Dent. Assoc., *60*:71, 1960.

54. Ross, M. R.: Hypersensitive teeth; effect of strontium chloride in a compatible dentifrice. J. Periodontol., 32:49, 1961.

55. Shira, R. B., Hall, R. J., and Guernsey, L. H.: Minor oral surgery during prolonged anticoagulant therapy. J. Oral Surg., 20:93, 1962.

56. Shuttleworth, C. W., and Gibbs, F. J.: Aetiological significance of Candida albicans in chronic angular cheilitis and its treatment with nystatin. Br. Dent. J., *108*:354, 1960.

57. Stahl, S. S., et al.: Gingival healing. III. The effects of periodontal dressings on gingivectomy repair. J. Periodontol., *40*:34, 1969.

58. Vargas, B., Collings, C. K., Polter, L., and Haberman, S.: Effects of certain factors on bacteremias resulting from gingival resection. J. Periodontol., *30*:196, 1959.

59. Wada, K., Tomizawa, M., and Sasaki, I.: Study on bacteremia in patients with pyorrhea alveolaris caused by surgical operations. Periodont. Abstr., *18*:27, 1970.

60. Waldrep, A. C., Jr., and McKelvey, L. E.: Oral surgery for patients on anticoagulant therapy. J. Oral Surg., 26:374, 1968.

61. Williams, L. F., Jr., and Wynne, G. F.: Fundamental Approach to Surgical Problems. Springfield, Ill., Charles C Thomas, Publisher, 1962, p. 127.

62. Williams, R. C., Jr., and Mahan, C. J.: Periodontal disease and diabetes in young adults. J.A.M.A., *172*:776, 1960.

63. Winslow, M. B., and Kobernick, S. D.: Bacteremia after prophylaxis. J. Am. Dent. Assoc., *61*:69, 1960.

64. Winslow, M. B., and Millstone, S. H.: Bacteremia after prophylaxis. Part II. J. Periodontol., 36:371, 1965.

65. Woodward, S. C., et al.: Histotoxicity of cyanoacrylate tissue adhesive in the rat. Ann. Surg., *162*:113, 1965.

66. Zimmerman, B.: The endocrine glands. *In* Textbook of Surgery. 8th ed. New York, Appleton-Century-Crofts, 1963, Chap. 39.

The Gingivectomy Technique

In a limited literal sense, the term *gingivectomy* means excision of the gingiva. In reality, it is a *two-stage operation* consisting of the *removal of diseased gingiva and the scaling and planing of the root surface.*

Gingivectomy derives its effectiveness from the following:

1. By removing the diseased pocket wall which obscures the tooth surface, it provides the visibility and accessibility that are essential for the complete removal of irritating surface deposits and thorough smoothing of the roots (Fig. 49–1).

2. By removing diseased tissue and local irritants, it creates a favorable environment for gingival healing and the restoration of physiologic gingival contour.

INDICATIONS AND CONTRAINDICATIONS

The gingivectomy technique is indicated in the following cases[9]: (1) Elimination of deep suprabony pockets in which the deposits on the root cannot be seen in their entirety when the pocket wall is deflected with a probe or blast of warm air. In deep or inaccessible pockets, calculus cannot be completely removed with any degree of

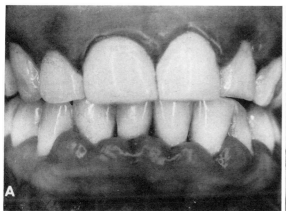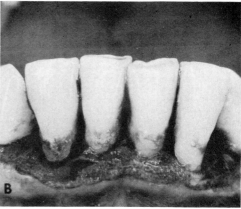

Figure 49–1   Visibility of and Accessibility to Calculus. *A,* Gingival enlargement. *B,* Removal of diseased gingiva exposes calculus. (Phase I therapy is sometimes omitted when the indication for a gingivectomy is obvious. It can never be omitted when a flap appears indicated.)

Before   After

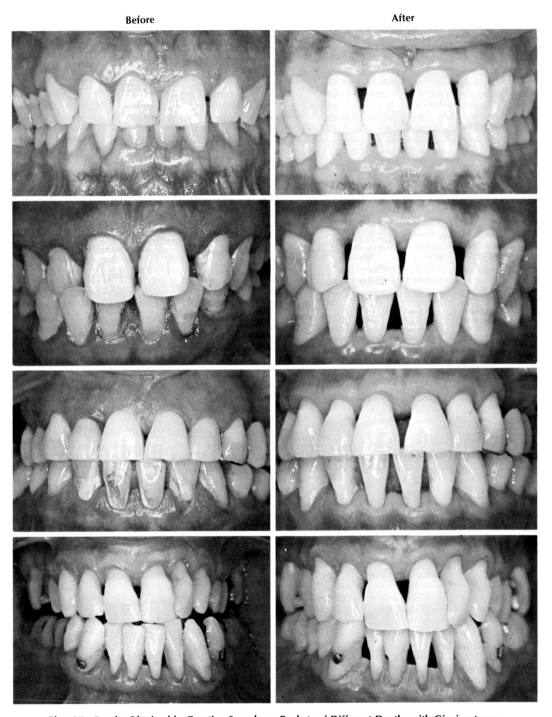

Plate VI   Results Obtained by Treating Suprabony Pockets of Different Depths with Gingivectomy.

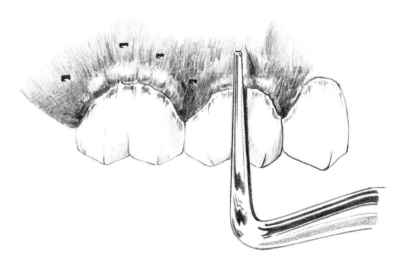

Figure 49–2 Pocket Marker No. 27G Makes Pin-Point Perforations which indicate pocket depth.

predictability by hand scalers if the operator must rely solely upon tactile sensation.[8] (2) Elimination of all suprabony pockets, regardless of their depth, if the pocket wall is fibrous and firm. Because fibrous gingival tissue does not shrink after scaling and curettage, some form of surgical treatment is necessary to eliminate the pocket. (3) Elimination of gingival enlargements. (4) Elimination of suprabony periodontal abscesses. Other techniques are also available for some of the above-mentioned indications (see Chap. 46).

The following two findings will contraindicate the gingivectomy technique: (a) The need for bone surgery or even for examination of the bone shape and morphology. (b) The location of the bottom of the pocket apical to the mucogingival junction.

When used for the purposes for which it is intended, the gingivectomy technique is a most effective form of treatment (see Color Plate VI).

A STEP-BY-STEP PROCEDURE FOR PERFORMING THE GINGIVECTOMY

Mark the Pockets

The pockets on each surface are explored with a periodontal probe and marked with a pocket marker. The instrument is held with the marking end in line with the vertical axis of the tooth. The straight end is inserted to the base of the pocket and the level marked by pressing the pliers together and producing a bleeding point on the outside surface (Figs. 49–2 and 49–3). The pockets are marked systematically, begin-

ning on the distal surface of the last tooth, then on the facial surface, proceeding anteriorly to the midline. The procedure is repeated on the lingual surface. Each pocket is marked in several areas so as to outline its course on each surface.

Resect the Gingiva

The gingiva may be resected with periodontal knives, a scalpel, or scissors. The

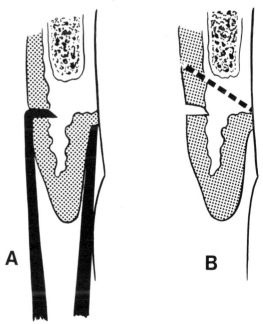

Figure 49–3 Marking the Depth of Suprabony Pocket. *A,* Pocket marker in position. *B,* Beveled incision extends apical to the perforation made by the pocket marker.

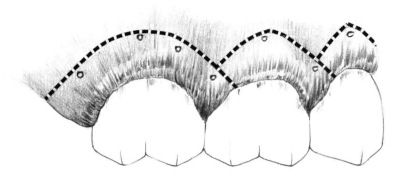

Figure 49–4 Discontinuous Incision apical to bottom of the pocket indicated by pinpoint markings.

removal of diseased gingiva is an important part of the gingivectomy, but the instrument with which it is done does not affect the outcome of treatment. The choice is based upon individual experience. The periodontal knives are used for incisions on the facial and lingual surfaces and distal to the terminal tooth in the arch. The interdental periodontal knives No. 22G and No. 23G are used for supplemental interdental incisions where necessary, and the Bard-Parker Blades No. 11 and No. 12 and scissors are used as auxiliary instruments.

Discontinuous and continuous incisions

Discontinuous or continuous incisions may be used, depending upon the operator's preference.

The *discontinuous incision* is started on the facial surface at the distal angle of the last tooth and carried forward, following the course of the pocket, and extending through the interdental gingiva to the distofacial angle of the next tooth (Fig. 49–4). The next incision is begun where the previous one

crosses the interdental space, and is carried to the distofacial angle of the next tooth. Individual incisions are repeated for each tooth to be operated (Fig. 49–5).

The *continuous incision* is started on the facial surface of the last tooth and carried forward without interruption, following the course of the pockets (Fig. 49–6). After the incisions have been made on the facial surface, the procedure is repeated on the lingual surface (Fig. 49–7). To avoid the blood vessels and nerve of the incisive canal and also to produce a better postoperative gingival contour, the incisions should be carried along the sides of the incisive papilla, not horizontally across it (Fig. 49–8).

The distal incision

After the facial and lingual incisions are completed, they are joined by an incision across the distal surface of the last erupted tooth. The distal incision is made with a periodontal knife inserted below the bottom of the pocket, and is beveled so that it blends with the facial and lingual incisions (Figs. 49–9 to 49–11).

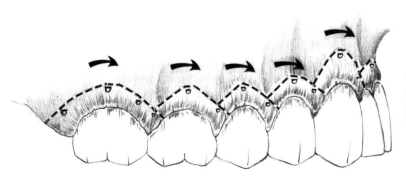

Figure 49–5 Quadrant Incised With Discontinuous Incision, which follows the outline of each pocket, apical to the pin-point markings.

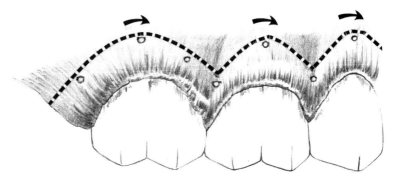

Figure 49-6 Continuous Incision begins on the molar and extends anteriorly without interruption.

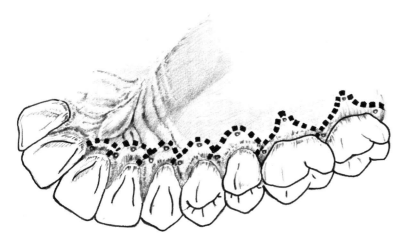

Figure 49-7 Discontinuous Incisions on the Palatal Surface follow the contours of deep periodontal pockets on the molars.

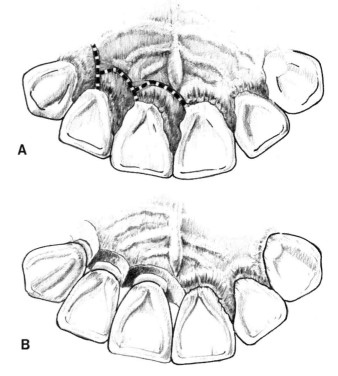

Figure 49-8 Incision Made Lateral to the Incisive Papilla. A, Discontinuous incision avoids cutting across incisive papilla. B, After pockets are removed.

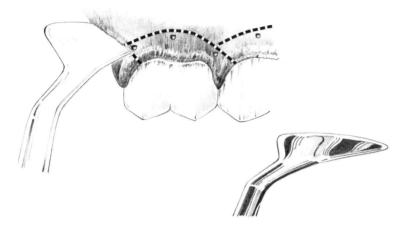

Figure 49–9 Beveled Distal Incision on the Maxilla with No. 20G periodontal knife.

How to make the incision

The incision is started apical to the points marking the course of the pockets[1, 30, 37] and directed coronally to a point between the base of the pocket and crest of the bone. **It should be as close as possible to the bone without exposing it so as to remove the soft tissue coronal to the bone.** Removal of the soft tissue between the bottom of the pocket and the bone is important, because (1) it provides the greatest likelihood of removing the entire junctional epithelium; (2) it ensures the exposure of all root deposits at the bottom of the pocket (Fig. 49–12); and (3) it eliminates excessive fibrous tissue which interferes with the attainment of physiologic contour when the gingiva heals

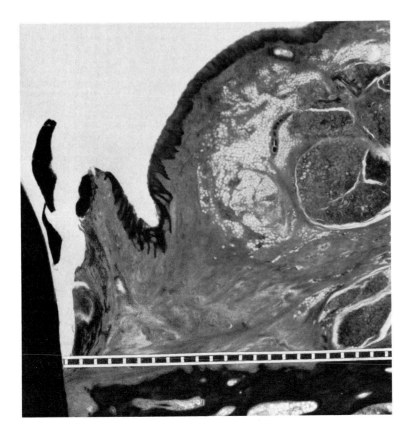

Figure 49–10 Retromolar Pad Behind Mandibular Third Molar. Fatty tissue and glands from bulbous pad behind periodontal pocket. Dotted line shows gingivectomy incision to resect the pocket and retromolar pad.

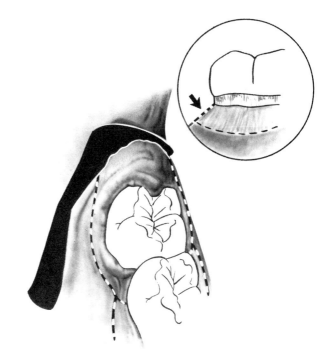

Figure 49–11 **Distal Incision on the Mandible Joins the Facial and Lingual Incisions** *(dotted lines). Inset,* The distal incision is beveled *(arrow)* to blend with the bevels on the facial and lingual surfaces.

(Fig. 49–13). Exposure of bone is undesirable. Should it occur, healing usually presents no problem if the area is adequately covered by the periodontal pack.

Some authors, however, recommend placing the incision 1 to 2 mm. coronal to the bottom of the pocket in order to reduce the potential post-healing root exposure and to limit the tissue destruction which occurs immediately below the line as part of tissue response to injury.[34]

The incision should be beveled at approximately 45 degrees to the tooth surface. This is most important where the pocket wall is enlarged and fibrous such as on the palatal surface in the molar area (Fig. 49–14). Failure to bevel leaves a broad fibrous plateau which takes more time than ordinarily required to develop physiologic contour. In the interim, plaque and food accumulation may lead to recurrence of pockets.

The incision should recreate the normal festooned pattern of the gingiva as far as possible, but not if it means leaving part of the pocket wall intact. The diseased pocket wall must be completely removed even if it requires departure from the regular outline of normal gingiva.

The incision should pass completely through the soft tissue to the tooth (Fig. 49–15). Incomplete incisions make it diffi-

cult to detach the pocket wall, and leave adherent tissue tabs that must be removed with a scissors or periodontal knife.

If in the course of the operation it becomes apparent that the incision is inadequate, it should be modified. The most common error is failure to make the incision

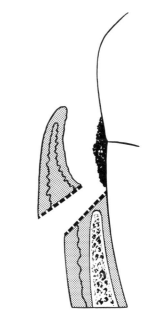

Figure 49–12 Complete removal of pocket wall assures exposure of calculus.

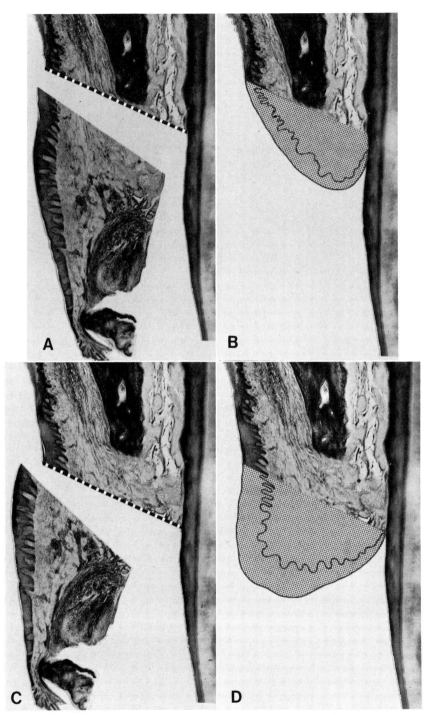

Figure 49–13   Incision Close to Bone Facilitates Healing Which Produces Physiologic Gingival Contour. *A,* Labial incision close beyond the pocket and close to the bone. *B,* Diagrammatic representation of healed gingiva with physiologic contour and normal sulcus. *C,* Incision is close to the bottom of the pocket but not deep enough. It leaves a remnant of epithelial attachment on the tooth and a wide band of inflamed fibrous connective tissue between the bottom of the pocket and the bone. *D,* Diagrammatic representation of bulbous gingiva and wide, deep sulcus formed on incompletely resected inflamed fibrous tissue.

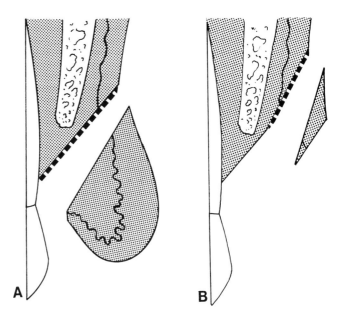

Figure 49–14 Beveled Incision for the Removal of Bulbous Fibrous Palatal Pocket. *A,* Bulbous gingiva on the palatal surface of maxillary first molar resected with a beveled incision. *B,* Corrective second incision sometimes required when proper contour cannot be obtained with single incision.

close enough to the bone. Very often, deep calculus is revealed after the incision is corrected.

Teeth adjacent to edentulous areas

For pockets on teeth adjacent to an edentulous area, the usual incisions are made on the facial and lingual tooth surfaces. In addition, a single incision is made across the edentulous ridge apical to the pockets on the teeth and close to the bone (Fig. 49–16). Pockets adjacent to edentulous spaces should not be excised as separate units, as this creates gingival troughs (Fig. 49–16) that complicate subsequent prosthesis.

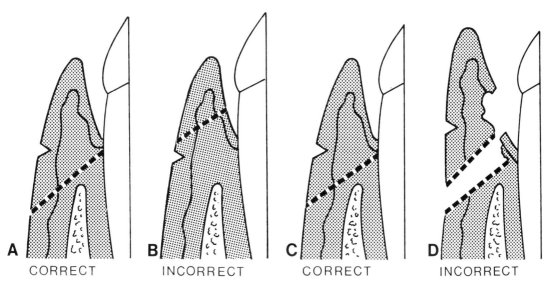

CORRECT   INCORRECT   CORRECT   INCORRECT

Figure 49–15   Correct and Incorrect Incisions. *A,* **Correct Incision** is apical to the bottom of the pocket, is beveled, and completely penetrates the soft tissue. The notch is made by the pocket marker at the level of the bottom of the pocket. *B,* **Incorrect Incision** is not deep enough, leaves part of pocket behind. *C,* **Correct Incision.** *D,* **Incorrect Incision** does not penetrate the soft tissues, leaves adherent tissue tab on the tooth.

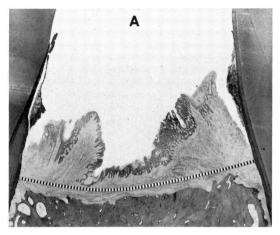

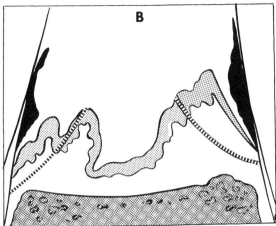

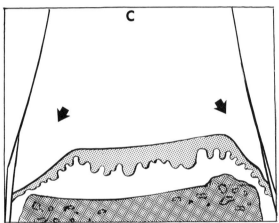

Figure 49–16 Incision Across Edentulous Space. *A,* Periodontal pockets adjacent to fibrous edentulous space. The proper incision is indicated by the dotted line. *B,* Incorrect incisions remove pockets separately, leaving fibrous mucosa intact. *C,* Troughs which result from improper incisions.

Remove the Marginal and Interdental Gingiva

Starting at the distal surface of the last erupted tooth, the gingival margin is detached at the line of incision with the No. 19G surgical hoe and the No. 3G and No. 4G scalers. The instrument is placed deep in the incision in contact with the tooth surface and moved coronally with a slow, firm motion (Fig. 49–17).

Appraise the Field of Operation

After the pocket wall is excised and the field is cleaned, the following features can be observed (Fig. 49–18A).

1. Bead-like granulation tissue.
2. Some calculus remnants that may extend close to where the pocket was attached. Calculus is **dark brown and slate-**

like in consistency, but some particles may be almost the same color as the root.

3. A band-like light zone on the root where the base of the pocket was attached.

Other features that may be noted at this time are softening of the root surface, indentations produced by cellular resorption, and cementum protuberances.

Remove the Granulation Tissue

The granulation tissue is removed before thorough scaling is attempted, so that hemorrhage from the granulation tissue will not obscure the scaling operation (Fig. 49–18B).

Curettes are used for this purpose. The curette is guided along the tooth surface and under the granulation tissue, separating it from the underlying bone. Removal of the

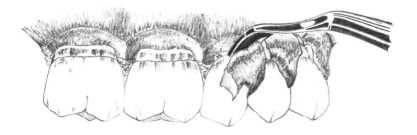

Figure 49–17 Detaching the Gingiva with a No. 19G Surgical Hoe. When the discontinuous incision is used, the marginal and interdental gingivae are removed as a unit.

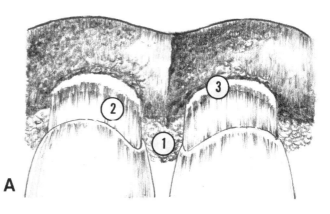

Figure 49–18 After the Pocket Wall Is Removed. *A,* Field of operation immediately after removing pocket wall. (1) Granulation tissue; (2) calculus and other root deposits; (3) clear space where bottom of the pocket was attached. *B,* Granulation tissue removed with curette to provide clear view of root surfaces. *C,* Root surfaces scaled and planed.

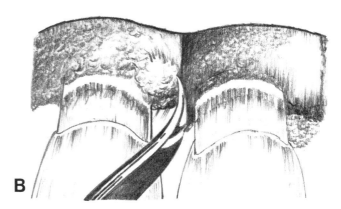

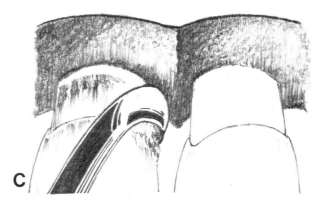

granulation tissue will reveal either the surface of the underlying bone or a covering band of fibrous tissue.

Remove the Calculus and Necrotic Root Substance

The calculus and necrotic cementum are removed and the root surface is smoothed, using scalers and curettes (Fig. 49–18C).

The success of the gingivectomy depends in large measure upon the thoroughness with which the root is scaled and planed. This should be done immediately after the granulation tissue is removed and not postponed to a subsequent visit for the following reasons:

1. The roots are most visible and accessible after the granulation tissue is removed.

2. The gingiva cannot heal properly if root deposits are permitted to remain until the next visit when they will be obscured by inflamed gingiva.

3. Postponement introduces an unnecessary extra operation.

Pre-pack Hygiene

Before placing the periodontal pack **each surface of every tooth** is checked for calculus or soft tissue remnants, after which the area is washed several times with warm water and covered with a gauze sponge folded in a U shape. The patient is instructed to bite on the sponge, which remains in place until the bleeding stops. Persistent bleeding interferes with adaptation and setting of the periodontal pack. It usually can be traced to a bleeding point partially covered with clot. The clot is cleaned away with a pledget of cotton saturated with hydrogen peroxide. **Pressure is then applied to the bleeding point with a pledget of cotton.** If the bleeding is interproximal, the cotton is wedged between the teeth.

The Blood Clot

The cut surfaces should be covered by clot before the pack is applied. The clot protects the wound and provides a scaffold-ing for the new blood vessels and connective tissue cells formed in healing. The clot should not be too bulky. Excessive clot interferes with retention of the periodontal pack. It is also an excellent medium for bacterial growth and increases the possibility of infection and delays healing. This permits downgrowth of epithelium onto the root which limits the height of connective tissue attachment.[20]

The Periodontal Pack

The different types of packs and the technique recommended for their application are described in detail in Chapter 48.

HEALING FOLLOWING GINGIVECTOMY

The initial response after gingivectomy is the formation of a protective surface clot; the underlying tissue becomes acutely inflamed with some necrosis. The clot is replaced by granulation tissue. After 12 to 24 hours, epithelial cells at the margins of the wound show an increase in glycogen[33] and DNA synthesis and migrate over the granulation tissue to separate it from the contaminated surface layer of the clot. Epithelial activity at the margins reaches a peak in 24 to 36 hours;[6] the new epithelial cells arise from the basal and deeper spinous layers of the wound edge epithelium and migrate over the wound over a fibrin layer that is later resorbed and replaced by a connective tissue bed.[15] The epithelial cells advance by a tumbling action, with the cells becoming fixed to the substrate by hemidesmosomes and a new basement lamina.[16] Surface epithelization is generally complete after five to 14 days. During the first four weeks after gingivectomy, keratinization is less complete than prior to surgery.

In experimental animals, the surgically removed junctional epithelium is reconstructed within two to three weeks.[12, 13, 17] Hemidesmosomes and basement lamina may be absent on the connective tissue side of the junctional epithelium. The outer surface of the gingival margin is healed by 14 days, but the epithelium of the gingival sulcus requires three to five weeks to heal.

In the initial 12 hours after gingivectomy, there are a slight reduction in cementoblasts and some loss of continuity of the osteoblastic layer on the outer aspect of the alveolar crest.[6] New bone formation occurs at the alveolar crest as early as the fourth day after gingivectomy,[28] and new cementoid appears at 10 to 15 days.[32]

By 24 hours, there is an increase in new connective tissue cells, mainly angioblasts, just beneath the surface layer of inflammation and necrosis; by the third day, numerous young fibroblasts are located in the area.[29] The highly vascular granulation tissue grows coronally, creating a new free gingival margin and sulcus.[25] Capillaries derived from blood vessels of the periodontal ligament migrate into the granulation tissue, and within two weeks they connect with gingival vessels.[38] Vasodilation and vascularity begin to decrease after the fourth day of healing and appear to be almost normal by the sixteenth day.[21] The connective tissue is still undergoing repair at the twenty-eighth day.

The flow of gingival fluid in humans is initially increased following gingivectomy and diminishes as healing progresses.[2, 31] The maximum is reached after one week, coinciding with the time of maximum inflammation.

The tissue changes that occur in postgingivectomy healing are the same in all individuals, but the time required for complete healing varies considerably, depending upon the area of the cut surface and interference from local irritation and infection. Gingival healing is affected by age[14] but not by sex or socioeconomic status.[33] In patients with physiologic melanosis, the pigmentation is diminished in the healed gingiva (Fig. 49–19).

Epithelization and re-formation of the junctional epithelium and re-establishment of the gingival and alveolar crest fiber system are slower in chemically created gingival wounds than in those produced by surgery.[36] Thirty-two days has been estimated as the average time required for complete repair of the epithelium following

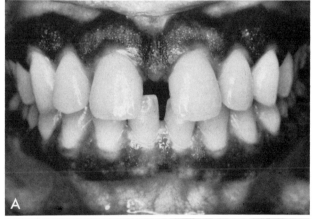
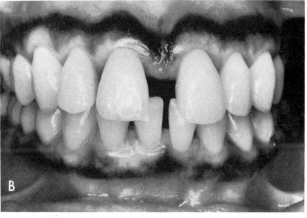

Figure 49–19 Physiologic Melanosis Diminished Following Gingivectomy. *A,* Before treatment— extensive physiologic pigmentation of the gingiva. *B,* One year after gingivectomy. Pigmentation is diminished; periodontal pockets are eliminated and physiologic gingival contour is restored.

gingivectomy and 49 days for the connective tissue.[35]

The following time sequence for healing following gingivectomy in humans has also been reported:[3]

TWO DAYS. Clot formed. Bone covered by proliferating connective tissue from the sides of the wound. Numerous leukocytes and fibrin shreds present.

FOUR DAYS. A portion of the clot remains adjacent to the tooth surface. Underlying portion of the clot replaced by granulation tissue. Epithelium without rete pegs extends over part of the surface. Dense inflammatory infiltration.

SIX DAYS. Entire wound covered by fairly well differentiated stratified squamous epithelium. There is consolidation of the granulation tissue, some collagen formation. Inflammation present.

SIXTEEN DAYS. Epithelium appears mature with new rete pegs. Connective tissue very collagenous. Slight chronic inflammatory exudate still present.

TWENTY-ONE DAYS. Epithelial rete pegs well developed, some thickening of the stratum corneum, hyperplasia and spongiosis of the epithelium. Increased collagenization of the connective tissue. Gingiva clinically normal.

Figure 49–20 shows the appearance of the gingiva before, during, and after treatment by gingivectomy. Figure 49–21 shows physiologic bone contouring one year after treatment by gingivectomy. Figure 49–22 is from a case in which gingivectomy of the entire mouth was performed in one session. Figure 49–23 shows the result of treatment of fibrous gingival enlargement with the gingivectomy technique.

GINGIVECTOMY BY CHEMOSURGERY

Several techniques have been described advocating the use of chemicals rather than a knife to remove the gingiva.[18, 22]

One technique entails the use of 5 per cent paraformaldehyde (trioxymethylene) incorporated in a modified zinc-oxide-eugenol paste and placed on the gingival margin and into the pocket.[22] Another technique suggests the use of potassium hydroxide.[18]

These methods have the following disadvantages: their depth of action cannot be controlled and therefore, healthy attached tissue underlying the pocket may be injured; gingival remodelling cannot be accomplished effectively.

GINGIVECTOMY BY ELECTROSURGERY

In periodontics, electrosurgery has been used for a variety of purposes:

The removal of gingival enlargements and gingivoplasty[23] are performed with the needle electrode supplemented by the small ovoid loop or diamond-shaped electrodes for festooning. A blended cutting and coagulating (fully rectified) current is used. In all reshaping procedures the electrode is activated and moved in a concise "shaving" motion.

In the treatment of acute periodontal abscesses, the incision to establish drainage can be made with the needle electrode without exerting painful pressure. The incision will remain open because the edges are sealed by the current. After the acute symptoms subside, the regular procedure for the treatment of the periodontal abscess is followed (Chapter 40).

For hemostasis, the ball electrode is used. Hemorrhage must be controlled by direct pressure (air, compress, or hemostat) first, then the surface lightly touched with a coagulating current. Electrosurgery is very helpful for the control of isolated bleeding points. Bleeding areas located interproximally are reached with a thin, bar-shaped electrode.

Frenum and muscle attachments can be relocated to facilitate pocket elimination, using a loop electrode. For this purpose, the frenum or muscle is stretched and sectioned with the loop electrode and a coagulating current.

For cases of **acute pericoronitis,** drainage may be obtained by incising the flap with a bent needle electrode. A loop electrode is used to remove the flap after the acute symptoms subside.

Electrosurgery is a convenient and effective method for cutting or eliminating tissue; it provides a clean operative field without hemorrhage.[24] However, **the heat generated by injudicious use can cause a serious risk of tissue damage and loss of periodontal support when it is used close to bone; this may seriously limit its useful-**

Text continued on page 824

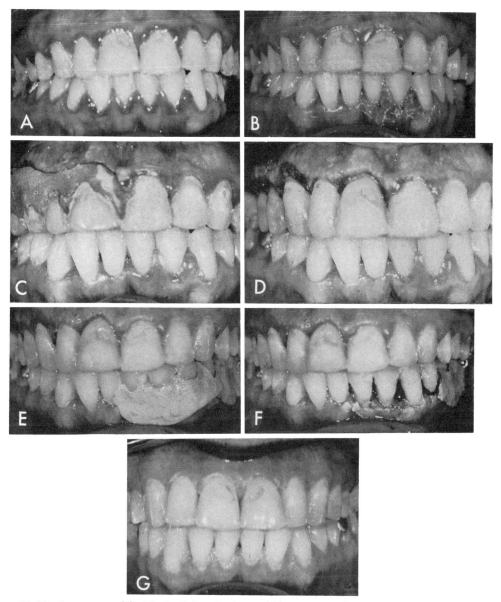

Figure 49–20   Appearance of the Gingiva Before, During, and After Treatment by Gingivectomy. *A,* Generalized chronic marginal gingivitis with deep periodontal pockets. *B,* Two weeks after gingivectomy in the mandibular quadrant *(left).* Note excellent gingival contour in relation to the treated central, lateral, and canine as compared with the inflammatory bulk of the gingiva in relation to the adjacent untreated anterior teeth. *C,* The patient returns one week after gingivectomy in the maxillary quadrant *(left).* The pack is still in position.

D, Immediately after the pack is removed; note the vascular appearance of the cut surface. *E,* The patient returns one week after gingivectomy in the mandibular quadrant *(right).* The pack is still in position. Note how the appearance of the gingiva in the maxilla *(left)* has changed as compared with the previous week *(D). F,* Immediately after the pack is removed from the mandible. The plaque-like material adherent to the gingiva is food debris which had seeped under the pack. *G,* Eighteen months after the generalized gingivectomy, note the excellent contour and position of the gingiva.

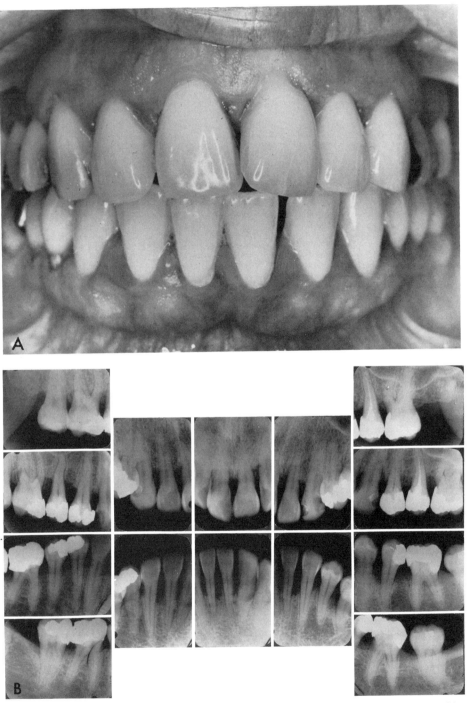

Figure 49–21 Bone Healing Following Gingivectomy. *A,* Generalized periodontal disease in 32-year-old patient. *B,* Extensive generalized bone loss. Note angular bone loss in mandibular incisor area.

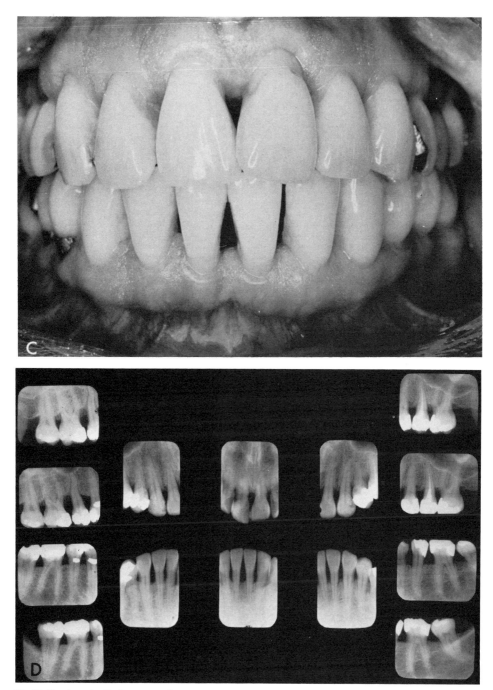

Figure 49–21 *Continued* C, One year after gingivectomy showing excellent condition of the gingiva. D, Radiographs after one year showing generalized smoothing of the interdental margins and filling in of bony defect in mandibular incisor area (compare with B).

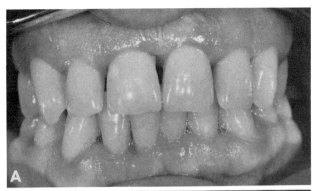

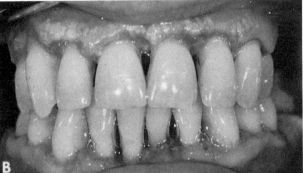

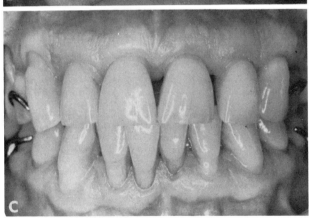

Figure 49–22 Complete-Mouth Gingivectomy. *A,* Generalized periodontal disease with fibrotic periodontal pockets. *B,* One week after operation. Note that the outline of the incision is irregular so as to follow the depth of individual pockets. *C,* After seven months. Physiologic contours restored by gingival healing. Note slight stain and calculus at recall visit.

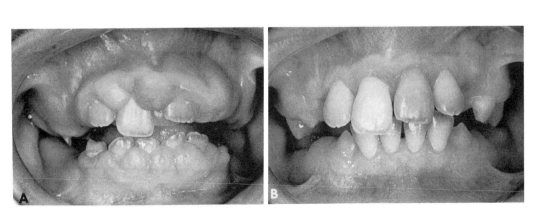

Figure 49–23 Gingival Enlargement in Child. *A,* Gingival enlargement associated with phenytoin therapy treated by complete-mouth gingivectomy. *B,* After healing.

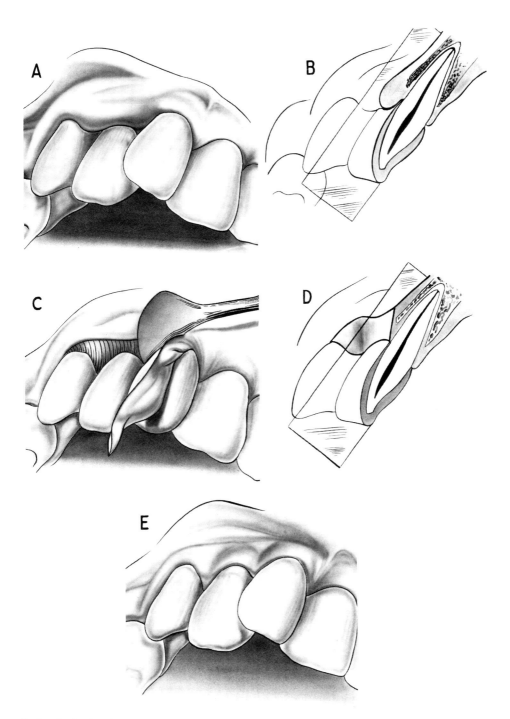

Figure 49–24   Reshaping the Gingiva With Gingivoplasty Incision. *A,* Fibrous chronic inflammatory gingival enlargement in relation to malposed anterior teeth. *B,* Diagram showing the relationship of the enlarged gingiva to the tooth. *C,* Removal of the gingiva with a fan-like incision. This resects the gingival margin and tapers the gingiva to desirable contour. The root surfaces are then thoroughly scaled and smoothed and periodontal pack is placed for a period of one week. *D,* Diagram showing the angle at which the gingiva is trimmed. *E,* After healing. The gingival disease is eliminated and physiologic contour is restored.

ness. It is valuable for superficial procedures such as the removal of gingival enlargement, gingivoplasty, relocating frenum and muscle attachments and incising periodontal abscesses and pericoronal flaps. It should not be used for procedures which involve proximity to the bone such as the treatment of infrabony pockets, flap operations, or mucogingival surgery.

HEALING FOLLOWING ELECTROSURGERY. Some investigators report no significant differences in gingival healing following resection by electrosurgery and periodontal knives;[5, 19] others find delayed healing, greater reduction in gingival height, and more bone injury.[26] There appears to be little difference in the results obtained following **shallow** gingival resection with electrosurgery and periodontal knives. However, when used for **deep resections close to bone**, electrosurgery reportedly can produce gingival recession,

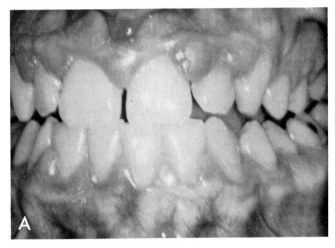

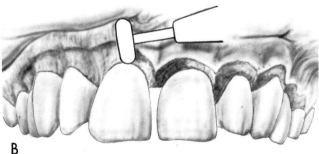

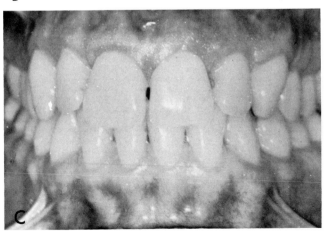

Figure 49–25 **Properly Contoured Gingivectomy Incision** produces same gingival architecture as improperly contoured gingivectomy incision followed by later gingivoplasty. A, Gingival enlargement. B, Patient's left side; maxilla and mandible treated by gingivectomy. Right side treated by gingivectomy followed by gingivioplasty with rotary diamond stones. C, After two months, the gingival contour is the same on both sides. In the early postoperative period healing was slower in the gingivoplasty quadrants.

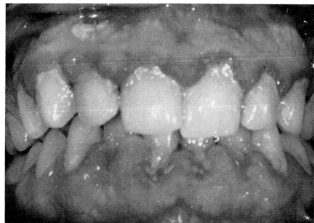

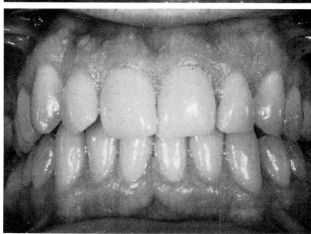

Figure 49–26 Attainment of Desired Gingival Contour by Properly Beveling the Gingivectomy Incision. Before treatment *(above)*. Pronounced gingival enlargement consisting of a combination of edematous and fibrous tissue. After treatment *(below)*. Gingival contour attained by properly beveling the incision in the regular gingivectomy technique.

bone necrosis and sequestration, loss of bone height, furcation exposure, and tooth mobility, which do not occur with the use of periodontal knives.[10]

GINGIVOPLASTY

Gingival and periodontal disease often produces deformities in the gingiva which interfere with normal food excursion, collect irritating plaque and food debris, and prolong and aggravate the disease process. Gingival clefts and craters, shelf-like interdental papillae caused by acute necrotizing ulcerative gingivitis, and gingival enlargement are examples of such deformities. *Artificially reshaping the gingiva to create physiologic gingival contours is termed gingivoplasty.*[11]

The gingivoplasty technique is similar to the gingivectomy technique; its purpose, however, is different. The gingivectomy technique is performed in order to eliminate periodontal pockets and includes reshaping as part of the technique. The gingivoplasty is done in the absence of pockets with the sole purpose of recontouring the gingiva (Fig. 49–24).

Gingivoplasty may be done with a periodontal knife, scalpel, rotary coarse diamond stones[7] (Fig. 49–25), or electrosurgery. It consists of procedures that resemble those performed in festooning artificial dentures—namely, tapering the gingival margin, creating an escalloped marginal outline, thinning the attached gingiva, and creating vertical interdental grooves and shaping the interdental papillae to provide sluiceways for the passage of food. Properly beveling the gingivectomy incision attains comparable results (Fig. 49–26).

REFERENCES

1. Ariaudo, A. A.: Symposium on the surgical approach to the periodontal problem. Procedure for gingivectomy. J. Periodontol., 28:62, 1957.
2. Arnold, R., Lunstad, G., Bissada, N., and Stallard, R.: Alterations in crevicular fluid flow during healing following gingival surgery. J. Periodont. Res., 1:303, 1966.
3. Bernier, J., and Kaplan, H.: The repair of gingival tissue after surgical intervention. J. Am. Dent. Assoc., 35:697, 1947.
4. Donnenfeld, O. W., and Glickman, I.: A biometric study of the effects of gingivectomy. J. Periodontol., 37:447, 1966.
5. Eisenmann, D., Malone, W. F., and Kusek, J.: Electron microscopic evaluation of electrosurgery. Oral Surg., 29:660, 1970.
6. Engler, W. O., Ramfjord, S., and Hiniker, J. J.: Healing following simple gingivectomy. A tritiated thymidine radioautographic study. I. Epithelialization. J. Periodontol., 37:298, 1966.
7. Fox, L.: Rotating abrasives in the management of periodontal soft and hard tissues. Oral Surg., 8:1134, 1955.
8. Frisch, J., Levin, M. P., and Bhaskar, S. N.: Calculus removal: Effectiveness of scaling. J. S. Calif. Dent. Assoc., 38:36, 1970.
9. Glickman, I.: The results obtained with the unembellished gingivectomy technic in a clinical study in humans. J. Periodontol., 27:247, 1956.
10. Glickman, I., and Imber, L. R.: Comparison of gingival resection with electrosurgery and periodontal knives—A biometric and histologic study. J. Periodontol., 41:142, 1970.
11. Goldman, H. M.: The development of physiologic gingival contours by gingivoplasty. Oral Surg., 3:879, 1950.
12. Henning, F.: Epithelial mitotic activity after gingivectomy. Relationship to reattachment. J. Periodont. Res., 4:319, 1969.
13. Henning, F.: Healing of gingivectomy wounds in the rat: Reestablishment of the epithelial seal. J. Periodontol., 39:265, 1968.
14. Holm-Pedersen, P., and Löe, H.: Wound healing in the gingiva of young and aged individuals. J. Periodont. Res., 2:245, 1967.
15. Innes, P. B.: An electron microscopic study of the regeneration of gingival epithelium following gingivectomy in the dog. J. Periodont. Res., 5:196, 1970.
16. Krawczyk, W. S.: A pattern of epithelial cell migration during wound healing. J. Cell Biol., 49:247, 1971.
17. Listgarten, M. A.: Electron microscopic features of the newly formed epithelial attachment after gingival surgery. J. Periodont. Res., 2:46, 1967.
18. Löe, H.: Chemical gingivectomy. Effect of potassium hydroxide on periodontal tissues. Acta Odontol. Scand., 19:517, 1961.
19. Malone, W. F., Eisenmann, D., and Kusck, J.: Interceptive periodontics with electrosurgery. J. Pros. Dent., 22:555, 1969.
20. Morris, M. L.: Healing of human periodontal tissues following surgical detachment from vital teeth: The position of the epithelial attachment. J. Periodontol., 32:108, 1961.
21. Novaes, A. B., Kon, S., Ruben, M. P., and Goldman, H.: Visualization of the microvascularization of the healing periodontal wound. III. Gingivectomy. J. Periodontol., 40:359, 1969.
22. Orban, B.: New methods in periodontal treatment. Bur, 42:116, 1942.
23. Oringer, M. J.: Electrosurgery for definitive conservative modern periodontal therapy. Dent. Clin. North Am., 13:53, 1969.
24. Oringer, M. J.: Electrosurgery in Dentistry. 2nd ed. Philadelphia, W. B. Saunders Company, 1975.
25. Persson, P. A.: The healing process in the marginal periodontium after gingivectomy with special regard to the regeneration of epithelium (an experimental study on dogs). Odont. T., 67: 593, 1959.
26. Pope, J. W., Gargiulo, A. W., Staffileno, H., and Levy, S.: Effects of electrosurgery on wound healing in dogs. Periodontics, 6:30, 1968.
27. Prandi, E. C., Blitzer, B., and Carranza, F. A., Jr.: Evaluación biométrica de la técnica de gingivectomia en humanos. Rev. Asoc. Odont. Argent., 57:84, 1969.
28. Ramfjord, S., and Costich, E. R.: Healing after simple gingivectomy. J. Periodontol., 34:401, 1963.
29. Ramfjord, S. P., Engler, W. D., and Hiniker, J. J.: A radiographic study of healing following simple gingivectomy. II. The connective tissue. J. Periodontol., 37:179, 1966.
30. Ritchey, B., and Orban, B.: The periodontal pocket. J. Periodontol., 23:199, 1952.
31. Sandalli, P., and Wade, A. B.: Alterations in crevicular fluid flow during healing following gingivectomy and flap procedures. J. Periodont. Res., 4:314, 1969.
32. Stahl, S. S.: Soft tissue healing following experimental gingival wounding in female rats of various ages. Periodontics, 1:142, 1963.
33. Stahl, S. S., Witkin, G. J., Cantor, M., and Brown, R.: Gingival healing. II. Clinical and histologic repair sequences following gingivectomy. J. Periodontol., 39:109, 1968.
34. Stahl, S. S.: Periodontal surgery, biologic basis and technique. Springfield, Ill., Charles C Thomas, Publisher, 1976.
35. Stanton, G., Levy, M., and Stahl, S. S.: Collagen restoration in healing human gingiva. J. Dent. Res., 48:27, 1969.
36. Tonna, E., and Stahl, S.: A polarized light microscopic study of rat periodontal ligament following surgical and chemical gingival trauma. Helv. Odont. Acta, 11:90, 1967.
37. Waerhaug, J.: Depth of incision in gingivectomy. Oral Surg., 8:707, 1955.
38. Watanabe, Y., and Suzuki, S.: An experimental study in capillary vascularization in the periodontal tissue following gingivectomy or flap operation. J. Dent. Res., 42:758, 1963.

The Periodontal Flap

A periodontal flap is a section of gingiva and/or mucosa surgically separated from the underlying tissues to provide visibility and access to the bone and root surface. The flap also allows the gingiva to be positioned in a different location in cases of mucogingival involvement.

The basic steps for the flap technique were described early in the 20th century by several clinicians;[6, 15, 21, 22] with some modifications and refinements they consti-

tute the techniques utilized today. The flap operation is used in many different situations and varies according to the degree of flap reflection, the amount of tissues reflected, the types of incisions utilized, and the final position of the flap.

CLASSIFICATION OF FLAPS

Periodontal flaps are classified as either full thickness (mucoperiosteal) or partial thickness (mucosal) flaps (Fig. 50–1). In *full thickness flaps,* all of the soft tissue, including the periosteum, is reflected to expose the underlying bone. This complete exposure and access to the underlying bone is indicated if osseous surgery is contemplated. The full thickness flap is reflected by means of a blunt dissection. A periosteal elevator is used to separate the mucoperiosteum from the bone by moving it mesially, distally, and apically until the desired reflection is accomplished.

The *partial thickness flap* includes only the epithelium and a layer of the underly-

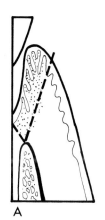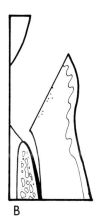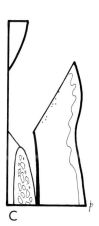

Figure 50–1   Different Types of Flaps.
A, Crevicular and internal bevel incisions are made to reflect either a mucosal or partial thickness flap (*B*) or a mucoperiosteal or full thickness flap (*C*).

A   B   C

ing connective tissue. The bone remains covered by a layer of connective tissue including the periosteum. Sharp dissection is necessary to reflect a partial thickness flap. A surgical scalpel (No. 15 or 11) is utilized to separate the flap carefully. The partial thickness flap is indicated when the flap is to be positioned apically or when the operator does not desire to expose bone.

There are some conflicting data regarding the advisability of uncovering the bone when this is not actually needed. Some writers have shown that marginal bone loss occurs when bone is stripped of its periosteum and that this loss is prevented when the periosteum is left on the bone.[5] Others have shown results that suggest that differences may not be clinically significant.[9] Therefore, the use of the partial thickness flap may be necessary only in cases where the crestal bone margin is very thin and will be exposed when the flap is placed apically. The periosteum left on the bone may also be used in suturing the flap when it is positioned apically.

DESIGN OF THE FLAP

The design of the flap will be dictated by the surgical judgment of the operator and may depend on the objectives of the operation. The degree of access to the underlying bone and root surfaces necessary and the final position of the flap must be considered in designing the flap. Preservation of good blood supply to the flap is a very important consideration.

INCISIONS

Periodontal flaps utilize horizontal and vertical incisions. *Horizontal incisions* are directed along the margin of the gingiva in a mesial or distal direction. Two types of incisions have been recommended: the *crevicular incision*, which starts at the bottom of pocket and is directed to the bone margin, and the *internal bevel incision*,[8] which starts about 1 mm. from the gingival margin and is also aimed at the bone crest. The latter will automatically remove most of the granulation tissue contained in the lateral wall of the pocket, whereas the

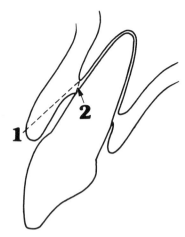

Figure 50–2 Different Horizontal Incisions. *1,* Internal bevel incision. *2,* Crevicular incision.

crevicular incision requires trimming and curetting the flap. When both incisions are made they circumscribe a wedge of tissue that contains the lateral wall of the pocket (Fig. 50–2).

Flaps can be reflected using only the horizontal incision if sufficient access can be obtained by this means and if apical, lateral, or coronal positioning of the flap is not anticipated. If no vertical incisions are made the flap is called an *envelope flap*.

Vertical or oblique releasing incisions can be utilized either on one end of the horizontal incision or on both, depending on the design and purpose of the flap. The vertical incision is necessary at both ends if the flap is to be repositioned. Vertical incisions must extend beyond the mucogingival line, reaching the alveolar mucosa, to allow for the release of the flap to be repositioned.

As a general rule, vertical incisions on the lingual and palatal areas are avoided. Facial vertical incisions should not be made in the center of the interdental papilla or over the radicular surface of a tooth. Incisions should be made at the line angles of a tooth either to include the papilla in the flap or to avoid it completely. The design of the vertical incision should also be such that short (mesial-distal) flaps with long, apically directed horizontal incisions be avoided, since blood supply to the flap could be jeopardized.

The following incisions are recommended.

The horizontally directed incision is

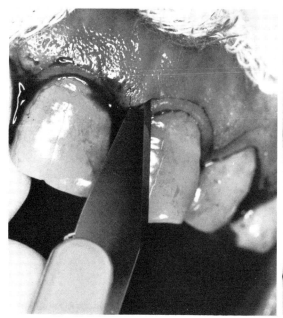

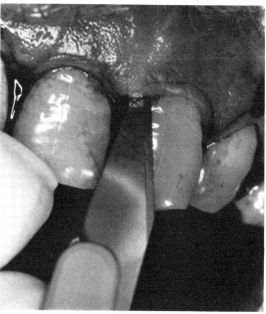

Figure 50–3   Position of Knife in Performing Internal Bevel Incision.

Figure 50–4   Position of Knife in Performing Crevicular Incision.

made using the internal bevel approach (Fig. 50–3). A surgical scalpel (No. 15 or 11) is used to incise slightly away from the gingival margin to the crest of the bone. The ulcerated epithelium lining the pocket and the underlying inflamed connective tissue lies on the tooth side of this incision. A crevicular incision is then made from the base of the pocket to the crest of the bone to release the wedge-shaped tissue between the two incisions (Fig. 50–4). The

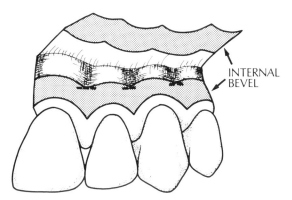

Figure 50–5   After the flap has been elevated, a wedge of tissue remains on the teeth, attached by the base of the papillae. An interdental incision along the horizontal lines seen in the interdental spaces will sever these connections.

gingiva is then reflected either by a blunt or sharp dissection, depending on whether the flap is to be full or partial thickness. The internal bevel incision allows the operator to retain the maximum amount of keratinized gingiva while removing the soft tissue pocket wall. The edge of the flap created by this incision is sharp, and thin and adapts well when placed over the bone.

An *interdental incision* performed after the flap has been elevated will sever the apical connections of the tissue wedge in the interdental spaces and thereby permit an easier and cleaner removal of the tissue (Figs. 50–5 and 50–6).

The internal bevel incision can be *scalloped* or *straight* according to the purpose of the operation. Scalloped incisions allow for complete coverage of the bone and are indicated particularly when reconstructive bone surgery is contemplated. An exaggerated scalloping in the palatal surfaces is suggested in order to obtain a better interproximal flap adaptation. When the purpose of the operation is apical positioning, the scalloping in the facial surfaces loses some of its importance since the flap displacement will make complete wound closure impossible.

Several authors[1, 2, 16, 19] have proposed the

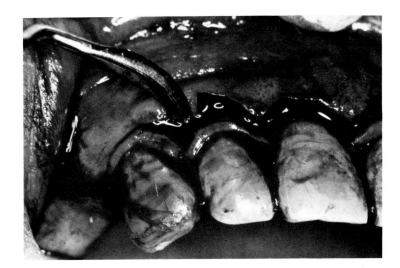

Figure 50–6 Interdental Incision Being Performed. Note the wedge of tissue still attached by its base.

so-called "internal denudation procedure" that consists of horizontal internal bevel incisions removing the gingival papillae and denuding the interdental space. This technique completely eliminates the inflamed interdental areas, which will heal by secondary intention and result in excellent gingival contour. It is contraindicated when bone implants will be used.

MANAGEMENT OF BULBOUS TUBEROSITIES AND RETROMOLAR PADS

The treatment of periodontal pockets on the distal surface of terminal molars is frequently complicated by the presence of bulbous fibrous tissue over the maxillary tuberosity or prominent retromolar pads in the mandible. The most direct approach to pocket elimination in such cases is to resect the bulbous tissue and the pocket wall with a gingivectomy incision (Fig. 50–7). To assure complete removal of the bulbous tissue, the incision is started on the distal surface of the tuberosity and carried forward to the distal surface of the tooth apical to the base of the pocket.

When there is little attached gingiva or there is an infrabony pocket with an osseous defect, it is desirable to reduce the bulbous tissue rather than remove it, for the following reasons: to produce attached gingiva, to provide access to the osseous

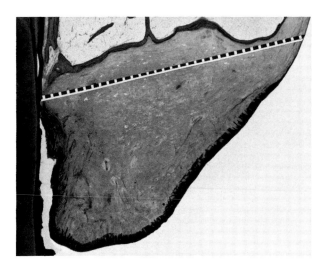

Figure 50–7 Removal of Bulbous Fibrous Tissue over Maxillary Tuberosity with Gingivectomy Incision.

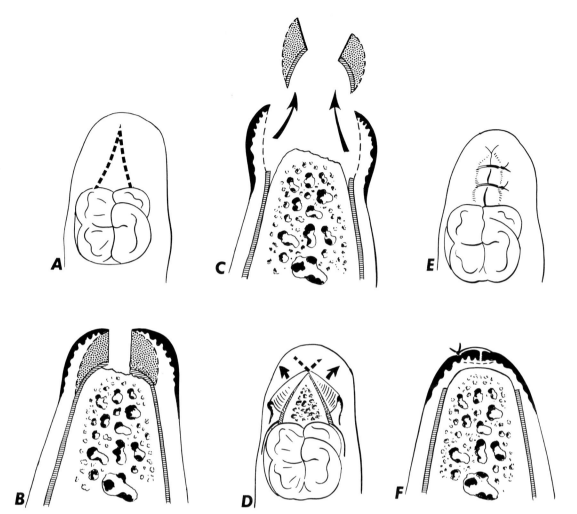

Figure 50–8 Distal Wedge Operation for Reduction of Fibrous Maxillary Tuberosity Pad and Treatment of Osseous Defect. *A,* Distal wedge outlined by triangular incisions. *B,* Section of bulbous fibrous tissue removed, including the periosteum over osseous defect. Additional tissue to be removed is shown in dotted areas. *C,* Fibrous pads removed, including the periosteum (*lined area*), exposing osseous defect and creating thin palatal and buccal flaps. *D,* Releasing incisions (*dotted lines*) provide greater access to underlying bone. Flap extended onto the buccal and palatal surfaces of the molar. *E,* Flaps replaced and sutured after tooth is scaled and smoothed and bone is contoured. *F,* Cross section showing buccal and palatal flaps sutured and bone contoured.

defect, and to preserve mucosa for protection of the healing wound. Reduction of bulbous tuberosity pads or retromolar pads entails removing the central core of tissue responsible for the bulk and preserving the mucosal walls to serve as covering flaps.

Operations for this purpose were described by Robinson[20] and Braden.[3] They may be modified according to individual requirements. The following is a representative procedure.

Step 1. Cut a triangular wedge in the bulbous tuberosity or retromolar pad, extending from the distal surface of the tooth (the base of the triangle) to the distal border of the soft tissue and from the external surface to the periosteum. The facial and lingual incisions should be extended anteriorly for a short distance on the tooth to provide access to the entire distal surface (Fig. 50–8 *A*) and for additional periodontal surgery, if necessary.

Step 2. Deflect the facial and lingual walls of the fibrous pad and, with a periodontal knife, resect the central core of tissue at its base, including the periosteum if recontouring of bone is intended (Fig. 50–8 A).

Step 3. With reverse bevel incisions, undermine the walls of the flaps to the width of the underlying bone. Remove the resected tissue, leaving twin buccal and palatal flaps (Fig. 50–8 B). Separate the flaps and the periosteum from the buccal and lingual surfaces of the tuberosity to increase visibility and access to the bone (Fig. 50–8 C). If necessary, make an oblique releasing incision at the distal end of each flap to avoid tension on the tissues (Fig. 50–8 D).

Step 4. Scale and plane the root surface. If an osseous defect is present, curette the inner walls to remove intact fibers, which interfere with vascularization and healing.

Step 5. Cleanse the area with warm water. Apply pressure with 2 by 2 inch gauze pads until a clot is formed, and remove the excess. Adapt the buccal and lingual flaps over the bone, trimming the edges to avoid overlapping, and suture (Fig. 50–8 E).

PALATAL FLAPS

Osseous defects are frequently corrected more effectively and with less tissue loss when approached from the palate than from the facial surface. Palatal flaps are used for osseous correction and for the reduction of bulbous fibrous tissue. The palatal flap operation consists of resecting the inner aspect of the periodontal pockets with an internal bevel from the tip of the gingival margin to a point apical to the crest of the palatal bone (Fig. 50–9 A). Another approach to thinning palatal flaps is shown in Fig. 50–9 B.

Figure 50–10 shows the steps in a clinical case. After an internal bevel incision, a full thickness flap is separated from the bone to provide access for bone corrective procedures (Fig. 50–10 A, B, and C). The inner aspect of the pockets is removed, the roots are scaled and planed, and the osseous defects are corrected. The flap is replaced, sutured (Fig. 50–10 D), and covered with periodontal pack.

SUTURING TECHNIQUES

There are many types of sutures, suture needles and materials;[7,13] the following methods, using a 3/8 circle reverse cutting needle and 4-0 black braided silk, fill most needs in periodontal surgery.

Interdental Ligation (Figs. 50–11 and 50–12)

Two types of interdental ligation can be used: the direct or loop suture and the figure eight suture.

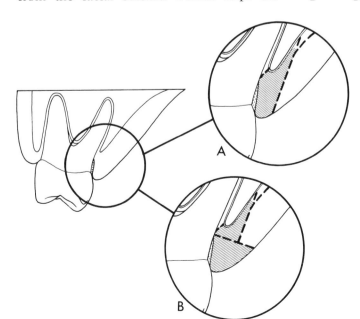

Figure 50–9 Different Types of Incisions for Palatal Flaps. *A,* Internal bevel incision, followed by crevicular incision and removal of wedge of tissue (*shaded*). Note that internal bevel incision is not aimed at bone crest but at a point apical to it depending on thickness of palatal tissue. *B,* Gingevectomy incision followed by internal incision thinning the remaining tissue.

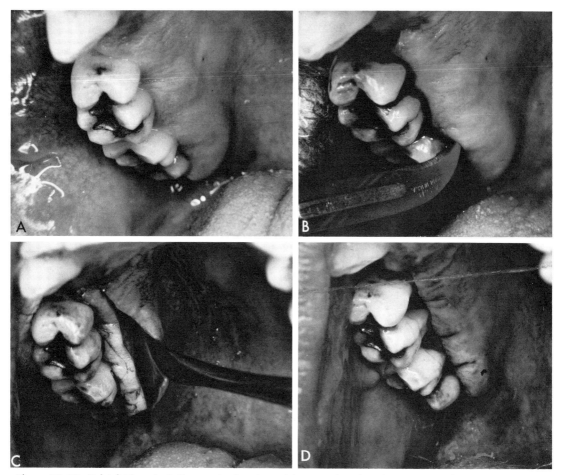

Figure 50–10   Palatal Flap. *A,* Bulbous palatal pad overlying periodontal pockets. *B,* Internal bevel incision resects inner pocket wall and thins palatal gingiva. *C,* Palatal tissue separated from inner pocket wall along line of incision. *D,* Bone is contoured, teeth are scaled and planed and thinned palatal tissue is sutured.

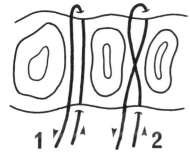

Figure 50–11   Types of Interdental Ligation. *1,* Direct or loop suture. *2,* Figure eight suture. *Arrowheads* indicate direction of tissue penetration during suturing.

The *direct* interdental suture is made by inserting the needle through the facial aspect of the facial flap through the interdental space to penetrate the lingual flap from its inner surface (Fig. 50–12) *A* and *B*). The suture is then passed under the contact point back to the facial side, where it is tied (Fig. 50–12 *C* and *D*).

The so-called *figure eight* interdental suture consists of inserting the needle through the facial aspect of the facial flap through the interdental space to penetrate the lingual flap from its outer surface. It is tied on the facial side. In the figure eight suture, there is thread between the two flaps. It will therefore be used when the

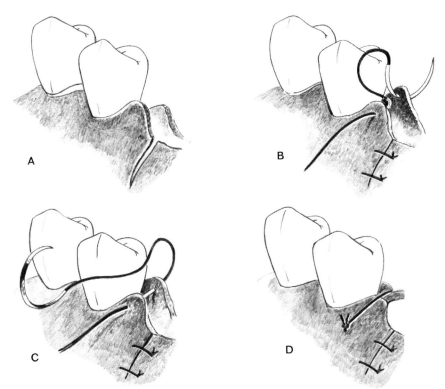

Figure 50–12 Interdental Ligation. *A,* Facial and lingual flaps to be sutured. *B,* The vertical incision is closed by simple, interrupted sutures. To suture interdentally, the needle is inserted through the facial aspect of the facial papilla and through the lingual papilla from its inner side. *C,* The needle is reversed through the same interdental space. *D,* A tie is made on the facial side.

flaps are not in close apposition, because of apical positioning or unscalloped incisions. It is simpler to do than the direct ligation.

The direct suture will permit a better closure of the interdental papillae and is to be performed when bone grafts are used or close apposition of the scalloped incision is required.

Sling Ligation (Fig. 50–13)

Sling ligation can be used for a flap on one surface of a tooth, involving two interdental spaces. The needle is passed from the lingual side, through one of the interdental spaces, beneath the contact point to pierce the facial flap from its inner aspect and emerge on the facial side (Fig. 50–13 *B*). The needle is returned through the same interdental space, the thread passing over the facial flap and then looping around the lingual surface of the tooth

(Fig. 50–13 *C* and *D*). It is then passed through the other interdental space to pierce the facial flap from its inner aspect (Fig. 50–13 *B* and *D*). The needle is reversed through the same interdental space, the thread passing over the facial papilla and the needle emerging on the lingual side (Fig. 50–13 *E*), where the tie is made. The suture is started on the facial side for a lingual flap.

Vertical Mattress Suture (Fig. 50–14)

This suture is used when there is a flap on the facial or lingual surface and another procedure such as gingivectomy on the other. The suture is started in the attached gingiva of the flap, and a vertical "bite" is taken with the needle beneath the interdental papilla (Fig. 50–14 *A* and *B*). The needle is then passed through the interdental space, around the lingual surface of the tooth, and through the next interdental

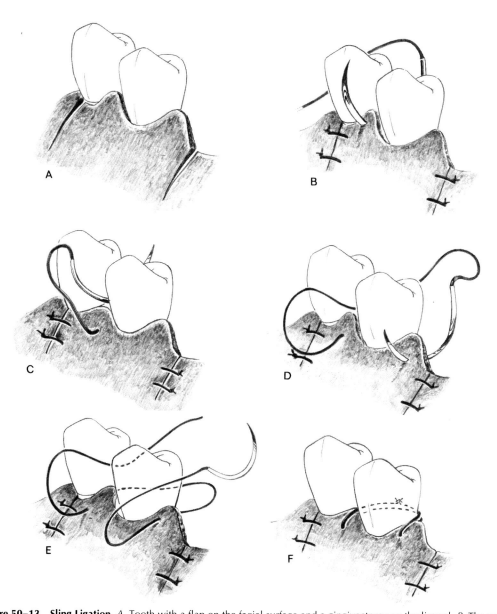

Figure 50–13 Sling Ligation. *A,* Tooth with a flap on the facial surface and a gingivectomy on the lingual. *B,* The vertical incisions are closed by simple, interrupted sutures. The needle is passed through the interdental space from the lingual to the facial side and pierces the flap from its inner aspect. *C,* The needle is returned over the edge of the flap through the same interdental space to the lingual side. *D,* The thread is looped around the lingual surface of the tooth, and the needle is passed through the adjoining interdental space from the lingual side to pierce the flap from its inner aspect. *E,* The needle is reversed through the same interdental space to the lingual side. (Dotted lines show thread on the lingual surface.) *F,* A tie is made on the lingual surface of the tooth (shown in dotted lines).

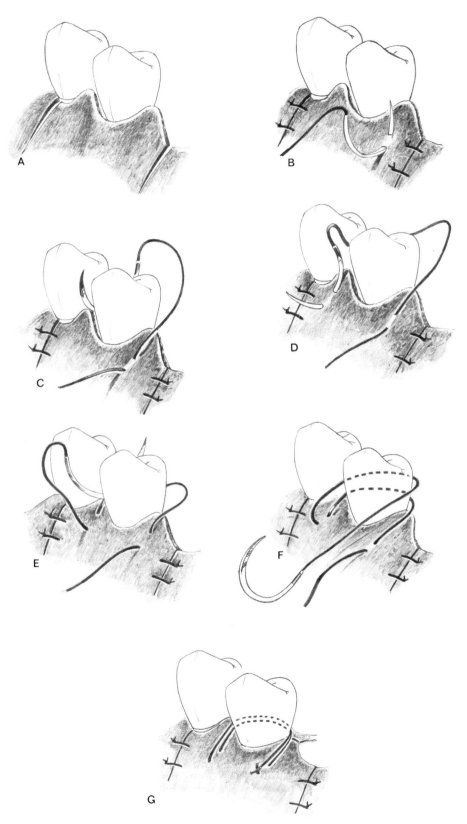

See opposite page for legend.

space to emerge on the facial surface. A vertical "bite" is taken with the needle on the facial surface of the flap beneath the interdental papilla (Fig. 50–14 C and D). The needle is then reversed through the same interdental space (Fig. 50–14 E), around the lingual surface, and through the other interdental space onto the facial surface (Fig. 50–14 F), where a tie is made (Fig. 50–14 G).

Continuous Sling Suture

Type I (Fig. 50–15)

This is used when there is a flap involving many teeth on one surface with another procedure such as gingivectomy on the other surface. The suture closely adapts the flap to the bone and fixes it at the desired level in relation to the bony crest. When suturing a flap on the facial surface, the needle is passed through the corners of the flap distal to the last tooth and tied at the end to hold it there (Fig. 50–15 A). The thread is looped around the distal surface of the tooth and onto the lingual and the needle is passed through the interdental space to emerge on the facial surface. The needle is then reversed, pierces the facial flap from its external aspect, and is returned through the same interdental space (Fig. 50–15 B). The thread is hooked around the lingual surface of the adjacent tooth, and the previous procedure is repeated until the next to last tooth in the group is reached (Fig. 50–15 B). The lingual loop on this tooth is left loose. The needle is then passed through the interdental space to the facial surface. It pierces the flap from the external aspect and is returned through the same interdental space to the lingual surface. A tie is made with the loose loop of thread that was left on the lingual surface (Fig. 50–15 C and D).

Type II (Fig. 50–16)

This is another type of suture that can be used when there is a flap involving many teeth on one surface with another procedure such as gingivectomy on the other surface. For a flap on the facial surface, the needle is started from the lingual side and engages the outer surface of the distogingival corner of the flap. The needle is passed through the flap, leaving a long end on the lingual side which is to be used later for a tie (Fig. 50–16 A). The thread is looped around the distal and lingual surfaces of the last tooth, and the needle is passed through the interdental space to the facial side. It engages the facial flap from its outer aspect, penetrates it and passes back through the same interdental space. This process is continued until the entire flap is sutured (Fig. 50–16 B). The needle is carried through the final interdental space onto the lingual surface, where a tie is made with the long end of the suture initially left there (Fig. 50–16 C and D).

SURGICAL CURETTAGE (MODIFIED WIDMAN FLAP)

The Widman flap, described early in modern periodontal literature, has recently been revised with several refinements. Morris in 1965 described it as "unrepositioned mucoperiosteal flap." He incorporated the internal bevel incision and described the importance of firm apposition of gingival tissue to the root as a prerequisite for success. In 1974, Ramfjord and Nissle[18] described the so-called "modified Widman flap," which was investigated in detail in a longitudinal study. The main advantage of this technique over the closed curettage procedure is that it offers the possibility of establishing an intimate postoperative adaptation of healthy collagenous connective tissue and normal epithelium to

Figure 50–14 **Vertical Mattress Suture.** *A,* Tooth with a facial flap and a lingual gingivectomy. *B,* Vertical incisions are closed by simple, interrupted sutures. Mattress suture is started in the flap by taking a vertical "bite" with the needle. *C,* The needle is then passed through the first interdental space, around the lingual surface of the tooth and through the adjoining interdental space in the direction of the facial surface. *D,* A vertical "bite" is taken with the needle through the external surface of the flap. *E,* The needle is reversed through the second interdental space. *F,* The thread is carried around the lingual surface and the needle is passed through the first interdental space to emerge on the facial side. Dotted lines represent the thread on the lingual surface. *G,* A tie is made on the facial side.

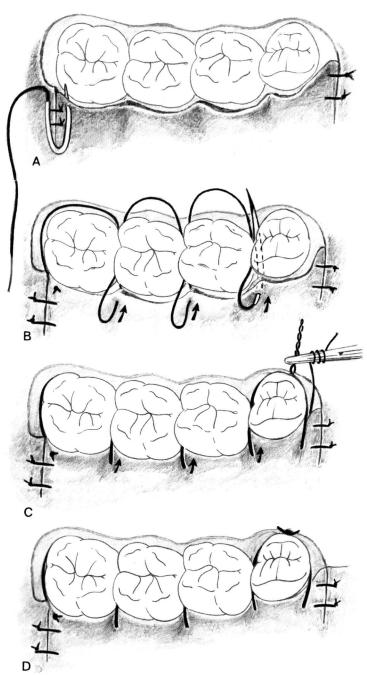

Figure 50–15 Continuous Sling Suture, Type I. *A,* Section of the mouth with flap operation on the facial surface and gingivectomy on the lingual. Vertical incisions are closed with interrupted sutures. The needle is inverted into the disto-gingival corner of the flap for an initial tie. *B,* The needle is being returned to the lingual side of the interdental space, after penetrating the flap from its outer aspect. *C,* Loose loop of thread left on the lingual surface of the premolar is twisted and tied with the other end of the suture. *D,* Tie is made on the lingual surface of the premolar.

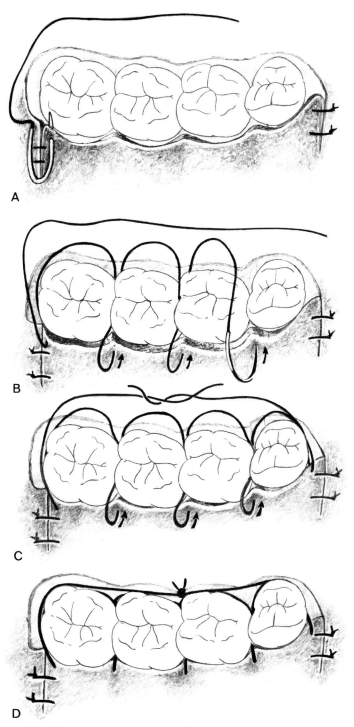

Figure 50–16 Continuous Sling Suture, Type II. *A,* Section of the mouth with flap on the facial surface and gingivectomy on the lingual. The two vertical incisions are closed with interrupted sutures. The needle has been passed from the lingual surface to the external surface of the facial flap and through the distogingival corner of it. One end of the thread is left on the lingual side. *B,* The thread passes around the distal and lingual surfaces and the needle is passed through the interdental space to the facial side. It engages the facial flap from its outer aspect and is passed back through the same interdental space to the lingual. *C,* Suturing is completed on the mesial aspect of the second premolar and the suture is tied with the end of the thread initially left on the lingual side. *D,* Lingual tie is completed.

tooth surfaces.[17] The modified Widman flap provides access for adequate instrumentation of the root surfaces and immediate closure of the area. The following is a step-by-step description of the procedure (Fig. 50–17).

1. The initial incision is a scalloped internal bevel incision to the alveolar crest and 1 to 2 mm. away from the gingival margin (Fig. 50–17 C). Care should be taken to insert the blade in such a way that the papilla is left with similar thickness as the remaining facial flap. Vertical relaxing incisions are usually not needed.

2. The gingiva is reflected with a periosteal elevator (Fig. 50–17 E).

3. A crevicular incision is made from the bottom of the pocket to the bone, circumscribing the triangular wedge of tissue containing the pocket wall (Fig. 50–17 D).

4. A third incision is made in the interdental spaces coronal to the bone with a curette or an interproximal knife, and the gingival collar is removed (Fig. 50–17 F and G).

5. Tissue tags and granulation tissue are removed with a curette. The root surfaces are checked and scaled and planed if needed (Fig. 50–17 H). Residual peridontal fibers attached to the tooth surface should not be disturbed.

6. Bone architecture is not corrected except when it prevents good tissue adaptation to the necks of the teeth. Every effort is made to adapt the facial and lingual interproximal tissue adjacent to each other so that no interproximal bone remains exposed at the time of suturing (Fig. 50–17 I). The flaps may be thinned to allow for close adaptation of the gingiva around the entire circumference of the tooth and to each other interproximally.

7. Interrupted direct sutures are placed in each interdental space (Fig. 50–17 J) and covered with Achromycin ointment and with periodontal surgical pack.

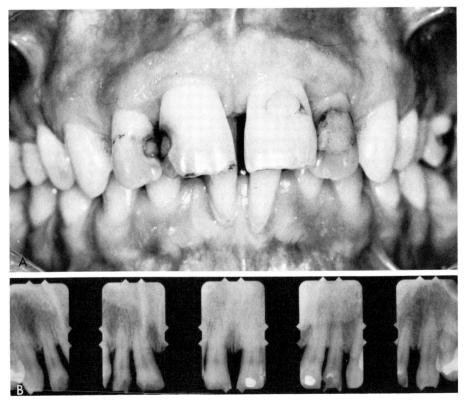

Figure 50–17 The Modified Widman Flap Technique. *A,* Facial view before surgery. Probing of pockets revealed interproximal depths ranging from 4 to 8 mm. and facial and palatal depths of 2 to 5 mm. *B,* Radiographic survey of area. Note generalized horizontal bone loss.

(Illustration continued on the opposite page)

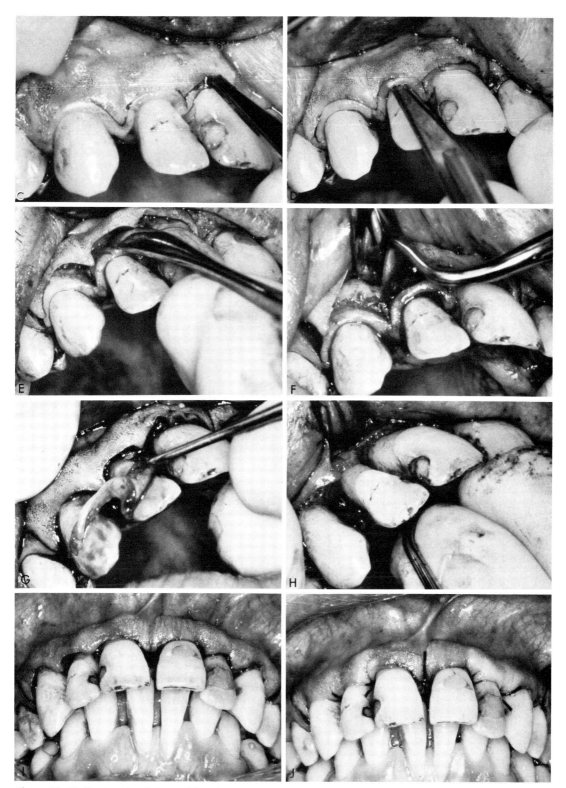

Figure 50–17 *Continued.* *C,* Internal bevel incision. *D,* Crevicular incision. *E,* Elevation of the flap leaving a wedge of tissue still attached by its base. *F,* Interdental incision sectioning the base of the papilla. *G,* Removal of tissue. *H,* Exposure of root surfaces and marginal bone; root planing and removal of remaining calculus. *I,* Replacement of flap in its original position. *H,* Interdental sutures in place. (Courtesy of Dr. Raul G. Caffesse, Ann Arbor, Michigan.)

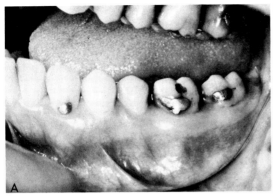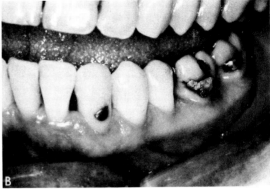

Figure 50–18   A case before (A) and after (B) treatment by means of Widman flaps. Note the reduction in gingival height and concomitant pocket depth. (Courtesy of Dr. Raul G. Caffesse, Ann Arbor, Michigan.)

Ramfjord and coworkers[17] have performed a longitudinal study comparing the Widman procedure, as modified by them, with the curettage technique and the pocket elimination methods that include bone contouring when needed. The techniques were selected at random and results analyzed yearly up to seven years post-therapy. They reported approximately similar results with the three methods tested. Pocket depth was initially similar for all methods but was maintained shallower with the Widman flap (Fig. 50–18); the attachment level remained higher with the Widman flap.

REFERENCES

1. Barkann, L.: A conservative surgical technique for the eradication of pyorrhea pockets. J. Am. Dent. Assoc., 26:61, 1939.
2. Beube, F. E.: Interdental tissue resection: an experimental study of a surgical technique which aids in repair of the periodontal tissues to their original contour and function. Oral Surg., 33:497, 1947.
3. Braden, B. E.: Deep distal pockets adjacent to terminal teeth. Dent. Clin. North Am., 161, 1969.
4. Carranza, F. A., Sr.: Tratamiento Quirurgico de la Paradentosis (Piorrea Alveolar). Thesis, University of Buenos Aires, 1935.
5. Carranza, F. A., Jr., and Carraro, J. J.: Effect of removal of periosteum on postoperative result of mucogingival surgery. J. Periodontol., 34:223, 1963.
6. Cieszynski, A.: Bemerkungen zur radikal-chirurgischen Behandlung der sogennante Pyorrhea Alveolaris. Deutsche Monatschr. für Zahnh., 32:376, 1914.
7. Dahlberg, W. H.: Incisions and suturing: some basic considerations about each in periodontal flap surgery. Dent. Clin. North Am., 149, 1969.
8. Friedman, N.: Mucogingival surgery: the apically repositioned flap. J. Periodontol., 33:328, 1962.
9. Hoag, P. M., Wood, D. L., Donnenfeld, O. W., and Rosenfeld, L. D.: Alveolar crest reduction following full and partial thickness flaps. J. Periodontol., 43:141, 1972.
10. Kirkland, O.: The suppurative periodontal pus pocket: its treatment by the modified flap operation. J. Am. Dent. Assoc., 18:1462, 1931.
11. Levine, H. L., and Stahl, S. S.: Repair following periodontal flap surgery with the retention of gingival fibers. J. Periodontol., 43:99, 1972.
12. Matelski, D. E., and Hurt, W. C.: The corrective phase: the modified Widman flap. In W. C. Hunt (Ed.): Periodontics in General Practice. Springfield, Illinois, C C Thomas, 1976.
13. Morris, M. L.: Suturing techniques in periodontal surgery. Periodontics, 3:84, 1965.
14. Morris, M. L.: The unrepositioned mucoperiosteal flap. Periodontics 3:141, 1965.
15. Neumann, R.: Die Alveolar-Pyorrhea und ihre Behandlung. Berlin: H. Meusser, 1912.
16. Prichard, J. F.: Present state of the interdental denudation procedure. J. Periodontol. 48:566, 1977.
17. Ramfjord, S. P.: Present status of the modified Widman flap procedure. J. Periodontol., 48:558, 1977.
18. Ramfjord, S. P., and Nissle, R. R.: The modified Widman flap. J. Periodontol., 45:601, 1974.
19. Ratcliff, P. A., and Raust, G. T.: Interproximal denudation: a conservative approach to osseous surgery. Dent. Clin. North Am., 121, 1964.
20. Robinson, R. E.: The distal wedge operation. Periodontics, 4:256, 1966.
21. Widman, L.: The operative treatment of pyorrhea alveolaris. A new surgical method. Sven. Tandlak. Tidskm. (special issue), Dec. 1918.
22. Zentler, A.: Suppurative gingivitis with alveolar involvement. J.A.M.A., 71:1530, 1918.

Chapter 51

Osseous Surgery

TREATMENT OF INFRABONY POCKETS

The infrabony pocket differs from the suprabony pocket in that it is situated in an osseous defect with its base apical to the margin of the alveolar bone rather than coronal to it. An infrabony pocket is initiated, like any other pocket, by an inflammatory reaction due to the irritation derived from bacterial plaque.

The defect underlying an infrabony pocket is vertical or angular rather than horizontal; trans-septal fibers in infrabony pockets are oblique rather than horizontal, extending from the cementum beneath the base of the pocket, along the bone, and over the crest to the cementum of the adjacent tooth.

One or more of the following factors may act so that a pocket becomes infrabony (1) trauma from occlusion; (2) food impaction; and (3) anatomical characteristics of underlying bone in the area (wide alveolar ridges) that maintain their height in a region far from the tooth side.

Classification of Infrabony Pockets

The classification of infrabony pockets is discussed in Chapter 14.

Detection and Diagnosis of Infrabony Pockets

The type of pocket should be established in the initial session(s) devoted to diagnosis and treatment planning so that their prognosis can be determined and the techniques necessary for their eradication selected.

Radiographic examination can reveal the existence of angular bone losses in the interdental spaces, and these usually coincide with infrabony pockets. The radiograph will not show the number of bony walls of the defect, nor will it determine with any degree of accuracy the presence of angular bony defects in facial or lingual surfaces. Clinical examination and probing will determine the presence and depth of periodontal pockets in any surface of any tooth; but it does not show whether the pocket is suprabony or infrabony. Both examinations, clinical and radiographic, can suggest the presence of infrabony pockets when the following are found:

1. Angular bone losses.
2. Irregular bone losses.
3. Pockets of irregular depth in adjacent areas of the same tooth or in adjacent teeth.

None of the above mentioned techniques will show the number of bony walls of a vertical defect or its general morphology.

Under local anesthesia, the underlying osseous morphology can be ascertained by probing from the bottom of the pocket both apically and laterally to the alveolar bone. Lateral "sounding" from the gingival surface can also be helpful. Because anesthesia is required, this technique is of limited use.

Infrabony pockets can appear in any surface of any tooth. A study of human skulls has shown that three-wall angular bone loss

843

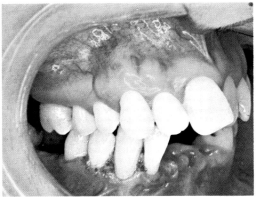

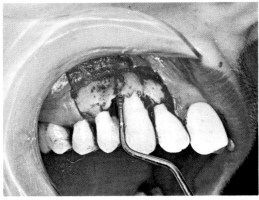

A, Before treatment.

B, Deep three wall infrabony defect with measuring probe inserted.

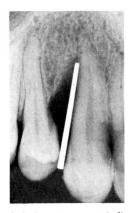

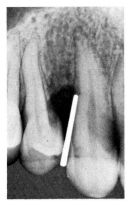

C, Radiograph before treatment indicates angular osseous defect. Gutta percha point extends to base of pocket.

D, Nine months after treatment. Radiograph indicates repair of osseous defect. Gutta percha point shows new level of sulcus.

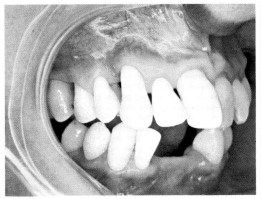

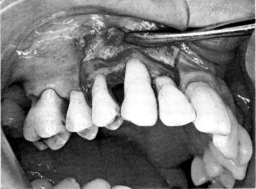

E, Nine months after treatment. Gingiva healed with physiologic contour.

F, Elevation of flap confirms radiographic appearance of repaired bone defect and reattachment of periodontium to tooth.

Plate VII   Flap Operation for Infrabony Pocket.

(intrabony lesions) is most common on the mesial surface of the maxillary and mandibular second and third molars. In some areas, such as the facial aspect of upper incisors, the bone plate is usually very thin and is lost completely, but the bony plate becomes thicker close to the apex, and an angular pattern of bone loss can then be produced.

Modes of Treatment

The periodontal pocket and the osseous defect are interrelated. Successful treatment requires that both be eliminated, because the persistence of one leads to the recurrence of the other.

Osseous defects associated with infrabony pockets may be corrected: (1) by *regeneration of the alveolar crest;* that is, by filling in with new bone and reattachment of new periodontal fibers to the root, or (2) by *surgically remodeling the defect,* that is, trimming the walls of the defect to eliminate it. Alveolar regeneration is the more desirable; it occurs often and in response to different treatment techniques, but not consistently enough to be predictable.[68] The healing process fills in the osseous defect and restores smooth physiological bone contours (Color Plate VII). Nature reduces sharp bony margins, eliminates abrupt inconsistencies between the bone levels interdentally and on the roots, and reduces the facial and lingual walls of interdental craters while filling in the depressed craters with new bone

The likelihood of obtaining "bone fill" depends in large measure on the architec-

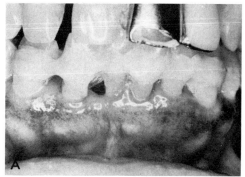
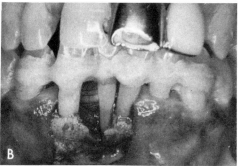
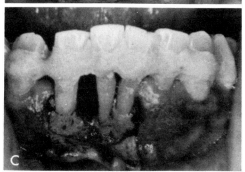
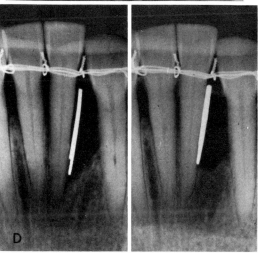

Figure 51–1   Flap Operation Followed by Repair of Two and One-Half Wall Infrabony Defect. (Part of a clinical experiment. Patur and Glickman.[68]) *A,* Mandibular teeth splinted with wire ligature covered with acrylic. *B,* Before treatment, flap reveals two and one-half wall osseous defect. It consists of a lingual wall, proximal wall, and one-half wall on the facial surface.

C, Eight and one-half months after treatment without artificially reshaping the bone. Bone defect filled and bone recontoured by the natural healing process. *D, Left,* Before treatment. Bone defect with silver point at base of pocket. *Right,* After eight and one-half months bone defect repaired. Clinical measurements indicate 3.5 mm. increase in bone height and 4.5 mm. soft tissue reattachment.

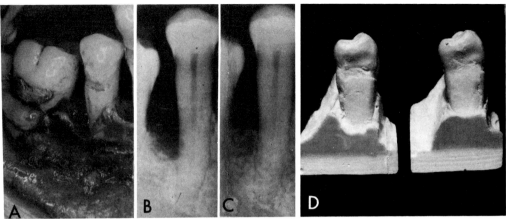

Figure 51–2 Repair of Two-Wall Osseous Infrabony Defect Following Flap Operation (Patur and Glickman). *A,* Flap reveals two-wall defect on distal surface of second premolar. It consists of a lingual wall and a proximal wall. *B,* Before treatment. Radiographs of defect shown in *A. C,* Seven and one-half months after treatment without osseous surgery. The bone is repaired; there is a 4 mm. increase in bone height and 4.5 mm. soft tissue reattachment. (Bone repair occurred despite fact that proximal contact was not restored because of conditions of clinical experiment in which this case was treated.)

D, Models from impressions taken of the bone distal to the premolar before treatment and after seven and one-half months. Note that the crater has been filled in and recontoured by natural healing process.

ture and the number of bony walls in the defect.[70] Broad, shallow defects are less likely to be filled in with bone than narrow, deep ones. The prognosis is best in three-wall osseous defects; two and two-and-one-half wall defects also undergo satisfactory repair but less consistently (Figs. 51–1 and 51–2). One-wall osseous defects tend to persist after treatment; there may be a slight reduction in the height of the osseous wall and an increased radiopacity of the inner surface, but the pocket generally recurs.

Selection of treatment technique

The morphology of the osseous defect will to a great extent determine the treatment technique to be followed. One-wall angular defects usually will have to be recontoured surgically.

Three-wall defects, particularly if they are narrow and deep, can be successfully treated by techniques aiming at reattachment and bone regeneration. Two-wall angular defects can be treated by either method depending on their depth, width, and general configuration.

Therefore, except for one-wall defects, infrabony pockets are treated with the objective of obtaining optimal repair of natural healing processes.

Since the general morphology of the underlying bone cannot be adequately determined by the radiograph, a definitive re-evaluation and final decision will have to be made after surgical exposure. The technique of choice for treating vertical defects will therefore be the flap operation, since it is the only method that will permit a clear visual examination of the defect. Sometimes, however, other techniques (curettage, gingivectomy) may be attempted, particularly if the defect is included in an area that will be treated with those methods.

REATTACHMENT AND BONE REGENERATION

Four critical areas are basic to all techniques for treating infrabony pockets and their associated osseous defects (Fig. 51–3): (1) the soft tissue pocket wall, (2) the root surface, (3) the periodontal fibers covering the bone surface, and (4) the walls of the osseous defect.

MANAGEMENT OF THE SOFT TISSUE POCKET WALL. The soft tissue wall consists of the epithelial lining of the pocket, the junctional epithelium, and the adjacent granulation tissue. The epithelial structures must be removed to make it possible for new connective tissue fibers to reattach to the tooth surface (Fig. 51–3*B*). If the

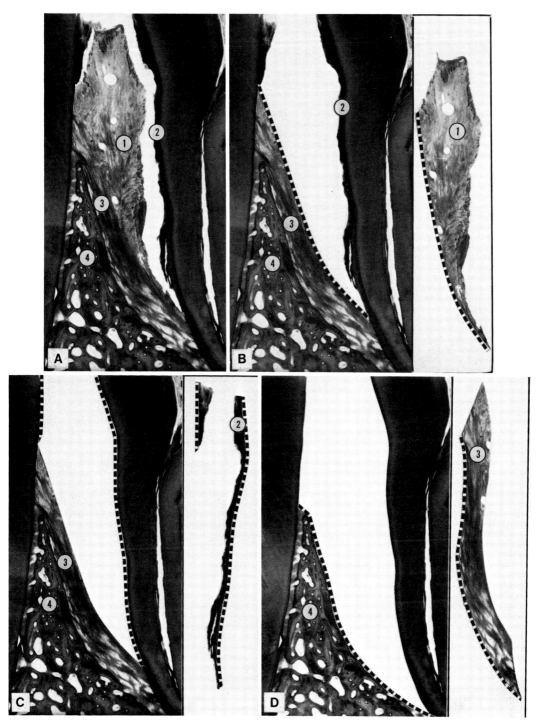

Figure 51–3 Four Critical Areas in the Treatment of Infrabony Pockets. *A,* (1) The soft tissue pocket wall. (2) The root surface. (3) The periodontal fibers that cover the bone surface. (4) The walls of the osseous defect. *B,* The inner lining of the pocket wall (1) is removed. *C,* The calculus (2) is removed and the roots are planed. *D,* The periodontal ligament fibers (3) are removed from the bone, leaving the scarified walls of the osseous defect (4).

junctional epithelium is permitted to remain, it will be joined by proliferating epithelium from the adjacent gingiva and will form an epithelial barrier between the healing connective tissue and the tooth. This will re-create the pocket, obstruct the connective tissue from reaching the root, and prevent filling in of the osseous defect (Fig. 51–4).

MANAGEMENT OF THE ROOT SURFACE. The root surface should be prepared for the deposition of new cementum and the embedding of new periodontal ligament fibers. It must be meticulously

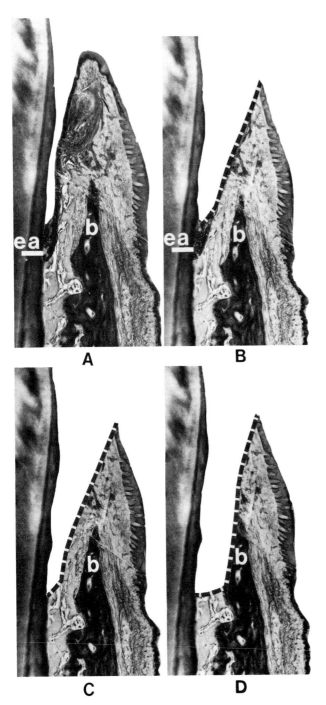

A   **B**

C   **D**

Figure 51–4   Removal of the Junctional Epithelium in the Treatment of Infrabony Pockets (A Composite Illustration). *A,* Infrabony pocket on the facial surface, showing the relationship of the junctional epithelium (ea) at the bottom of the pocket to the bone (b). *B,* Incomplete removal of pocket lining (*dotted line*) leaves the junctional epithelium on the tooth. *C,* Complete removal of the junctional epithelium (*dotted line*) creates the possibility of reattachment of new periodontal ligament fibers. *D,* Removal of periodontal ligament fibers from the bone surface (*dotted line*) facilitates migration of osteogenic cells from the bone into the defect.

scaled and planed to remove all deposits, softened tooth structure, and adherent remnants of the junctional epithelium (Fig. 51–3C).

MANAGEMENT OF PERIODONTAL FIBERS COVERING THE BONE SURFACE. In infrabony pockets, periodontal ligament fibers extend in an angular course over the surfaces of the osseous defects. One of the effects of abnormal occlusal forces upon the periodontium is to alter the alignment of the transseptal fibers (interproximally) and the alveolar crest fibers (facially and lingually). When infrabony pockets are formed, the walls of the angular (vertical) bone defects are covered with these fibers, and both the bone surface and fibers are aligned perpendicular to the direction of the injurious force. The fibers must be removed to permit the flow of blood and osteogenic cells into the osseous defect (Fig. 51–4D). Intact fibers must be firmly curetted from the bone surface. When inflamed, the fibers undergo degeneration and are partially or completely replaced by granulation tissue, which is more easily removed.

MANAGEMENT OF THE WALLS OF THE OSSEOUS DEFECT. The walls of the osseous defect should be curetted to form a clean surface with numerous small bleeding points. In some long-standing pockets, condensation of bone has produced a comparatively dense cortical wall. If necessary, perforations may be made in the bone surface with a small round bur[63] to facilitate passage of blood and osteogenic cells from the bone into the osseous defect.

Techniques for Reattachment and Bone Regeneration

Reconstruction of the periodontium destroyed by inflammatory periodontal disease is one of the major goals of periodontal therapy. Recently, a vast number of human and animal studies have been devoted to the concept of restoration of destroyed periodontium rather than removal of irregularities through osseous resection. A serious attempt has been made to find an organic or inorganic material and a technique that will rebuild defects caused by periodontal disease. Therefore, in order to avoid bone recontouring and the subsequent loss of bony support, various surgical methods aimed at eliminating the intrabony defects through regeneration of new bone, cementum, and fibrous attachment have been proposed. This solution affords the ideal result of periodontal therapy, i.e., a fully restored, functionally healthy periodontium.

The term *reattachment* is often used to express the objective of reconstructive periodontal surgery. The term *new attachment* has been suggested.[72] Both terms are used interchangeably in this text.

Reconstructive periodontics can be subdivided into two major areas. Non-graft associated new attachment and graft associated new attachment.

Traditionally, the earliest reattachment experiments were carried out using subgingival curettage. Observations in humans[85, 103] have indicated that a reduction in the depth of periodontal pockets may occur with subgingival curettage (see Chapter 47). A shallower pocket following curettage may be due in part to re-establishment of a connective tissue attachment in the bottom of the pocket, and in part to shrinkage of the inflamed tissue.[5] Radiographic evidence of bone regeneration has also been shown after subgingival curettage.[15, 16, 39, 73, 85, 103]

EXCISIONAL NEW ATTACHMENT PROCEDURE (ENAP)

Past results indicate, however, that soft tissue curettage may not be a reliable procedure for gaining new attachment. The technical problems of execution, particularly access to and visualization of the root surface and proper management of the soft tissue wall, may be partially to blame. Accordingly, the excisional new attachment procedure (ENAP), which is definitive subgingival curettage performed with a knife, was developed to accomplish proper soft tissue preparation, gain better access to the root surface, and take advantage of new understanding of wound healing mechanisms. The ENAP has been used in the Navy Dental Corps for more than eight years with clinically satisfactory results but has not been adequately documented or experimentally evaluated.[91]

The ENAP is indicated when there is

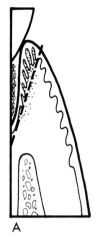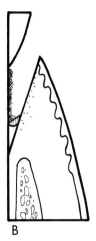

Figure 51–5   Excisional New Attachment Procedure. *A,* Internal bevel incision to point below bottom of pocket. *B,* After excision of tissue, scaling and root planing are performed.

shallow to moderate pocket depth coronal to the mucogingival junction. It is particularly applicable in the anterior region, where appearance is a consideration.

TECHNIQUE.[69] Once the patient has established plaque control and phase I therapy is complete:

1. Anesthetize the area.

2. Measure pocket depth with a probe and penetrate the gingival tissue at this distance with the probe.

3. Make a reverse bevel (internally beveled) incision with a surgical blade from the margin of the free gingiva apically to a point below the depth of the pocket (Fig. 51–5).

4. Carry the incision interproximally on both the facial and the lingual sides, attempting to retain as much interproximal tissue as possible. The intention is to cut the inner portion of the soft tissue wall of the pocket, all around the tooth. No attempt is made to break through the mucogingival junction.

5. Remove the excised tissue with a curette.

6. Carefully root plane all cementum that has been exposed to the oral cavity to a smooth, hard consistency. Preserve all connective tissue fibers that remain attached to the root surface.

7. Rinse the area with normal saline solution and examine the root surface to en-

sure that no calculus remains and that no large clots are present.

8. Approximate the wound edges. If the edges do not meet passively, contour the bone until good adaptation of wound edges is achieved. Healing of the wound edges by secondary intention is imperative.

9. Suture interproximally with interrupted or vertical mattress sutures.

10. Apply pressure to the operative site for two or three minutes from both facial and lingual aspects with saline-soaked gauze in order to permit only a thin clot to form between the tissue and the tooth.

11. Place a periodontal dressing over the site without forcing the dressing between the tooth and the tissue.

12. Remove the sutures in seven days and polish the area. Carefully review plaque control of the area with the patient. Advise the patient to brush and floss the area carefully but meticulously. Success is dependent on the patient's ability to control plaque during the critical first three or four weeks of healing.

13. Do not probe for three months in order to permit complete attachment of connective tissue fibers.

Clinical studies in humans[106] and animals[105] using this technique have shown considerable reduction in pocket depth. Histological study using monkeys[105] revealed a long thin junctional epithelium with a minimum amount of inflammation in the subjacent densely collagenous lamina propria.

ACID DEMINERALIZATION OF THE ROOT SURFACE

Recently, Register[74-76] has put considerable emphasis on the induction of new attachment through demineralization of root surfaces. This hypothesis is based on animal experiments by Urist[10, 101, 102] and Bang[3] demonstrating bone induction properties of intramuscular implants of dentin demineralized in vitro.

The technique consists of simply rubbing exposed root surfaces with a cotton applicator soaked in citric acid at pH 1.0 for two minutes. The teeth must be planed to remove cementum prior to demineralization. An effort should be made to avoid contact with surrounding periodontium during root dentin demineralization by suctioning away excess acid at the apical border of the wound. When demineralization is completed, teeth are suctioned to remove the remaining acid but should not be rinsed. The flaps are replaced.

Though human studies as well as animal experiments[74-76, 97] have been undertaken, the effectiveness and predictability of this technique have not been established, and further study is necessary.

Graft Materials and Procedures

Traditionally, periodontal reconstruction using non-graft material is best accomplished in the three-wall pocket[40] and the periodontal and endodontal abscess.[44, 63] However, the defects left by most periodontal diseases are not of three-wall configuration. Therefore, numerous other therapeutic grafting modalities for restoring these defects have been investigated and attempted. Several authors have advocated that in new attachment attempts employing a flap procedure, bone grafts should be inserted into the angular defects in order to improve bone regeneration and achieve a greater amount of new connective tissue attachment.[17, 46, 64, 65, 79, 80, 88]

Periodontal defects as sites for bone transplantation differ from osseous cavities surrounded by bony walls. Saliva and bacteria may easily penetrate along the root surface, and epithelial cells may proliferate into the defect, resulting in contamination and possible exfoliation of the grafts. Therefore, the principles established to govern transplantation of bone into closed osseous cavities may not be fully applicable to transplantation of bone into periodontal defects.[29]

The considerations that govern the selection of a material have been defined by Schallhorn:[91]

1. Biological acceptability.
2. Predictability.
3. Clinical feasibility.
4. Minimal operative hazards.
5. Minimal postoperative sequelae.
6. Patient acceptance.

Naturally, it is difficult to find a material that encompasses all these characteristics, and to date there is no "ideal" material or technique.

Once the material is placed in the bony defect it may act in a number of ways. It may have no effect, it may act only as a scaffolding material for the host to lay down new bone, it may actively induce bone formation, or through its own viability it may deposit new bone in the defect.

Graft materials have been developed and tried in many complex forms. To familiarize the reader with various types of graft material as defined by either the technique or the material used, a brief discussion of each is provided.

AUTOGENOUS BONE AUTOGRAFTS

Bone from intra-oral site

Nabers and O'Leary[64] were among the first in the contemporary literature to describe the use of intraoral donor sites for periodontal bony defect transplants. They used cortical shavings of bone from various intraoral sites to augment periodontal bony defects. If the bony walls of the defects were dense, multiple perforations were made into the bone with a small round bur to facilitate vascularization of the graft. Other sources of bone include healing extraction wounds,[47] edentulous ridges,[79] bone trephined from within the jaw without damaging the roots, newly formed bone in wounds especially created for the purpose,[42] and bone removed during osteoplasty and ostectomy. The last has received great popularity largely due to the technique by Robinson.[78]

OSSEOUS COAGULUM. Robinson[78] described a technique using a mixture of bone dust and blood that he termed *osseous coagulum* for repair of bony defects. The technique uses small bony particles ground from cortical bone. The advantage of the particle size is that it provides additional surface area for interaction of cellular and vascular elements. The technique may be described as follows:

Step 1. Preparing the recipient site. After presurgical scaling and occlusal adjustment as required, the defect is exposed by elevating a mucoperiosteal flap with an internal bevel. Root deposits and granulation tissue are removed, the root is planed, and the bony walls of the defect are perforated with a small round bur or a stainless steel cowhorn explorer.

Step 2. Obtaining the implant. Sources of the implant material include the lingual ridge on the mandible, exostoses, edentulous ridges, the bone distal to a terminal tooth, bone removed by osteoplasty or ostectomy, and the lingual surface of the mandible or maxilla at least 5 mm. from the roots. Bone is removed with a carbide bur, No. 6 or No. 8, at speeds between 5000 and 30,000 r.p.m. The coagulum formed by mixing the bone particles and blood is placed in a sterile dappen dish or amalgam cloth.

Step 3. Placing the implant. The coagulum is placed in the defect a little at a time, starting at the bottom and packing and drying with moist gauze until there is a considerable excess. The flap is replaced over the coagulum, sutured, compressed with moist gauze for three minutes, and covered with appropriate periodontal dressing. Appropriate antibiotics are recommended for three to seven days beginning the evening before surgery, and the sutures and pack are removed after a week. The patient follows up with plaque control. (Fig. 51–6).

The obvious advantage of this technique is the ease of obtaining bone from already exposed surgical sites. This technique is also very quick to accomplish and can be done in areas without great preparation. In addition, it complements osseous resective techniques needed in the area.

The disadvantages of the technique are centered on relatively low predictability[34] and inability to procure adequate material for large defects. The major criticism of this technique has been its nearly total

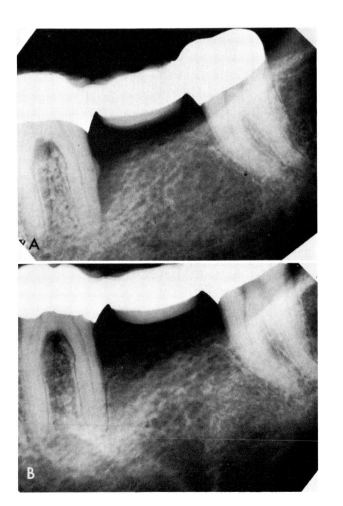

Figure 51–6 Bony Defect on Distal Root of First Molar Treated With Osseous Coagulum Implants. *A,* Before treatment. *B,* One year after treatment. (Courtesy of Dr. R. Earl Robinson, San Mateo, California.)

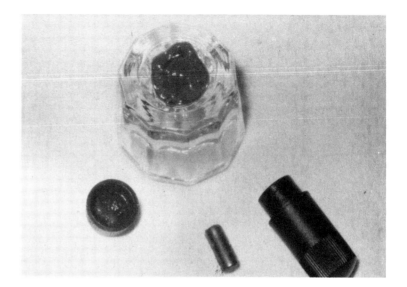

Figure 51–7 The sterile capsule shown above is used to produce the soft pliable osseous mass present in the top of dappen dish.

reliance on cortical bone for graft material. Although notable success has been obtained by many individuals in conservative defects, studies documenting the technique's efficacy are still inconclusive.[18, 34, 36, 77]

BONE BLEND. Some disadvantages of using osseous coagulum derive from the inability to use the aspiration during accumulation of the coagulum as well as the unknown quantity and quality of the bone fragments in the collected material. To overcome these problems, Diem, Bowers, and Moffett[20] have proposed the so-called "bone blend" technique.

The bone blend technique uses an autoclaved plastic capsule and pestle. Bone is removed from a predetermined site (extraction socket, exostosis, edentulous area, region of defect) by chisels or rongeur forceps. The pestle and bone fragments are placed in the capsule and a few drops of sterile saline are added. The capsule is closed, wrapped in sterile gauze, and placed in the triturator. The bone is triturated for 60 seconds. A dense mass of bone, such as that removed from an exostosis, may require more blending time. After trituration the bone blend is observed clinging to the walls of the capsule and to the pestle. It is removed from the capsule with a spoon-shaped instrument. Trituration reduces the bone fragments to a workable, plastic-like osseous mass, similar to slushy amalgam in consistency, which can be "packed" or molded into bony defects (Fig. 51–7).

Froum[36-38] has studied this technique extensively by comparing it to iliac autografts and open curettage and found osseous coagulum–bone blend procedures to be at least as effective.

INTRAORAL CANCELLOUS BONE MARROW TRANSPLANTS. Hiatt and Schallhorn[47] have described the use of cancellous bone obtained from the maxillary tuberosity, edentulous areas, and healing sockets.

The maxillary tuberosity frequently contains a good amount of cancellous bone, particularly if the third molars are not present; also, foci of red marrow are occasionally observed. After a ridge incision distally from the last molar, bone is removed with a curved and cutting rongeur. Care should be taken not to extend the incision too far distally to avoid sectioning the tendons of the palatine muscle; also, the location of the maxillary sinus has to be analyzed in the radiograph in order to avoid opening into it.

Edentulous ridges can be approached with a flap, and cancellous bone and marrow are removed with curettes. Healing sockets are allowed to heal for eight weeks, and the apical portion is utilized as donor material. The particles are reduced to small pieces. (Figs. 51–8 and 51–9).

The recipient site is opened with a full

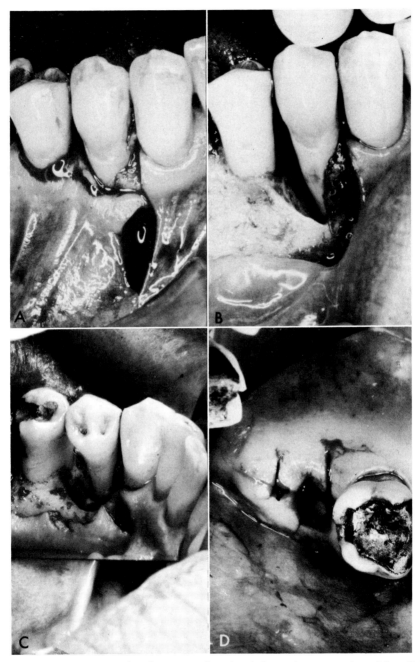

Figure 51–8   Autogenous Bone Transplant from Extraction Site. *A,* Separating mucoperiosteal flap. *B,* Buccal view of angular defect on the distal surface of the first premolar. *C,* Elevating lingual mucoperiosteal flap and view of angular defect. *D,* Bone obtained from six week old extraction site.

(Illustration continued on opposite page)

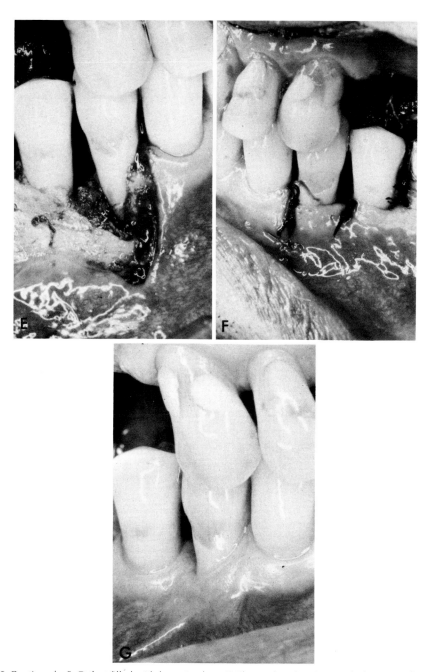

Figure 51–8 *Continued* E, Defect filled with bone implant. F, Flap replaced and sutured. G, Two and one-half months after treatment. Note excellent gingival contour. (Courtesy of Dr. Edward S. Cohen, West Newton, Mass.)

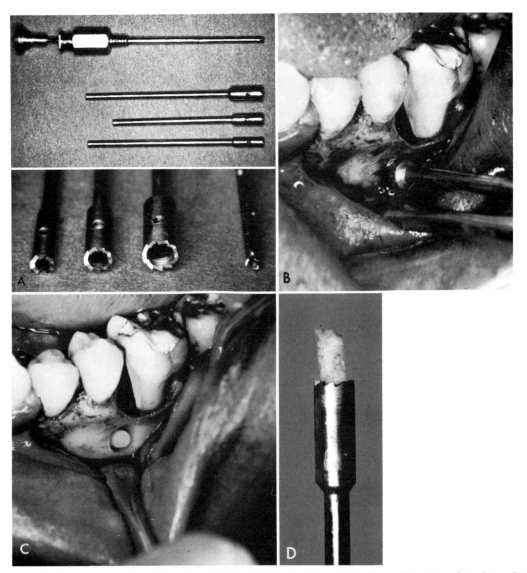

Figure 51–9 Autogenous Bone Transplant Obtained With Trephine. *A,* Trephines. *Top,* Manual trephine. *Center,* Different-sized power trephines No. 2, No. 4 and No. 6. *Bottom,* Orifices of trephines. *B,* Mucoperiosteal flap elevated, showing osseous defect on the mesial surface of the first molar. Trephine inserted into bone distal to the second molar. *C,* Bone separated by trephine. *D,* Bone transplant; the cancellous portion is used, the cortical layer is removed.

(Illustration continued on opposite page)

thickness flap, retaining all marginal tissues, and granulation tissue is eliminated by curettage. After the transplant has been placed, the flap is reapproximated and sutured, fully covering the graft site.[47]

The authors report a mean fill of 3.44 mm. in 166 sites studied.

BONE SWAGING. Ewen[31] and Ross et al.[81] proposed bone swaging or contiguous osseous grafts as another intraoral technique for the treatment of angular defects. This technique requires that bone from the edentulous area adjacent to the defect be pushed into contact with the root surface without fracturing the bone from its base. If the transposition can be carried out without interrupting the blood supply, theoretically the graft should remain viable.

For defects adjacent to edentulous space, the following procedure is used.

Step 1. Preparing the recipient site. Mu-

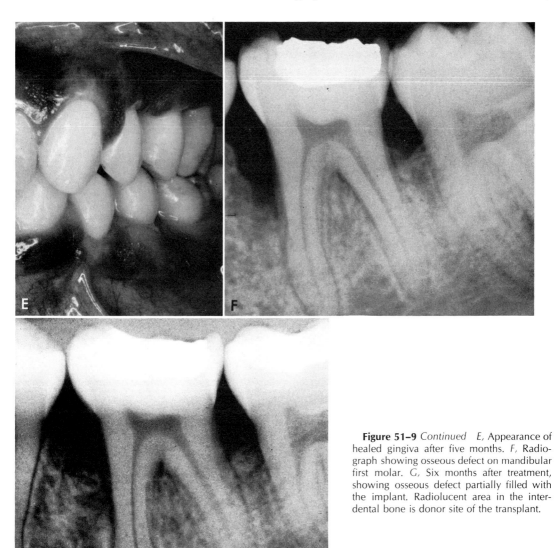

Figure 51–9 Continued   E, Appearance of healed gingiva after five months. F, Radiograph showing osseous defect on mandibular first molar. G, Six months after treatment, showing osseous defect partially filled with the implant. Radiolucent area in the interdental bone is donor site of the transplant.

coperiosteal flaps are elevated, granulation tissue is removed from the defect, and the roots are scaled and planed.

Step 2. Transferring the bone. The dimension of the required bone transfer is determined, and it is separated from the bone bordering the defect with a thin linear bur cut. A thin, blunted surgical chisel is inserted into the cut, and the bone is pushed into the defect with a mallet (Fig. 51–10*B* and *C*).

The flaps are returned over the area, sutured, and covered with periodontal pack. Sutures and pack are removed in a week, and the pack is replaced for another week if necessary.

Interdental craters may be filled by forcefully collapsing the facial and lingual walls inward using the same general principles.

This technique is complicated by varying degrees of elasticity of the bone. Bone with a greater cancellous composition is more flexible. Bone without adequate can-

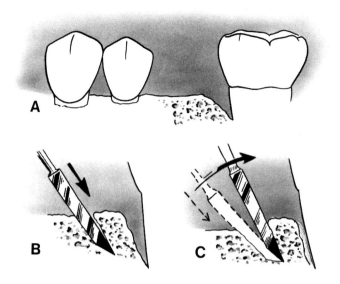

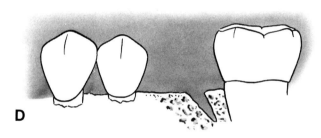

Figure 51–10 Bone Swaging to Fill Infra-bony Defect. *A,* Infrabony defect of the mesial of the mandibular molar. *B,* Chisel separate section (*arrow*). *C,* Bone swaged into infra-bony defect (*arrow*). *D,* Infrabony defect filled with bone.

cellous material tends to fracture from the alveolus, providing a noncontiguous bone graft. Bone swaging is therefore technically difficult, and its use is limited by the need for a substantially cancellous composition to the bone and the presence of an edentulous area adjacent to the defect being grafted.

Bone from extra-oral sites

ILIAC AUTOGRAFTS. The use of fresh or preserved iliac cancellous marrow has been extensively investigated. This material has been used by orthopedic surgeons for years. Schallhorn[87-90] and others[6, 11, 19, 21-23, 41] have been instrumental in providing data from human and animals studies to support the use of autogenous iliac grafts. This technique has been proved successful in bony defects with various numbers of walls, in furcations, and even supracres-

tally to some extent. In comparison with other known techniques, it also provides the greatest potential for success. Problems have also been associated with its use, however. Schallhorn[89] has observed postoperative sequelae of infection, exfoliation and sequestration, varying rates of healing, root resorption and rapid recurrence of the defect. The last two, which of course have the most lasting effects, have been observed by other authors.[11, 23]

Techniques for Iliac Bone Graft. Numerous authors have described techniques of obtaining bone marrow from both the posterior and anterior iliac crest. Dragoo and Irwin[21, 30, 99] gave an excellent description of a technique utilizing a modified Turkel trephine needle (Fig. 51–11). Briefly, the technique requires the patient to be placed in the supine position or in a lateral decubitus position. The area of the anterior crest is surgically prepared and

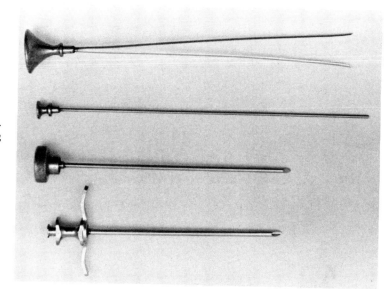

Figure 51–11 Modified Turkel Trephine Needle. Used for obtaining bone marrow from iliac crest.

draped. A point 3 to 4 cm. dorsal to the anterior spine and in the center of the iliac crest is the point of entry. This point is anesthetized with a subcutaneous injection of 1 per cent lidocaine. The skin is then punctured with a No. 11 blade to introduce the outer needle and stylet. The cutting tip of the stylet is placed through the skin into the periosteum and rotated to penetrate approximately 2 mm. into the bone. This provides a secure rest for the outer needle, which should be parallel to a line from the pubic bone to the anterior iliac spine. The stylet is removed and the inner needle is inserted. The inner needle is then withdrawn with the cancellous bone in its shaft (Fig. 51–12A and B). The outer needle remains in place, allowing re-entry at various angulations for multiple marrow cores. After the desired number of cores is obtained, the outer needle is removed and pressure bandage is placed. Suturing is seldom necessary. The biopsied material may then be used fresh or frozen. Fresh material has been associated with root resorption[89] (Fig. 51–13). The reason

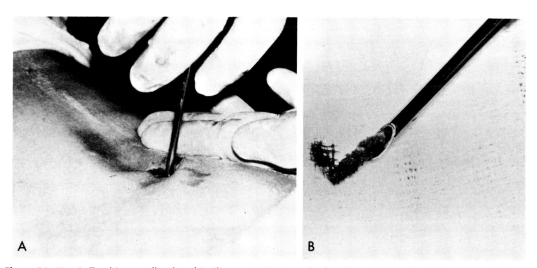

A   B

Figure 51–12   *A,* Trephine needle placed in iliac crest. *B,* One cylinder of material obtained. Numerous cylinders can be obtained through one skin perforation.

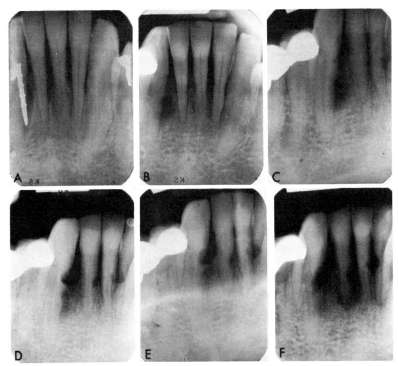

Figure 51–13 *A,* November 1973, radiograph of a patient immediately prior to the placement of a fresh iliac autograft. *B,* Two months later, bone repair is evident. Note the early radiolucent areas on the mesial aspect of the canine. *C,* After seven months bone "fill" is occurring but obvious root resorption is present. *D,* April 1975. Root resorption is now apparent on all grafted teeth. Note the obvious degree of "fill" of the original bony defects. *E,* February 1976. Further involvement. *F,* October 1977. Four years later, root resorption has progressed into the pulp on the lateral incisor causing a periosteal-endosteal complication.

for this occurrence is still unknown. Ellegaard[29] concluded that the osteogenic potential of fresh iliac bone marrow cannot be utilized in new attachment procedures until methods of preventing root resorption and ankylosis are developed. Therefore, stored material is usually preferred.

Various cryopreservation techniques have been discussed by Sottosanti and Bierly.[96] A commonly used method described by Schallhorn, Hiatt, and Boyce[88] requires the storage of marrow in Minimum Essential Media with glycerol in a refrigerator at 4°C. More elaborate and expensive techniques of program freezing also have been developed to maintain cell viability.[4, 8]

Most authors[22, 26, 79, 88] agree that careful case selection and preparation are necessary for the successful placement of the marrow into periodontal defects.

In preparing the implant site, care should be taken to preserve as much covering tissue as possible (Fig. 51–14). A full or partial thickness flap is reflected without an internal bevel incision at the margin. Care must be taken to maintain the blood supply and integrity of the gingival tissue to cover the graft material. This principle applies to all materials or techniques used. The intact gingival tissue is thought to provide nourishment to the grafted material and prevent intraoral contamination.

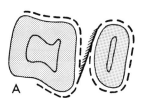

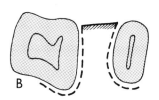

Figure 51–14 Interdental Incisions for Greater Tissue Conservation. *A,* When interdental space permits, a diagonal incision is made across the papillary area. The effective amount of tissue can be increased by beveling the incision (shown by the cross-hatched lines). *B,* If larger interdental areas are available, a "flag"-type incision can be utilized to provide complete interdental coverage.

After the area is exposed, granulation tissue is removed and the roots are scaled and planed (Fig. 51–15*B* and *C*). The cortical bone in the walls of the osseous defect is perforated with a small round bur in several areas, to permit vascularization of the implant.

The cores of marrow and cancellous bone are placed snugly into the defect, which is overfilled if possible (Fig. 51–15*D*). The flaps are returned over the area, sutured, and covered with dry foil and periodontal dressing. Antibiotics are used prophylactically, beginning the evening before surgery and continuing for several days postoperatively. Healing is usually uneventful, with normal gingival contours restored within two months (Fig. 51–15*E*).

Schallhorn, Hiatt, and Boyce[88] described the results of a clinical study of 182 transplants in 52 patients. Freshly frozen hip autografts were used in all cases. Evaluations were performed for from 5 to 24 months. The results indicated the most fill was in three-wall defects, but complete fill was obtained in 33 two-wall defects (4.18 mm. average fill). The overall average of fill was approximately 3.0 mm. In one-wall defects and inter-radicular lesions, new attachment was obtained to a smaller extent. However, ankylosis and root resorption were noted in some cases. Hiatt and Schallhorn[47] found that hip marrow grafts result in greater supracrestal bone apposition and fill of furcation defects than with grafts from intraoral sites.

Ellegaard[26, 27] compared the effect of fresh iliac crest marrow in new attachment procedures in inter-radicular and three-wall vertical defects in monkeys. A total of 107 bifurcation defects and 94 vertical defects were created in 17 Rhesus monkeys. Eight to ten weeks after creation of the defects, new attachment attempts were made. Autogenous young cancellous bone and fresh or frozen iliac bone marrow were transplanted into the defects. Regeneration of periodontal tissues took place to the greatest extent with autogenous bone transplants in inter-radicular lesions, whereas no difference was observed in three-wall vertical defects treated with or without bone grafts. Transplantation of fresh iliac bone marrow resulted in a high degree of bone formation but with ankylosis and resorption of the root surface.

Dragoo and Sullivan[22, 23] provided additional information by evaluating histologically the results of treating one- and two-wall vertical defects and suprabony pockets with iliac bone marrow in four patients. They found an average apposition of supracrestal bone of 0.7 mm. and an average supracrestal new attachment area of 1.03 mm.

Prevention of epithelial migration

Despite the gratifying results achieved with the various autogenic techniques previously described, the results of bone grafting have not been as predictable as demanded by many therapists. Postoperative inflammation and/or epithelial migration into the defects have been blamed by Ellegaard, Karring, Davies, and Loe[27] as important factors limiting bone augmentation. In an attempt to decrease one of these factors, epithelial migration, Ellegaard[25, 27, 28, 29] developed the following technique.

On the facial and lingual aspects of vertical defects, a split flap procedure was performed. Granulation tissue was removed from the defects, and following transplantation of the autogenous bone grafts, the defects were covered with a free palatal graft (Fig. 51–16) (see Chapter 53). Ellegaard and associates have found an increased degree of connective tissue attachment and less residual pocket formation with this technique as compared with the standard flap procedure described earlier. This technique is contrary to the carefully engineered primary closure flap technique previously described, and its value is still a matter of further investigation.

ALLOGRAFTS

Although most data indicate that autografts of cancellous bone and marrow offer the greatest potential for success,[14, 19, 29] xenografts[1, 9, 57, 95] and allografts[2, 52, 53, 55, 58, 61, 62, 66, 83, 86] have provided some successful results.

Unfortunately, obtaining donor material for autograft purposes necessitates inflicting surgical trauma on another part of the patient's body. Obviously, it would be to

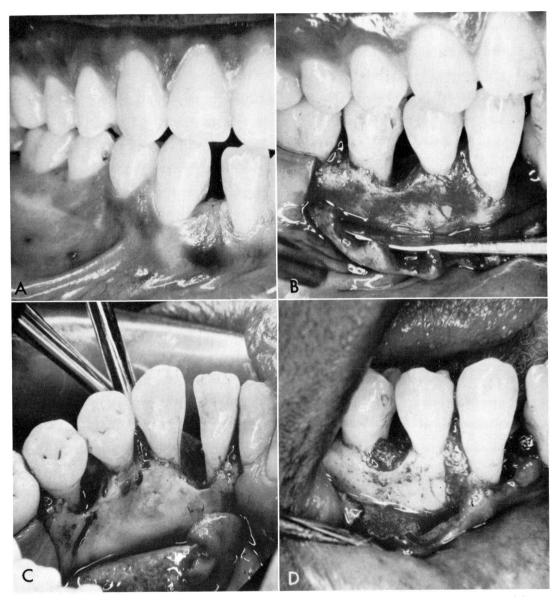

Figure 51-15 Autogenous Hip Marrow Implant. A, Before treatment. B, Mucoperiosteal flap reveals osseous defect on the second premolar. C, Lingual view of infrabony defect revealed by periosteal flap. (Note the defect between the canine and lateral.) D, Hip marrow implant in premolar osseous defect.

(Illustration continued on opposite page)

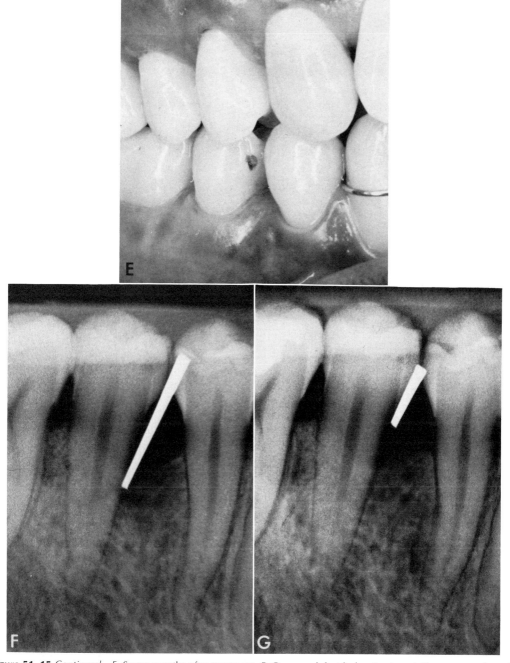

Figure 51–15 *Continued E,* Seven months after treatment. *F,* Osseous defect before treatment. The gutta percha point is at the base of the pocket. *G,* Seven months after treatment. The bone is repaired. The gutta percha point is at the base of the healed sulcus which is now attached higher on the root. (Courtesy of Dr. Edward S. Cohen, West Newton, Mass.)

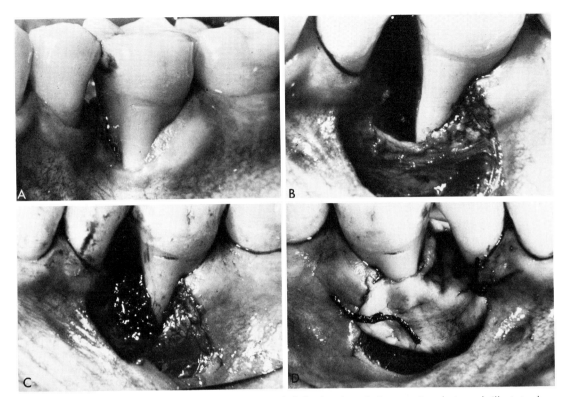

Figure 51–16 Ellegaard's Technique for Preventing Epithelial Migration: *A,* Preoperative photograph illustrates bony defect on mesial aspect of molar. *B,* Area is debrided of connective tissue. *C,* Osseous material is placed in defect. *D,* A free gingival graft is placed over osseous material and secured with interrupted sutures.

the patient's as well as the therapist's advantage if a suitable substitute could be utilized for grafting purposes which would offer similar potential for repair and not require the additional surgical removal of donor material. However, both allografts and xenografts are foreign to the organism and therefore have the potential to provoke an immune response. The principal antigenic component in these grafts seems to be contained in the red marrow, although bone devoid of marrow has also been shown to exert antigenic effect.[12, 13]

Attempts have been made to suppress the antigenic potential of allografts and xenografts by means of radiation, freezing, or chemical treatment.[10]

ILIAC MARROW ALLOGRAFTS. On the basis of dog studies,[45] Hiatt and Schallhorn[46, 90] established a rationale and methodology involving the banking and utilization of allogeneic iliac material.

Cancellous bone with its marrow was removed from the iliac crests of "living cadavers" being used for major organ transplant therapy following brain death. The material was stored in sterile vials, as with autografts, in Minimum Essential Medium with 15 per cent glycerol as a cryoprotective agent. The vials were then frozen, and the material was tested for sterility. Freezing reduces the antigenic potential of the material, thereby rendering the graft more acceptable to the host.[13, 46, 90]

Patients were selected and matched with recipients for major blood grouping and human lymphocyte antigens (HLA). No more than two incompatible donor lymphocyte antigens were present in any materials used. Thus, the rationale for using allografts of bone and marrow is based on immunologic testing parameters and the body of knowledge acquired in organ transplant therapy. A total of 194 sites consisting of furcations, one-, two- and three-wall defects, and suprabony pockets in 20 patients were treated by the same technique described for using auto-grafts of human iliac crest material.[90] Although perfect crossmatching was never achieved and 2 of the 20 patients developed cytotoxin antibodies to lymphocyte antigens, no rejection of the allografts was observed. Coronal regeneration of bone was determined by preoperative and postoperative measurements. An average bone apposition of 3.6 mm. was found in a combined total of three-, two-, and one-walled 121 defects. In 5 furcation defects the average augmentation of bone was 3.3 mm., and in 68 supracrestal defects apposition was 2.06 mm. These results are similar to those obtained by the same investigators in a study using fresh and frozen iliac autografts or autografts from intraoral sites.[47, 48] However, numerous problems associated with tissue incompatibilities must be solved before this approach can be utilized clinically.

FREEZE-DRIED ILIAC ALLOGRAFTS. Promising work on freeze-dried allografts has been undertaken at the Navy Tissue Bank. The material is obtained under sterile conditions from a cadaver that has met the rigid criteria for tissue donation established by the Navy Tissue Bank.[61] The bone is frozen, and the tissue water is removed by lyophilization. This process, commonly referred to as freeze-drying, is carried out under vacuum at a low temperature ($-40°C$). Mellonig et al.[61] reported a longitudinal clinical study involving many periodontists who used freeze-dried crushed cortical bone as a graft material in human periodontal defects. Results of the study to date indicate that of the 97 defects treated, 23 manifested complete bone regeneration, 39 showed better than 50 per cent and 24 showed less than 50 per cent osseous repair. Twelve defects, of which nine were furcation involvements, failed to demonstrate any bony regeneration. This study provides strong evidence that freeze-dried bone allografts may have definite potential as grafting material in certain defects; however, the limitations of the study are obvious, and better-controlled investigations are needed.

A preliminary controlled study in rats[35] showed that freeze-dried fine particled bone allografts in extraoral sites may induce the differentiation of osteoblasts from host cells under some circumstances.

XENOGRAFTS. *Calf bone*, treated by detergent extraction, sterilization, and freeze-drying, has been used to formulate a material (Boplant) for treatment of osseous defects.[2] Although some studies were promising,[92, 93] Boplant was withdrawn from the market because immunological complications developed after its use.[48]

Kiel Bone, which is calf or oxbone that is denatured with 20 per cent hydrogen peroxide, dried with acetone, and sterilized with ethylene oxide, has also been studied. However, data are not sufficient for complete evaluation.

Anorganic bone is ox bone from which the organic material has been extracted by means of ethylenediamine and sterilized by autoclaving. Melcher has used anorganic bone for obtaining new attachment in vertical defects.[59, 60] However, he warned against the use of anorganic bone, because of protracted sequestration of the graft particles and slow resorption.

Nonbone graft material

SCLERA. In addition to bone graft materials, many different nonbone graft materials have been tried for restoration of the periodontium. Among them are dura,[28] cartilage,[7, 83, 84] cementum,[86] dentin,[3, 94, 101] plaster of Paris,[54, 95] ceramics,[9, 56, 57] and sclera.[51–53, 67, 100] In recent years, Klingsberg[51–53] has promoted the use of sclera as an allogeneic nonbone material to rebuild the attachment apparatus forming a fibrous attachment to bone and/or gingiva.[53] Sclera was originally utilized in periodontal procedures because it is a dense fibrous connective tissue with poor vascularity and minimal cellularity. This provides a low incidence of antigenicity or other untoward reactions.[49] In addition, it was thought that sclera may provide a barrier for apical migration of the junctional epithelium and serve to protect the blood clot during the initial healing period.

Utilization of sclera was demonstrated by Klingsberg,[51–53] and the technique for preparation and preservation was described by Feingold and Chasens.[32] Sclera may be obtained from eyes donated to eye banks. These eyes are enucleated at autopsy by aseptic technique and then stored in various antibiotic solutions and tested for sterility. The specific procedure followed will depend on the protocol of the eye bank used. The sclera is stored in anhydrous glycerin solution with a molecular sieve—a series of absorbents composed of sodium and calcium alumina silicates which are capable of removing water to an extremely low vapor pressure (Fig. 51–17).[50]

Sclera appropriately preserved can be stored indefinitely at room temperature. When dehydrated, sclera becomes translucent but not transparent. Scleral tissue should be rejected if it has a rubbery consistency or if any of the tissue components resist separation, because this may indicate degenerative changes due to improper preservation techniques.[53] However, Hassard[43] found no difference in preserved, nonviable tissue and fresh scleral homografts when used in cats.

At the time of implantation, the length and width of the scleral graft must be measured. The sclera should overlap the facial and lingual walls by 3 to 4 mm. No more than two layers of sclera should be used, because the graft material must be

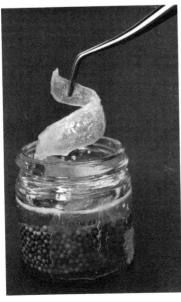

Figure 51–17 Scleral tissue being removed from anhydrous glycerin storage solution. The small beads in the bottom of vial compose the molecular sieve.

in contact with viable tissue on at least one surface. Just prior to implantation, the graft is placed for 20 minutes in a disposable sterile petri dish containing the first of two fresh solutions of Neosporin. The graft is then scraped smooth and placed in the second solution of Neosporin. The amount of scraping and tissue removal depends in the early preparation by the eye bank. Some sclera have considerable muscle and pigment attached. This must be removed or the tissue must be discarded.

Sclera exhibits tissue memory, so the natural curvature of the globe should be utilized in the layering procedure. If not carefully sectioned and situated, sclera tends to return to its original shape, and this places additional tension on the sutured tissue which may result in the loss of the graft.

Although some studies[33] show that sclera is well accepted by the host and sometimes invaded by host cells and capillaries and replaced by dense connective tissue, it does not appear to induce osteogenesis or cementogenesis.[62, 67, 100] It may, however, be useful for its scaffolding effect (Fig. 51–18).

CARTILAGE. Cartilage has been used for repair studies in monkeys and for treatment of periodontal defects in humans.[83, 84] It served as a scaffolding around which new bone was formed, and some new attachment was obtained in 60 out of 70 cases. It has received only limited evaluation, however.

PLASTER OF PARIS. Although plaster of Paris was found useful in one uncontrolled clinical study,[1] others reported that it does not induce bone formation.[95] Its usefulness, therefore, appears questionable.

CERAMICS. Porous ceramics in powder form have been suggested as substitutes for bone grafts in the treatment of periodontal defects. This material seems to be well tolerated by the organism, and bone apposition occurs directly on the ceramic lattice.[56, 57] The results of this technique have not yet been clearly evaluated.

SUMMARY

In summary, the subject of grafting has received a great deal of attention, owing to its obvious importance in improving the

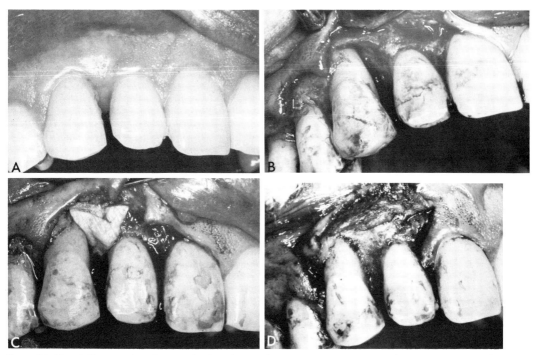

Figure 51–18 *A*, Preoperative photograph of a sclera graft area. *B*, An incision is made to conserve gingival tissue, and the area is debrided. Note the vertical defect on the mesial aspect of the canine. *C*, Sclera is placed over defect. *D*, Re-entry shows apparent remodeling of defect. (Courtesy of Dr. Jules Klingsberg, New York.)

results of therapy. The clinician should make an effort to differentiate between those materials that have been studied in depth and with acceptable results and others that, although promising, are still experimental. Research papers must be given critical evaluation, considering the adequacy of controls, selection of cases, methods of evaluation, and long-range postoperative results.

The following methods can be recommended on the basis of available information: autogenous bone implants obtained from intraoral sites, particularly extraction sockets, edentulous areas, and tuberosity areas; osseous coagulum–bone blend technique, and frozen iliac bone and marrow autogenous transplants. The clinician should also remember that careful curettage, open or closed, has been shown to result in bone regeneration without the use of bone-inducing agents. Caution in the adoption of new, as yet not fully proven, methods is recommended.

REFERENCES

1. Alderman, N. E.: Sterile plaster of Paris as an implant in the infrabony environment: a preliminary study. J. Periodontol., *40*:11, 1969.
2. Arrocha, R., Wittwer, J., and Gargiulo, A.: Tissue response to heterogenous bone implantation in dogs. J. Periodontol., *39*:162, 1968.
3. Bang, G., and Urist, M. R.: Bone induction in excavation chambers in matrix of decalcified dentin. Arch. Surg., *94*:781, 1967.
4. Barkin, M., and Newman, N.: Ultrastructure of bone marrow prior to and after programmed freezing. Oral Surg., *33*:341, 1972.
5. Beube, F. E.: Radiographic and histologic study of reattachment. J. Periodontol., *23*:158, 1952.
6. Bierly, J. A., Sottosanti, J. S., Costley, J. M., and Cherrick, H. M.: An evaluation of the osteogenic potential of marrow. J. Periodontol., *46*:277, 1975.
7. Boyne, P. J., and Cooksey, D. E.: Use of cartilage and bone implants in restoration of edentulous ridges. J. Am. Dent. Assoc., *71*:1426, 1965.
8. Boyne, P. H., and Yeager: An evaluation of the osteogenic potential of frozen marrow. Oral Surg., *28*:764, 1969.
9. Bump, R. L., Salimeno, T., Hooker, S. P., and Wilkinson, E. G.: Grafting one-wall infrabony

pockets with woven ceramic fabric. I.A.D.R. Abstracts 1974, p. 98.

10. Buring, K., and Urist, M. R.: Effects of ionizing radiation on the bone induction principle in the matrix of bone implants. Clin. Orthop. Rel. Res., 55:225, 1967.

11. Burnette, W. E.: Fate of the iliac crest graft. J. Periodontol., 43:88, 1972.

12. Burwell, R. G., and Gowland, G.: Studies in the transplantation of bone III. The immune responses of lymph nodes draining components of fresh homologous cancellous bone treated by different methods. J. Bone Joint Surg., 44:131, 1962.

13. Burwell, R. G., Gowland, G., and Dexter, F.: Studies in the transplantation of bone VI. Further observations concerning the antigenicity of homologous cortical and cancellous bone. J. Bone Joint Surg., 45:597, 1963.

14. Burwell, R. G.: Studies in the transplantation of bone VII. J. Bone Joint Surg., 46:110, 1964.

15. Carranza, F. A., Sr.: A technic for reattachment. J. Periodontol., 25:272, 1954.

16. Carranza, F. A., Sr.: A technique for treating infrabony pockets so as to obtain reattachment. Dent. Clin. North Am., March, 1960, p. 75.

17. Carraro, J. J., Sznajder, N., and Alonso, C. A.: Intraoral cancellous bone autografts in treatment of infrabony pockets. J. Clin. Periodontol., 3:104, 1976.

18. Coverly, L., Toto, P., and Gargiulo, A.: Osseous coagulum: a histologic evaluation. J. Periodontol., 46:596, 1975.

19. Cushing, M.: Autogenous red marrow grafts: potential for induction of osteogenesis. J. Periodontol., 40:492, 1969.

20. Diem, C. R., Bowers, G. M., and Moffitt, W. C.: Bone blending: a technique for osseous implants. J. Periodontol., 43:295, 1972.

21. Dragoo, M. R., and Irwin, R. K.: A method of procuring cancellous iliac bone utilizing a trephine needle. J. Periodontol., 43:82, 1972.

22. Dragoo, M. R., and Sullivan, H. C.: A clinical and histologic evaluation of autogenous iliac bone grafts in humans: Part I. Wound healing after 2 to 8 months. J. Periodontol., 44:599, 1973.

23. Dragoo, M. R., and Sullivan, H. C.: A clinical and histologic evaluation of autogenous iliac bone grafts in humans: Part II. External root resorption. J. Periodontol., 44:614, 1973.

24. Ellegaard, B., and Löe, H.: New attachment of periodontal tissues after treatment of intrabony lesions. J. Periodontol., 42:648, 1971.

25. Ellegaard, B., Karring, T., and Löe, H.: Retardation of epithelial migration in new attachment attempts in intrabony defects in monkeys. J. Clin. Periodontol., 3:23, 1976.

26. Ellegaard, B., Karring, T., Listgarten, N., and Löe, H.: New attachment after treatment of interradicular lesions. J. Periodontol., 44:209, 1973.

27. Ellegaard, B., Karring, T., Davies, R., and Löe, H.: New attachment after treatment of intrabony defects in monkeys. J. Periodontol., 45:368, 1974.

28. Ellegaard, B., Nielsen, I. M., and Karring, T.: Lyodura grafts in new attachment procedures. J. Dent. Res., 55: Special issue B, B-304, 1976.

29. Ellegaard, B.: Bone grafts in periodontal attachment procedures. J. Clin. Periodontol., 3(5):5, 1976.

30. Ellis, L. D., Jensen, W. N., and Westermann, M. P.: Needle biopsy of bone and marrow. Arch. Intern. Med., 114:214, 1964.

31. Ewen, S. J.: Bone swaging. J. Periodontol., 36:57, 1965.

32. Feingold, J. P., and Chasens, A. I.: Preserved scleral allografts in periodontal defect in man. I. Preparation, preservation and use. J. Periodontol., 48:1, 1977.

33. Feingold, J. P., Chasens, A. I., Doyle, J., and Alfano, M. C.: Preserved scleral allografts on periodontal defects in man. II. Histologic evaluation. J. Periodontol., 48:4, 1977.

34. Freeman, E., and Turnbull, R. S.: The value of osseous coagulum as a graft material. J. Periodontol. Res., 8:299, 1973.

35. Freeman, E., and Turnbull, R. S.: Short communication: Histologic evaluation of freeze-dried fine particles bone allografts. Preliminary observation. J. Periodontol., 48:288, 1977.

36. Froum, S. J.: Comparison of different autograft material for obtaining bone fill in human periodontal defects. J. Periodontol., 45:240, 1974.

37. Froum, S. J., Thaler, R., Scoop, I. W., and Stahl, S. S.: Osseous autografts I. Clinical responses to bone blend or hip marrow grafts. J. Periodontol., 46:515, 1975.

38. Froum, S. J., Thaler, R., Scoop, I. W., and Stahl, S. S.: Osseous autografts II. Histologic responses to osseous coagulum–bone blend grafts. J. Periodontol., 46:656, 1975.

39. Goldman, H.: A rationale for the treatment of the intrabony pocket, one method of treatment—subgingival curettage. J. Periodontol., 20:83, 1949.

40. Goldman, H. M., and Cohen, D. W.: The infrabony pocket: classification and treatment. J. Periodontol., 29:272, 1958.

41. Haggerty, P. C., and Maeda, I.: Autogenous bone grafts: a revolution in the treatment of vertical bone defects. J. Periodontol., 42:626, 1971.

42. Halliday, D. G.: The grafting of newly formed autogenous bone in the treatment of osseous defects. J. Periodontol., 40:511, 1969.

43. Hassard, D. T. R.: Scleral grafting. Can. J. Ophthal., 2:292, 1967.

44. Hiatt, W. H.: Periodontal pocket elimination by combined endodontic-periodontic therapy. J. Periodontol., 1:153, 1963.

45. Hiatt, W. H.: The induction of new bone and cementum formation III. Utilizing bone and marrow allografts in dogs. J. Periodontol., 4:596, 1970.

46. Hiatt, W. H., and Schallhorn, R. G.: Human allografts of iliac cancellous bone and marrow in periodontal osseous defects I. Rationale and methodology. J. Periodontol., 42:642, 1971.

47. Hiatt, W. H., and Schallhorn, R. G.: Intraoral transplants of cancellous bone and marrow in periodontal lesions. J. Periodontol., 44:194, 1973.

48. Hjorting-Hansen, E.: Studies on implantation of anorganic bone in cystic jaw lesions. Thesis. Munksgaard, Copenhagen, 1972.

49. Johnson, W., et al.: Transplantation of homografts of sclera: experimental study. Am. J. Ophthal., *54*:1019, (June) 1962.

50. King, J. H., Metique, J. W., and Meryman, H. T.: Preservation of cornea. Am. J. Ophthal., 53: 445, 1962.

51. Klingsberg, J.: Scleral allografts in the repair of periodontal osseous defects. N. Y. State D. J., *38*:418, 1972.

52. Klingsberg, J.: Preserved sclera in periodontal surgery. J. Periodontol., *43*:634, 1972.

53. Klingsberg, J.: Periodontal scleral grafts and combined grafts of sclera and bone: two year appraisal. J. Periodontol., *45*:262, 1974.

54. Kornbleuth, J.: Histologic evaluation of plaster as a seal for bone autografts. I.A.D.R. Abstracts, 1972, p. 184.

55. Kromer, H.: Transplantation in Surgical Treatment of Cysts of the Jaw and Periodontal Pockets. Oslo University Press, 1960.

56. Levin, M. P., Getter, L., Adrian, J., and Cutright, D. E.: Healing of periodontal defects with ceramic implants. J. Periodontol., *1*:197, 1974.

57. Levin, M. P., Getter, L., and Cutright, D. E.: A comparison of iliac marrow and biodegradable ceramic in periodontal defects. J. Biomed. Mater. Res., 9:183, 1975.

58. Libin, B. M., Ward, H. L., Fishman, L. L.: Decalcified lyophilized bone allografts for use in human periodontal defects. J. Periodontol., *46*:51, 1975.

59. Melcher, A. H.: The use of heterogenous anorganic bone in periodontal bone grafting: a preliminary report 1. Dent. Assoc. So. Africa, *13*:80, 1958.

60. Melcher, A.: The use of heterogenous anorganic bone as an implant material in oral procedures. Oral Surg., *15*:996, 1962.

61. Mellonig, J. T., Bowers, G. M., et al.: Clinical evaluation of freeze-dried bone allografts in periodontal osseous defects. J. Periodontol., *47*:125, 1976.

62. Moskow, B. S., Gold, S. I., and Gottsegen, R.: Effects of scleral collagen upon the healing of experimental osseous wounds. J. Periodontol., *47*:596, 1976.

63. Nabers, J. M., Meador, H. L., Nabers, C. L., and O'Leary, T. J.: Chronology, an important factor in the repair of osseous defects. Periodontics, 2:304, 1964.

64. Nabers, C. L., and O'Leary, T. J.: Autogenous bone transplants in the treatment of osseous defects. J. Periodontol., *36*:5, 1965.

65. Nabers, C. L., and O'Leary, T. J.: Autogenous bone grafts: case report. Periodontics, 5:251, 1967.

66. Narang, R., and Wells, H.: Bone induction in experimental periodontal bone defects in dogs with decalcified allogenic bone matrix grafts: a preliminary study. Oral Surg., *33*:306, 1972.

67. Passell, M. S., and Bissada, N. F.: Histomorphologic evaluation of scleral grafts in experimental bony defects. J. Periodontol., *46*:629, 1975.

68. Patur, B., and Glickman, I.: Clinical and roentgenographic evaluation of the post-treatment healing of infrabony pockets. J. Periodontol., *33*:164, 1962.

69. Periodontics Syllabus, NAVED P–5110, pp. 113–115. U.S. Naval Dental Corps., 1975.

70. Prichard, J. F.: The intrabony technique as a predictable procedure. J. Periodontol., *28*:202, 1957.

71. Prichard, J.: Regeneration of bone following periodontal therapy. Oral Surg., *10*:247, 1957.

72. Ramfjord, S. P., Kerr, D. A., and Ash, M. M.: World Workshop in Periodontics. American Acad. Periodont. and Univ. Michigan, 1966.

73. Ramfjord, S. P., Nissle, R. R., Schick, R. A., and Cooper, H., Jr.: Subgingival curettage versus surgical elimination of periodontal pockets. J. Periodontol., *39*:167, 1968.

74. Register, A. A.: Bone and cementum induction by dentin, demineralized in situ. J. Periodontol., *44*:49, 1973.

75. Register, A. A., and Burdick, F. A.: Accelerated reattachment with cementogenesis to dentin, demineralized in situ. J. Periodontol., *46*:497, 1976.

76. Register, A. A., and Burdick, F. A.: Accelerated reattachment with cementogenesis to dentin, demineralized in situ: I. Optimum range. J. Periodontol., *46*:646, 1975.

77. Rivault, A. F., Toto, P. D., Levy, S., and Gargiulo, A. W.: Autogenous bone grafts: osseous coagulum and osseous retrograde procedures in primates. J. Periodontol., *42*:787, 1971.

78. Robinson, R. E.: Osseous coagulum for bone induction. J. Periodontol., *40*:503, 1969.

79. Rosenberg, M. M.: Free osseous tissue autografts as a predictable procedure. J. Periodontol., *42*:195, 1971.

80. Rosenberg, M. M.: Reentry of an osseous defect treated by a bone implant after a long duration. J. Periodontol., *42*:360, 1971.

81. Ross, S. E., Malamed, E. H., and Amsterdam, M.: The contiguous autogenous transplant—its rationale, indications and technique. Periodontics, 4:246, 1966.

82. Ross, S. E., and Cohen, D. W.: The fate of a free osseous tissue autograft a clinical and histologic case report. Periodontics, 6:145, 1968.

83. Schaffer, E. M.: Cartilage transplants into periodontium of rhesus monkeys. Oral Surg., *11*: 1233, 1956.

84. Schaffer, E. M.: Cartilage grafts in human periodontal pockets. J. Periodontol., *29*:176, 1958.

85. Schaffer, E. M., and Zander, H. A.: Histologic evidence of reattachment of periodontal pockets. Parodontologie, 7:101, 1953.

86. Schaffer, E. M.: Cementum and dentine implants in a dog and a rhesus monkey. J. Periodontol., *28*:125, 1957.

87. Schallhorn, R. G.: The use of autogenous hip marrow biopsy implants for bony crater defects. J. Periodontol., *39*:145, 1968.

88. Schallhorn, R. G., Hiatt, W. H., and Boyce, W.: Iliac transplants in periodontal therapy. J. Periodontol., *41*:566, 1970.

89. Schallhorn, R. G.: Postoperative problems associated with iliac transplants. J. Periodontol., *43*:3, 1972.

90. Schallhorn, R. G., and Hiatt, W. H.: Human allografts of iliac cancellous bone and marrow in periodontal osseous defects II. Clinical observations. J. Periodontol., *43*:67, 1972.

91. Schallhorn, R. G.: Osseous grafts in the treatment of periodontal osseous defects. Periodontal Surgery, S. Sigmund Stahl (Ed.). Springfield, Illinois: Charles C Thomas, 1976.

92. Scoop, I. W., Morgan, F. H., Dooner, J. J., Fredrics, H. J., and Heyman, R. A.: Bovine bone (Boplant) implants for infrabony oral lesions (clinical trials in humans). Periodontics, 4:169, 1966.

93. Scoop, I. W., Kassouny, D. Y., and Morgan, F. H.: Bovine bone (Boplant). J. Periodontol., 37:400, 1966.

94. Scoop, I. W., Kassouny, D. Y., and Register, A. A.: Human bone induction by allogenic dentin matrix. I.A.D.R. Abst. 1970, p. 100, no. 105.

95. Shaffer, C. D., and App, G. R.: The use of plaster of Paris in treating infrabony periodontal defects in humans. J. Periodontol., 42:685, 1971.

96. Sottosanti, J. S., and Bierly, J. A.: The storage of bone marrow and its relation to periodontal grafting procedures. J. Periodontol., 46:162, 1975.

97. Stahl, S. S., and Froum, S. J.: Human clinical and histologic repair responses following the use of citric acid in periodontal therapy. J. Periodontol., 48:261, 1977.

98. Sugarman, E. F.: A clinical and histological study of the attachment of grafted tissue to bone and teeth. J. Periodontol., 40:381, 1969.

99. Tarrow, A. B., Turkel, H., and Thompson, M. S.: Infusion via the bone marrow and biopsy of bone marrow. Anesthesiology, 13(5):501, 1952.

100. Turnbull, R. S., Freeman, E., and Melcher, A. H.: Histological evaluation of the osteogenic capacity of sclera. J. Dent. Res., 55:972, 1976.

101. Urist, M. R.: Bone histogenesis and morphogenesis in implants of demineralized enamel and dentin. Oral Surg., 29:88, 1971.

102. Urist, M. R., et al.: Bone induction principle. Clin. Orthop., 53:243, 1967.

103. Waerhaug, J.: The gingival pocket. Odont. Tidskr., 60:suppl. 1, 1952.

103. Wilderman, N. M., and Wentz, F. M.: Repair of a dentogingival defect with a pedicle flap. J. Periodontal., 36:218, 1965.

105. Yukna, R. A.: A clinical and histologic study of healing following the excisional new attachment procedure in rhesus monkeys. J. Periodontol., 47:701, 1976.

106. Yukna, R. A., Bowers, G. M., Lawrence, J. J., and Fedi, P. F.: Clinical study of healing in humans following the excisional new attachment procedure. J. Periodontol., 47:696, 1976.

CORRECTION OF OSSEOUS DEFECTS BY BONE RESECTION AND REMODELING

The procedures used to correct osseous defects have been classified in two groups:[7] *osteoplasty* and *osteoectomy*. *Osteoplasty refers to reshaping the bone without removing tooth-supporting bone. Osteoectomy includes removal of tooth-supporting bone.*

There is considerable difference of opinion regarding the wisdom of artificially remodeling bone in the treatment of periodontal disease. It is a severe form of therapy that involves more than just the mechanical reshaping of a structure; biologic processes involved in the bone response may produce more severe alterations in bone morphology than the therapist intended.

The decision to reshape bone to an idealized form is based on the assumption that if defects are permitted to persist following periodontal treatment, they will cause deformity of the overlying gingiva followed by retention of bacterial plaque and debris and recurrence of pockets. However, in healing following periodontal surgery the gingiva does not necessarily follow the contour of the underlying bone; rather, the morphology of the interdental gingiva depends more on the shape and contour of the proximal tooth surfaces.[17] On the facial and lingual surfaces, the level of attachment and the contour of the gingiva are often unrelated to the height or shape of the underlying radicular bone.[9]

Osteoplasty and osteoectomy are used in association with pocket elimination procedures. Most bone defects under suprabony pockets are remodeled by osteoclastic and osteoblastic activity in normal posttreatment healing (Fig. 51-19). Osseous defects associated with infrabony pockets are a more serious problem, but every effort should be made to obtain natural remodeling and filling in of the defects before resorting to bone resection. Removing facial and lingual bone and soft tissue to the level of interproximal craters in an attempt to eliminate interproximal pockets may result in undesirable reductions in the level of gingival attachment.[15]

When used with mucoperiosteal periodontal flaps, bone recontouring by grinding increases the post-treatment loss in bone height.[6] Slight reshaping with chisels is reportedly followed by complete restoration of bone in experimental animals.[2] The post-treatment contour of the facial bone under periodontal flaps is also affected by the occlusion.[9]

Grinding with stones causes bone degeneration and necrosis on the bone surface, where tissue viability is required for healing. It retards healing because of the additional time required for cellular and

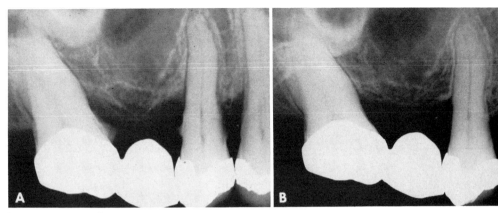

Figure 51–19   Angular Bone Defects Repaired by Healing Without Osseous Surgery. *A,* Angular bone defects under bridge. *B,* Three years after pocket elimination and occlusal adjustment. (Courtesy of Dr. Carl Stoner, New London, Connecticut.)

enzymatic removal of the injured tissue before the reconstruction phase of repair occurs. New bone can form in vascular spaces adjacent to necrotic zones produced by grinding; it is more likely to occur in areas cut with high-speed rather than low-speed rotary instruments.[1] The thickness of the bone affects the results produced by grinding. Interdental septa may retain the shapes artificially created for them,[11] but grinding thin radicular bone produces bone necrosis which, despite attempts at repair, results in loss of bone and unpredictable morphology.[10] Reducing the crest of thick cancellous facial bone by osteoectomy and osteoplasty is followed by repair and restoration of presurgical levels, but further

reduction of height occurs if the bone is thin.[14]

Despite the risk it entails, there are instances in which recontouring of the bone is required. In patients with exostoses, when it can be anticipated that the bone deformity will interfere with the attainment of satisfactory post-treatment oral hygiene and gingival health, the bone is reshaped when the pockets are eliminated (Fig. 51–20). In other situations, the bone should not be artificially remodeled until other treatment procedures combined with conscientious patient cooperation fail to achieve the desired results. Experienced clinicians, however, can anticipate the results and include bone remodeling as

Figure 51–20   Patient with Exostoses on Maxilla and Mandible. Note the scuffing caused by toothbrushing.

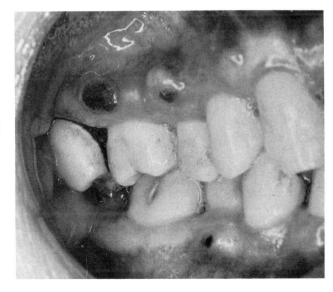

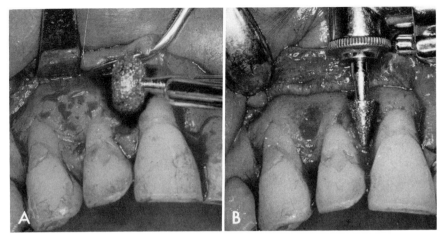

Figure 51–21   Bone Contoured with Diamond Stone. *A,* Round stone used to reduce prominence of labial bone. *B,* Tapered stone used to create interdental sluiceways.

part of the first surgical intervention to avoid subjecting the patient to a second corrective operation.

Techniques for Remodeling Bone

Bone can be remodeled with coarse mounted diamond stones (Fig. 51–21), bone files, rongeurs, chisels, or large round burs. If diamond stones or burs are used, the area is bathed in a stream of warm water to minimize injury from frictional heat.

CORRECTION OF ONE-WALL VERTICAL DEFECTS. To eliminate one-wall infrabony defects on the facial or lingual surface, the margin of the bone is reduced to the level of the base of the defect and then

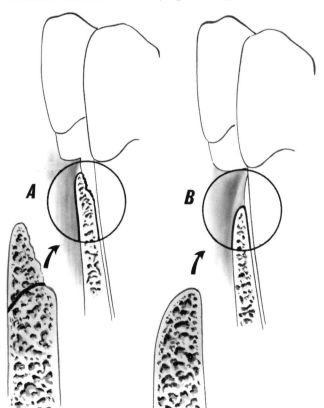

Figure 51–22   Bone Recontoured to Correct One Wall Infrabony Defect. *A,* Angular defect in the facial bone on a premolar is shown in the circle and in enlarged view. The dark line shows the level to which the bone is reduced to correct the defect. *B,* Recontoured bone shown in the circle and in enlarged view.

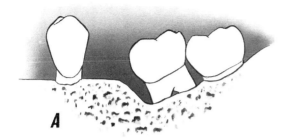

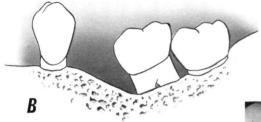

Figure 51–23   Reduction of One Wall Infrabony Angular Defect. *A*, Angular bone defect mesial to tilted molar. *B*, Defect reduced by "ramping" angular bone.

Figure 51–24   Infrabony Pockets on Mesial and Distal Surfaces of Same Interdental Septum. *Above*, Before treatment. One wall osseous defects on proximal surfaces of molars and premolar. *Below*, Seven months after treatment of infrabony pockets without artificially remodeling the osseous defects are corrected by natural healing.

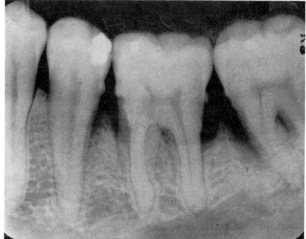

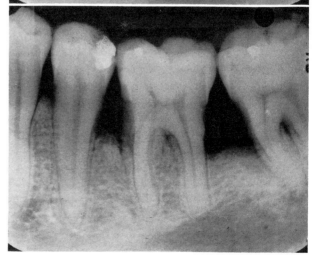

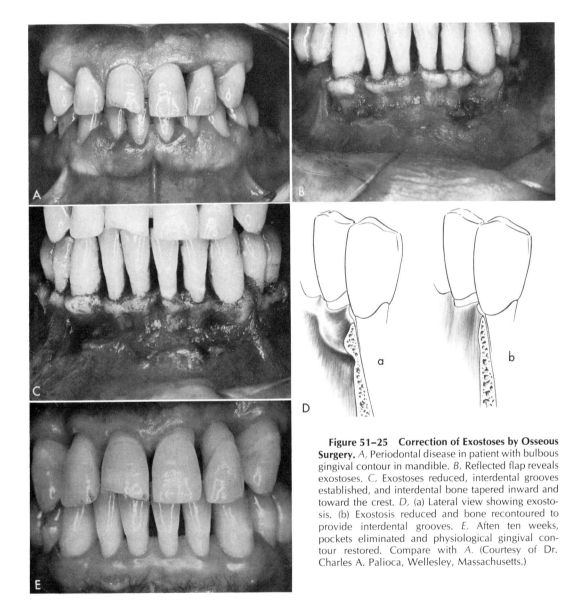

Figure 51-25   Correction of Exostoses by Osseous Surgery. A, Periodontal disease in patient with bulbous gingival contour in mandible. B, Reflected flap reveals exostoses. C, Exostoses reduced, interdental grooves established, and interdental bone tapered inward and toward the crest. D, (a) Lateral view showing exostosis. (b) Exostosis reduced and bone recontoured to provide interdental grooves. E, Aften ten weeks, pockets eliminated and physiological gingival contour restored. Compare with A. (Courtesy of Dr. Charles A. Palioca, Wellesley, Massachusetts.)

rounded[3, 4, 8] (Fig. 51–22). Interproximally, one-wall defects often produce a hemiseptum formed by the remnant of the interdental bone. In the treatment of this condition, the bone is reduced to the level of the defect, and facial and lingual surfaces are thinned and tapered toward the crown. In one-wall defects adjacent to edentulous spaces, the edentulous ridge is reduced to the level of the osseous defect (Fig. 51–23). Artificial remodeling of bone is not required when one-wall infrabony defects are "back to back" on the same interdental septum. Treatment of the pockets without alteration of the bone is generally followed by resorption of the intervening bony septum, which also eliminates the one-wall defects on both sides of it (Fig. 51–24).

CORRECTION OF EXOSTOSES. Make a vertical incision from the gingival margin to the mucobuccal fold mesial and distal to the involved area, and raise a gingival flap, including the periosteum of the bone (Fig. 51–25). With a coarse rotating diamond stone, under a stream of water, reduce the bulk of the bone and reshape it in conformity with the prominence of the roots, creating interdental grooves, tapering the interproximal bone inward toward the crest, and eliminating marginal irregularities. Remove all tissue debris, replace the flap, suture and cover with periodontal pack.

CORRECTION OF INTERDENTAL CRATERS. Interdental craters may be corrected by reducing the facial or lingual wall or both inward and toward the crown (Fig. 51–26). To preserve the facial bone in the anterior maxilla[3] and avoid bone loss and denudation of the buccal roots of the maxillary molars, the major correction is done on the lingual surface (Fig. 51–27).[13] The lingual wall of the crater is reduced, and the bone is ramped and tapered toward the tooth.

CORRECTION OF THICK BONY LEDGES. Persistent, thick, shelf-like marginal ledges, which interfere with the maintenance of gingival health in furcations, are thinned and tapered inward (Fig. 51–28). Crater-like defects that undermine bulbous marginal bone are caused by removing the overlying bony ledge (Fig. 51–29). Abrupt irregularities in the bone margin are reduced in order to create continuity between the interdental and radicular bone (Fig. 51–30).

Text continued on page 880

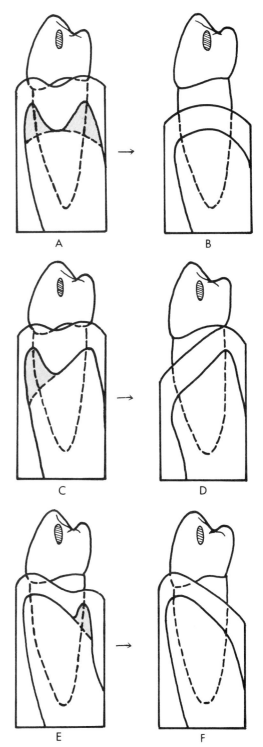

Figure 51–26 Different Methods of Bone Contouring in an Interdental Bony Crater. *A,* Crater to be corrected by reduction of both facial and lingual wall; *B,* After removal of both walls. *C,* Crater to be corrected by reduction of facial wall; *D,* After correction. *E,* Crater to be corrected by reduction of lingual wall; *F,* After correction.

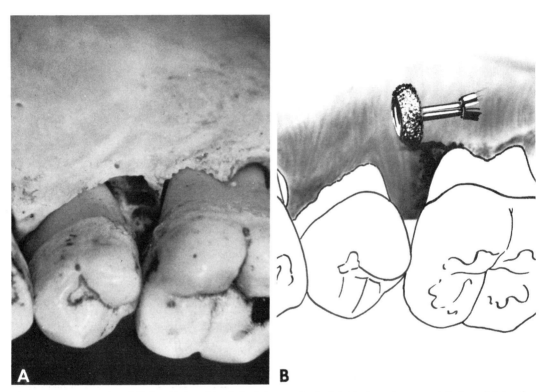

Figure 51–27 Interdental Defect Reduced by Palatal Approach. *A,* Palatal view of osseous defect on distal surface of maxillary second premolar. *B,* Palatal wall of crater reduced and tapered with diamond stone.

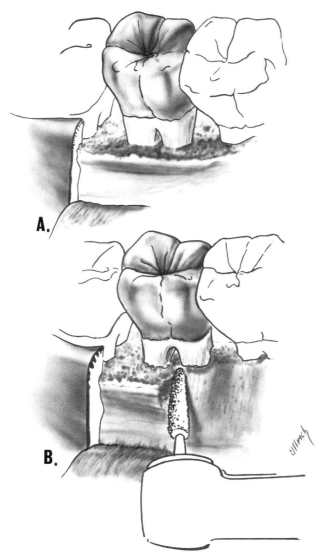

Figure 51–28   A, Remodeling of Bulky Bony Margins. *A,* Bony ledge interferes with proper healing of bifurcation area. *B,* Bone reshaped and tapered with diamond stone to eliminate shelf-like margin.

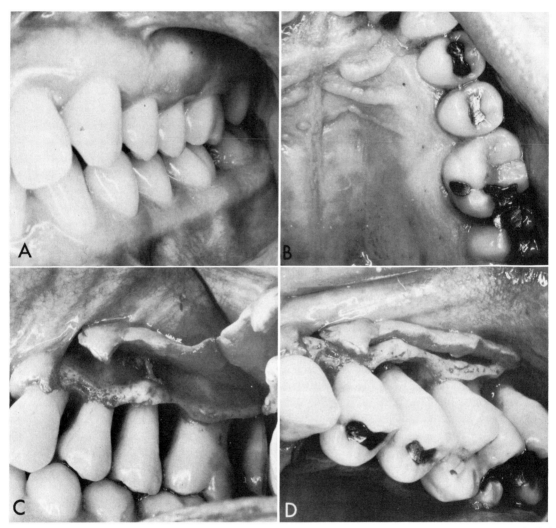

Figure 51–29   Osteoplasty for Reduction of Bulbous Bone Undermined by Craters. *A,* Before treatment. Note the bulbous contour in the premolar area. *B,* Before treatment. Bottom of pockets marked on the palate. *C,* Elevation of full thickness flap reveals irregular bulbous bony ledge. *D,* Craters under bulbous bony ledge.

(Illustration continued on opposite page)

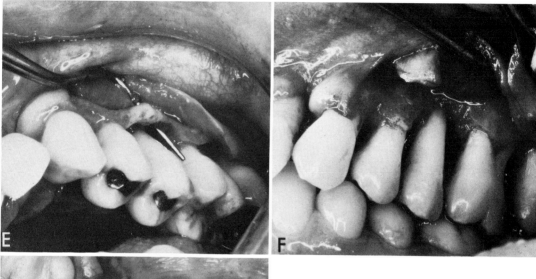

Figure 51–29 *Continued* *E,* Probe demonstrates dehiscence in the bone. *F,* Bony ledge and craters removed by osseous surgery. *G,* Palatal flap sutured to flap on the facial surface. (Courtesy of Dr. Edward S. Cohen, West Newton, Mass.)

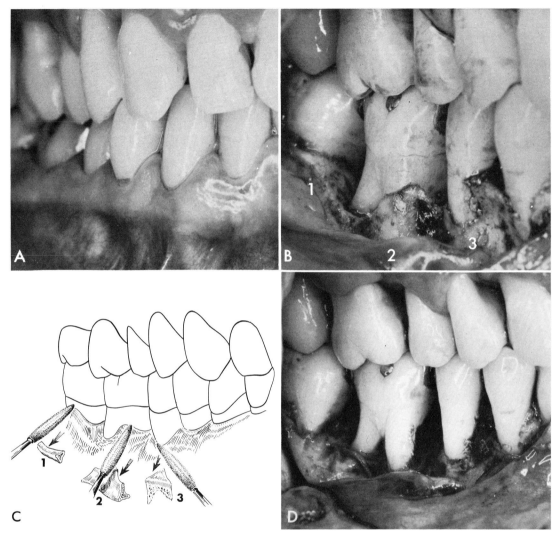

Figure 51–30   Bone Recontoured by Osteoplasty. *A,* Patient with deep periodontal pockets and bone loss. *B,* Elevation of full thickness flap reveals broad osseous plateau (1) and bone irregularities (2 and 3). *C,* Osseous deformities (1, 2 and 3) recontoured by osteoplasty. *D,* After correction of osseous deformities. (*A, B* and *D* courtesy of Dr. Edward S. Cohen, West Newton, Mass.)

REFERENCES

1. Boyne, P. J.: Histologic response of bone to sectioning by high-speed rotary instruments. J. Dent. Res., *45*:270, 1966.
2. Caffesse, R. G., Ramfjord, S. P., and Masjleti, C.: Reverse bevel periodontal flaps in monkeys. J. Periodontol., *39*:219, 1968.
3. Carranza, F. A., Sr.: When and why the elimination of bone is necessary in the treatment of periodontal disease. Anales Del Ateneo del Instituto Municipal de Odontologia (Buenos Aires), *3*:311, 1941.
4. Carranza, F. A., Sr., and Carranza, F. A., Jr.: The management of the alveolar bone in the treatment of the periodontal pocket. J. Periodontol., *27*:29, 1956.
5. Donnenfeld, O. W., and Glickman, I.: A biometric study of the effects of gingivectomy. J. Periodontol., *37*:447, 1966.
6. Donnenfeld, O. W., Hoag, P. M., and Weissman, D. P.: A clinical study in the effects of osteoplasty. J. Periodontol., *41*:131, 1970.
7. Friedman, N.: Periodontal osseous surgery: osteoplasty and osteoectomy. J. Periodontol., *26*:257, 1955.
8. Fröhlich, von, E.: Grundsätzliche Fragen der chirugische Behandlung der marginalen Perodontitis. Deutsche Zahnartzl. Zschr., *8*:523, 1953.
9. Glickman, I., Smulow, J. B., O'Brien, T., and Tannen, R.: Healing of the periodontium following mucogingival surgery. Oral Surg., *16*:530, 1963.

10. Lobene, R., and Glickman, I.: The response of alveolar bone to grinding with rotary diamond stones. J. Periodontol., *34*:105, 1063.
11. Matherson, D. G., and Zander, H. A.: An evaluation of osseous surgery in monkeys. I.A.D.R. Abst. #325, 1963, p. 116.
12. Ochsenbein, C.: Osseous resection in periodontal surgery. J. Periodontol., *29*:15, 1958.
13. Ochsenbein, C., and Bohannan, H. M.: The palatal approach to osseous surgery. I. Rationale. J. Periodontol., *34*:60, 1963.
14. Pennel, B. M., King, K. O., Wilderman, M. H., and Barron, J. M.: Repair of the alveolar process following osseous surgery. J. Periodontol., *38*:426, 1967.
15. Ramfjord, S. P., Nissle, R. R., Schick, R. A., and Cooper, H., Jr.: Subgingival curettage versus surgical elimination of periodontal pockets. J. Periodontol., *39*:167, 1968.
16. Schluger, S.: Osseous resection: a basic principle in periodontal surgery. Oral Surg., *2*:316, 1949.
17. Zander, H. A., and Matherson, D. G.: The effect of osseous surgery on interdental tissue morphology in monkeys. I.A.D.R. Abstr. #236, 1963, p. 117.

Chapter 52

Treatment of Furcation Involvement; and Combined Periodontal-Endodontic Therapy

The prognosis of teeth with furcation involvement is governed by the same factors that determine the prognosis of single-rooted teeth with comparable periodontal destruction. Multirooted teeth have, however, the advantage of added stability provided by the extra root anchorage and the disadvantage of being less accessible to the treatment procedures performed by the operator and to oral hygiene performed by the patient. Prognosis is better in teeth with widely separated roots since accessibility is better in these cases. The principles governing the treatment of furcations are the same as those applicable to periodontal disease in general, with certain special procedural considerations which are presented here.

CLASSIFICATION OF FURCATION INVOLVEMENT

The following classification of furcation involvement, based on severity of destruc-

tion, provides one of the criteria for treatment in individual cases; the types of pockets and the presence or absence of osseous defects are additional important diagnostic considerations.

Grade I involvement (incipient)

Involvement of the periodontal ligament in the furcation without gross or radiographic evidence of bone loss (Fig. 52–1).

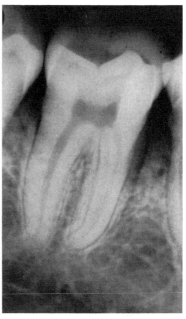

Figure 52–1 Grade I Bifurcation Involvement (Incipient). No marked radiographic change in the bifurcation area.

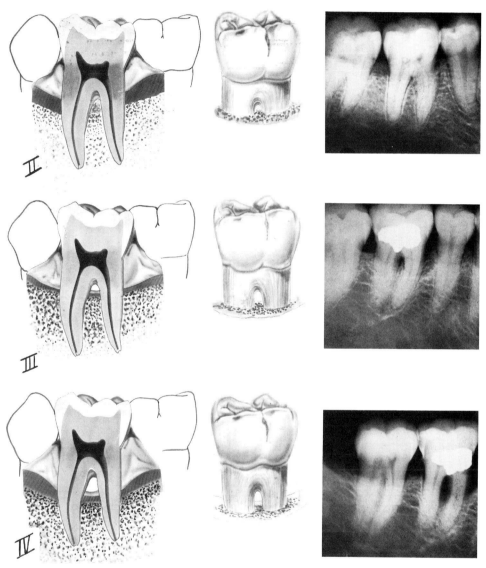

Figure 52–2   *II*, **Grade II Bifurcation Involvement.** Radiograph reveals a small area of radiolucence. A remnant of bony wall is still present in the bifurcation area. *III*, **Grade III Bifurcation Involvement.** Radiograph reveals distinct triangular area of radiolucence. A probe can be passed buccolingually through the bifurcation. *IV*, **Grade IV Bifurcation Involvement.** Radiograph reveals pronounced bone loss. There is clinically obvious exposure of the bifurcation area.

Grade II involvement

In these cases (Fig. 52–2), bone is destroyed on one or more aspects of the furcation, **but a portion of the alveolar bone and periodontal ligament remains intact.** The intact periodontal structures permit only partial penetration of the furcation with a blunt probe.

Grade III involvement

In these cases (Fig. 52–2), the furcation is occluded by gingiva, but the bone has been destroyed to such a degree as to permit the complete passage of a probe faciolingually or mesiodistally.

Grade IV involvement

The periodontium has been destroyed to such a degree that the furcation is open and exposed (Fig. 52–2).

TREATMENT OF FURCATION INVOLVEMENT

Furcations are treated by scaling and curettage, gingivectomy, flap operation, or

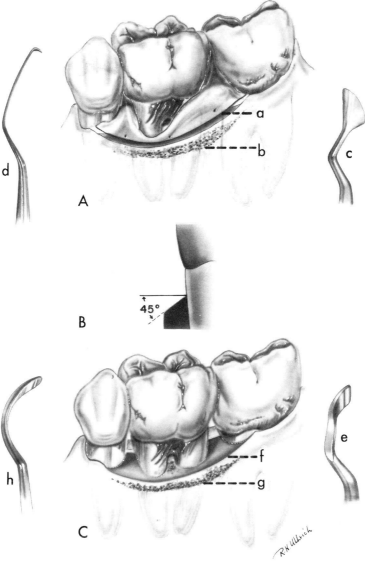

Figure 52–3   Gingivectomy Technique for the Treatment of Bifurcation Involvement. *A,* (a) Line of incision for removing the gingiva. (b) The level of the underlying bone. *B,* The gingiva is cut at a 45° angle to the tooth. *C,* Appearance of the area after the diseased gingiva is removed. (f) The cut surface. (g) The level of the underlying bone.

root resection, depending on the severity of involvement and the architecture of the destructive process. Suprabony pockets without osseous deformities are treated by scaling and curettage or gingivectomy; furcations with infrabony pockets and osseous defects are treated with the flap operation. Furcation involvement may be confined to a single tooth, but very often several teeth are affected. The furcations are treated as they are encountered in the systematic care of the mouth[4].

Treatment of grade I involvement (with suprabony pockets)

Early furcation involvement usually presents suprabony pockets, which are treated by scaling and curettage or gingivectomy, depending on pocket depth and fibrosity of the pocket walls. Since the destructive process is in its incipient stages, it is not necessary to enter the furcation during the treatment process. Elimination of the

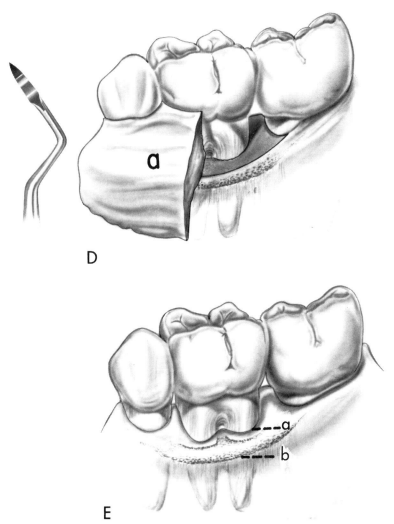

Figure 52–3 *Continued   D,* The pack (a) in position. Part of the field is uncovered to show the relationship of the pack to the furcation. This part is also covered with pack. *E,* The healed lesion showing the contour of the gingiva (a) and the level of the bone (b). **Compare with Treated Cases shown in Figure 52–4.**

pocket is followed by resolution of inflammation and repair of the periodontal ligament and adjacent bone margin.

Treatment of grade II involvement (with suprabony pockets)

Under local anesthesia, each tooth surface is probed down to the bone to determine the pattern of periodontal destruction. One aspect of the furcation is intact in grade II involvement; treatment is from the most extensively involved side and is usually gingivectomy or an apically positioned flap.

Figure 52–3 shows diagrammatically a case solved by gingivectomy. A gingivectomy incision is made through the pinpoint markings, conforming to the outline of the underlying bone margin (Fig. 52–3A). The incision is made with periodontal knives or a Bard-Parker scalpel No. 12 and is beveled at approximately a 45 degree angle to the tooth (Fig. 52–3B). The resected gingiva is detached, exposing underlying bead-like granulation tissue, which is removed with curettes. The root is scaled and planed.

The area is cleaned with warm water, and strips of periodontal pack are placed on the facial and lingual surfaces and pressed together so that they join interproximally for retention (Fig. 52–3D). The pack is removed after one week.

When the pack is removed, the area is cleaned and the roots are checked for small particles of calculus and for smoothness. The patient is instructed in plaque control in the furcation area. Interdental cleansers such as Prox-a-Brush, Stimudents, and Perio-aids should be used in these areas.

Treatment of grade III and grade IV involvement (with suprabony pockets)

In these conditions, interradicular tissue destruction permits a probe to pass freely through the furcation. The gingiva is resected just coronal to the bone or displaced to the same level to provide visibility and access from all directions so that the involved root surfaces may be thoroughly planed and smoothed without disturbing the bone. The periodontal pack is placed for one week except when patient comfort requires repacking for an additional week.

POST-TREATMENT GINGIVAL CONTOUR

Removal of all root deposits, planing of all exposed root surfaces, and fastidious patient care are essential for obtaining optimal post-treatment gingival contour in the furcation areas (Fig. 52–4). Bulging of the gingival margin and recurrence of pockets invariably can be traced to calculus, roughness of the root, or inadequate plaque control. In the treatment of early bifurcation involvement, the buccal groove is sometimes eliminated by reshaping the tooth (**odontoplasty**) to reduce post-treatment accumulation of irritating plaque and debris[5.]

TREATMENT OF FURCATION INVOLVEMENT COMPLICATED BY PERIODONTAL ABSCESS

When furcation involvement is complicated by periodontal abscess formation, the abscess is eradicated as part of the treatment of the furcation (Fig. 52–5).

TREATMENT OF FURCATION INVOLVEMENT COMBINED WITH INFRABONY POCKETS AND OSSEOUS DEFECTS

When infrabony pockets and osseous defects are part of the clinical picture of furcation involvement, the treatment of choice is the flap operation. Adjunctive procedures usually used for these conditions are described in Chapters 50 and 51.

To preserve as much bony support as possible in the furcation area, these lesions are treated without removing bone from the osseous defects (Fig. 52–6). The aim of the approach is to obtain bone repair and recontouring by the natural healing processes (Fig. 52–7). Autogenous bone implants may be used to obtain bone repair in the osseous defect. However, bone grafts in furcation areas have limited chances of success. If bone repair is not obtained after nine months to one year, the osseous defects may be eliminated by reshaping the bone.

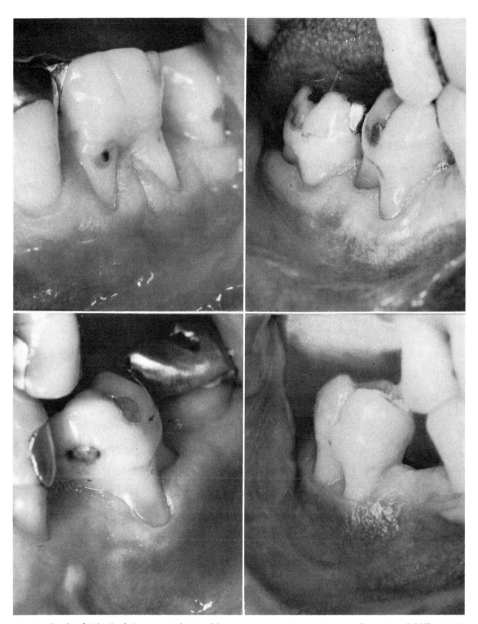

Figure 52–4 Optimal Gingival Contour Obtained by Treatment of Furcation Involvement of Different Severity.

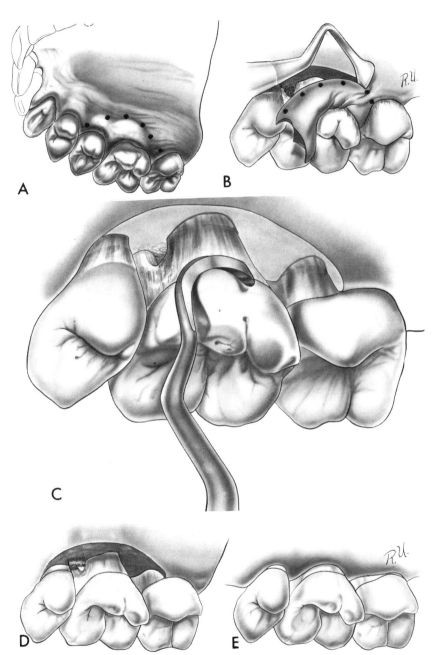

Figure 52–5 Gingivectomy for the Treatment of Furcation Involvement Complicated by Periodontal Abscess. *A,* Periodontal abscess outlined by pinpoint markings. *B,* Abscess excised apical to the markings. *C,* After the calculus is removed, the roots are planed with a curette. Note the exposed trifurcation. *D,* Furcation cleansed before inserting periodontal pack. *E,* Area healed.

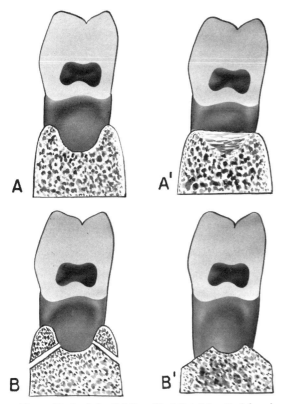

Figure 52–6   Potential Benefit of Retaining Facial and Lingual Bone in the Treatment of Osseous Defects in the Furcation Area. *A,* Faciolingual view showing crater in bifurcation of mandibular molar *A',* Undisturbed facial and lingual plates provide scaffolding for filling in of the defect by healing process. *B,* When the facial and lingual plates are artificially reshaped the potential height obtainable by healing is reduced (*B'*).

Occlusal adjustment in the treatment of furcations with infrabony pockets and osseous defects

Furcation involvement is not of itself indicative of the presence of trauma from occlusion; inflammation may be the only responsible destructive factor. **However, of all the areas of the periodontium, the furcation is most susceptible to injury from excessive occlusal forces.** When furcation involvement is complicated by infrabony pockets and osseous defects, or if the tooth is excessively mobile, checking the occlusion and adjusting it, if necessary, are essential. If the treated teeth are used as abutments for restorations, every effort should be made to align the occlusal forces in the vertical axis of the teeth in order to attain optimal bone repair (Fig. 52–8).

ROOT RESECTION AND HEMISECTION IN THE MANAGEMENT OF FURCATION INVOLVEMENT

Under special circumstances, a root may be resected or a tooth may be sectioned in half (**hemisection**), to preserve teeth with furcation involvement.[1, 8] These forms of treatment are resorted to if it is not possible to obtain success by other methods.

Root resection and hemisection should be

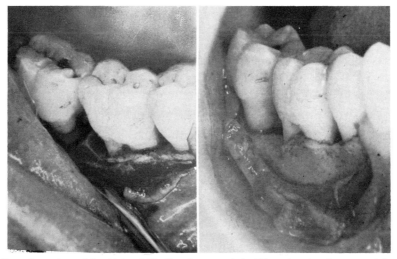

Figure 52–7   Bone Recontoured by Natural Healing Process. *Left,* Bifurcation involvement of the first and second molars with crater-like interdental bony defect and bony shelf. *Right,* One year after treatment without reshaping the bone, the area was re-entered to examine the bone. Note that the buccal ledge has been recontoured and the interdental defect has been eliminated by the natural healing process.

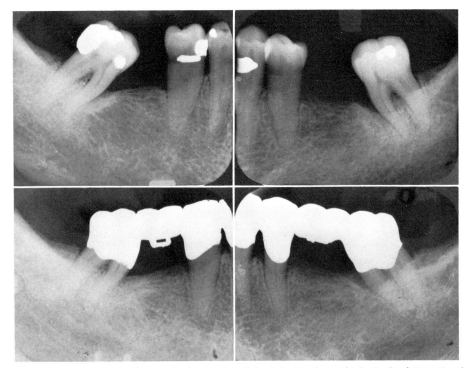

Figure 52–8 Alignment of Occlusal Forces in the Vertical Axis of the Teeth to Obtain Optimal Bone Repair of Furcation Involvement. *Above,* Furcation involvement of mandibular molars with angular osseous defects on the mesial surface. *Below,* Eight years after treatment. The teeth have been reshaped with crowns to direct the occlusal forces toward the vertical axis. Note the improvement in the appearance of the bone. (Restorations by Dr. R. Sheldon Stein, Boston, Massachusetts.)

restricted to firm teeth. They are indicated when the bone destruction is concentrated around one root.

Root resection

This procedure may be used on any root of a multirooted maxillary tooth, but the mesiobuccal or distobuccal root of the maxillary molars is the most suitable. A clinical study[7] has shown that removal of one of the buccal roots of a maxillary molar does not increase the mobility of the tooth in normal function; splinting is not always necessary.

Technique for root resection

This procedure consists of filling the root canals, resecting the root, and sometimes placing a restoration in the severed root canal (Fig. 52–9).

STEP 1. Endodontic therapy is performed first, with the involved root only partially filled. In this way, the patient is spared the discomfort that may occur if the root is resected and there is a time lapse before endodontic therapy.

STEP 2. Under local anesthesia, probe the area to determine the extent and outline of alveolar bone destruction around the root to be removed (Fig. 52–10A).

STEP 3. Make vertical or oblique incisions in the gingiva and mucosa mesial and distal to the involved tooth, and elevate a mucoperiosteal flap (Fig. 52–10B and C).

STEP 4. With a contra-angle handpiece and a cross-cut bur, sever the root where it joins the crown (Fig. 52–10D). Remove the root (Fig. 52–10E).

STEP 5. With a stone or diamond point, smooth the resected root stump and contour the tooth to create an easily cleansable area (Fig. 52–10F).

STEP 6. Scale and plane root surfaces, which become visible and more accessible when the root is removed. This is a most critical part of the treatment.

STEP 7. Clean the area, replace the flap, suture, and cover with periodontal pack.

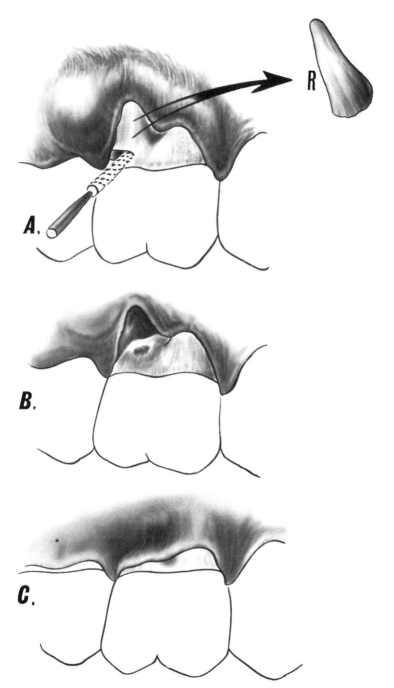

Figure 52–9   Root Resection in the Treatment of Trifurcation Involvement. A, Distobuccal root resected and removed (R). B, Tooth surface smoothed, showing the root canal which was filled before the resection. C, After healing.

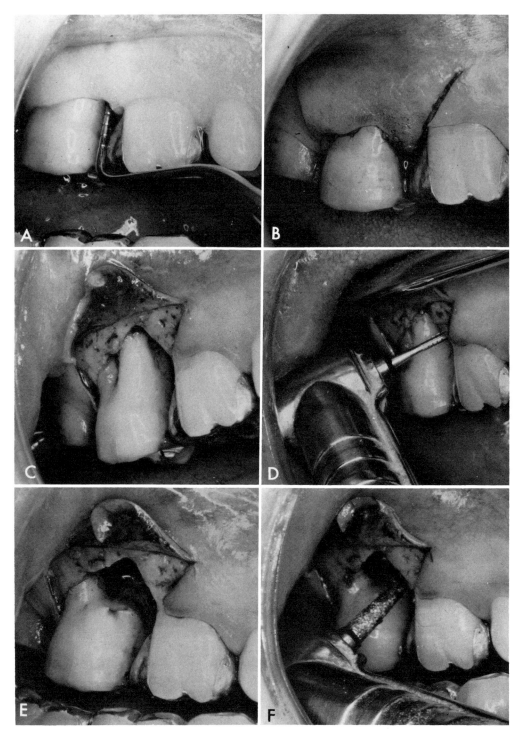

Figure 52–10   Resection of the Mesiobuccal Root of a Molar with Furcation Involvement. *A,* Probing the extent of periodontal destruction. *B,* Incisions for a flap. *C,* Mucoperiosteal flap elevated, revealing extensive bone loss and osseous defect on mesiobuccal root. *D,* Root resected with cross-cut bur. *E,* Root removed; sharp stump remains. *F,* Sharp stump planed and tooth contoured to prevent food entrapment.

(Illustration continued on opposite page)

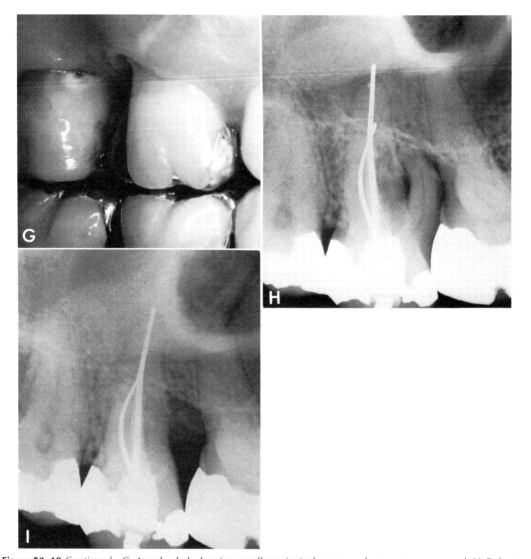

Figure 52–10 *Continued*   *G,* Area healed, showing excellent gingival contour where root was removed. *H,* Before treatment. Radiograph shows extensive bone loss around mesiobuccal root. *I,* Nine months after treatment, showing bone repair where root was removed.

Remove the pack and suture after one week. Physiologic gingival contour is usually restored by two months (Fig. 52–10*G*), and bone repair is detectable radiographically by nine months (Figs. 52–10*H* and *I*).

Hemisection

Hemisection involves the same technique as that used for root resection, except that half the crown is removed along with one of the roots of a mandibular molar. The retained mesial or distal half serves as a useful abutment for a dental restoration (Fig. 52–11).

COMBINED PERIODONTAL-ENDODONTIC THERAPY

Periodontics and endodontics are separate specialties, but the periodontium is not

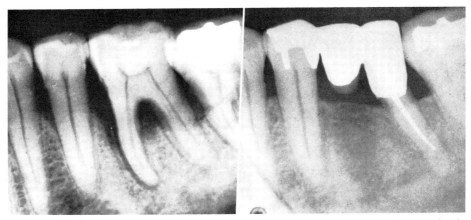

Figure 52–11   Hemisection. *Left,* Bifurcation involvement of first molar. *Right,* Two years and three months after resection of the mesial half of the first molar. (Courtesy of Dr. John Cane, Philipsburg, New Jersey.)

similarly divided into periodontal and periapical halves; the periodontium is a continuous unit. As inflammation spreads from the gingiva into the alveolar bone and periodontal ligament, it may reach the pulp through the root apices or accessory pulp canals near the apex or in the furcation. Periapical destruction caused by pulpal infection may spread along the root and cause a retrograde periodontitis, [9] or inflammation in the pulp may spread through accessory canals and cause inflammation and periodontal destruction in the furcation.[10] There are, therefore, many occasions when the survival of a tooth depends upon combined periodontal and endodontic approaches to treatment.[6]

Indications

Combined periodontal-endodontic therapy is indicated when there is continuity of destruction between the gingival margin and the periapical region. The diagnosis is made by probing the periodontal pocket to the root apex; radiographs with gutta percha points are helpful diagnostic aids (Fig. 52–12). The pulp in such cases is usually nonvital.

Combined periodontal-endodontic therapy is also sometimes indicated for **teeth with periodontal destruction that extends close to but does not reach the periapical area.** Such teeth often resist repeated attempts at periodontal treatment. The pulp usually responds to vitalometer and other tests. However, repair of the periodontal lesion is strikingly improved after endodontic therapy.

The prognosis of combined periodontal-endodontic therapy depends upon the degree of mobility and the severity and distribution of bone loss. Best results are obtained on firm teeth with bone loss

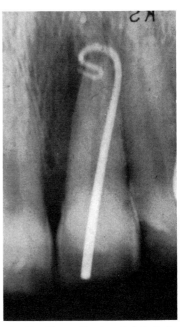

Figure 52–12 Gutta Percha Point Indicates that Periodontal Pocket Extends to the Apex of Maxillary Central Incisor.

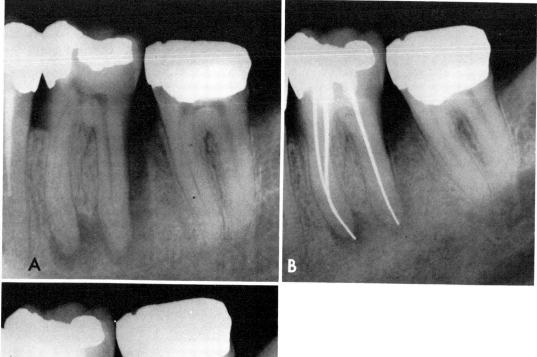

Figure 52-13 Combined Periodontal-Endodontic Therapy. *A,* Before treatment, showing vertical radiolucent zone from the margin to the periapical region of the distal root of the first molar and a radiolucent area on the mesial root. *B,* One year after combined periodontal-endodontic treatment, showing considerable improvement. *C,* Three years after treatment, showing further improvement.

confined to one root surface or one root of a multirooted tooth. Prognosis is improved by consideration of the occlusion and correction when necessary.

Sequence of combined treatment

The types of periodontal and endodontic therapy used vary in individual cases; properly performed, they produce gratifying results (Fig. 52-13). Since the healing responses of the periodontium to both forms of therapy are interrelated, they should be performed together. If they are done at different times, there is no rule regarding which should be first. Treating the periodontal pocket first might benefit periapical healing by shutting off bacterial flow from the oral cavity. Treating the root canal first could force toxic bacterial products and chemical irritants through the dentinal tubules, injuring the cementum[3] and interfering with the outcome of periodontal treatment. Relief of pain often governs the sequence of treatment in these cases.

REFERENCES

1. Amen, C. R.: Hemisection and root amputation. Periodontics, *4*:197, 1966.
2. Basaraba, N.: Root amputation and tooth hemisection. Dent. Clin. North Am. *13*:121, Jan. 1969.
3. Erausquin, J., and Muruzabál, M.: Necrosis of cementum induced by root canal treatments in the molar teeth of rats. Arch. Oral Biol., *12*:1123, 1967.
4. Ericsson, I., and Nyman, S.: Treatment of molar furcation involvement. Tandlakart., 65:252, 1973.
5. Goldman, H. M.: Therapy of the incipient bifurcation involvement. J. Periodontol., 29:112, 1958.

6. Hiatt, W. H.: Periodontic pocket elimination by combined endodontic-periodontic therapy. Periodontics, *1*:152, 1963.
7. Klavan, N.: Clinical observations following root amputations in maxillary molar teeth. J. Periodontol., *46*:1, 1975.
8. Messinger, T. F., and Orban, B.: Elimination of periodontal pockets by root amputation. J. Periodontol., 25:213, 1954.
9. Simring, M., and Goldberg, M.: The pulpal pocket approach: retrograde periodontitis. J. Periodontol., 35:22, 1964.
10. Winter, G. B., and Kramer, I. R. H.: Changes in periodontal membrane and bone following experimental pulpal injury in deciduous molar teeth in kittens. Arch. Oral Biol., *10*:279, 1965.

Mucogingival Surgery

Mucogingival surgery consists of plastic surgical procedures for the correction of gingivo—mucous membrane relationships that complicate periodontal disease and may interfere with the success of periodontal treatment.

OBJECTIVES

Mucogingival surgery is performed as an adjunct to regular pocket elimination procedures for the following purposes:

1. **To widen the zone of attached gingiva or create a new zone of attached gingiva when periodontal pockets extend close to or beyond the mucogingival junction (Fig. 53–1) or into the alveolar mucosa (Fig. 53–1).** This is the most common purpose for which mucogingival surgery is performed. The procedure is based upon the premise that a minimum width of attached gingiva is required to support the gingival fibers which brace the marginal gingiva and prevent it from being deflected from the tooth during mastication.

The width of the attached gingiva varies in different individuals and on different teeth. It is generally greatest in the incisor region (3.5 to 4.5 mm. in the maxilla and 3.3 to 3.9 mm. in the mandible) and less in the posterior segments, with the least width in the first premolar area (1.9 mm. in the maxilla and 1.8 mm. in the mandible).[1] No minimum width of attached gingiva has been established as a standard necessary for gingival health; even as little as 1 mm. may create no problems in a patient with excellent oral hygiene.[15] It has been reported that the width of attached gingiva increases with age[1a] and in supraerupted teeth.[1b]

The following are useful guides for determining whether mucogingival surgery is required for correction of the attached gingiva:

If the base of periodontal pockets is apical to the mucogingival line, some attached gingiva must be created to separate the healed gingival sulcus from the alveolar mucosa and prevent pockets from recurring.

If the base of periodontal pockets is close to the mucogingival line, the functional adequacy of the post-treatment attached gingiva can be predicted by the following *tension test.* Retract the cheeks and lips laterally with the fingers. If such tension pulls the marginal gingiva from the teeth, the attached gingiva is too narrow and should be widened along with the treatment of the pockets.

2. **To relocate frena and muscle attachments that encroach upon periodontal pockets and pull them away from the tooth surface.** Tension from such attachments (a) distends the gingival sulcus and fosters the accumulation of irritants that lead to gingivitis and pocket formation, and (b) aggravates the progress of periodontal pockets and causes their recurrence after

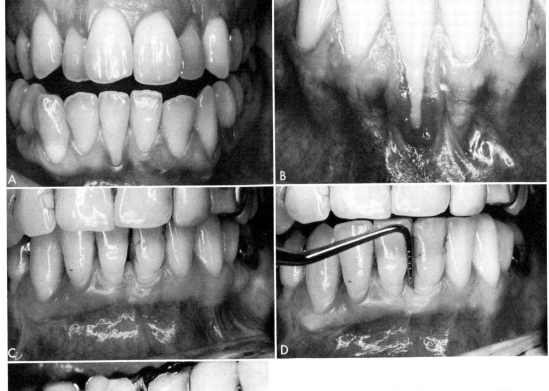

Figure 53–1 Periodontal Pockets with Little or no Attached Gingiva. *A,* Pocket on mandibular incisor extends into alveolar mucosa. *B,* Pocket on mandibular incisor extends into alveolar mucosa. Note pronounced inflammation. *C,* Periodontal pockets in mandibular area. *D,* Probe indicates 4 mm. pocket on the mesial surface of the central incisor reaches to the mucogingival line. *E,* Extreme exposure of the mesiobuccal root of the mandibular first molar.

treatment (Fig. 53–2). The problem is more common on the facial surface, but it occasionally occurs on the lingual surface (Fig. 53–3).

3. **To cover denuded root surfaces.** Root surfaces denuded by gingival disease and recession are functional and esthetic problems. The tension test should also be used in cases of progressive gingival recession to check the effect of soft tissue tension on the gingival margin. Gingiva may be transplanted onto exposed roots by plastic operations and may become so adherent to the root that it does not permit the entrance of a periodontal probe. Reattachment involves the formation of new cementum and the embedding of new connective fibers into the root. Some reattachment (3.5 mm.)[102, 103] on exposed roots has been reported in artificially created defects in experimental animals,[115] and in isolated clinical studies in humans,[99] but the likelihood of obtaining it is not predictable.

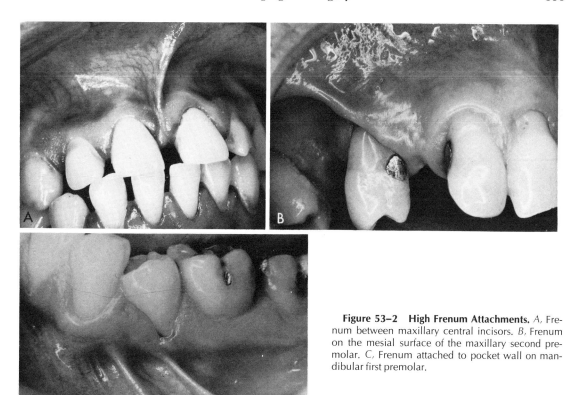

Figure 53–2 High Frenum Attachments. *A*, Frenum between maxillary central incisors. *B*, Frenum on the mesial surface of the maxillary second premolar. *C*, Frenum attached to pocket wall on mandibular first premolar.

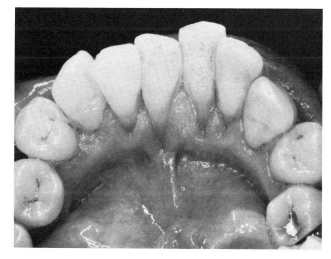

Figure 53–3 Frenum attached to pocket wall on lingual surface of incisor.

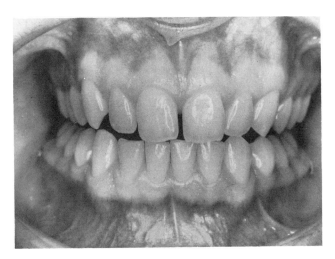

Figure 53-4 Normal Relationship of the Marginal and Attached Gingiva to the Mucogingival Line which demarcates the gingiva from the alveolar mucosa. Also shown are the oral vestibule, the vestibular fornix, and frena attachments in the incisor and premolar areas.

It should be noted that deepening of the vestibule is not important in relation to periodontal therapy.[7] Increasing the depth of the vestibule is very important in surgical preparation of edentulous ridges.

FACTORS THAT AFFECT THE OUTCOME OF MUCOGINGIVAL SURGERY

Anatomical Structures

The structures involved in mucogingival surgery are the marginal and attached gingiva, mucogingival line (junction) (Figs. 53-4 and 53-5), alveolar mucosa, periodontal ligament, cementum, alveolar bone and alveolar periosteum, regional blood vessels, lymphatics and nerves, muscle and frenum attachments, and fornix of the oral vestibule. The reader is referred to Chapters 1 to 4 for a review of these structures, except for muscle and frenum attachments and the mental nerve, which are discussed here.

MUSCLE ATTACHMENTS. Tension from high muscle attachments interferes with mucogingival surgery by postoperative reduction in vestibular depth and width of attached gingiva. To prevent this, muscle attachments in the operative field must be separated from the bone (Fig. 53-6). The following muscles may be encountered in mucogingival operations:

1. The mentalis: Originates on the facial surface of the alveolar process in the inci-

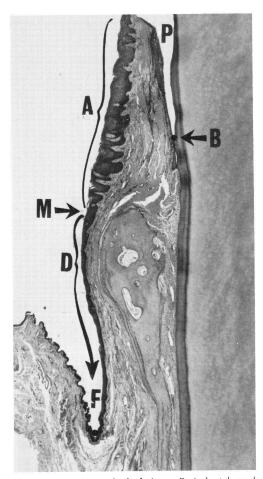

Figure 53-5 Mucogingival Area. Periodontal pocket (P) encroaches upon the mucogingival line (M). The bottom of the pocket is at B. Part of the attached gingiva (A) forms the wall of the pocket. Also note the alveolar mucosa (D), and vestibular fornix (F).

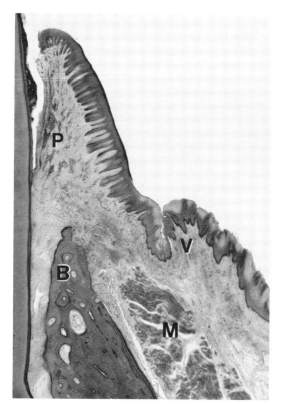

Figure 53–6   Muscle Attachment (M) close to vestibular fornix (V) and crest of the facial bone (B) in an autopsied jaw with periodontal disease. P, Periodontal pocket.

sive fossa and is inserted into the skin of the chin (Fig. 53–7).

2. The incisivus labii inferioris: Originates on the alveolar process close to the border in the mandibular lateral incisor area and passes to the lower lip (Fig. 53–7).

3. The depressor labii inferioris: Originates on the oblique line of the mandible between the symphysis and the mental foramen and passes upward and medially into the lower lip, where it blends with the orbicularis oris and fibers of the opposite side (Fig. 53–7).

4. The depressor anguli oris (triangularis): Originates on the oblique line of the mandible to be inserted into the angle of the mouth.

5. The incisivus labii superioris: Originates from the alveolar process close to the border in the maxillary lateral incisor area and passes to the upper lip (Fig. 53–7).

6. Levator anguli oris (caninus): Arises from the canine fossa below the infraorbital foramen and inserts into the angle of the mouth (Fig. 53–7).

7. The buccinator muscle: Attaches along the apical portion of the alveolar process from the maxillary first molar to

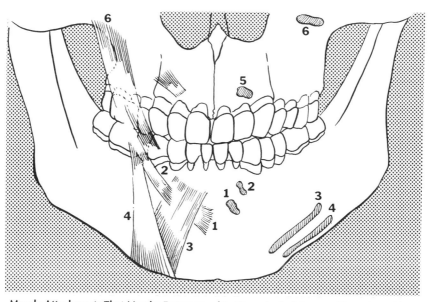

Figure 53–7   Muscle Attachments That May be Encountered in Mucogingival Surgery. The origin of the muscle is shown on the right; the insertion on the left. 1. Mentalis. 2. Incisivus labii inferioris. 3. Depressor labii inferioris. 4. Depressor anguli oris (triangularis). 5. Incisivus labii superioris. 6. Levator anguli oris (caninus).

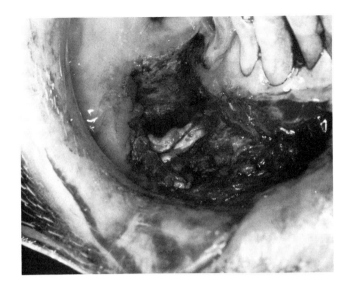

Figure 53–8   Mental Nerve. Emerging From the Foramen in the Premolar Area.

the posterior portion of the maxilla and on the mandible in the lower end of the retromolar fossa and in the external oblique line.

THE MENTAL NERVE. Trauma to the mental nerve can produce uncomfortable paresthesia of the lip, which recovers slowly. Familiarity with the location and appearance of the mental nerve reduces the likelihood of injuring it. The mental nerve emerges from the mental foramen located apical to the first and second mandibular premolars and usually divides into three branches (Figs. 53–8, 53–9, and 53–10). One turns forward and downward to the skin of the chin. The other two course anteriorly and upward to supply the skin and mucous membrane of the lower lip and the mucosa of the labial alveolar surface.

Irregularity of Teeth

Abnormal tooth alignment is an important cause of gingival deformities that require corrective surgery and is an important factor in determining the outcome of treatment. The location of the gingival margin, the width of the attached gingiva, and alveolar bone height and thickness are all affected by tooth alignment. On teeth that are tilted or rotated labially, the labial bony plate is thinner and located further apically than on the adjacent teeth, and

the gingiva is receded so that the root is exposed.[118] On the lingual surface of such teeth, the gingiva is bulbous and the bone margins are closer to the cemento-enamel junction. The level of gingival attachment on root surfaces and the width of attached gingiva following mucogingival surgery are affected as much, or more, by tooth alignment as by variations in treatment procedures (Fig. 53–11).

Orthodontic correction is indicated when mucogingival surgery is performed on malposed teeth in an attempt to widen the attached gingiva or to restore the gingiva over denuded roots. If orthodontic treatment is not feasible, the prominent tooth should be ground to within the borders of the alveolar bone with special care taken to avoid pulp injury.

Roots covered with thin bony plates comprise a hazard in mucogingival surgery. Even the simplest type of flap (partial thickness) creates the risk of bone resorption on the periosteal surface.[48] Resorption in amounts that ordinarily are not significant may cause loss of bone height when the bony plate is thin or tapered at the crest.

The Mucogingival Line (Junction)

Normally, the mucogingival line in the incisor and canine areas is located approximately 3 mm. apical to the crest of the

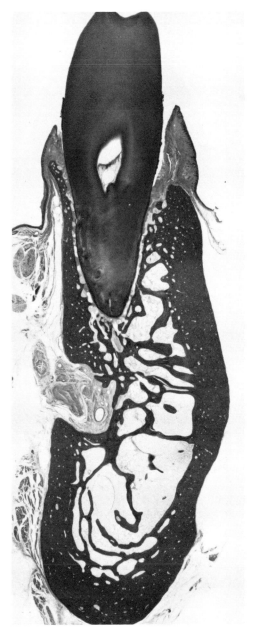

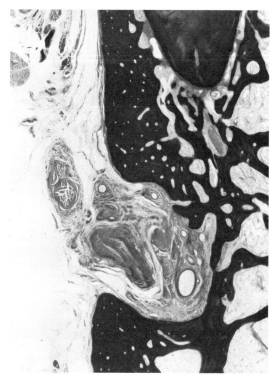

Figure 53–10 Detailed View of Mental Nerve and Blood Vessels in the Mental Foramen. Note Relationship to Premolar Root.

Figure 53–9 Mental Nerve and Blood Vessels in Mental Foramen. Note the relationship of the mental foramen to the apex of the second premolar and the oral vestibule.

alveolar bone on the radicular surfaces and 5 mm. interdentally.[98] In periodontal disease and on malposed disease-free teeth, the bone margin is located further apically and may extend beyond the mucogingival line.

The distance between the mucogingival line and the cemento-enamel junction before and after periodontal surgery is not necessarily constant. After inflammation is eliminated, there is a tendency for the tissue to contract and draw the mucogingival line in the direction of the crown.[32]

MUCOGINGIVAL OPERATIONS

In the first half of this century, periodontal surgery was confined to eliminating disease and arresting tissue destruction; in the last three decades there has been considerable clinical experimentation with mucogingival procedures. Unfortunately, in an attempt to broaden the scope of periodontal therapy and increase the longevity of the natural dentition, operations have been performed before the research had determined their usefulness and limitations. Before surgical procedures are performed on a patient, there should be acceptable evidence that the operation is likely to solve the problem, and the extent

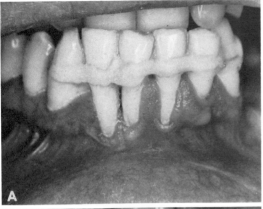

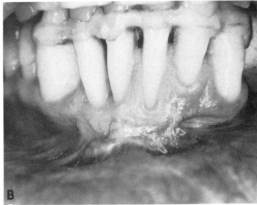

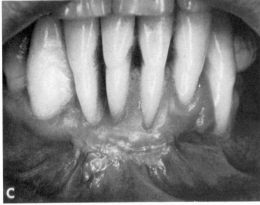

Figure 53–11 **Gingival Recession and Narrow Band of Attached Gingiva Persist Around Labially Positioned Roots After Mucogingival Surgery.** *A,* Before treatment, showing gingival recession with narrow band of attached gingiva around labially prominent teeth. *B,* Three months after mucogingival surgery. The attached gingiva around the central and lateral incisors has been widened. *C,* Five months after surgery. Recession is increased and the attached gingiva is narrowed around the prominent roots. Compare the patient's left canines in *B* and *C.*

to which it is experimental should be made clear to the patient.[108]

Descriptions of those operations that have been shown in human and animal studies to be useful, with their accomplishments and limitations, are presented in the remainder of this chapter. Research findings in some instances are inconclusive or conflicting. This is to be expected for many reasons, such as subtle differences in the way the same operation is performed by different operators; the difficulty of obtaining histological material to corroborate what appears to be obvious clinical results; differences between postoperative healing of artificially created and naturally occurring periodontal lesions; differences in tissue response among animal species, between animals and humans, and among different individuals; differences in oral hygiene among humans; and the difference between pretreatment and post-treatment *impressions* gathered from clinical observations and photographs and

facts based on measurements subjected to statistical analysis.

Initially, the operation that was advocated was a partial thickness flap with the purpose of deepening the vestibular fornix, increasing the width of the attached gingiva and relocating frenum attachments. It consisted of (1) a gingivectomy incision apical to the base of the pockets, even if this entailed incising into the alveolar mucosa; (2) resection of the pockets; (3) vertical incisions from the gingival margin into the fornix, outlining the area where the increased depth was desired; (4) placing a No. 15 Bard-Parker blade flat against the gingiva to separate a flap, dissecting it away from the underlying tissue; and finally, (5) insertion of the periodontal pack. Variations of this technique included using a full thickness (mucoperiosteal) flap or a combined full thickness flap in the coronal portion and a partial thickness flap in the apical portion; this was based on the assumption that the level to which the

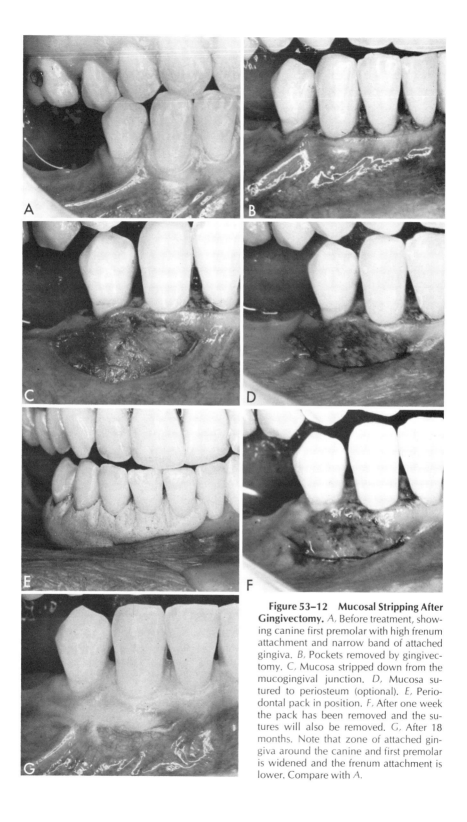

Figure 53–12 Mucosal Stripping After Gingivectomy. *A,* Before treatment, showing canine first premolar with high frenum attachment and narrow band of attached gingiva. *B,* Pockets removed by gingivectomy. *C,* Mucosa stripped down from the mucogingival junction. *D,* Mucosa sutured to periosteum (optional). *E,* Periodontal pack in position. *F,* After one week the pack has been removed and the sutures will also be removed. *G,* After 18 months. Note that zone of attached gingiva around the canine and first premolar is widened and the frenum attachment is lower. Compare with *A.*

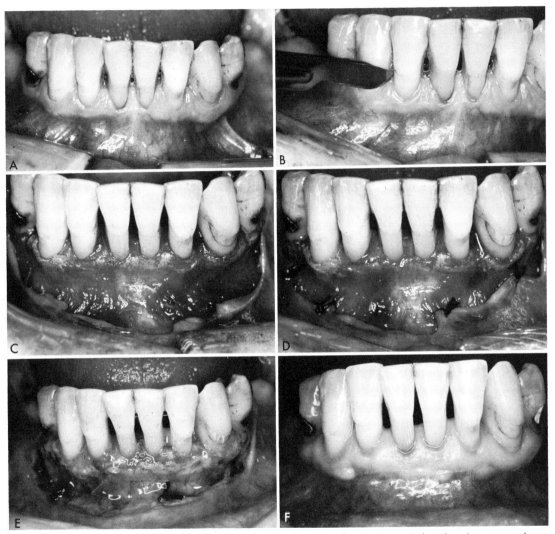

Figure 53–13   Mucosal Stripping with Internal Bevel. *A,* Before treatment, showing periodontal pockets, exposed roots, and narrow band of attached gingiva. *B,* Inner surface of periodontal pockets resected with internal bevel. *C,* Mucosa has been separated away, leaving the bone covered with periosteum. The inner pocket walls have been removed from the teeth, and the roots are scaled. *D,* The mucosa is sutured to the periosteum (optional). *E,* After one week, the periodontal pack has been removed. The sutures will also be removed. *F,* After eight months, the pockets are eliminated and there is a widened zone of attached gingiva. (Compare with *A.*)

bone was denuded would determine the post-treatment width of the attached gingiva (Figs. 53–12 and 53–13).

The postoperative course with these techniques was stormy, sometimes including painful ulcerations or numbness of the lower lip. Results were not favorable. Increased vestibular depth created with partial thickness operations shrunk during the healing process and practically disappeared in a few months. Increased depths created with full thickness operations tended to be more stable, but a significant marginal bone loss occurred.[22] Combination methods had the disadvantages of both techniques with none of their virtues. From these unsuccessful attempts, however, some of the currently used techniques evolved.

Gingival Extension Procedures

Two types of procedures are currently performed in order to widen the zone of attached gingiva:

1. The *gingival extension operations*, which consist of the surgical deepening of the mucogingival line. In order to prevent the mucogingival line from creeping back coronally during the postoperative healing, two methods have proved useful, the so-called *fenestration procedure* and the placement of a *free mucosal autograft*. The latter is more predictable and heals with fewer problems in spite of the two surgical sites needed. It is therefore preferred.

2. The *apical displacement* of *the existing pocket wall*, which by this method becomes attached to the cementum and/or bone and takes on the appearance and function of attached gingiva.

Fenestration procedure[29, 80, 82, 83]

This operation is designed to widen the zone of attached gingiva with a minimum loss of bone height. It has also been called periosteal separation.[29] It utilizes a partial thickness flap, except in a rectangular area at the base of the operative field, where the periosteum is elevated and the bone is exposed (Fig. 53–14). This is the area of fenestration. Its purpose is to create a scar

that is firmly bound to the bone and will prevent separation from the bone and narrowing of the width of the attached zone.

PROCEDURE. *Step 1: Eliminate the Periodontal Pockets.* With a No. 15 Bard-Parker blade, make a shallow, vertical incision from the gingival margin to the vestibular fornix at each end of the operative field. With a gingivectomy incision, resect the periodontal pockets; remove the calculus and plane the root surfaces (Fig. 53–14A).

Step 2: Elevate a Partial Thickness Flap. A partial thickness flap consists of epithelium and a thin underlying layer of connective tissue. The periosteum is left intact as a protective covering for the bone. To start the flap, hold a No. 15 Bard-Parker blade flat against the facial surface and insert it on the field (Fig. 53–14B). Make a shallow incision along the mucogingival line.

Hold the corners of the mucosa with fine forceps and insert the Bard-Parker blade midway between the epithelial surface and the periosteum. Slowly incise across the operative field, gently separating a partial thickness flap with the forceps. If the periodontal pockets extend into the alveolar mucosa and no attached gingiva remains after they are resected, the flap is started from the cut mucosal surface (Figs. 53–14E and F, and 53–15).

Extend the dissection apically (Fig. 53–14C) to a level approximately twice the desired width of the new attached gingiva. With a scissors, remove irregularities in the flap margin. Slide the flap apically until the edge is at the newly created level of the vestibule.

Step 3: Cleanse the Periosteum. At this stage, there is a wide area of bone covered by periosteum and a thin layer of connective tissue. With a scissors, remove all muscle fibers and soft tissue from the periosteum until the surface is smooth and firm.

Step 4: Fenestration. At the deepest level in the vestibule, make an incision through the periosteum to the labial plate along the length of the operative field. Bluntly dissect the periosteum and overlying tissue from the bone (a fenestration) across the operative field (Fig. 53–14D). The margin of the flap may be sutured to the periosteum at the lower border of the fenestrated area, but this is not necessary.

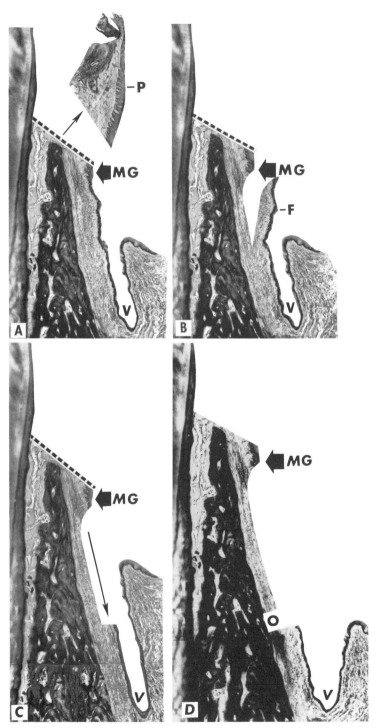

Figure 53–14   Fenestration. *A,* Periodontal pocket (P) resected with gingivectomy incision. MG, Mucogingival junction. V, Vestibular fornix. *B,* Incision at mucogingival junction separates partial thickness flap, (F), leaving periosteum and layer of connective tissue on the bone. *C,* Partial thickness flap moved apically, deepening the oral vestibule (V). *D,* Fenestration (O) cut through the periosteum, leaving the bone exposed.

,Illustration continued on opposite page.

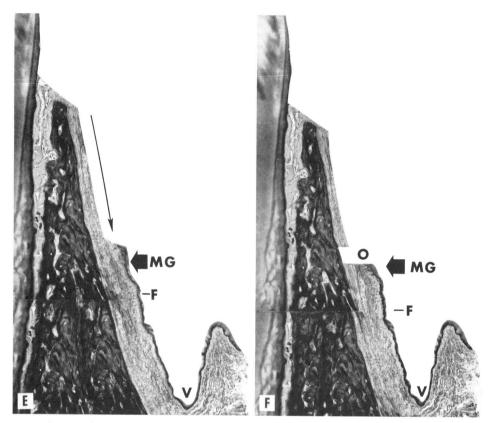

Figure 53–14 *Continued* *E,* Variation of operation when little or no attached gingiva remains following gingivectomy. Partial thickness flap is separated at the cut gingival margin and moved apically (F), deepening the oral vestibule (V) in the process. *F,* Fenestration (O) cut through the periosteum, exposing the bone.

Apply pressure with 2″ × 2″ gauze pads until the bleeding stops; remove excess clot; then insert a periodontal pack (Fig. 53–15). Replace the pack after two weeks and twice again at weekly intervals. If sutures are used, remove them after one week.

ACCOMPLISHMENTS OF THE FENESTRATION OPERATION. The fenestration produces an increase in the width of attached gingiva and in vestibular depth approximately one half of that created at the time of operation.

In the fenestration area, a scar forms that ultimately develops microscopic features resembling those of attached gingiva.[73, 82] The scar is initially firmly attached to the underlying bone[21] and prevents narrowing of the new zone of attached gingiva (Fig. 53–15G). The binding effect lasts about four weeks;[3] by three months the width of

attached gingiva is reduced by approximately 28 per cent[79] and remains that way for approximately a year, after which the width is usually further reduced. **Post-treatment shrinkage of the attached gingiva is anticipated at the time of operation by providing space for twice the desired width of attached gingiva.**

The tendency of repositioned muscle attachments to return to their original position is an important limiting factor in vestibular extension operations. The most lasting results are obtained when minimal invasion of musculature is required in order to create increased space for attached gingiva.[73]. Muscle attachments encountered in the course of deepening the vestibule must be removed to reduce the likelihood of their return. Contraction of the scar also tends to reduce post-treatment vestibular depth.[93]

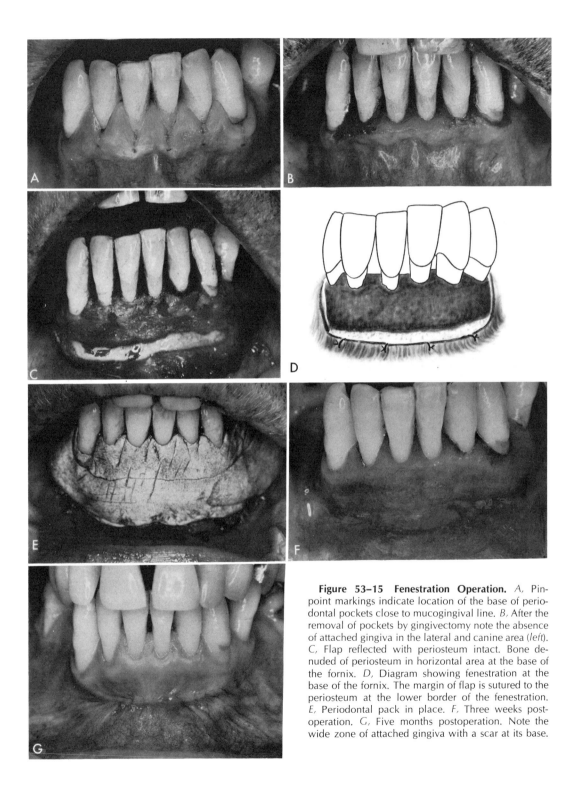

Figure 53-15 Fenestration Operation. *A,* Pinpoint markings indicate location of the base of periodontal pockets close to mucogingival line. *B,* After the removal of pockets by gingivectomy note the absence of attached gingiva in the lateral and canine area (*left*). *C,* Flap reflected with periosteum intact. Bone denuded of periosteum in horizontal area at the base of the fornix. *D,* Diagram showing fenestration at the base of the fornix. The margin of flap is sutured to the periosteum at the lower border of the fenestration. *E,* Periodontal pack in place. *F,* Three weeks postoperation. *G,* Five months postoperation. Note the wide zone of attached gingiva with a scar at its base.

Free gingival autografts[11, 66, 75, 92]*

Free gingival grafts are used to create a widened zone of attached gingiva. They have also been tried for covering denuded roots.

PROCEDURE. *Step 1: Eliminate the Pockets.* With a gingivectomy incision, resect the periodontal pockets and scale and plane the root surfaces.

Step 2: Prepare the Recipient Site. The purpose of this step is to prepare a firm connective tissue bed to receive the graft. The recipient site can be prepared by incising at the existing mucogingival junction with a No. 15 Bard-Parker knife to a little more than the desired depth, blending the incision on both ends with the existing mucogingival line. Periosteum should be left covering the bone.

Another technique consists of outlining the recipient site with two vertical incisions from the cut gingival margin into the alveolar mucosa (Fig. 53–16A and B). Extend the incisions to approximately twice the desired width of the attached gingiva, allowing for 50 per cent contraction of the graft when healing is complete. The amount of contraction depends upon the extent to which the recipient site penetrates the muscle attachments. The deeper the recipient site, the greater is the tendency for the muscles to elevate the graft and reduce the final width of the attached gingiva. The periosteum along the apical border of the graft is sometimes penetrated in an effort to prevent postoperative narrowing of the attached gingiva.[17]

Insert a No. 15 Bard-Parker blade along the cut gingival margin and separate a flap consisting of epithelium and underlying connective tissue without disturbing the periosteum. Extend the flap to the depth of the vertical incisions. Suture the flap where the apical position of the free graft will be placed.

If a narrow band of attached gingiva remains after the pockets are eliminated, it should be left intact and the recipient site

*A better name is probably "free mucosal autografts," since the donor site is usually the palatal mucosa.

started by inserting the blade at the mucogingival junction, instead of at the cut gingival margin.

Prepare the recipient bed for the graft by removing extraneous soft tissue with a curved scissors or tissue nippers, leaving a firm connective tissue surface. Control the bleeding with a 2″ × 2″ sponge and pressure, and protect the area with a sponge moistened with saline. Make a tinfoil or wax template of the recipient site to be used as a pattern for the graft (Fig. 53–16C and D).

Grafts can also be placed directly on bone tissue. For this technique the flap has to be separated by blunt dissection with a periosteal elevator. Reported advantages of this variant to the technique are less postoperative mobility of the graft, less swelling and better hemostasis; a healing lag is observed for the first two weeks, however.[34]

Step 3: Obtain the Graft from Donor Site. A partial thickness graft is used; the sites from which it is obtained are, in order of preference, attached gingiva, masticatory mucosa from an edentulous ridge, and palatal mucosa. The graft should consist of epithelium and a thin layer, approximately 3 mm., of underlying connective tissue. Proper thickness is important for survival of the graft. It should be thin enough to permit ready diffusion of nutritive fluid from the recipient site, which is essential in the immediate post-transplant period. A graft that is too thin may shrivel and expose the recipient site.[75] If the graft is too thick, its peripheral layer is jeopardized because of the excessive tissue that separates it from new circulation and nutrients.[40]

Place the template over the donor site, and make a shallow incision around it with a No. 15 Bard-Parker blade. Insert the blade to the desired thickness at one edge of the graft. Elevate the edge and hold it with a tissue forceps. Continue to separate the graft with the blade, lifting it gently as separation progresses to provide visibility. Placing sutures at the margins of the graft helps control it during separation and transfer and simplifies placement and suturing to the recipient site.[6]

After the graft is separated, remove loose tissue tabs from the undersurface. Thin the edge to avoid bulbous marginal and inter-

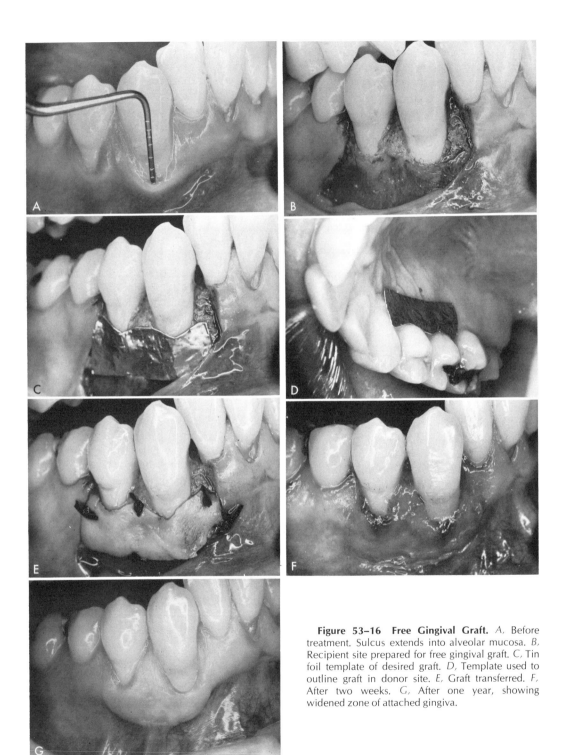

Figure 53–16 Free Gingival Graft. *A,* Before treatment. Sulcus extends into alveolar mucosa. *B,* Recipient site prepared for free gingival graft. *C,* Tin foil template of desired graft. *D,* Template used to outline graft in donor site. *E,* Graft transferred. *F,* After two weeks. *G,* After one year, showing widened zone of attached gingiva.

dental contours. Special precaution must be taken with grafts from the palate. The submucosa in the posterior region is thick and fatty and should be trimmed so that it will not interfere with vascularization. Grafts tend to re-establish their original epithelial structure, so mucous glands may occur in grafts obtained from the palate.

Step 4: Transfer and Immobilize the Graft. Remove the sponge from the recipient site; reapply with pressure if necessary until bleeding is stopped. Clean away excess clot. A thick clot interferes with vascularization of the graft;[70] it is also an excellent medium for bacteria and increases the risk of infection.

Position the graft and adapt it firmly to the recipient site. Space between the graft and the underlying tissue (dead space) will retard vascularization and jeopardize the graft. Suture the graft at the lateral borders and to the periosteum to secure it in position (Fig. 53–16E). Before suturing is complete, elevate the unsutured portion and cleanse the recipient bed beneath it with an aspirator to remove clot or loose tissue fragments. Press the graft back into position and complete the sutures. Be sure the graft is immobilized, because movement interferes with healing. Avoid excessive tension, which will warp the graft and may pull it away from the underlying surface. **Respect for tissue is essential for success.** Use every precaution to avoid injury to the graft. Use tissue forceps delicately to avoid crushing it. Use a minimum number of sutures to avoid unnecessary tissue penetration. The graft can survive some injury, but abuse may damage it beyond recovery.

Cover with periodontal pack for one week when the sutures are removed (Fig. 53–16F). Repack for another week.

Step 5: Protect the Donor Site. Cover the donor site with periodontal pack for one week and repeat if necessary. Retention of the pack on the donor site is sometimes a problem. If facial attached gingiva was used, the pack may be retained by locking it through the interproximal spaces onto the lingual surface. If there are no open interdental spaces, the pack can be covered by a plastic stent wired to the teeth. A modified Hawley retainer is useful to cover the pack on the palate and over edentulous ridges.

THE FATE OF THE GRAFT. The success of the graft depends upon survival of the connective tissue (Fig. 53–16G). Sloughing of the epithelium occurs in most cases, but the extent to which the connective tissue withstands the transfer to the new location determines the fate of the graft. Fibrous organization of the interface between the graft and the recipient bed occurs within two to several days.[95]

The graft is initially maintained by a diffusion of fluid from the host bed, adjacent gingiva, and alveolar mucosa.[40] The fluid is a transudate from the host vessels and provides nutrition and hydration essential for the initial survival of the transplanted tissues. During the first day, the connective tissue becomes edematous and disorganized and undergoes degeneration and lysis of some of its elements. As healing progresses, the edema is resolved and degenerated connective tissue is replaced by new granulation tissue.

Revascularization of the graft starts by the second[16] or third day.[60] Capillaries from the recipient bed and from periodontal ligament included in the recipient site proliferate into the graft to form a network of new capillaries and anastomose with pre-existing vessels.[60] Many of the graft vessels degenerate and are replaced by new ones, and some participate in the new circulation. The central section of the surface is the last to vascularize, but it is complete by the tenth day.

The epithelium undergoes degeneration and sloughing, with complete necrosis occurring in some areas.[19, 70] It is replaced by new epithelium from the borders of the recipient site. A thin layer of new epithelium is present by the fourth day, with rete pegs developing by the seventh day. In skin grafts, the basement membrane remains in situ, disengaged from the overlying epithelium and attached to the underlying connective tissue. New epithelial cells migrate over the basal membrane and appear to be guided by it. The plasma membrane of the cells thickens and forms hemidesmosomes that attach to the basement membrane, and the regenerating epithelium synthesizes new basement membrane.[41]

The fact that heterotopically placed grafts maintain their structure (keratinized epithelium) even after the grafted epithelium has become necrotic and replaced from neighboring areas of nonkeratinized epithelium has suggested that there exists a genetic predetermination on the specific character of the oral mucosa dependent on stimuli that originate in the connective tissue.[62] It has been shown in clinical studies that the width of keratinized gingiva can be extended by means of grafts composed of only connective tissue obtained from

areas where it is covered by keratinized epithelium.[18, 36]

As seen microscopically, healing of a graft of intermediate thickness (0.75 mm.) is complete by ten and one half weeks; thicker grafts (1.75 mm.) may require 16 weeks or longer.[46]

The gross appearance of the graft reflects the tissue changes within it. At the time of transplantation, the graft vessels empty and the graft is pale. The pallor

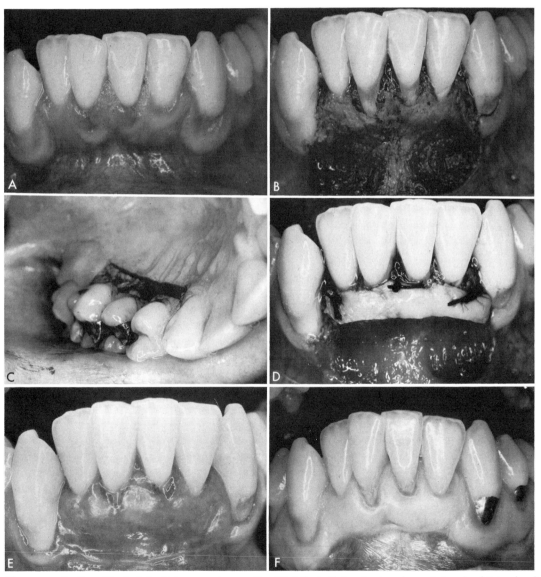

Figure 53–17   Free Gingival Graft (same patient as Fig. 53–16). A, Before treatment—pockets extend into alveolar mucosa. B, Recipient site prepared for graft. C, Graft obtained from the palate. D, Graft sutured in position. E, After two weeks. F, After one year. Note the widened zone of attached gingiva.

changes to an ischemic gray-white during the first two days, until vascularization begins and pink color appears. The plasmatic circulation accumulates and causes softening and swelling of the graft, which is reduced when the edema is removed from the recipient site by the new blood vessels. Loss of epithelium leaves the graft smooth and shiny. New epithelium creates a thin, gray, veil-like surface which develops normal features as the epithelium matures.

Functional integration of the graft occurs by the seventeenth day, but the graft is morphologically distinguishable from surrounding tissue for months. It may eventually blend with adjacent tissues, but more often, although it is pink, firm and healthy, it tends to be somewhat bulbous (Figs. 53–17 and 53–18). This ordinarily presents no problem, but if it traps irritating plaque or is esthetically unacceptable, thinning of the graft may be necessary.

THINNING BULBOUS GRAFTS. Paring

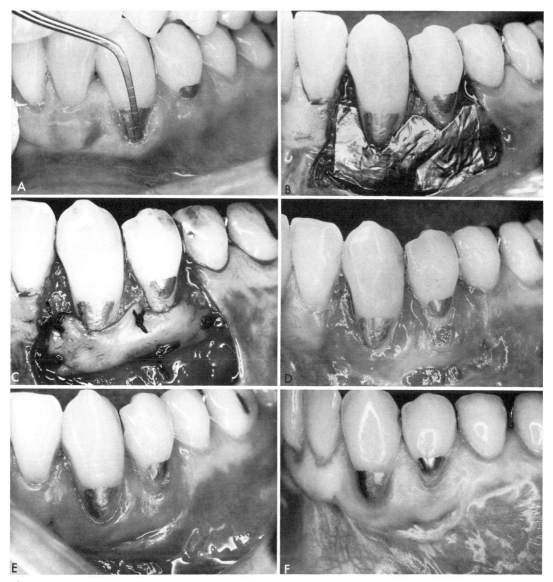

Figure 53–18   Free Gingival Graft (same patient as Figs. 53–16 and 53–17). *A,* Before treatment—periodontal pocket in the canine extends into the alveolar mucosa. *B,* Recipient site prepared and template made for desired graft. *C,* Graft sutured in place. *D,* After two weeks. *E,* After nine weeks. *F,* After one year. Note the widened zone of healthy attached gingiva. Compare with *A.*

down the surface will not reduce the bulbous condition, because the surface epithelium tends to proliferate again. The graft should be thinned as follows:

Step 1. With a No. 15 Bard-Parker blade, make vertical incisions along the lateral border of the graft to the gingival margin. If the graft does not extend to the gingival margin, make the incisions along three of the borders.

Step 2. Elevate the graft from the underlying periosteum, and thin it by removing tissue from the undersurface.

Step 3. Replace the graft and suture.

ACCOMPLISHMENTS OF FREE GINGIVAL GRAFTS. Free gingival grafts effectively widen the attached gingiva and deepen the oral vestibule. Compared with other operations for the same purposes, they entail involvement of an additional operative site (the donor site). Some feel that grafts protect the underlying bone,[106] in that they cause less osteoclastic activity and stimulate osteoblastic activity and thickening of the bone.[16] If this were so, it would be advantageous to use grafts for widening attached gingiva when the facial bone is thin.

Other materials have been used to replace gingival tissue in gingival extension operations. Attempts with lyophilized dura mater[63, 86] and with sclera[68a] have not been satisfactory; the use of irradiated free gingival allografts showed satisfactory results,[85] but further research is necessary before they can be considered for clinical use.

Free gingival grafts and denuded roots

Roots denuded by gingival defects are unattractive and are commonly the sites of plaque accumulation and persistent gingival disease. The incentive for experimenting with procedures that offer promise of restoring the gingiva on denuded roots is great. Grafts placed over exposed roots generally shrink, re-exposing part of the root but covering a portion of it, particularly when the gingival defect is long and narrow.

Since the vascular bed is required for preservation of a free gingival graft, it cannot be expected to correct extensive root exposure.[55, 95] However, if the gingival defect is narrow, collateral circulation from the connective tissue around the margins of the recipient site aids survival of the graft over the root.[100] The graft may be firmly adherent and resist separation from the tooth by a periodontal probe,[66] but the extent to which it is reattached to the root by new fibers embedded into new cementum has not been established. Reattachment of free gingival grafts has been reported on artificially exposed roots in animals,[71] but the results in humans are as yet inconclusive.[99, 101]

Free autogenous gingival grafts have been found useful to cover "nonpathologic" dehiscences and fenestrations; "nonpathologic" refers to openings of the bone through to the tooth surface not previously exposed to the oral environment and found in the course of flap surgery.[35]

Vestibule extension operation

This technique, originally described by Edlan and Mejchar,[37] produces statistically significant widening of attached nonkeratinized tissue. This increase in width in the mandibular area reportedly persists in patients observed for periods of up to five years.[37, 87, 107]

PROCEDURE. *Step 1: Outline the Operative Field* (Fig. 53–19A). Starting at the junction of the gingival margin and attached gingiva, make a vertical incision at each end of the operative field, extending approximately 12 mm. from the alveolar margin into the vestibule. Join the vertical incisions with a horizontal incision.

Step 2: Reflect a Flap (Fig. 53–19B). Separate a mucosal flap and elevate it to expose the periosteum of the bone.

Step 3: Separate the Periosteum from the Bone (Fig. 53–19C). Starting at the crest of the facial bone, just under the elevated flap, separate the periosteum and attached muscle fibers from the bone and transpose them to the lip.

Step 4: Replace the Mucosal Flap (Fig. 53–19D). Fold the mucosal flap down over the bone and suture it to the inner surface of the periosteum. The fornix of the vestibule is now formed by the junction of the mucosal flap and the transposed periosteum.

Step 5: Suture the Periosteum (Fig. 53–19E). The upper edge of the periosteum is

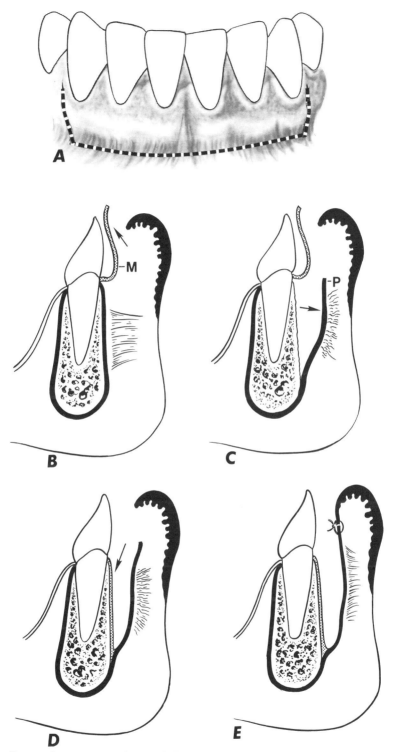

Figure 53–19   Edlan-Mejchar Operation for Vestibular Deepening. *A,* The operated field is outlined by two vertical incisions from the junction of the marginal and attached gingiva to approximately 12 mm. from the alveolar margin into the vestibule. The vertical incisions are joined by a horizontal incision. *B,* A mucosal flap (M) is elevated, exposing the periosteum of the bone. *C,* The periosteum (P) is separated from the bone, starting from the line of attachment of the mucosal flap; the periosteum, including muscle attachments, is transposed to the lip. *D,* The mucosal flap is folded down over the bone (*arrow*) and sutured to the inner surface of the periosteum. *E,* The periosteum is transposed to the lip and sutured where the initial horizontal incision was made.

sutured to the mucosa of the lip or vestibule where the horizontal initial incision was made. According to Edlan and Mejchar, the periosteum is covered with epithelium within seven to ten days, and the mucous membrane attaches to the bone in two to three weeks. Figure 53–20 shows the steps in a clinical case.

The Apically Positioned Flap[4, 5, 38, 39, 67, 68]

Positioned flaps are used to correct mucogingival deformities without some of the limitations of vestibular extension operations, and with less extensive surgical interference. This operation utilizes the apically positioned flap, partial thickness or

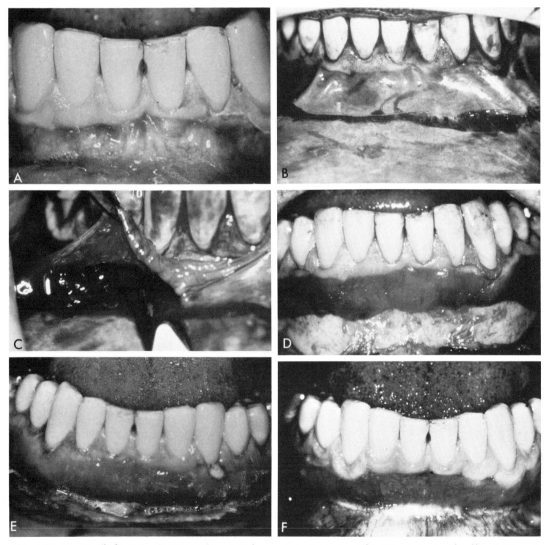

Figure 53–20 Vestibular Extension Operation. *A,* Before surgery. *B,* Horizontal incision in inner side of lip. *C,* Dissection of flap. *D,* After separation of periosteum and muscle fibers, flap is folded down over the bone. *E,* Results one week after operation. *F,* Results one year after operation. Note the nonkeratinized attached tissue. (Courtesy of Dr. Max O. Schmid, Los Angeles.)

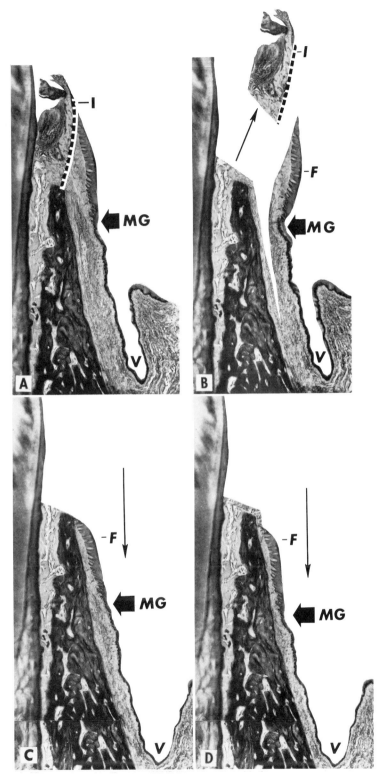

Figure 53–21   Apically Positioned Partial Thickness Flap. *A,* Internal incision (I) separates inner wall of periodontal pocket. MG, Mucogingival junction. V, Vestibular fornix. *B,* Partial thickness flap (F) separated away, leaving periosteum and layer of connective tissue on the bone. Inner wall of periodontal pocket (I) is removed and the tooth scaled and planed. *C,* Partial thickness flap (F) positioned apically with the edge of the flap at the crest of the bone. Note that the vestibular fornix is also moved apically. *D,* Partial thickness flap (F) positioned apically with the edge of the flap several millimeters below the crest of the bone.

full thickness, for the combined purposes of eliminating pockets, widening the zone of attached gingiva, deepening the oral vestibule, and relocating frena apically. The partial thickness (mucosal) flap is generally used to avoid exposure of bone and the accompanying risks of bone resorption and aggravation of bone dehiscences and fenestrations.[84, 94] The full thickness (mucoperiosteal) flap is indicated when access to the bone for recontouring purposes is also desired.

The apically positioned partial thickness flap

There are three distinguishing features of this operation: (1) the internal (reverse) bevel incision for removing the inner aspect of periodontal pockets (2) the partial thickness flap, and (3) the location of the flap (Figs. 53–21, 53–22, and 53–23).

PROCEDURE. *Step 1: Vertical Incisions.* Make a vertical incision from the gingival margin into the fornix of the vestibule at each end of the operative field. The incisions should be placed at the distofacial angle of the terminal teeth rather than interproximally to avoid unequal shrinkage and notching of the interdental papillae. The incision should penetrate to the periosteum but not through it.

Step 2: The Internal Bevel Incision. With a Bard-Parker blade, make an incision from the tip of the gingival margin to the crest of the labial plate (Fig. 53–21A). This incision differs from the gingivectomy incision in that it removes the diseased inner aspect of the pocket and retains the outer gingival wall. The outer gingival wall is important in this operation because it contributes to the increased width of the attached gingiva. To avoid bulky gingival contours, the internal bevel should thin the pocket wall at the same time that it removes the diseased inner portion.

Step 3. Insert a No. 15 Bard-Parker blade into the internal incision, and separate the outer wall of the periodontal pockets. Continue with the blade under the attached gingiva, separating a flap consisting of epithelium and a thin layer of underlying connective tissue from the periosteum (Fig. 53–21B). Progressively dissect the flap toward the fornix of the vestibule. Be sure to separate the flap far enough into the fornix to provide space for the flap to be positioned apically without "buckling." If the space is inadequate, the healed gingiva will have a "ruffled" surface which requires several months to become smooth (Fig. 53–22).

Step 4. Remove the inner wall of the periodontal pockets from the teeth; scale the root surfaces free of all deposits and plane.

Step 5. Position the flap apically. Trim the edge of the flap to conform to the contour of the bone margin and place it on the labial plate. The edge of the flap may

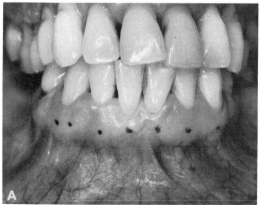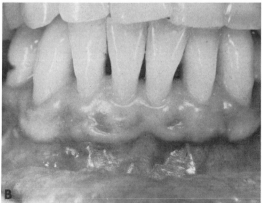

Figure 53–22 Deep Periodontal Pockets Encroach Upon Mucogingival Line. *A,* Marks inserted to show location of the base of deep periodontal pockets in relation to the mucogingival line. *B,* Two months after apically repositioned flap operation. The attached gingiva is ruffled because the flap was not separated deep enough in the fornix.

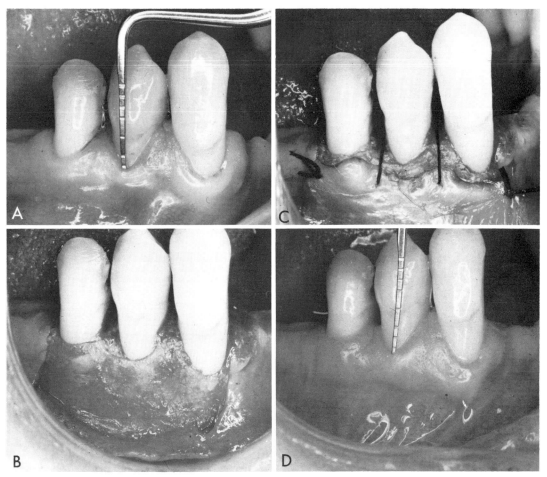

Figure 53–23   Apically Positioned Partial Thickness Flap. *A,* Before treatment, the base of pocket extends to the mucogingival line. *B,* Mucosal flap separated from the periosteum, teeth scaled and smoothed. *C,* Flap replaced below the crest of the bone. *D,* Eight months after treatment. Note the shallow sulcus and widened zone of attached gingiva. Compare with *A.*

be located in three possible positions in relation to the bone: (1) **Slightly coronal to the crest of the bone,** in an attempt to preserve the attachment of supracrestal fibers. This location may also result in thick gingival margins and interdental papillae with deep sulci, and may create the risk of recurrent pockets. (2) **At the level of the crest of the labial plate** (Fig. 53–21C). This provides satisfactory gingival contour, provided the flap is adequately thinned. (3) **Two millimeters short of the crest** (Fig. 53–21D). This position produces the most desirable gingival contour and the same post-treatment level of gingival attachment as is obtained by placing

the flap at the crest of the bone.[42] New tissue will cover the crest of the bone to produce a firm, tapered gingival margin. Placing the flap short of the crest increases the risk of a slight reduction in bone height,[30] but this is compensated for by the advantages of a well-formed gingival margin.

Step 6. Secure the flap. Remove excess clot; be sure the flap rests firmly on the underlying tissue and suture it with interrupted suspensory and lateral sutures with 4–0 silk.

Step 7. Protect the flap. Apply a gauze sponge until bleeding stops, and cover the area with periodontal pack. Remove the

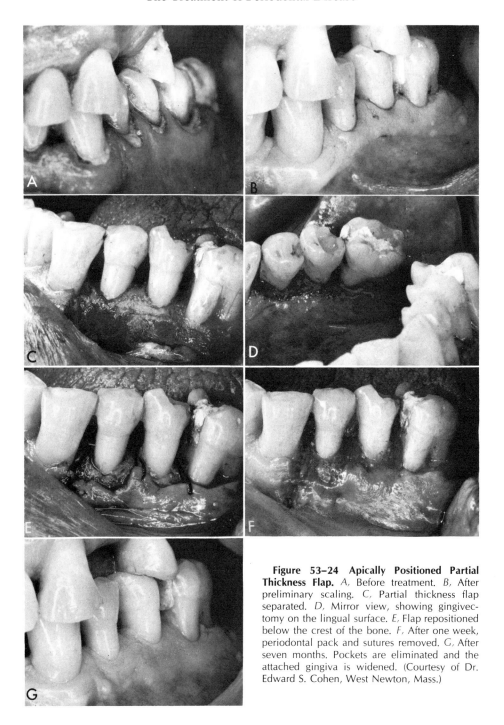

Figure 53–24 Apically Positioned Partial Thickness Flap. *A,* Before treatment. *B,* After preliminary scaling. *C,* Partial thickness flap separated. *D,* Mirror view, showing gingivectomy on the lingual surface. *E,* Flap repositioned below the crest of the bone. *F,* After one week, periodontal pack and sutures removed. *G,* After seven months. Pockets are eliminated and the attached gingiva is widened. (Courtesy of Dr. Edward S. Cohen, West Newton, Mass.)

pack and sutures after one week. Repacking is not usually necessary.

ACCOMPLISHMENTS. The apically positioned full thickness flap operation increases the width of attached gingiva and relocates the fornix of the vestibule and frena apically. It results in less postoperative discomfort and heals more rapidly than vestibular extension procedures.[56] The width of the attached gingiva is increased by approximately half the pretreatment depth of the pockets.[33] The post-treatment width can be estimated before the operation by using the following formula:

Estimated post-treatment width of attached gingiva =

$$\frac{\text{Pretreatment depth of pockets}}{2} + \frac{\text{Pretreatment width of attached gingiva}}{}$$

This is applicable if the flap is positioned at the crest. Since the pocket wall contributes to the increase in attached gingiva, the operation is best suited for patients with deep pockets who require additional attached gingiva. The final width of attached gingiva may be increased by placing the flap further apically from the crest (Figs. 53–23 and 53–24).

The apically positioned full thickness flap

This is the same operation as the apically positioned partial thickness flap, except that it employs a full thickness (mucoperiosteal) flap (Fig. 53–25). It is used when the bone is to be recontoured as part of the total operation. It should not be used when bone dehiscence or fenestration is suspected, which is more likely on labially prominent teeth.[84]

The procedure is the same as that described above for the apically positioned flap, except that in Step 3 the periosteum is included when the flap is elevated, leaving the bone exposed (Fig. 53–26).

Comparison of results obtained with partial thickness (mucosal) and full thickness (mucoperiosteal) apically positioned flaps

Both operations eliminate periodontal pockets and correct mucogingival deformities with some limiting side effects.

Elevating any type of flap results in inflammation and bone resorption and introduces the risk of thinning of bone and loss in bone height,[43, 97, 104, 114] particularly over the roots; some of the damaged tissue undergoes repair. Full thickness flaps produce more bone loss and gingival recession than the partial thickness (mucosal) type,[22, 25, 31, 33, 76, 96, 104, 111, 113, 116] and healing is slower. Mucoperiosteal flaps may create a deeper vestibule, but the gain in width of attached gingiva at the apical end is more than offset by the added gingival recession.[25] Some hold different opinions regarding the relative merits of these flaps[77, 117] and note that they may heal at the same rate[8-10] or that full thickness flaps heal more rapidly, with less vascular congestion or tissue necrosis.[105]

Laterally (Horizontally) Positioned Flap-Pedicle Graft[50, 52]

PURPOSE. The purpose of this operation is to cover root surfaces denuded by a gingival defect or periodontal disease and widen the zone of attached gingiva.

PROCEDURE. *Step 1: Prepare the Recipient Site.* Make a rectangular incision, resecting the periodontal pockets or gingival margin around the exposed root (Figs. 53–27A and B, and 53–28B). The incision should extend to the periosteum and include a border of 2 to 3 mm. of bone mesial and distal to the root to provide a connective tissue base to which the flap can attach. The rectangle should extend apically for a sufficient distance into the alveolar mucosa to provide space for the zone of attached gingiva.

Remove the resected soft tissue without disturbing the narrow zone of periosteum around the root, and scale and plane the root surface (Fig. 53–27B).

Step 2: Prepare the Flap. The periodontium of the donor site should be healthy, with a satisfactory width of attached gingiva and minimal loss of bone, and without dehiscences or fenestrations. Malposed or rotated teeth should be avoided. Inflammation should be eliminated before the flap operation is undertaken. A full thickness or partial thickness flap may be used, but the latter is preferable because it offers the advantage of more rapid healing in the donor site[10] and reduces the risk of loss of facial bone height, particularly if the bone is thin or dehiscence or fenestration is suspected. However, if the gingiva is thin, partial thickness may not be sufficient for flap survival.

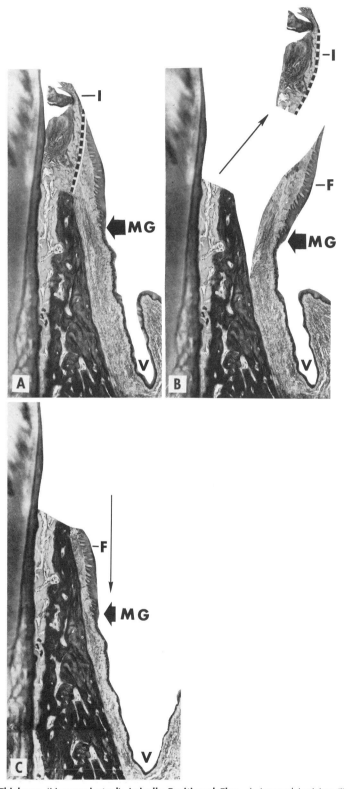

Figure 53–25   Full Thickness (Mucoperiosteal) Apically Positioned Flap. *A,* Internal incision (I) separating inner wall of periodontal pocket. MG, Mucogingival junction. V, Vestibular fornix. *B,* Full thickness flap (F), including periosteum, is separated from the bone. Inner wall of periodontal pocket removed. Tooth scaled and planed. *C,* Flap positioned apically on the bone with the edge of the flap at the bony crest.

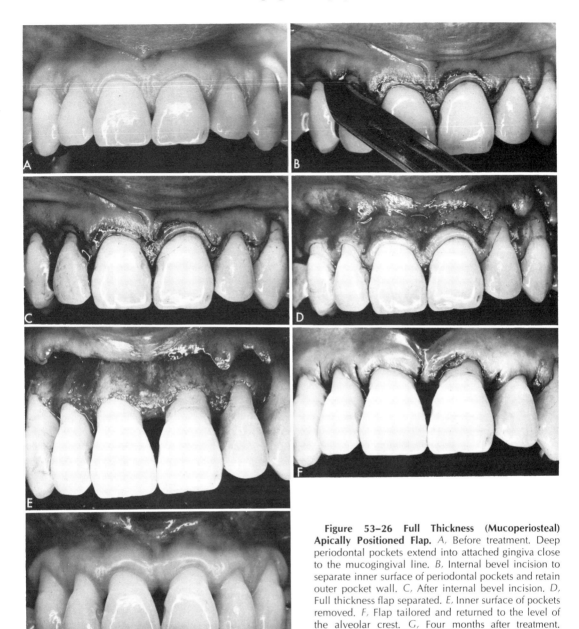

Figure 53–26 Full Thickness (Mucoperiosteal) Apically Positioned Flap. *A,* Before treatment. Deep periodontal pockets extend into attached gingiva close to the mucogingival line. *B,* Internal bevel incision to separate inner surface of periodontal pockets and retain outer pocket wall. *C,* After internal bevel incision. *D,* Full thickness flap separated. *E,* Inner surface of pockets removed. *F,* Flap tailored and returned to the level of the alveolar crest. *G,* Four months after treatment. Pockets eliminated with healthy zone of attached gingiva.

With a No. 15 Bard-Parker blade, make a vertical incision from the gingival margin to outline a flap adjacent to the recipient site. Incise to the periosteum of the bone and extend the incision into the oral mucosa to the level of the base of the recipient site (Fig. 53–27B). The flap should be sufficiently wider than the recipient site to cover the root and provide a broad margin

for attachment to the connective tissue border around the root. The interdental papilla at the distal end of the flap or a major portion of it should be included to secure the flap in the interproximal space between the donor and recipient teeth.

Make a vertical incision along the gingival margin and interdental papilla. Insert a No. 15 Bard-Parker blade into the incision

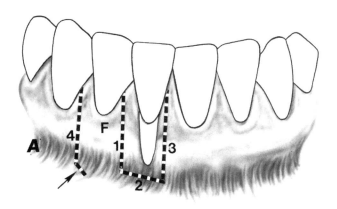

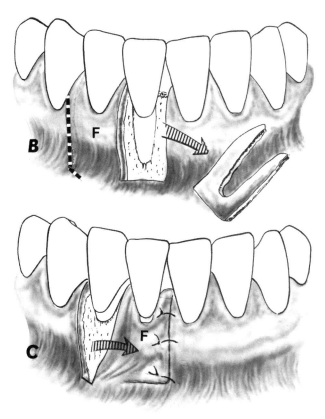

Figure 53–27 Laterally Positioned Flap. *A,* Incisions (1,2,3) made around gingival defect on central incisor. A vertical incision (4) at the distal of the lateral outlines the flap (F) to be positioned. A small angular releasing incision (*arrow*) relieves tension when flap is moved. *B,* Diseased gingival tissue removed from around central incisor (*arrow*), including the periosteum. Tooth scaled and planed. *C,* Flap (F), including periosteum, is transferred from the lateral incisor onto the central.

and, directing the blade apically, separate away a flap consisting of epithelium and a thin layer of connective tissue, leaving the periosteum on the bone. Hold the edge of the flap with a tissue forceps, and continue the dissection to the desired depth in the oral vestibule. Tailor the margin of the flap to conform to the recipient site, and thin it if necessary so that it will not be bulbous.

It is sometimes necessary to make a *releasing incision* to avoid tension on the base of the flap, which impairs the circulation when the flap is moved. To do this, make an oblique incision into the alveolar mucosa at the distal corner of the flap, pointing in the direction of the recipient site (Fig. 53–27B).

Step 3: Transfer the Flap. Slide the flap laterally onto the adjacent root, making sure that it lies flat and firm without excess tension on the base. Fix the flap to the adjacent gingiva and alveolar mucosa with interrupted sutures. A suspensory suture may be made around the involved tooth to prevent the flap from slipping apically (Fig. 53–27C).

Step 4: Protect the Flap and Donor Site. Cover the operative field with a soft periodontal pack, extending it interdentally and onto the lingual surface to secure it. Remove the pack and sutures after one week, and repack twice at weekly intervals.

VARIATIONS.[52] There are many variations in the incisions for this operation. A common one is the use of converging oblique incisions over the recipient site and a vertical or oblique incision at the distal end of the donor site (Fig. 53–29) so that the transposed flap is slightly wider at its base. In another modification, the marginal attachment in the donor site is preserved to reduce the likelihood of recession and marginal bone resorption, but this requires a donor site with a wide zone of attached gingiva.[49]

ACCOMPLISHMENTS. Attainment of a functionally satisfactory zone of attached gingiva in the recipient site is not a problem (Figs. 53–28 and 53–30). Some cellular degeneration and necrosis is associated with the transfer of the flap, but this is followed by repair. The morphologic features of the transplanted tissues do not change.[89-91]

Coverage of the exposed root surface is a less definitive matter. The flap attaches to the connective tissue bordering the root and bridges over the formerly denuded root surface. It appears to be attached and may adhere so firmly to the root as to resist insertion of a periodontal probe.[2] There is some shrinkage of the flap with time, but the root remains partially covered. Better results are obtained with narrow, long gingival defects than with broad, shallow ones.

The extent to which the flap "reattaches" to the root with the formation of new cementum and the embedding of new connective tissue fibers has not been settled. Reattachment on artificially denuded roots in experimental animals[115] and in some clinical studies in humans has been reported,[99, 102, 103] but it does not occur consistently enough to be predictable.

In the donor site, there is uneventful repair and restoration of gingival health and contours, with some loss of radicular bone (0.5 mm.) and recession (1.5 mm.) reported with full thickness flaps.

Double laterally positioned flaps

The laterally positioned flap is most often used on single teeth. However, when two adjacent roots are exposed, twin flaps are used to correct the condition. The procedure is the same as that for a single lateral flap, except that there are two teeth in the recipient site and there are two donor sites, one on each side of the involved area. The results are the same as those following laterally positioned flaps on single teeth.

Double papillae positioned flaps[27, 54]

The purposes of this operation are (1) to restore the zone of attached gingiva and (2) to attempt to cover roots denuded by isolated gingival defects with a flap formed by joining two interdental papillae. It is recommended when the areas bordering the gingival defect are unsatisfactory for a laterally positioned flap because of insufficient attached gingiva or deep periodontal pockets. These problems are overcome by utilizing the contiguous halves of the adja-

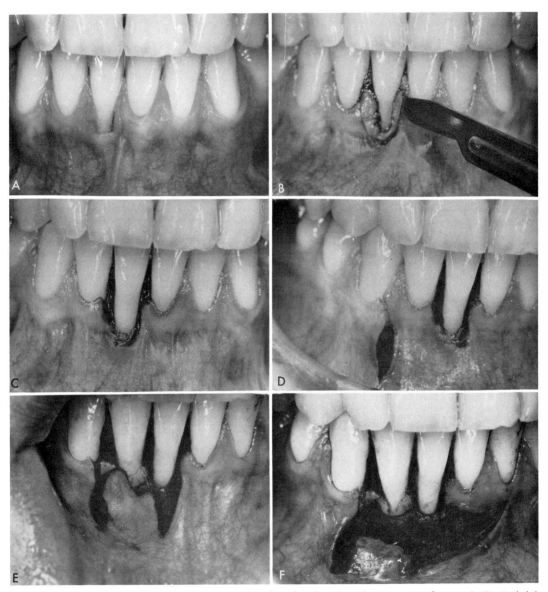

Figure 53–28   Horizontally Repositioned Flap Combined With Relocation of Frenum Attachment. *A,* Gingival defect of central incisor. *B,* Defect incised. *C,* Gingiva removed and tooth scaled and planed. *D,* Vertical incision on canine for sliding flap. *E,* Sliding flap detached. Note high frenum attachment between the central incisors. *F,* Frenum detached and resected to level of vestibular fornix.

(Illustration continued on opposite page)

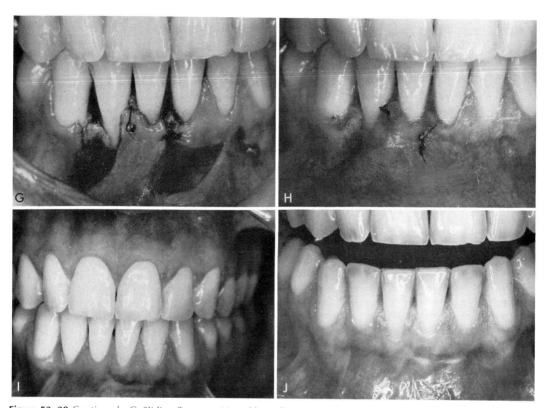

Figure 53–28 *Continued* G, Sliding flap repositioned laterally on central incisor and fixed lateral and suspensory suture. H, One week postoperation, sutures to be removed. I, Five weeks after operation. J, Seven years after treatment. Note the preservation of gingival position and contour.

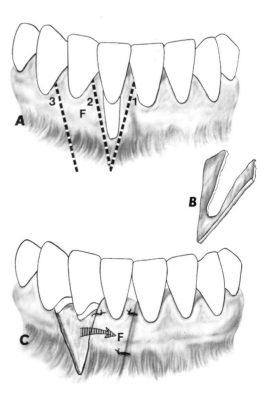

Figure 53–29 Lateral Sliding Flap Using Oblique Incisions. A, Oblique incisions (1 and 2) to remove gingiva around exposed incisor root. Parallel incision (3) to outline flap (F) which is transferred onto root. B, Gingiva removed from around root. C, Partial thickness flap (F) transferred onto incisor root and sutured.

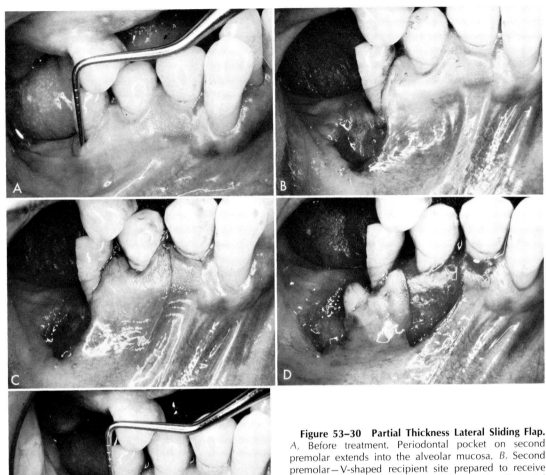

Figure 53–30   Partial Thickness Lateral Sliding Flap.
A, Before treatment. Periodontal pocket on second premolar extends into the alveolar mucosa. B, Second premolar—V-shaped recipient site prepared to receive the flap. C, Flap outlined on the first premolar. D, Partial thickness flap transferred to second premolar. E, Seven months after treatment, showing shallow gingival sulcus and widened zone of attached gingiva. Compare with A. (Courtesy of Dr. Edward S. Cohen, West Newton, Mass.)

cent interdental papillae. The interdental papillae provide a zone of attached gingiva that is usually wider than on the radicular surface and also reduce the risk of loss in radicular bone height because the bone is thicker interdentally than on the roots. Results with this technique are frequently poor, probably because the two flaps are sutured over the root surface.

PROCEDURE. *Step 1: Prepare the Recipient Site.* With periodontal knives or a No. 15 Bard-Parker blade, make a V-shaped incision and resection the diseased gingiva

around the involved root. Scale and plane the root surfaces (Fig. 53–31A and B).

Step 2: Prepare the Flaps. With a No. 15 Bard-Parker blade, start at the gingival margin lateral to the mesial and distal interdental papillae and make a slightly oblique incision into the oral vestibule to the level of the V-shaped incision on the involved root. This will outline the flaps, each of which consists of part of the interdental papillae on both sides of the root (Fig. 53–31B). Each flap is broader at its base than at the gingival margin. Make a horizontal incision across the tip of each interdental papilla. Separate a partial thickness flap on each side of the root by inserting a No. 15 Bard-Parker blade into the oblique incision beneath the alveolar mucosa and moving it to the tip of the interdental papilla. Thin the edge of the flap to avoid a bulky gingival margin after healing.

Step 3: Transfer and Secure the Flaps. Move the flaps together until they meet over the root surface (Fig. 53–31C). The outer epithelium of one section is sometimes removed so that the flaps can be overlapped with two connective tissue surfaces in contact. Suture the flaps together on the bone with interrupted sutures secured to the periosteum to prevent the flaps from

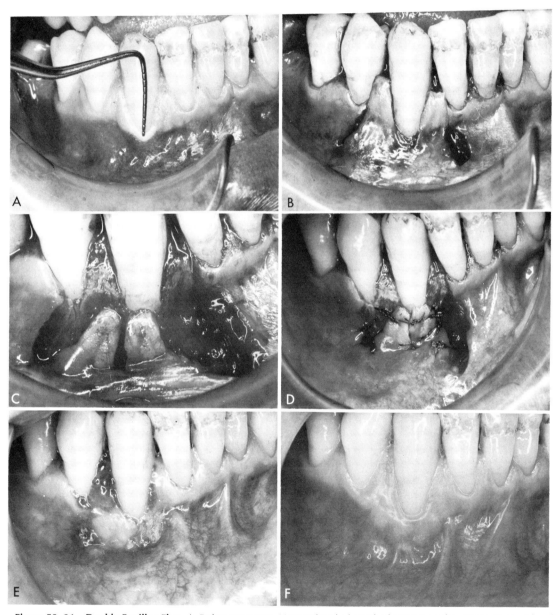

Figure 53–31 Double Papillae Flap. *A,* Before treatment. Narrow band of attached gingiva on the canine. *B,* Mesial and distal papillae separated. *C,* Papillae transferred to the canine. *D,* Papillae placed on bony plate and sutured to the periosteum. *E,* After one week. *F,* After seven months. Note the widened zone of attached gingiva. Compare with *A.* (Courtesy of Dr. Edward S. Cohen, West Newton, Mass.)

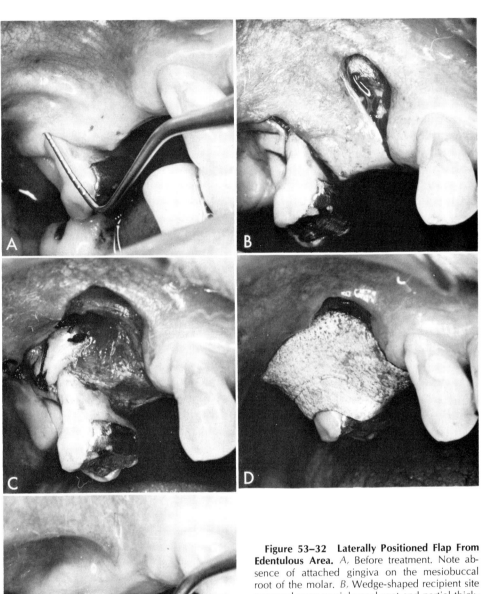

Figure 53–32   Laterally Positioned Flap From Edentulous Area. *A,* Before treatment. Note absence of attached gingiva on the mesiobuccal root of the molar. *B,* Wedge-shaped recipient site prepared over mesiobuccal root and partial thickness flap outlined in edentulous area. *C,* Flap transferred to bone over mesiobuccal root and sutured. *D,* Periodontal pack in position. *E,* After eight months. Note the zone of attached gingiva on the mesiobuccal root. Compare with *A.* (Courtesy of Dr. Edward S. Cohen, West Newton, Mass.)

slipping apically (Fig. 53–31D). A suspensory suture through the margin of the joined flaps and around the neck of the tooth may also be used for this purpose.

Step 4: Protect the Flaps. Cover the operative field with a soft periodontal dressing for one week. Remove the sutures and repack for another week (Fig. 53–31E and F).

Sliding partial thickness flap from an edentulous area (pedicle graft)

The purpose of this operation is to restore attached gingiva on teeth adjacent to edentulous spaces with denuded roots and a small vestibular fornix, often complicated by tension from a frenum.[28] A partial thickness flap of masticatory mucosa from the adjacent edentulous ridge is used.

Procedure. *Step 1: Prepare the Recipient Site.* With a No. 15 Bard-Parker blade, make a V-shaped incision from the gingival margin mesial and distal to the involved tooth into the alveolar mucosa apical to the root apex or apices (Fig. 53–32A and B). Include frenum attachments in the resected area. Elevate the tip of the tissue wedge outlined by the incision with a tissue forceps, and dissect away the wedge of tissue with a No. 15 Bard-Parker blade. Leave the periosteum and covering connective tissue on the bone, except in areas where bone is to be recontoured. Remove the loose strands or clumps of tissue from the connective tissue surface to provide a firm base for the transferred flap.

Step 2: Scale and Plane the Root Surfaces.

Step 3: Prepare the Flap. Make an incision along the crest of the edentulous ridge from the proximal tooth surface for a distance equal to or slightly longer than the width of the recipient site. From the end of the incision make a vertical incision from the crest of the ridge into the alveolar mucosa to the level of the base of the wedge-shaped recipient site, outlining a flap that is wider at the base (Fig. 53–32B). Insert a periodontal knife into the incision at the crest of the ridge, and separate away a partial thickness flap of masticatory mucosa, leaving the periosteum on the bone. Con-

tinue the separation into the alveolar mucosa.

If the mucogingival junction is high on the edentulous ridge and the buccal masticatory mucosa is narrow, masticatory mucosa from the lingual surface is included in the graft. The initial incision is made on the

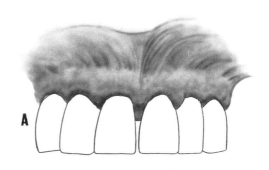

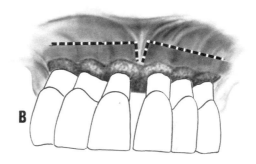

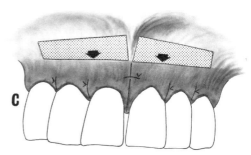

Figure 53–33 Coronally Positioned Pedicle Flap. *A,* Patient with deep periodontal pockets. *B,* Periodontal pockets removed and roots scaled and planed. Mucoperiosteal flaps are outlined by horizontal and vertical incisions indicated by dotted lines. *C,* Flaps drawn down over the root surfaces as indicated by arrows and joined and sutured in position over the roots. The bone in the stippled areas is denuded.

lingual surface close to, but not at, the mucogingival junction.

Step 4: Transfer the Flap. To facilitate free movement of the flap without stretching or twisting the pedicle and interfering with the circulation, a short, oblique releasing incision may be made at the base in the direction the flap is to be moved. Check the recipient site to be sure bleeding has stopped, and remove excessive clot from the surface.

Move the flap laterally and place it firmly on the recipient surface with the free end of the flap at the margin of the bone. Suture one margin of the flap to the adjacent cut tissue surface and the other to the periosteum (Fig. 53–32C). A suspensory suture may be made through the free margin of the flap around the tooth to prevent the flap from slipping apically. Cover the area with a

periodontal pack, which is removed with the sutures after one week (Fig. 53–32D). Repack two more times at weekly intervals (Fig. 53–32E).

Coronally Positioned Pedicle Graft (Kalmi, Moscor, Goranov[61])

Of historical interest is an operation developed in an effort to improve the appearance of patients with teeth denuded by advanced periodontal disease. It consists of covering denuded roots of maxillary anterior teeth by sliding pedicle flaps from adjacent uninvolved gingiva and alveolar mucosa as follows (Fig. 53–33).

Periodontal pockets are resected by gingivectomy, and the roots are scaled and planed. A mucoperiosteal flap as wide as

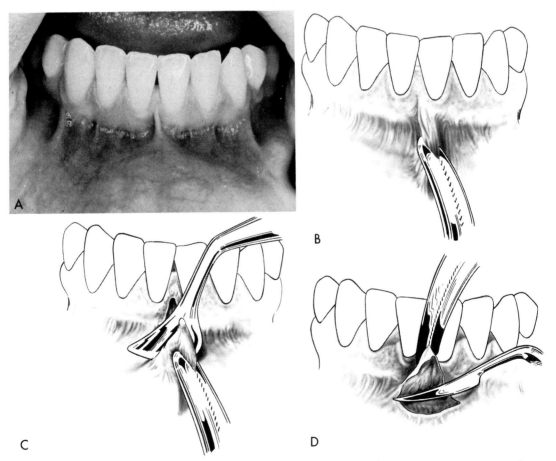

Figure 53–34 Relocating the Frenum. *A,* Frenum attached close to the gingival margin. *B,* Hemostat engages frenum. *C,* Incision along the upper border of the hemostat. *D,* Incision along the lower border of the hemostat removes a wedge-shaped section of the frenum.

(Illustration continued on opposite page)

the exposed root surface and outlined by a horizontal incision across the anterior maxilla is elevated from the bone (Fig. 53–33A and B). The flap is divided in two by a midline V-shaped incision at the frenum, and the two flaps are moved onto the roots and sutured. Reattachment of the flaps to the exposed roots has been reported in experimental animals,[56] but not in humans.[72]

Coronally Positioned Flap[53]

The purposes of this operation are (1) to eliminate periodontal pockets and (2) to attempt to obtain reattachment of the gingiva to root surface previously denuded by disease.

PROCEDURE. The inner wall of the periodontal pockets is separated from the outer wall, and a mucoperiosteal flap is laid back, exposing the diseased area. The inner walls of the pockets are removed, and the tooth surfaces are scaled free of deposits and planed.

The flap is returned and sutured in place at a level coronal to the pretreatment position. The area is covered with periodontal pack, which is removed along with sutures after one week. The pack is repeated for an additional week if necessary.

Frenectomy or Frenotomy

A frenum is a fold of mucous membrane, usually with enclosed muscle fibers, that attaches the lips and cheeks to the alveolar mucosa and/or gingiva and underlying periosteum. A frenum becomes a problem if its attachment is too close to the marginal gingiva. It may then pull on a healthy gingival margin and invite the accumulation of irritants; it may deflect the wall of a periodontal pocket and aggravate its severity; or it may interfere with post-treatment healing, prevent close adaptation of the gingiva and lead to pocket formation, or interfere with proper brushing of the teeth.

PURPOSES. The terms *frenectomy* and *frenotomy* represent operations that differ

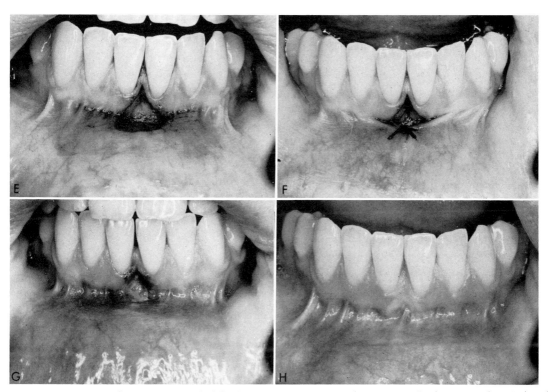

Figure 53–34 *Continued   E,* After removal of the frenum. *F,* Mucosa sutured in position. *G,* After one week, periodontal pack and suture removed. *H,* After six months, frenum relocated at the mucogingival line.

in degree. *Frenectomy is complete removal of the frenum, including its attachment to underlying bone, such as may be required in the correction of an abnormal diastema between maxillary central incisors. Frenotomy is partial removal of the frenum.* Both are used, but frenotomy generally suffices for periodontal purposes, namely relocating the frenum attachment so as to create the zone of attached gingiva between the gingival margin and the frenum. Frenectomy or frenotomy is usually performed in conjunction with other periodontal treatment procedures but occasionally is done as a separate operation.

Frenum problems occur most often on the facial surface between the maxillary and mandibular central incisors and in the canine and premolar areas,[112] and, less frequently, on the lingual surface of the mandible.

PROCEDURE. If the vestibule is deep enough, the operation is confined to the frenum, but it is often necessary to deepen the vestibule to provide space for the repositioned frenum. This is accomplished as follows:

1. Anesthetize the area.

2. Engage the frenum with a hemostat inserted to the depth of the vestibule (Fig. 53–34A and B).

3. Incise along the upper surface of the hemostat, extending beyond the tip (Fig. 53–34C).

4. Make a similar incision along the under surface of the hemostat (Fig. 53–34D).

5. Remove the triangular resected portion of frenum with the hemostat. This exposes the underlying brush-like fibrous attachment to the bone.

6. Make a horizontal incision, separating the fibers, and bluntly dissect to the bone.

7. If necessary, extend the incisions laterally and suture the labial mucosa to the apical periosteum (Fig. 53–34F).

8. Clean the field of operation and pack with gauze sponges until bleeding stops.

9. Insert the periodontal pack. First, pack the marginal area, as is ordinarily done following gingivectomy. Then, using the marginal pack as a stable base, add thin strips on the edge to the depth of the incision.

10. Remove the pack after two weeks and repack if necessary. One month from the time of operation is usually required for the formation of an intact mucosa with the frenum attached in its new position.

High frenum attachments on the lingual surface are uncommon. To correct these without involving the structures in the floor of the mouth, approximately 2 mm. of the attachment is separated from the mucosa with a periodontal knife at weekly intervals until the desired level is reached. The area is covered with periodontal pack in the intervals between treatments.

REFERENCES

1. Ainamo, J., and Löe, H.: Anatomical characteristics of gingiva. A clinical and microscopic study of the free and attached gingiva. J. Periodontol., 37:5, 1966.

1a. Ainamo, J., and Talari, A.: The increase with age of the width of attached gingiva. J. Periodontal Res., 11:182, 1976.

1b. Ainamo, A., and Ainamo, J.: The width of attached gingiva on supraerupted teeth. J. Periodontal Res., 13:194, 1978.

2. Albano, E. A., Caffesse, R. C., and Carranza, F. A., Jr.: A biometric analysis of laterally displaced pedicle flaps. Rev. Asoc. Odontol. Argent., 57:351, 1969.

3. Allen, D. L., and Shell, J. H.: Clinical and radiographic evaluation of a periosteal separation procedure. J. Periodontol., 39:290, 1968.

4. Ariaudo, A. A., and Tyrrell, H. A.: Elimination of pockets extending to or beyond mucogingival junction. Dent. Clin. North Am., March 1960, p. 67.

5. Arnold, N. R., and Hatchett, C. M., Jr.: A comparative investigation of two mucogingival surgical methods. J. Periodontol., 33:129, 1962.

6. Becker, N. G.: A free gingival graft utilizing a pre-suturing technique. Periodontics, 5:194, 1967.

7. Bergenholtz, A., and Hugoson, A.: Vestibular sulcus extension surgery in cases with periodontal disease. J. Periodont. Res., 2:221, 1967.

8. Bhaskar, S. N., Beasley, J. D. III, Cutright, D. E., and Perez, B.: Free mucosal grafts in miniature swine and men. J. Periodontol., 42:322, 1971.

9. Bhaskar, S. N., Cutright, D. E., Beasley, J. D. III, Perez, B., and Hunsuck, R. E.: Healing under full and partial thickness mucogingival flaps in the miniature swine. J. Periodontol., 41:675, 1970.

10. Bhaskar, S. N., Cutright, D. E., Perez, B., and Beasley, J. D. III.: Full and partial thickness pedicle grafts in miniature swine and man. J. Periodontol., 42:66, 1971.

11. Björn, H.: Free transplantation of gingiva propria. Sveriges Tandlak. T., *22*:684, 1963.

12. Bohannan, H. M.: Studies in the alteration of vestibular depth. I. Complete denudation. J. Periodontol., *33*:120, 1962.

13. Bohannan, H. M.: Studies in the alteration of vestibular depth: II. Periosteum retention. J. Periodontol., *33*:354, 1962.

14. Bohannan, H. M.: Studies in the alteration of vestibular depth: III. Vestibular incision. J. Periodontol., *34*:209, 1963.

15. Bowers, G. M.: A study of the width of attached gingiva. J. Periodontol., *34*:201, 1963.

16. Brackett, R. C., and Gargiulo, A. W.: Free gingival grafts in humans. J. Periodontol., *41*:581, 1970.

17. Bressman, E., and Chasens, A. I.: Free gingival graft with periosteal fenestration. J. Periodontol., *39*:298, 1968.

18. Broome, W. C., and Taggart, E. J., Jr.: Free autogenous connective tissue grafting. J. Periodontol., *47*:580, 1976.

19. Caffesse, R. G., Carraro, J. J., and Carranza, F. A., Jr.: Injertos gingivales libres en perros; estudio clinico y histologico. Rev. Asoc. Odont. Argent., *60*:465, 1972.

20. Caffesse, R. G., Albano, E., and Plot, C.: Injertos gingivales fibres en perros; analisis biometrico. Rev. Asoc. Odont. Argent., *60*:517, 1972.

21. Carranza, F. A., Jr., Carraro, J. J., Dotto, C. A., and Cabrini, R. L.: Effect of periosteal fenestration in gingival extension operations. J. Periodontol., *37*:335, 1966.

22. Carranza, F. A., Jr., and Carraro, J. J.: Effect of removal of periosteum on postoperative result of mucogingival surgery. J. Periodontol., *34*:223, 1963.

23. Carranza, F. A., Jr., and Carraro, J. J.: Mucogingival techniques in periodontal surgery. J. Periodontol., *41*:294, 1970.

24. Carranza, F. A., Jr., Carraro, J. J., and Albano, E.: Mucogingival surgery. *In* S. S. Stahl (Ed.): Periodontal Surgery, Biologic Basis and Technique. Springfield, Illinois: Charles C Thomas, 1976.

25. Carraro, J. J., Carranza, F. A., Jr., Albano, E. A., and Joly, G.: Effect of bone denudation in mucogingival surgery in humans. J. Periodontol., *35*:463, 1964.

26. Chacker, F. M., and Cohen, D. W.: Regeneration of gingival tissues in non-human primates. J. Dent. Res., *39*:743, 1960.

27. Cohen, D. W., and Ross, S. E.: The double papillae repositioned flap in periodontal therapy. J. Periodontol., *39*:65, 1968.

28. Corn, H.: Edentulous area pedicle grafts in mucogingival surgery. Periodontics, *2*:229, 1964.

29. Corn, H.: Periosteal separation—its clinical significance. J. Periodontol., *33*:140, 1962.

30. Costich, E. R., and Ramfjord, S. P.: Healing after exposure of periosteum and labial bone in periodontal surgery. J. Dent. Res., *43*:791 (Suppl.), 1964 (Abst.).

31. Costich, E. R., and Ramfjord, S. P.: Healing after partial denudation of the alveolar process. J. Periodontol., *39*:127, 1968.

32. Donnenfeld, O. W., and Glickman, I.: A biometric study of the effects of gingivectomy. J. Periodontol., *37*:447, 1966.

33. Donnenfeld, O. W., Marks, R., and Glickman, I.: The apically repositioned flap: a clinical study. J. Periodontol., *35*:381, 1964.

34. Dordick, B., Coslet, J. G., and Seibert, J. S.: Clinical evaluation of free autogenous gingival grafts placed on alveolar bone. Part I. Clinical predictability. J. Periodontol., *47*:559, 1976.

35. Dordick, B., Coslet, J. G., and Seibert, J. S.: Clinical evaluation of free autogenous gingival grafts placed on alveolar bone. Part II. Coverage of non-pathologic dehiscences and fenestrations. J. Periodontol., *47*:568, 1976.

36. Edel, A.: Clinical evaluation of free connective tissue grafts used to increase the width of keratinized gingiva. J. Clin. Periodontol., *1*:185, 1974.

37. Edlan, A., and Mejchar, B.: Plastic surgery of the vestibulum in periodontal therapy. Int. Dent. J., *13*:593, 1963.

38. Friedman, N.: Mucogingival surgery: the apically repositioned flap. J. Periodontol., *33*:328, 1962.

39. Friedman, N., and Levine, H. L.: Mucogingival surgery: current status. J. Periodontol., *35*:5, 1964.

40. Gargiulo, A. W., and Arrocha, R.: Histo-clinical evaluation of free gingival grafts. Periodontics, 5:285, 1967.

41. Giacomatti, L., and Parakkal, P. F.: Skin transplantation: orientation of epithelial cells by the basement membrane. Nature, 223:514, 1969.

42. Glickman, I., Smulow, J. B., Ellinger, H. A., and Foulke, C. N.: Healing of apically positioned mucosal flaps and free gingival grafts. I.A.D.R. Abst., #468, 1971, p. 169.

43. Glickman, I., Smulow, J. B., O'Brien, T., and Tannen, R.: Healing of the periodontium following mucogingival surgery. Oral Surg., 16:530, 1963.

44. Glickman, I., Smulow, J., Vogel, G., and Passamonti, G.: The effect of occlusal forces on healing following mucogingival surgery. J. Periodontol., *37*:319, 1966.

45. Goldman, H. M.: Periodontia. 3rd ed. St. Louis, C. V. Mosby Co., 1953, pp. 552–561.

46. Gordon, H. P., Sullivan, H. C., and Atkins, J. H.: Free autogenous gingival grafts. II. Supplemental findings—histology of the graft site. Periodontics, 6:130, 1968.

47. Gottsegen, R.: Frenum position and vestibule depth in relation to gingival health. Oral Surg., 7:1069, 1954.

48. Grant, D. A.: Experimental periodontal surgery: sequestration of alveolar bone. J. Periodontol., *38*:409, 1967.

49. Grupe, H. E.: Modified technique for the sliding flap operation. J. Periodontol., *37*:491, 1966.

50. Grupe, H. E., and Warren, R. F., Jr.: Repair of gingival defects by a sliding flap operation. J. Periodontol., *27*:92, 1956.

51. Guinard, E. A., and Caffesse, R. G.: Localized gingival recessions: I. Etiology and prevalence. J. Western Soc. Periodont. 25:3, 1977.

52. Guinard, E. A., and Caffesse, R. G.: Localized gingival recessions. II. Treatment J. Western Soc. Periodont. 25:10, 1977.

53. Harvey, P. M.: Management of advanced periodontitis. Part I. Preliminary report of a method of surgical reconstruction. New Zeal. Dent. J., 61:180, 1965.

54. Hattler, A. B.: Mucogingival surgery—utilization of interdental gingiva as attached gingiva by surgical displacement. Periodontics, 5:126, 1967.

55. Hawley, C. E., and Staffileno, H.: Clinical evaluation of free gingival grafts in periodontal surgery. J. Periodontol., 41:105, 1970.

56. Helburn, R. L., Cohen, D. W., and Chacker, F. M.: Healing of repositioned mucogingival flaps in monkeys. I.A.D.R. Abst., 41:116, 1963.

57. Hileman, A. C.: Surgical repositioning of vestibule and frenums in periodontal disease. J. Am. Dent. Assoc., 55:676, 1957.

58. Hilming, F., and Jervoe, P.: Surgical extension of vestibular depth on the results in various regions of the mouth in periodontal patients. Tandlaegebladet, 74:329, 1970.

59. Ivancie, G. P.: Experimental and histological investigation of gingival regeneration in vestibular surgery. J. Periodontol., 28:259, 1957.

60. Janson, W. A., et al.: Development of the blood supply to split-thickness free gingival autografts. J. Periodontol., 40:707, 1969.

61. Kalmi, J., Moscor, M., and Goranov, Z.: The solution of the aesthetic problem in the treatment of periodontal disease of anterior teeth: gingivoplastic operation. Paradentologie, 3:53, 1949.

62. Karring, T., Ostergaard, E., and Löe, H.: Conservation of tissue specificity after heterotopic transplantation of gingiva and alveolar mucosa. J. Periodont. Res. 6:282, 1971.

63. Köster, H. D., and Flores de Jacoby, L.: Vergleicheride Untersuchungen von Schleimhanttransplantaten und lyophilisierter Dura., Dtsch. Zahaertzl. Z., 28:1229, 1973.

64. Klingsberg, J.: Periodontal scleral grafts and combined grafts of sclera and bone; two year appraisal. J. Periodontol., 45:262, 1974.

65. Morris, M.: The unrepositioned muco-periosteal flap. Periodontics, 3:147, 1965.

66. Nabers, J.: Free gingival grafts. Periodontics, 4:243, 1966.

67. Nabers, C. L.: Repositioning the attached gingiva. J. Periodontol., 25:38, 1954.

68. Nabers, C. L.: When is gingival repositioning an indicated procedure? J. Western Soc. Periodont., 5:4, 1957.

68a. Neacy, K.: The use of allogenic sclera and autogenous gingiva as free gingival grafts. Thesis, University of California at Los Angeles, 1978.

69. Ochsenbein, C.: Newer concepts of mucogingival surgery. J. Periodontol., 31:175, 1960.

70. Oliver, R. C., Löe, H., and Karring, T.: Microscopic evaluation of the healing and revascularization of free gingival grafts. J. Periodontol., 3:84, 1968.

71. Oliver, R. C., and Woofter, C.: Healing and revascularization of free mucosal grafts over roots. I.A.D.R. Abst., #469, 1971, p. 170.

72. Patur, B., and Glickman, I.: Gingival pedicle flaps for covering root surfaces denuded by chronic destructive periodontal disease—a clinical experiment. J. Periodontol., 29:50, 1958.

73. Pennel, B., King, K. O., Higgason, J. D., Towner, J. D., Fritz, B. D., and Sadler, J. F.: Retention of periosteum in mucogingival surgery. J. Periodontol., 36:39, 1965.

74. Pennel, B. M., King, K. O., Wilderman, M. H., and Barron, J. M.: Repair of the alveolar process following osseous surgery. J. Periodontol., 38:426, 1967.

75. Pennel, B. M., Tabor, J. C., King, K. O., Towner, J. D., Fritz, B. D., and Higgason, J. D.: Free masticatory mucosa graft. J. Periodontol., 40:162, 1969.

76. Pfeifer, J. S.: The reaction of alveolar bone to flap procedures in man. Periodontics, 3:135, 1965.

77. Ramfjord, S. P., and Costich, E. R.: Healing after exposure of periosteum on the alveolar process. J. Periodontol., 39:199, 1968.

78. Ramfjord, S. P., Nissle, R. R., Schick, R. A., and Cooper, H., Jr.: Subgingival curettage versus surgical elimination of periodontal pockets. J. Periodontol., 39:167, 1968.

79. Redondo, V. F., Bustamante, A., and Carranza, F. A., Jr.: Evaluación biometrica de la tecnica de extensión gingival con fenestración periostica. Rev. Asoc. Odont. Argent., 56:346, 1968.

80. Robinson, R. E.: Periosteal fenestration in mucogingival surgery. J. West. Soc. Periodont., 9:107, 1961.

81. Robinson, R. E.: The distal wedge operation. Periodontics, 4:256, 1966.

82. Robinson, R. E., and Agnew, R. G.: Periosteal fenestration at the mucogingival line. J. Periodontol., 34:503, 1963.

83. Rosenberg, M. M.: Vestibular alterations in periodontics. J. Periodontol., 31:231, 1960.

84. Roth, H.: Some speculations as to predictable fenestrations prior to mucogingival surgery. Periodontics, 3:29, 1965.

85. Rubinstein, H. S., Ruben, M. P., Levy, C., and Peiser, C.: Evidence for successful acceptance of irradiated free gingival allografts in dogs. J. Periodontol., 46:195, 1975.

86. Schoo, W. H., and Copes, L.: Use of palatal mucosa and lyophilized dura mater to create attached gingiva. J. Clin. Periodontol., 3:166, 1976.

87. Schmid, M. O.: The subperiosteal vestibule extension—literature review, rationale and technique. J. Western Soc. Periodont., 24:89, 1976.

88. Seibert, J. S.: Technique for the stabilization of soft tissue flap employing chrome-cobalt alloy tissue tacks. J. Periodontol., 32:283, 1961.

89. Simaan, G.: Histology study of the so-called attached gingiva following the deepening of

the vestibulum by the mucosal flap technique. Czas. Stomat., 69:91, 1969; Periodont. Abstr., 17:116, 1969.

90. Smith, R. M.: A study of the intertransplantation of alveolar mucosa. Oral Surg., 29:328, 1970.

91. Smith, R. M.: A study of the intertransplantation of gingiva. Oral Surg., 29:169, 1970.

92. Snyder, A. J.: A technic for free autogenous gingival grafts. J. Periodontol., 40:702, 1970.

93. Spengler, D. E., and Hayward, J. R.: Study of sulcus extension wound healing in dogs. J. Oral Surg., 22:413, 1964.

94. Staffileno, H.: Palatal flap surgery: mucosal flap (split thickness) and its advantages over the mucoperiosteal flap. J. Periodontol., 40:547, 1969.

95. Staffileno, H., and Levy, S.: Histologic and clinical study of mucosal (gingival) transplants in dogs. J. Peridontol., 40:311, 1969.

96. Staffileno, H., Levy, S., and Gargiulo, A.: Histologic study of cellular mobilization and repair following a periosteal retention operation via split thickness mucogingival flap surgery. J. Periodontol., 37:117, 1966.

97. Staffileno, H., Wentz, F., and Orban, B.: Histological study of healing of split thickness flap surgery in dogs. J. Periodontol., 33:56, 1962.

98. Strahan, J. D.: The relation of the mucogingival junction to the alveolar bone margin. D. Practit. & D. Rec., 14:72, 1963.

99. Sugarman, E. F.: A clinical and histological study of the attachment of grafted tissue to bone and teeth. J. Periodontol., 40:381, 1969.

100. Sullivan, H. C., and Atkins, J. H.: Free autogenous gingival grafts. I. Principles of successful grafting. Periodontics, 6:5, 1968.

101. Sullivan, H. C., and Atkins, J. H.: The role of free gingival grafts in periodontal therapy. Dent. Clin. North Am., 13:133, 1969.

102. Sullivan, H. C., Carman, D., and Dinner, D.: Histological evaluation of laterally positioned flap. I.A.D.R. Abst. #467, 1971, p. 169.

103. Sullivan, H. C., Dinner, D., and Carman, D.: Clinical evaluation of the laterally positioned flap. I.A.D.R. Abst., No. 466, 1971, p. 169.

104. Tavtigian, R.: The height of the facial radicular alveolar crest following apically positioned flap operations. J. Periodontol., 41:412, 1970.

105. Tisot, R. J., and Sullivan, H. C.: Evaluation of the survival of partial thickness and full thickness flaps. I.A.D.R. Abst. #470, 1971, p. 170.

106. Vande Voorde, H. E.: Gingival grafting and gingival repositioning. J. Am. Dent. Assoc., 79:1415, 1969.

107. Wade, A. B.: Vestibular deepening by the technique of Edlan and Mejchar. J. Periodont. Res., 4:300, 1969.

108. Waerhaug, J.: Review of Cohen: "Role of Periodontal Surgery." J. Dent. Res., 50:219, 1971.

109. Waltzer, R. E., and Halik, F. J.: Repositioning of the frenum in periodontal involvement. J. Oklahoma Dent. Assoc., 43:10, 37, 1954.

110. Ward, A. W.: The surgical eradication of pyorrhea. J. Am. Dent. Assoc., 15:2146, 1928.

111. West, T. L., and Bloom, A.: A histologic study of wound healing following mucogingival surgery. J. Dent. Res., 40:675, 1961.

112. Whinston, G. J.: Frenotomy and mucobuccal fold resection utilized in periodontal therapy. N.Y. Dent. J., 22:495, 1956.

113. Wilderman, M. N.: Exposure of bone in periodontal surgery. Dent. Clin. North Am., March, 1964, p. 23.

114. Wilderman, M. N.: Repair after a periosteal retention procedure. J. Periodontol., 34:487, 1963.

115. Wilderman, M. N., and Wentz, F. M.: Repair of a dentogingival defect with a pedicle flap. J. Periodontol., 36:218, 1965.

116. Wilderman, M. N., Wentz, F. M., and Orban, B. J.: Histogenesis of repair after mucogingival surgery. J. Periodontol., 31:283, 1960.

117. Wood, D. L., Hoag, P. L., Donnenfeld, O. W., and Rosenfeld, L. D.: Alveolar crest reduction following full and partial thickness flaps. J. Periodontol., 43:141, 1972.

118. Woofter, C.: The prevalence and etiology of gingival recession. Periodont. Abstr., 17:45, 1969.

Chapter 54

Treatment of Gingival
Enlargement

Treatment of gingival enlargement is based upon an understanding of the etiology and underlying pathological changes (see Chapter 10). Enlargements caused by inflammation alone can be treated effectively by local procedures. When systemic or unknown conditions are partly or entirely responsible, local treatment will only reduce the enlargement by the extent to which inflammation contributes to it. Because gingival enlargements differ in etiology, their treatment is best considered under separate headings.

TREATMENT OF CHRONIC INFLAMMATORY GINGIVAL ENLARGEMENT

Scaling and curettage

Chronic inflammatory enlargements, which are soft and discolored and are caused principally by edema and cellular infiltration, are treated by scaling and curettage, provided the size of the enlargement does not interfere with complete removal of deposits from the involved tooth surfaces.

Gingivectomy

Since most chronic inflammatory gingival enlargements consist of a significant fibrotic component that will not undergo shrinkage following scaling and curettage, or are of such size that they obscure deposits on the tooth surfaces and interfere with access to them, gingivectomy (Chapter 49) is the treatment of choice. (See Color Plate VIII). **The location and bevel of the incision are particularly critical.** The following procedure is used:

After the area is anesthetized, the junction of the enlarged gingiva with the adjacent mucosa is probed and outlined with pinpoint markings (Fig. 54–1A). The incision is made **apical to the markings and sufficiently close to the bone to assure complete removal of the enlarged tissue and complete exposure of all root deposits. No extraneous fibrous tissue should be left on the bone, because it interferes with the attainment of normal gingival contour.** The mucosa adjacent to the enlargement should be tapered by beveling the incision (Fig. 54–1B). The teeth are scaled and planed, and a periodontal pack is inserted for one week.

Tumor-like inflammatory enlargement

Tumor-like inflammatory enlargements are treated by gingivectomy as follows:

Under local anesthesia the tooth surfaces beneath the mass are scaled to remove calculus and other debris (Fig. 54–2). The lesion is separated from the mucosa at its base with a No. 12 Bard-Parker blade (Fig. 54–2). If the lesion extends interproximally, the interdental gingiva is included in the

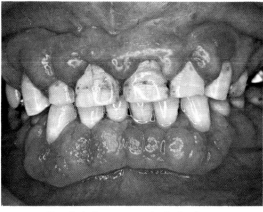

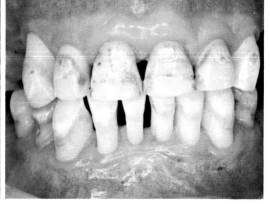

A. **Chronic inflammatory gingival enlargement.**

B. **After treatment**

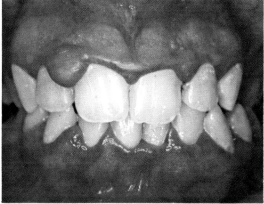

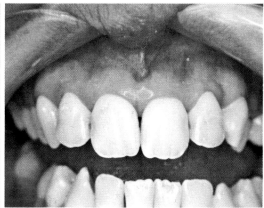

C. **Chronic inflammatory enlargement associated with mouth breathing.**

D. **After treatment.**

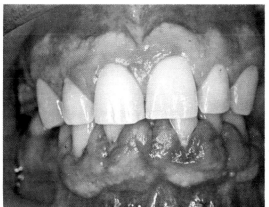

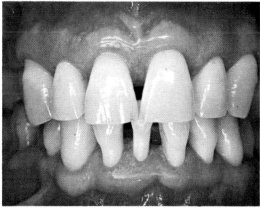

E. **Gingival enlargement associated with Dilantin therapy.**

F. **After treatment.**

Plate VIII

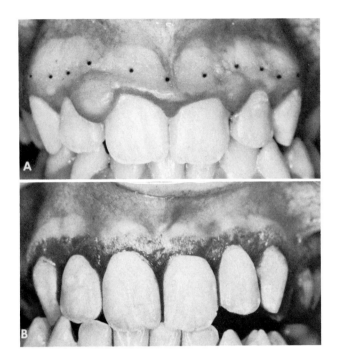

Figure 54–1 Gingivectomy Incision for Gingival Enlargement. *A,* Chronic inflammatory gingival enlargement with tumor-like area. Pinpoint markings outline extent of the enlargement. *B,* Enlarged gingiva removed. Note the bevelled incision. (For the pre- and post-treatment appearance see Color Plate VIII *C* and *D.*)

Figure 54–2 Treatment of Tumor-like Inflammatory Gingival Enlargement. *A,* Appearance of the lesion between the maxillary central and lateral incisors. *B,* The nature of attachment of the lesion is explored and the superficial calculus removed with a scaler. *C,* The lesion is excised with a No. 12 Bard-Parker blade. *D,* After the lesion is removed, calculus deposits are noted on the root surfaces. *E,* The tooth surfaces are scaled and planed. *F,* Appearance of the area one month after treatment. (Compare with *A.*)

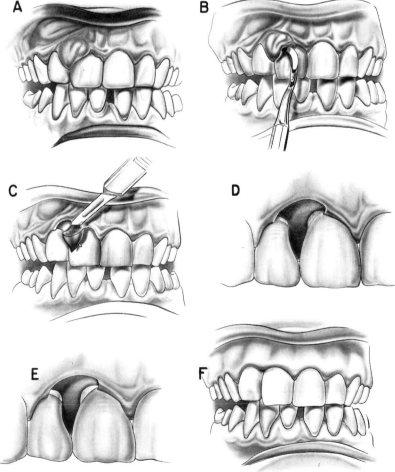

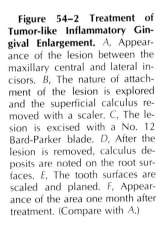

incision to ensure exposure of irritating root deposits. After the lesion is removed, the involved root surfaces are scaled and planed, and the area cleansed with warm water. A periodontal pack is applied and removed in a week, at which time the patient is instructed in plaque control.

TREATMENT OF THE GINGIVAL ABSCESS

In contrast with a periodontal abscess, which involves the supporting periodontal tissues, the *gingival abscess is a lesion of the marginal or interdental gingiva, usually produced by an impacted foreign object.* It is treated as follows:

Under topical anesthesia, the fluctuant area of the lesion is incised with a Bard-Parker blade, and the incision is gently widened to permit drainage. The area is cleansed with warm water and covered with a gauze pad. After bleeding stops, the patient is dismissed for 24 hours and instructed to rinse every two hours with a glass of warm water.

When the patient returns, the lesion is generally reduced in size and symptom-free. Topical anesthetic is applied and the area is scaled and curetted. If the residual size of the lesion is too great, it is removed surgically.

TREATMENT OF GINGIVAL HYPERPLASIA ASSOCIATED WITH PHENYTOIN (DILANTIN) THERAPY

Gingival enlargement does not occur in all patients receiving phenytoin; when it does occur, it may be of three types:

Type I. **Noninflammatory hyperplasia caused by the phenytoin** (Fig. 54–3A). Discontinuing the phenytoin is the only method of eliminating it. This is usually not feasible, but if it is done, the enlargement disappears after a few months.

Type II. **Chronic inflammatory enlargement entirely unrelated to the phenytoin** (Fig. 54–3B). The enlargement is caused entirely by local irritants and resembles inflammatory enlargement in patients not receiving phenytoin. It can be treated successfully by gingivectomy and fastidious plaque control, without recurrence.

Type III. **Combined enlargement is a combination of hyperplasia caused by phenytoin plus inflammation caused by local irritation** (Fig. 54–3). **This is the most common type of enlargement in patients treated with phenytoin** (Fig. 54–3C). It is treated by gingivectomy and elimination of all sources of local irritation, plus fastidious plaque control by the patient. The enlarged gingiva is removed with periodontal knives, or electrosurgery.

The initial treatment of combined enlargement presents no difficulty; the problem is with recurrence. Recurrence can be kept to a minimum by periodic scaling and diligent plaque control by the patient (see Color Plate VIII).[6] A hard natural rubber fitted bite guard worn at night sometimes assists in the control of recurrence.[1, 2]

Local treatment is very effective; it keeps patients comfortable and without disfigurement for years,[3, 5, 7] but it does not keep them entirely free of enlargement.[8, 9] It prevents the return of that part of the enlargement caused by inflammation (Fig. 54–4); it does not usually prevent the recurrence of the hyperplastic component of the enlarge-

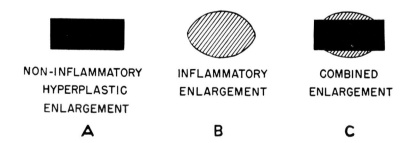

NON-INFLAMMATORY HYPERPLASTIC ENLARGEMENT   INFLAMMATORY ENLARGEMENT   COMBINED ENLARGEMENT

A   B   C

Figure 54–3   Types of Gingival Enlargement in Patients Under Phenytoin Therapy. *A,* Non-inflammatory hyperplastic enlargement caused by the phenytoin alone. *B,* Inflammatory enlargement caused by local irritation without phenytoin-induced hyperplasia. *C,* Combined enlargement that results from inflammation superimposed upon phenytoin-induced hyperplasia.

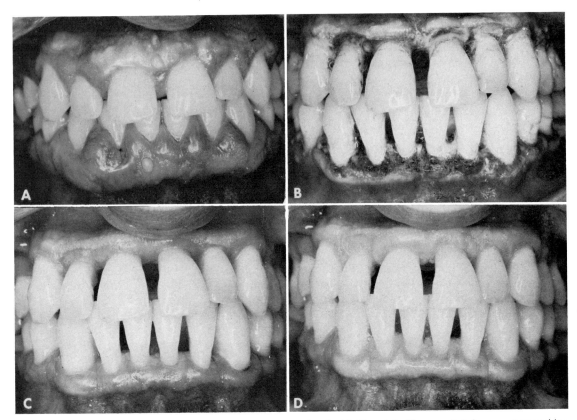

Figure 54–4 Combined Type of Gingival Enlargement Associated with Phenytoin Therapy. A, Enlargement caused by phenytoin combined with superimposed inflammation. B, Appearance at time of pack removal, one week after complete mouth gingivectomy. C, After four months. D, After five years. There is some hyperplasia caused by the phenytoin, but its size has been kept to a minimum by periodic scalings and diligent plaque control, which prevent inflammation from recurring.

ment caused by the phenytoin, although it has been reported to do so in some cases.[4, 6] In patients treated with phenytoin whose gingival enlargement is caused by local irritation alone, with no drug-induced hyperplasia, recurrence is totally preventable by local measures.

TREATMENT OF LEUKEMIC GINGIVAL ENLARGEMENT

Leukemic enlargement occurs in acute or subacute leukemia and is uncommon in the chronic leukemic state. The medical care of leukemic patients is often complicated by gingival enlargement with superimposed painful acute necrotizing ulcerative gingivitis, which interferes with eating and creates toxic systemic reactions. The bleeding and clotting times and platelet count of the patient are checked and the hematologist is consulted before periodontal treatment is instituted.

Treatment of the acute gingival involvement is described in Chapter 41. After the acute symptoms subside, attention is directed to correction of the gingival enlargement. The rationale is to remove the local factors in order to control the inflammatory component of the enlargement.

The enlargement is treated by scaling and curettage carried out in stages under topical anesthesia. The initial treatment consists of gently removing all loose accumulations with cotton pellets, superficial scaling, and instruction in oral hygiene procedures for plaque control. Oral hygiene is extremely important in these cases and should be performed by the nurse, if necessary.

Progressively deeper scalings are carried out at subsequent visits. Treatments are confined to a small area to facilitate control of bleeding. Antibiotics are administered systemically the evening before and for 48 hours after each treatment to reduce the risk of infection.

TREATMENT OF GINGIVAL ENLARGEMENT IN PREGNANCY

Treatment requires elimination of all local irritants that are responsible for precipitating the gingival changes in pregnancy. **Elimination of local irritants early in pregnancy is a preventive measure against gingival disease, which is preferable to treatment of gingival enlargement after it occurs.**

Marginal and interdental gingival inflammation and enlargement are treated by scaling and curettage (see Chapters 42 and 47). Treatment of **tumor-like gingival enlargements** consists of surgical excision plus scaling and planing of the tooth surface. **The enlargement will recur unless all irritants are removed.** Food impaction is a frequent factor.

When to treat

The lesion should be treated as soon as it is detected. It should not be permitted to remain until the pregnancy terminates, on the assumption that it will disappear spontaneously. This invites the possibility of increased growth of the lesion during pregnancy, with added patient discomfort. It also misleads the patient into thinking that parturition will solve her gingival problem. **Gingival enlargements do shrink after pregnancy, but they do not disappear.** There is a residual area of local irritation and inflammation which, if untreated, may cause progressive destruction of the periodontal tissues.

In pregnancy the emphasis should be upon (1) preventing gingival disease before it occurs, and (2) treating existing gingival disease before it becomes worse. All patients should be seen as early as possible in pregnancy. Those without gingival disease should be checked for potential sources of local irritation, and should be instructed in plaque control procedures (see Chap. 43). Those with gingival disease should be treated promptly, before the conditioning

effect of pregnancy upon the gingiva becomes manifest.

Every pregnant patient should be scheduled for periodic dental visits, and their importance as a preventive against serious periodontal disturbances should be stressed.

TREATMENT OF GINGIVAL ENLARGEMENT IN PUBERTY

Gingival enlargement in puberty is treated by scaling and curettage, removal of all sources of irritation, and plaque control. Gingivectomy may be required in severe cases. The problem in these patients is recurrence because of poor oral hygiene.

DRUGS IN THE TREATMENT OF GINGIVAL ENLARGEMENT

Gingival enlargement can be reduced by escharotic drugs, but this is not a recommended form of treatment. The destructive action of the drugs is difficult to control; injury to healthy tissue and root surfaces, delayed healing, and excessive postoperative pain are complications that can be avoided when the gingiva is removed with the use of periodontal knives, scalpels, or electrosurgery. Removal of the enlarged gingiva by any method must be accompanied by elimination of local irritants.

RECURRENCE OF GINGIVAL ENLARGEMENT

Recurrence following treatment is the most common problem in the management of gingival enlargement. Residual local irritation and systemic or hereditary conditions that cause noninflammatory gingival hyperplasia are the responsible factors.

Recurrence of chronic inflammatory enlargement immediately after treatment indicates that all irritants have not been removed. Contributory local conditions, such as food impaction and overhanging margins of restorations, are factors that are commonly overlooked. If the enlargement recurs after healing is complete and normal contour is attained, inadequate plaque control by the patient is the most common cause.

Recurrence during the healing period appears as red, bead-like granulomatous masses which bleed upon slight provocation. This is a proliferative vascular inflammatory response to local irritation, usually a fragment of calculus on the root. The condition is corrected by removing the granulation tissue and planing the root surface.

Familial, hereditary, or *idiopathic* gingival enlargement recurs after surgical removal even if all local irritants have been removed. The enlargement can be maintained at minimal size by preventing secondary inflammatory involvement.

REFERENCES

1. Aiman, R.: The use of positive pressure mouthpiece as a new therapy for Dilantin gingival hyperplasia. Chron. Omaha Dent. Soc., *131*:244, 1968.
2. Babcock, J. R.: The successful use of a new therapy for Dilantin gingival hyperplasia. Periodontics, 3:196, 1965.
3. Bergmann, C. L.: Dilantin: its effect on the gingival tissue, Dent. Dig., *73*:63, 1967.
4. Ciancio, S. G., Yaffe, S. J., and Catz, C. C.: Gingival hyperplasia and diphenylhydantoin. J. Periodontol., *43*:411, 1972.
5. Ginwalla, T. M., et al.: Management of gingival hyperplasia in patients receiving Dilantin therapy. J. Indian Dent. Assoc., 39:124, 1967.
6. Hall, W. B.: Dilantin hyperplasia: a preventable lesion. J. Periodont. Res., *4*:36, 1969.
7. Miller, F. D.: Multipronged attack against Dilantin gingival hyperplasia. Dent. Survey, *42*:51, 1966.
8. Russell, B., and Bay, L.: The effect of toothbrushing with chlorhexidine gluconate toothpaste on epileptic children (Abs.). J. Dent. Res., *54*:Special issue A, L 114, 1975.
9. Staple, P. H., Reed, M. J., Mashimo, P. A., Sedransk, N., and Umemoto, T.: Diphenylhydantoin gingival hyperplasia in *Macaca arctoides*. Prevention by inhibition of dental plaque deposition. J. Periodontol., *49*:310, 1978.

Occlusal Adjustment

Occlusal adjustment is the establishment of functional relationships favorable to the periodontium by one or more of the following procedures: reshaping the teeth by grinding, dental restoration, tooth movement or tooth removal. **There is a tendency to identify occlusal adjustment solely in a negative sense – namely, as a method of eliminating injurious occlusal forces, which indeed it should do. But its equally important purpose is to provide the functional stimulation necessary for the preservation of periodontal health, a positive dimension that occlusal adjustment adds to the practice of all phases of dentistry.**

ENVIRONMENTAL CONTROL AND THE PERIODONTIUM

The local environment of the periodontium and periodontal health

The local environment of the periodontium consists of two principal factors: (1)

the saliva with its microbial population, and (2) the occlusion. Two environmental pollutants adversely affect the periodontium: (1) dental plaque formed by oral bacteria, which leads to destructive periodontal inflammation, and (2) injurious occlusal forces, which damage the supporting periodontal tissues.

The establishment of a satisfactory local environment is essential in the treatment of periodontal disease and in the preservation of periodontal health. The urgency of controlling plaque is well recognized; occlusal adjustment to eliminate injurious forces and create forces favorable to the periodontium is equally important.

THE RATIONALE OF OCCLUSAL ADJUSTMENT

Occlusal adjustment is based upon the premises that tissue damage and excessive tooth mobility[35, 68] caused by unfavorable occlusal forces undergo repair when the injurious forces are corrected,[27] and that realigning occlusal forces by creating unobstructed functional contacts provides trophic stimulation beneficial to the periodontium, the muscles, and the temporomandibular joints.

For which patients is the occlusion adjusted?

The occlusion is adjusted for patients with evidence of microtrauma manifested in one or more of the following ways: (1) **periodontal injury** (excessive tooth mobility, angular thickening of the periodontal ligament, angular [vertical] bone destruction, infrabony pockets, some instances of furcation involvement, and migration of maxillary anterior teeth); (2) **muscular dysfunction;** and (3) **temporomandibular joint disorders.**

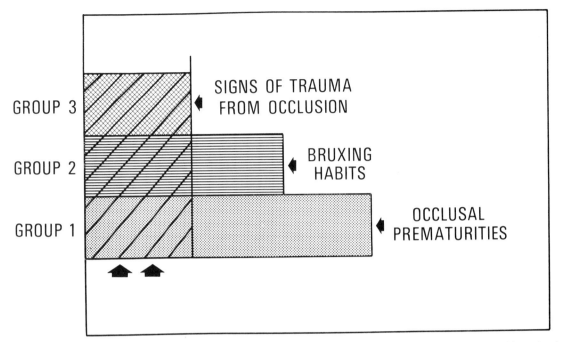

Figure 55–1   Occlusal Adjustment for Patients with Signs of Trauma from Occlusion. Group 1, Patients with occlusal prematurities. Group 2, Patients with prematurities who develop bruxing habits or abnormal function. Group 3, Patients with bruxing habits who develop trauma from occlusion. Occlusal adjustment is for patients in the cross-hatched vertical column (*double arrow*).

Most of the population has retrusive prematurities in the permanent[4, 8, 19, 59] and deciduous[20] dentition, and prematurities in the intercuspal position (habitual occlusion) are also extremely common (Fig. 55–1, Group 1). Not all patients with occlusal prematurities have trauma from occlusion. It is assumed that trauma from occlusion is caused by repetitive parafunctional forces (bruxism, clamping, and clenching) more than by chewing and swallowing. This is because it has been estimated that teeth are in functional contact for approximately 17.5 minutes[15] in a 24-hour period, which would leave ample time for the periodontium to recover if it were injured by functional occlusal forces.

Occlusal prematurities are inciting causes of bruxism. Of the many people with occlusal prematurities, only some develop parafunctional habits (Fig. 55–1, Group 2). Bruxism* is common, but only some patients who brux develop trauma from occlusion (Fig. 55–1, Group 3).

———————————
*Used throughout the chapter to include clamping and clenching habits.

The occlusion is adjusted for patients with occlusal prematurities who brux and present evidence of trauma from occlusion (the vertical crosshatched column in Fig. 55–1).

Preventive occlusal adjustment

We do not recommend preventive occlusal adjustment—the correction of what appear to be abnormal occlusal relationships in patients without signs of trauma from occlusion, for the ostensible purpose of preventing future damage. It is the tissue response in the periodontium, masticatory musculature, and temporomandibular joints that determines whether an occlusion is traumatic; the determination is not made by the alignment of the teeth and the presence or absence of occlusal prematurities. The absence of tissue injury means that the occlusal forces are acceptable to the tissues despite the fact that the alignment and relationship of the teeth may appear abnormal. Changing the occlusion in anticipation of future injury, without any indication that it will necessarily occur, may upset the present satisfactory balance between the occlusion and the tissues. The occlusion must satisfy the needs of the periodontium, the musculature and the temporomandibular joints, not the desires of the therapist.

When to adjust the occlusion in the sequence of periodontal treatment

We are often confronted with patients suffering from both inflammation and trauma from occlusion: it would be best to eliminate both at the same time. This is not always feasible, and when a choice must be made **the occlusion is usually adjusted after gingival inflammation and periodontal pockets have been eliminated, for the following reasons:**

1. Evidence related to the pathogenesis and healing aspects of trauma from occlusion[39, 40] suggests that the benefits of occlusal adjustment are not complete if inflammation is not eliminated first.

2. Teeth with periodontal disease often migrate. After the inflammation is eliminated, the teeth shift again, often in the direction of their original position (Fig. 55–2). If the occlusion is adjusted before the inflammation is alleviated, it will have to be readjusted after gingival health is restored.

The usual sequence of treatment is modified under the following conditions: **In infrabony pockets, excessive occlusal forces are important in determining the pattern of the osseous defects.** To provide optimal conditions for repair of the bony defect with or without the use of osseous and marrow implants, the occlusion is adjusted before or along with the pocket elimination procedures.[52] In mucogingival surgery, because occlusal forces affect the post-treatment contour of the facial bony plate[14] and in cases of excessive tooth mobility in which trauma from occlusion is a major causative factor, the occlusion is adjusted before or along with the treatment of the inflammation.

TECHNIQUES OF OCCLUSAL ADJUSTMENT*

There are many methods of occlusal adjustment, most of which fall into one of three categories:

1. **"Functional method"** (active jaw movement).[13, 16, 22, 24, 25] Functional movements made by the patient disclose the contacts to be reshaped or removed. This meth-

---

*For detailed presentations of this subject, see Arnold, N. R., and Frumker, S. C.[2]; Dawson, P. E.,[10] Ramfjord, S. P.,[43] and Shore, N. A.[56]

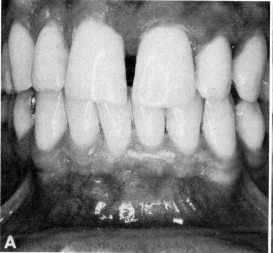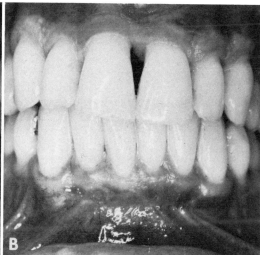

Figure 55–2 Change in Tooth Position Following Periodontal Treatment. *A,* Before treatment. Note the diastema between the maxillary central incisors. *B,* In the course of treatment the teeth return to their normal position following resolution of inflammation.

od develops intercuspal closure at the *muscular contact position* (**MCP**)† which in most cases is synonymous with the *intercuspal position* (**ICP**) and anterior to the *retruded contact position* (**RCP**). *The main feature of this technique is its dependence on the patient's neuromuscular control for determining the optimal occlusal position.*

2. **Schuyler method** (passive jaw manipulation).[53, 54] The dentist manipulates the mandible to disclose interferences at lateral and retrusive border positions and especially at the retruded contact position (RCP). This method develops a new ICP coincident with RCP or at some point slightly anterior and sagittal to RCP. The postoperative ICP may be more *cranial* than the original one. *The main feature of this technique is its dependence upon the stability and alignment of the temporomandibular joints to achieve an optimal occlusal position.*

3. **Myomonitor method**‡ (transcutaneous neural stimulation)[23]: The masticatory muscles are "pulsed" by intermittent electrical stimulation, resulting in repetitive mandibular contact with the maxillary teeth (myocentric contact position). This method is reported to develop a new intercuspal position anterior to both RCP and the previous ICP.[3, 26, 30, 45, 61] *This technique relies upon the effect of an artificially induced polymuscular contraction to achieve the prescribed occlusal (myocentric) position.*

Which technique of occlusal adjustment should be selected?

Mandibular positions obtained with the *Myomonitor technique* have been compared with other reference positions in several studies.[3, 26, 30, 45, 61] These investigations reported that "myocentric" mandibular position was anterior to both the retruded position and the intercuspal position. On the basis of these studies, the myomonitor technique appears questionable since myocentric records position the condyles and the teeth anterior and inferior with respect to those intercuspal rela-

tionships[59] found in otherwise normal individuals.

Some authors favor *functional adjustment* to a neuromuscular closure (coordination of MCP and ICP) without attention to border positions, which they consider nonphysiological parafunctional movements rather than regular features of chewing and swallowing.[17, 25] The advocates of the functional adjustment claim that correction of prematurities at ICP and elimination of retrusive prematurities are sufficient to inhibit bruxing and dysfunctional habits (evidence is unsupported or inconclusive). Some advocates of the "functional method" do not adjust the retrusive range (RCP).

The advocates of the *Schuyler method* take a more comprehensive approach and recommend adjustment of lateral and protrusive excursions which are often taken up by the bruxing patient. In this technique, minimal attention is given to the coordination of MCP and ICP. Whereas the functional method emphasizes intraborder adjustment (ICP), the Schuyler method emphasizes the adjustment of border excursions and the development of a stable RCP. Dentists using either method routinely correct gross interferences such as extruded or tipped teeth, plunger cusps, uneven marginal ridges, and enlargement of flat areas due to occlusal wear.

Both methods appear to have some advantages; that is, **both intraborder and border adjustment are desirable.** *Intraborder* adjustment is logical, since there seems little doubt that the intercuspal position is the most commonly used functional occlusion of the dentition.[13] *Border position* adjustment is practical because excursive interferences during gnashing and grinding of the teeth are traumatic (parafunctional).[44] The occlusal adjustment technique suggested in this chapter consists of a combined approach that can be progressively utilized to accomplish both limited and comprehensive occlusal adjustment. **The goal of this technique is to minimize occlusal interferences and to insure that both the joints and the teeth are stabilized at a common functional end-point at or centered slightly anterior to the retruded contact position (RCP).**[42] The occlusal alterations include stabilization of RCP and a coordination of the pathway between RCP

---

†See Chapter 28 for definitions of nomenclature.
‡Myotronics Inc., Seattle, Washington.

and ICP. Also, smooth, interference-free lateral and protrusive excursions are facilitated from both RCP and ICP. Mediotrusive (balancing) interferences are reduced or eliminated. These features are expected to strengthen the adaptive capacity of individuals with a low tolerance to occlusal interferences or with occlusions weakened by bone loss.

RECOMMENDED TECHNIQUE FOR OCCLUSAL ADJUSTMENT

Objectives for Occlusal Adjustment

The practical objective of occlusal adjustment is to mechanically eliminate occlusal interferences involved in function and parafunction. Positive actions resulting from occlusal adjustment are:[29]

1. A change in the pattern and degree of afferent impulses.

2. A decreased tooth mobility, since stabilization of tooth position helps control the occlusal sensory input.

3. The creation of a multiple simultaneous contact spread over the occlusal scheme in order to create *occlusal stabilization* of the mandible (i.e., decrease *muscular stabilization*).

4. A change in the pattern of chewing or swallowing function.

5. The establishment of multidirectional mandibular movement patterns.

Casts and Occlusal Analysis

Casts should be made before the teeth are altered by occlusal adjustment. These records are useful during the procedure and for reference at follow-up visits. *When occlusal adjustment is to be performed in the mouth a reasonable prediction of the biomechanical result by this approach is required.* Mounting the casts on a semi-adjustable articulator using a facebow transfer and a retruded position intermaxillary record is an aid in reaching this objective.[9] Many clinicians find that trial carving of the casts allows them to proceed with the intraoral occlusal adjustment with greater confidence and efficiency.

Armamentarium

It is best to employ the combined use of various products for identifying and marking tooth contact. Selected products are listed in Table 55–1 with recommendations for specific application in the occlusal adjustment process. Marking ribbon and marking paper mark best on a dry tooth surface. Therefore, these products should be used in combination with adequate isolation. Blotting paper* and cotton rolls are useful for this purpose. The rec-

---

*Dri-Angles, Tru-Eze Mfg. Co., Temecula, CA 92390.

TABLE 55–1 RECOMMENDED MATERIALS FOR IDENTIFYING AND MARKING TOOTH CONTACT AND CONTACT MOVEMENT

Product	Suggested Application of Product			
	ICP Contact	*RCP Contact*	*Protrusive and Lateral Contact*	*Intensity/Area of Contact*
Occlusal registration strips[a]	x		x	x
Occlusal indicator wax[b]	x	x		x
Marking ribbon[c] — red, green; blue Mylar ribbon[d]	x	x	x	
Articulating paper — blue[e]	x			

[a]Artus Corp., Englewood, NJ
[b]Kerr Corp., Romulus, MI
[c]Columbia Ribbon, Cucamonga, CA
[d]Parkel, Farmingdale, NJ 11735
[e]Holg Mark-Rite Interstate Dental Co., New Hyde Park, NY 11140

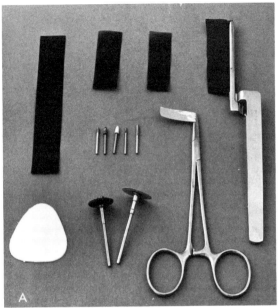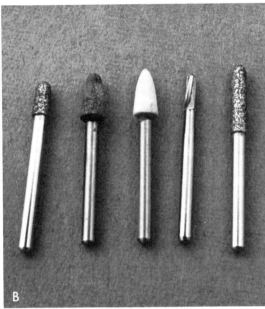

Figure 55–3 Instruments and Materials Used in Performing Occlusal Adjustment. *A,* (Clockwise) Mylar strip in hemostat, abrasive disc and wheel, blotting paper to reduce salivary flow, inked marking ribbon in ribbon holder, and (center) friction grip burs and stones. *B,* **Cutting and Abrasive Burs Used in Performing Occlusal Adjustment.** (Left to right) diamond, green stone, polystone, fluted carbide, elongated diamond.

ommended armamentaria are shown in Fig. 55–3*A* and *B.*

Classification of Supracontacts (Prematurities, Interferences)

Excursive interferences are classified according to the mandibular movement that caused the contact in question to take place (See Figure 55–4*A* and *B*). The reference point for this movement is the intercuspal position (ICP). For example, supracontacts occurring under retrusive excursion are called *retrusive* supracontacts. Supracontacts occurring under laterotrusion are termed *laterotrusive* supracontacts. *Note that excursive contacts are named exactly according to the way each functional segment of the mandible moves from ICP (Fig. 55–4A).*

Static prematurities at the intercuspal position (ICP) are not related to horizontal mandibular movements. They are identified as contact relationships in the frontal plane and are classified as follows:

CLASS I PREMATURITY. The buccal inclines of the buccal cusps of the mandibular molars and premolars, against the lingual inclines of the buccal cusps of the

maxillary molars and premolars (Fig. 55–5); and the facial surfaces of the mandibular anterior teeth, against the lingual surfaces of their maxillary antagonists.

CLASS II PREMATURITY. The lingual inclines of the lingual cusps of the maxillary molars and premolars, against the buccal inclines of the lingual cusps of the mandibular molars and premolars (Fig. 55–5).

CLASS III PREMATURITY. The buccal inclines of the lingual cusps of maxillary molars and premolars, against the lingual inclines of the buccal cusps of the mandibular molars and premolars (Fig. 55–5).

How to Correct Supracontacts (Prematurities, Interferences)

The correction of occlusal prematurities after they have been located and marked on the teeth is a technique in itself. The objective is to reduce the prematurities so as to create unobstructed closure of cusps into fossae, while restoring and preserving original tooth anatomy. *It is not simply a matter of grinding down premature contacts,* which creates flattened planes that

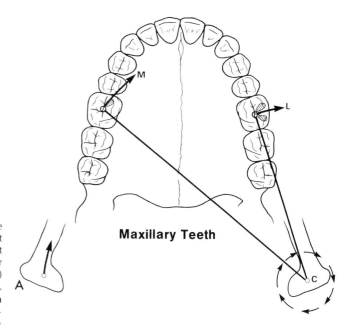

Figure 55–4 Excursive Interferences. These are named after the mandibular movement that caused them to come into contact. *A,* Note that the potential for interferences occurs over pathways determined by the rotating (working) condyle (C). *M,* mediotrusive interference. *L,* laterotrusive interference. *B,* **The Four Main Occlusal Interferences.** *R,* Retrusive. *P,* Protrusive. *L,* Laterotrusive. *M,* Mediotrusive. Open circle denotes the intercuspal position (ICP) contact area.

Maxillary Teeth

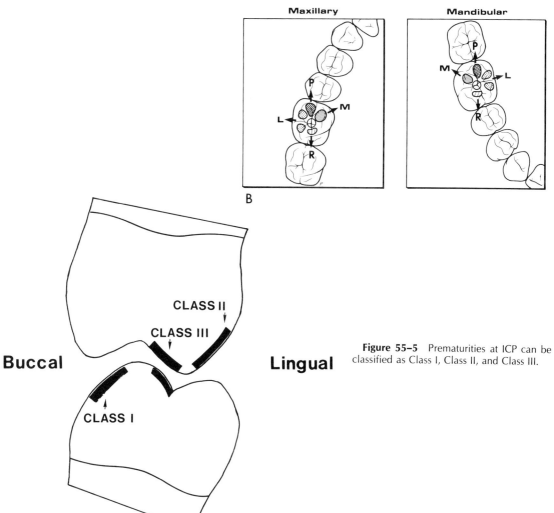

Figure 55–5 Prematurities at ICP can be classified as Class I, Class II, and Class III.

953

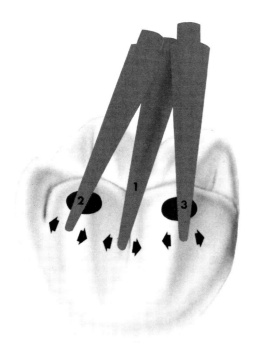

Figure 55–6   Grooving to Restore the Depth of Developmental Grooves on Worn Tooth Surfaces. A tapered diamond stone (1) is rotated slowly in the groove as indicated. After the desired depth is attained, the stone is moved (2 and 3) to spheroid the adjacent tooth surface.

will further disrupt the occlusion. The correction of occlusal prematurities consists of: (1) **grooving**, (2) **spheroiding**, and (3) **pointing.**

Grooving consists of restoring the depth of developmental grooves made shallow by occlusal wear. It is done with a tapered cutting tool until the desired depth is attained (Fig. 55–6).

Spheroiding consists of reducing the prematurity and restoring the original tooth contour. Starting 2 or 3 mm. mesial or distal to the prematurity, the tooth is recontoured from the occlusal margin to a distance 2 or 3 mm. apical to the marking (Figs. 55–6 and 55–7). This is done with a light "paintbrush" stroke, gradually blending the area of prematurity with the adjacent tooth surface. A special effort is made to preserve the occlusal height of the cusps (Figs. 55–8 and 55–9).

The purpose of spheroiding is not simply to narrow occlusal surfaces. When teeth are flattened by wear, the buccolingual diameter of the occlusal surface is increased. Spheroiding restores the buccolingual width of the occlusal surface to what it was before wear occurred (Fig. 55–10).

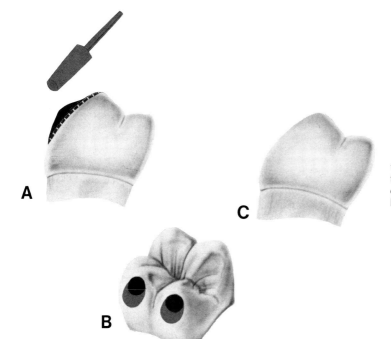

A

B

C

Figure 55–7   Spheroiding to Restore the Original Tooth Contour. *A,* Recontouring prematurity. *B,* Recontouring extends several millimeters below the black marking. *C,* Corrected contour.

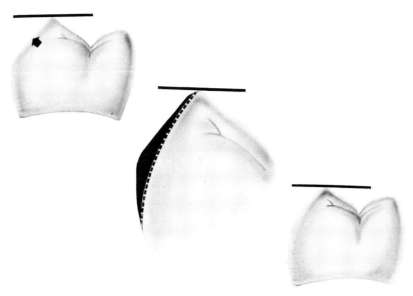

Figure 55–8 Correct Method of Spheroiding (*broken line*) and preserving the height of the buccal cusp (*horizontal line*). *Arrow* points to the prematurity.

Pointing consists of restoring cusp point contours (Fig. 55–11). It is done by reshaping the tooth with rotating cutting tools.

As a general rule, Class I prematurities are corrected on mandibular teeth. Class II and Class III prematurities are adjusted where feasible on both the maxillary and mandibular teeth. If doing all the correction on one jaw would entail mutilation of tooth anatomy, the opposing teeth are included in the correction process. The emphasis is always upon restoring and preserving tooth anatomy.

Schedule for Occlusal Adjustment

Occlusal adjustment can be accomplished using a variety of different sequences. A step-by-step approach is pre-

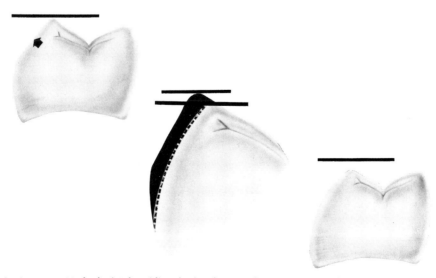

Figure 55–9 Incorrect Method of Spheroiding (*broken line*) results in excessive reduction in buccal cusp height (*horizontal line*). The arrow points to the prematurity.

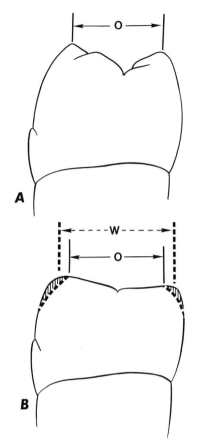

Figure 55–10 Flattened Occlusal Surface Restored to 'Jnworn Width. *A,* Occlusal diameter (O) of unworn mandibular molar. *B,* Widened occlusal diameter (W) of worn molar restored to diameter of unworn surface (O) by recontouring (*shaded areas*).

TABLE 55–2 SCHEDULE OF OCCLUSAL ADJUSTMENT

Step 1.	Explain; create positive patient acceptance.
Step 2.	Remove retrusive prematurities and eliminate the deflective shift from RCP to ICP (the retrusive pathway prematurities are eliminated).
Step 3.	Adjust ICP to achieve stable, simultaneous, multi-pointed, widely distributed contacts.
Step 4.	Test for excessive contact (fremitus) on the incisor teeth.
Step 5.	Remove posterior protrusive interferences and establish contacts bilaterally distributed on the anterior teeth.
Step 6.	Remove or lessen mediotrusive (balancing) interferences.
Step 7.	Reduce excessive cusp steepness on the laterotrusive (working) contacts.
Step 8.	Eliminate gross occlusal disharmonies.
Step 9.	Recheck tooth contact relationships.
Step 10.	Polish all rough tooth surfaces.

plished over two or more appointments, with each visit limited to a half-hour of adjustment. The number and duration of sessions may vary according to patient tolerance, but the sequence should not be changed.

Many situations in periodontal therapy require occlusal adjustment of only one or two teeth. Obviously, comprehensive occlusal adjustment is not warranted. In these cases, localized occlusal adjustment is often limited to intraborder reduction of Class I, II, and III supracontacts on the involved teeth (steps 1,3, and 4).

THE TEN STEPS OF OCCLUSAL ADJUSTMENT

Step 1. Explain occlusal adjustment and create positive patient acceptance

Patients may be concerned that grinding their teeth will change their appearance,

sented here for clarity, even though experienced operators tend to blend the steps together.

The occlusion is adjusted systematically according to the schedule in Table 55–2. The series of steps normally is accom-

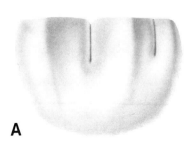
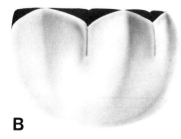

A   **B**

Figure 55–11   Pointing. *A,* Buccal margin of mandibular molar flattened by wear. *B,* Tooth recontoured to restore cusp points.

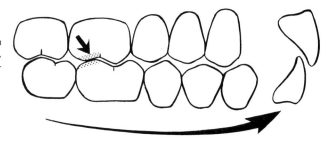

Figure 55–12 Shift from RCP to ICP. When contact is located on terminal hinge closure (RCP), prematurities may cause the mandible to glide mesially into the intercuspal position.

cause tooth decay, and increase tooth sensitivity. The operator should explain that the teeth are not going to be "ground down" but rather *reshaped* so that they will function better. The reshaping is done in areas where tooth decay rarely occurs. It should also be made clear that adjusting the occlusion is a necessary part of the total periodontal treatment, which benefits the periodontal tissues and prolongs the life of the teeth. The appearance of the teeth will not be spoiled; if anything, they may look better and feel more comfortable. Above all, the patient should understand that occlusal adjustment is not permanent, that the teeth and the occlusion change with time, and that the occlusion will be checked at periodic recall visits, at which time minor adjustments will be made, if necessary.

Step 2. Remove retrusive prematurities and eliminate the deflective shift from RCP to ICP

The purpose of this step is to eliminate prematurities that interfere with hinge closure of the mandible to a stable retruded contact position (**RCP**). When contact is located on terminal hinge closure, prematurities may cause the mandible to glide mesially into the intercuspal position (ICP). This glide is termed the **shift from RCP to ICP** (Fig. 55–12). Retrusive adjustment will result in the elimination of the deflective RCP to ICP shift; particularly it will neutralize or remove *asymmetrical shifts from RCP to ICP* (Fig. 55–13A and B). The normal areas of contact at RCP or ICP are referred to as *vertical (or centric) stops.*

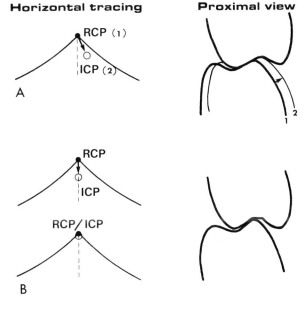

Figure 55–13 RCP to ICP Shift. *A,* Before occlusal adjustment. Mandibular teeth shift from point 1 to point 2 (asymmetrical shift). The same movement is seen in the arrow point tracing in the horizontal plane. *B,* After occlusal adjustment. Asymmetrical shift from RCP to ICP is removed and resulting intercuspal position is nearer or identical to RCP.

How to locate the retruded contact position. **Locating the retruded contact position is the key to controlled occlusal adjustment.** Begin by placing the patient in the supine position, which has been shown to reduce the activity of the protruder muscles most completely.[12, 31, 36] Test and rehearse hinge closure to RCP. Some patients allow their mandibles to be passively retruded quite easily; other patients defy experts! *Arriving at RCP is dependent upon specific verbal and motor actions by the operator.* Figure 55–14 shows two hand grasp methods that have proved effective for manipulation of the mandible.[10, 43] A common error is to grab the chin and nervously order the patient to "relax!" Ideally, the patient's mandible will fall passively to the retruded position—the operator's main function is to create an arcing terminal hinge movement.

Experience has shown that certain specific statements are better than others in obtaining the desired result:

1. With very light pressure, encourage small hinge movements and say, "*Let your mouth drop open.*"

2. As the jaw falls downward and backward to the retruded position, exert more pressure and seek out the ligamentous resistance of the temporomandibular joints. You may encounter muscular resistance; when you sense this, remove your hands completely and begin the manipulation again. Talk in low tones, using repetitious phrases, e.g., "*Just let it go.*" At this point you should have the jaw arcing. Then say, "*Let your jaw come together . . . just so you first touch.*"

3. After the initial contact is perceived say, "*Squeeze.*" The shift from RCP to ICP, if present, should be apparent. *Remember:*

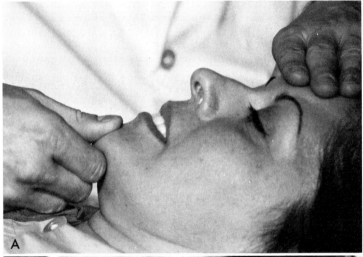

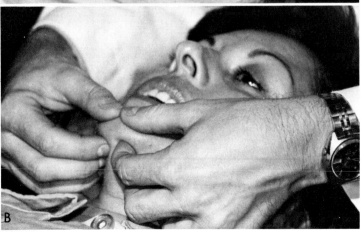

Figure 55–14　Method of Locating RCP. *A,* Patient is supine. Forefinger and thumb are "butted" against the chin, with the other hand stabilizing the head. *B,* Dawson[10] method. All four fingers of each hand are placed on the lower border of the mandible. This places an upward pressure on the condyle during the manipulation. The thumbs are placed in the notch over the symphysis exerting a downward pressure. The thumbs should touch each other.

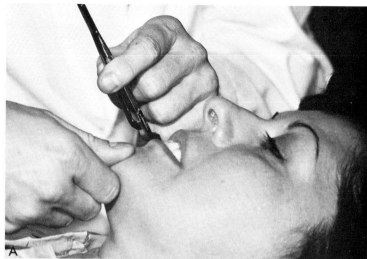

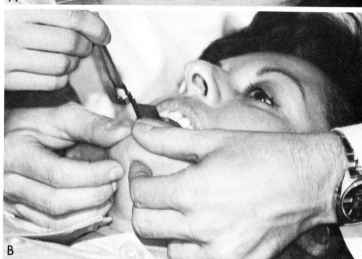

Figure 55–15 Technique for Marking RCP Contacts on the Teeth. *A,* Chin grasp technique. *B,* Technique after Dawson.[10]

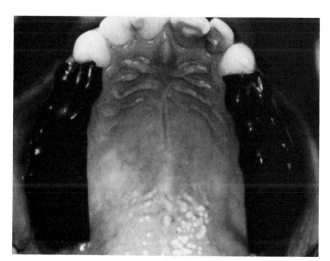

Figure 55–16 Wax Strips on the Maxillary Premolars and Molars. The anterior teeth are not covered.

The location of RCP is dependent upon your ability to detect the "ligamentous signal" from the patient. A stiff wrist and forearm will improve your receptibility to the "ligamentous signal." Generally, if you cannot manipulate the mandible to RCP, an occlusal adjustment in the retruded position should not be attempted. Removable interocclusal splints are indicated for reducing the neuromuscular antagonism prior to occlusal adjustment.

4. Retrusive prematurities can be

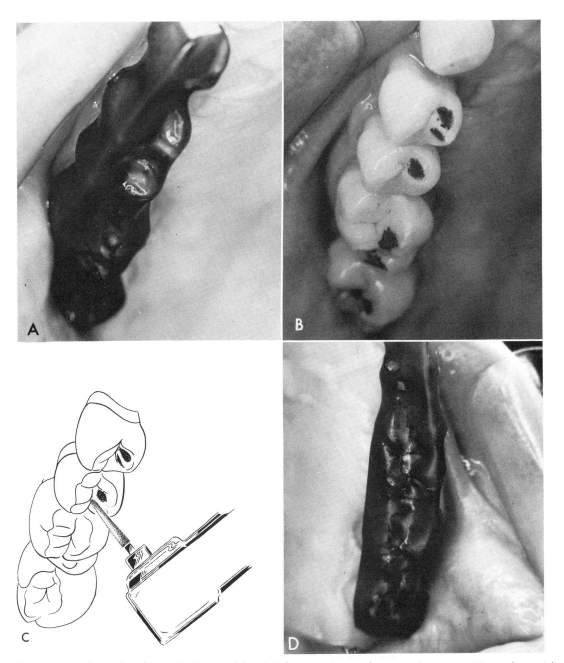

Figure 55–17   Correction of Retrusive Prematurities. *A,* Indentations in wax show retrusive prematurities on the mesial inner inclines of the maxillary lingual cusps. *B,* Retrusive prematurities marked on the teeth. *C,* Prematurities corrected with diamond point. *D,* After correction, wax shows evenly distributed contact on cusp tips and fossae.

(Illustration continued on opposite page)

marked with either green wax or red marking ribbon. Red ribbon should be placed in a ribbon forceps* and inserted between the desired teeth after they are properly dried (Fig. 55–15). Occlusal registration wax is first placed on the maxillary or mandibular posterior quadrant, with the adhesive (shiny) surface pressed against the teeth (Fig. 55–16). The occlusal surface of the wax is moistened with a wet finger to prevent adherence of the opposing teeth. The mandible is manipulated to strike against the wax in short, interrupted closures. Mobile teeth are stabilized with the fingers so that prematurities will not be pushed aside. If there are no supracontacts on retruded closure of the jaw, the wax will be uniformly transparent at the contact areas. Severe prematurities will cause perforation of the wax. The prematurities are marked on the teeth through the wax with a pencil, and the wax strips are removed (Fig. 55–17).

5. Question the patients as to which teeth seem to "hit first" as the jaws close. The patient's impression is often useful in locating the areas of premature contact. Common sites of prematurities are the mesial inclines of the lingual cusps and marginal ridges of the maxillary molars and premolars and their opposing tooth surfaces. The mesial inner incline of the lingual cusp of the maxillary first premolars is the most common initial prematurity.

*Miltex Instrument Company, New York, NY 10010.

PRINCIPLES THAT SHOULD NOT BE VIOLATED IN THE RETRUSIVE OCCLUSAL ADJUSTMENT.

1. Remove the inclines that cause interferences when the mandible moves from RCP to ICP. Do not remove the vertical stop or supporting cusp tip, only the incline between these two areas (Fig. 55–17C, D, and E). These inclines, which are called retrusive prematurities, are usually found on *mesial facing inclines of the maxillary teeth and distal facing inclines of the mandibular teeth* (MUDL Rule).

2. Strive to achieve vertical stops at RCP on each tooth. Avoid losing them when grinding excursive interferences. If the vertical cusps are not aligned within the desired opposing fossa, corrections are made on the cusp slope or incline to place the cusp more nearly within the fossa. If the cusp and fossa are in alignment, either the fossa is deepened or the cusp is shortened—whichever element is most out of harmony with the other like elements in the arch.[46]

3. Reshape, if possible, at the expense of the fossa, ridges, or cusp inclines. Preserve the marginal ridges; adjust the cusp tip as a last resort. Adjust worn facets to achieve point-to-surface rather than surface-to-surface contact.

4. Mobile teeth are stabilized with the fingers so that prematurities will be accurately registered and not be pushed aside. To avoid excessive grinding of one dental arch, do part of the correction on the other arch.

5. *Removing the lateral thrust in the RCP to ICP Shift.* In lateral shifts, the significant retrusive markings on the maxillary teeth face in the direction to which the

Figure 55–17 *Continued E,* Correction of retrusive interferences involves flat reduction (a) and (b) but should be followed by spheroiding (c).

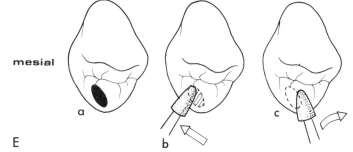

mandible shifts from RCP to ICP. Adjustment of these prematurities will eliminate the lateral component of the shift. This simple observation can be of great help in rapidly achieving the end point in retrusive range adjustment.

6. Continue to adjust the RCP vertical stops so that they approach the same vertical level as the previous ICP. If the RCP stops appear stable but still require reduction to approach the same level as ICP, use the following guidelines: (a) reduce the cusp tip when supracontacts in excursions are associated with that movement of that cusp; (b) otherwise, reduce the fossa, especially if it appears too shallow. Both the cusps and the fossae may eventually require adjustment to obtain RCP and ICP at the same level. Once this relationship is obtained, both the cranial and lateral components of the RCP-ICP shift are removed. The therapeutic result is to allow sagittal movement between RCP and ICP at the same level; alternatively, RCP may be made slightly cranial to the preoperative ICP, in which case RCP and ICP may be nearly synonymous after occlusal adjustment.

7. The retrusive range adjustment is complete when the following conditions are achieved: (a) The contact pattern is bilateral with many-pointed contacts; (b) the deflective shift from RCP to ICP has been eliminated; (c) both RCP and ICP approach the same vertical dimension of occlusion, (d) the pathway from RCP to ICP, if present, is smooth and gliding; and (e) repeated closure of the teeth together in the hinge position produces a sharp, resonant sound.

Step 3. Adjustment of the intercuspal position (ICP)

A task common to many dental procedures is the localized adjustment of ICP contacts on one or more teeth. The adjustment of ICP is also a major step involved with comprehensive occlusal adjustment. The purpose of this step is to achieve a stable ICP and to refine occlusal table relationships. **The main feature of this step is that the prematurities are identified without guidance of the operator's hand.** The reshaping is accomplished by progressive adjustment of class I, II, and III prematurities during one or more visits. The posterior teeth are adjusted first, followed by the anterior teeth.

HOW TO LOCATE PREMATURITIES IN ICP. Instruct the patient, *"Tap your back teeth together, both sides at the same time, slow and hard."* Have the patient repeat this process once or twice; the teeth normally will meet in the same position. This is the intercuspal position (ICP) or habitual occlusion. Since relatively heavy muscular force is used, the choice of marking medium is less critical. The combined use of more than one medium for cross-comparison is advantageous. Occlusal indicator wax, blue marking paper,

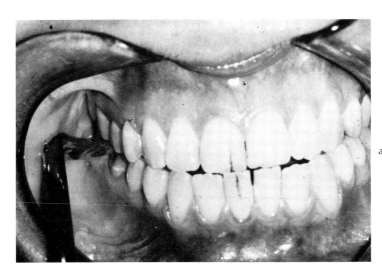

Figure 55–18 Mylar occlusal strips are used in confirming areas of contact.

or marking ribbon work equally well. Actual ICP contact can be assessed by using Mylar occlusal indicator strips inserted between the closed teeth and tested with a "tugging" motion (Fig. 55–18). If wax is used, it is placed on the occlusal and incisal surfaces of the mandibular teeth (Fig. 55–19), and the patient is asked to open and close again as before. The translucent areas are marked on the mandibular teeth with a pencil, and the wax is removed.

Correction of Class I prematurities (Fig. 55–20) is started on the posterior teeth with contouring on the facial surface of the molars (Fig. 55–21), followed by spheroiding and pointing of the molars and premolars (Fig. 55–22). After the posterior segments are corrected, attention is directed to the anterior teeth (Fig. 55–23). The fa-

cial surfaces are spheroided mesiodistally to relieve the prematurities and at the same time to reduce the width of the worn incisal edges. Extruded teeth are reduced in the adjustment procedure (Fig. 55–24). Wax strips are placed on the teeth again, and correction is repeated until light transparencies appear only on the cusp tips and incisal edges (Fig. 55–23C). This usually requires several applications of wax strips. It may be necessary to complete the correction on the opposing maxillary surfaces in order to avoid excessive reduction of the mandibular teeth. After the prematurities are eliminated. the teeth are smoothed and the patient is dismissed.

Teeth tend to right themselves and to erupt into the spaces created by the correction of Class I prematurities (Fig. 55–

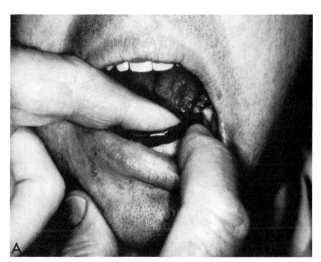

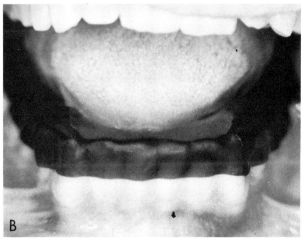

Figure 55–19 Correcting Prematurities in the Intercuspal Position (ICP). *A,* Placing the wax on the mandibular teeth. *B,* Wax in position.

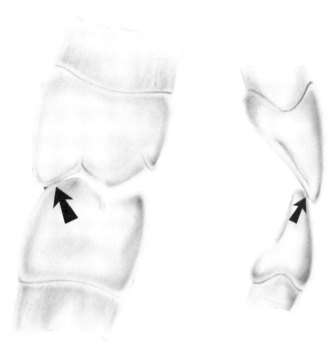

Figure 55–20 Class I Prematurities in the Intercuspal Position. Class I prematurities on the facial surface of the mandibular anterior and posterior teeth indicated by *arrows*.

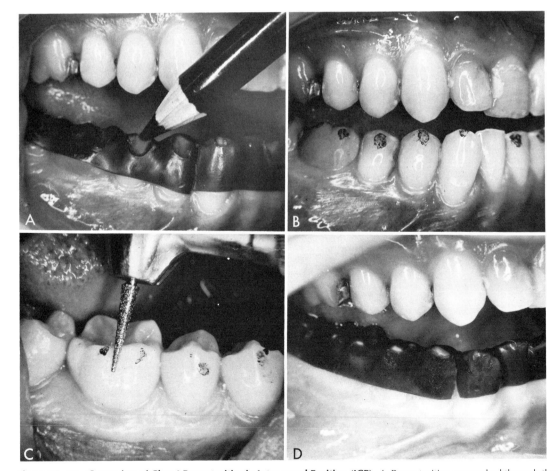

Figure 55–21   Correction of Class I Prematurities in Intercuspal Position (ICP). *A,* Prematurities are marked through the wax onto the teeth. *B,* Prematurities marked on the teeth. *C,* Grooving the buccal surface with a tapered diamond. *D,* After correction, contact is shown on the cusp tips.

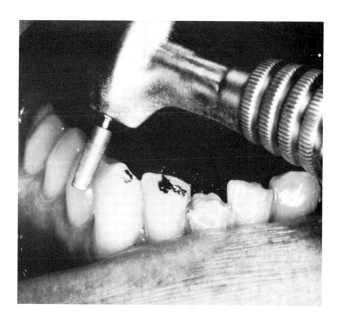

Figure 55–22 Spheroiding the Facial Surface of a Mandibular Premolar to Correct a Class I prematurity in ICP.

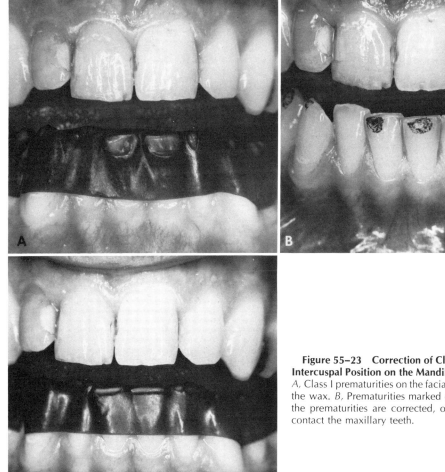

Figure 55–23 Correction of Class I Prematurities in Intercuspal Position on the Mandibular Anterior Teeth. *A,* Class I prematurities on the facial surface registered in the wax. *B,* Prematurities marked on the teeth. *C,* After the prematurities are corrected, only the incisal edges contact the maxillary teeth.

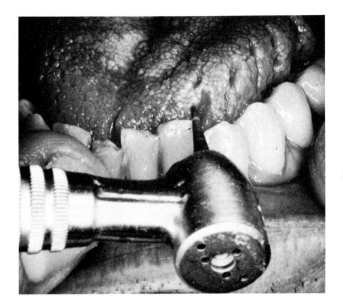

Figure 55–24   Reduction of Extruded Mandibular Incisors.

25). This reduces lateral stresses and redirects occlusal forces in the long axis of the teeth, but often creates new Class I prematurities, which are corrected at the next visit.

To locate *Class II prematurities* (Fig. 55–26) in ICP, the wax is applied to the maxillary posterior teeth (Fig. 55–27A). The patient again closes in habitual occlusion, and Class II prematurities are registered on the lingual surface of the lingual cusps (Fig. 55–27B and C). Prematurities are corrected by grooving and spheroiding (Fig. 55–27D), which are repeated until

only the tips of the lingual cusps register in the wax (Fig. 55–27E).

To locate *Class III prematurities* (Fig. 55–28) in ICP, wax is placed on the maxillary posterior teeth. The patient closes in the intercuspal position, and the Class III prematurities are registered in the wax on the buccal surface of the lingual cusps. The class III prematurities in ICP are corrected by grooving and pointing procedures described for correcting retrusive prematurities in the retruded position. It is desirable to achieve cross-tooth vertical stops in ICP wherever possible (Fig. 55–29).

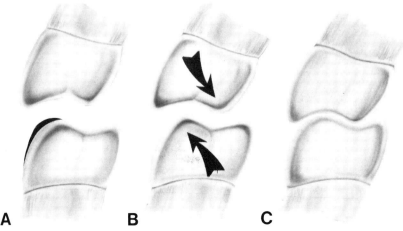

A   B   C

Figure 55–25   Eruption and Uprighting of Teeth After Correction of Class I Prematurities. *A,* Class I prematurity indicated in black. *B,* Direction of tooth movement after correction of prematurity. *C,* Teeth in adjusted position.

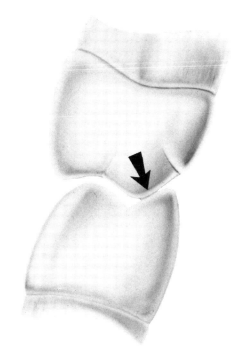

Figure 55–26 Class II Prematurity in the Intercuspal Position (ICP) on the Lingual Surface of Maxillary Molar indicated by *arrow.*

Step 4. Test for excessive contact on the incisor teeth in ICP

The incisor teeth should be slightly out of contact or in light contact. The firmness of contact can be detected by using Mylar occlusal strips held by a hemostat. The Mylar strip should just slip through the incisor teeth when the patient clenches firmly in ICP. In addition, closing contacts should be tested for **fremitus**, *a vibration or displacement, perceptible on palpation of the facial tooth surface with a moistened forefinger during repeated, firm closure to ICP.* If a supracontact is present, it may be marked with wax or marking ribbon and reduced (see Figure 55–23). No fremitus should be detectable on firm, intercuspal closure of the teeth.

The ICP adjustment is complete when the following conditions are achieved:

1. The contact pattern is bilateral, stable and many-pointed (Fig. 55–30*A* and *B*).

2. Each posterior vertical stop holds a Mylar occlusal strip with equal resistance.

3. Sharp resonant sounds are heard when the patient taps his teeth together in ICP (stethoscope placed over the infraorbital skin area[69]). (Fig. 55–31.)

4. Patient responds negatively to the following test: "Tap on your back teeth, slow and hard—do you feel any difference between the two sides?"

Step 5. Remove posterior protrusive interferences—obtain bilateral protrusive glide on the anterior teeth

Protrusive excursion refers to the path of the mandible as it moves anteriorly or posteriorly between the intercuspal position (ICP) and the edge-to-edge relationship of the anterior teeth. The latter is called the **protrusive position.** Protrusive position and excursion are corrected separately.

CORRECTION OF PROTRUSIVE POSITION. The objective of this step is to attain bilateral, well-distributed contact on the incisal edges of the maxillary and mandibular incisor teeth. This is done as follows: From ICP contact, instruct the patient to protrude his mandible slowly. There should be bilateral contact in this segment with little or no deviant shift of the mandible. A deviant shift usually is caused by a molar interference or an asymmetrical incisal plane. Use finger pressure to help guide the patient's jaw along a

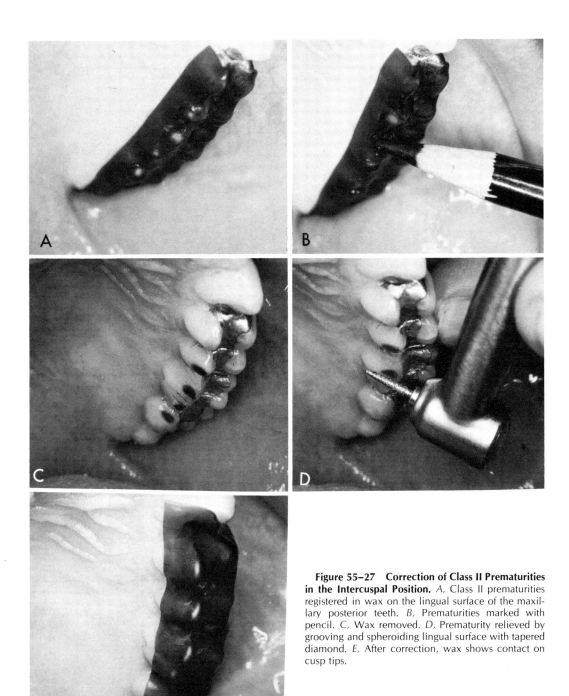

Figure 55–27　Correction of Class II Prematurities in the Intercuspal Position. *A,* Class II prematurities registered in wax on the lingual surface of the maxillary posterior teeth. *B,* Prematurities marked with pencil. *C,* Wax removed. *D,* Prematurity relieved by grooving and spheroiding lingual surface with tapered diamond. *E,* After correction, wax shows contact on cusp tips.

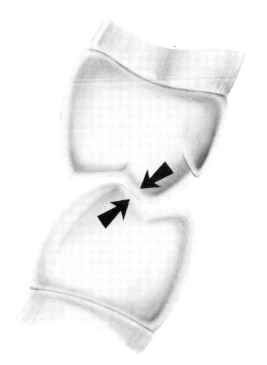

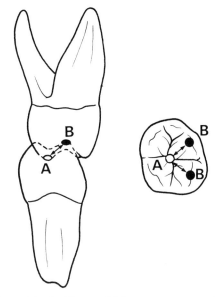

Figure 55–29 The establishment or preservation of cross-tooth contacts is a desirable goal in occlusal adjustment. Cross-tooth contacts (A–B) are shown above in proximal and occlusal views.

Figure 55–28 Class III Prematurity in the Intercuspal Position (ICP). The buccal surface of the lingual cusp of the maxillary molars and premolars, with the lingual aspect of the buccal cusps of the mandibular teeth.

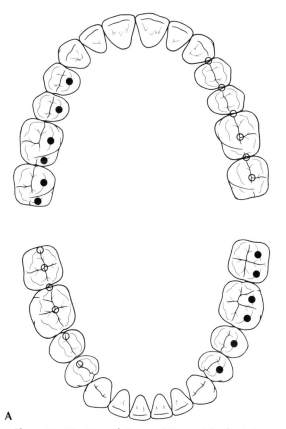

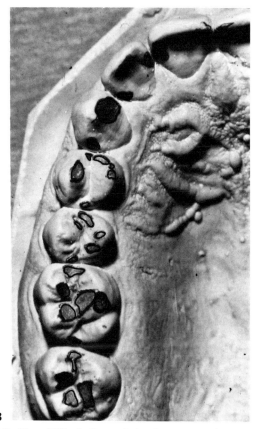

A   B

Figure 55–30 Normal Zones of Contact in the Intercuspal Position (ICP). *A,* Open circles denote vertical (centric) stops; black circles denote centric cusps. *B,* Zones of contact in a natural dentition.

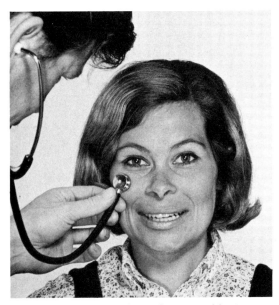

Figure 55–31 Occlusal sounds are tested by instructing the patient to tap *slowly* and *firmly* in ICP. Ideally, the sounds should be sharp. Dull or mixed sounds are the result of discrepancy between the muscular contact position (MCP) and the intercuspal position (ICP).[69] MCP-ICP discrepancies can be caused by occlusal prematurities or muscle imbalance or both.

precise, symmetrical excursion until the protrusive position is reached (Fig. 55–32A). The patient is instructed to open and close on this position with marking ribbon or wax strips between the teeth. Progressive adjustment of the marked areas permits the unmarked incisal edges to come into contact (Fig. 55–32B to E). Wherever possible, adjustment is confined to the maxillary teeth. The mandibular teeth are ground (a) when, because of pain, proximity to the pulp, or for esthetic reasons, the limit of grinding of the maxillary teeth has been reached, and (b) when individual mandibular teeth protrude either incisally or facially. It is important *not* to grind the mandibular teeth so that they would be out of contact in the various mandibular excursions. If such contact is not maintained, the mandibular teeth tend to extrude and re-create prematurities.

The production of flat broad incisal surfaces by grinding should be avoided. After the maximum number of anterior teeth are in contact, the width of the incisal edges is reduced by grinding the facial margin of the maxillary teeth and the lingual margin on the mandible. Caution should be exercised in reshaping the anterior tooth merely to improve esthetics. *The ideal result of correction of protrusive position is several contact points equally distributed between the right and left anterior teeth.* This may not be fully attainable in cases of tooth irregularity.

CORRECTION OF PROTRUSIVE EXCURSION. If any posterior teeth interfere or contact in the protrusive excursion, remove tooth structure from the offending cusps until all articulating contacts between the posterior teeth have been eliminated. Harmonious protrusive contact occurring during the first millimeter of jaw movement is permissible. Protrusive interferences are on the *distal facing* inclines of the maxillary teeth and the *mesial facing* inclines of the mandibular teeth. A practical method for marking excursive contact is the **two-color method.** The protrusive contacts are first marked by drying and isolating the teeth, inserting **red** marking ribbon, and having the patient produce several protrusive glides. The vertical stops are then marked with **blue** marking paper by having the patient tap his teeth together in ICP. As a result, the unwanted protrusive (RED) interferences are clearly distinguished from the vertical stops (BLUE) which are to be preserved. *It is important not to disturb the cusp tips and vertical stops required for maintenance of the intercuspal position.* Mobile teeth should be stabilized by the operator's fingers to prevent them from moving away from the forces of contact. Confirm the absence of posterior protrusive interferences by the use of occlusal Mylar strips.

The lingual surfaces of the maxillary teeth also are marked using the two-color method (protrusive gliding contacts in red; ICP stops, if present, in blue). The protrusive contacts are reduced to provide a bilateral, smooth contact glide along the path approaching the previously established protrusive position. Attempts should be made to limit the protrusive glide adjustment to the lingual surfaces of the maxillary teeth in most cases.

There are several types of problems that require the use of clinical judgment in the protrusive excursion adjustment. Occasion-

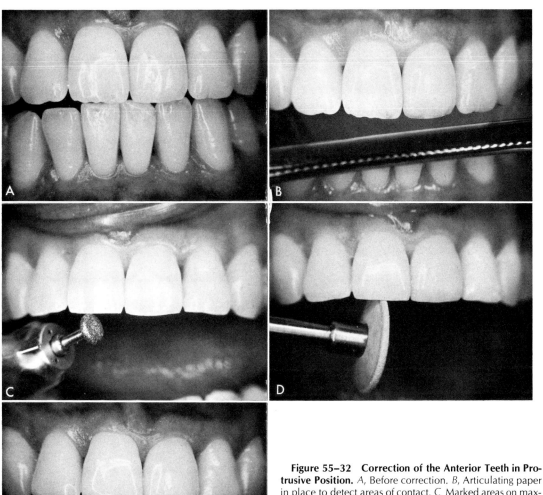

Figure 55–32 Correction of the Anterior Teeth in Protrusive Position. *A,* Before correction. *B,* Articulating paper in place to detect areas of contact. *C* Marked areas on maxillary teeth reduced. *D,* Smoothing the ground surfaces with rubber wheel. *E,* Multipointed, bilateral contact of anterior teeth in protrusive position.

ally, an open-bite situation will not permit edge-to-edge contact of the anterior teeth. The posterior teeth then must be recruited to play a role in the protrusive guidance, i.e., the preservation of smooth protrusive posterior contact.

Similarly, the anterior teeth may not be suitable for use as sole discluders of the teeth on protrusive excursion because of loss of bony support. In such instances, the anterior and posterior teeth should be brought into contact during the protrusive glide (especially the first two mm. of

contact movement). Attempts should also be made to evaluate habitual incisal "lock and key" bruxism facets. Any significant facets on teeth in the anterior segment should be rounded over without shortening the clinical crowns.

Step 6. Remove or lessen mediotrusive (balancing) interferences

Mediotrusive (balancing) interferences complicate the correction of the laterotru-

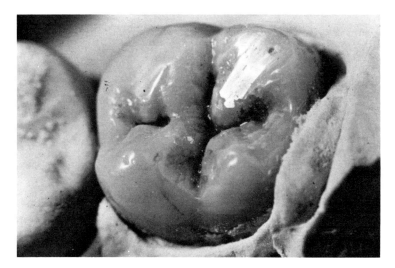

Figure 55–33 Mediotrusive (Balancing) Interferences appear as oblique facets on the molar teeth. Example shows extracted mandibular tooth set in dental cast.

sive (working) guidance. They even may prevent laterotrusive side guidance. Mediotrusive interferences are routinely observed as oblique facets on the first and second molar teeth (inner inclines of the mandibular buccal cusps and the inner inclines of the maxillary lingual cusps, Fig. 55–33). *Mediotrusive interferences should be lessened or removed to facilitate a dominant disclusion on the laterotrusive side.* It is recommended that both habitual excursion and passive (border) manipulation of the mandible be employed in order to detect mediotrusive interferences originating both from ICP and RCP. To record for reduction, mark the mediotrusive contact with red marking ribbon, then locate the ICP stops with blue marking paper (two-color method). Often, reduction is achieved by grinding new groove or shallow depression for the opposing cusp pathway (Fig. 55–34). The effect of the reduction can intermittently be checked by the insertion of Mylar occlusal strips.

Care should be taken, because the complete elimination of mediotrusive interferences may disrupt ICP contact. Therefore, one must weigh the advantages of complete removal of all mediotrusive interferences in relation to the effect of this adjustment on the overall mandibular stability in ICP.

It should be stressed that all mediotrusive contact is not necessarily pathological. It could hardly be, since the probability of observing a mediotrusive contact on at least one side in healthy young adults[21] is 84 per cent. It is probable that the traumatic potential of mediotrusive interferences is related to *intensity* of contact combined with the lack of adequate cross-arch canine guidance. Thus, correct adjustment of mediotrusive interferences may involve reducing them so that they conform to smooth, interference-free functional contact. A functional chewing test is helpful in making this assessment. The test is conducted as follows: Place a strip of adhesive occlusal registration wax over the mandibular quadrant in question. Give another strip of folded occlusal registration wax to the patient, and instruct him to chew the wax on

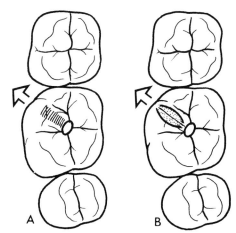

Figure 55–34 Adjustment of Mediotrusive (Balancing) Interference often involves grooving to allow freedom for the opposing cusp movement.

the opposite side 3 to 5 times. If there are significant mediotrusive interferences, oblique perforations of the applied wax strip will be observed. Repeat the test following adjustment for comparison and evaluation.

When the mediotrusive interferences have been dealt with on one side, the laterotrusive interferences are adjusted for the opposite side (step 7). Thus, the lateral excursion of one laterotrusive (working) side and its corresponding mediotrusive (balancing) side is completely corrected before the other lateral excursion is treated.

Step 7. Reduce interferences on the laterotrusive (working) side

Lateral guidance is dominated by the canine and first premolar teeth (termed the canine segment) in healthy young adults. The canine tooth is most frequently involved in disclusion.[21, 51] The disclusion scheme is likely to include more posterior teeth with advancing age and accelerated wear. The lack of adequate guidance in the

canine area brings on *single-tooth molar interferences* that have traumatic potential during function and parafunction. The first two millimeters of excursive guidance from ICP and RCP are important because maximum force can be applied near the closed position.

The positional availability of teeth as discluders and the periodontal status of all potential discluder teeth should be clinically assessed. Laterotrusive discluding contact should be on the ipsilateral canine and, frequently, on the first premolar, unless these teeth are weakened periodontally. In the case of mobile canines, all the teeth on the laterotrusive side, except the second molar, should assist in lateral guidance. *An attempt should be made to remove or neutralize single-tooth interferences on the molar teeth.* Contact area may be reduced on the canine and premolars if severe surface-to-surface faceting predominates. Existing "lock and key" facets on laterotrusive cusps should be rounded over without shortening the clinical crown.

In lateral function, whether canine segment or group, the discluding angle should

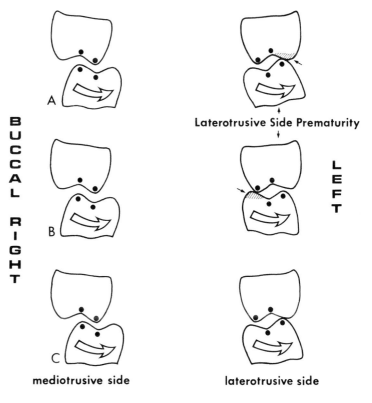

Figure 55–35 Correction of Laterotrusive Interferences (Hatched Areas) on Posterior Teeth to Gain Smooth Contact Movement Patterns. Mandibular movement indicated by *arrows. A,* Laterotrusive interference on buccal cusps. *B,* Laterotrusive interference on lingual cusps. *C,* Unrestricted glide after correction of laterotrusive interferences. Note absence of contact on the mediotrusive side.

BUCCAL RIGHT

A

B

C

mediotrusive side

Laterotrusive Side Prematurity

LEFT

laterotrusive side

be great enough to prevent mediotrusive contact on the contralateral side and a definite separation of the ipsilateral molar teeth (Fig. 55–35). Normally, very little reduction is done on the canine and premolar teeth, as these contacts are considered to be important for disclusion of the molar teeth in lateral movement. *Unrestricted smooth contact movement in laterotrusion is more important than the number of contacts that are brought into lateral function.*

Laterotrusive contacts can be marked with the two-color method described previously. Reshape the inner inclines of the maxillary buccal cusps, if possible, as grinding of the mandibular buccal cusps could interfere with ICP vertical stops. Always grind to the point of the ICP vertical stop. Never include it in the reduction. Adjustment of the inclines often can be achieved through the process of grooving. As customary with this technique, all reductions should result in spherical or grooved surfaces. *Avoid creating flat planes.* Check your adjustment by the use of Mylar occlusal strips.

Step 8. Eliminate gross occlusal disharmonies

At this point all occlusal disharmonies involving tooth contact or contact movement will have been removed or lessened. However, other occlusal disharmonies harmful to the periodontal structures may remain; these should be modifed. Care should be taken to avoid changing or removing previously attained occlusal contact relationships. Elimination of gross occlusal disharmonies at the beginning of the occlusal adjustment may be tempting, and indeed is permissible. Early gross adjustment should only be done to the extent that tooth contacts important to the future stability of the occlusion are not destroyed in the process.

EXTRUDED TEETH. Extruded teeth are reduced to the level of the occlusal plane by grinding and reshaping within the limits permitted by the position of the pulp. If large areas are exposed by grinding, a dental restoration in conformity with the corrected occlusal relationship is indicated. Extruded unopposed third molars may irri-

tate the mucosa of the opposing jaw, interfere with closure in centric occlusion, and deflect the mandible. Food impaction is also common between extruded third molars and the second molar. Extruded molars should be extracted or reduced to the occlusal plane and splinted to the second molar.

When an unopposed maxillary third molar is removed, the interdental space between the first and second molars should be watched for evidence of food impaction. Distal thrusts produced on occlusal contact may momentarily break the contact between the maxillary first and second molars and permit impaction of food (Fig. 55–36). At the first sign of such impaction, ICP contacts should be evaluated and adjusted if their incline contact relationships promote distal movement of the second molar. If subsequent adjustment fails to result in

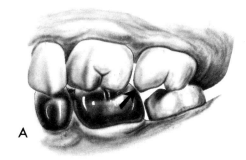

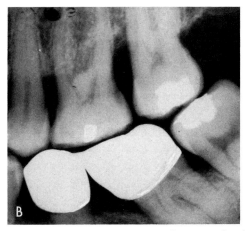

Figure 55–36   Displacement of Maxillary Second Molar in the Absence of Distal Support. *A,* Impact of mandibular first molar (*arrow*) leads to displacement of maxillary second molar and creates area of food impaction. Note absence of contact between the mandibular molars. *B,* Radiograph showing accentuated bone loss in area of food impaction on mesial surface of maxillary second molar.

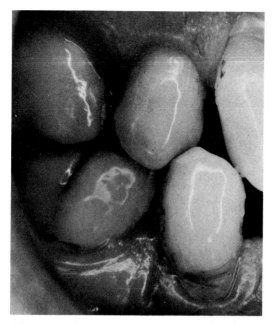

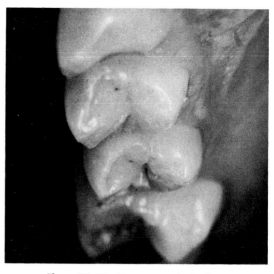

Figure 55-38 Uneven marginal ridges.

Figure 55-37 **Plunger Cusp on the Maxilla.** The premolar forces food between the mandibular teeth, causing gingival inflammation.

closure of the contact, it may be necessary to splint the first and second molars together.

PLUNGER CUSPS. Plunger cusps are cusp points that wedge into the interproximal spaces between opposing teeth and cause food impaction (Fig. 55-37). Distolingual cusps of maxillary molars often are plunger cusps. The cusp points should be rounded and shortened, and if this does not suffice, the opposing interproximal space can be protected by splinting the teeth adjacent to it.

UNEVEN ADJACENT MARGINAL RIDGES. Differences in the height of adjacent marginal ridges may cause food impaction and should be corrected by either

reducing the height of the comparatively high marginal ridge or increasing the height of the lower one with a restoration (Fig. 55-38). Extreme differences are overcome by using both procedures. In grinding the marginal ridges the natural tooth contour should be preserved. *The marginal ridge should not be reduced if this entails sacrifice of occlusal contact.*

ROTATED, MALPOSED, AND TILTED TEETH. Teeth that are rotated or tilted facially or lingually may interfere with functional movement of the mandible and cause food accumulation and impaction. Depending on their severity, such conditions can be reshaped by grinding or cor-

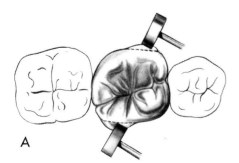

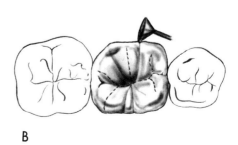

A

B

Figure 55-39 **Reshaping Slightly Rotated Tooth by Grinding.** *A,* Slightly rotated molar. Areas removed by grinding indicated by dotted lines. *B,* Occlusal surface recontoured (*dotted lines*) and buccal grooves relocated.

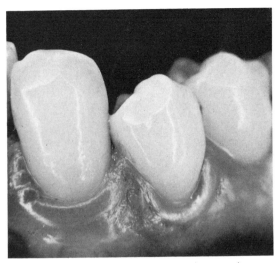

Figure 55–40   Prominent facets on the premolars.

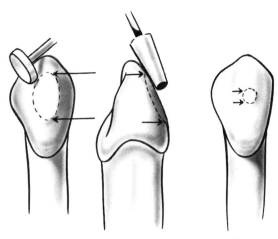

Figure 55–41   Reduction of Facet by Grinding. The dimensions of the facet before and after reduction are indicated by the *arrows*.

rected by orthodontic procedures (Chapter 57) or restorations that conform to the corrected occlusal and proximal relationship of the dentition (Fig. 55–39).

FACETS AND FLAT OCCLUSAL WEAR. Facets are flattened planes produced by wear on a convex tooth surface,[64] which vary in size and outline (Fig. 55–40.) They are detected by examination after the teeth have been dried. Study casts are also

helpful. Occlusal contact at the periphery of broad facets may create lateral or tipping forces potentially injurious to the periodontium and should be adjusted so that only a small area remains in occlusal contact (Fig. 55–41).

FLAT OCCLUSAL WEAR. When excessive wear produces broad, flat or cupped-out occlusal surfaces, forces applied at the periphery are directed outside the confines

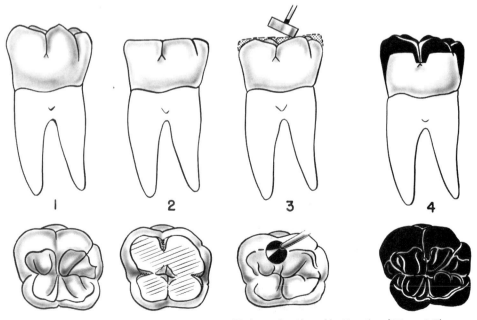

Figure 55–42   Reshaping the Occlusal Surface of a Mandibular Molar Altered by Functional Wear. *1*, The unworn molar crown. *2*, The molar crown altered by wear. *3*, Reshaping the molar crown to reduce the area of the occlusal surface and restore cuspal inclines and marginal ridges. (The outlined stippled area is the portion of the tooth surface removed.) *4*, The use of a restoration to reshape a worn molar crown where correction by grinding is not feasible. (After S. C. Miller.)[34]

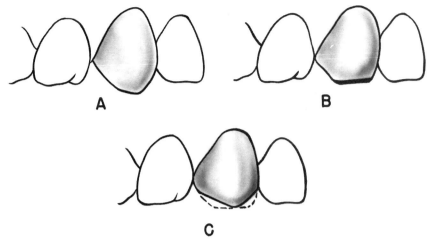

Figure 55–43   Recontouring Canine Altered by Incisal Wear. A, Contour of unworn maxillary canine. B, Facet frequently seen at incisal edge of canine. C, Correction of facet. Areas of tooth removed are indicated by the broken line.

of the root and may create tipping forces injurious to the periodontium. The occlusal surface is modified by grinding to restore the normal faciolingual and mesiodistal diameters, cuspal anatomy, grooves, and marginal ridges (Fig. 55–42). Proximal contact relationships must be maintained. If the desired correction is not attainable by grinding, the use of a restoration is indicated (Fig. 55–42). Incisal edges flattened by excessive occlusal wear are also reshaped by grinding (Fig. 55–43).

Step 9. Recheck tooth contact relationships

Tooth relationships in all positions and movements are rechecked to verify that the following *seven* criteria are met:

1. There is no asymmetrical shift from RCP to ICP. If a shift is present, it is smooth, symmetrical, and less than 1 mm. in magnitude.

2. The completed adjustments have light contact or none between the incisor teeth and firm contact between as many posterior teeth as possible.

3. The patient perceives "even" (bilateral) contact when closing the teeth to ICP.

4. Sharp occlusal sounds are produced when the patient taps slowly and firmly into ICP.

5. Molar excursive interferences are eliminated or significantly reduced so that unrestricted glide paths are available for the posterior cusps.

6. Tooth guidance under lateral and protrusive excursions is smooth and without effort.

7. The displacement of mobile teeth is minimized under closure and gliding movements.

The above criteria also can serve as guidelines to help determine the *feasibility* of achieving a satisfactory result by means of occlusal adjustment. There are many instances when restorative or prosthetic treatments are necessary, sometimes in combination with orthodontic and surgical intervention. In questionable cases, a trial carving of articulated casts is the best means by which to judge the fulfillment of the foregoing criteria.

Step 10. Polish all rough occlusal surfaces

The occlusal surfaces are smoothed and polished so that they feel "comfortable" for the patient.

Special Problems (Crossbite)

Crossbite is a reversal of the normal buccolingual relationship of the maxillary and mandibular teeth. When only a few teeth are involved, orthodontic corrective measures should be employed. When a large segment of the arch is in crossbite

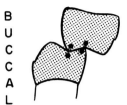

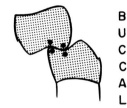

B
U
C
C
A
L

CROSSBITE

Figure 55–44 Crossbite showing reversal of normal buccolingual cuspal relationships. Large black dots indicate the areas of centric maintenance.

relationship, special techniques must be employed in adjusting the occlusion. In crossbite, the tips of the buccal cusps of the maxillary teeth and the tips of the lingual cusps of the mandibular teeth and the areas into which they occlude are the vertical stops (Fig. 55–44). The cusp surfaces relieved in adjusting the occlusion in crossbite are the reverse of those in patients with a normal buccolingual relationship. The prognosis for achieving a stable postoperative occlusion is less favorable when dealing with crossbite relationships.

Maintenance of Occlusal Stability

There is evidence that the method of occlusal adjustment recommended here will remain stable for the short term.[67] Teeth and dental restorations wear with use, however, and as a result, the occlusion changes over longer periods. No method of occlusal adjustment creates a permanent occlusal relationship. The occlusion must be checked periodically for minor adjustments, and the patient should be advised accordingly.

TREATMENT OF BRUXISM

Bruxism* is common, but all patients with the habit are not necessarily injured by it. Those who are suffer from microtrauma in the periodontium, musculature,[5–7, 37] and temporomandibular joints. Occlusal prematurities, excessive muscle tension, and emotional factors, singly or together, are the accepted causes of bruxism, but opinions differ as to which is the primary or most critical factor. (For more discussion of bruxism, see Chapter 27.)

---

*Includes clamping and clenching habits

There are three general modalities by which the patient with bruxism can be treated. The **behavioral modality** is initiated by the dentist through *explanation* and *arousal* of the patient to the habit. Specific behavioral therapies such as biofeedback, hypnosis, and negative practice may be prescribed.[48] The **emotional modality** may be initiated in the form of psychological guidance.[37, 49, 55, 63] The **interceptive modality** consists of prescribing a bite guard appliance (maxillary stabilization splint) to protect the tooth surfaces and to dissipate forces built up in the musculoskeletal system through bruxism.[41] There is evidence that these appliances effect a significant decrease in the bruxism habit of some individuals.[57] In application, the bite guard is more practical for *nocturnal* bruxism than for daytime clenching habits.

Occlusal adjustment plays a role in treating bruxism when prematurities are obvious, especially when they occur in connection with recently placed dental restorations. More invasive occlusal alterations are sometimes necessary in the form of reconstruction or orthodontic treatment.

Occlusal therapies, even when combined with psychological guidance and behavioral therapies, may not be effective in all patients. In these patients bite guards become more significant in the management of the destructive effects of bruxism.

TREATMENT OF TEMPOROMANDIBULAR JOINT DISORDERS

Except for conditions caused by other recognizable joint[50] and myofascial disease, **temporomandibular pain and dysfunction can usually be treated by allowing normalization of what is essentially an acute or poorly healed traumatic injury.** The notion that most temporomandibular joint disorders are caused solely by occlusal factors should be viewed with caution. The probability that a given patient will present with dysfunctional symptoms is clearly dependent upon a staggering number of factors, many of which are not well understood. The one cause–one disease–one treatment concept must therefore be discarded in favor of the more applicable polytherapeutic concept (several therapeutic factors act upon an organ system at the same time).[49] *It should be realized that some of these patients will not get well despite the use of treatments that have been successful for others.* This is especially true in patients with long-standing pain. Chronic pain associated with temporomandibular joint disorders eventually complicates management and can potentiate emotional disturbances and untoward behavioral changes in some individuals. In effect, these patients will continue to have intermittent or chronic musculoskeletal rheumatism. For these patients, data gathering and patient monitoring techniques take on added importance, as does the need to attain a practical end-point in therapy.[62]

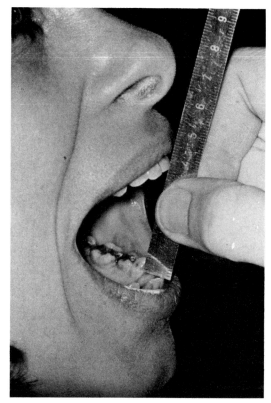

Figure 55–45 Maximum Mouth Opening Measured Interincisally. Less than 40 mm. is considered abnormal. (*From* Clark, J. [ed.]: Clinical Dentistry, Vol. II, Chapter 35. New York: Harper and Row, 1976.)

Clinical History and Examination

The *history* should focus on the categorical complaints seen in temporomandibular pain and dysfunction: (1) **decreased mobility of the mandible,** (2) **joint incoordination,** and (3) **muscle and joint pain.** The relationship of these symptoms to macrotrauma, dental treatment, or bruxism should be noted. Symptoms aggravated by emotional stress are significant.[32] Pre-auricular pain is characteristic of peri-articular problems, whereas masseter pain is more apt to be associated with bruxism.

Muscle and joint function is examined first; then these findings are correlated with features of the occlusion.[29, 60] *Mouth opening* is measured (<40 mm., abnormal range[1]), and the path of opening is observed (Fig. 55–45). Protrusive and lateral test excursions are made (<8mm., abnormal range[1]). If the mandible deviates to the side of the painful joint, malfunction of the muscles or condyle on that side may be responsible. Pre-auricular pain when the mandible is moved to the contralateral side

could be caused by inflammation of the temporomandibular joint or the lateral pterygoid muscle. If the mandible deviates to the side opposite the painful joint, malfunction of the medial pterygoid may be the cause. Simultaneous shortening of the masseter and medial pterygoid on the same side restricts mandibular movement without deflection. In evaluating *joint incoordination,* the forefingers are placed *lightly* over the joint area, and an attempt is made to detect clicking or crepitation (grating) on opening and closing of the mouth. Crepitation is correlated with osteoarthritis.[60] Early clicks on opening are more significant than clicks at full mouth opening, which are more easily treated by avoidance. Early, reciprocal clicks (those occurring repeatedly on opening and closing) are associated with anterior disc displacement. Closed locking is a form of

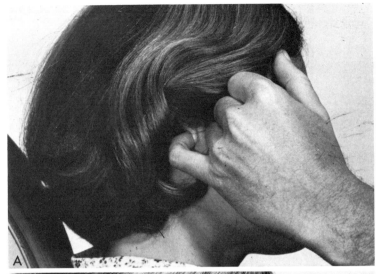

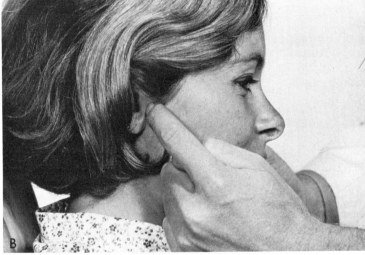

Figure 55-46 *A,* Posterior capsular tenderness suggests that **periarticular inflammation** is present. *B,* Lateral tenderness may be temporomandibular joint inflammation or may result from the lateral pterygoid muscle spasm. (*B* is *From:* Clark, J. [ed.]: Clinical Dentistry, Vol. II, Chapter 35. New York: Harper and Row, 1976.)

unresolved disc displacement and may also result from adhesions within the joints.

In testing for *tenderness*, the temporomandibular joints are palpated bimanually with point pressure on the lateral and dorsal (posterior) aspects of the joint capsule (Fig. 55-46). Posterior tenderness (Fig. 55-46*A*) suggests peri-articular inflammation. The masticatory muscles generally are palpated near their musculo-tendinous junctions. The posterior cervical, trapezius, and sternocleidomastoid muscles are included in the muscle palpation, as these muscles refer pain to the ear, temporomandibular joint, and head.[65] It is helpful if a diagram is used (Fig. 55-47) to chart tenderness.

The main feature of the occlusal examination should involve testing the zones of *ICP contact, occlusal instability,* or *bite collapse,* and *asymmetrical relationships between RCP and ICP.* Interferences disturbing free and smooth gliding contact movement should also be identified, in addition to gross features involving occlusal plane, overjet, and overbite. An effort should be made to detect active facet patterns caused by bruxism.

Radiographic Examination

Radiographs of the joints are useful but show only the position and structure of the subchondral bony parts. Since many of the

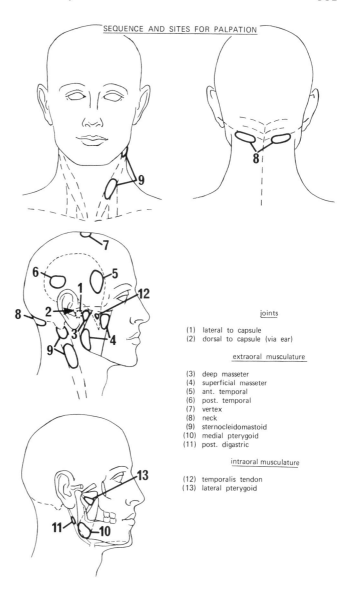

SEQUENCE AND SITES FOR PALPATION

Figure 55–47 Suggested Areas for Muscle and Joint Palpation.

joints

(1) lateral to capsule
(2) dorsal to capsule (via ear)

extraoral musculature

(3) deep masseter
(4) superficial masseter
(5) ant. temporal
(6) post. temporal
(7) vertex
(8) neck
(9) sternocleidomastoid
(10) medial pterygoid
(11) post. digastric

intraoral musculature

(12) temporalis tendon
(13) lateral pterygoid

problems of clinical temporomandibular pain and dysfunction involve noncalcified tissues of the joint, radiographs are not conclusive. Indeed, most appear remarkably normal. There are many special techniques for joint radiographs.[11, 47, 71] Orthopantomograms (e.g., Panorex) are useful for identifying gross pathologic conditions of the condyle. The lateral oblique transcranial projections[38] are the most common projections taken on the temporomandibular joints. Tomography,[11, 28, 38] however, is most reliable for detecting changes in structure and condyle position. Lateral views of the temporomandibular joints are best made

with the teeth fully together and at maximum jaw opening.

Osteoarthritis (degenerative joint disease) of the temporomandibular joints involves chiefly the articulating surface of the temporal bone and the articular disc. Osteoarthritis is correlated with the clinical symptom of crepitus (grating).[18] Remodeling (deviation in form) is most common in the condyle.[18] For this reason, radiographic changes (flattening and lipping) seen in the condyle do not necessarily imply the condition of osteoarthritis.[18] Asymmetrical condyle-fossa relationships are frequently associated with clinical temporomandibular joint dysfunction.[33, 70] Some clinicians treat these condyle malrelationships by altering the mandibular occlusal position.[72] Frequently, this is accomplished by means of a splint (repositioning splint).

Recently, arthrography of the temporomandibular joint has been employed as a means of identifying disorders of the articular disc.[73] In this technique, radioopaque contrast medium is injected into the upper and lower joint compartments, allowing visualization of the articular parts. Perforation, hyperplasia, and anterior displacements are the most common findings reported from arthrographic investigations.[73] Clinically, these conditions have been associated with clicking, subluxation, and closed locking. Investigations on several aspects of temporomandibular joint conditions suggest that intracapsular pathology is more common in patients with "TMJ syndrome" than previously thought.

Diagnosis

Diagnosis of temporomandibular pain and dysfunction includes the delineation of potential problems within the *temporomandibular joints* and the *masticatory muscles*, and *referred pain from the neck muscles*. Conditions commonly encountered in patients with facial pain and mandibular dysfunction are categorized in Table 55–3. These are also discussed in Chapter 27.

TABLE 55–3 CONDITIONS COMMONLY ENCOUNTERED IN PATIENTS WITH FACIAL PAIN AND MANDIBULAR DYSFUNCTION.*

I. Traumatic and Degenerative Disorders
 A. Temporomandibular Joints
  1. Traumatic derangement (clicking, subluxation, and closed locking)
  2. Traumatic capsulitis (pain, contracture, no history of clicking or locking)
  3. Degenerative joint disease (crepitation)
  4. Open dislocation (luxation)
  5. Fibrosis
 B. Myofascial Structures
  1. Myofascitis (interstitial myofibrositis)
   (a) Latent myofascial tenderness
   (b) Active myofascial trigger points and referred pain
    (1) masticatory muscles
    (2) neck muscles
  2. Contracture (fibrosis, mechanical shortening)
  3. Dyskinesia (weakness, incoordination)
  4. Muscle spasm (acute muscle splinting)
 C. Oro-dental Structures
  1. Accelerated tooth wear, uncontrolled migration of teeth.
  2. Trauma from occlusion.
  3. Trauma to the lips, cheeks, and tongue.

II. Atypical (Idiopathic) Symptoms Affecting the Head and Neck
 A. Chronic facial pain (emotional and behavior problems prominent)
 B. Positive occlusal sense (uncomfortable bite)
 C. Atypical facial neuralgias.

III. Arthritis
 A. Polyarthritis (rheumatoid arthritis)
 B. Infectious
 C. Other

*Does not include pathological entities such as cranial nerve neuralgias, organ-related disease (sinuses, ears), regional tumors, headache (vascular, migraine) fracture, or bony impingement.

TABLE 55–4 TEMPOROMANDIBULAR AND MYOFASCIAL DISORDERS: THREE-PART TREATMENT PROGRAM

	Problem	Treatment Goal
1. Neutralization	a. Abrupt condyle translation	Prescribed condyle rotation
	b. Neuromuscular tension	Graded relaxation; coordinated motion
	c. Chronic overuse	Neutralization of habits
2. Mobilization	a. Myofascial referred pain (active trigger points) Muscles shortened	Desensitize trigger points. Stretch muscles to physiologic resting length.
	b. Inelastic muscles and capsular tissues	Range-of-motion exercises
	c. Uncoordinated movement	Symmetrical coordinated motion
	d. Weakened muscles	Prescribe strengthening exercises.
*3. Stabilization**	a. Muscular stabilization	Occlusal stabilization
	b. Asymmetrical joint relationships	Symmetrical condylar relationships
	c. Disturbed closure	One functional end-point of closure

*Axial tomographic radiographs may reveal obvious condyle malpositioning. Decision to reposition condyle(s) by altering normal ICP closure position on splint may be made immediately or following evaluation of standard splint therapy. This type of splint is termed a *repositioning splint.*

Treatment

Conservative treatment of temporomandibular and myofascial pain is formulated using the three part conceptual treatment program outlined in Table 55–4. Overall, **this program aims at eliminating abnormal function and does no more than provide conditions favorable for the normal processes of repair and resolution.** Using this system, the best prognosis can be given when treatment is started before irreversible pathological changes have occurred in the musculoskeletal or dental structures. The three-part treatment is an approach of *escalation*, which begins with generalized therapy, mobilization techniques, and removable splints. Temporomandibular joint surgery, intracapsular injections, or irreversible "spot grinding," intended as a quick solution to temporomandibular pain and dysfunction, can result in unnecessary problems and generally should be considered only after conservative, reversible therapy has been attempted.

Part 1. Neutralizing self-destructive behavior

Undoubtedly, the most important and universal treatment for controlling temporomandibular pain and dysfunction is some form of arousal and behavior modification.[49] The patient is made aware of excessive and inappropriate oral habits. This orientation sets the stage for the patient to relearn specific behavior that will allow the tissues to normalize. The axis-opening exercise is the basis for retraining or relearning mandibular movements.[74] This exercise involves making symmetrical opening and closing movements with the jaw in a centered hinge position. When appropriate, ample time should be taken to discuss the role of emotional stress in creating muscle tension in the gnathic system. In so doing, the dentist demonstrates that healing and health maintenance depend upon the patient's input and willingness to actively participate in the therapy process. Diazepam (Valium) may be prescribed to induce muscle relaxation and decrease anxiety. The dosage should be individualized (2 to 10 mg. two to four times per day) and prescribed for short durations.

Part 2. Mobilization

Many physical modalities have a beneficial effect on abnormal muscular and capsular tissues, e.g., heat, cold, medications, electrostimulation, acupuncture, and vapocoolant sprays. Even though these modalities soothe the muscles and joints, they do not give physiological restoration of function and therefore are not sufficient in themselves.[58, 65] *Therapeutic mobilization is the key to restoring and perpetuating normal musculoskeletal function.* The *spray-stretch technique*[66] is a common method for mobilization of muscles and joints. Fluori-Methane* is sprayed on the skin over the tender area, resulting in momentary desensitization of muscles and joints (Fig. 55–48). During this period the jaws are actively or passively stretched to gain increased opening. This technique is based on the rationale that muscles brought to their physiological resting length will cease to be painful. Continuous joint and muscle pains are relieved at home by applying moist heat by means of a towel soaked in hot water for 15 minutes, two or three times a day. Prescribed retraining exercises or gentle range-of-motion stretching should follow the application of moist heat. With recovery, the muscles should be exercised under light to moderate loads (resistance exercises). The chief causes of failure of the correct spray-stretch procedure are inability to secure full muscle length because of subordination of the reflex mechanisms of trigger point pain to fibrosis or some other pathologic condition of the temporomandibular joint.

Part 3. Stabilization:

The majority of patients with temporomandibular pain and dysfunction are helped by prescribing removable full-arch maxillary stabilization splints (Fig. 55–49). The purpose of the splint is threefold: (1) to allow the muscles of mastication to function without spasm at their proper physiological length from origin to insertion; (2) to allow normalization of tem-

---

*Gebauer Chemical Co., Cleveland, Ohio 44104.

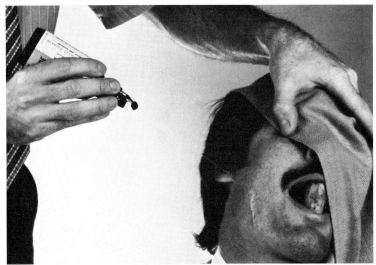

Figure 55–48 Fluori-Methane spray is used to desensitize the skin and underlying muscle trigger points temporarily. Following application, the muscles are put on stretch.

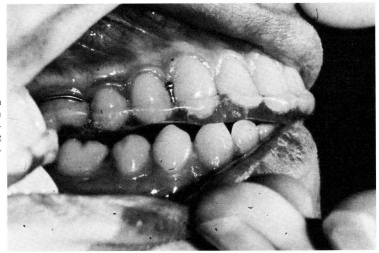

Figure 55–49 Removable Full-Arch Stabilization Splint used for bruxism patients and patients with temporomandibular joint disorders. The splint may be constructed for either the maxillary or the mandibular arch.

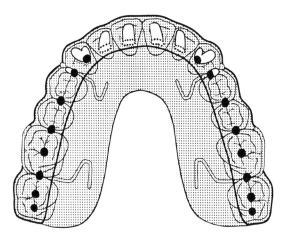

Figure 55–50 The Occlusal Contact Scheme Established for the Maxillary Full-Arch Stabilization Splint. Large *black dots* denote posterior vertical stops of positive ICP contact. Dotted lines denote light incisal contact. Clear areas are the pathways of protrusive and lateral guidance. Note that there is freedom from lateral or protrusive posterior contact. If heavy lateral and protrusive facets are observed at the follow-up visit, these areas should be reduced. Wrought-wire ball clasps (between canines are premolars) and retentive arms (molars) are used to aid retention.

TABLE 55–5 CRITERIA FOR MAXILLARY STABILIZATION SPLINT

Occlusal Criteria

1. *Appliance:* stable.
2. *RCP, ICP:* stable, multi-pointed, widely distributed contacts.
3. *ICP:* posterior vertical stops in firm contact; incisor teeth in slight infracontact.
4. *RCP–ICP relationship:* RCP and ICP in same sagittal plane; ICP and RCP are nearly identical.
5. Smooth gliding contact in all excursions (incisal and/or canine disclusion optional).
6. *MCP:* stable, repeatable.

Technique for Verification of Criteria

Criterion 1 (Splint Stability)	No hint of movement to tipping forces.
Criterion 2 (RCP)	Red inked ribbon on dry surface.
Criterion 3 (Vertical Stops)	Mylar strips held firmly by telling subject, "Close your back teeth, both sides at the same time."
Criterion 4 (RCP–ICP)	No slide from RCP to ICP.
Criterion 5 (Guidance)	Use full arch red-blue paper. Mark excursion in RED, then vertical stops in BLUE.
Criterion 6 (MCP)	"Solid" MCP tapping by patient in upright position; patient verifies "even" contact.

poromandibular joint derangements, particularly those related to disc-condyle malrelationships and synovitis; and (3) to achieve a precise functional end-point of closure compatible with joint and occlusal harmony. The occlusal criteria for splinting are summarized in Table 55–5. The prescribed contact scheme is seen in Figure 55–50.

Occlusal adjustment without prior splint therapy is performed only when an obvious connection can be made between the symptoms and recent occlusal changes (e.g., dental treatment, tooth migration). If initial occlusal adjustment is done, the patient should be forewarned of the possibility that a removable splint may be necessary at a later date.

The splint is placed and carefully adjusted according to the criteria in Table 55–5. The patient is instructed to wear the splint constantly, day and night, even when eating. The patient is seen at two or three week intervals for evaluation and adjustment of the splint. When symptoms disappear, an evaluation of the occlusion will reveal discrepancies from the muscu-

loskeletal readjustment. The dentist must use judgment in determining: (1) whether immediate permanent occlusal adjustment is advisable, (2) whether the splint should be worn indefinitely at night, or (3) whether the splint therapy should be stopped with no occlusal change. To repeat, *occlusal therapy following splint therapy is not mandatory unless clear-cut occlusal problems are evident.*[75] The evident multifactorial causes for temporomandibular pain and dysfunction argue against such dogmatic treatment methods.[49]

Subluxation of the Temporomandibular Joint

It is within the range of normal for the condyle to move anterior to the articular eminence. However, if the condyle becomes momentarily locked open in this position, the condition is referred to as subluxation or, when persistent, open dislocation (luxation). Subluxation of the mandible is self-reducing, incomplete dislocation of the temporomandibular articulation. Acute trauma, previous dislocation of the mandible, or excessive manipulation of the jaw during a dental procedure may cause abnormal looseness of the capsule and recurrent subluxation or luxation. Reduction of acute dislocation of the mandible often may be accomplished by applying pressure downward on the mandibular buccal shelf while applying upward pressure under the chin. Unresolved cases may be relieved by local anesthetics, immobilization, or surgical arthroplasty.

REFERENCES

1. Agerberg, G.: On Mandibular Dysfunction and Mobility. Umea University Odontological Dissertation. Abstract No. 3, 1974.
2. Arnold, N. R., and Frumker, S. C.: *Occlusal Treatment.* Philadelphia: Lea & Febiger, 1976.
3. Azarbal, M.: Comparison of myo-monitor centric position to centric relation and centric occlusion. J. Pros. Dent., 38:331, 1977.
4. Bell, D. H., Jr.: Sagittal balance of the mandible. J.A.M.A., 64:486, 1962.
5. Christensen, L. V.: Facial pain from the masticatory system induced by experimental bruxism. Tandlaegebladet, 71:1171, 1967.
6. Christensen, L. V.: Facial pain from experimental tooth clenching. Tandlaegebladet, 74:175, 1970.

7. Christensen, L. B.: Facial pain in negative and positive work of human jaw muscles. Scand. J. Dent. Res., 84:327, 1976.

8. Clark, T. D., Perachio, A., and Mahan, P.: A neurophysiological study of bruxism in the rhesus monkey. I.A.D.R. Abstr., #566, 1970, p. 190.

9. Clayton, J. A., Kotowicz, W. E., and Zahler, J. M.: Pantographic tracings of mandibular movments and occlusion. J. Pros. Dent., 25:389, 1971.

10. Dawson, P. E.: Evaluation, Diagnosis, and Treatment of Occlusal Problems. St. Louis: C. V. Mosby Co., 1975, p. 56.

11. Eckerdal, O.: Tomography of the temporomandibular joint. Acta Radiologica, Supp. 329, Stockholm, 1973.

12. Federick, D. R., Pameijer, C. H., and Stallard, R. E.: A correlation between force and distalization of the mandible in obtaining centric relation. J. Periodontal., 45:70, 1974.

13. Glickman, I., Pameijer, J. H., Roeber, F. W., and Brion, M. A. M.: Functional occlusion as revealed by miniaturized radio transmitters. Dent. Clin. North Am., 13:666, 1969.

14. Glickman, I., Smulow, J. B., Vogel, G., and Passamonti, G.: The effect of occlusal forces on healing following mucogingival surgery. J. Periodontol., 37:319, 1966.

15. Graf, H.: Bruxism. Dent. Clin. North Am., 13:659, 1969.

16. Grove, C. J.: Trauma produced by occlusion, due to horizontal stress. J. Am. Dent. Assoc., 11:813, 1924.

17. Haddad, A. W.: The functioning dentition. In J. Kawamura (Ed.): Frontiers of Oral Physiology, Physiology of Oral Tissues. Basel: S. Karger, 1976.

18. Hansson, T.: Temporomandibular Joint Changes: Occurrence and Development. Dissertation, University of Lund, 1977.

19. Ingervall, B.: Retruded contact position of mandible. A comparison between children and adults. Odontol. Rev., 15:130, 1964.

20. Ingervall, B.: Retruded contact position of mandible in the deciduous dentition. Odontol. Rev., 15:414, 1964.

21. Ingervall, B.: Tooth contacts on the functional and non-functional side in children and young adults. Archs. Oral Biol., 17:191, 1972.

22. James, A. F.: A discussion by correspondence. Dent. Items Int., 45:584, 1923.

23. Jankelson, B., et al.: Neural conduction of the myo-monitor stimulus. A quantitative analysis. J. Prosthet. Dent., 34:245, 1975.

24. Jankelson, B.: A Technique for obtaining optimum functional relationship for the natural dentition. Dent. Clin. North Am., March 1960, p. 131.

25. Jankelson, B.: Physiology of human dental occlusion. J. Am. Dent. Assoc., 50:664, 1955.

26. Kantor, M. E., Silverman, S. I., and Garfinkel, M. A.: Centric-relation recording techniques. A comparative investigation. J. Prosthet. Dent., 28:593, 1972.

27. Karlsen, K.: Traumatic occlusion as a factor in the propagation of periodontal disease. Inter. Dent. J. 22:387, 1972.

28. Klein, I. E., Blatterfein, L., and Miglino, J. C.: Comparison of the fidelity of radiographs of mandibular condyles made by different techniques. J. Prosth. Dent., 24:419, 1970.

29. Krogh-Poulsen, W. G., and Olsson, A.: Management of the occlusion of the teeth. In L. S. Schwartz and C. M. Chayes (Eds.): Facial Pain and Mandibular Dysfunction. Philadelphia: W. B. Saunders Co., 1968.

30. Lundeen, H. C.: Centric relation records: the effect of muscle action. J. Pros. Dent., 31:244, 1974.

31. Lund, P., Nishiyama, T., and Moller, E.: Postural activity in the muscles of mastication with the subject upright, inclined, and supine. Scand. J. Dent. Res., 78:417, 1970.

32. Lupton, D.: Psychological aspects of temporomandibular joint dysfunction. J. Am. Dent. Assoc., 79:131, 1969.

33. Marcovic, M. A., and Rosenberg, H. M.: Tomographic evaluation of 100 patients with temporomandibular joint symptoms. Oral Surg., 42:838, 1976.

34. Miller, S. C.: Textbook of Periodontia, 3rd ed. Philadelphia: The Blakiston Co., 1950, p. 343.

35. Mühlemann, H. R., Herzog, H., and Rateitschak, K. H.: Quantitative evaluation of the therapeutic effect of selective grinding. J. Periodontal., 28:11, 1957.

36. Möller, E., Sheik-Ol-Eslam, A., and Lous, I.: Deliberate relaxation of the temporal and masseter muscles in subjects with functional disorders of the chewing apparatus. Scand. J. Dent. Res., 78:478, 1971.

37. Nadler, S.: The importance of bruxism. J. Oral Med., 23:142, 1968.

38. Omnell, K–A, and Petersson, A.: Radiography of the temporomandibular joint utilizing oblique lateral transcranial projection. Odont Rev., 27:77, 1976.

39. Polson, A. M., Meitner, S. W., and Zander, H. A.: Trauma and progression of marginal periodontitis in squirrel monkeys, III. Adaptation of interproximal alveolar bone to repetitive injury. J. Periodont. Res., 11:279, 1976.

40. Polson, A. M., Meitner, S. W., and Zander, H. A.: Trauma and progression of marginal periodontitis in squirrel monkeys, IV. Reversibility of bone loss due to trauma alone and trauma superimposed upon periodontitis. J. Periodont. Res., 11:290, 1976.

41. Posselt, V., and Wolff, I. B.: Treatment of bruxism by bite guards and bite plates. J. Can. Dent. Assoc., 29:773, 1963.

42. Ramfjord, S. P.: Occlusion. Indent., 1:20, 1973.

43. Ramfjord, S. P., and Ash, M. M.: Occlusion, 2nd Ed., Philadelphia: W. B. Saunders Co., 1971, p. 206.

44. Ramfjord, S. P.: Bruxism, a clinical and electromyographic study. J. Am. Dent. Assoc., 62:21, 1961.

45. Remien, J. C., and Ash, M. M.: Myo-monitor centric: an evaluation. J. Pros. Dent., 31:137, 1974.

46. Reynolds, J. M.: Occlusal Adjustment. Pamphlet. Augusta, Ga. 1975.

47. Ricketts, R. M.: Laminagraphy in the diagnosis of

temporomandibular joint disorders. J. Am. Dent. Assoc., *46*:620, 1953.

48. Rugh, J. D., and Solberg, W. K.: Electromyographic evaluation of bruxist behavior before and after treatment. Ca. Dent. Assoc. J., *3*:56, 1975.

49. Rugh, J. D., and Solberg, W. K.: Psychological implications in temporomandibular pain and dysfunction. Oral Sci. Rev. 7, 1976.

50. Sarnat, B. G., and Laskin, D. M.: Diagnosis and surgical management of diseases of the temporomandibular joint. Springfield, Ill.: Charles C Thomas, 1962.

51. Scaife, R. R., Jr., and Holt, J. E.: Natural occurrence of cuspid guidance. J. Prosthet. Dent., *22*:225, 1969.

52. Scharer, P., Butler, J., and Zander, H.: Die heilung parodontaler Knochentaschen bei okklusalar Dysfunktion. Schweiz. Mschr. Zahnheik., *79*:244, 1969.

53. Schuyler, C. H.: Factors contributing to traumatic occlusion. J. Pros. Dent., *11*:708, 1961.

54. Schuyler, C. H.: Fundamental principles in the correction of occlusal disharmony, natural and artificial. J. Am. Dent. Assoc., *22*:1193, 1935.

55. Shapiro, S., and Shannon, J.: Bruxism—as an emotional reactive disturbance. Psychosomatics, *6*:427, 1965.

56. Shore, N. A. Temporomandibular Joint Dysfunction and Occlusal Equilibration, 2nd ed. Philadelphia: J. B. Lippincott Company, 1976.

57. Solberg, W. K., Clark, G. T., and Rugh, J. D.: Nocturnal electromyographic evaluation of bruxism patients undergoing short term splint therapy. J. Oral Rehab., *2*:215, 1975.

58. Solberg, W. K.: Myofascial pain and dysfunction. *In* J. Clark (Ed.): Clinical Dentistry, Hagerstown, Md.: Harper and Row, Vol. II, Chapter 37, 1976.

59. Solberg, W. K., Woo, M. W., and Houston, J. B.: Prevalence of mandibular dysfunction in young adults. J.A.D.A. 98:25, 1979.

60. Solberg, W. K.: Occlusion related pathosis and its clinical evaluation. *In* J. Clark (Ed.): Clinical Dentistry. Hagerstown, Md.: Harper and Row, Vol. II, Chapter 35, 1976.

61. Strohaver, R. A.: A comparison of articulator mountings made with centric relation and myocentric position records. J. Prosthet. Dent., *28*:379, 1972.

62. Taylor, R. C., Ware, W. H., and Horowitz, M. J.: The importance of determining the end point in treatment of patients with temporomandibular joint syndrome. J. Oral Med., *22*:3, 1967.

63. Thaller, J. L., Rosen, G., and Saltzman, S.: Study of the relationship of frustration and anxiety to bruxism. J. Periodontol., *38*:193, 1967.

64. Thomas, B. O. A., and Gallagher, J. W.: Practical management of occlusal dysfunctions in periodontal therapy. J. Am. Dent. Assoc., *46*:18, 1953.

65. Travell, J.: Myofascial trigger points: clinical view. *In* J. Bonica and DeAlbe-Fessards (Eds.): Advanced Pain Research and Therapy. New York: Raven Press, 1976.

66. Travell, J.: Temporomandibular joint pain referred from muscles of the head and neck. J. Pros. Dent., *10*:745, 1960.

67. Vale, J. D. F., and Ash, M. M., Jr.: Occlusal stability following occlusal adjustment. J. Prosthet. Dent., *27*:515, 1972.

68. Vollmer, W. H., and Rateitschak, K. H.: Influence of occlusal adjustment by grinding on gingivitis and mobility of traumatized teeth. J. Clin. Periodont, *2*:113, 1975.

69. Watt, D.: A study of the average duration of occlusal sounds in different age groups. Br. Dent. J., *138*:385, 1975.

70. Weinberg, L. A.: Posterior bilateral condylar displacement; its diagnosis and treatment. J. Prosthet. Dent., *36*:426, 1976.

71. Weinberg, L. A.: Technique for temporomandibular joint radiographs. J. Prosthet. Dent., *27*:284, 1972.

72. Weinberg, L. A.: Temporomandibular joint function and its effect on centric relations. J. Prosthet. Dent., *30*:176, 1972.

73. Wilkes, C. H.: Alterations in structure and function of the temporomandibular joint in patients with the TMJ syndrome. Accepted for publication, Minn. Med., 1978.

74. Yavelow, I., Forster, I., and Winniger, M.: Mandibular relearning. Oral Surg., *36*:632, 1973.

75. Yemm, R.: Some experimental evidence of the aetiology and pathology of masticatory dysfunction. J. Dent. Assoc. S. Afr., *30*:213, 1975.

Part VI

Reconstructive Phase

Chapter 56

Restorative–Periodontal Interrelationships

Dental restorations and periodontal health are inseparably interrelated. Technical excellence is important in restorative dentistry. The adaptation of the margins, the contours of the restoration, the proximal relationships, and the surface smoothness fulfill critical biological requirements of the gingiva and supporting periodontal tissues. Dental restorations therefore play a significant role in maintaining periodontal health.

Gingival and periodontal disease must be eliminated before restorative procedures are begun, for the following reasons:

Tooth mobility and pain interfere with mastication and function of restorative dentistry.

Inflammation of the periodontium impairs the capacity of abutment teeth to meet the functional demands of restorative dentistry. Restorations constructed so as to provide beneficial functional stimulation to a healthy periodontium become a destructive influence when superimposed upon existing periodontal disease, shortening the life span of the teeth and the restoration.

The position of teeth is frequently altered in periodontal disease. Resolution of inflammation and regeneration of periodontal ligament fibers following periodontal treatment cause the teeth to move again, often in the direction of their original position. Restorations designed for

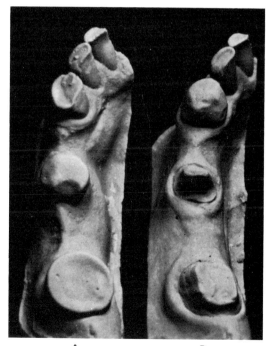

A　　　　　　　**B**
Figure 56–1　Change in Contour of Edentulous Mucosa Following Resolution of Inflammation. *A,* Before treatment. Note the pyramidal contour of the edentulous mucosa. *B,* After resolution of inflammation. The teeth are in process of preparation.

989

teeth before the periodontium is treated may produce injurious tensions and pressures on the treated periodontium.

Partial prostheses constructed on casts made from impressions of diseased gingiva and edentulous mucosa will not fit properly when periodontal health is restored. When the inflammation is eliminated, the contour of the gingiva and adjacent mucosa is altered (Fig. 56–1). Shrinkage creates spaces beneath the pontics of fixed bridges and the saddle areas of removable prostheses. Resultant plaque accumulation leads to inflammation of the mucosa and gingiva of the abutment teeth.

To locate the gingival margin of restorations properly, the position of the healthy gingival sulcus must be established before the tooth is prepared. Margins of restorations hidden behind diseased gingiva will be exposed when the inflamed gingiva shrinks following periodontal treatment.

PREPARATION OF THE PERIODONTIUM FOR RESTORATIVE DENTISTRY

In patients with mutilated dentitions and extensive periodontal disease, the usual treatment sequence is changed, and a temporary prosthesis is constructed before the periodontal pockets are eliminated. The teeth are prepared with provisional margins, which are relocated after the tissues heal. This provides improved occlusal relationships and splinting during the healing period. Approximately two months after periodontal treatment, when gingival health is restored and the location of the gingival sulcus is established, the preparations are modified to relocate the margins in proper relation to the healthy gingival sulcus, and a final restoration is constructed.

The aims of periodontal treatment are not limited to the elimination of periodontal pockets and restoration of gingival health. Treatment should also create the gingival mucosal environment necessary for the proper function of fixed and removable partial prostheses. Preparation of the mouth for restorative dentistry consists of soft tissue corrective measures performed as part of periodontal treatment.

Phase I Therapy

The procedures contained in phase I therapy are directed toward one specific goal, i.e., the control of active dental disease (see Chapters 42 and 43). Therefore, when initial therapy is completed, patients should be in a state of dental health with active caries no longer occurring and with active destruction of the periodontium under control. This will result in elimination of the acute inflammatory response associated with periodontal destruction. Thus, the status of gingival tissues should be such that further restorative procedures of a more complex nature can be carried out without undue detrimental effects from unhealthy gingiva.

In some patients, periodontal surgery will be necessary. These periodontal surgical procedures should also be carried out with due regard to the restorative needs of the patient. Therefore, the final level of the periodontium should allow good access to all restorative marginal regions, and any necessary increase in clinical crown length should be obtained by the postsurgical positioning of the periodontal tissues. If restorative procedures are going to necessitate the resolution of mucogingival inadequacies, the appropriate surgical procedure should be completed before the restorative therapy is begun.

Obtaining control of periodontal inflammation during phase I therapy will result in restorative procedures of a much higher quality than what they would be if they were carried out in an environment of gingival inflammation. The presence of an acute inflammatory response in the gingiva results in ulceration of the epithelium that lines the gingival pocket and an increase of vascularity and edema of the tissues immediately under this epithelium. There is a possibility of continual bleeding and exudation of inflammatory tissue fluid into the gingival crevice and into the environment where restorative dental procedures are carried out. Therefore, it is of utmost importance that all areas of the gingiva that show hemorrhage and significant amounts of inflammatory exudate be brought to an improved state of health before any restorative procedures other than emergency control of dental pain are carried out.

The removal of etiological factors causing gingival inflammation will result in a return to a more healthy state of the gingiva within one or two weeks. Thus, plaque control, calculus removal, and the removal of any inadequate restorative dentistry in the gingival environment should be important first-order procedures in initial therapy.

Periodontal Surgery

The routine procedures of periodontal surgery aimed at correction of periodontal defects and the correction of mucogingival defects are described in previous chapters. However, there are some surgical procedures which are modified because restorative dentistry or prosthodontic therapy is combined with the periodontal surgical procedure.

Pockets adjacent to edentulous regions

Periodontal pockets frequently occur on the proximal surfaces adjacent to edentulous regions. The corrections of these

periodontal defects should occur before any fixed or removable prosthodontic appliance is placed in these areas. The general principles involved in pocket elimination are similar to those used in other areas, but some special procedures are necessary in order to take into account the special needs of the edentulous space.

Periodontally involved teeth adjacent to edentulous spaces present two problems, which must be treated together: (1) elimination of the pockets, and (2) management of the edentulous mucosa. Inflammation from the periodontal pockets extends for varying distances into the adjacent edentulous mucosa (Fig. 56–2) and alters its color, consistency, and shape. The edentulous mucosa affected by inflammation may present various degrees of discoloration and edema with a smooth glistening surface, depending upon the relative predominance of cellular and fluid exudate or fibrosis. If principally fibrotic, it is pink, firm, and enlarged, with a lobulated surface.

The contour of the edentulous mucosa and gingiva is affected by mechanical factors as well as inflammation from adjacent pockets. The edentulous mucosa may con-

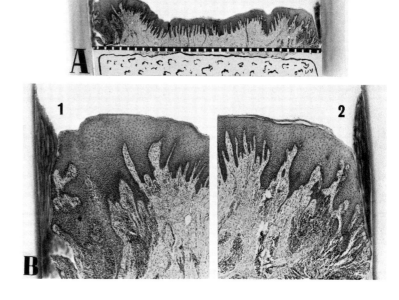

Figure 56–2 Preparation of the Mouth for Prosthesis. *A,* Edentulous mucosa with periodontal pockets (*1* and *2*) on the adjacent teeth. The location of the necessary incision is indicated by the dotted line. *B,* Inflammation from the periodontal pockets (*1* and *2*) extends into the edentulous mucosa.

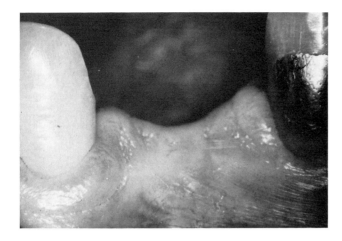

Figure 56–3 "Pyramiding" of Edentulous Mucosa and Adjacent Gingiva. The gingiva and mucosa are contoured by pressure from the tongue and food excursion.

form to the shape of the underlying bone, it may be swollen and rounded faciolingually, or lateral pressure from the tongue and cheek and food excursion may cause a pyramiding of the mucosa to form an elongated triangular ridge (Fig. 56–3). Because of the absence of the normal protective action of the embrasure, the gingiva is often similarly deformed.

The deformed edentulous mucosa reduces the vertical height available for prosthetic replacements. It does not provide a reliable base for the support of saddle areas or the proper design of pontics. The triangular mucosa is unsatisfactory for the placement of pontics. In an effort to overcome the problem, short pontics with a deep V-shaped base, which

straddles the ridge, are used. These are unsatisfactory, because food wedges between the mucosa and the pontics and the accumulation of plaque causes inflammation that jeopardizes retention of the bridge (Fig. 56–4).

Management of pockets and edentulous mucosa

The area is prepared for the prosthesis with the following objectives:

1. To establish a healthy gingival sulcus. The pontics adjacent to the natural teeth can be designed to create the gingival embrasure necessary for preservation of gingival health.

2. To eliminate extraneous mucosal tis-

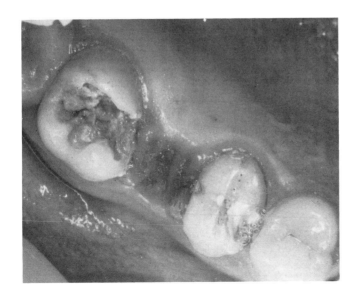

Figure 56–4 Chronic Inflammation of Edentulous Mucosa. Under bridge with ridge-lap type of pontic.

sue so as to permit adequate vertical space for the replacements.

3. To provide a firm, healthy mucosal base for placement of saddles or pontics.

In some situations, when pocket depth occurs in areas adjacent to edentulous areas, a *gingivectomy* may be used to eliminate these pockets and at the same time provide a maintainable contour of the edentulous ridge region (Fig. 56–5). The gingivectomy incision is continued from the gingival tissues into the edentulous area in such a way that the resulting tissue contour will form a firm and thin band of keratinized tissue across the saddle areas. This incision should be made so that the final contour of the saddle areas blends into the adjacent gingival contours and the edentulous ridge has a rounded,

smooth contour. The procedure will also result in the removal of inflamed tissues in the submucosa so that the final tissue will have a thin yet dense submucosa bound tightly to the periosteum and covered by an intact keratinized epithelium.

Because of the importance of maintaining a keratinized epithelium over the edentulous area, the gingivectomy procedure cannot be used in places where it would result in the complete removal of all keratinized tissue. In these situations, where the gingivectomy would result in the nonkeratinized oral mucosa forming the edentulous ridge or marginal gingival area, a *flap procedure* is indicated. In those areas where the pockets on the proximal surfaces of the teeth adjacent to the edentulous area are of the infrabony type,

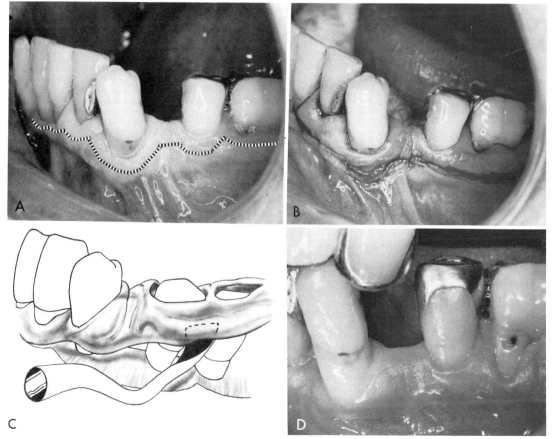

Figure 56–5   Preparation for Prosthesis. *A,* Deformed edentulous mucosa and adjacent periodontal pockets. The incision is indicated by the dotted line. *B,* The incision. *C,* Inflamed gingiva and edentulous mucosa removed. *D,* Mucosa and gingiva healed with deformity corrected.

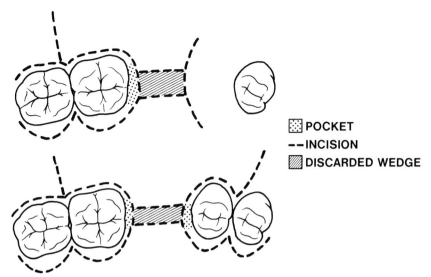

POCKET
-- INCISION
DISCARDED WEDGE

Figure 56–6 Flap Surgery in Edentulous Areas. Incisions for pockets adjacent to edentulous regions. The dotted line marks the initial incisions. Vertical incisions may be used at the interproximal spaces, or the excision may be continued as an envelope flap design.

a flap procedure is also needed. The incisions normally made around the adjacent teeth are carried into the edentulous area in the form of parallel buccal and lingual incisions that run across the crest of the ridge so that an adequate band of keratinized gingiva is maintained on both buccal and lingual portions of the flap. These incisions across the edentulous area are made so that the flap is undermined (Fig. 56–6). The inflamed tissue between the buccal and lingual incisions is removed. The undermining of the buccal and lingual flaps leaves a thin band of tissue that will lie close to the underlying bone once the flap is sutured back into position at completion of the operation. The undermining and subsequent repositioning of the flap will result in an apical positioning of the soft tissue covering the edentulous area.

By means of the parallel incisions over the edentulous area, access is obtained to any osseous defects on the adjacent teeth. These periodontal osseous defects can be recontoured in order to eliminate the pockets. The flaps will provide tissue to cover these corrected osseous defects completely so that the healing that follows will be uneventful and of short duration (Fig. 56–7).

Management of mucogingival problems

It is often necessary to carry out a free soft tissue autograft in patients who have a mucogingival defect associated with gingival inflammation and require a dental restoration in the immediate environment of the gingiva (Fig. 56–8). The procedure for carrying out this free soft tissue autograft has been covered in Chapter 53 and need not be further discussed here. Mucogingival surgery should be carried out at least two months prior to the completion of the dental restoration. This will allow time for mature tissue to be formed in the gingival margin so that restorative procedures will not cause a return of clinical inflammation. Augmentation of keratinized gingiva provides stability of the free gingival margin and surrounding gingival tissues so that the dental restoration can be placed in an environment where gingival health can be maintained.

PERIODONTAL ASPECTS OF FIXED AND REMOVABLE PROSTHESES

In addition to esthetics, the purposes of fixed and removable prostheses include

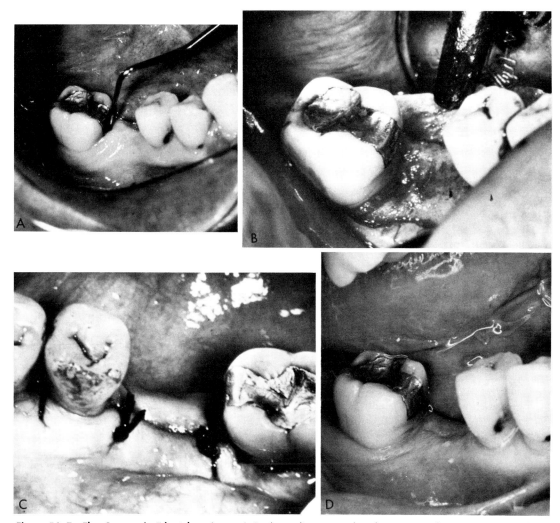

Figure 56–7 Flap Surgery in Edentulous Areas. *A,* Pockets adjacent to edentulous region. There is a 6-mm. pocket on the mesial aspect of the lower second molar, and additional crown length is required for abutment preparation. *B,* Wedge-shaped tissue removed. The exposed tooth surfaces are root planed, and any necessary osseous recontouring is carried out. *C,* Closure of flaps. Lingual view of interrupted sutures used to close the flaps and to hold tissue in an apical position. *D,* Three months postoperation. The gingival tissue is established at a more apical level on the tooth. Pocket depth is now 2 mm. on mesial aspect of second molar. Additional crown length is available for abutment preparation.

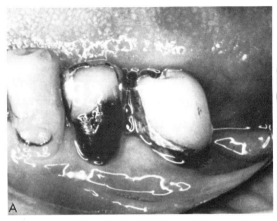
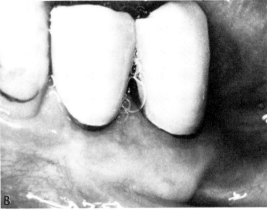

Figure 56–8   Mucogingival Problems. *A,* Preoperative mucogingival problem. There is inadequate gingiva in the region where a crown margin is to be placed. The presence of a plaque-enhancing margin necessitates the development of an adequate band of gingiva. *B,* Postoperative soft tissue autograft. Six months after mucogingival surgery and placement of restoration. Note the adequate band of gingiva.

the improvement of masticatory efficiency and the prevention of tilting and extrusion of teeth with resultant disruption of the occlusion and food impaction.

Occlusal Adjustment Before Prostheses

Traumatic occlusal relationships should be eliminated before restorative procedures are begun, and restorations should be constructed in conformity with the newly established occlusal patterns. If this is not done, the prosthesis perpetuates occlusal relationships injurious to the periodontium.

The harmful effects of occlusal trauma are not confined to the teeth involved in the restoration and their antagonists. Other areas of the dentition are secondarily affected by an occlusal disharmony created or perpetuated by an inlay or bridge. Delaying occlusal adjustment until the restorations are inserted often necessitates grinding through the occlusal surface of the newly constructed restorations.

The occlusion must be checked at regular intervals after a prosthesis is inserted. Occlusal relationships change with time as the result of wear of restorative materials and settling of saddle areas of removable prostheses, especially those without distal support.

Tooth Preparation in Relation to the Gingival Margin

The first requirement for proper location of the gingival margin of a crown or other restoration close to the gingiva is a healthy gingival sulcus. Preparation is not complete until the gingiva is healthy and its position on the root has been established. Periodontal pockets should not be permitted to remain undisturbed for the ostensible purposes of "keeping the root covered" or "hiding the margins of the restorations." When the gingiva is treated, as it eventually must be, the denuded root and margins of the restoration that were "hidden" by the inflamed gingiva become visible. In the interim, the patient has suffered unnecessary destruction of the periodontium, and the longevity of the tooth and restoration has been jeopardized.

Treatment of the gingiva, final tooth preparation, and impression taking should not be attempted in one operation, for this does not allow time for the gingiva to heal, and the location of the margin of the restoration in relation to the healed gingival sulcus can only be estimated.

Dental restorations should be kept away from the gingiva whenever possible. Extension of cavity margins into the gingival sulcus should only occur in those situations where there is a definite indication for introducing restorative materials into the subgingival environment. If the restorative margin is placed subgingivally, it is more difficult for the patient's oral hygiene procedures to control the bacteria that colonize this area.

There are some clinical situations in which it is advisable to carry the margin of the restoration into the gingival sulcus, e.g., the existence of a previous restoration extending into the gingival area, the presence of rampant caries or caries that extends apically into the gingival environment, the need for apical extension in order to obtain adequate retention of the restoration, and the advantage of placing the restoration subgingivally on the labial surface of upper anterior teeth in those patients to whom appearance is of primary importance. In *all* other cases, dental restorations should be kept away from the gingival third of the tooth.

Once a decision has been made to place restorative dental materials into the gingival crevice, the level at which the margin should be placed is of critical importance. It is advisable to keep the restorations in the coronal half of the gingival crevice. Thus, all subgingival margins should be placed within one or two millimeters of the free gingival margin wherever possible (Fig. 56–9). This allows access to the margin for oral hygiene procedures and will give better access for refining the margin during cavity preparation and impression taking. The coronal half of the gingival sulcus has a much thicker protective layer of epithelium (the oral sulcular epithelium) than does the apical half of the sulcus, where the junctional epithelium is just a few cells thick. This coronal region therefore has better resistance to the toxic products of dental plaque than does the region of the junctional epithelium.

It should be recognized that placing a margin in the gingival crevice at the time of completion of a restoration does not guarantee that this relationship of the gingiva to the margin will maintain itself. There is no reliable way to predict accurately what the movement of the gingival margin over time will be. In patients with an adequate level of oral hygiene associated with a nontraumatic toothbrushing technique, there is much less risk of apical migration of the gingival margin than

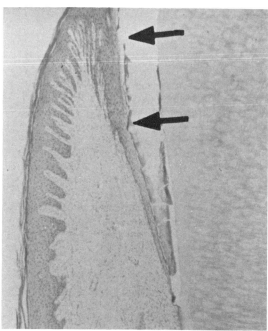

Figure 56–9 Position of Gingival Margins. In those cases in which subgingival margins are indicated, the most ideal position for the margin is the coronal half of the gingival sulcus (*arrows*). In this region the thick band of oral sulcular epithelial cells provides a better barrier to penetration of bacterial products than does the narrow junctional epithelium found in the apical half of the sulcus. Cavity preparation, impression taking, and cementation of restorations are all more likely to be ideal when good access to the margin is made possible by positioning it in the coronal half of the gingival sulcus.

there is in patients with ineffective and/or traumatic oral hygiene techniques utilizing hard toothbrushes. All clinical signs of gingival inflammation should be resolved before restorations are placed, as the shrinkage associated with the resolution of gingival inflammation will frequently cause the healthy gingival margin to be positioned apical to its position when the gingiva was inflamed.

"Avoid the Gingival Third"

The full crown is extremely useful because it fulfills requirements that can be met by no other type of restoration (Fig. 56–10). However, even when ideally constructed in relation to the gingival sulcus, the full crown introduces the risk of gingival inflammation. Crowns substitute a

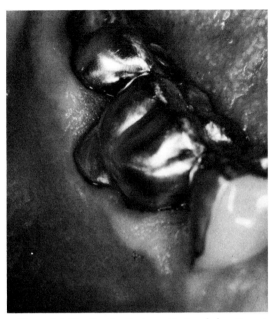

Figure 56–10 Tooth Contour Restored by Crown. Note the excellent condition of the gingiva in the bifurcation area.

foreign substance such as gold, acrylic, or porcelain for the natural tooth wall of the gingival sulcus. The materials are not irritating, but plaque can accumulate on these surfaces, and this irritates the gingiva. If not removed within 24 to 48 hours, this plaque may undergo calcification and develop into calculus. The junction of the crown and the tooth also presents a problem. Even with perfect marginal fit, an extremely thin cement line, which attracts plaque,[56] is unavoidable.

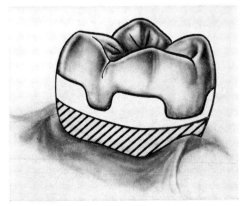

Figure 56–11 "Avoid the Gingival Third." Inlay constructed without involving the gingival third of the crown.

The risk of irritation to the gingiva is reduced by restorations that terminate coronal to the gingival margin,[49] encroaching upon the gingival third of the tooth (Fig. 56–11).[53] Wherever possible, inlays,[48] pinledges, and three-quarter crowns should be used as individual restorations and retainers for fixed prostheses. This is not a matter of substituting other restorations for purposes that can only be fulfilled by crowns. However, when there is a choice and high caries incidence is not a problem, the gingival third of the tooth should not be involved in the restoration.

Gingival Retraction for Taking Impressions

When using elastic impression materials, it is often necessary to retract the gingiva to gain access to the gingival margin of the preparation. Several methods of accomplishing this are described below. These are methods for retracting healthy gingiva. They are not for the removal, displacement, or shrinkage of inflamed, swollen gingival tissue. The gingiva must be healthy and its position on the tooth established before the impression is taken.

Methods of retracting the gingiva

SURGERY. Surgical resection of the gingiva is the preferred method for providing access to the margin of the preparation. Under local anesthesia the gingiva is excised apical to the margin of the preparation with periodontal knives or a No. 11 or No. 12 Bard-Parker blade (Fig. 56–12). Bleeding is controlled with a cotton pellet under pressure, moistened with epinephrine if necessary. The gingiva will regenerate and be restored to its normal position, provided it was healthy when the preparation was started. If the gingiva is diseased when the tooth is prepared, resection of the gingiva or inadvertent removal of plaque and calculus during tooth preparation would affect shrinkage in the pocket wall and exposure of tooth surface beyond the margin of the preparation (Fig. 56–13). The recession is sometimes erroneously attributed to the surgery.

ELECTROSURGERY. The gingiva may also be retracted by electrosurgery without

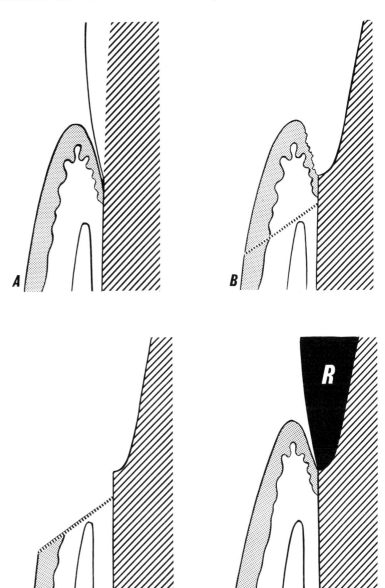

Figure 56–12 Marginal Gingiva Removed to Provide Access for Taking Impressions. *A,* Normal dento-gingival relationship before tooth is prepared. *B,* Champfer-type tooth preparation. The gingival margin is slightly lacerated during preparation. Gingiva incised at dotted line. *C,* Gingival margin removed by periodontal knife or electrosurgery. *D,* Restoration (*R*) in position at the base of the healed gingival sulcus.

the problem of bleeding. Electrosurgery may be used for gingival retraction in some situations in which access to margins is required. It should be carried out so as to minimize tissue damage, and the current should be adapted so that electrosection is used rather than coagulation. The use of equipment that provides fully rectified current and an undamped wave form results in the least amount of tissue damage.[27] Several studies have shown that the careful use of electrosurgery in the super-

ficial part of the gingival crevice results in little if any residual damage to the gingiva.[9, 18] Recent reports have emphasized the dangers of electrosurgery when the cutting instrument is allowed to be in close proximity to the base of the crevice and cementum.[36, 60] In patients in whom there is a thin covering of gingiva and alveolar bone over the root, electrosurgery should not be used, as the loss of tissue from the internal or crevicular surface can result in gingival recession. In these cases

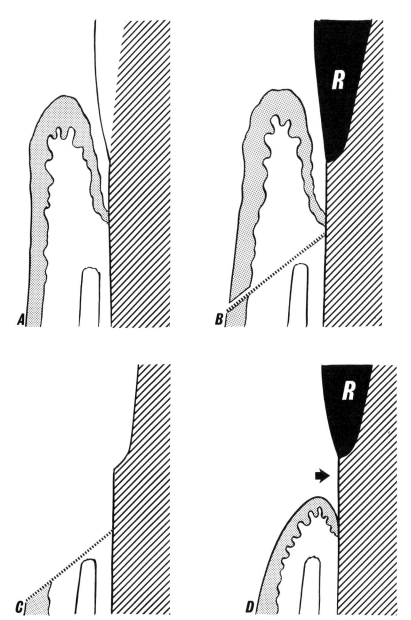

Figure 56–13   Recession Following Restoration of Tooth with Untreated Periodontal Disease. *A,* Periodontal pocket present before tooth preparation. *B,* Restoration (*R*) erroneously inserted in tooth with untreated periodontal pocket. Dotted line shows incision required for elimination of pocket. *C,* Diseased gingiva removed. *D,* Gingiva heals, revealing the root surface (*arrow*), which had been denuded by periodontal disease before restoration was inserted.

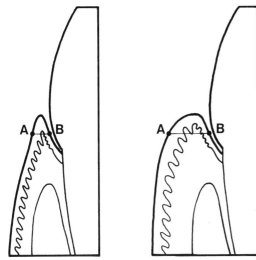

Figure 56–14 Electrosurgery for Retraction. The use of electrosurgery in patients in whom the gingival tissue is thin buccolingually (i.e., A–B on the *left* diagram) will result in destruction of almost all the gingival tissue, causing postoperative gingival recession. In these situations retraction cords are the method of choice for obtaining access to the gingival margins. When a thick covering of gingiva is present (i.e., A–B on the *right* diagram), it is possible to use electrosurgical techniques for gingival retraction.

the gingiva should be retracted with retraction strings (Fig. 56–14).

RETRACTION STRINGS. Strings impregnated with chemicals are used for gingival retraction. Among the types of chemicals for this purpose are vasoconstrictors (8 per cent racemic epinephrine),[19] which cause rapid transient elevation in blood pressure and blood sugar and are contraindicated in patients with coronary disease, hyperthyroidism, or diabetes. They also produce local ischemia, which may be injurious to the gingiva. Also used are corrosives (zinc chloride 8 per cent, tannic acid 10 per cent, and trichloracetic acid 10 per cent) and astringents (aluminum sulfate 14 per cent).

Impregnated strings will cause the gingiva to wilt away from the tooth and expose the margin of the preparation. The gingiva will ordinarily return to its proper position, provided it was healthy at the outset and the string is not permitted to keep the gingiva separated long enough to permit disease-producing plaque to accumulate in the sulcus. Impregnated strings should not be used on diseased gingiva; pocket walls temporarily retracted from the root will return and jeopardize the tooth and restoration (Fig. 56–15). Because the effects of the chemicals cannot be controlled, pressure retraction of the gingiva with chemical-free strings or other methods of retraction is preferred.

The use of retraction strings can result in tissue tearing and inflammation if these strings are kept dry.[2] The epithelial lining of the gingival sulcus adheres to the dry string and is torn when the string is removed prior to taking impressions. It is advisable to moisten impression retraction strings with saline while they are placed in the gingival crevice, in order to limit tearing of the epithelium. Tearing of the epithelium will make taking of an accurate impression difficult or even impossible, as it will result in immediate hemorrhage into the area of the gingival sulcus (Fig. 56–16).

There have been reports of periodontal abscesses associated with impression material left in the gingival environment following the taking of impressions for fixed prosthodontic appliances.[36, 41] Immediately after an impression is removed from the mouth, it should be carefully checked to make sure that no pieces have been torn from it and left in the gingival environment. The gingival sulcus should also be carefully inspected to ensure that no residual pieces of impression material are left in the gingival tissues.

Even with extreme care the gingiva is often lacerated in the course of tooth preparation. If the gingiva is healthy before the restoration is started, it will regenerate and return to its previous position on the tooth,[21, 22] provided the area to which it was attached is not cut away and included in the preparation.

Temporary Coverage

Temporary restorations are often a cause of periodontal inflammation and gingival recession.[12] All temporary restorations should be constructed so that they minimize the damage done to the gingiva during the time they are in the mouth. It is important that the marginal integrity of

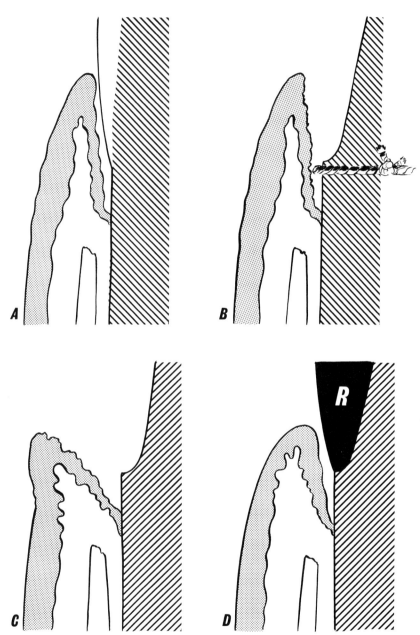

Figure 56–15   Periodontal Pocket Persisting after Retraction. *A,* Periodontal pocket present before tooth is prepared. *B,* Tooth prepared, retraction string placed to retract diseased gingiva. *C,* Diseased gingiva temporarily retracted to provide access to tooth for impression. *D,* Restoration (R) inserted. The periodontal pocket has returned.

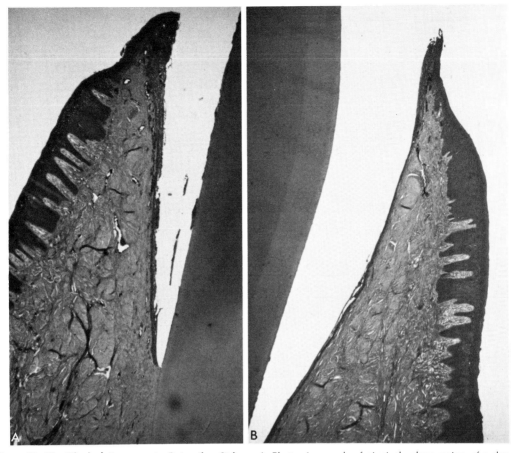

Figure 56–16   Gingival Response to Retraction Strings. *A,* Photomicrograph of gingival sulcus region of a dog after removal of gingival retraction cord that had been placed in the sulcus for 7 minutes. In this case the cord was dried prior to placement and the sulcus was air dried during the time the cord was in place. Note the tearing of the sulcular epithelium and the initial acute inflammatory reaction in the connective tissue of the gingiva, with dilatation of blood vessels. There is evidence of bleeding into the gingival crevice. *B,* Photomicrograph of gingival sulcus region of a dog after removal of gingival retraction cord that had been placed in the sulcus for 7 minutes. In this case the cord was moistened with saline prior to placement, and the gingival sulcus was bathed with saline during the time the cord was in place. Note the intact epithelium, the absence of acute inflammation, and the lack of hemorrhage.

temporary restorations be as good as is technically possible, and the surface of these temporary restorations should be made highly polished so that plaque accumulation on them is minimized. The contour of these restorations should also be compatible with gingival tissues. In those cases where a temporary restoration is to be in place for more than a few days, the requirements of contour polish and fit should be the same as for the final restoration. Such long-term restorations should not be called temporary but should be regarded as provisional or treatment res-

torations that may remain in place for many months. Provisional or treatment restorations allow the dentist to assess the effect of the final restoration on the periodontium. The contour of the restorations, the occlusal pattern, and the patient's oral hygiene procedures may be modified while provisional restorations are in place, so that optimal periodontal health is obtained. The final restorations can duplicate the provisional restorations, providing some certainty about the long-term effect of the restorations on the periodontium (Fig. 56–17).

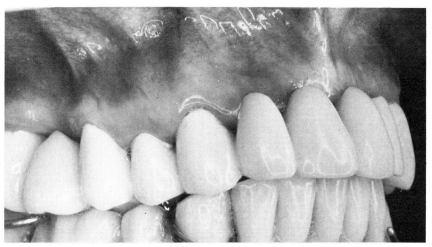

Figure 56-17   Provisional Restorations. Provisional restorations provide an opportunity to evaluate the patient's response to the final restorations. The esthetics can be modified, but more importantly, the contour of the restorations can be changed so that the gingival tissues can be kept healthy. When previous restorations have caused gingival inflammation, a provisional restoration can become a treatment restoration as it provides an environment for the gingiva to return to health. These restorations should be made of heat-cured acrylic, should have accurate marginal adaption, and should be contoured and polished so as to duplicate the form of the natural teeth. (Courtesy of Dr. John Flocken, Los Angeles.)

The Embrasures

When teeth are in proximal contact, the spaces that widen out from the contact are known as embrasures. The interdental space is divisible into a facial and lingual embrasure (Fig. 56–18), an occlusal or incisal embrasure that is coronal to the contact area (Fig. 56–19A), and a gingival embrasure, which is the space between the contact area and the alveolar bone.[4, 58] The gingival embrasure is filled with soft tissue, but in periodontal disease (Fig. 56–19B), spaces are created in the gingival embrasure.

THE GINGIVAL EMBRASURE. Embrasures are critical considerations in restorative dentistry. Proximal surfaces of dental restorations are important because they create the embrasures essential for gingival health (Fig. 56–20). From the periodontal viewpoint, the gingival embrasure is the most significant. Periodontal disease causes tissue destruction, which reduces the level of the alveolar bone, increases the size of the gingival embrasure, and creates open interdental spaces. Restorations may be constructed so as to preserve the morphology of the crown and root and retain the enlarged embrasure and the open interdental space (Fig. 56–21A and B), or the teeth may be reshaped by the restorations so as to relocate the gingival embrasure close to the new level of the gingiva. This is accomplished by changing the contour of the proximal surfaces and locating the contact areas more apically (Fig. 56–21C). The interdental gingiva will assume its normal shape by filling the new embrasure provided for it, which must be adequate in all dimensions.

The following dimensions of the gingival embrasure are important to the preservation of gingival health:

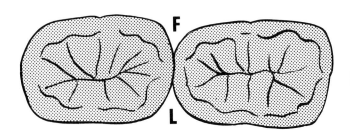

Figure 56-18   Occlusal View of Mandibular Molars showing facial (F) and lingual (L) embrasures.

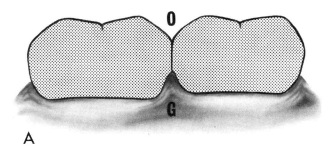

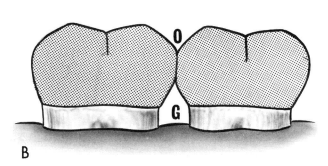

Figure 56–19 Occlusal (O) and Gingival (G) Embrasures. *A,* Interdental gingiva fills gingival embrasure (G). *B,* Open gingival embrasure (G) in patient with periodontal disease.

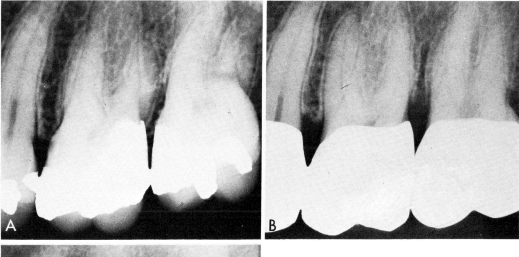

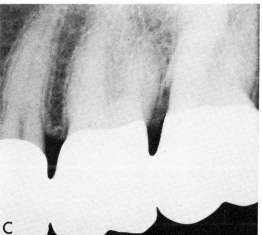

Figure 56–20 Contour of Restoration Corrected to Provide Proper Gingival Embrasures. *A,* Improperly contoured restorations on the molars; the gingival embrasure is too narrow. *B,* New restorations; the gingival embrasure between the molars is now wider at its base but too narrow beneath the contact area. *C,* Proper gingival embrasure created by widening the space beneath the molar contact area.

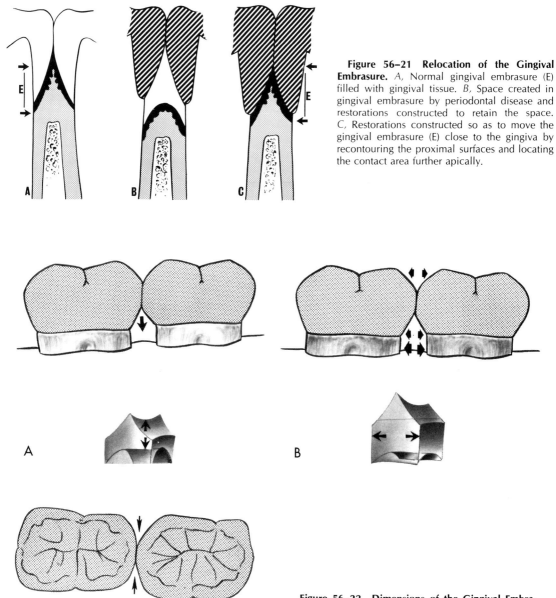

Figure 56–21 Relocation of the Gingival Embrasure. A, Normal gingival embrasure (E) filled with gingival tissue. B, Space created in gingival embrasure by periodontal disease and restorations constructed to retain the space. C, Restorations constructed so as to move the gingival embrasure (E) close to the gingiva by recontouring the proximal surfaces and locating the contact area further apically.

A

B

C

Figure 56–22 Dimensions of the Gingival Embrasure (indicated by arrows). A, Height. B, Mediodistal width. C, Faciolingual depth.

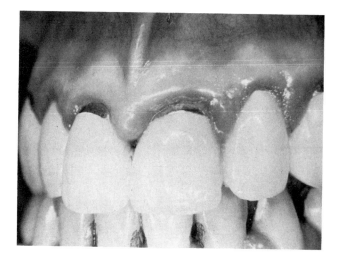

Figure 56–23 Inadequate gingival embrasures lead to gingival disease.

Height. The distance between the contact area and the bone margin (Fig. 56–22*A*). When the contact area is too close to the cervical line of the tooth, the embrasure is shortened.

Width. The distance mesiodistally between the proximal surfaces (Fig. 56–22*B*).

Depth. The distance faciolingually from the contact area to a line joining the proximofacial or proximolingual angles (Fig. 56–22*C*).

The proximal surfaces of crowns should taper away from the contact area—facially, lingually, and apically. Excessively broad proximal contact areas and inadequate contour in the cervical region crowd out the facial and lingual gingival papillae. The prominent papillae lead to gingival inflammation and pocket formation (Fig. 56–23).

Restorative dental procedures too often result in the restorative material taking up space that is normally occupied by the interdental papilla. This problem has been accentuated since the advent of restorations in which metal is bonded to porcelain. The problem begins with underpreparation of the tooth, so that the technician is left with no choice except to place an excessive amount of restorative material into the interproximal space. During the preparation of dies for cast restorations, the technician first removes all the replicated gingival tissue in order to get access to the margins; thus it is impossible to visualize the space available for the dental restoration in the interproximal embrasure area. If two models are poured from the same impression and the second one is used as an indicator of how much space is currently occupied by the gingival tissues, the technician can have a much better understanding of what the contour of the final restorations should be.

Overcrowding of the interdental space results in a narrowed embrasure area so that oral hygiene is difficult. The space available for gingival tissues is reduced, also, so that a thin strand of collagen is often all that can occupy this space. This reduction in the space available for gingiva means that the ability of the collagen to form an efficient seal in association with the junctional epithelium is diminished. This increases the risk of periodontal destruction and will eventually lead to pocket formation and destruction of the support of the tooth (Fig. 56–24).

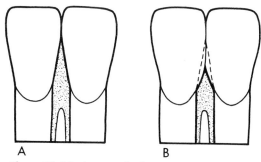

A   B

Figure 56–24 Interproximal Crown Contours. Overcontouring of crowns in the interdental region results in encroachment upon the space available for gingival tissue. *A,* Normally available space. *B,* Excess mesio-distal width of crowns and excess length of contact points results in compression of gingival tissue and predilection to inflammation. Access for oral hygiene is also much more difficult when embrasure spaces are over-filled with restorative materials.

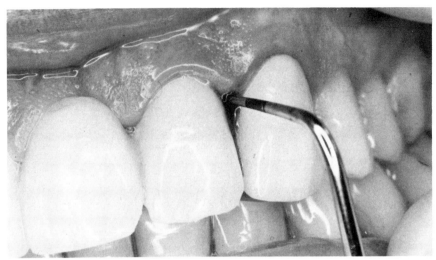

Figure 56–25 Excessive Contact Area. Soldered point carried too far apically. The periodontal probe is at the apical level of the solder joint. There is a 7-mm. pocket in the adjacent interproximal periodontium.

In fixed bridgework the soldered joint is frequently carried too far in an apical direction and so invades the embrasure space from its coronal aspect. This also results in inadequate space for the interdental gingiva and leads to inflammation and destruction of periodontal tissues (Fig. 56–25). For those patients who require increased strength in a soldered joint, it is best obtained by extending the soldered joint buccally and lingually, rather than coronally and apically.

The responsibility for determining the size of the soldered joint should rest with the dentist, not with the technician. Frequently the technician will decide the position and size of the solder joint without being aware of how much gingival tissue is present in the interproximal embrasure. These problems of the interproximal embrasure space being encroached upon by restorative materials is maximized in those patients whose gingival tissue fully occupies the embrasure space. In patients in whom periodontal surgery or gingival recession has resulted in recession of the interdental papilla, the problems of encroachment into the space are minimized. The principles that determine the size and form of the solder joint apply equally to the size and form of contact points associated with all interproximal restorations (Fig. 56–26).

Contours of Restorations

The facial and lingual contours of restorations are also important in the preservation of gingival health.

The most common error in re-creating the contours of the tooth in dental restorations is over-contouring of the facial and lingual surfaces. In one study approximately 80 per cent of full gold crowns were wider than the tooth they were replacing, and all porcelain bonded to metal crowns were too wide buccolingually.[37] This over-contouring generally occurs in the gingival third of the crown and results in an area where oral hygiene procedures are unable to control plaque accumulation. Consequently, plaque bacteria accumulate in the

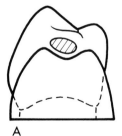 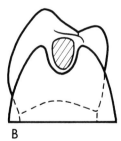

A   B

Figure 56–26 Size and Shape of Contact Areas. A, Correct shape of solder joint or contact area. B, Incorrect shape with excessive apical extension of solder joint or contact area. This results in the gingival col being disrupted, and the interproximal tissue is forced to take on a morphology in which the buccal and lingual portions of the papilla are split. This interproximal tissue is less able to maintain its health because of its form and because of the inaccessibility of the midproximal gingival sulcus region to oral hygiene procedures.

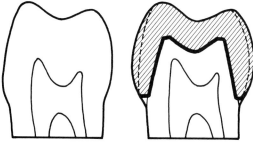

Figure 56–27 Buccolingual Crown Contours. Over-contouring of crowns in the buccolingual dimension is frequently due to inadequate removal of dentin during cavity preparation. The original contour of the tooth on the left diagram cannot be reproduced in the crown (shaded area in the right diagram) because there is not enough space for porcelain and metal in the gingival third.

tion,[27, 30, 38, 45, 61] but under-contouring has little if any effect on gingival health[26, 38] (Fig. 56–27).

Over-contouring on the buccal or labial surfaces frequently occurs in metal bonded to porcelain crowns owing to the technician's attempt to obtain a thickness of porcelain adequate to mask the underlying metal and provide the most esthetic appearance for the crown. Frequently the technician has no choice but to put excess porcelain in this area, as removal of tooth material in the crown during cavity preparation has been inadequate. It is important to remove enough tooth material to allow adequate width for the metal and porcelain so that the resulting crowns will not bulge beyond the space normally occupied by the anatomical crown of the tooth. A minimum space of 2.0 mm. is required.

In those patients in whom periodontal destruction and/or periodontal surgery causes the gingival margin to be in a much more apical position than it was during health, the facial lingual contours become even more significant. In these cases the bulge on the facial contour of the crown, which normally would be subgingival, now appears supragingival. This makes the portion of the exposed root immediately apical to the bulge less accessible for oral hygiene, with resultant plaque accumulation and periodontal inflammation. In these cases it is frequently necessary to recontour existing restorations or even ex-

gingival area and the gingiva becomes inflamed.

Over-contouring of restorations is a result of the mistaken belief that all natural teeth have a pronounced supragingival bulge in the gingival third of the clinical crown. In fact, much of the bulge that is present on natural teeth occurs in the area of the gingival crevice and does not have the function normally ascribed to it, i.e., deflecting food away from the gingiva. Apparently, under-contouring is not nearly as damaging to the gingiva as over-contouring. Evidence from studies on animals and humans demonstrates that over-contouring is a significant factor in gingival inflamma-

Figure 56–28 Facial Contour of Crowns in Relation to Gingiva. *A,* The gingival margin is normally coronal to the facial bulge of the anatomical crown. *B,* When the gingiva recedes, the gingiva is overprotected by the contour of the crown, so plaque accumulation is facilitated. *C,* The crown of the tooth is reshaped so that the gingiva is accessible for proper oral hygiene procedures. This should be carried out in areas where gingival recession is associated with gingival inflammation.

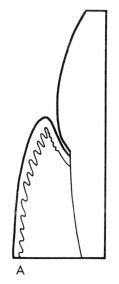

A

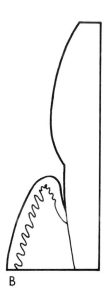

B

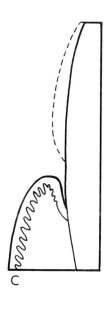

C

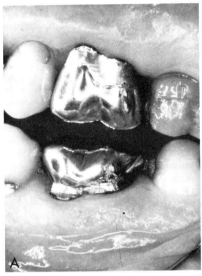

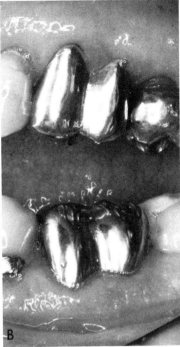

Figure 56–29 Recontouring of Crowns in Periodontally Involved Teeth. A, Preoperative photograph of molar region. There were 6-mm. pockets interproximally between the molars and a Class I furcation involvement of both upper and lower first molars. B, Following periodontal surgery the crowns have been replaced by crowns with accentuated grooves in the furcation region. Note the development of pyramidal gingiva in the midfacial region.

isting natural crowns in order to facilitate oral hygiene procedures. This problem is especially important in the area of the facial furcations of upper and lower molars and in the area of the lingual furcations of lower molars (Fig. 56–28).

In those situations where the furcation has been exposed by periodontal surgical procedures or by gingival recession, it is important that the crown be contoured in such a way as to facilitate access for oral hygiene. In these cases it is important to emphasize the midfacial groove of the crown so that this groove is confluent with the furcation. It is equally important to remove the apical bulge of the crown, thereby eliminating any plaque traps apical to the cemento-enamel junction. These crown contours should be mirrored in the contours in the underlying bone in those cases where osseous surgery is carried out. Thus the midfacial groove that runs apically in the bone covering the molar roots is continued in a groove running occluso-apically in the crown preparation and in the completed restoration in the area of the furcation (Fig. 56–29).

The Occlusal Surface

Occlusal surfaces should be designed so as to direct forces along the long axis of the teeth. They should restore occlusal dimensions and cuspal contours in harmony with the remainder of the natural dentition—after occlusal abnormalities have been eliminated by occlusal adjustment. The occlusal surfaces of the teeth should not be arbitrarily narrowed. Proper occlusal relationships are more important than the width of the occlusal table in the attainment of physiological occlusal forces. The anatomy of the occlusal surface should provide well-formed marginal ridges and occlusal sluiceways to prevent interproximal food impaction.

The Effect of Surface Finish of Restorative Materials on the Periodontium

The surface of restorations should be as smooth as possible in order to limit plaque accumulation. Roughened tooth surfaces and roughened surfaces in the subgingival region result in increased plaque accumulation and increased gingival inflammation.[50, 56]

In the clinical situation, porcelain, highly polished gold, and highly polished acrylic all result in similar plaque accumulation.[7, 25, 40] There is evidence that porcelain may accumulate less plaque than gold in dogs, and it has been suggested that this is due to differences in the inherent properties of these materials, but the surface roughness of these materials seems to be the most important factor in humans.[7] The surface roughness of vacuum-fired porcelain is 1.262 microinches, of highly polished gold 1.085 microinches, and of highly polished acrylic 1.015 microinches.[7] (Fig. 56–30) This compares to a surface roughness of 4.0 microinches on amalgam restorations polished with xxx silex and tin oxide[6] and a surface roughness of 4.7 and 3.8 microinches for dentine polished with pumice and zircate respectively.[54] Composite restorative materials have a much rougher surface of 8.0 microinches, and polishing and finishing of these restorations results in an even rougher surface of

40.0 microinches with pumice and 28.0 microinches with aluminum oxide.[57] Plaque accumulation occurs very quickly on composite restorations that have a rough surface due to finishing procedures.

The exact relationship between the degree of surface roughness and plaque accumulation is as yet undetermined. There is evidence that the amount of plaque accumulating in patients with relatively poor oral hygiene is not affected to a significant degree by minor changes in root surface configuration.[44] In patients with rough dental restorations, however, one can expect that the surface configuration may play an important role in plaque accumulation.[28, 57] Therefore, all restorative materials placed in the gingival environment should have as high a polish as is possible on their surface.

Pontics

A pontic should meet the following requirements: it should (a) be esthetically acceptable; (b) provide occlusal relation-

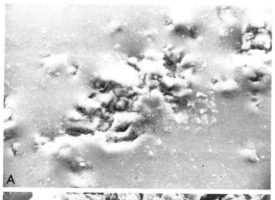
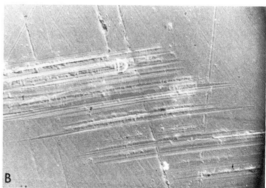
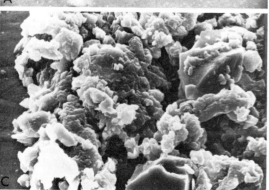

Figure 56–30 Surface of Restorations. A, Scanning electron micrograph of surface of vacuum-fired porcelain (original magnification ×1100). Note the irregular surface with roughness of approximately 1 microinch. B, Scanning electron micrograph of cast gold restoration (original magnification ×1100). The surface was given a final polish with rouge on a felt wheel. The surface irregularities are approximately 1 microinch. C, Scanning electron micrograph of composite restoration (original magnification ×1100). Note the extreme irregularity of the surface, which would facilitate plaque accumulation.

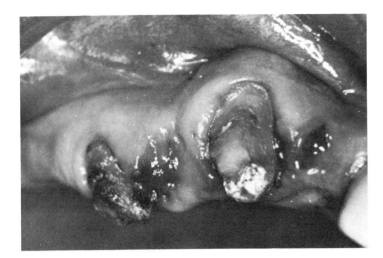

Figure 56–31 Poor Pontic Design. Chronic inflammation of edentulous mucosa under bridge with ridge-lap type of pontic.

ships that are favorable to the abutment teeth and opposing teeth and the remainder of the dentition; (c) restore the masticatory effectiveness of the tooth it replaces; (d) be designed to minimize accumulation of irritating dental plaque and food debris and to permit maximum access for cleansing by the patient; and (e) provide embrasures for passage of food.

Plaque, which causes inflammation of the mucosa under pontics and the gingiva around abutment teeth, tends to accumulate around fixed prostheses because special effort is required to keep them clean.

The health of the tissues around fixed prostheses depends primarily upon the patient's oral hygiene; the materials of which pontics are constructed appear to make little difference, and pontic design is important only to the extent that it enables the patient to keep the area clean. Plaque accumulates to an equal degree upon pontics made of glazed and unglazed porcelain,[20] polished gold, and polished acrylic resin,[41, 52] despite the finding that the surfaces of the latter two are smoother.[7]

The principles of contours of crowns apply equally well to pontics, but with

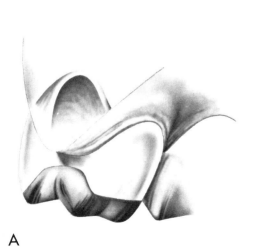

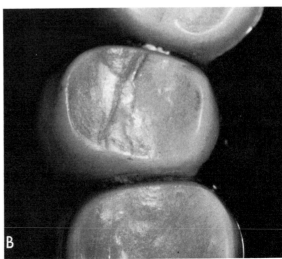

Figure 56–32 Saddle-Type Pontics. A, Diagrammatic view of saddle-type pontic in position. B, Undersurface of saddle-type pontic. Note the irregularities that conform to surface of the underlying mucosa and trap food debris.

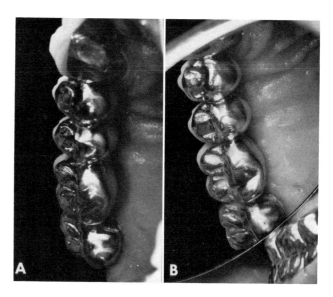

Figure 56–33 Replacement of Saddle-Type Pontics by Bullet-Shaped Pontics Leads to Resolution of Mucosal Inflammation. *A,* Bullet-shaped pontics inserted in area previously covered by saddle-type pontics. Note the inflammation where the saddle-type pontics had been. *B,* After several months, note the excellent condition of the mucosa under the bullet-shaped pontics.

pontics there is an additional concern associated with the contour of the tissue facing surface. In general, this surface should be kept as convex as possible, and all concavities should be eliminated. The convexity of the tissue surfaces of pontics allows oral hygiene procedures to be effective in keeping the tissue of the edentulous ridge healthy. Concavities in the tissue surfaces of pontics result in plaque trap areas where accumulation of dental bacteria will lead to inflammation of the adjacent edentulous tissues (Figs. 56–31 through 56–34).

The bullet-shaped spheroidal pontic (Fig. 56–35) is the most hygienic next to the sanitary type, (Fig. 56–36). The proximal surfaces are tapered to create spaces between adjoining pontics for self-cleansing passage of food and stimulation of the edentulous mucosa by food excursion and for cleansing with toothbrush and dental floss. It should also re-create spaces adjacent to the abutment teeth that approach the shape and dimension of the natural embrasure to protect the marginal gingiva (Fig. 56–34). A pontic no larger than a premolar may be cantilevered off the end of a multi-unit bridge to prevent extrusion of the opposing teeth. Proper contour of such terminal pontics is especially important (Fig. 56–34E), because the absence of protection from a proximal tooth increases the risk of food accumulation under the pontic.

In the posterior segments of the mouth, the bullet-shaped pontic is the most appropriate. In the anterior segments, where esthetics is of primary consideration, the modified ridge lap design may be used (Fig. 56–37). This pontic design should have a convex surface in its tissue facing surface, and the tip of the pontic should just barely contact the edentulous mucosa. Casts should not be scraped or scored in an attempt to seat the pontic into the mucosa, as this creates a depression around the pontic that makes it very difficult to get access for plaque removal. The pontic follows the facial contour of the ridge to the crest where it joins the lingual surface. The lingual surface of the pontic should follow the normal tooth form for a distance of approximately half its occluso-gingival length, then taper in a convex line to meet the facial portion at the crest of the ridge.[59]

The least damaging pontic design is the sanitary or hygienic pontic. This pontic should be designed so that there is at least a 3-mm. space between the undersurface of the pontic and the edentulous ridge; this allows the tongue and cheeks to remove any food particles that may lodge in this area. It is often necessary to use a design other than the hygienic pontic for esthetic reasons.

Saddle type pontics, which straddle the ridge and have a concave tissue facing surface, are the least desirable type of pontic design and should be avoided. Sad-

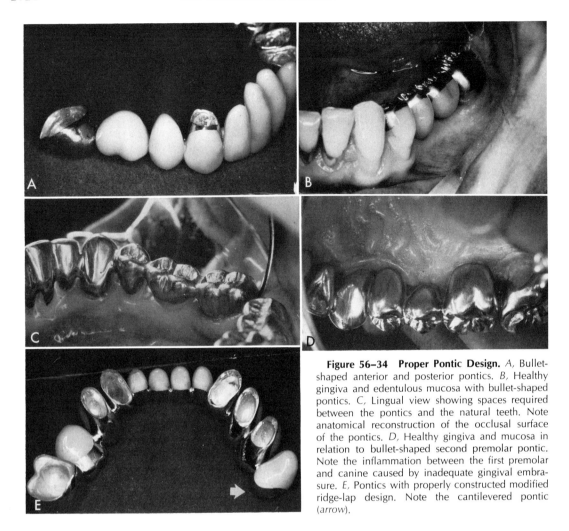

Figure 56–34   Proper Pontic Design. *A,* Bullet-shaped anterior and posterior pontics. *B,* Healthy gingiva and edentulous mucosa with bullet-shaped pontics. *C,* Lingual view showing spaces required between the pontics and the natural teeth. Note anatomical reconstruction of the occlusal surface of the pontics. *D,* Healthy gingiva and mucosa in relation to bullet-shaped second premolar pontic. Note the inflammation between the first premolar and canine caused by inadequate gingival embrasure. *E,* Pontics with properly constructed modified ridge-lap design. Note the cantilevered pontic (*arrow*).

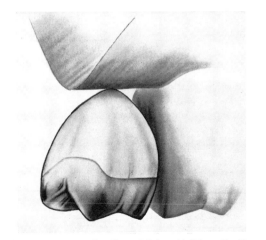

Figure 56–35   Bullet-Shaped Spheroidal Type Pontic.

dle type pontics make it impossible for the patient to control plaque and inevitably result in inflammation of the tissues with which they are in contact.

The natural teeth should guide the design of the occlusal surface of pontics. The width of the occlusal surface should not be narrowed to less than that of the tooth being replaced. The assumption that reduced occlusal width provides occlusal forces more favorable to the periodontium of the abutment teeth has not been proved.

Narrowing the proximal contact areas of posterior teeth causes recession and inflammation of the interdental gingiva. Restoring the width of the contact area leads

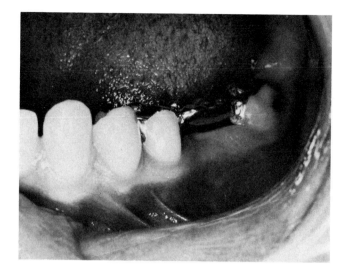

Figure 56–36 Sanitary-Type Fixed Bridge with Healthy Gingiva and Edentulous Mucosa.

to resolution of the inflammation and keratinization of the interdental gingiva. Abnormally shaped spaces between narrowed pontics and broad proximal surfaces of adjacent natural teeth create food impaction problems (Fig. 56–38). Occlusal width is also necessary to shunt the food laterally so that it is not forced into the tissue around the base of the pontic; the gingiva of abutment teeth is especially vulnerable to inflammation and pocket formation.[14]

The functional relationships of the cusps are the most critical consideration in the design of the occlusal surface of pontics. The cusps should be in harmony with the functional pattern of the entire dentition. Abnormal occlusal relationships jeopardize the opposing teeth and the remainder of

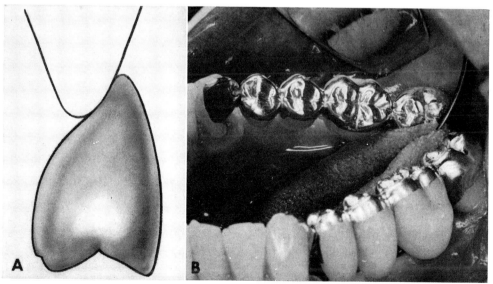

Figure 56–37 Modified Ridge-lap Pontic for Esthetics. *A,* Bullet-shaped pontic extended onto the facial aspects of the edentulous ridge. *B,* Modified ridge-lap type of pontic replacing the first molar. The premolars are bullet-shaped. Note the excellent condition of the mucosa made possible by adequate spaces for food passage.

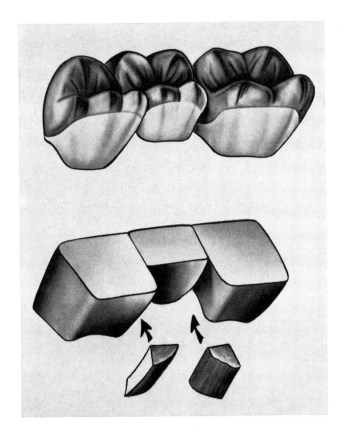

Figure 56–38 Occlusal Width of Pontics. *Above,* Pontic with narrow occlusal width creates food impaction problems. *Below,* Occlusal width required to provide proper proximal relations between pontic and adjacent teeth.

the dentition as well as the periodontium of the abutment teeth.

Cementation

Retained cement particles irritate the gingiva and should be removed. Removal of cement from the interproximal joints of pontics and abutments can be facilitated by coating the exterior surfaces of the prosthesis with mineral oil prior to cementation.

The dentition should be evaluated periodontally, and the teeth to be included in the prosthesis should be determined before the prosthesis is designed. Permanent cementation should not be postponed indefinitely for the ostensible purpose of "testing" questionable teeth.

Failure to finalize cementation of prostheses is contraindicated for several reasons:

1. It interferes with adaptation of the gingiva to the margin of the restorations.

2. Seepage under temporarily cemented restorations may lead to caries and pulp involvement that escape detection, particularly if patients do not adhere to the schedule of periodic removal and recementation.

3. It encourages diagnostic indecision.

4. It is an unnecessary burden to the patient, who is never finished with treatment, while the dentist is repeatedly confronted with a problem case.

5. The technical excellence required for a permanent restoration is often unwittingly compromised by the thought that required corrections can be made "the next time."

REMOVABLE PARTIAL DENTURE PROSTHESES

At the present time, available clinical data show that even with advanced periodontal disease and extensive tooth loss, fixed bridges combined with periodontal therapy including vigorous maintenance therapy can result in periodontal health.[34]

From the periodontal viewpoint, fixed prostheses are the restorations of choice for replacement of missing teeth, but there are some clinical situations where removable partial prostheses are the only possible way to restore the lost function of the dentition. There have been studies on the effect of removable prosthetic appliances on gingival and periodontal health.[5, 46, 55] It has been shown that the teeth that are included in the design of a partial denture have significantly more periodontal destruction than those teeth that are not included in the design.[5] It has also been shown that those patients who have removable prosthetic appliances have worse periodontal health than their counterparts who have a similar dental situation but whose missing teeth have not been replaced.[46] There is increased caries and increased mobility associated with teeth used as abutments for removable prosthodontic appliances.[5, 46] The detrimental effects of caries and periodontal destruction are accentuated in those patients who have poor oral hygiene; therefore, it is unwise to consider a removable partial denture in patients whose oral hygiene is inadequate. A major part of the treatment plan for patients requiring removable partial prostheses is the establishment of a satisfactory level of oral hygiene.[46] The presence of a partial denture increases plaque formation around the remaining teeth,[1] so oral hygiene must receive great emphasis in these patients.

Many different design approaches have been suggested for removable prosthodontic appliances. However, there is no experimental evidence to suggest that one particular design has any great advantage over any other. The choice of an appropriate design is based on clinical judgments and inferences gained from clinical experience.

From the periodontal viewpoint, therefore, a fixed prosthesis is the restoration of choice, but a removable partial prosthesis may also be extremely effective. Its usefulness in the total treatment of periodontal problems should not be minimized.[16] The periodontal implications of removable partial prostheses must be understood so that they will benefit the periodontium and not

cause periodontal destruction and tooth mobility.[13, 32, 35, 46]

Design

To provide maximum stability for removable partial prostheses, every effort should be made to retain posterior teeth for the distal support of the saddle areas.

Some partial denture designs include the use of metal plates as connectors; these plates are positioned so that they cover the gingival tissues.[30, 31] Other designs have suggested that the gingival tissues should be left uncovered as part of the partial denture design and that bars be used as the major connectors.[11] The advocates of covering the gingiva suggest that this minimizes food impaction and calculus formation on the tooth surface. Those who suggest leaving the gingiva free point out the advantages of access to the gingiva by the tongue and muscles of mastication. There is no experimental evidence to support either point of view, and the question of whether the gingiva should be covered or not is unanswered at this stage.

The relationship of the partial denture framework to the distal surface of abutment teeth in a bilateral distal extension partial denture is also an area of controversy. There is some support for the concept of having the metal framework tightly adapted to the distal surface and the gingiva of this tooth,[30, 31] whereas others suggest that this area should be relieved and that no impingement of the denture framework should occur here.[11] Again, there is no real evidence to prove which method is more beneficial to the gingiva, and one must rely on subjective clinical observations in order to justify one or the other of these design philosophies.

Recent clinical research has shown that many patients who were previously treated with removable prosthodontic appliances, e.g., those with bilateral edentulous areas, can be treated with fixed appliances using multiple cantilevered pontics.[34] This controversial approach to the treatment of edentulous areas in patients with advanced periodontal disease has been carefully documented and fol-

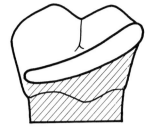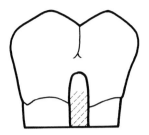

Figure 56–39 Effect of Clasp Design. The amount of gingiva affected by the change in tooth contour associated with a circumferential clasp is much greater than that associated with an I-bar infrabulge clasp.

lowed in many patients over a period of six years. There seems to be no doubt that, if patients are treated for periodontal destruction and then placed on a strict oral hygiene program, distally extending cantilevered pontics can be used in conjunction with fixed prosthodontic appliances. In these cases the occlusal pattern was established by an intraoral technique for developing a functionally generated path over a period of many months in provisional restorations. This type of occlusal pattern is apparently the least destructive to the abutment teeth when they are used as support for multiple pontics.

Clasps

It has been generally accepted that clasps should be passive and exert no force on the teeth when the denture is at rest.[51] Recent research shows that the use of a supra-bulge or circumferential clasp exerts a great deal of force on the abutment tooth[8]—force beyond that required for orthodontic movement even when a wrought wire clasp is used. Such nonfunctional force against the tooth causes the increased mobility that has been reported following the insertion of removable partial dentures. Apparently, after a period of eighteen months to two years, the abutment teeth either move or are able to develop a stronger periodontal support so that their mobility often returns to the denture level of mobility.[42] It has been suggested that the use of an infra-bulge or I-bar design clasp may alleviate the traumatic forces associated with circumferential clasps.[30, 51] However, in one laboratory study the I-clasp design resulted in more movement of abutment teeth than circumferential and back-action clasps. In the

clinical situation, the use of guide planes and I-clasps is associated with a modification of fitting surfaces so that there is equilibration of forces in the abutment teeth—this may result in less force being applied to these teeth. The I-bar clasp has the advantage of producing a minimal change in the buccal surface of the tooth on which it is placed as compared with the circumferential clasp, which affects the buccal contour of the entire surface.[30, 31] The over-contouring of the buccal surface associated with a circumferential clasp on the tooth surface may result in increased gingival inflammation in much the same way as does over-contouring of artificial crowns (Fig. 56–39).

Stress breakers, which connect the retainer and saddle areas by flexible and movable joints, are sometimes used to prevent excessive occlusal forces on abutment teeth. However, comparisons have revealed no advantage of stress breakers over rigid connectors in this respect.[3] With rigid connectors between clasps and saddle areas, the resilience of the mucosa acts as a stress breaker. It permits controlled movement of the prosthesis so that the tissue-borne sections take the initial occlusal stress and prevent sudden impact on the periodontium of the natural teeth.

Occlusal rests

Occlusal rests should be designed to direct the forces along the vertical axis of the tooth. To accomplish this, the rest is seated in a spoon-shaped preparation in the abutment tooth with the floor inclined so that the deepest point is toward the vertical axis of the tooth[24] (Fig. 56–40). This purpose is also accomplished by extending occlusal rests beyond the central

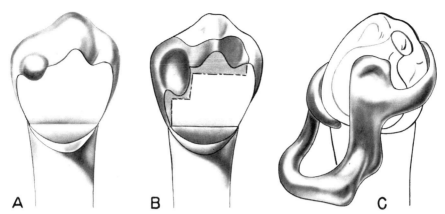

Figure 56–40 Occlusal Rests in Line with Vertical Axis. *A,* Properly constructed lug rest in a premolar without a restoration. *B,* Properly constructed lug rest in a restoration in a premolar. *C,* Clasp in position on a premolar with a lug rest in a restoration (After Dr. Irving R. Hardy, Boston.)

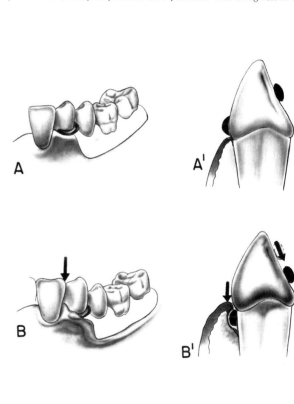

Figure 56–41 "Setting" of a Lingual Bar with an Inadequate Lug Rest on the Canine. *A,* Lingual bar in position. *A¹,* Labiolingual view showing cross-section of labial and lingual arms of the clasp. *B,* Lingual bar settles in direction indicated by *arrow.* *B¹,* Labial arm digs into gingiva; lingual arm slides down along inclined plane of lingual surface. *C,* View of distal surface of canine showing recession of gingiva and marginal gingival disease resulting from settling of partial denture.

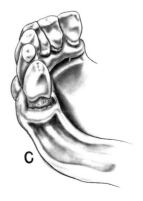

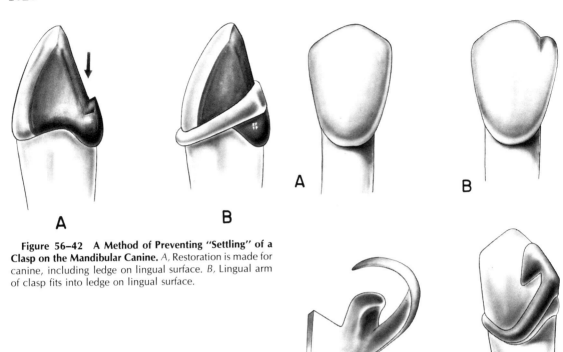

Figure 56–42 A Method of Preventing "Settling" of a Clasp on the Mandibular Canine. *A,* Restoration is made for canine, including ledge on lingual surface. *B,* Lingual arm of clasp fits into ledge on lingual surface.

Figure 56–43 Incisal Stop on Anterior Tooth. *A,* Mandibular canine. *B,* Notch is cut in incisal edge. *C,* View of clasp with incisal rest. *D,* Clasp in position on tooth. (After Dr. Irving R. Hardy, Boston.)

zone of the occlusal surface of premolars or covering the occlusal surface overlying one of the roots of the molars.[39]

Lug rests on inclined lingual surfaces of anterior teeth tend to be spread by occlusal forces so that the denture settles. The facial and lingual arms of the clasp then impinge upon the gingiva, and the connecting bar digs into the lingual mucosa. Pockets form, and the roots are denuded (Fig. 56–41). Spreading of lug rests on anterior teeth can be prevented by constructing a restoration on the abutment teeth with a horizontal ledge on the lingual surface into which the clasp fits (Fig. 56–42). The floor of the ledge should be sloped so as to direct the forces axially. An incisal stop will also prevent settling of clasps (Fig. 56–43). The notch is cut for a slight distance into the tooth substance, at a point approximately one third from the disto-incisal angle. The incisal rest fits into the notch and is tapered to terminate in a point on the facial surface.

Removable partial prostheses should always be constructed with occlusal rests. Rests are sometimes omitted for the osten-sible purpose of reducing axial load on teeth with weakened periodontal support. Such dentures jeopardize the teeth because they settle and cause gingival and periodontal disturbances.

Precision attachments

Precision attachments are used for esthetic reasons and to direct occlusal forces axially rather than laterally. There are many types of precision attachments, and advantages have been demonstrated for some.[23] They cause greater stress and displacement on the abutment teeth of free-end saddle prostheses than is produced by conventional back-action clasps.[47] More evidence is required to establish the relative merits of precision attachments and clasps in terms of their effects upon the periodontium.

Multiple abutments

Multiple abutments reduce injurious lateral and torsional stresses on abutment teeth and should be standard procedure in

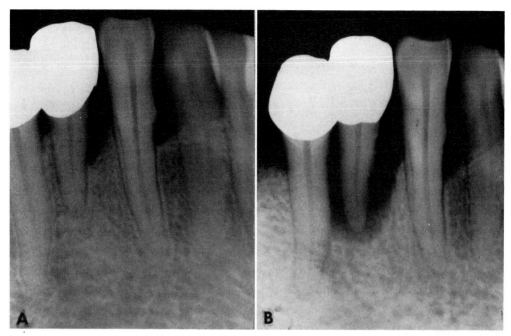

Figure 56–44 Weakened Tooth Splinted to Single Firm Tooth. *A*, First premolar with weakened periodontal support splinted to firm second premolar. *B*, After 3 years, periodontal condition is worse, second premolar is also denuded of bone, and both premolars are mobile.

patients with reduced periodontal support. Multiple abutments are made by connecting inlays or crowns or clasping abutment and adjacent teeth in sequence. When the terminal tooth is periodontally weak, more than one adjacent tooth should be used for added support. Joining a weakened tooth to a strong one is just as likely to weaken the strong tooth as it is to strengthen the weakened one (Fig. 56–44). It is always advisable to consider whether the long-term interest of the patient would be better served by extracting the prospective weak abutment tooth and making a multiple abutment of two adjacent teeth that are relatively well-supported. In patients who have had generalized periodontal involvement, all teeth should be joined together by the partial denture, either by clasping or by inclusion in continuous clasps.

Combined Fixed and Removable Partial Prostheses

Isolated teeth with reduced periodontal support are particularly vulnerable to periodontal injury and loosening when used as abutments in removable partial prostheses. They lack mesial and distal buttressing action to assist in withstanding forces transmitted by the denture. In such cases, fixed and removable prostheses should be combined. The isolated teeth should be joined to their nearest neighbors by a fixed bridge (Fig. 56–45) and can then be used as abutments for removable prostheses.

The use of blade implants as a distal abutment in patients whose natural molar teeth are totally missing has had relatively wide clinical acceptance (Fig. 56–46). However, when reproducible methods are used to follow these cases it is found that the use of such therapeutic approach must be regarded as experimental at this time. There is evidence that the design of many of the blade implants used will prevent the detection of destruction of the tissues surrounding the posts when a periodontal probe is used clinically, even though large amounts of destruction can be detected histologically and radiographically.

Another procedure that has been widely used clinically but remains untested from the standpoint of its effect on periodontal health is the use of overdentures. These full dentures are designed to receive additional support from strategically placed

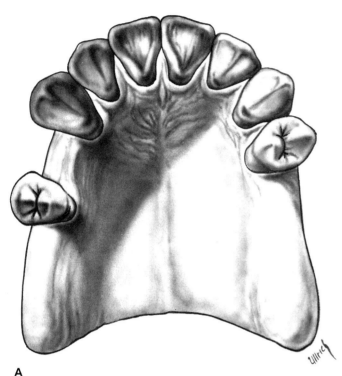

A

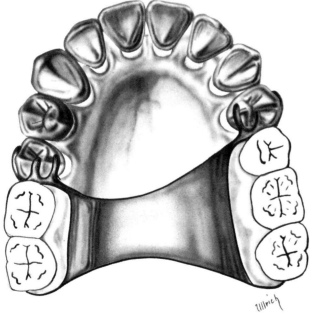

B

Figure 56–45   Combined Fixed and Removable Partial Prosthesis. *A,* Prosthesis required for mouth with isolated second premolar. *B,* Isolated second premolar included in fixed prosthesis before palatal bar is constructed. First premolar is replaced by a pontic.

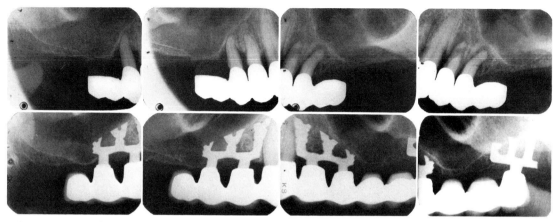

Figure 56–46 Endo-osseous Blade Implant Used as Distal Abutment for Fixed Prosthesis. *Top,* Before. Radiographs showing periodontal and periapical involvement of maxillary premolars with cantilevered distal pontics. *Bottom,* Endo-osseous blade implants replacing two premolars (*left*) and replacing two premolars and providing a distal abutment for the fixed prosthesis (*right*). The entire restoration is a single unit.

teeth, which are prepared in such a way that a dome-like crown is left surrounding the edentulous tissue. It is obvious that oral hygiene is extremely critical when overdentures are installed, and that maintenance of periodontal health in these patients requires special attention to fastidious techniques of dental plaque control.

PERIODONTAL SPLINTING

A splint is an appliance for the immobilization or stabilization of injured or diseased parts. Teeth may be splinted as part of phase I therapy, before periodontal surgery, utilizing temporary or provisional splints. Permanent splints utilizing cast restorations may be placed as part of the restorative phase of therapy.

Splinting of periodontally involved teeth should not be the sole method of obtaining tooth stability. One must always find the etiology for the increased tooth mobility or for the pathological migration of the teeth. Frequently the cause is an abnormal occlusal pattern, i.e., a deflective occlusal contact resulting in nonaxial forces on teeth and/or excessive occlusal forces associated with parafunction (Fig. 56–47). It is imperative that occlusal stability and control of excessive occlusal forces be obtained first, before splinting is applied. Frequently, the modification of occlusal forces will eliminate the need for a splint, as teeth will become less mobile and more stable in their position.

Occlusal forces applied to splints are shared by all teeth within the splint even if the force is applied only to one section

Figure 56–47 Transmission of Forces in a Splint. Excessive occlusal force applied only to second molar (*large arrow*) injures periodontium of all splinted teeth, and in comparable locations. *Small arrows* indicate areas of injury. Location of injury depends upon direction of occlusal force.

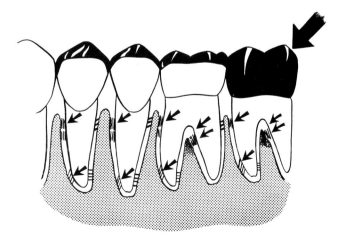

of the splint.[17] The rigidity of a splint allows it to act as a lever, so that the forces applied to some teeth in the splint may be much greater than before splinting.[17] Therefore, the inclusion of a mobile tooth in a splint does not completely relieve it of the burden of occlusal forces, nor does it guarantee against injury from excessive occlusal forces. If one tooth in a splint is in a traumatic occlusal relationship, the periodontal tissues of the remaining teeth may also be injured (see Figure 56–44). Therefore it is of primary importance to stabilize the occlusion prior to splinting.

The use of splinting in periodontal therapy is controversial.[32] There is little evidence to support the much quoted rationale that splinting of mobile teeth enhances the resistance to further periodontal breakdown and improves the healing response.[10, 33] Therefore, the indications for splinting are more limited than many authors believe. Splinting in almost all cases should be of a temporary or provisional type, and permanent splints should only be used where it is necessary for obtaining occlusal stability or for replacement of missing teeth. Permanent splinting does not necessarily reduce the effect of damaging forces on mobile teeth, nor does it predictably reduce mobility.[43]

The two major indications for periodontal splinting are:

1. To immobilize excessively mobile teeth so that the patient can chew more comfortably.

2. To stabilize teeth in their new position after orthodontic movement.

Although there is no agreement as to what degree of tooth mobility is pathological, the use of splints to make patients comfortable when chewing should only be considered for teeth with mobility of 2 or more on a scale of 3. Immediately after periodontal surgery, there is an increase in mobility, which may necessitate the use of a provisional splint during the first six postoperative months. The two procedures of most significance for temporary or provisional stabilization are:

1. The wire and acrylic splint for use in posterior teeth (Fig. 56–48).

2. The acid etch–resin splint for use in anterior teeth (Fig. 56–49).

The introduction of splints into the dental arch generally makes oral hygiene procedures more complex. Therefore, it is important that patients receive special instruction in the techniques required for control of interproximal plaque (see Chapter 43). When an interdental papilla completely fills the embrasure space, the best method of interdental plaque removal is the use of dental floss together with a threader. When the interdental papilla does not fill the embrasure space, the best method for plaque removal is the use of an interdental brush.[15]

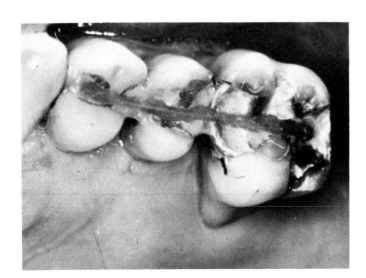

Figure 56–48 Posterior Splint. Wire and acrylic splint. This splint is used for temporary or provisional splinting in posterior teeth with existing amalgam restorations.

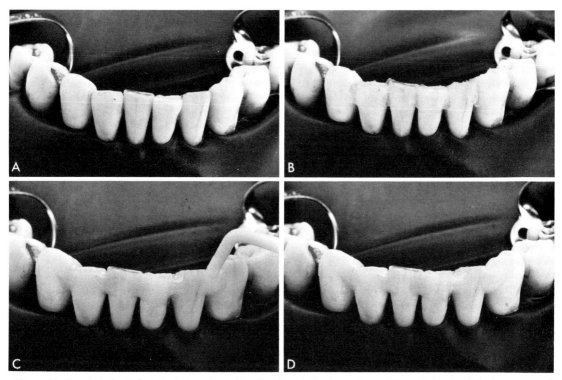

Figure 56–49   Anterior Splint. Technique for acid etch splint. *A,* Teeth are thoroughly scaled and polished to remove all deposits. *B,* Enamel surface is etched with an acid gel for 2 minutes. *C,* Polymerizing resin restorative material is placed on prepared teeth. *D,* Completed splint.

REFERENCES

1. Addy, M., and Bates, J. F.: The effect of partial dentures and chlorhexidine on plaque accumulation in the absence of oral hygiene. J. Clin. Periodontol., *4*:41, 1977.
2. Al Hamadane, K. K., and Crabb, H. S. M.: Marginal adaptation of composite resins. J. Oral. Rehab., *2*:21, 1975.
3. Barkann, L.: The case for metal ligatures in periodontia. J. Sec. District D. Soc. (N.Y.), *31*:341, 1945.
4. Bryan, A. W.: Some common defects in operative restorations contributing to the injury of the supporting structures. J. Am. Dent. Assoc., *14*:1486, 1927.
5. Carlsson, G., Hedegard, B., and Koivumaa, K.: Final results of a 4 year longitudinal investigation of dentogingivally supported partial dentures. Study IV. Acta. Odont. Scand., *23*:443, 1965.
6. Charbeneau, G. T.: A suggested technic for polishing amalgam restorations. J. Mich. State. Dent. Assoc., *47*:320, 1965.
7. Clayton J., and Green, E.: Roughness of pontic materials and dental plaque. J. Pros. Dent., *23*:407, 1970.
8. Clayton, J. A., and Jaslow, C.: A measurement of clasp forces on teeth. J. Pros. Dent., *25*:21, 1971.
9. Coelho, D. H., Cavallaro, J., and Rothschild, E. A.: Gingival recession with electrosurgery for impression making. J. Pros. Dent. *33*:422, 1975.
10. Cross, W.: The importance of immobilization in periodontology. Paradontologie, *8*:119, 1954.
11. Derry, A., and Bertram, U.: A clinical survey of removable partial dentures after 2 years usage. Acta. Odont. Scand., *28*:581, 1970.
12. Donaldson, D.: Gingival recession associated with temporary crowns. J. Periodontol., *44*:691, 1973.
13. Fenner, W., Gerber, A., and Mühlemann, H. R.: Tooth mobility changes during treatment with partial denture prosthesis. J. Pros. Dent., *6*:520, 1956.
14. Fröhlich, Von E.: Zahnfleischrand und Künstliche Krone in pathologisch-anatomischer Sicht. Dtsch. Zahn. Ztschr., *22*:1252, 1967.
15. Gjermo, P., and Flotra, L.: The effect of different methods of interdental cleaning. J. Periodont. Res., *5*:230, 1970.
16. Glickman, I.: The periodontal structures and removable partial denture prostheses. J. Am. Dent. Assoc., *37*:311, 1948.
17. Glickman, I., Stein, R. S., and Smulow, J. B.: The effect of increased functional forces upon the periodontium of splinted and nonsplinted teeth. J. Periodontol., *32*:290, 1961.

18. Glickman, I., and Imber, T.: Comparison of gingival resection with electrosurgery and periodontal knives. J. Periodontol., 41:142, 1970.
19. Goransson, P., and Nyman, L.: Review of methods for exposing the gingival margin. Sci. Ed. Bull. Int. Col. Dent., 2:24, 1969.
20. Henry, P. J., Johnston, J. F., and Mitchell, D. F.: Tissue changes beneath fixed partial dentures. J. Pros. Dent., 16:937, 1966.
21. Hildebrand, G. Y.: The problem of the cervical preparation. Proc. Swed. Dent. Soc., 1927, S.T.T., p. 14.
22. Hildebrand, G. Y.: Studies in Dental Prosthetics. Stockholm: Aktiebolaget Fahlcrantz Boktryckeri, 1937, p. 226.
23. Homma. S., Homma, M., and Nakamura, Y.: Dynamic study of attachments. (Abst.) J. D. Res., 40:228, 1961.
24. Ito, H., Inoue, Y., and Yamada, M.: Three dimensional photoelastic studies on the clasp-rest and tooth extraction. (Abst.) J. Dent. Res., 38:203, 1959.
25. Kaqueler, J. C., and Weiss, M. B.: Plaque accumulation on dental restorative materials. I.A.D.R. Abst., 1970, Abst. 615, p. 202.
26. Karlsen, K.: Gingival reactions to dental restorations. Acta. Odont. Scand., 28:895, 1970.
27. Kelly, W. J., and Harrison, J. D.: Laboratory experimental evaluation of efficiency of clinical electrosurgical techniques. In: M. J. Oringer (Ed.): Electrosurgery in Dentistry, 2nd ed., Philadelphia: W. B. Saunders, 1975.
28. Knowles, J. W., and Snyder, D. T.: The effect of roughness on supragingival and subgingival plaque formation. I.A.D.R. Abst., 1970, Abst. 345, p. 135.
29. Koivumaa, K. K., and Wennstrom, A.: A histologic investigation of the changes in gingival margins adjacent to gold crowns. Sart. UR. Odont. Tska., 68:373, 1960.
30. Kratochvil, F. J.: Influence of occlusal rest position and clasp design on movement of abutment teeth. J. Pros. Dent., 13:114, 1963.
31. Kratochvil, F. J.: Maintaining supporting structures with a removable partial prosthesis. J. Pros. Dent., 26:167, 1971.
32. Krogh-Poulsen, W.: Partial denture design in relation to occlusal trauma and periodontal breakdown. Int. Dent. J., 4:847, 1954.
33. McCune, R. J., Phillips, R. W., Swartz, M. L., and Mumford, G.: The effect of occlusal venting and film thickness on the cementation of full cast crowns, J. South. Cal. Dent. Assoc., 39:36, 1971.
34. Nyman, S., Lindhe, J., and Lundgren, D.: The role of occlusion for the stability of fixed bridges in patients with reduced periodontal support. J. Clin. Periodontol., 2:53, 1975.
35. Osborne, J., Brills, N., and Lammie, G. A.: Partial dentures. Int. Dent. J., 7:26, 1957.
36. O'Leary, T. M., Standish, S. M., and Coomer, R. S.: Severe periodontal destruction following impression procedures. J. Periodontol., 44:43, 1973.
37. Parkinson, C. F.: Excessive crown contours facilitate endemic plaque niches. J. Pros. Dent., 35:424, 1976.
38. Perel, M.: Axial crown contours. J. Pros. Dent., 25:642, 1971.
39. Plitzner, J.: Role of occlusal rest lug as transmitter of masticating stress. Dent. Reform., 42:77, 1938.
40. Podshadley, A. G.: Gingival response to pontics. J. Pros. Dent., 19:51, 1968.
41. Price, C., and Whitehead, F. J. H.: Impression material as foreign bodies. Br. Dent. J., 133:9, 1972.
42. Rateitschak, K. H.: The therapeutic effect of local treatment on periodontal disease assessed upon evaluation of different diagnostic criteria. I. Changes as to mobility. J. Periodontol., 34:540, 1963.
43. Renggli, H. H.: Splinting of teeth an objective assessment. Helv. Odontol. Acta, 15:129, 1971.
44. Rosenberg, R., and Ash, M. M.: The effect of root roughness on plaque accumulation and gingival inflammation. J. Periodontol., 45:146, 1974.
45. Sacket, B. P., and Gildenhuys, R. R.: The effect of axial crown overcontour on adolescents. J. Periodontol., 47:320, 1976.
46. Seemann, S. K.: Study of the relationship between periodontal disease and the wearing of partial dentures. Australian Dent. J., 8:206, 1963.
47. Shohet, H.: Relative magnitudes of stress on abutment teeth and different retainers. J. Pros. Dent., 21:267, 1969.
48. Shooshan, E. D.: A pin-ledge casting technique—its application in periodontal splinting. Dent. Clin. North Am., March 1960, p. 189.
49. Silness, J.: Treated with dental bridges III. The relationship between the location of the crown margin and the periodontal condition. J. Periodontol. Res., 5:225, 1970.
50. Sotres, L. S., Van Huysen, G., and Gilmore, H. W.: A histologic study of gingival response to amalgam silicate and resin restorations. J. Periodontol., 40:543, 1969.
51. Steffel, V. L.: Clasp partial dentures, J. Am. Dent. Assoc., 66:803, 1963.
52. Stein, R. S.: Pontic-residual ridge relationship: a research report. J. Pros. Dent., 16:251, 1966.
53. Stein, R. S., and Glickman, I.: Prosthetic considerations essential for gingival health. Dent. Clin. North Am., March, 1960, p. 177.
54. Taylor, S. M.: The polishing effectiveness of zircate, silex, and pumice on curetted root surfaces. Thesis. Ann Arbor: University of Michigan School of Dentistry, 1967.
55. Tomlin, M., and Osborne, J.: Cobalt-chromium partial dentures: a clinical survey. Br. Dent. J., 110:307, 1961.
56. Waerhaug, J.: Effect of rough surfaces upon gingival tissues. J. Dent. Res., 35:323, 1956.
57. Weitman, R. T., and Eames, W. B.: Plaque accu-

mulation on composite surfaces after various finishing procedures J. Am. Dent. Assoc., *91*: 101, 1975.

58. Wheeler, R. C.: A Textbook of Dental Anatomy and Physiology. 3rd ed. Philadelphia: W. B. Saunders Co., 1958, pp. 64–65.

59. Wing, C.: Pontic design and construction in fixed bridgework. Dent. Prac. Dent. Rec., *12*:390, 1962.

60. Wilhelmsem, N. R., Ramfjord, S. P., and Blankenship, J. R.: Effects of electrosurgery on the gingival attachment in rhesus monkeys. J. Periodontol., *47*:160, 1976.

61. Yuodelis, R. A., Weaver, J. D., and Sapkos, S.: Facial and lingual contours of artificial complete crowns and their effect on the periodontium. J. Pros. Dent., *29*:61, 1973.

Chapter 57

Periodontal–Orthodontic Interrelationships

ORTHODONTIC PROCEDURES IN PERIODONTAL TREATMENT

Orthodontic procedures to restore satisfactory functional relationships[1, 8, 14, 15] are sometimes required in periodontal therapy. The advisability of undertaking orthodontic correction depends upon the following factors: (1) the severity of the occlusal problem and its correctability by orthodontics, (2) the level of the remaining bone, and (3) the possibility of the periodontal and occlusal conditions worsening without orthodontic correction. Reduced bony support caused by periodontal disease does not contraindicate orthodontic treatment unless the remaining bone is insufficient to withstand ordinary functional requirements. **Repositioning teeth in the bone so as to direct occlusal forces in the vertical axis increases the longevity of teeth with reduced bony support.**

Gingival inflammation interferes with the effectiveness of orthodontic appliances and should be eliminated before orthodontic treatment is begun. Inflammation causes degeneration of periodontal ligament fibers and impairs their ability to transmit external forces to the bone. This dissipates the orthodontic forces and delays the desired bone response and tooth movement.

Teeth can often be repositioned in relatively uncomplicated mechanotherapy with the Hawley appliance, grassline or wire ligatures, or rubber dam elastics, either singly or in combination. **No tooth movement should be undertaken before the patient's problem has been thoroughly analyzed.** Supposedly "minor" tooth movement may lead to unexpected complications unless it is planned in conformity with the overall pattern of forces involved in the maintenance of tooth-to-tooth and arch-to-arch relationships.

Correction of Pathological Migration

The following factors should be considered when orthodontic correction of migrated teeth is contemplated:

1. The availability of space for the teeth to be repositioned.

2. The absence of interference from teeth in the opposing arch.

3. The extent to which loss of posterior tooth support, reduced vertical dimension, and accentuated anterior overbite complicate tooth movement.

4. The availability of sufficient anchorage from which forces can be applied.

5. Habits that may interfere with the desired tooth movement.

Hawley appliance for the correction of pathological migration

The Hawley appliance is a removable tissue-borne appliance with an anterior wire frame extension or labial bow. It may be modified in a variety of ways for moving individual teeth (Fig. 57–1) and is most often used on the maxilla. The tissue-borne portion covers the palate, is usually constructed of acrylic, and may have clasps on the posterior teeth for added retention. To prevent irritation to the gingiva it should cover approximately one-third the length of the crowns. The margin is cut away when necessary to create space for the desired tooth movement.

The labial bow is embedded in the acrylic and extends through the interproximal spaces between the canines and premolars onto the facial surfaces of the anterior teeth (Fig. 57–1). When used on the mandible, the tissue-borne portion is horseshoe-shaped and may be made of acrylic or metal, depending on the strength required.

To correct pathological migration of maxillary anterior teeth, the wire labial bow or rubber dam elastics attached to hooks embedded in the acrylic at the distal surface of each canine are used. The appliance should be worn at all times until the desired tooth movements are effected (Fig. 57–2).

When excessive overbite interferes with

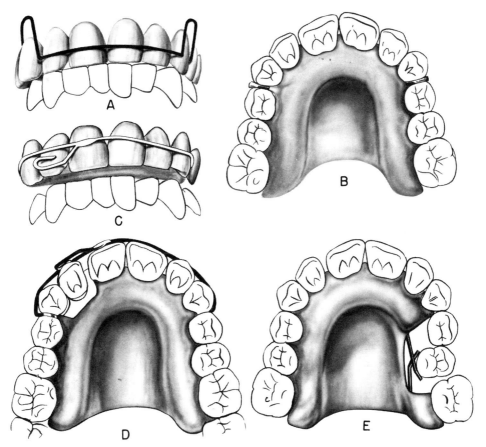

Figure 57–1 The Hawley Appliance. *A,* Hawley appliance with labial bow. *B,* Acrylic tissue-borne portion covers approximately one third of the length of the crowns. *C,* Wire soldered to labial bow to move lateral incisor. The palatal acrylic is used as an anterior bite palate. *D,* Palatal view showing acrylic cut away to provide space for the lateral incisor. *E,* Wire spring embedded in acrylic to move the second premolar buccally. If necessary, the proximal tooth surfaces are stripped to provide space.

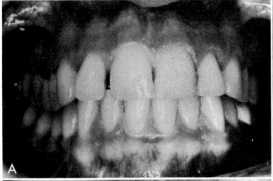
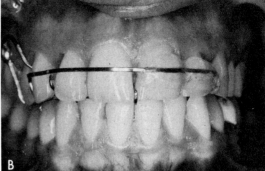
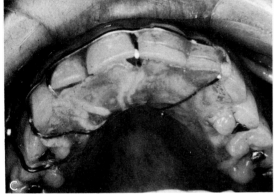

Figure 57–2 Correction of Pathological Migration. A, Pathological migration of maxillary lateral incisor. B, Hawley appliance with wire spring on distal surface of lateral accomplishes desired movement. C, Lingual view of labial bow with wire spring to lateral incisor.

the movement of the anterior teeth, the acrylic may be brought onto the occlusal surfaces of the posterior teeth to create enough space anteriorly to permit the lingual movement of the maxillary anterior teeth (Fig. 57–3). After the desired anterior tooth movement is attained, the Hawley appliance is replaced by a prosthesis on the posterior teeth to retain the vertical dimension.

When the mandibular anterior teeth are procumbent so that there is insufficient overjet to permit lingual movement of the maxillary teeth, the mandibular teeth are retracted to provide the necessary space.

Stabilization of migrated anterior teeth

After migration has been corrected, an effort is made to create an environment in which the teeth will be stable without artificial retention. The entire occlusion is adjusted to eliminate prematurities that would tend to displace the teeth. Grinding the anterior teeth alone may leave the pa-

tient with posterior prematurities that deflect the mandible anteriorly against the maxillary teeth and cause them to migrate again. Tongue-thrusting habits, grinding, and clenching also tend to displace the teeth, particularly those with weakened periodontal support.

If the teeth tend to separate after the occlusion is adjusted, they should be stabilized with fixed internal retention. The teeth are brought back into position and splinted from first premolar to first premolar with inlays, which require a minimal loss of tooth structure.

Correction of Malposed Teeth

Grassline ligatures and rubber dam elastics[9] are useful for the correction of malposed individual teeth. With grassline ligatures, tooth movement is effected by contraction of the ligature after it absorbs moisture from the mouth. The dry ligature is applied in such a manner that the force created by contraction is in the direction

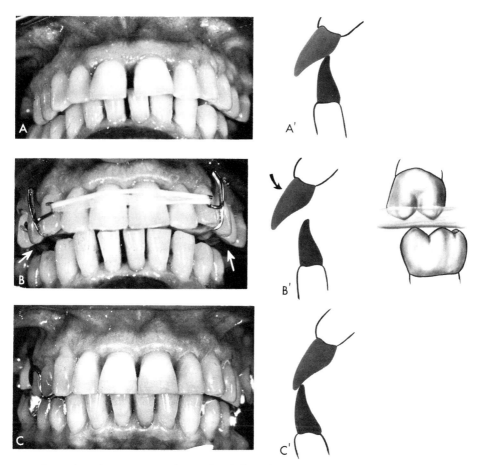

Figure 57–3 Correction of Excessive Overbite and Pathological Migration by Combining Orthodontic and Prosthetic Procedures. *A,* Excessive anterior overbite and spacing of anterior teeth in patient with periodontal disease. *A',* diagrammatic representation of anterior overbite. *B,* Hawley appliance used to correct migration of anterior teeth, using elastics. The acrylic portion of the appliance is extended over the occlusal surfaces of the posterior teeth (*arrows*) to increase the vertical dimension and permit lingual movement of maxillary anterior teeth. The appliance is constructed of clear acrylic, which is not visible on the photograph. *B',* Space created between anterior teeth by using posterior acrylic bite plane. *C,* Prosthesis constructed to retain newly established vertical dimension. *C',* Newly established relationships of anterior teeth.

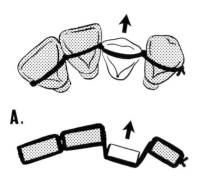

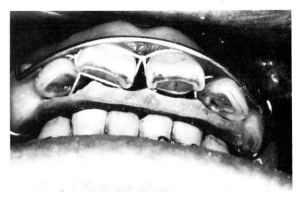

Figure 57–5 Grassline Ligature used in conjunction with bite plate to correct rotated teeth.

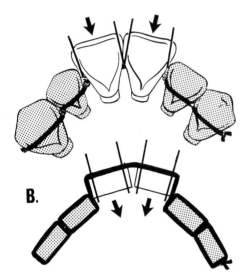

Figure 57–4 Grassline Ligature to Correct Malposition. *A,* Repositioning of lingually placed lateral incisor. *B,* Two labially placed central incisors are brought into proper alignment. The proximal surfaces of the incisors may be trimmed (*vertical lines*) to fit into available space.

of desired tooth movement. Particular care must be taken to include a sufficient number of teeth for anchorage (Figs. 57–4 and 57–5). **The ligature should be placed close to the contact points, incisal to the cingulum, to prevent slipping and irritation of the gingiva.** Ligatures are usually replaced weekly until the desired tooth movement is attained.

Teeth can be moved more rapidly with rubber dam elastics, but risk of damage to the supporting tissues is greater. Rootward sliding of the band with injury to the periodontium and extrusion of teeth are infrequent complications of the use of rubber dam elastics.

Crowded mandibular anterior teeth

Crowded and malposed teeth frequently present a problem from both the periodontal and orthodontic viewpoints (Fig. 57–6). The gingiva around teeth in labial version is often attached apical to the level on the adjacent teeth. On teeth in lingual version, the labial gingiva is often enlarged and attracts irritating plaque and debris. Orthodontic correction of malposed teeth creates gingival contours more conducive to periodontal health.

A tooth may be extracted to correct crowding (Fig. 57–7), provided the extraction creates sufficient space for proper alignment of the teeth that remain. Another consideration when tooth extraction is being contemplated is the degree of overbite. Normally, the mandibular teeth are "contained within" the maxillary arch. Extraction of a mandibular incisor may result in "closing in" of the arch with increase in the overbite and the possibility of undesirable periodontal sequelae.

Another consideration when tooth extraction is contemplated is the mechanics required to realign the remaining teeth without proximal tipping. Improper proximal contacts create areas of potential food impaction. Where possible, it is preferable to avoid tooth extraction by judicious grinding of the proximal surfaces to create space for the crowded teeth (Fig. 57–8).

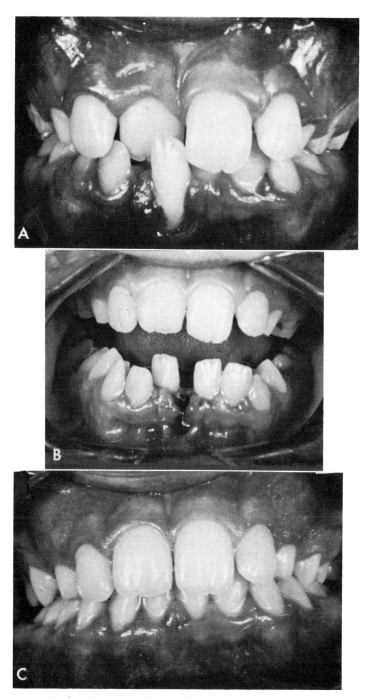

Figure 57–6   Improvement in the Gingival Condition Following Correction of Crowding in the Mandibular Anterior Region. *A,* Marked gingival disease associated with malocclusion. *B,* Central incisor removed. *C,* Improved condition of the gingiva associated with improvement in the tooth relationship after orthodontic treatment. (Courtesy Dr. Coenraad F. A. Moorrees, Forsyth Dental Center.)

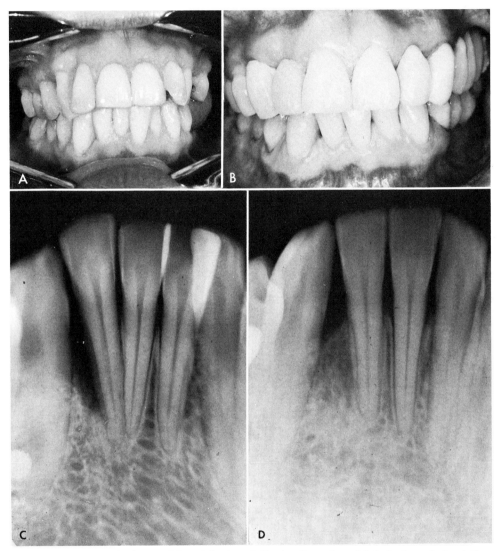

Figure 57–7   Improvement in the Condition of the Bone Following Correction of Anterior Irregularity. A, Crowding of mandibular teeth with left central incisor in labial version. B, After treatment, which included extraction of the right lateral incisor, alignment of the anterior teeth, and prosthesis. C, Before treatment. Note the angular bone defect. D, Three years after treatment. Note improvement in the bone. (Restorations by Dr. Philip Williams, Lynn, Mass.)

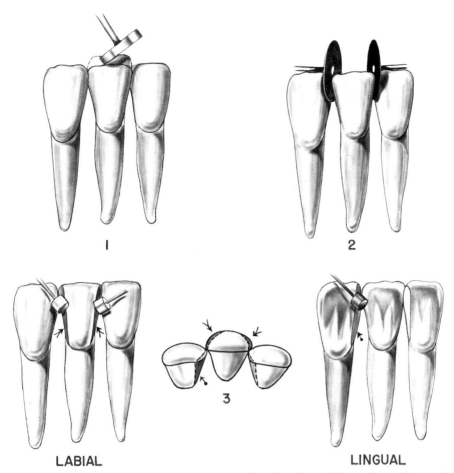

I   2

LABIAL   LINGUAL

Figure 57–8   Grinding as an Adjunct to the Treatment of Malposed and Extruded Anterior Teeth. *1,* Reduction of the incisal edge of a prominent mandibular anterior tooth. *2,* Grinding of the proximal surfaces of a mandibular tooth in labial version as well as the proximal surfaces of the adjacent teeth to provide space for proper alignment. *3,* Where space cannot be provided by grinding the proximal surfaces as illustrated in (2), the mesial and distal aspects of the labial surface of the malposed tooth are reduced along with the marginal ridges on the lingual surfaces of the adjacent teeth.

Crossbite relationship

Crossbite relationships often result in food impaction and trauma from occlusion. A comparatively simple procedure may be used effectively to correct single teeth in facial, or lingual version if space in the arch permits. The malposed tooth on each arch is banded with a hook on the facial surface of the tooth in facial version and the lingual surface of its antagonist. A "cross" elastic attached to the hooks results in the restoration of proper alignment (Fig. 57–9). The occlusion should then be adjusted.

Occasionally, an anterior crossbite occurs in patients with a pseudoprognathic mandibular relationship. The maxillary teeth are in lingual version, but the anterior teeth are edge-to-edge when the mandible is retruded (Fig. 57–10A and B). The condition may sometimes be corrected with a Hawley appliance by temporarily opening the bite and pushing the maxillary anterior teeth forward, but comprehensive mechanotherapy on both jaws is often required (Fig. 57–10C).

Correction of Anterior Open Bite

An anterior open bite may impair periodontal health if attended by inadequate functional stimulation to the gingiva and the supporting tissues. Some of the unde-

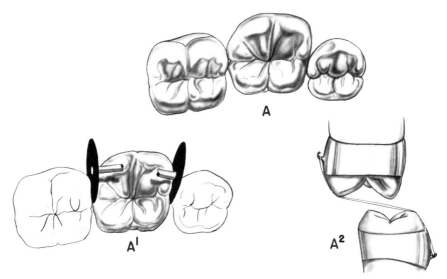

Figure 57–9 Crossbite Relationship of First Molars Corrected by Intermaxillary Elastics. *A,* Mandibular first molar in buccal version. *A¹,* Reduction of the mesiodistal diameter to permit the molar to fit into the available space. *A²,* Orthodontic bands and intermaxillary elastic in position.

sirable sequelae include accumulation of plaque and food debris with resultant chronic gingivitis, atrophy of the alveolar bone around the anterior teeth, and trauma to the periodontium of the posterior teeth. Bites that are slightly open anteriorly may be reduced by judiciously grinding the posterior teeth, but if this is not feasible, orthodontic therapy is indicated.

OCCLUSAL ADJUSTMENT IN ORTHODONTIC THERAPY

Occlusal forces created by orthodontically corrected dentitions affect the condition of the periodontium upon which the stability of the renovated occlusion depends. The anatomical and esthetic goals of orthodontics have been expanded to include the attainment of satisfactory occlusal relationships, and occlusal adjustment has become an integral part of orthodontic therapy.

Occlusion During Active Orthodontic Treatment

The periodontal tissues cannot differentiate between the forces of occlusion and those created by orthodontic appliances. Both types of forces are transmitted to the periodontium together, and tooth movement results from their combined effect rather than from the appliances alone.[11] Injurious occlusal forces in the course of tooth movement detract from the efficiency of orthodontic appliances. Unfavorable occlusal forces may be unavoidable during tooth movement, but the damage they produce should be minimized by checking the occlusion each time appliances are adjusted and correcting gross prematurities in retruded contact position and in intercuspal position (for occlusal adjustment, see Chapter 55).

Occlusion During and After the Retention Period

Orthodontic therapy is incomplete so long as the dentition functions so as to injure the periodontium. The occlusion should be adjusted before and during the retention period for several reasons: injurious occlusal forces during the retention period interfere with the maturation of bone and the stabilization of tooth position and may defeat the purpose of the retaining device. Teeth held firmly in a retain-

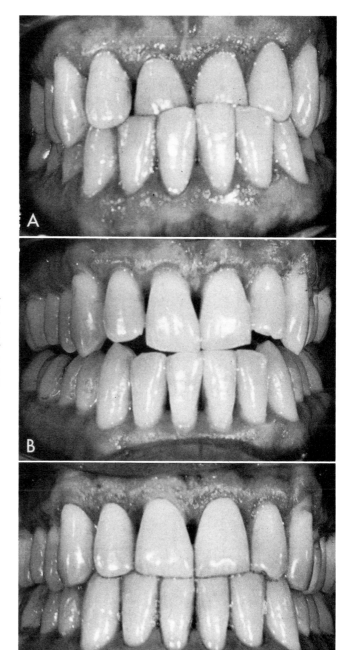

Figure 57–10 Anterior Crossbite Relationship. *A,* Patient with anterior crossbite and associated periodontal disease. *B,* Determination of centric indices that the crossbite is a "habitual" occlusion and that the anterior teeth are edge to edge when the mandible is in centric. *C,* After periodontal treatment which includes orthodontic correction (compare with *A*).

ing device are more vulnerable to trauma from occlusion because they cannot move away from injurious forces.

After retainers are removed, **uncontrolled drifting of the teeth ("settling in") cannot be relied upon to provide satisfactorily functioning occlusion.** Teeth may "settle into" positions that are esthetically acceptable and meet the requirements of static jaw relationships, but the dentition must be checked in function. "Settling in" should be accompanied by occlusal adjustment to avoid trauma that injures the periodontium and increases the risk of collapse of the newly created occlusion.

Hawley appliances should not be used as permanent retainers in orthodontically treated patients; they are periodontally contraindicated. The appliances are usually worn at night with the result that the periodontium is injured and the teeth become loosened as a result of the in-terplay between daytime pressures in one direction and nighttime pressures in the other. Young adults who do not wear their appliance until spaces reappear between their teeth create greater periodontal damage when they try to force the teeth back into the retainer.

For teeth with a persistent tendency toward migration after orthodontic therapy, the interest of the periodontium is best served by adjusting the entire occlusion and splinting the offending teeth into the adjusted occlusion.

PERIODONTAL PROBLEMS ASSOCIATED WITH ORTHODONTIC THERAPY

RETENTION OF PLAQUE. Orthodontic appliances tend to retain bacterial plaque and food debris, resulting in gingivitis (Fig. 57–11). Patients should be taught

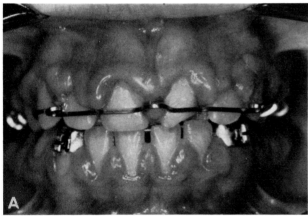

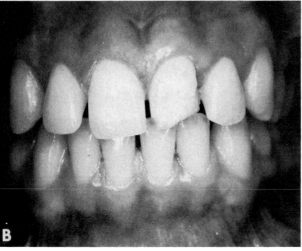

Figure 57–11 Gingival Inflammation and Enlargement Associated with Orthodontic Appliance and Poor Oral Hygiene. A, Gingival disease with orthodontic appliance in place. B, After removal of the appliance and periodontal treatment.

proper oral hygiene methods when appliances are inserted, and their importance should be stressed. The condition of the periodontium should be checked regularly during orthodontic treatment and periodontal care should be instituted at the earliest sign of disease. Water irrigation under pressure is a helpful oral hygiene aid for these patients.

IRRITATION FROM ORTHODONTIC BANDS. Orthodontic treatment is often started at a stage of tooth eruption when the junctional epithelium is still on the enamel. The bands should not extend into the gingival tissues beyond the level of attachment. Forceful detachment of the gingiva from the tooth followed by apical proliferation of the junctional epithelium results in the increased gingival recession sometimes seen in orthodontically treated patients.[12] If gingival inflammation is present, the gingival margin is prevented from following the migrating epithelium, and pocket formation results.

TISSUE RESPONSE TO ORTHODONTIC FORCES. Orthodontic tooth movement is possible because the periodontal tissues are responsive to externally applied forces.[13, 15] The bone is remodeled by an increase in osteoclasts and bone resorption in areas of pressure, and by increased osteoblastic activity and bone formation in areas of tension. Orthodontic forces also produce vascular changes in the periodontal ligament that may influence the bone resorptive and bone formative patterns.[4, 7]

Radioautographic and histochemical studies indicate that cellular proliferation in the periodontal ligament may be related to the magnitude of orthodontic forces,[17] that alkaline phosphatase in periodontal ligament cells is decreased in areas of pressure,[17] and that oxidative enzyme activity is intensified in the periodontium in areas of orthodontically induced bone resorption and formation.[5]

TISSUE INJURY FROM ORTHODONTIC FORCES. From the periodontal viewpoint, it is important to avoid excessive forces and too rapid tooth movement in orthodontic treatment. Excessive force may produce necrosis of the periodontal ligament and adjacent alveolar bone, which ordinarily undergo repair. However, destruction of the periodontal ligament at the crest of

the alveolar bone may lead to irreparable damage. If the periodontal fibers beneath the junctional epithelium are destroyed by excessive force and the epithelium is stimulated to proliferate along the root by local irritants, **the epithelium will cover the root and prevent reembedding of the periodontal fibers in the course of repair. Absence of functional stimulation from the periodontal fibers may result in atrophy of the crest of the alveolar bone.** Excessive orthodontic forces also increase the risk of apical root resorption.[19]

It has been reported that the marginal and attached gingiva are "pulled" when teeth are orthodontically rotated,[6] and that relapse of the occlusion after orthodontic treatment can be reduced by surgical resection or removal of free gingival fibers, combined with a brief retention period.[3, 10] Temporary separation of the reduced enamel epithelium of the tension side of orthodontically moved teeth and displacement and folding of the interdental papillae on the pressure side have also been noted.[2]

REFERENCES

1. Alexander, P. C.: Orthodontic procedures in periodontal therapy. J. Periodontol., 28:46, 1957.
2. Atherton, J. D., and Kerr, N. W.: Effect of orthodontic tooth movement upon the gingivae. Br. Dent. J., 124:555, 1968.
3. Brain, W. E.: The effect of surgical transsection of free gingival fibers on the regression of orthodontically rotated teeth in the dog. Am. J. Orthodont., 55:50, 1969.
4. Castelli, W. A., and Dempster, W. T.: The periodontal vasculature and its responses to experimental pressures. J. Am. Dent. Assoc., 70:891, 1965.
5. Deguchi, T., and Mori, M.: Histochemical observations on oxidative enzymes in periodontal tissues during experimental tooth movement in the rat. Arch. Oral Biol., 13:49, 1968.
6. Edwards, J. G.: A study of the periodontium during orthodontic rotation of teeth. Am. J. Orthodont., 54:441, 1968.
7. Gianelly, A. A.: Force-induced changes in the vascularity of the periodontal ligament. Am. J. Orthodont., 55:5, 1969.
8. Granerus, R.: Some orthodontic-therapeutic aspects of the treatment of periodontal diseases. Sveriges Tandlak. Forb. Tidn., 47:455, 1955.
9. Hirschfeld, L., and Geiger, A.: Minor tooth movement in general practice. St. Louis, C. V. Mosby Co., 1966.
10. Moffett, B. C.: Remodeling changes of the facial

sutures, periodontal and temporomandibular joints produced by orthodontic forces in Rhesus monkeys. Bull. Pacif. Coast Soc. Orthodont., 44:46, 1969.

11. Parodi, R. J., Carranza, F. A., Jr., and Cabrini, R. L.: Combined effect of trauma from occlusion and orthodontic movement in periodontal bone response. (Abs.) J. Dent. Res., 48:1082, 1969.

12. Pearson, L. E.: Gingival height of lower central incisors, orthodontically treated and untreated. Angle Orthodont., 38:337, 1968.

13. Reitan, K.: Tissue changes following experimental tooth movement as related to the time factor. Dent. Rec., 73:559, 1953.

14. Rothenberg, S., and Shapiro, E.: The orthodontic management of functional problems in periodontal therapy. Dent. Clin. North Am., March, 1960, p. 143.

15. Schwartz, A. M.: Tissue changes incidental to orthodontic tooth movement. Ortho., Oral Surg., Rad., Int. J., 18:331, 1932.

16. Shapiro, M.: Orthodontic procedures in the care of the periodontal patient. J. Periodontol, 27:7, 1956.

17. Takimoto, K., Deguchi, T., and Mori, M.: Histochemical detection of acid and alkaline phosphatases in periodontal tissues after experimental tooth movement. J. Dent. Res., 47:340, 1968.

18. Tayer, B. H., Gianelly, A. A., and Ruben, M. P.: Visualization of cellular dynamics associated with orthodontic tooth movement. Am. J. Ortho., 54:515, 1968.

19. Tirk, T. M., Guzman, C. A., and Nalchajian, R.: Periodontal tissue response to orthodontic treatment studied by panoramix. Angle Ortho., 37:94, 1967.

Maintenance Phase

Maintenance Care

Preservation of the periodontal health of the treated patient requires as positive a program as the elimination of periodontal disease. After treatment is completed, patients are placed on a program of periodic recall visits for maintenance care to prevent recurrence of the disease.

Transfer of the patient from active treatment status to a maintenance program is a definitive step in total patient care that requires time and effort on the part of the dentist and staff. Patients must be made to understand the purpose of the maintenance program, with emphasis on the fact that preservation of the teeth is dependent upon it. In fact, a recent study has found that tooth loss in treated cases is three times as great in patients who do not return for regular recall.[3] It is meaningless simply to inform patients that they are to return for periodic recall visits without pinpointing their significance and without describing what is expected of the patients between visits.

THE MAINTENANCE PROGRAM

Periodic recall visits form the foundation of a meaningful long-term prevention program. The interval between visits is set initially at three months but may be varied according to the patient's needs.

Periodontal care at each recall visit consists of two phases. The first is concerned with examination and evaluation of the patient's current oral health. The second phase of the recall appointment involves the necessary maintenance treatment and oral hygiene reinforcement.

Examination and evaluation

The recall examination is similar to the initial evaluation of the patient discussed in Chapter 32. However, since the patient is not new to the office, the dentist will primarily be looking for changes that have occurred since the last evaluation. Analysis of the current oral hygiene status of the patient is essential. Updating of changes in the medical history and evaluation of restorations, caries, prostheses, occlusion, tooth mobility, gingival status, and periodontal pockets are important parts of the recall appointment. The oral mucosa should be carefully inspected for pathologic conditions.

A complete series of intra-oral radiographs is taken every two to four years, depending on the initial severity of the case and the findings at the recall visit. These are compared with previous radiographs in order to check the bone height, the repair of osseous defects, signs of trauma from occlusion, periapical pathology, and caries.

Checking plaque control

Plaque control in the patient's mouth should be checked with disclosing agents (see Chapter 42). It is helpful to store patients' toothbrushes and interdental cleansers in the dental office in individual plastic boxes for use at recall visits. Plaque control must be reviewed and corrected until the patient demonstrates the necessary proficiency, even if it requires additional instruction sessions. Patients instructed in plaque control have less plaque and gingivitis than uninstructed patients.[1, 4–15]

Treatment phase

The required scaling and root planing are performed followed by an oral prophylaxis (see Chapter 44).

RECURRENCE OF PERIODONTAL DISEASE

Occasionally, lesions may recur. This can usually be traced to inadequate plaque control on the part of the patient. It should be realized, however, that it is the dentist's responsibility to teach, motivate, and control the patient's oral hygiene technique and that the patient's failure is our failure. Surgery should not be undertaken unless the patient has shown proficiency and willingness to cooperate by performing adequately his or her part of therapy.[13]

Other causes for recurrence are the following:

1. Inadequate or insufficient treatment that has failed to remove all the potential factors favoring plaque accumulation. Incomplete calculus removal in areas with difficult access is a common source of problems.

2. Inadequate restorations placed after the periodontal treatment was completed.

3. The patient's not coming for periodical check-ups. This may be due to the patient's conscious or unconscious decision not to continue treatment or to the dentist and staff's not having emphasized the need for periodic examinations.

4. Some systemic diseases that may affect host resistance to previously acceptable levels of plaque.

A failing case can be recognized by:

1. Recurring inflammation discovered by gingival changes and bleeding of the sulcus upon probing.

2. Increasing depth of sulci leading to recurrence of pocket formation.

3. Gradual increases in bone loss, recognized by the radiograph.

4. Gradual increases in tooth mobility as ascertained by clinical examination.

The decision to re-treat a periodontal patient should not be made at the preventive maintenance appointment but should be postponed for one or two weeks.[2] Often the mouth will look a great deal better at that time, owing to resolution of edema and improved tone of the gingiva. A summary of

TABLE 58–1 SYMPTOMS AND CAUSES OF RECURRENCE OF DISEASE

Symptom	Possible Causes
Increased Inflammation	Poor oral hygiene. Subgingival calculus. Deteriorating or inadequate restorations. Deteriorating or poorly designed prostheses. Systemic disease modifying host response to plaque.
Recession	Toothbrush abrasion. Inadequate attached gingiva
Increased Mobility with No Change in Pocket Depth and No Radiographic Change	Occlusal trauma due to lateral occlusal interference. Bruxism. High restoration. Poorly designed or worn-out prosthesis. Poor crown-to-root ratio.
Increased Pocket Depth with No Radiographic Change	Poor oral hygiene. Infrequent recall. Subgingival calculus. Poorly fitting partial dentures. Mesial drifting into edentulous space. Failure of new attachment surgery.
Increased Pocket Depth with Increased Radiographic Bone Loss	Poor oral hygiene. Subgingival calculus. Infrequent recall. Inadequate or deteriorating restorations. Poorly designed prosthesis. Inadequate surgery. Systemic disease modifying host response to plaque.

the symptoms of recurrence of periodontal disease and the probable causes can be found in Table 58–1.

CLASSIFICATION OF POST-TREATMENT PATIENTS

The first year following periodontal therapy is important in terms of indoctrinating the patient in a recall habit pattern and reinforcement of oral hygiene. In addition, it may take several months to evaluate the results of some periodontal surgery procedures accurately. Consequently, some areas may have to be re-treated because results

TABLE 58–2 RECALL INTERVALS FOR VARIOUS CLASSES OF RECALL PATIENTS

Classification	Characteristics	Recall Interval
Class A	First-year patient. Routine therapy. Uneventful healing.	3 months
	First-year patient. "Difficult" case. Complicated prosthesis, furcation involvement, questionable patient cooperation.	1 to 2 months
Class B	Excellent results maintained well for one or more years. Patient displays good oral hygiene, minimal calculus, no occlusal problems, and no complicated prostheses.	6 months to 1 year
Class C	Generally *good* results maintained reasonably well for one or more years, but patient displays *some* of the following negative factors: 1. Inconsistent or poor oral hygiene. 2. Heavy calculus formation. 3. Systemic disease that predisposes to periodontal breakdown. 4. Some remaining pockets. 5. Occlusal problems. 6. Complicated prostheses. 7. Ongoing orthodontic therapy. 8. Recurrent dental caries.	3 to 4 months (Decide on recall interval on the basis of the number and severity of negative factors. Consider re-treating some areas.)
Class D	Generally *poor* results following periodontal therapy and/or *several* negative factors from the following list. 1. Inconsistent or poor oral hygiene. 2. Heavy calculus formation. 3. Systemic disease that predisposes to periodontal breakdown. 4. Remaining pockets. 5. Occlusal problems. 6. Complicated prostheses. 7. Recurrent dental caries. 8. Periodontal surgery indicated but not performed because of medical, psychological, or financial reasons. 9. Condition too far advanced to be improved by periodontal surgery.	1 to 3 months (Decide on recall intervals on the basis of the number and severity of negative factors. Consider re-treating some areas or extracting several involved teeth.)

are not optimum. Furthermore, the first-year patient will often present etiological factors that may have been overlooked and that may be more amenable to treatment at this early stage. Because of the above reasons, the recall period for the first-year patients should be not more than three months.

The patients who are on a periodontal recall schedule are a most varied group.

Table 58–2 lists several categories of maintenance patient and a suggested recall interval for each. One must realize that patients can improve or relapse to a different classification with reduction or exacerbation of periodontal disease. When one dental arch is worse than the other, the patient is classified by the arch that is in the worse condition.

REFERENCES

1 Axelsson, P., and Lindhe, J.: The effect of a preventive programme on dental plaque, gingivitis and caries in school children. J. Clin. Periodontol. *1*:126, 1974.

2. Chace, R.: Retreatment in periodontal practice. J. Periodontol., *48*:410, 1977.

3. Lietha-Elmer, E.: Langsfristige Ergebnisse regelmässig betreuter und unbetreuter Parodontosepatienten. Schweiz. Mschr. Zahnheilkt., *87*:613, 1977.

4. Lightner, L. M., O'Leary, J. T., Drake, R. B., Crump, P. O., and Allen, M. F.: Preventive periodontic treatment procedures: results over 46 months. J. Periodontol., *42*:555, 1971.

5. Lindhe, J., and Koch, G.: The effect of supervised oral hygiene on the gingiva of children. J. Periodont. Res., *1*:260, 1966.

6. Lindhe, J., and Koch, G.: The effect of supervised oral hygiene on the gingiva of children. Lack of prolonged effect of supervision. J. Periodontol. Res., *2*:215, 1967.

7. Lindhe, J., and Nyman, S.: The effect of plaque control and surgical pocket elimination on the establishment and maintenance of periodontal health. A longitudinal study of periodontal therapy in cases of advanced disease. J. Clin. Periodontol., *2*:67, 1975.

8. Nyman, S., Rosling, B., and Lindhe, J.: Effect of professional tooth cleaning on healing after periodontal surgery. J. Clin. Periodontol., *2*:80, 1975.

9. Ramfjord, S. P., Knowles, J. W., Nissle, R. R., Burgett, F. G., and Shick, R. A.: Results following three modalities of periodontal therapy. J. Periodontol., *46*:522, 1975.

10. Rosling, B., Nyman, S., and Lindhe, J.: The effect of systematic plaque control on bone regeneration in infrabony pockets. J. Clin. Periodontol., *3*:38, 1976.

11. Rosling, B., Nyman, S., Lindhe, J., and Jern, B.: The healing potential of the periodontal tissues following different techniques of periodontal surgery in plaque-free dentitions. J. Clin. Periodontol., *3*:233, 1976.

12. Stahl, S. S., et al.: Gingival healing. IV. The effects of home care on gingivectomy repair. J. Periodontol., *40*:264, 1969.

13. Sternlicht, H. C.: Evaluating long-term periodontal therapy. Texas Dent. J., Oct. 1974.

14. Suomi, J. D., Greene, J. C., Vermillion, J. R., Doyle, J., Chang, J. J., and Leatherwood, E. C.: The effect of controlled oral hygiene on the progression of periodontal disease in adults: Results after the third and final year. J. Periodontol., *42*:152, 1971.

15. Suomi, J. D., West, J. D., Chang, J. J., and McClendon, B. J.: The effect of controlled oral hygiene procedures on the progression of periodontal disease in adults: radiographic findings. J. Periodontol., *42*:562, 1971.

Results of Periodontal Treatment

The prevalence of periodontal disease and the high tooth mortality due to this disease raise an important question: Is periodontal treatment effective in preventing and stopping the progressive destruction of periodontal disease? Evidence that periodontal therapy is effective in preventing the disease, slowing the destruction of the periodontium, and reducing tooth loss is now overwhelming.

TREATMENT AND PREVENTION OF GINGIVITIS

For many years, the belief that good oral hygiene is necessary for the successful prevention and treatment of gingivitis has been widespread among periodontists. In addition, world-wide epidemiological studies have confirmed a close relationship between the incidence of gingivitis and lack of oral hygiene.[2, 3]

Conclusive evidence on the relation of oral hygiene and gingivitis in healthy dental students was shown by Löe and co-workers.[10, 24] After 9 to 21 days without oral hygiene, experimental subjects with previously excellent oral hygiene and healthy gingivae developed heavy accumulations of plaque and generalized mild gingivitis. When oral hygiene was reinstituted, the plaque in most areas disappeared in one or two days, and the gingival inflammation in these areas disappeared one day after the plaque had been removed. Gingivitis is therefore reversible and can be resolved by daily effective plaque removal.

A number of long-term studies have shown that gingival health can be maintained by a combination of effective oral hygiene and dental scaling. The combined effect of subgingival scaling and controlled oral hygiene was evaluated over a period of five years in a group composed of 1428 men and women working in a factory in Oslo, Norway.[12] Gingival conditions were carefully recorded prior to treatment and after its conclusion. Treatment consisted exclusively of meticulous subgingival scaling at three- to six-month intervals along with oral hygiene instructions. The average reduction in gingivitis was about 60 per cent at the end of five years. The investigators speculated that the reduction in gingival inflammation might have been even greater had they resorted to surgical techniques in the areas with deep pockets.

A three-year study on 1248 General Telephone workers in California was conducted to determine whether the progression of gingival inflammation is retarded in an oral environment in which high levels of hygiene are maintained.[22, 23] Experimental and control groups were computer matched on the basis of periodontal and oral hygiene status, past caries experience, age, and sex. During the study period, several procedures were instituted to insure that the oral hygiene status of the experimental group was maintained at a high level. They were given a series of frequent oral prophylaxis, combined with oral hygiene instruction. Subjects in the control groups received no attention from the study team except for annual examinations. They were advised to continue with their usual daily practices and visits for professional care. After three years, the increase in plaque and debris in the control group was four times as great as in the experimental group. Similarly, gingivitis scores were much higher in the controls than in the matching experimental group.

Several other studies have produced similar results in regard to the reduction of gingivitis.[1, 5, 7] **It is therefore an established fact that chronic marginal gingivitis can be controlled by oral hygiene and dental prophylaxis.**

PREVENTION AND TREATMENT OF LOSS OF ATTACHMENT

Modern techniques of periodontal therapy have been employed for more than fifty years. It is only within the last ten years, however, that a number of studies have been conducted to determine the effect of treatment on reducing the progressive loss of periodontal support for the natural dentition.

Prevention of Loss of Attachment

A four-year study on 470 Air Force Academy students was conducted to determine the relationship between the frequency of oral hygiene procedures and gingival health.[7] Mean loss of tissue attachment in a group receiving four preventive treatments per year with brushing instruction was less than half that of the control group, which received one treatment per year without oral hygiene in-

structions. The information on loss of attachment secured after four years shows that frequent preventive treatments and toothbrushing instruction are effective in retarding attachment loss.

In the previously discussed study on General Telephone workers in California, loss of attachment was measured clinically, whereas alveolar bone loss was measured radiographically.[22, 23] After three years, the control group showed loss of attachment at a rate more than 3.5 times as high as its matching experimental group during the same period (Fig. 59–1). In addition, subjects who received frequent oral prophylaxis and were instructed in good oral hygiene practices showed less bone loss radiographically after three years than did the controls. **It is clear that loss of attachment can be reduced by good oral hygiene and frequent dental prophylaxis.**

Treatment of Loss of Attachment

Thus far, the studies cited involved treatment of populations without extensive periodontal disease. The following investigation on loss of attachment was done on patients with moderate to advanced periodontal disease, in order to determine which approach to periodontal therapy gives the best long-term results with regard to maintenance or gain of attachment.[16–19] This report is based on 104 patients who had been treated during a ten-year period. The limiting criteria for acceptance of patients for the project were (1) that they had one or more periodontal

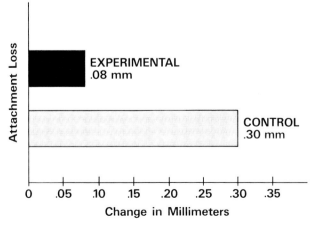

Figure 59–1 Change in mean attachment level from base-line to third-year examination for experimental and control groups. (*From* Suomi, John D., et al.[22])

pockets extending 4 mm. or more apical to the cemento-enamel junction and (2) that they were interested and willing to come when called for examination and treatment. All degrees of severity of periodontal disease were treated, including advanced disease with bifurcation and trifurcation involvement. After initial scaling and oral hygiene, a "split mouth" design was adopted, using one side of the mouth for curettage and the other for surgical pocket elimination on a random basis. The results showed that the progression of periodontal disease was stopped for a period of three years postoperatively regardless of modality of treatment. Even for long-term observations, the average loss of attachment was only 0.3 mm. over seven years.[17] These results indicated a more favorable prognosis for treatment of advanced periodontal lesions than previously assumed.

Another study was conducted on 75 patients with advanced periodontal disease to determine the effect of plaque control and surgical pocket elimination on the establishment and maintenance of periodontal health.[9] This study showed that no further alveolar bone loss occurred during the five-year observation period. The meticulous plaque control practiced by the patients in this study was considered a major factor in the excellent results produced.

The rate of destruction for untreated periodontal disease is unknown. The data from young, healthy patients who are not receiving optimum prophylactic care show about 0.1 mm. loss of attachment for each tooth surface per year.[22, 23] For ethical reasons, patients with moderate to advanced periodontal disease cannot be followed as a control group while their dentition deteriorates. Therefore, there are no adequate controls on these studies. However, the studies that involved advanced periodontal disease showed minimal loss of attachment (between 0 and 0.04 mm. per surface per year) for five to seven years after treatment. It is logical to conclude, therefore, **that treatment is very effective in reducing loss of attachment.**

TOOTH MORTALITY

The ultimate test for the effectiveness of periodontal treatment is whether or not the loss of teeth can be prevented. There are now enough studies both from private practice and research institutions to document that loss of teeth is retarded or prevented by therapy.

In the group of 1428 factory workers in Norway previously referred to, the combined effects of three- to six-month subgingival scaling and controlled oral hygiene was evaluated over a period of five years.[12] The loss of teeth for all age groups was very low. The figures were compared with those for the "normal" loss of teeth that could be calculated from the data of the initial examination. As a consequence of the scheme, tooth loss was reduced by at least half as compared with "normal" tooth loss. In fact, in the group with good oral hygiene, tooth loss was reduced 64 per cent (Table 59–1).

A study on patients with advanced periodontal disease was undertaken to evaluate the results of different types of

TABLE 59–1 AVERAGE LOSS OF TEETH DURING FIVE-YEAR PERIOD AS COMPARED WITH "NORMAL" LOSS OF TEETH IN 1428 MEN AND WOMEN AGES 20 THROUGH 59

| | Grade of Oral Hygiene | | |
	Good	Fairly Good	Not Good
"Normal" loss of teeth. Estimate based on the data recorded at the initiation of the period.	1.1	1.4	1.8
Actual loss of teeth during the five-year period	0.4	0.6	0.9

(From: Lovdal, A., Arno, A., Shei, O., and Waerhaug, J.[12])

TABLE 59–2   TOOTH MORTALITY FOLLOWING TREATMENT OF
ADVANCED PERIODONTITIS IN 104 PATIENTS WITH 2604 TEETH
TREATED OVER A TEN-YEAR PERIOD

Teeth Lost	Reason
2	Pulpal disease
3	Accidents
4	Prosthetic considerations
14	One patient wanted a maxillary denture for cosmetic reasons
30	Periodontal
53 total	**All reasons**

2 per cent of the teeth were lost during the study period.

(Adapted from data in Ramfjord, S., et al.[19])

treatment (Table 59–2).[16–19] The 104 patients in the study had 2604 teeth, of
which 53 were lost during the study (one
to seven years following initial treatment).
Two of these teeth were lost strictly because of pulpal disease; 3 by accident; 4
for prosthetic considerations; and 14 by
one patient who, after periodontal treatment, desired a maxillary denture for cos-
metic reasons. The remaining 30 teeth
were extracted because of periodontal or
combined periodontal and pulpal disease
resulting in discomfort. Thirty-two teeth
were lost during the first and second year
after initiation of treatment. The remaining
21 teeth were lost in a random pattern
over the next six years. The loss of teeth
due to advanced periodontal disease following treatment was, therefore, minimal
(2 per cent).

Another study was undertaken to test
the effect of periodontal therapy on cases

of advanced disease.[9] The subjects were
75 patients who had lost 50 per cent or
more of their periodontal support (Fig.
59–2 and Table 59–3). Treatment consisted of oral hygiene, scaling, extraction
of untreatable teeth, periodontal surgery,
and prosthetics where indicated. After
completion of periodontal treatment, there
followed a five-year period during which
none of the patients showed any further
loss of periodontal support. No teeth were
extracted in the five-year post-treatment
period. It should be pointed out that the
patients in this study were selected because of their capacity to meet high requirements of plaque control following repeated   instruction   in   oral   hygiene
techniques. This fact does not detract from
the validity of the study but tends to show
the   etiological   importance   of   bacterial
plaque. The results show that periodontal
surgery   coupled   with   a   detailed   plaque

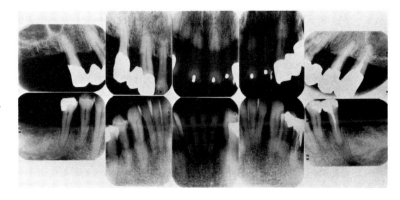

**Figure 59–2   Radiographs Taken
5 Years after Treatment of a Typical
Case.** (*From* Lindhe, Jan, and Nyman,
Sture.[9])

TABLE 59–3 TOOTH MORTALITY

75 patients aged 26 to 72
1620 teeth treated with advanced periodontitis
134 of these teeth had bifurcation or trifurcation involvement
All teeth maintained for 5 years

(Adapted from data of Lindhe, J., and Nyman, S.[20])

control program not only will temporarily cure the disease but also will prevent further progression of periodontal breakdown—even in patients with severely reduced periodontal support.

There have been three private-practice studies that have attempted to measure tooth loss following periodontal therapy. In one study, 180 patients who had been treated for chronic destructive periodontal disease were evaluated.[20] The average age of the patients before treatment was 43.7 years. From the beginning of treatment to the time of the survey, the majority of patients lost no teeth (Fig. 59–3). A total of 141 teeth were lost. Three patients out of 180 (1.7 per cent) lost 35 teeth or approximately 25 per cent of the teeth lost.

Twelve additional patients lost 46 teeth or 32.6 per cent of the teeth lost. Many patients in the study had advanced alveolar bone loss including extensive furcation involvements. A relatively small number (141) of the teeth were lost in the study group of 180 patients between the beginning of periodontal treatment and the time of the study. The teeth were lost for several reasons, including periodontal disease as well as caries and other nonperiodontal causes. The length of time after treatment varied from 2 to 20 years with an average of 8.6 years. Of considerable significance is the fact that a large number of teeth (81 teeth or 57.5 per cent) were lost by a few patients (15 patients or 8.4 per cent). Even when this group is considered with the

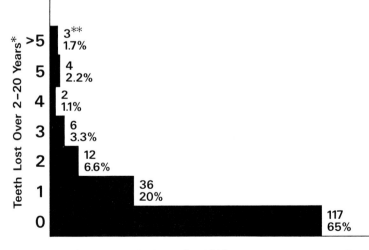

Figure 59–3 Tooth Mortality. (Adapted from Ross, I. F., Thompson, R. H., and Gold, M.[20])

Number of Patients (n=180) with Percentage of Total

*Average of 8.6 years.
**3 patients lost 35 teeth.

The average tooth lost per patient was 0.9 per 10 years.

TABLE 59–4 TOOTH MORTALITY IN 442 PERIODONTAL PATIENTS TREATED OVER A PERIOD OF TEN YEARS

Reason for Loss	Number Lost per Patient over 10.1 Years
Periodontal disease	0.40
Caries	0.10
Other	0.22
All reasons	**0.72**

Courtesy of Dr. R. G. Oliver, University of Minnesota, School of Dentistry.

remaining 165 patients, it may be seen that the periodontal care provided helped to retain most teeth, as the average patient lost slightly less than one tooth (0.9) over ten years following treatment.

In another study, all the patients in a practice who had been treated five or more years previously and had received regular preventive periodontal care since that time were included.[14, 15] There were 442 patients included, with an average length of time since treatment of 10.1 years. Two thirds of the patients were over age 40 at the time of treatment. These patients had been seen every 4.6 months on the average for their preventive perio-

dontal care, which consisted of oral hygiene instruction and prophylaxis (Table 59–4 and Figures 59–4 and 59–5).

The total tooth loss due to periodontal disease was 178 teeth out of just over 11,000 teeth available for treatment. More importantly, 78 per cent of the patients did not lose a single tooth following periodontal therapy and 11 per cent lost only one tooth. When one considers that over 600 teeth had furcation involvements at the time of the original treatment and well over 1000 teeth had less than half of the alveolar bone support remaining, the tooth loss was very low. During the same average ten-year period following periodontal therapy, only 45 teeth were lost through caries or pulpal involvement. Even more surprising are the statistics over an average ten-year period for teeth with less than optimum prognoses.

Only 85 (14 per cent) of a total of 601 teeth with furcation involvement were lost, and 117 (11 per cent) of 1039 teeth with half or less of the bone remaining were lost. Of the teeth listed as having a guarded prognosis for any reason by the clinician performing the initial exam, only 126 (12 per cent) of 1043 were lost over this ten-year average period. When one looks at these figures from the standpoint of the average tooth mortality per patient, one finds that 0.72 teeth are lost per patient per ten years.

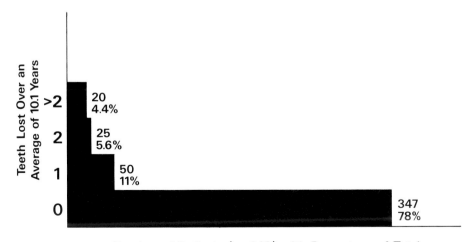

Number of Patients (n = 442) with Percentage of Total

Figure 59–4   **Tooth Mortality in 442 Periodontal Patients Treated over a Period of Ten Years.** (Courtesy of Dr. R. G. Oliver, University of Minnesota School of Dentistry.)

Furcation Involvement

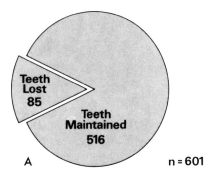

A   n = 601

Teeth Lost 85

Teeth Maintained 516

One-half Bone Lost

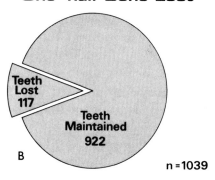

B   n = 1039

Teeth Lost 117

Teeth Maintained 922

Guarded Prognosis

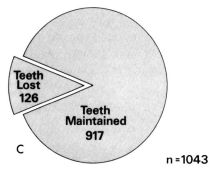

C   n = 1043

Teeth Lost 126

Teeth Maintained 917

Figure 59–5 Tooth Mortality in 442 Periodontal Patients Treated over a Period of Ten Years. (Courtesy of Dr. R. G. Oliver, University of Minnesota School of Dentistry.)

TABLE 59–5 DATA FROM 600 PATIENTS

Years of Treatment	Number of Patients
15 to 19	260
20 to 24	184
25 to 29	96
30 to 34	33
35 to 39	8
40 to 44	8
45 to 49	7
50 to 53	4
Average: 22 years	

Courtesy of Dr. L. Hirschfeld, New York.

follow-up period (22 years average), a total of 1312 teeth were lost owing to all causes. Of this number, 1110 were lost for periodontal reasons. The average tooth mortality per patient was 2.2 teeth; when this is converted to a ten-year rate, an average of one tooth was lost per ten years in each patient. During this period of observation, 666 questionable prognosis teeth were lost out of a total of 2141. This means that 31 per cent of the questionable prognosis teeth were lost over 22 years of treatment. A total of 1464 teeth with furcation involvement were treated and 31.6 per cent were lost during the period of study. Eighty-three per cent of the patients lost less than three teeth over the 22-year average treatment period and were classified as well-maintained. The remaining 17 per cent of patients were divided into two groups identified as either downhill (4 to 9 teeth lost) or extreme downhill (10 to 23 teeth lost). This 17 per cent of the patients studied accounted for 69 per cent of the teeth lost owing to periodontal causes. This study also showed that

In a third private-practice study, 600 patients were followed over a period between 15 and 53 years after periodontal therapy Tables 59–5 and 59–6; Figs. 59–6 and 59–7).[4] The majority (76.5 per cent) were advanced periodontal cases at the start of treatment. There were 15,666 teeth present, an average of 26 teeth per patient. During the

TABLE 59–6 TOOTH MORTALITY IN PRIVATE PRACTICE STUDIES

Author of Study	Average Number of Teeth Lost per 10 Years with Periodontal Treatment
Hirschfeld[12]	1.0
Oliver[32]	0.72
Ross[43]	0.9

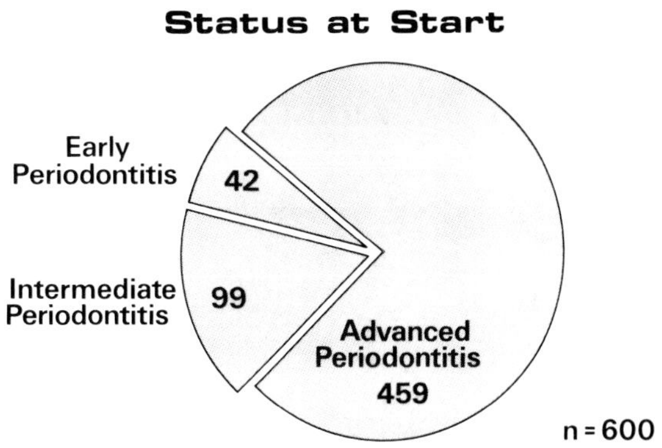

Status at Start

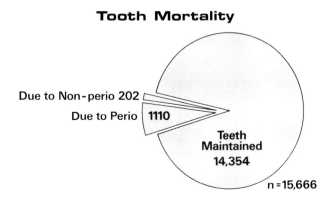

Early Periodontitis 42

Intermediate Periodontitis 99

Advanced Periodontitis 459

n = 600

Figure 59–6 Data from 600 Patients. (Courtesy of Dr. L. Hirschfeld, New York.)

relatively few teeth are lost following periodontal therapy. Secondly, relatively few of the guarded prognosis teeth, including teeth with furcation involvement, are lost. And finally, a small percentage of patients are losing most of the teeth.

Comparison of these tooth mortality studies with other epidemiological surveys is hazardous, since few involve treatment and few are longitudinal. Marshall-Day and associates reported an average tooth loss of 5.2 teeth per ten years after the age of 35 due to all causes.[13] In patients over age 40, the rate increased to 6 teeth per ten years. The United States Public Health Service surveys indicate that about 4.3 teeth are lost per ten years after the age of 35 in the general population.[3, 8] It is obvious that the tooth loss in the general-population epidemiological studies far exceeds that in the treated periodontal patients.

In summary, the prevalence of periodontal disease and the high tooth mortality due to the disease have raised the need for effective treatment. **Treatment is now available that is effective in preventing the disease and stopping the progress of bone destruction once periodontitis is present. In addition, there is overwhelming evidence that periodontal therapy greatly reduces tooth mortality. Every dental practitioner should be familiar with the philosophy and techniques of periodontal therapy.** Failure to diagnose and treat or make periodontal treatment available to our patients will cause unnecessary dental problems and tooth loss.

Tooth Mortality

Due to Non-perio 202

Due to Perio 1110

Teeth Maintained 14,354

n = 15,666

Figure 59–7 Data from 600 Patients. (Courtesy of Dr. L. Hirschfeld, New York.)

After 15 - 53 years. Average of 22 years.

REFERENCES

1. Bay, I., and Møller, I. J.: The effect of a sodium monofluorophosphate dentifrice on the gingiva. J. Periodontol., Res., 3:103, 1968.
2. Greene, J. C.: Periodontal disease in India: report of an epidemiological study. J. Dent. Res., 39:302, 1960.
3. Greville, T. N. E.: United States Life Tables by Dentulous or Edentulous Condition, 1971, and 1577–58. Dept. of Health Education and Welfare, publication No. (HRA) 75–1338, August, 1974.
4. Hirschfeld, L., and Wasserman, B.: A long-term survey of tooth loss in 600 treated periodontal patients. J. Periodontol., 49:225, 1978.
5. Hoover, D. R., and Lefkowitz, W.: Reduction of gingivitis by toothbrushing. J. Periodontol., 36:193, 1965.
6. Ladavalya, M. R. N., and Harris, R.: A study of the gingival and periodontal conditions of a group of people in Chieng Mai province. J. Periodontol., 30:219, 1959.
7. Lightner, L. M., O'Leary, J. T., Drake, R. B., Crump, P. P., and Allen, M. F.: Preventive periodontic treatment procedures: results over 46 months. J. Periodontol., 42:555, 1971.
8. Linder, F. E., et al.: Decayed Missing and Filled Teeth in Adults. United States – 1960–1962. Public Health Service Publication No. 1000, Series 11, No. 23, February 1967.
9. Lindhe, J., and Nyman, S.: The effect of plaque control and surgical pocket elimination on the establishment and maintenance of periodontal health. A longitudinal study of periodontal therapy in cases of advanced disease. J. Clin. Periodontol., 2:67, 1975.
10. Löe, H., Theilade, E., and Jensen, S. B.: Experimental gingivitis in man. J. Periodontol., 36:177, 1965.
11. Löe, H., and Silness, J.: Periodontal disease in pregnancy. I. Prevalence and severity. Acta Odont. Scand., 21:533, 1976.
12. Lovdal, A., Arno, A., Schei, O., and Waerhaug, J.: Combined effect of subgingival scaling and controlled oral hygiene on the incidence of gingivitis. Acta Odont. Scand., 19:537, 1961.
13. Marshall-Day, C. D., Stephens, R. G., and Quigley, L. F.: Periodontal disease: prevalence and incidence. J. Periodontol., 26:185, 1955.
14. Oliver, R. C.: Tooth loss with and without periodontal therapy. Periodontal Abs., 17:8, 1969.
15. Oliver, R. C.: Personal communication, 1977.
16. Ramfjord, S. P., Nissle, R. R., Shick, R. A., and Cooper, H.: Subgingival curettage versus surgical elimination of periodontal pockets. J. Periodontol., 39:167, 1968.
17. Ramfjord, S. P., Knowles, J. W., Nissle, R. R., Shick, R. A., and Burgett, F. G.: Longitudinal study of periodontal therapy. J. Periodontol., 44:66, 1973.
18. Ramfjord, S. P., and Nissle, R. R.: The modified Widman flap. J. Periodontol., 45:601, 1974.
19. Ramfjord, S. P., Knowles, J. W., Nissle, R. R., Burgett, F. G., and Shick, R. A.: Results following three modalities of periodontal therapy. J. Periodontol., 46:522, 1975.
20. Ross, I. F., Thompson, R. H., and Galdi, M.: The results of treatment. A long term study of one hundred and eighty patients. Parodontologie, 25:125, 1971.
21. Russell, A. L.: Some epidemiological characteristics of periodontal diseases in a series of urban populations. J. Periodontol., 28:286, 1957.
22. Suomi, J. D., Greene, J. C., Vermillion, J. R., Doyle, J., Chang, J. J., and Leatherwood, E. C.: The effect of controlled oral hygiene on the progression of periodontal disease in adults: results after the third and final year. J. Periodontol., 42:152, 1971.
23. Suomi, J. D., West, J. D., Chang, J. J., and McClendon, B. J.: The effect of controlled oral hygiene procedures on the progression of periodontal disease in adults: radiographic findings. J. Periodontol., 42:562, 1971.
24. Theilade, E., Wright, W. H., Jensen, S. B., and Löe, H.: Experimental gingivitis in man II. J. Periodont. Res., 1:1, 1966.

INDEX

Note: Page numbers in *italics* indicate illustrations and "t" indicates a table. The expression "vs." denotes "differential diagnosis from."